MICROBIOLOGY
PRINCIPLES AND HEALTH SCIENCE APPLICATIONS

MICROBIOLOGY PRINCIPLES AND HEALTH SCIENCE APPLICATIONS

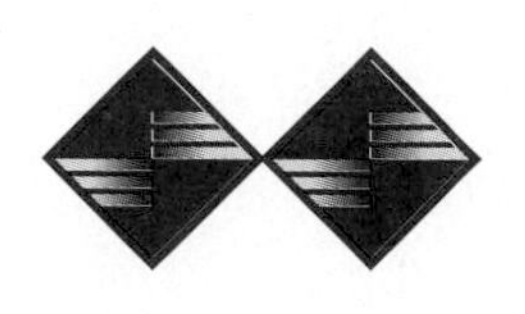

Lois M. Bergquist, PhD
Professor of Microbiology
Los Angeles Valley College
Van Nuys, California

Barbara Pogosian, MS
Professor, Biology Department
Golden West College
Huntington Beach, California

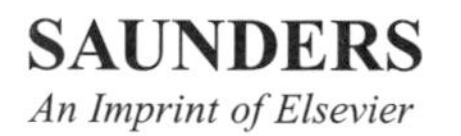

SAUNDERS
An Imprint of Elsevier

The Curtis Center
Independence Square West
Philadelphia, Pennsylvania 19106

Library of Congress Cataloging-in-Publication Data

Bergquist, Lois M.
Microbiology principles and health science applications/Lois M. Bergquist, Barbara Pogosian.

p. cm.

ISBN 0–7216–7663–4

1. Microbiology. 2. Medical microbiology. I. Title. II. Pogosian, Barbara.
[DNLM: 1. Microbiology. 2. Communicable Diseases—microbiology.
3. Host-Parasite Relations. QW 4 B499ma 2000]

QR41.2.B45 2000

579 21—dc21 99-040813

MICROBIOLOGY PRINCIPLES AND
HEALTH SCIENCE APPLICATIONS ISBN 0–7216–7663–4

Copyright © 2000 by Saunders

All rights reserved. No part of this publication may be reproduced or transmitted in any form or by any means, electronic or mechanical, including photocopy, recording, or any information storage and retrieval system, without permission in writing from the publisher.

Permissions may be sought directly from Elsevier's Health Sciences Rights Department in Philadelphia, USA: phone: (+1)215-238-7869, fax: (+1)215-238-2239, email: healthpermissions@elsevier.com. You may also complete your request on-line via the Elsevier Science homepage (http://www.elsevier.com), by selecting 'Customer Support' and then 'Obtaining Permissions'.

Printed in the United States of America.

Last digit is the print number: 9 8 7 6 5 4

To my teachers, who introduced me to the microbial world, and to my students, who continue to motivate me and give my life purpose

Lois M. Bergquist

For everyone who knows life is a web of visible and invisible interdependence, and for those who now embark on this path of discovery.

Barbara Pogosian

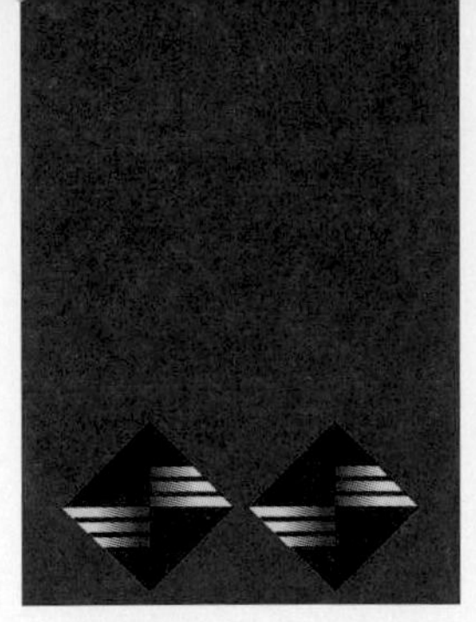

Reviewers

James E. Daly, MT(ASCP), BS, MEd
Lorain County Community College
Elyria, Ohio

DeAnna Davis, CDA, RDA, MEd
Program Director
Polaski Technical College
North Little Rock, Arkansas

Jeff D. Foster
Southern State Community College
Hillsboro, Ohio

Arthur S. Keehnle, MS, BS, MT(ASCP), CLS(NCA)
Medical Lab Technology Program
Beaufort County Community College
Washington, North Carolina

Frances M. Kittelmann, MS, MLT(ASCP), CLS-M(NCA)
Orange County Community College
Middletown, New York

Donna Leach, EdD, MT(ASCP)DLM
Winston-Salem State University
Winston-Salem, North Carolina

Rosemarie Marshall, PhD
Specialist, Clinical Microbiology
Professor, Department of Biology and Microbiology
California State University
Los Angeles, California

Cynthia A. Martine, MEd, MT(ASCP)
University of Texas Medical Branch
School of Allied Health Sciences
Galveston, Texas

Elizabeth F. McPherson, MS
Department of Microbiology
University of Tennessee
Knoxville, Tennessee

William C. Payne, MS, MT(ASCP)
Assistant Professor of Clinical Laboratory Science
Clinical Education Coordinator
Arkansas State University
Jonesboro, Arkansas

Richard G. Pendula, PhD
Biological Sciences
C.C.R.I.
Warwick, Rhode Island

Malcolm Slifkin, PhD
Diplomate of the American Board of Medical Microbiology in Public Health and Medical Laboratory Medicine
Allegheny University of the Health Sciences
Allegheny General Hospital
Pittsburgh, Pennsylvania

Ann C. Smith, PhD
University of Maryland
College Park, Maryland

Frank Christopher Sowers, BA, MS
Wilkes Community College
Wilkesboro, North Carolina

Preface

Many high-quality texts are available for students taking a first course in microbiology, so what would motivate two people to write yet another text? We wanted to create a text that could be used in a single quarter or semester course, to emphasize health science applications, and to share our enthusiasm for the diverse world of microorganisms.

Some students are required to take one class in microbiology as a prerequisite for entrance to professional schools of nursing, pharmacy, respiratory therapy, optometry, nutrition, dental hygiene, laboratory technology, and many others. This text assumes that students have taken no previous classes in biology or chemistry. For most health science majors, an introductory class in microbiology is their only exposure to microbiology, although microorganisms have an impact on most human activities. Students are usually not aware of their daily confrontations with the ubiquitous microorganisms or of the possible consequences of these confrontations. Learning about the activities of microorganisms should increase their awareness and be a prelude to personal and professional responsibility.

The text is organized into seven units: An Introduction to Microbiology; Growth, Metabolism, and Variation; Major Groups of Microorganisms; Host-Parasite Relationships; Infectious Diseases of Humans; Control of Microorganisms; and Environmental and Food Microbiology. Each chapter begins with a brief outline of contents and a list of learning objectives and contains periodic questions in sections entitled Micro Check for students to evaluate their comprehension. Sections entitled Focal Point in each chapter highlight information, expanding chapter content or offering unique insights into the history and current status of microbiology. At the end of each chapter, two sections entitled Understanding Microbiology and Applying Microbiology provide questions for review and comprehension of the chapter's main principles. Each chapter in Unit 5, Infectious Diseases of Humans, contains a case study of a pertinent disease taken from actual case files.

The appendices contain sections on prefixes, roots, and suffixes; temperature and metric system measurements; a pronunciation guide; and web sites. A comprehensive glossary contains concise definitions of the microbiological terms used in the text.

Illustrations, photographs, and tables are used to clarify concepts, to provide examples of concepts, and to illustrate the unseen world of microorganisms. Supplements include an instructor's manual provided for adopters of the text for classroom use and a student study guide containing practice questions, diagrams for labeling, and crossword puzzles to augment learning. Students are consistently encouraged to take responsibility for their own learning.

We have made a conscientious effort to limit the amount of material in the text and to focus on principles that relate to real-life situations. No doubt we have omitted topics of interest to some instructors and included some that others will think are unnecessary. The choice of topics was dictated by our own experience in teaching introductory microbiology classes over a span of more than twenty years.

LOIS M. BERGQUIST, PhD
BARBARA POGOSIAN, MS

Acknowledgments

We are thankful to our colleagues for their contributions and insights. We are most grateful to David M. Carlberg for his contributions to Chapter 7. We recognize Micheline Carr, illustrator extraordinaire, for her anatomic drawings, and Michele Paul for her unswerving dedication in preparing manuscript material.

We are appreciative of the reviewers' comments with suggestions on content and balance. We want to thank the staff of W.B. Saunders Company, especially our editors, Shirley A. Kuhn and Helaine A. Barron, for their roles as expeditors and for their expertise as problem solvers.

We acknowledge you, the readers, who have chosen to embark on the discovery trails of microbiology. We hope you have an enjoyable journey and that the information you learn will have a positive impact on your lives and enable you to be successful in your chosen professions.

The authors are especially indebted to the following individuals who shared their expertise in the basic principles and applications of the immune response contained in Chapters 13 and 14.

L.B. and B.P.

Sharyn M. Walker, PhD
Associate Professor of Molecular Microbiology and Immunology
University of Southern California School of Medicine
Division of Research Immunology/Bone Marrow Transplantation
Childrens Hospital Los Angeles
Los Angeles, California

Raymond J. Dorio, MD
Visiting Scientist
Division of Research Immunology/Bone Marrow Transplantation
Childrens Hospital Los Angeles
Los Angeles, California

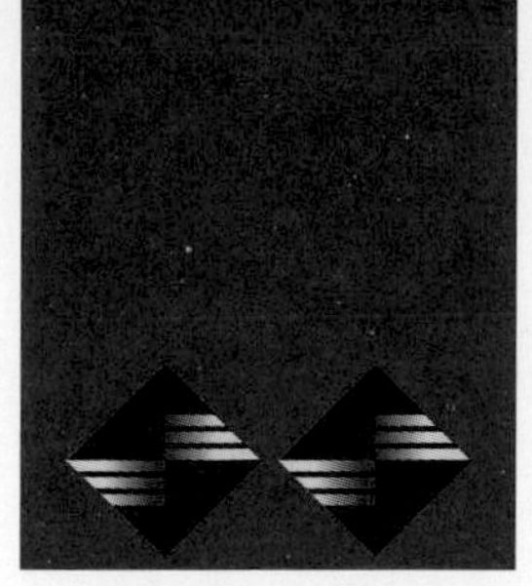

Contents

◆ Unit 7

Environmental and Food Microbiology

◆ Appendixes

Color Plates

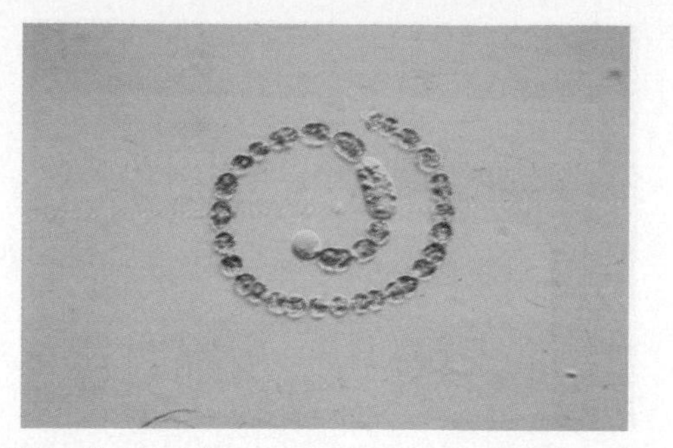

Color Plate 1 ◆ *Anabaena spiroides,* a cyanobacterium showing a chain of cells with heterocysts.

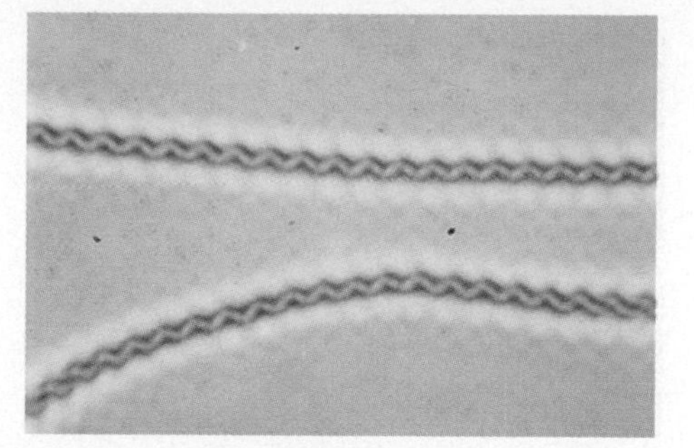

Color Plate 2 ◆ *Spirulina subsalva,* a cyanobacterium, showing chained cells.

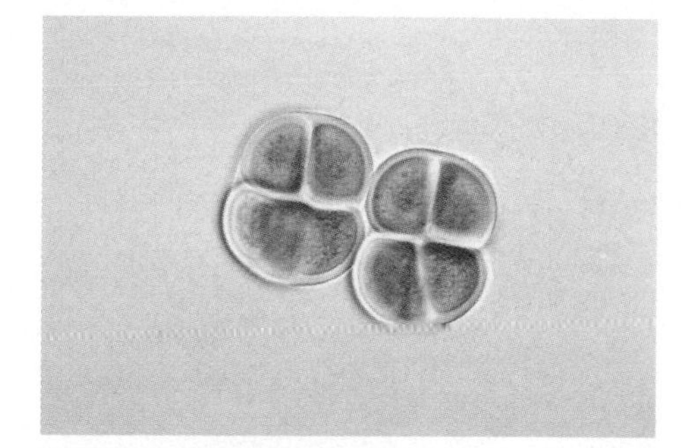

Color Plate 3 ◆ *Chroococcus turgidus,* cyanobacterial cells undergoing cell division.

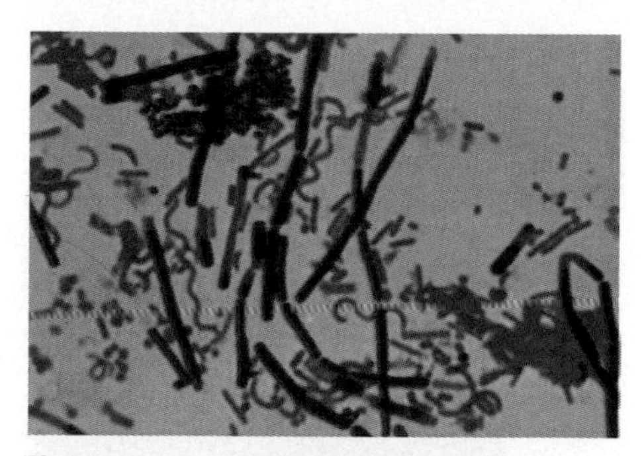

Color Plate 4 ◆ Three shapes of bacteria: rods, cocci, and spirals.

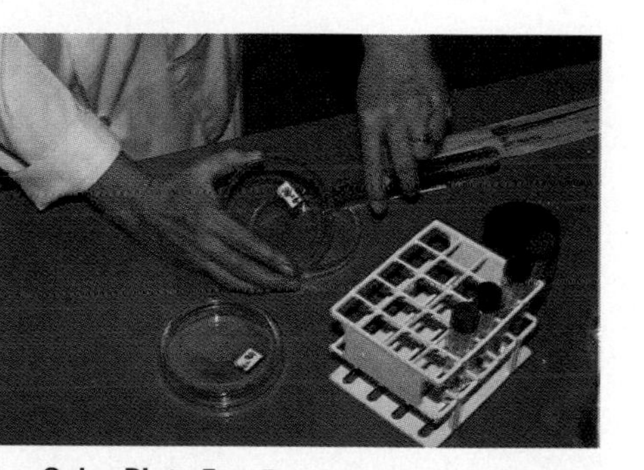

Color Plate 5 ◆ Pouring an agar plate.

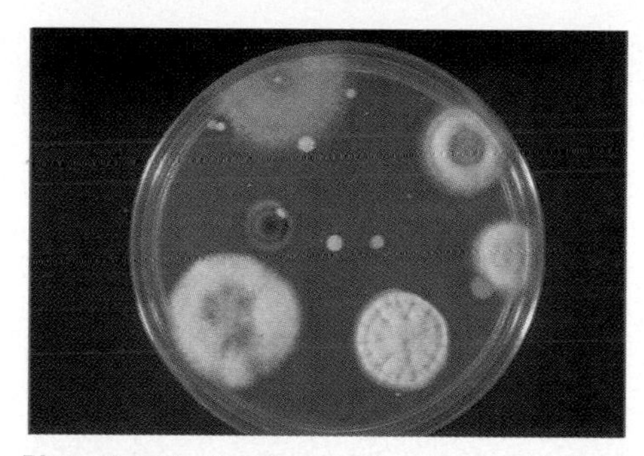

Color Plate 6 ◆ Surface bacterial and fungal colonies on a nutrient agar plate.

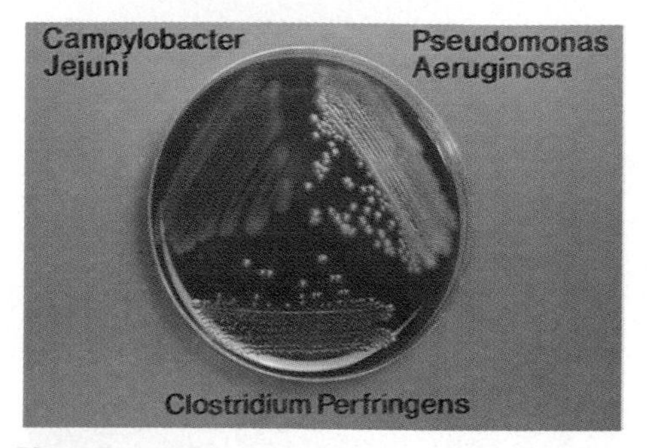

Color Plate 7 ◆ Three organisms growing under microaerophilic conditions.

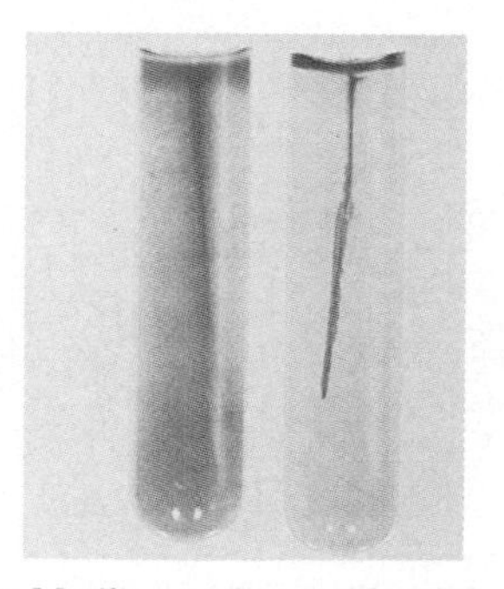

Color Plate 8 ◆ Motility medium with triphenyl tetrazolium chloride showing spreading growth of a motile organism (L) and a nonmotile organism (R).

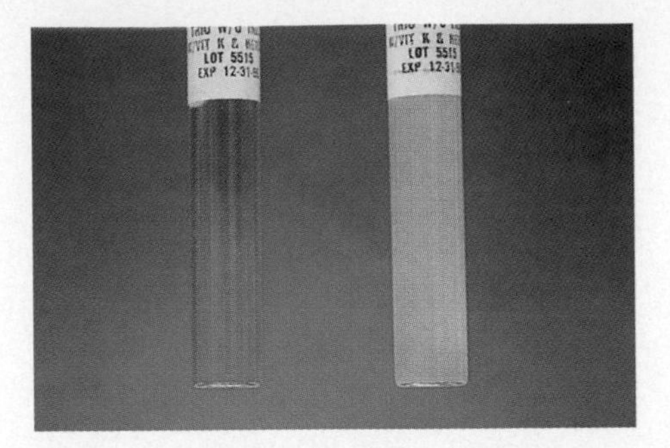

Color Plate 9 ◆ Inoculated tubes of broth showing no growth (L) and growth (R).

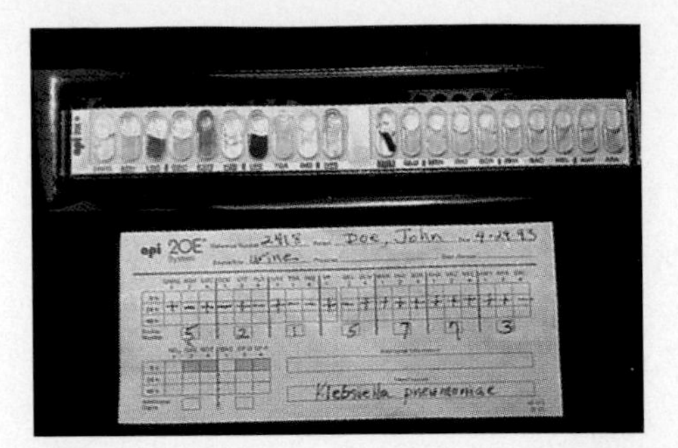

Color Plate 10 ◆ Biochemical test panel and organism identification code.

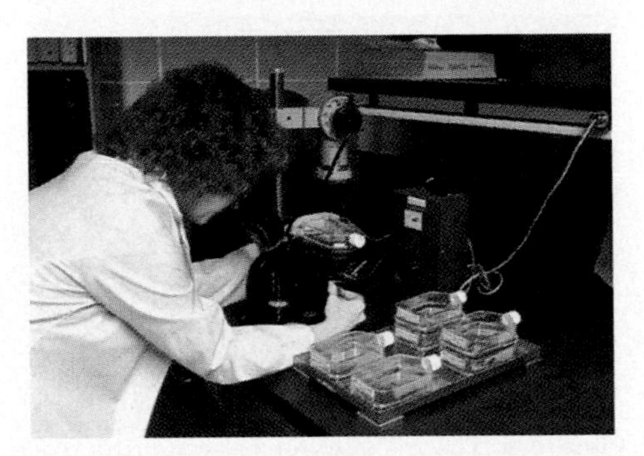

Color Plate 11 ◆ Inverted microscope used to examine bottles of animal cell monolayer cultures.

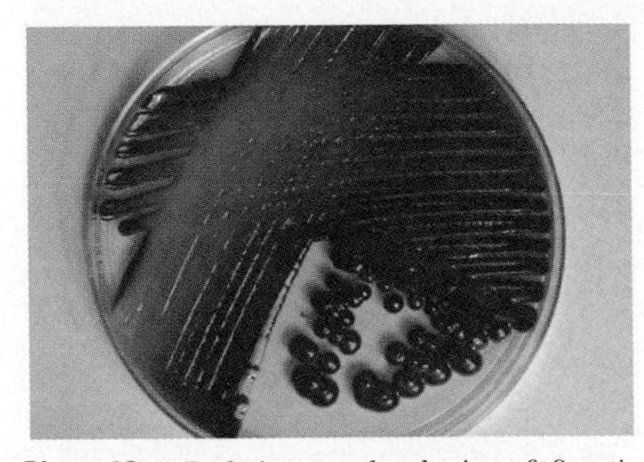

Color Plate 12 ◆ Red-pigmented colonies of *Serratia marcescens* on MacConkey agar.

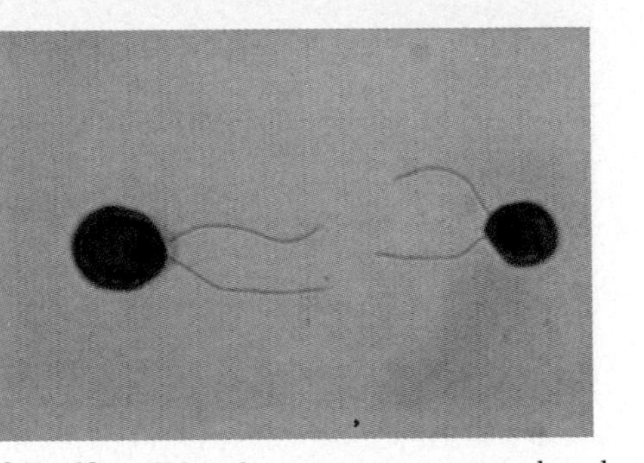

Color Plate 13 ◆ *Chlamydomonas* sp., a green alga showing flagella.

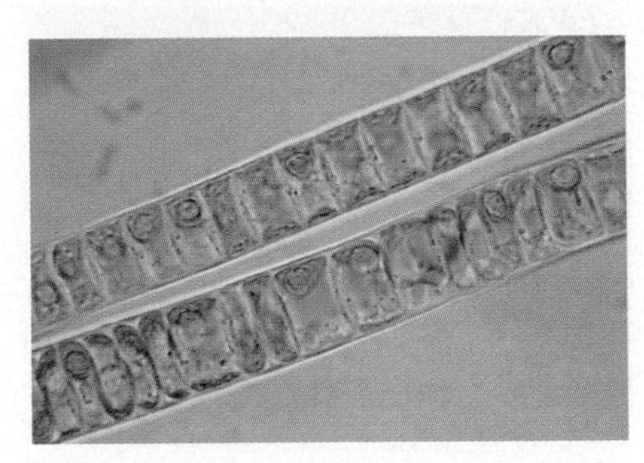

Color Plate 14 ◆ *Ulothrix* sp., a filamentous green alga.

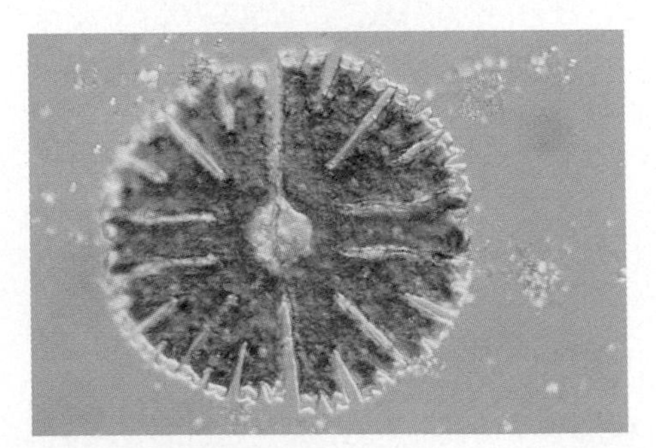

Color Plate 15 ◆ *Micrasterias* sp., a green alga.

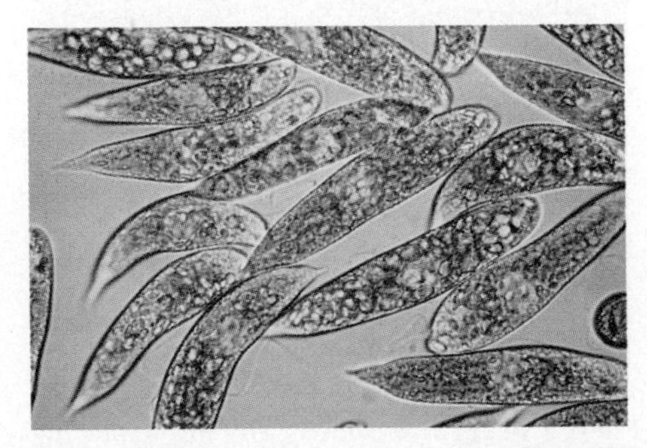

Color Plate 16 ◆ *Euglena* sp. has green chloroplasts and light-sensitive red eyespot.

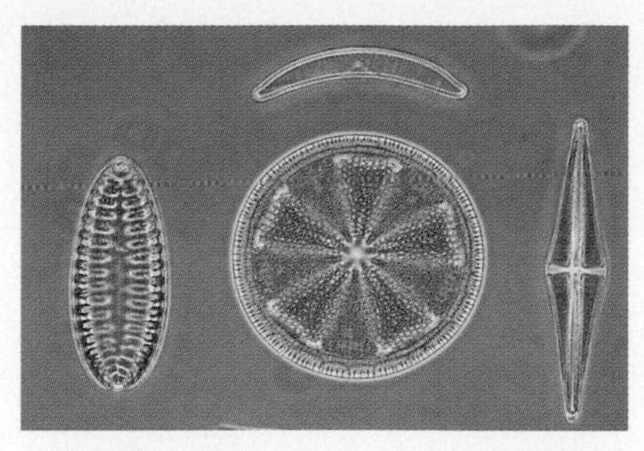

Color Plate 17 ◆ Diatoms, freshwater forms.

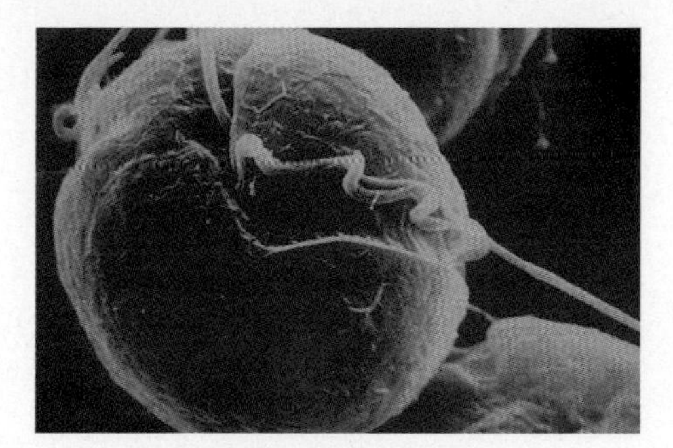

Color Plate 18 ◆ *Gonyaulax,* a dinoflagellate, commonly causes "red tide."

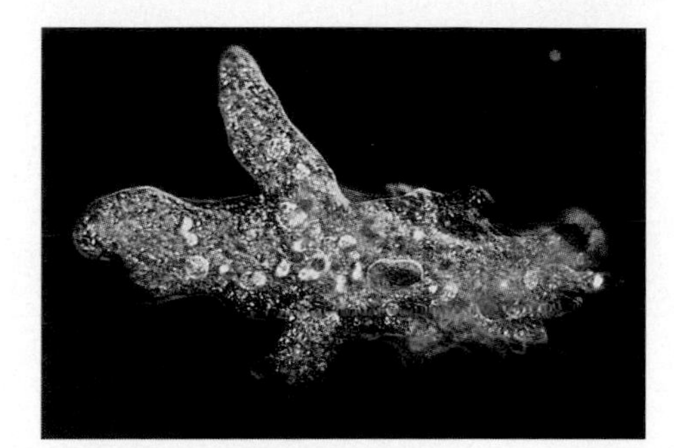

Color Plate 19 ◆ *Amoeba* sp., a protozoan showing intracellular granules.

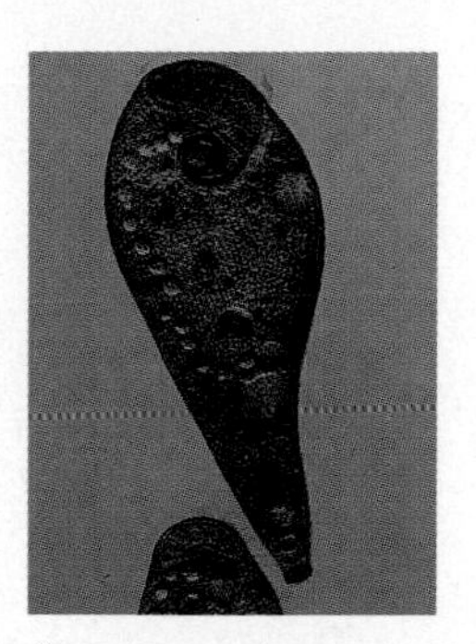

Color Plate 20 ◆ *Stentor* sp., a large protozoan showing nuclei, and cilia.

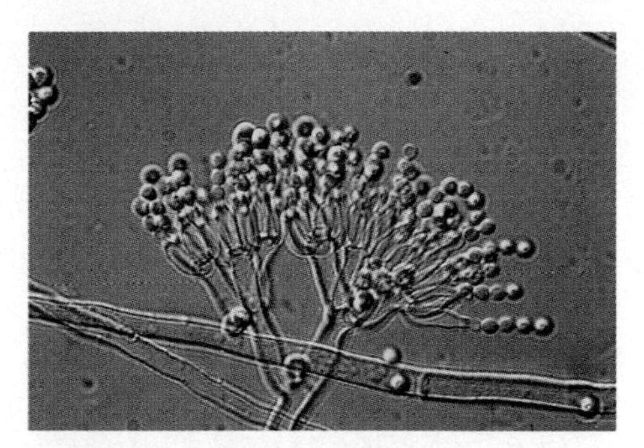

Color Plate 21 ◆ *Penicillium,* showing clear hyphae, distinct septa, and microconidia.

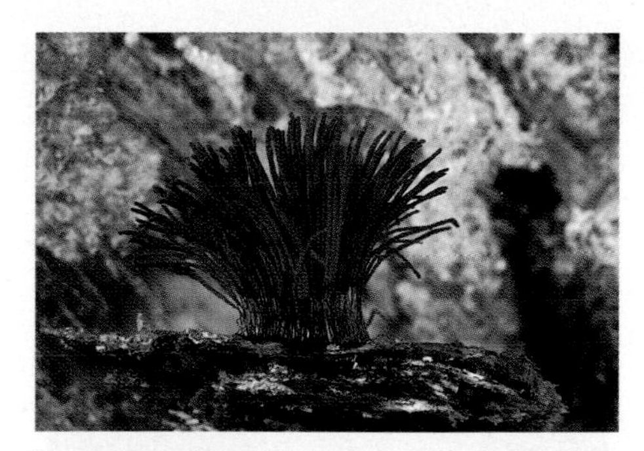

Color Plate 22 ◆ *Stemonitis splendens,* slime mold, on dead tree.

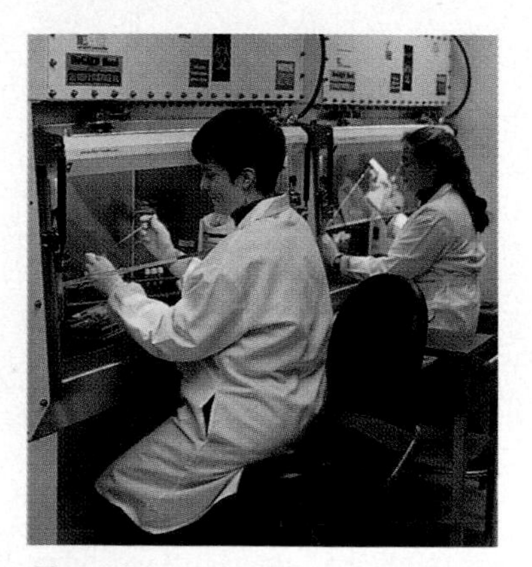

Color Plate 23 ◆ Biological safety cabinets used in maximum containment laboratories.

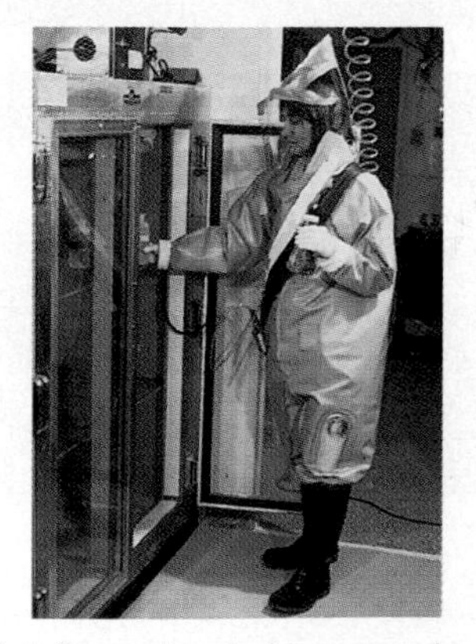

Color Plate 24 ◆ Protective clothing worn in maximum containment laboratory at Centers for Disease Control and Prevention.

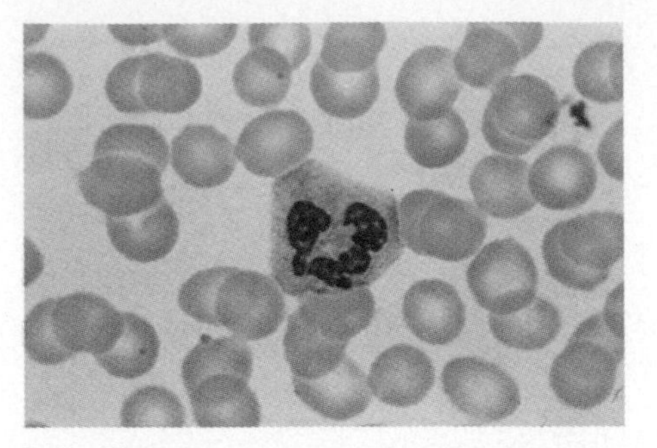

Color Plate 25 ◆ Neutrophil in a blood smear.

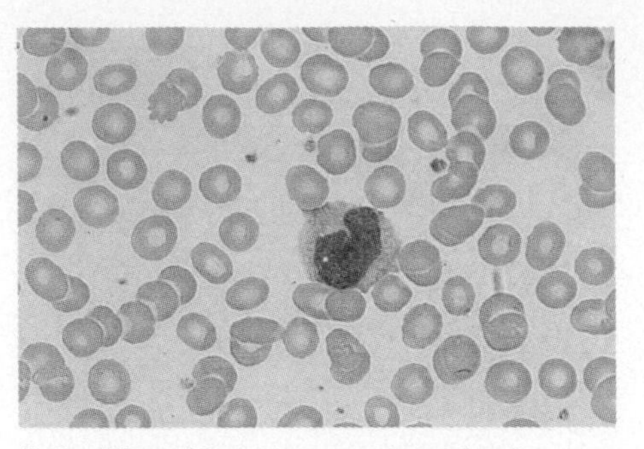

Color Plate 26 ◆ Monocyte in a blood smear.

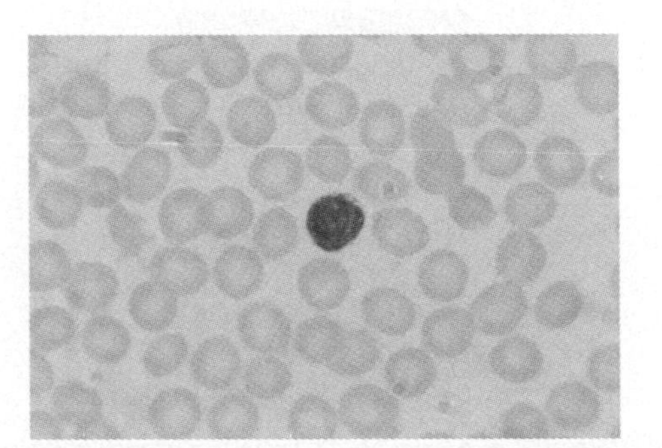

Color Plate 27 ◆ Peripheral blood smear showing erythrocytes and one lymphocyte.

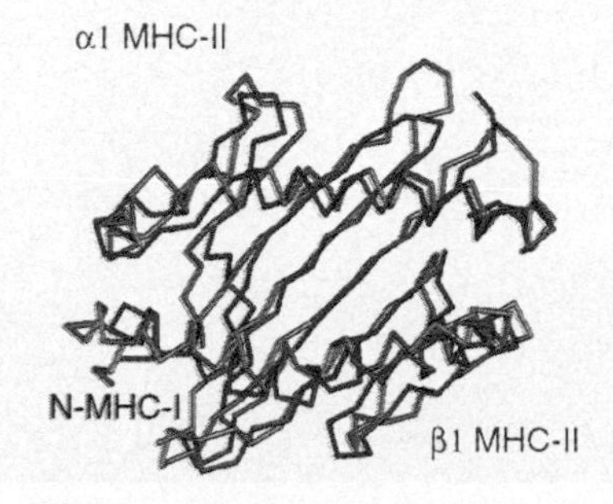

Color Plate 28 ◆ Superposition of an MHC class I molecule (in blue, with N-terminal end, N-MHC-1) on an MHC class II molecule (in red).

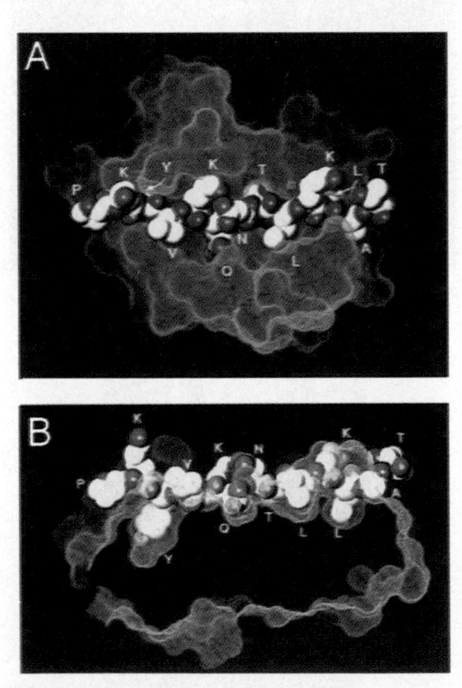

Color Plate 29 ◆ Influenza virus peptide antigen (colored circles represent amino acids in the peptide) presented by the MHC class II molecule (blue ribbons). (*A*) Top view. (*B*) Side view.

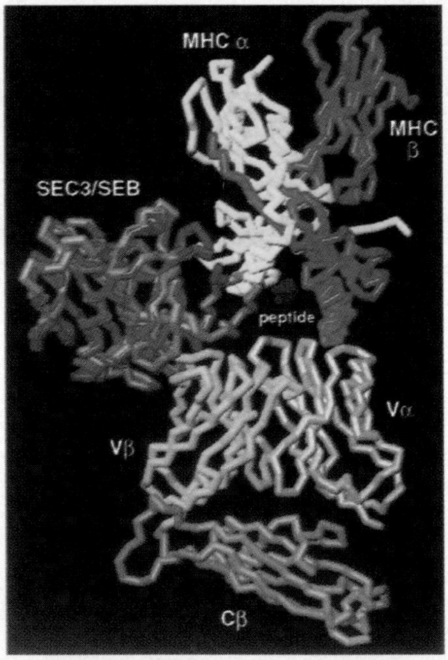

Color Plate 30 ◆ A model of the interaction of a staphylococcal enterotoxin superantigen (SEC3 and SEB) alongside the MHC class II molecule (teal blue and chartreuse) and the T cell receptor (pink, gray, orange) surrounding the peptide antigen (red).

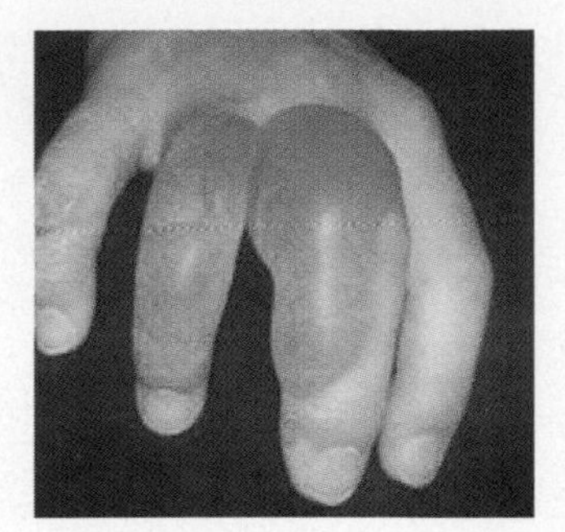

Color Plate 31 ◆ Contact dermatitis from poison ivy.

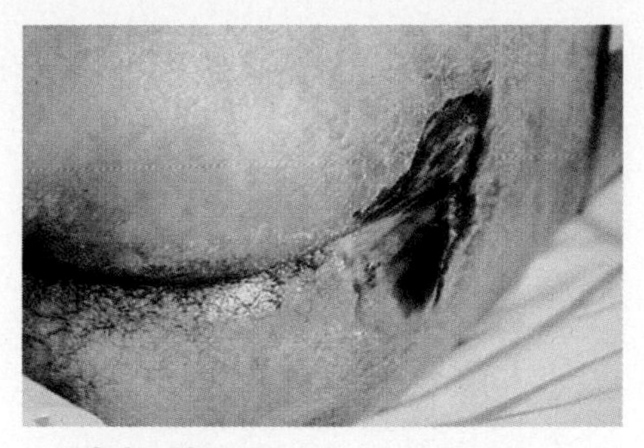

Color Plate 32 ◆ A sacral decubitus.

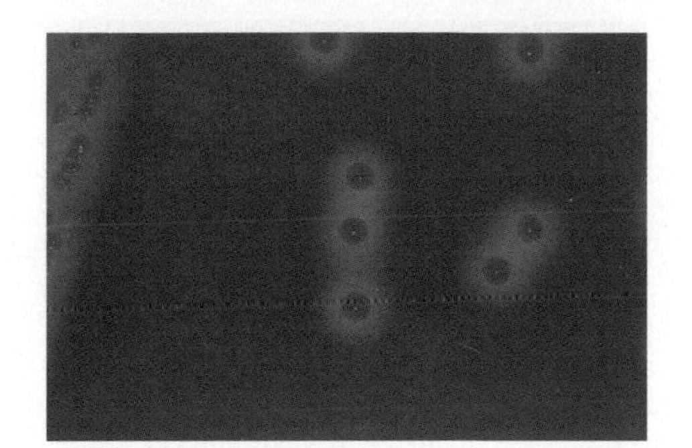

Color Plate 33 ◆ Beta-hemolytic streptococcal colonies on blood agar.

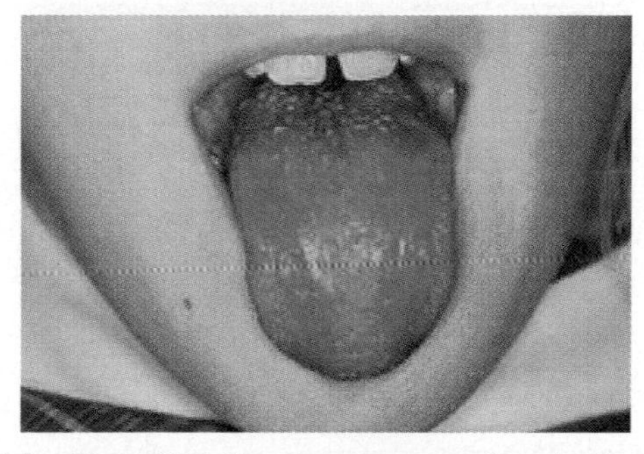

Color Plate 34 ◆ Strawberry tongue of scarlet fever.

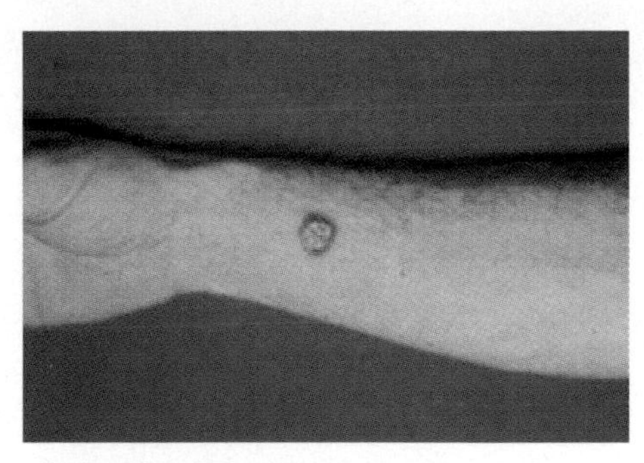

Color Plate 35 ◆ Cutaneous anthrax lesion.

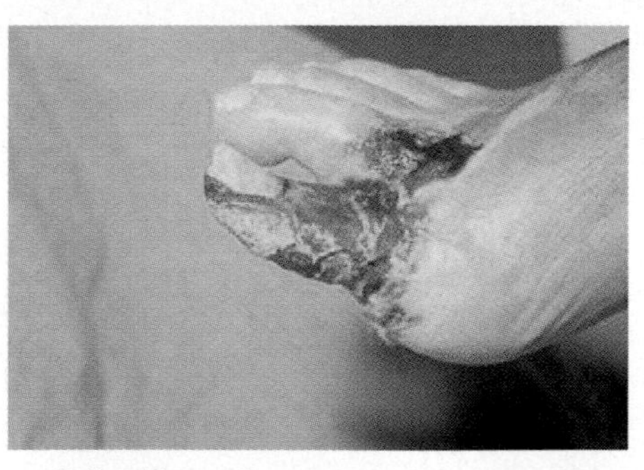

Color Plate 36 ◆ Gangrene of the toes.

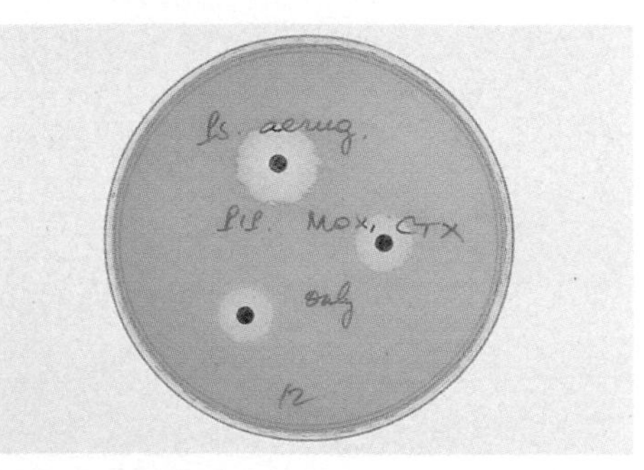

Color Plate 37 ◆ Blue-green pigmented growth of *Pseudomonas aeruginosa* on Mueller-Hinton medium.

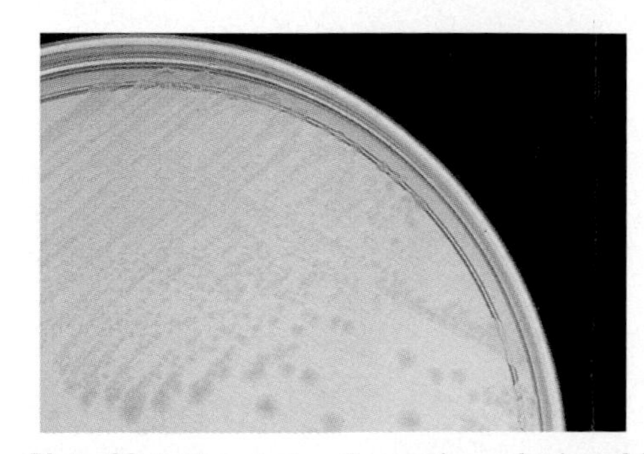

Color Plate 38 ◆ Non–lactose-fermenting colonies of *Pseudomonas aeruginosa* on MacConkey medium.

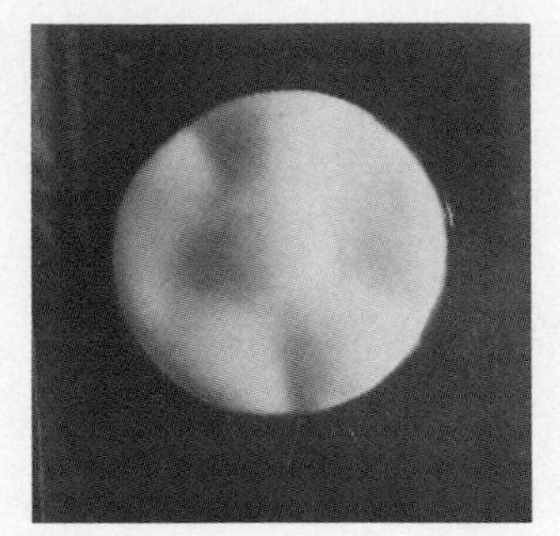

Color Plate 39 ◆ A colony of *Epidermophyton floccosum.*

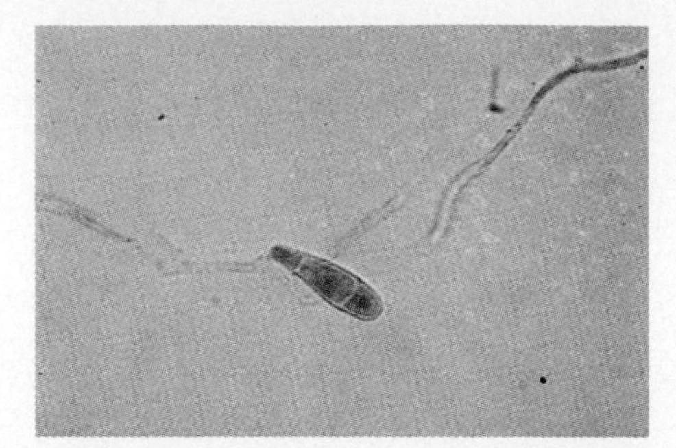

Color Plate 40 ◆ Microscopic view of *Epidermophyton floccosum.*

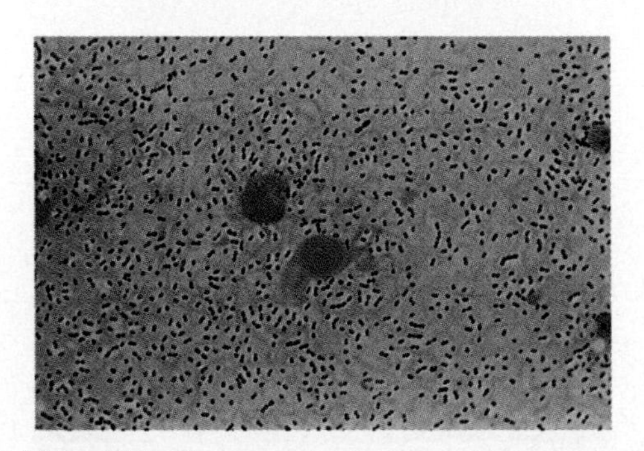

Color Plate 41 ◆ Direct smear of sputum from a patient with pneumonia stained by Gram stain showing *Streptococcus pneumoniae.*

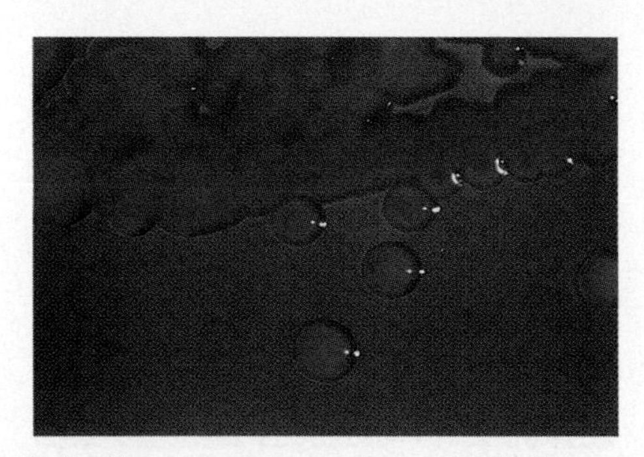

Color Plate 42 ◆ Mucoid appearance of *Klebsiella pneumoniae* colonies on MacConkey agar.

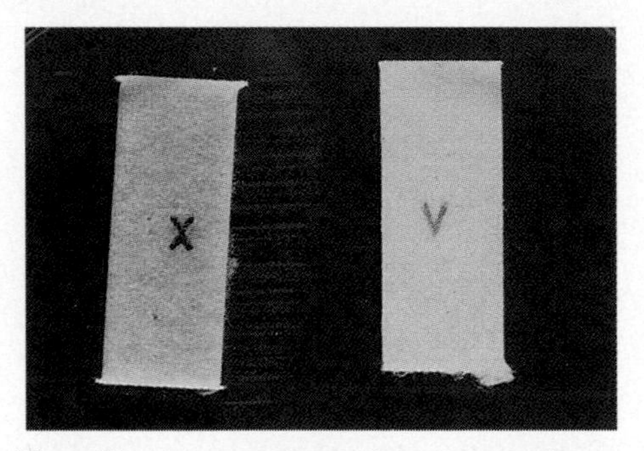

Color Plate 43 ◆ The growth of *Haemophilus influenzae* occurs only between the strips containing the X and V factors.

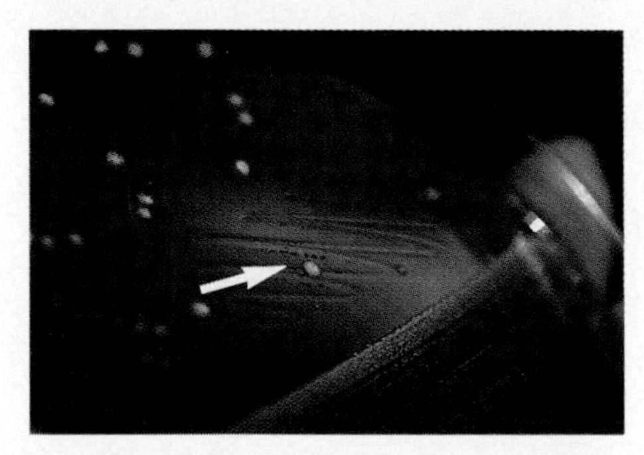

Color Plate 44 ◆ Satellite colonies of *Haemophilus influenzae (arrow)* around a colony of *Staphylococcus aureus.*

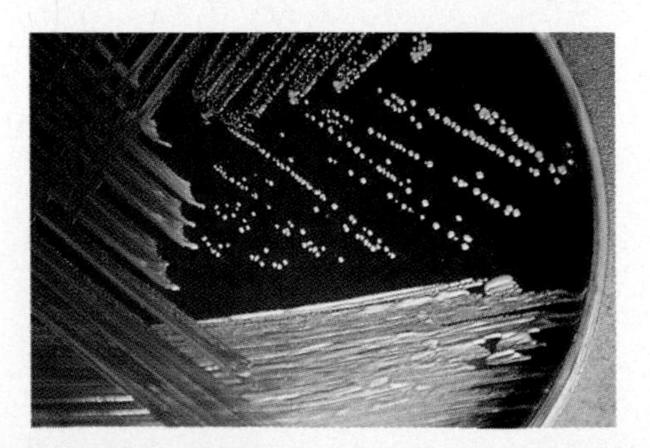

Color Plate 45 ◆ *Bordetella pertussis* colonies on Regan-Lowe medium.

Color Plate 46 ◆ Immunofluorescence of *Bordetella pertussis.*

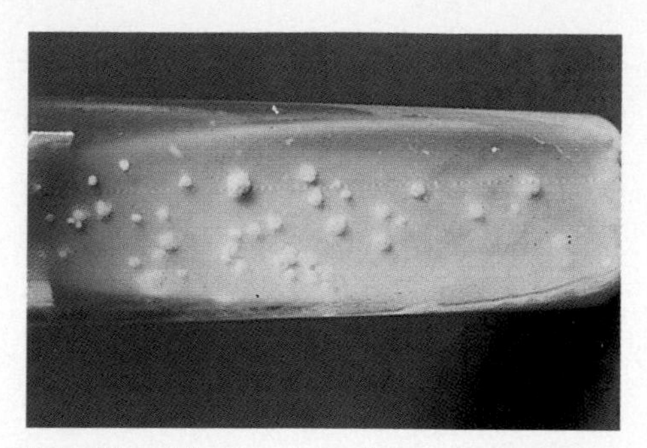

Color Plate 47 ◆ *Mycobacterium tuberculosis* growing on Löwenstein-Jensen medium.

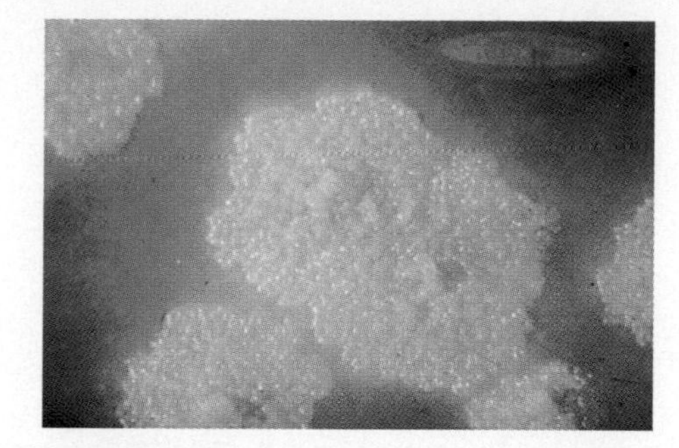

Color Plate 48 ◆ A view at higher magnification of *M. tuberculosis* colonies.

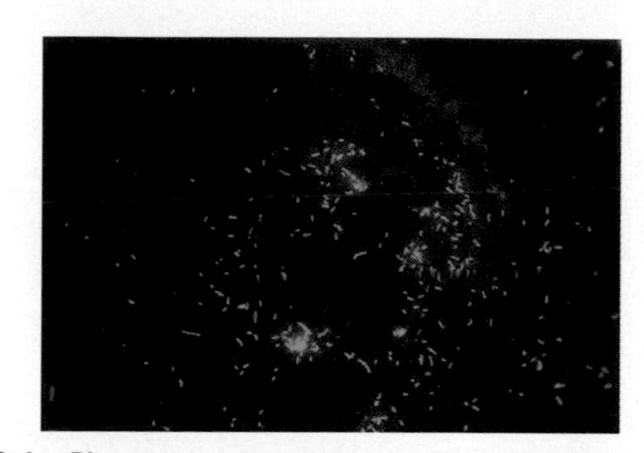

Color Plate 49 ◆ Immunofluorescence of *Legionella* sp.

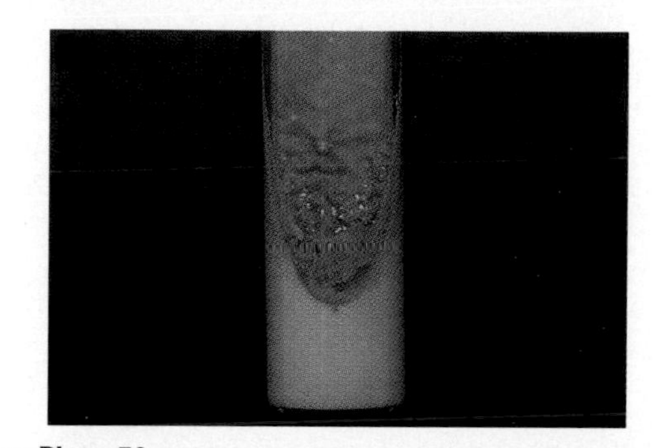

Color Plate 50 ◆ *Nocardia asteroides* colonies on Löwenstein-Jensen medium.

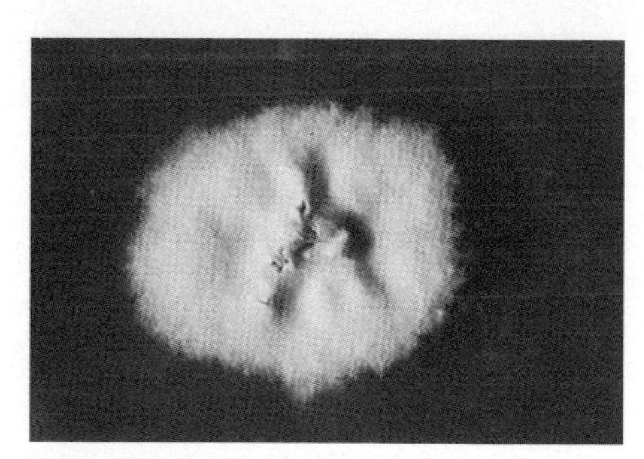

Color Plate 51 ◆ A colony of a dimorphic fungus, *Histoplasma capsulatum,* in its mold phase.

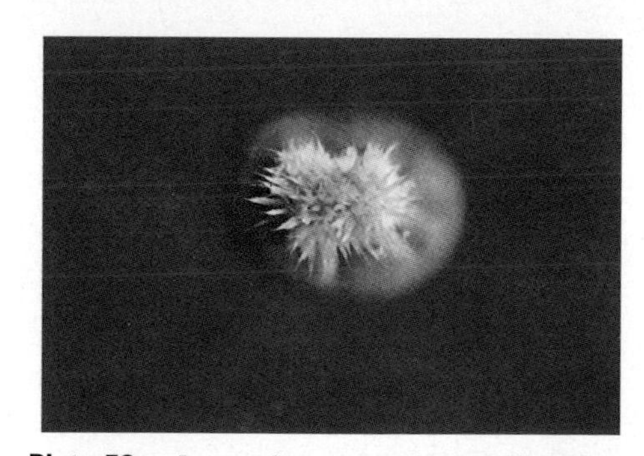

Color Plate 52 ◆ Incomplete conversion of *Histoplasma capsulatum* to its yeast phase as shown on the fringes of the colony.

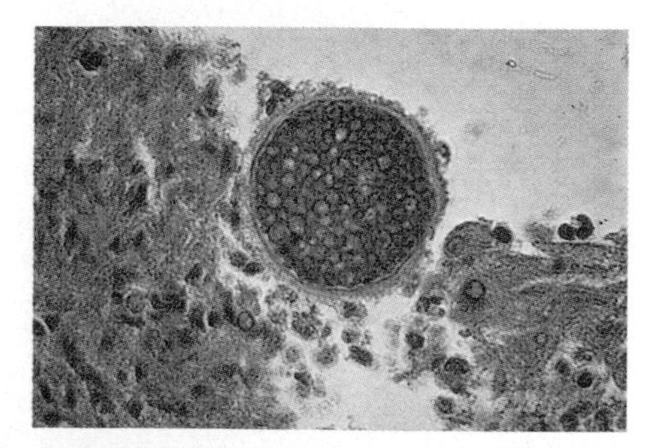

Color Plate 53 ◆ Spherules of *Coccidioides immitis* in tissue.

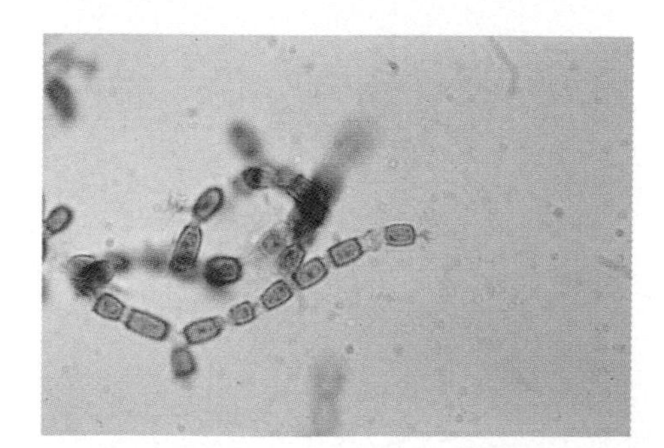

Color Plate 54 ◆ Arthroconidia of *Coccidioides immitis.*

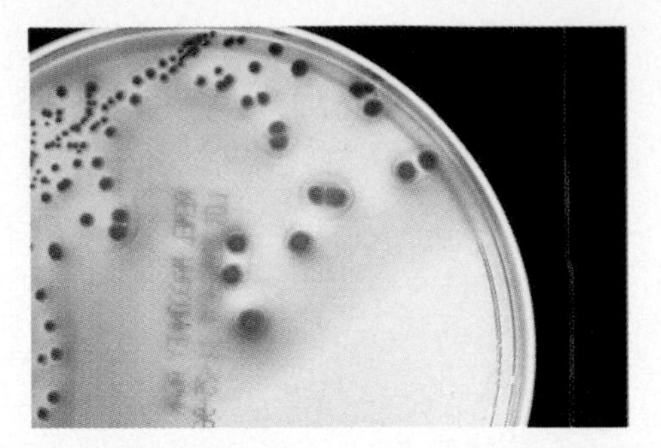

Color Plate 55 ◆ Lactose-fermenting colonies of *Escherichia coli* on MacConkey agar.

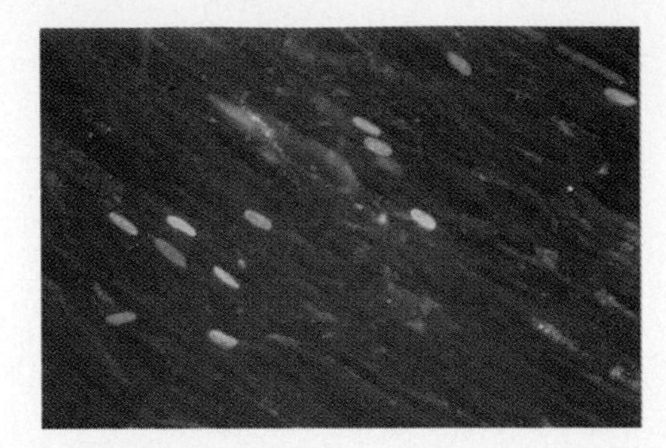

Color Plate 56 ◆ Typical fluorescing nuclei of fibroblast cells infected with cytomegalovirus.

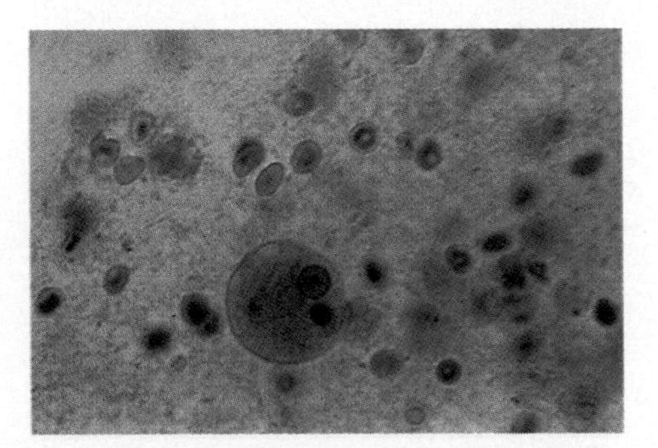

Color Plate 57 ◆ *Entamoeba histolytica* trophozoite with an ingested red blood cell (dark color) near the nucleus.

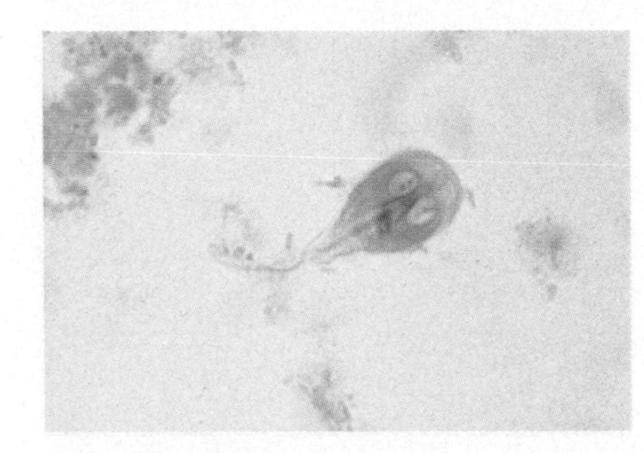

Color Plate 58 ◆ *Giardia lamblia,* trophozoite.

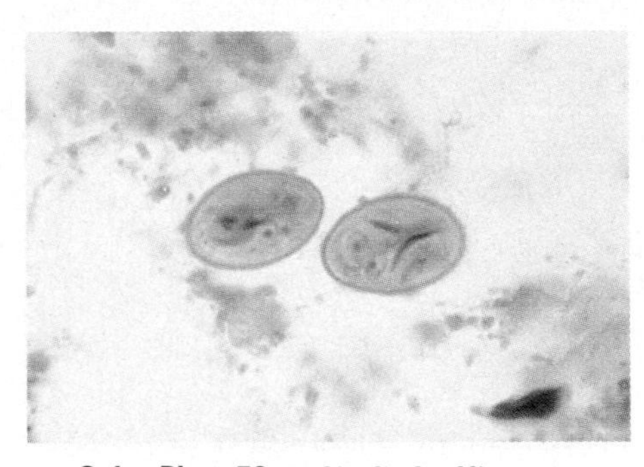

Color Plate 59 ◆ *Giardia lamblia,* cysts.

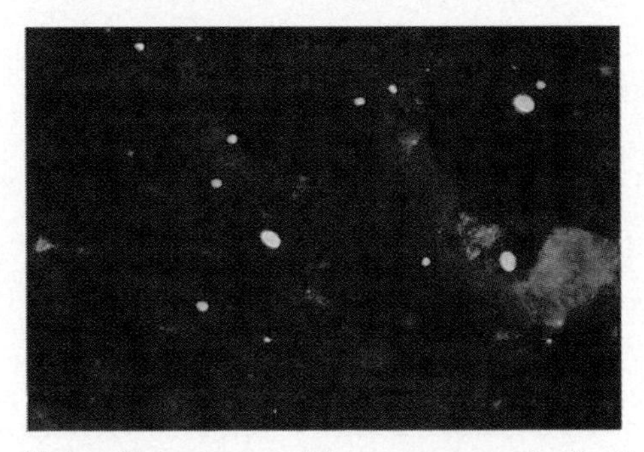

Color Plate 60 ◆ *Cryptosporidium* oocysts and *Giardia* cysts stained with monoclonal antibody conjugated reagent.

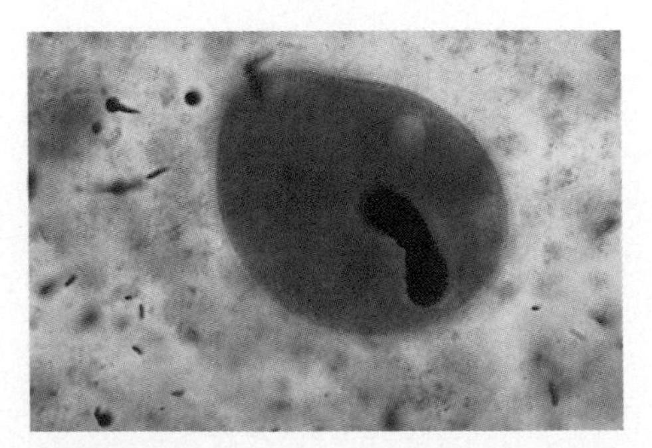

Color Plate 61 ◆ *Balantidium coli* trophozoite, iodine stain.

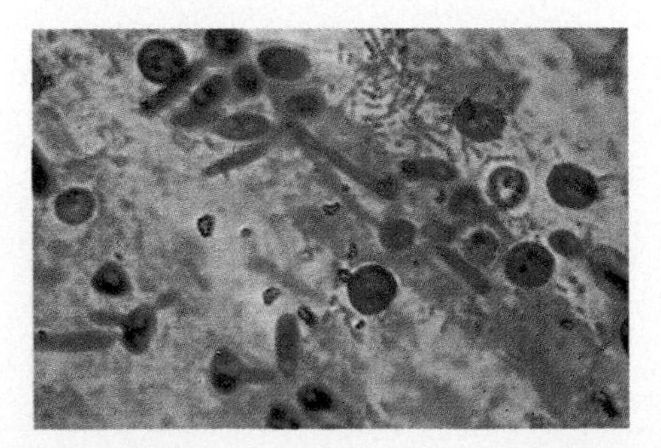

Color Plate 62 ◆ Acid-fast oocysts of *Cryptosporidium.*

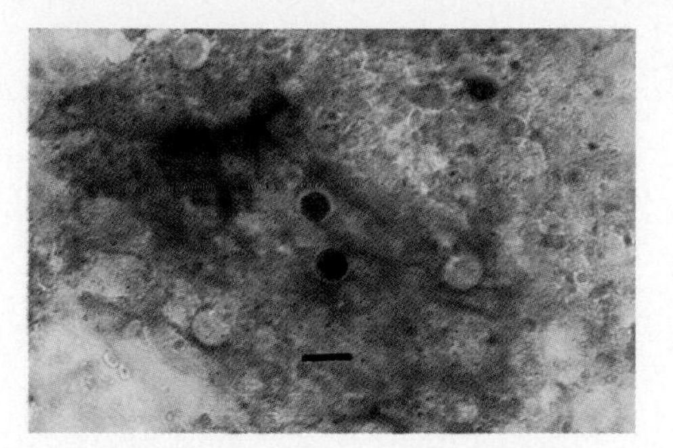

Color Plate 63 ◆ Purple to red oocysts of *Cyclospora* species, stained by Kinyoun's acid-fast method. Bar measures 10 μm.

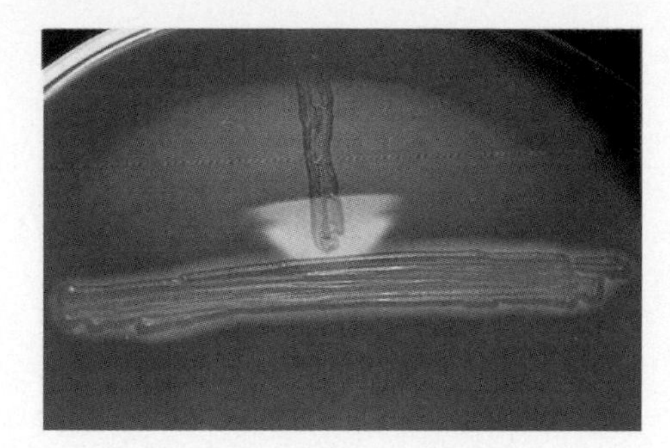

Color Plate 64 ◆ Presumptive identification of a group B *Streptococcus* by the CAMP test showing the classic arrow-shaped hemolysis near the *Staphylococcus* line of growth (center).

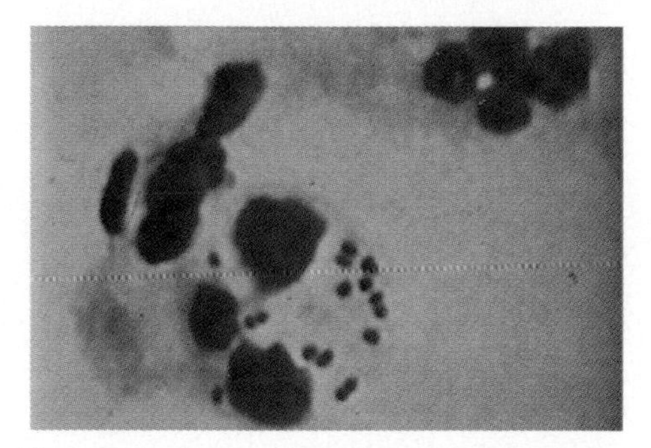

Color Plate 65 ◆ Intracellular *Neisseria gonorrhoeae* diplococci in phagocytic cells.

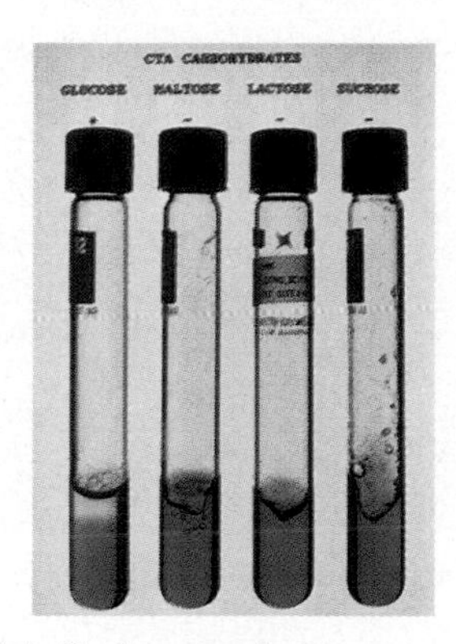

Color Plate 66 ◆ Cystine trypticase agar tubes with added sugar (1%) differentiate *Neisseria* species.

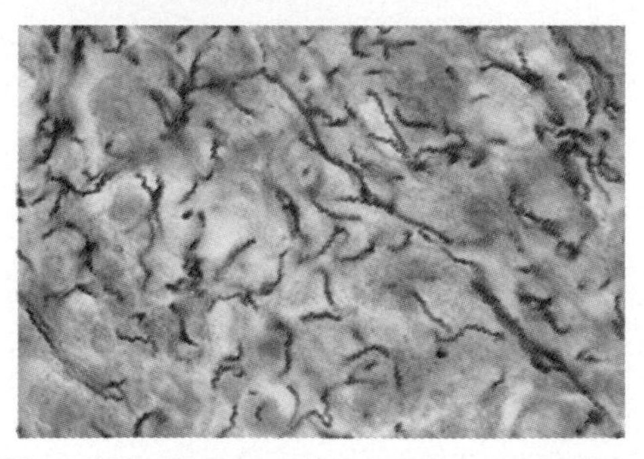

Color Plate 67 ◆ The spirochete *Treponema pallidum* in tissue stained by the silver nitrate method.

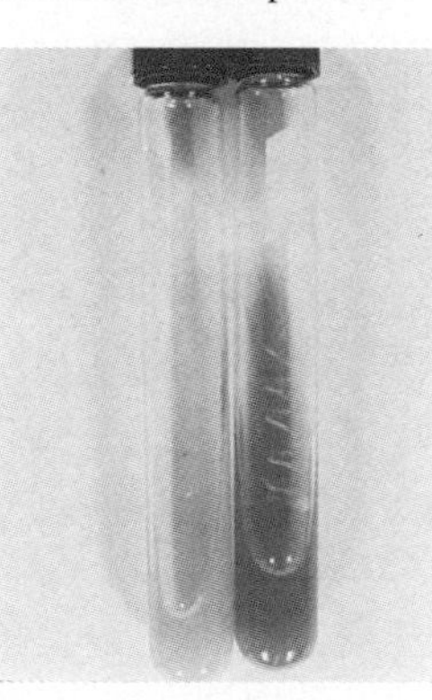

Color Plate 68 ◆ Uninoculated control (L) and urease production by *Cryptococcus neoformans* (R).

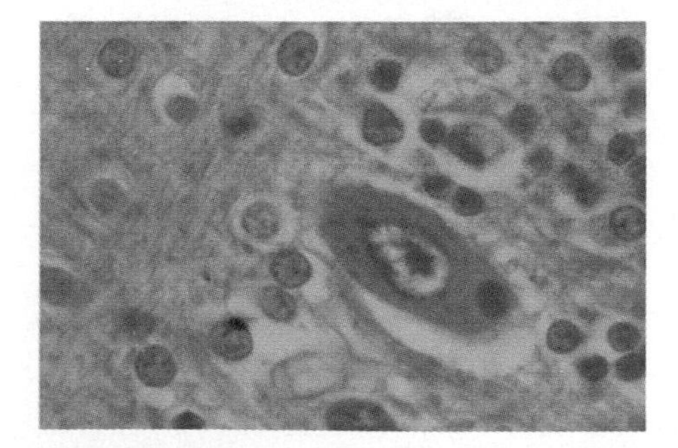

Color Plate 69 ◆ Hematoxylin-eosin–stained brain tissue showing large oval Negri body of rabies.

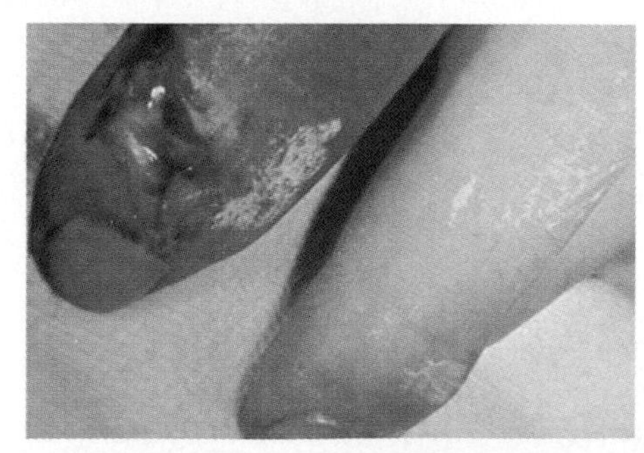

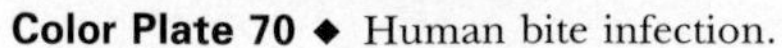

Color Plate 70 ◆ Human bite infection.

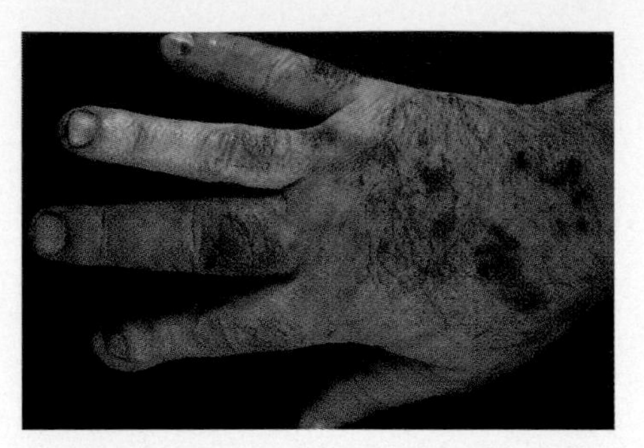

Color Plate 71 ◆ Classic Kaposi's sarcoma, an opportunistic disease of the acquired immunodeficiency syndrome.

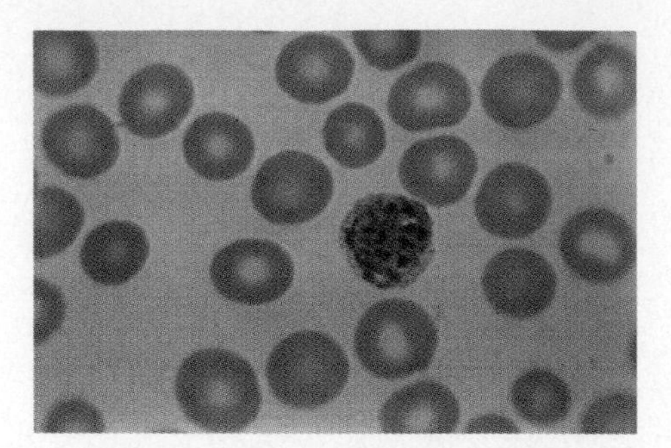

Color Plate 72 ◆ Immature schizont of *Plasmodium vivax.*

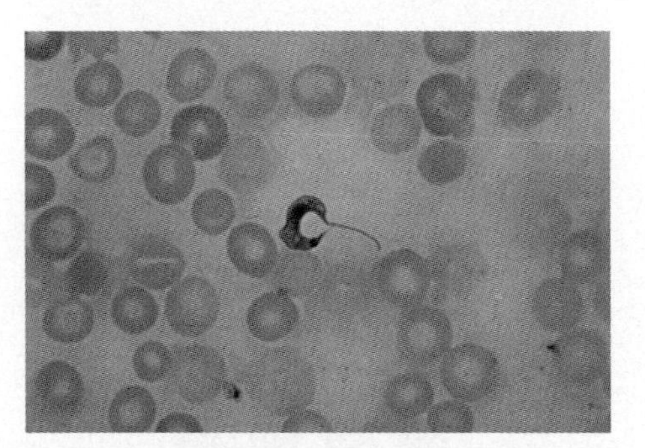

Color Plate 73 ◆ *Trypanosoma cruzi,* tryptomastigote stage, in blood.

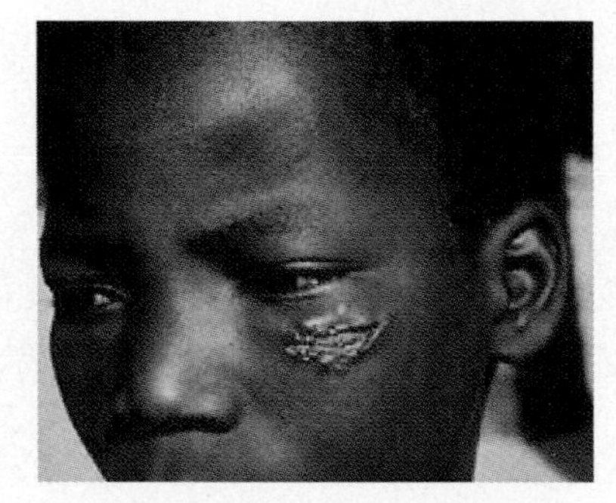

Color Plate 74 ◆ Cutaneous leishmaniasis.

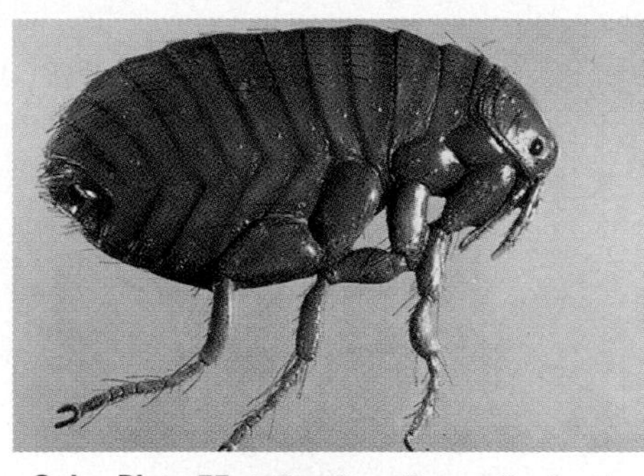

Color Plate 75 ◆ Rat flea, *Xenopsylla cheopis.*

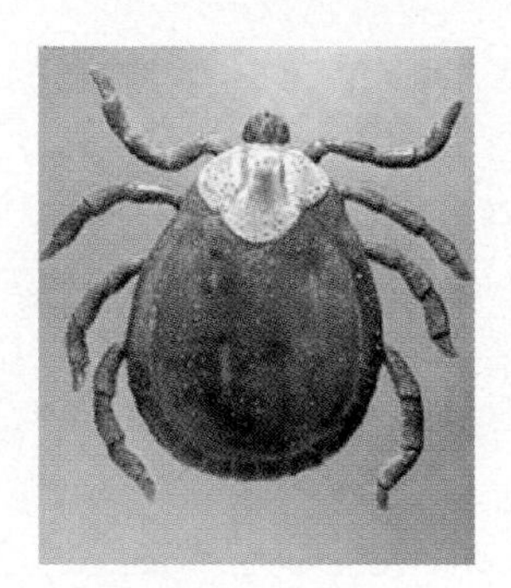

Color Plate 76 ◆ Wood tick, *Dermacentor andersoni.*

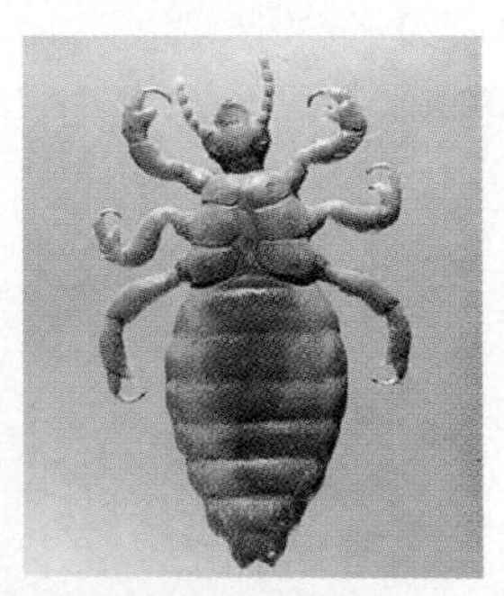

Color Plate 77 ◆ Body louse, *Pediculus humanus corporis.*

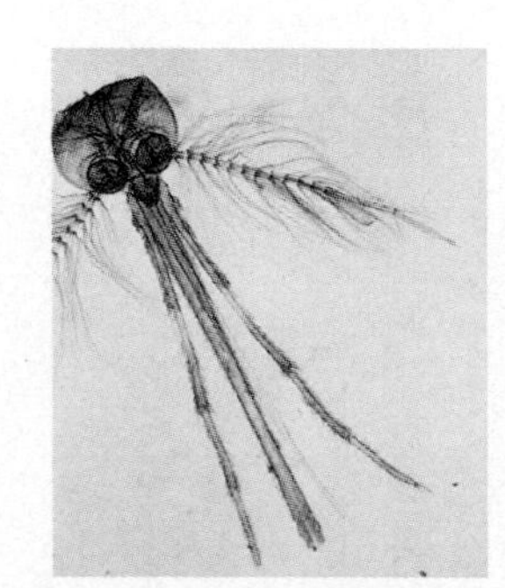

Color Plate 78 ◆ Mouth parts of the male mosquito *Aedes aegypti.*

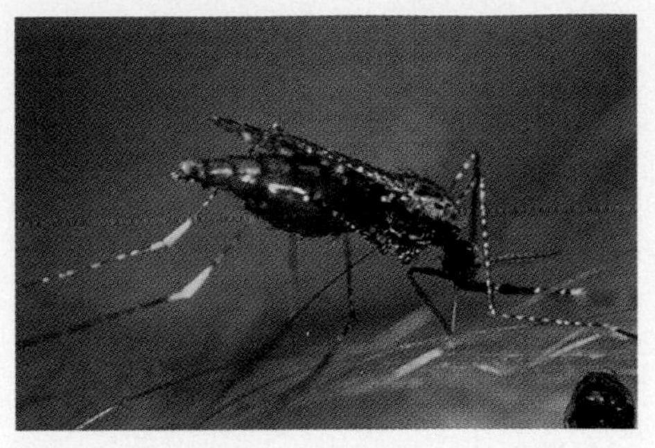

Color Plate 79 ◆ *Anopheles* mosquito obtaining a blood meal.

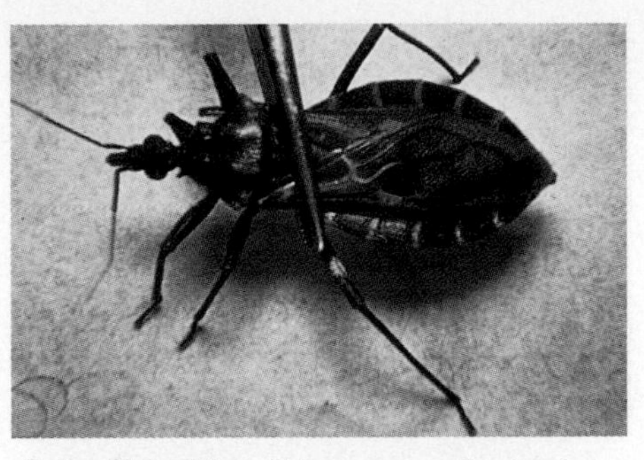

Color Plate 80 ◆ *Triatoma* sp. or kissing bug.

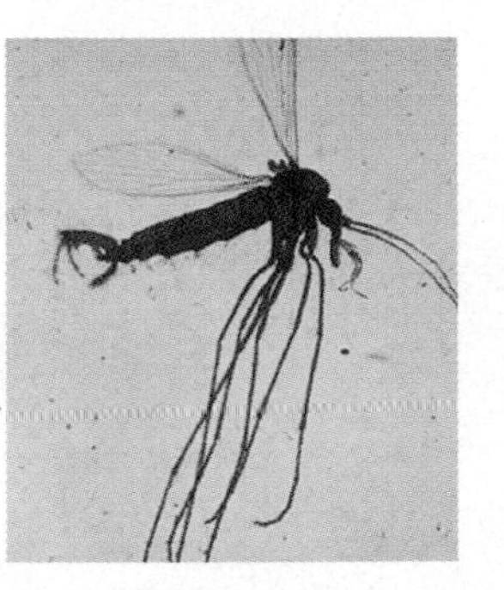

Color Plate 81 ◆ Sandfly belonging to the genus *Phlebotomus.*

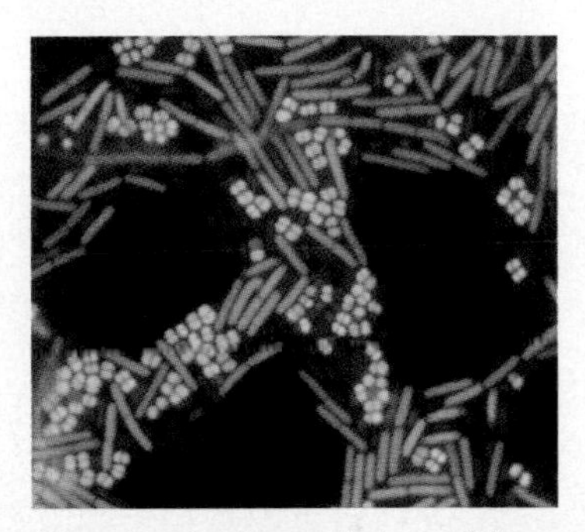

Color Plate 82 ◆ A mixed population of live and isopropyl alcohol–killed *Micrococcus luteus* and *Bacillus cereus* stained with the LIVE/DEAD *Bac*Light Bacterial Viability Kit. Bacteria with intact membranes exhibit the green fluorescence of SYTO 9 dye, which binds to nucleic acid in intact cells. The cells with damaged membranes exhibit the red fluorescence of propidium iodide, which binds to the nucleic acid in cells with damaged cell membranes.

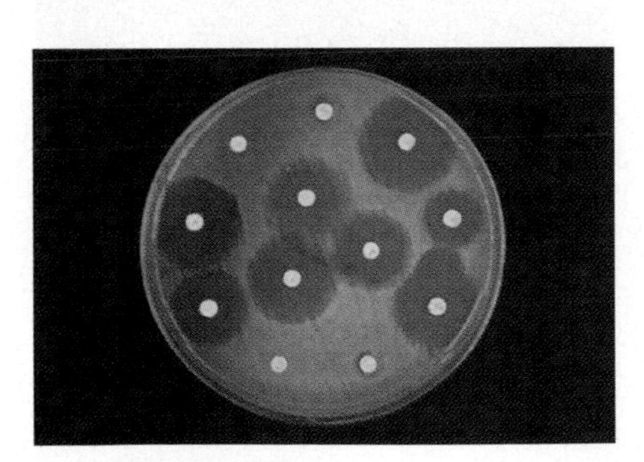

Color Plate 83 ◆ Disk diffusion method for antimicrobial susceptibility testing.

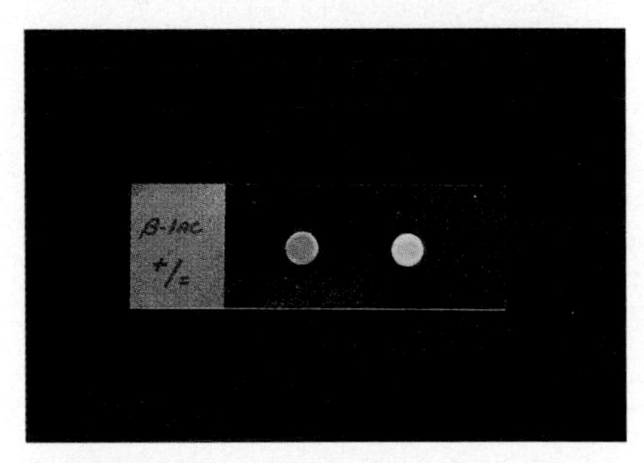

Color Plate 84 ◆ Disk test for β-lactamase. The disk on the left is pink, indicating the bacteria produce β-lactamase.

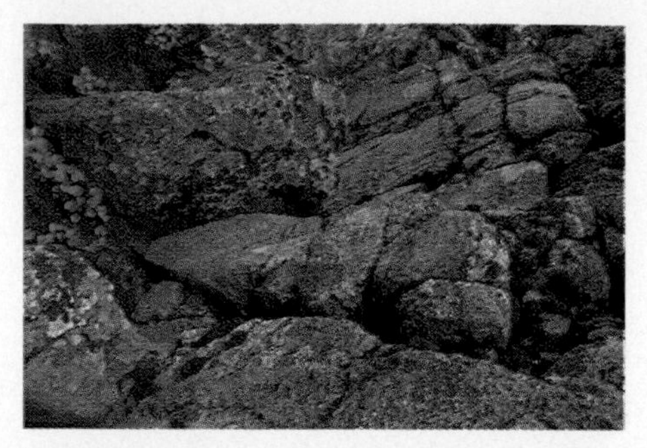

Color Plate 85 ◆ Crustose red-pigmented lichen growing on basalt rock.

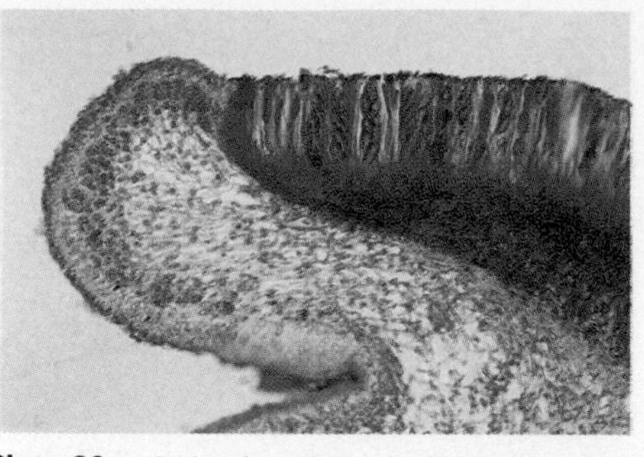

Color Plate 86 ◆ Stained section of a lichen showing its cup-shaped thallus (hyphal body) with algae cells and its asci with septate ascospores.

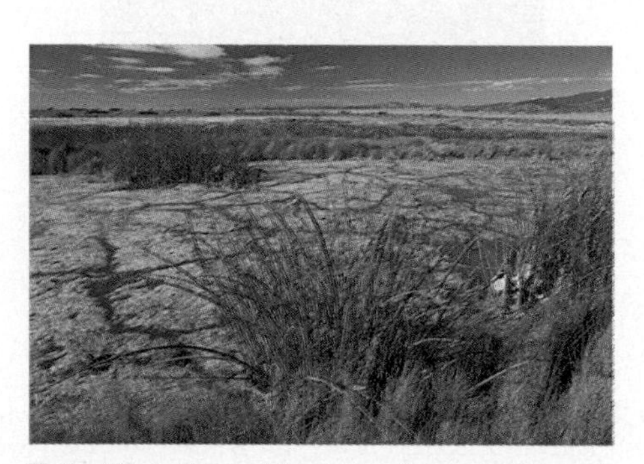

Color Plate 87 ◆ Eutrophication of a stream results when high concentrations of nitrogen and phosphorus feed algae and other green plants, producing an algal "bloom."

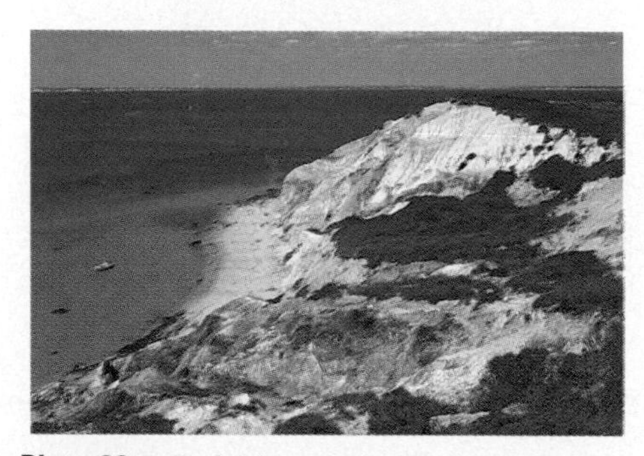

Color Plate 88 ◆ Red tide caused by a "bloom" of dinoflagellates in a California coastal bay.

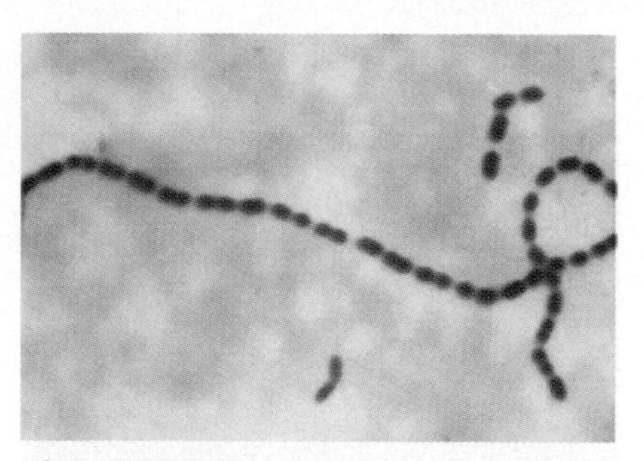

Color Plate 89 ◆ Chains of *Lactococcus lactis.*

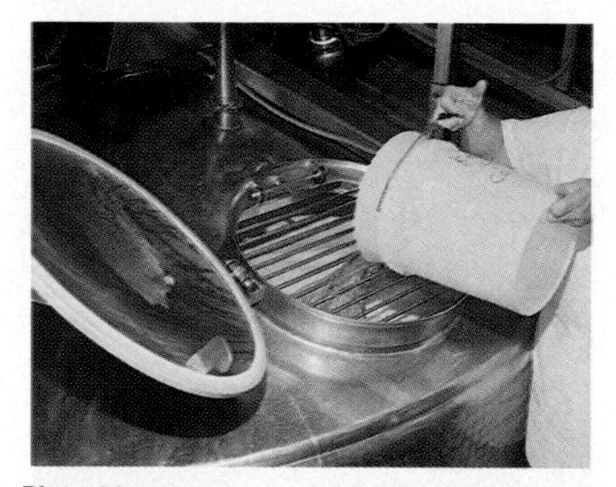

Color Plate 90 ◆ Rennin is added to milk to begin coagulating curds for cheese.

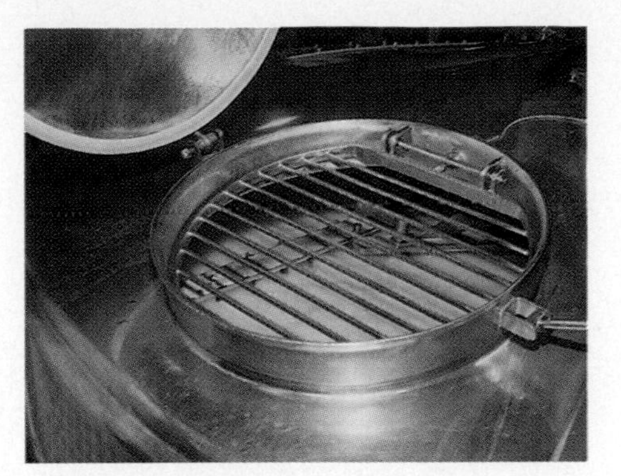

Color Plate 91 ◆ Bacteria ferment lactose in milk at 100°C, producing acids and more curds.

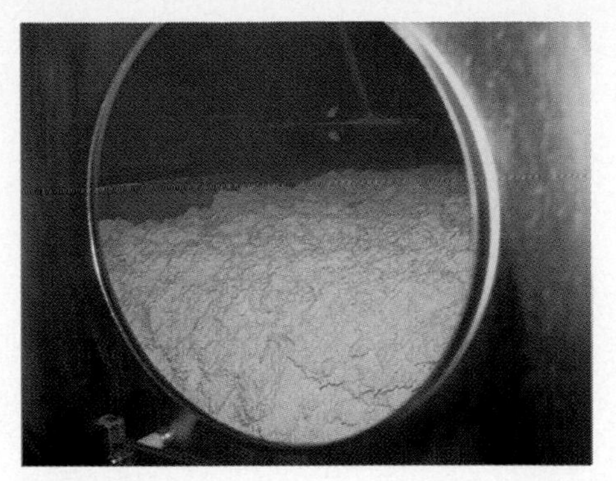

Color Plate 92 ◆ Liquid whey is removed, leaving cheese curds.

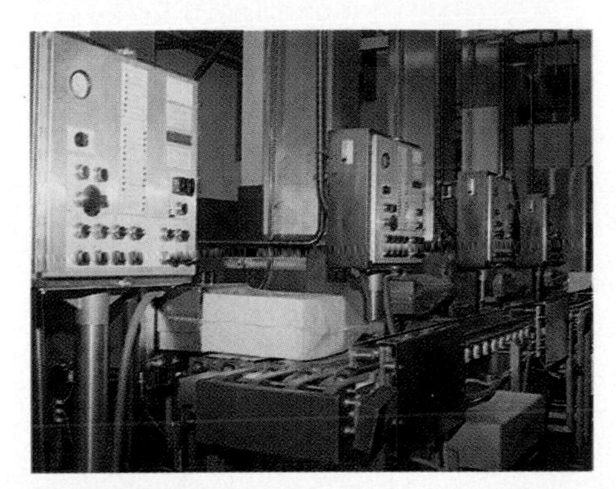

Color Plate 93 ◆ After salting curds, cheddar cheese is packed into 40-pound blocks for aging at least 60 days.

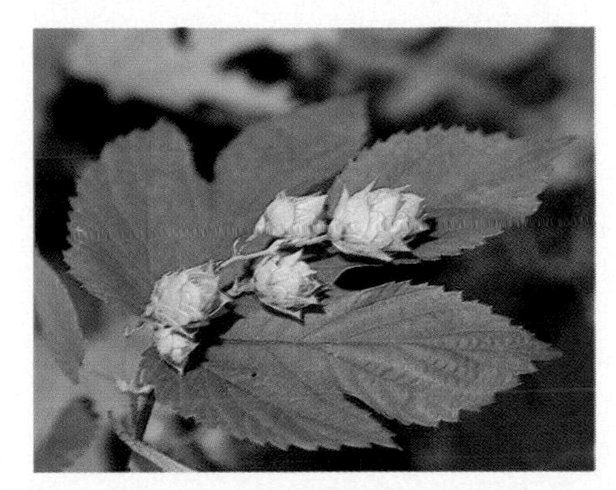

Color Plate 94 ◆ Female flowers of *Humulus* species, the hops plant, are used in making beer.

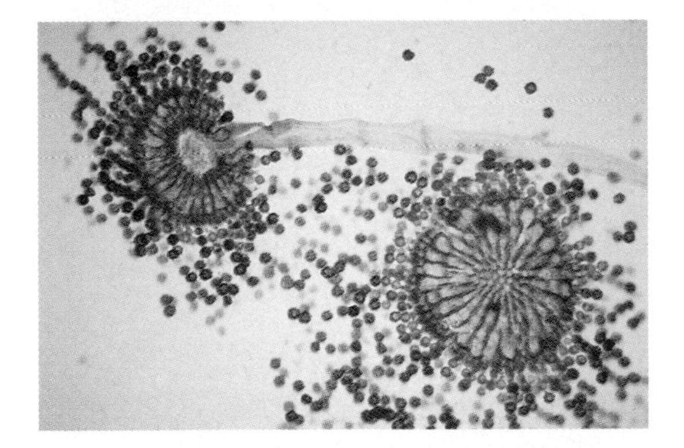

Color Plate 95 ◆ *Aspergillus* sp., a toxin-producing fungus in moldy grains.

Unit 1

An Introduction to Microbiology

Chapter 1

Discovery and Diversity of the Microbial World

Chapter Outline

- **THE ORIGIN OF LIFE**
- **THE CONTROVERSY OVER SPONTANEOUS GENERATION**
  - Redi's Experiment on Flies
  - Leeuwenhoek's "Animalcules"
  - The Continuing Controversy
  - Needham's and Spallanzani's Experiments
  - Pasteur Ends the Controversy
  - Tyndall's Discovery of Endospores
- **THE GERM THEORY OF DISEASE**
  - Contributions of Holmes and Semmelweis
  - Pasteur's Continuing Trail of Discovery
  - Lister's Attempt to Control Infection
- **THE DEVELOPING SCIENCE OF MICROBIOLOGY: KOCH'S TECHNIQUES**
- **THE BEGINNINGS OF IMMUNOLOGY**
  - Jenner and the First Vaccine
  - Pasteur's Attenuated Vaccines
  - Metchnikoff and Phagocytosis
  - Ehrlich and Serum Protective Factors
- **THE DISCOVERY OF ANTIMICROBIAL AGENTS**
  - Domagk and Sulfa Drugs
  - Fleming and Penicillin
- **MICROORGANISMS: THE NATURAL JEWELRY OF THE EARTH**
  - Classification and Nomenclature of Microorganisms
  - The Major Groups of Microorganisms

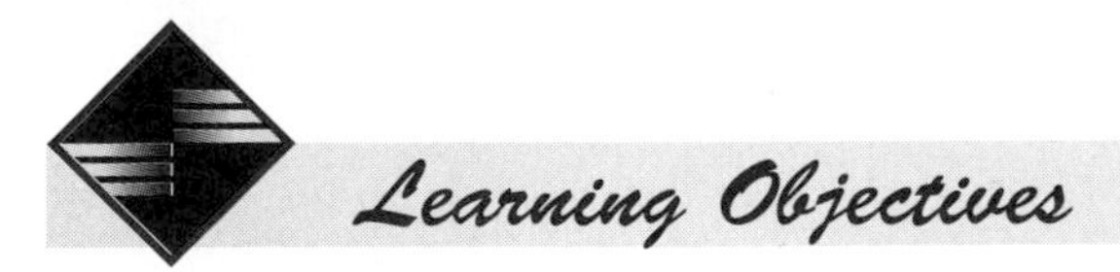

Learning Objectives

After you have read this chapter, you should be able to:

1. Explain the methods used to disprove the theory of spontaneous generation.
2. Describe the origin of the germ theory of disease.
3. Name the contributions of the early pioneers in microbiology.
4. Explain the basis of vaccination in prevention of infectious diseases.
5. Name the two patterns of cellular organization found in microorganisms.
6. Explain why acellular particles cannot be classified as procaryotes or eucaryotes.

The microorganisms on Earth have an impact on our lives from the time of our birth until the time of our death. Because of their microscopic nature we are usually unaware of their presence unless they cause us to be ill. Most of us can remember the intense itching caused by the lesions of chickenpox or the appearance of a pimple just before that important date. Few escape the discomfort of one or more common colds during the winter months. Others of us experience more exotic diseases, and even life-threatening illnesses, caused by our microbial enemies. The harmful microorganisms have gained more fame over the years than their beneficial counterparts. Some microorganisms of less renown are responsible for our very ability to exist on the planet.

We seldom associate the air we breathe or the food we eat with microbial populations. Yet microorganisms have the largest role in photosynthesis, which releases the oxygen required to sustain our cells. Some microorganisms, such as those used in production of flavorful cheeses and fine wines, provide us with tantalizing culinary delights. Still others are used in disposal of waste products, in fertilizing our soils, and in the production of drugs. We have time to relate only the highlights along the discovery trail to the science of microbiology as we know it today.

THE ORIGIN OF LIFE

The belief in the spontaneous generation of life from nonliving matter was introduced by Aristotle (384–322 BC) and remained unchallenged for over 2000 years. According to his theory, living things arose from muck, decaying food, warm rain, or even dirty shirts. Through the years a number of innovative recipes appeared which guaranteed the spontaneous generation of living things. One ingenious recipe for generating mice, proposed by the Flemish physician, Baptista van Helmont (1579–1644), consisted of placing a dirty shirt into a bin of wheat germ and allowing 20 days for the appearance of mice.

THE CONTROVERSY OVER SPONTANEOUS GENERATION

The theory of spontaneous generation was not universally accepted. Early biologists performed a number of experiments to prove or refute that explanation for the origin of life. Most biologists recognized that higher forms of life, such as sheep and cattle, arose from interaction between males and females, but lower forms of life were still widely believed to arise spontaneously.

Redi's Experiments on Flies

It had been known for a long time that white worms frequently were seen on spoiled meat or fish. It was Francesco Redi (1626–1698), an Ital-

FOCAL POINT

The Microscopic Zoo Within Us

A microscopic zoo is found in the many nooks and crannies of our bodies. Most of the time, we do not even know that the residents of the zoo, including protozoa, fungi, bacteria, and viruses, are there. Some microorganisms are permanent residents; others are transient residents that come and go. Microorganisms are found in the ears, eyes, armpits, groin, mucous membranes of the body, and intestines. The typical healthy colon harbors 10 billion microbes per gram of contents. These organisms make up the normal flora of the body. Within 12 hours after birth, the body becomes colonized with various kinds of bacteria. Most are beneficial to the infant in that they act as stimulants to the immune system and synthesize needed nutrients, such as biotin, pantothenic acid, pyridoxine, and vitamin B_{12}. They actually stake out territory that otherwise could be occupied by disease-producing organisms. When the numbers of normal-flora fall, it provides an opportunity for remaining residents or any entering harmful microorganisms to multiply. Should members of the normal flora venture into unfamiliar territory of the body, they may or may not cause trouble. If the common intestinal bacterium, *Escherichia coli,* migrates to the urinary bladder or gains access to the abdominal cavity, outside the intestines, an infection occurs. Certain human behavior can result in alterations in normal flora. For example, dietary patterns, smoking, and douching allow new microorganisms to gain entrance and become part of the microscopic zoo within us. A diet high in carbohydrates encourages growth of gas-producing fermentative bacteria. Smoking destroys protective cilia on cells lining the respiratory tract. The lower pH created by douching promotes entrance of cervical organisms into the uterus and fallopian tubes. By these and other behaviors, we can control in part the composition of our own microscopic zoos.

FDA Consumer 26:37–42, 1992

ian physician, who first challenged their spontaneous generation. He devised a very simple experiment to show that the worms actually developed from eggs that flies deposited on the decaying meat or fish. Redi placed samples of meat in each of two jars. He left one jar uncovered, but covered the other one with gauze. He observed that flies deposited eggs on the meat left uncovered and on the gauze covering the other jar (Fig. 1–1). Only the eggs deposited on the meat gave rise to worms, and ultimately, to new flies. Redi concluded that the flies were actually the parents of the white worms we know as maggots today. Redi's experiment temporarily resolved the questions on the origin of life.

Leeuwenhoek's "Animalcules"

In 1673 the idea of spontaneous generation was reopened once again. Antony van Leeuwenhoek (1632–1723), a Dutch merchant and amateur scientist, used a primitive microscope to observe stagnant water, hay infusions, and scrapings from the teeth. His microscope consisted of a small lens mounted between two thin plates of metal (Fig. 1–2). With the lens, which had a magnification of about 300, van Leeuwenhoek was able to see small forms of life he called "animalcules" (Fig. 1–3). Leeuwenhoek was a skilled observer, a diligent worker, and a man with a great deal of patience. After 20 years of careful observations, he reported his findings to the Royal Society of London. The almost universal presence of microscopic organisms from environmental sources seemed to support a spontaneous origin for life.

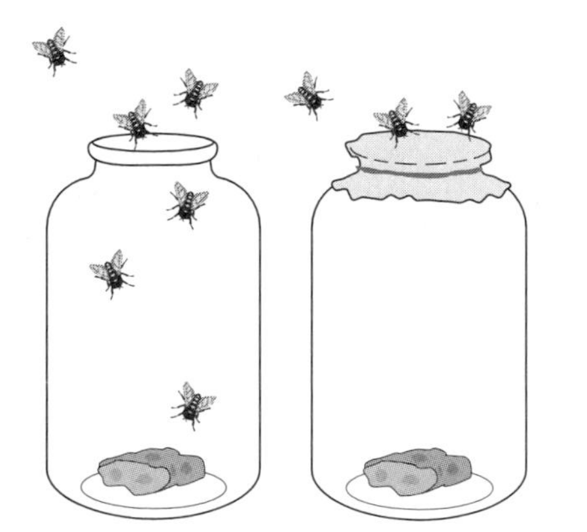

Figure 1–1 ◆ Francisco Redi's jars helped to resolve questions on the origin of life. Maggots did not develop in the jar the flies could not enter.

The Continuing Controversy

Several eighteenth century scientists and clergymen became interested in the presence of microorganisms in mixtures of plant or animal material and water. Such mixtures contain numerous microorganisms. It was suspected that the tiny life forms could be destroyed by heat.

Needham's and Spallanzani's Experiments

The demonstration of van Leeuwenhoek's "little animals" prompted an English priest, John Needham (1713–1781), and an Italian naturalist, Lazzaro Spallanzani (1729–1799), to try to discover the source of the small life forms. Needham boiled mutton broth in corked flasks for a short period of time in an attempt to kill the microorganisms. He found the broth was teeming with microbial life within a few days. Confident that the heat had killed the small forms of life, he concluded that the organisms arose spontaneously from the organic contents of the mutton broth.

Meanwhile, Spallanzani boiled a similar broth in airtight flasks for at least one hour. The turbidity associated with microbial growth never did appear. He concluded that prolonged heating and complete exclusion of air from flasks had destroyed the microorganisms. With Antoine Lavoisier's recognition of the importance of oxygen to life in 1775, the validity of Needham's and Spallanzani's conclusions were doubted. The lack of growth in Spallanzani's flasks was attributed to the lack of oxygen in the flasks.

Pasteur Ends the Controversy

It remained for the French chemist, Louis Pasteur (1822–1895) to disprove the theory of spontaneous generation and to associate living microorganisms with disease (Fig. 1–4). Pasteur designed the now famous swan-necked flasks for heating broths (Fig. 1–5). The tortuous pathway afforded by the bends in the glass prevented dust particles, laden with microorganisms of the air, from entering heated broths. Instead, dust particles settled by gravity in the bends of the long-necked flasks. No signs of life appeared in the heated broths kept in the flasks even over an extended period of time. When the top of a flask was removed, microorganisms once again ap-

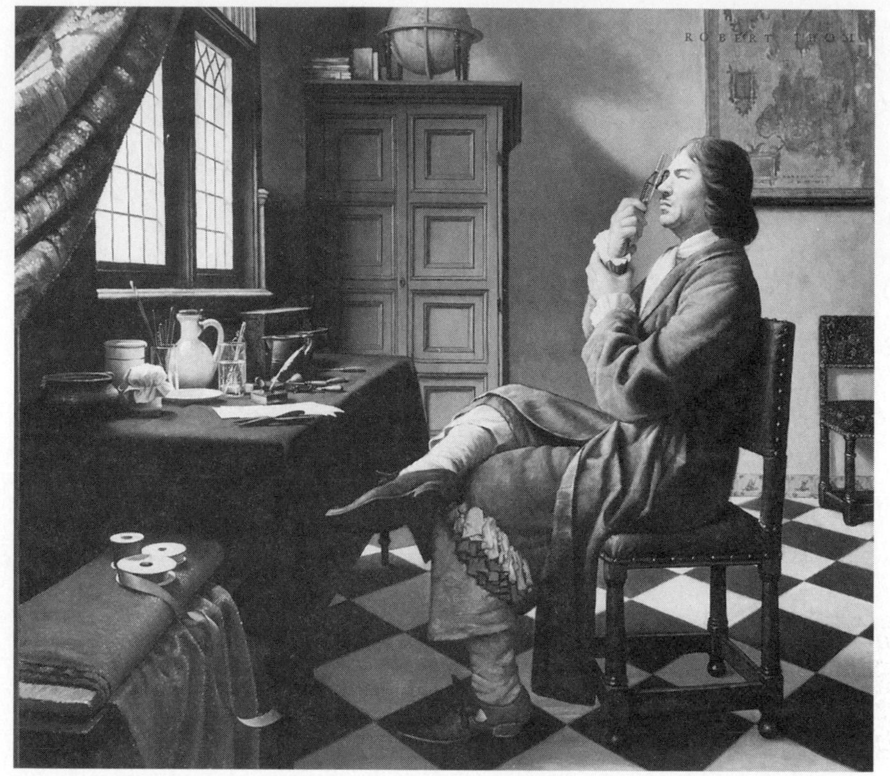

A

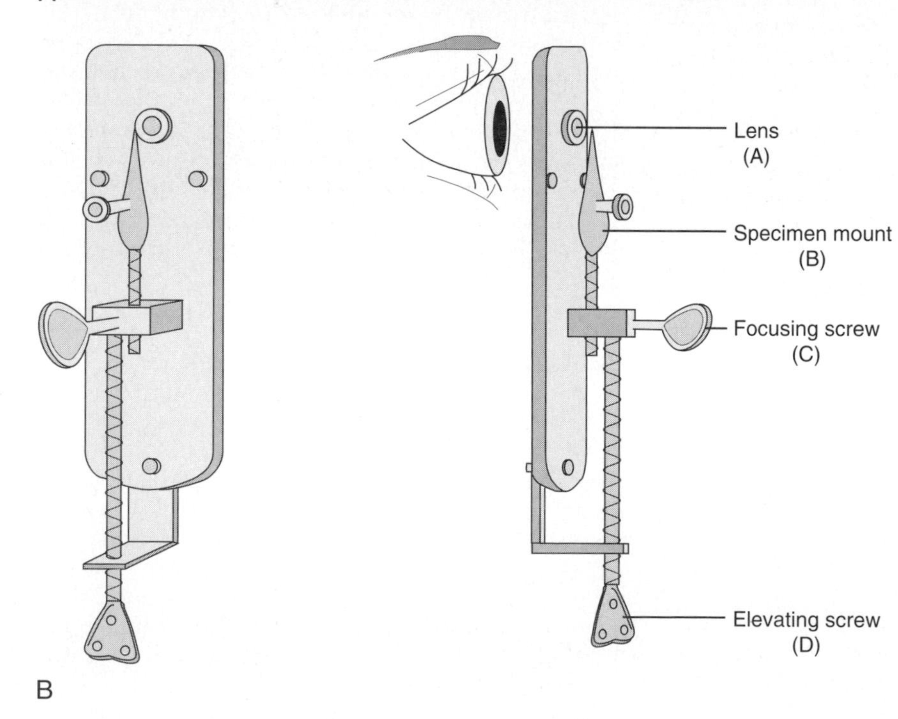

B

Figure 1–2 ◆ *A,* Antony van Leeuwenhoek observing microorganisms he called "animalcules" in his laboratory. *B,* Two views of van Leeuwenhoek's microscope showing the lens (A), specimen mount (B), focusing screw (C), and elevating screw (D).

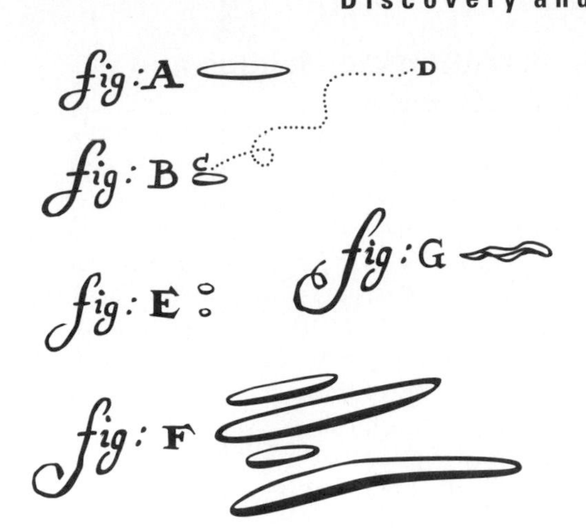

Figure 1–3 ◆ Drawings of "animalcules" of the human mouth from van Leeuwenhoek's original engravings showing variation in size and shape as well as the direction of movement for a motile microorganism.

peared in the liquid. Airborne microorganisms had made their way into the heated broths unless extraordinary means were taken to prevent their entrance. Pasteur's experiments put an end to the theory of spontaneous generation.

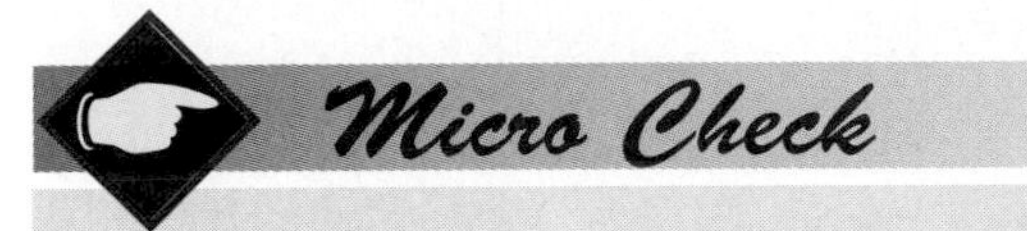

- Why is the design of any experiment so important?
- What were the major variables in Needham's and Spallanzani's experiments?
- How did swan-necked flasks help to end the controversy over spontaneous generation?

Tyndall's Discovery of Endospores

The English physicist John Tyndall (1820–1893), a contemporary of Pasteur's, was able to explain the need for prolonged heating to destroy microbial life in the broths. He discovered that some bacteria existed in two forms: a heat-stable form and a heat-sensitive form. It took either prolonged or intermittent heating to destroy the heat-stable forms. Intermittent heating, now called **tyndallization,** killed both forms. After the initial heating periods, the heat-stable forms changed to heat-sensitive forms, which were killed during subsequent heating. Almost simultaneously, the German botanist, Ferdinand Cohn

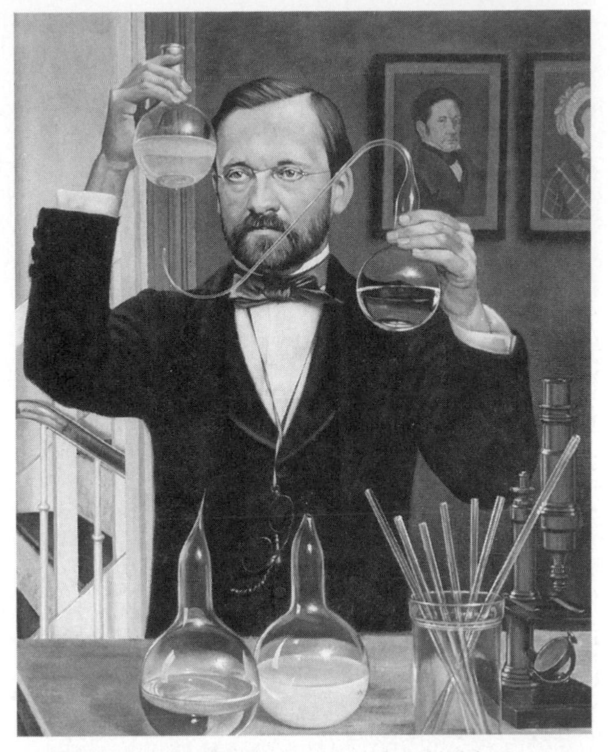

Figure 1–4 ◆ Louis Pasteur at work in his laboratory.

(1828–1898), described the heat-stable forms as **endospores.** We now know that endospores are formed during the life cycle of certain bacteria. The heat-stable endospores and the heat-sensitive bacteria were airborne and thus responsible for the appearance of microbial life in Needham's broths.

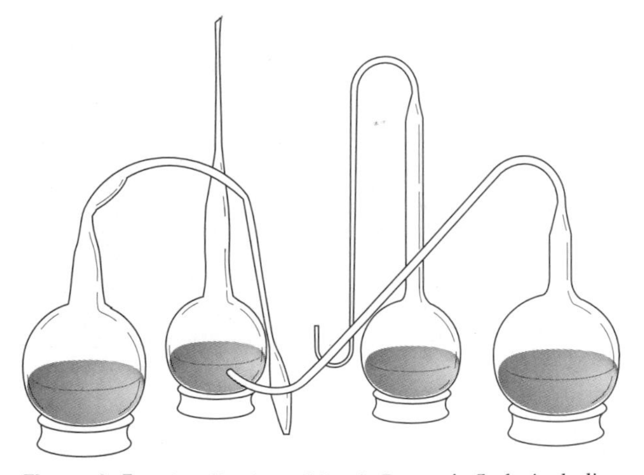

Figure 1–5 ◆ A collection of Louis Pasteur's flasks including the swan-neck flasks. The bends in the swan-neck flasks prevented microorganisms from entering the sterilized infusions.

The ability of some bacteria to form endospores turned out to be significant information. It was to be a key factor in determining the temperatures used to free materials from contaminating microorganisms. The process of destroying all forms of life is known as **sterilization.** Once the need for sterilization of surgical instruments, gloves, gowns, needles, syringes, and bandages was recognized, dramatic changes occurred in the practice of medicine.

THE GERM THEORY OF DISEASE

One of the first persons to propose a relationship between microorganisms and disease was Hieronymus Frascatorius (1484–1553). He speculated that syphilis, rabies, and plague were caused by living organisms. However, three centuries passed before a germ theory of disease was validated.

Contributions of Holmes and Semmelweis

The view that living things originated from nonliving sources diverted attention from humans as reservoirs of microorganisms. The observations made by two physicians in different parts of the world contributed significantly to the germ theory of disease. In the United States, Oliver Wendell Holmes (1809–1894) demonstrated that death following childbirth was often caused by material on the hands of midwives or attending physicians. The disease transmitted in that manner was called puerperal fever because it occurred in the **puerperium,** the period during or following delivery.

Meanwhile in Vienna, Ignaz Semmelweis (1818–1865), a Hungarian physician, noticed that death rates were higher in maternity wards staffed by medical students than in those at-

FOCAL POINT

The Scientific Method

OBSERVATION

HYPOTHESIS

EXPERIMENTATION

CONCLUSION

The foundations of microbiology, like those of other sciences, have been developed by application of the scientific method. That method consists of a series of steps necessary to support or reject a hypothesis as an explanation for an observation. It begins with one or more observations made over a period of time or made only once in a single setting. The next step is to develop a hypothesis to explain the observation. Once a hypothesis has been established, an experiment can be designed to test the validity of the hypothesis. It takes a knowledgeable scientist to plan experiments that take into consideration all possible variables. The experiment must be carefully designed to establish a single cause for the effect observed. All conditions under which the experiment is conducted must be kept constant except the experimental or **independent variable.** Good science requires the use of controls in which the independent variable is left out. This ensures that future observations are not due to anything other than that variable. The investigator must observe and record the **dependent variable** to see if a cause-and-effect relationship can be established. Numerical data obtained from experimentation can be subjected to statistical analyses. The results must be repeatable in the same laboratory and in the laboratories of other investigators. When enough data has been obtained, a conclusion can be drawn. That conclusion may or may not support the hypothesis. Sometimes it is necessary to revise the hypothesis and redesign the experiment. Only when the same conclusion, under identical circumstances, has been reached over and over again, is it possible to formulate a theory to explain the original observation.

Theories based on extensive experimentation differ substantially from the common use of the word theory. In everyday life the term "theory" is used to speculate on a reason for a happening. We may speculate that the reason our favorite football team lost the big game is because the star quarterback had been sidelined by an injury. Such a speculation may or may not be true, but it is impossible to prove the theory because the football game cannot be repeated. Scientific experiments are repeatable, and the theories developed from them stand the test of time. Their acceptance often constitutes major turning points in a science. Theories, based on experimentation, enable scientists to make predictions about the future and to develop new technologies.

tended by midwives. Furthermore, death rates went down in the wards during the summer when medical students were on vacation. Investigation revealed that medical students were coming immediately from the autopsy room to maternity wards without washing their hands. When the students were required to wash their hands in a solution of chlorine before entering the maternity wards and between patients, the number of infections and deaths was reduced. Semmelweis published his observations in 1847, but his recommendations for the prevention of puerperal fever were not widely accepted. He returned to his native Hungary and died in 1865 without receiving the recognition he so richly deserved for reducing death rates in maternity wards.

Pasteur's Continuing Trail of Discovery

Pasteur's contributions to the emerging germ theory of disease earned him the title Father of Microbiology. In 1863 Napoleon III solicited Pasteur's help on a problem of national importance. The flavorful wine, for which France had become so famous, was souring in many parts of the country. The activities of yeast cells were responsible for the alcoholic content of the wine. Pasteur saved the wine industry by showing that the spoiled vats contained acid-producing bacteria. The undesirable organisms could be destroyed at temperatures of 50° to 60°C in a short period of time. Ultimately, the heating of the grape juice to reduce the numbers of contaminating microorganisms became known as **pasteurization.**

In 1879 Pasteur discovered the microbial agent of puerperal fever in the bloodstream of infected patients. In 1880, in collaboration with Jules-Francois Joubert and Charles Chamberland, he described the causative agent of fowl cholera, a life-threatening disease of chickens.

Lister's Attempt to Control Infection

Joseph Lister (1827–1912), an English surgeon and contemporary of Pasteur's, was among the first to recognize the role of airborne microorganisms in postsurgical infections that often followed repair of compound fractures. He found that the number of infections could be reduced by applying carbolic acid to dressings and using an aerosol of carbolic acid during surgery (Fig. 1–6). Although we have better ways of preventing hospital-acquired infections today, Lister's contributions most certainly lowered the risk of infection following surgery.

Micro Check

- Why is handwashing so important in the prevention of infectious diseases?
- Of what importance are endospores in determining conditions necessary for sterilization?
- What products are pasteurized for consumer use today?

THE DEVELOPING SCIENCE OF MICROBIOLOGY: KOCH'S TECHNIQUES

While Pasteur vigorously pursued the discovery trail, many other scientists were attracted to the developing science of microbiology. There was no shortage of problems waiting to be solved. In 1865 France and Germany were ravaged by a disease of livestock known as anthrax. It was not only costly economically, but the disease was a threat to humans as well.

The devastating disease of anthrax captured the interest of Robert Koch (1843–1910), a physician in Germany. The young Koch provided both the techniques and discipline necessary to guide future microbiologists. Techniques developed in Koch's laboratories are still used today in the isolation of microorganisms. The need for a solid surface for growing bacteria led him to try gelatin as a support medium, but that experiment was a dismal failure. Not only did the gelatin melt at temperatures required for growth of some bacteria, but some organisms could digest the gelatin, causing it to become liquid. Fanny Angelina Hesse, a New Jersey native and wife of one of Koch's colleagues, recommended the use of agar, a product derived from a seaweed, as a solidifying agent. She had used agar in making jellies and jams. Not only did the agar not melt at the temperatures required for growth of microorganisms, but agar was not liquefied by bacteria. Various nutrients could be added to agar in order to accommodate requirements of

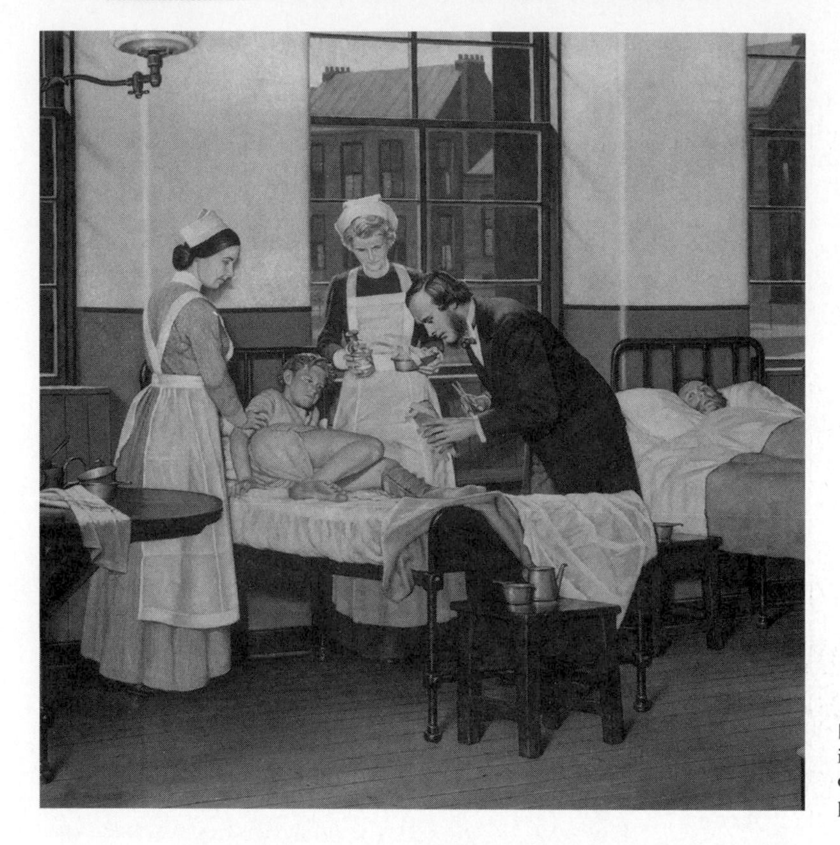

Figure 1–6 ◆ Joseph Lister's use of aerosolized carbolic acid during surgery. The spray destroyed atmospheric microorganisms and prevented postsurgical infections.

particular organisms. Agar is still used as a solidifying agent in growing many types of microorganisms.

Other major techniques originating in Koch's laboratories were the use of a two-part dish for growing bacteria and a technique for isolating pure colonies of bacteria (Fig. 1–7). The two-part dishes were named Petri plates after Julius Petri (1852–1921), the German bacteriologist. The application of the pure-culture technique led to the isolation of the causative organisms of the major bacterial diseases in the latter half of the nineteenth century.

In order to obtain proof that a specific microorganism caused a particular disease, Koch applied guidelines that became known as Koch's postulates. Those requirements, stated simply, are as follows:

1. The microbial agent must be found in every case of the disease.
2. The microorganism must be isolated and grown in pure culture.
3. The microorganism must cause the same disease when inoculated into a susceptible animal.
4. The same microbial agent must be recovered from the inoculated animal.

Koch's postulates cannot be met if a particular disease occurs only in humans or if the disease can be caused by more than one organism. Cholera, gonorrhea, and AIDS are examples of diseases found only in humans. Pneumonia and dysentery are examples of diseases caused by more than one infectious agent. Koch's postulates also cannot be fulfilled if an organism will not grow in the laboratory. The bacterial organisms causing leprosy and syphilis infect humans, but grow only in specific animal hosts. Armadillos will support the growth of the bacterium that causes leprosy. Several animal hosts, including rabbits, have been used to maintain the microbial agent of syphilis in the laboratory. How does one obtain the proof needed to demonstrate that a specific microorganism causes a particular disease in such instances? The demonstration of protective factors in the blood formed in response to a suspected microbial agent can implicate a microbial agent as the cause of a disease. Sometimes this is done in retrospect, such as in the mysterious outbreak of a respiratory infection occurring in

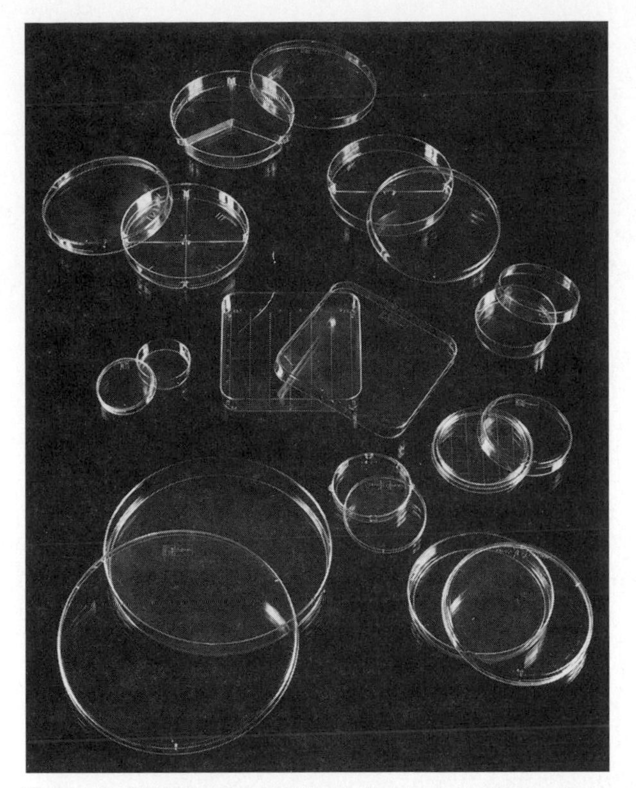

Figure 1–7 ◆ An array of plastic Petri plates. Some of the plates are partitioned so that one type of medium may be used in each separate compartment. Other plates contain grid markings for ease of counting colonies.

members of the American Legion in 1976. Once the organism was isolated in the absence of an animal model, the blood of the survivors implicated the same microorganism.

THE BEGINNINGS OF IMMUNOLOGY

There is evidence that both the Chinese and the Turks recognized that material from lesions of infectious disease could be used to promote resistance. Voltaire described the ancient Chinese custom of placing dried smallpox crusts in the nose to prevent the feared disease. Around 1717 Lady Worley Montague, the wife of the English ambassador to Turkey, reported inoculating material from a smallpox lesion into a vein. Lady Montague permitted her own son to receive the injection. The child, along with hundreds of Turkish infants, apparently received life-long immunity against smallpox.

Jenner and the First Vaccine

The English physician Edward Jenner (1749–1823) is usually credited with introducing use of scabs from cowpox lesions to prevent smallpox. Jenner noticed that milkmaids did not get smallpox if they had already contracted cowpox (Fig. 1–8). Acting on that observation, Jenner made incisions or punctures with cowpox material on the arms of human subjects to prevent the dreaded smallpox. At first Jenner's peers doubted both the safety and the efficiency of his methods. By the time of his death, the value of the cowpox inoculum was recognized. One can only imagine Jenner's thoughts today if he could know that smallpox has been completely eradicated in the

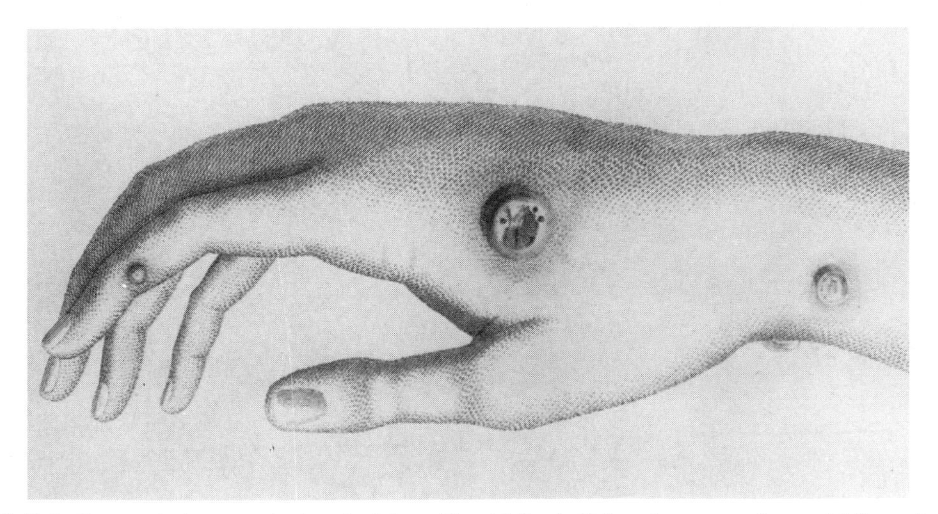

Figure 1–8 ◆ Cowpox lesions on the hand of the milkmaid Sarah Nelms. Jenner used material from the lesions to protect individuals from smallpox by a procedure to become known as vaccination.

world (Fig. 1–9). That feat was made possible by a massive immunization program conducted by the World Health Organization and succeeded because humans were the only reservoir for the infectious agent.

Pasteur's Attenuated Vaccines

It was observed that individuals who recovered from an infectious disease were often immune to any future attack. The reasons for that type of resistance were not understood, but it meant that an initial contact with a particular organism or, in the case of smallpox, a similar one, could prevent the disease. That realization prompted Pasteur to seek a means of preventing fowl cholera in chickens. When Charles Chamberland, a colleague of Pasteur's, postponed planned inoculations of the deadly cholera organisms into a group of chickens, a remarkable discovery followed.

The organisms, left to grow under laboratory conditions while Chamberland was off on a holiday, no longer could cause the dreaded disease. Instead, inoculation with the neglected cultures made chickens immune to fowl cholera. The organisms had been weakened or **attenuated** by leaving them on laboratory media for an extended period. It became apparent that bacteria could differ in their capacity to cause disease. However, that change did not affect their ability to promote resistance in a host. The discovery was the beginning of the triumph of medicine over many infectious diseases. It became the foundation for the branch of microbiology now known as immunology.

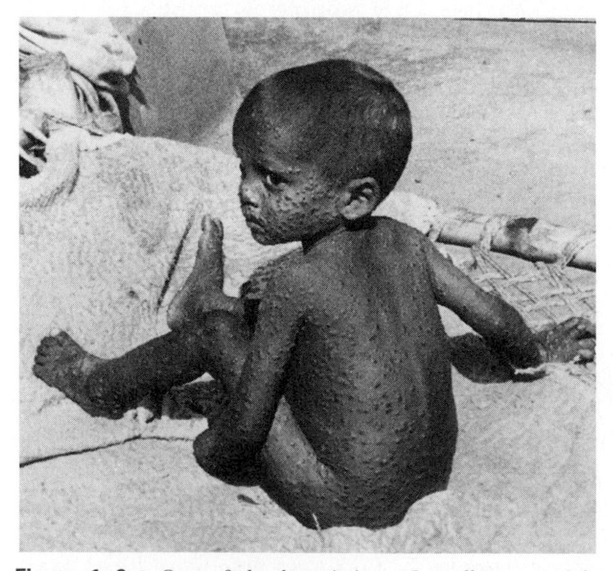

Figure 1–9 ◆ One of the last victims of smallpox—a sight the world will never see again.

Pasteur was also able to modify the microorganism that caused anthrax. The microbes kept at temperatures of 42° to 43°C lost their ability to produce disease. Furthermore, animals inoculated with the attenuated bacilli were protected against future attacks of anthrax. Pasteur honored Jenner by calling his own inoculation procedures **vaccinations.** The term is derived from the word vaccinia, the other name for cowpox.

Perhaps the success that brought Pasteur the greatest satisfaction and recognition was the preparation of the first vaccine for rabies, the animal disease that was invariably fatal. Without ever isolating the virus of rabies, he was able to infect rabbits by inoculating them with a preparation from the medulla of rabid dogs. The viruses migrated to the spinal cord and brain of the rabbits. He maintained the organism by successive inoculations in rabbits (Fig. 1–10). He inoculated dogs with dried, powdered rabbit medulla, suspended in broth, to prevent rabies.

In 1885 a distraught mother brought her young son, who had been bitten numerous times by a rabid dog, to Pasteur. Fearing that her son was facing certain death, she begged Pasteur to try the rabies vaccine on him. The boy, Joseph Meister, received 13 injections in 10 days. He survived the administration of the animal vaccine and did not develop rabies. Joseph Meister later became the gatekeeper at the Pasteur Institute built by a grateful country in Pasteur's honor in 1888.

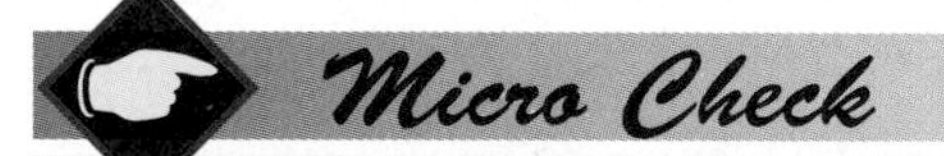

- What problems might be encountered in preparing a vaccine of attenuated organisms?
- Is it likely that infectious diseases, other than smallpox, can be eradicated?
- What are the major obstacles preventing eradication of infectious diseases?

Metchnikoff and Phagocytosis

The way in which the body resisted infectious disease, with or without benefit of vaccinations,

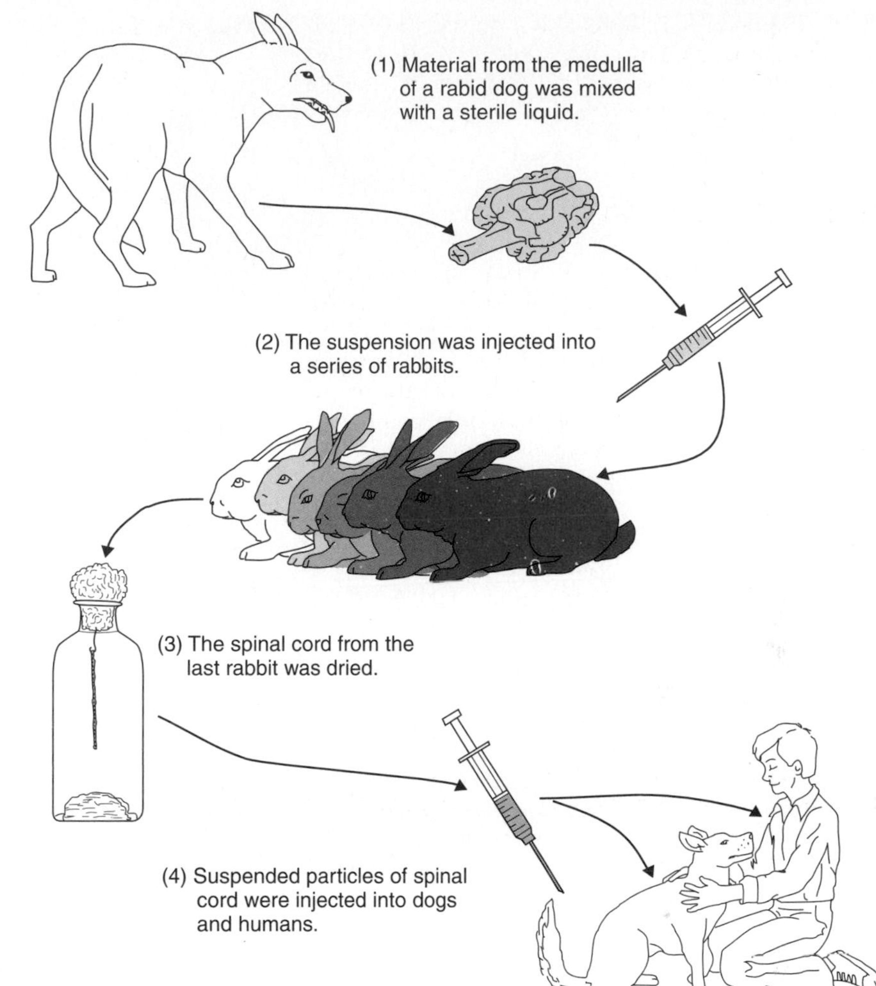

Figure 1–10 ◆ Pasteur's technique for "taming" the rabies virus. The term "virus" was used in Pasteur's time for any infectious agent.

was a subject of controversy. In 1884 Elie Metchnikoff (1845–1916) used the common water flea, *Daphnia,* to study microbial diseases (Fig. 1–11). The tiny crustacean was particularly susceptible to a disease caused by a yeast. The invasive process could be studied quite easily under a microscope. Metchnikoff observed that certain blood cells were able to ingest and destroy invading microorganisms. He called those cells **phagocytes** (cell eaters).

Ehrlich and Serum Protective Factors

Almost simultaneously in Germany, Paul Ehrlich (1854–1915), a colleague of Koch's, proposed that immunity could be explained by components of the fluid portion of the blood. The research of Emil von Behring (1854–1917), a Prussian bacteriologist, and Shibasaburo Kitasato (1856–1931), a Japanese bacteriologist, showed that protective factors for tetanus and diphtheria were contained in an acellular component of the blood of immune rabbits and mice. The protective factors were able to neutralize the harmful products, or **toxins,** made by the causative agents of those diseases. The discovery would not have been possible without the use of the animals.

The dispute over the importance of phagocytes and the acellular protective factors in the defense against microbial diseases lasted more than 60 years. Today we know that the protective factors, now called **antibodies,** are of vital importance in immunity. Some antibodies are not long lasting, but some antibody-producing cells have a

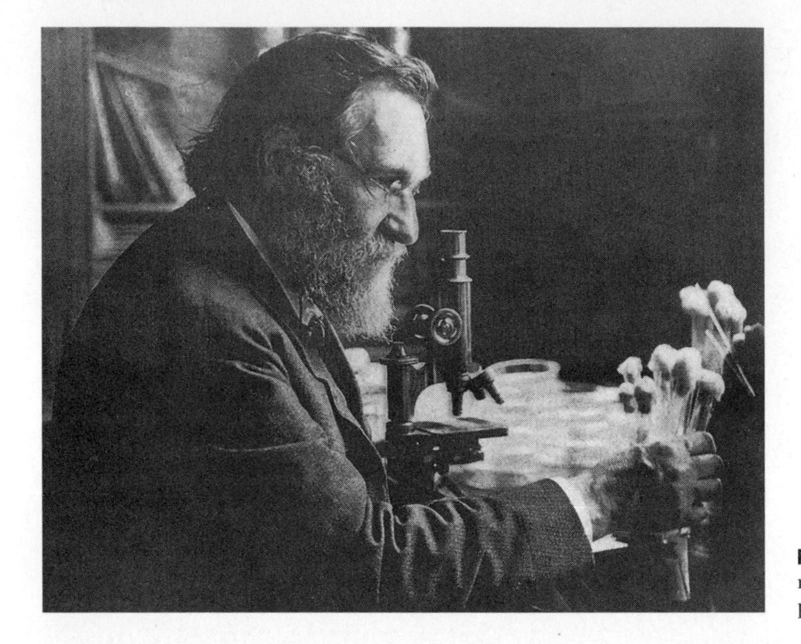

Figure 1–11 ◆ Elie Metchnikoff, a pioneer of microbiology who validated the process of phagocytosis.

memory enabling them to set into motion the machinery for making more antibodies against microbial intruders. Phagocytes do destroy large numbers of some invading microorganisms, but still other cells release chemicals that interfere with the reproduction or survival of invading microorganisms. Immune factors and their interactions are discussed in Chapter 13.

Micro Check

- Of what importance are animals in microbiological research?
- What are the first types of cells to react to invasion by microbial enemies?
- What is the origin of the protective factors found in the fluid component of blood?

THE DISCOVERY OF ANTIMICROBIAL AGENTS

It is difficult to imagine a world without antimicrobial agents to treat infectious diseases. Ehrlich's early work on the selectivity of dyes for staining microorganisms led him to search for chemicals that could be beneficial in the treatment of infectious diseases. Most chemicals that would kill microorganisms were also highly toxic to humans. In 1906 he announced the discovery of an arsenic-containing compound **salvarsan** or 606, sometimes called the "magic bullet." It was the 606th compound tested that finally yielded favorable results. The drug was active against the causative agent of syphilis, but was not without toxic effects on patients. Ehrlich likened the new form of a treatment to "a chemical knife" for, like surgical procedures, it was not without risk. The discovery earned Ehrlich the title Father of Chemotherapy. Ehrlich's contributions had a tremendous impact, for they paved the way for research on other compounds with antimicrobial activity. Moreover, the use of chemicals to combat infectious diseases was an alternative to immunological intervention.

Domagk and Sulfa Drugs

It was not until 1935 that a group of drugs, known as the sulfonamides or **sulfa drugs,** were shown to be effective against a large number of bacteria. Gerhard Domagk (1895–1964), a German chemist, found that the dye **Prontosil** could be used to treat streptococcal infections in mice. A sulfonamide portion of the molecule was found to be the active ingredient. Many derivatives of the original drug Prontosil quickly appeared on the market. Sulfonamides received worldwide attention when one of the drugs was credited with saving the life of Sir Winston

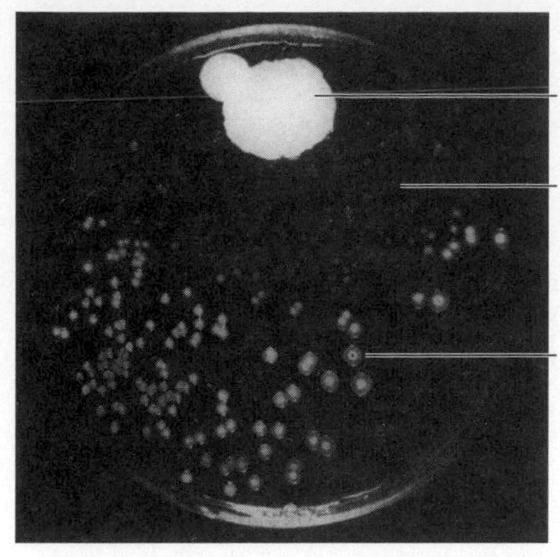

Figure 1–12 ◆ The original plate showing dissolution of staphylococcal colonies by a colony of the mold *Penicillium notatum,* as observed by Alexander Fleming in 1929.

Churchill. Churchill had contracted pneumonia when he visited the Allied troops in Algeria during World War II.

Fleming and Penicillin

The testing of another antimicrobial agent was proceeding in the laboratory of Alexander Fleming (1881–1955), a British bacteriologist. During experimentation on bacteria known as staphylococci in 1928, Fleming observed that some of the bacterial colonies were disappearing on plates contaminated with an airborne mold (Fig. 1–12). The colonies were actually being dissolved by a product of the mold. Fleming extracted a compound from the mold that was responsible for the destruction of the bacterial colonies. The product of the mold was called penicillin after the *Penicillium* mold from which it was derived.

Penicillin was purified a decade later by Howard Florey (1898–1968) and Ernst Chain (1906–1979). The purified product was only mildly toxic to patients, but it was not made in large quantities until World War II. A devastating fire in a Chicago nightclub provided an opportunity to test penicillin against staphylococcal skin infections in fire victims. The "miracle drug" was used to treat Allied troops wounded in action. Today physicians have a large number of antibiotics available for treating infectious diseases. The impetus for the discovery of the additional antimicrobial agents came from the initial observation by Fleming that something was destroying his staphylococcal colonies.

Would you recognize a microorganism if you saw one? Do you know where they live? Do you know the names of any microorganisms? The next section will introduce you to the major groups of microorganisms, their habitats, and some of their special activities.

MICROORGANISMS: THE NATURAL JEWELRY OF THE EARTH

The microbial world is made up of a diverse population of organisms. The noted protozoologist John Corliss called microorganisms the "natural jewelry of the Earth." Intricate architectural patterns may be observed in many microorganisms. The majority of microorganisms contribute immeasurably to the biosphere, but some, as we have seen, cause serious disease. Many microorganisms consist of single cells; some are multicellular; still others lack cellular organization.

Microorganisms are measured in units known as **micrometers** (μm) or **nanometers** (nm). One micrometer is 0.0001 (10^{-4}) of a centimeter (cm) or 0.000001 (10^{-6}) of a meter. One nanometer is 0.0000001 (10^{-7}) of a centimeter or 0.001 (10^{-3}) of a micrometer. The diameter of a microscopic field using low power with an ocular lens that magnifies 10 times is 1.5 μm or 1500 nm. Human red blood cells measure 6.0 to 8.0 μm in diameter; white blood cells range from 12 to 20 μm in diameter. Protozoa, like a paramecium, often attain lengths of 200 μm. Most rod-shaped bacteria are 1.0 to 3.0 μm in length and 0.5 μm or less in width. One thousand bacteria could occupy the head of a single pin. It is more convenient to express the size of viruses in nanometers. The virus that causes AIDS is only 100 nm in diameter and can be seen only with the powerful electron microscope.

Classification and Nomenclature of Microorganisms

Many of the "little animals" observed by van Leeuwenhoek were not animals at all, but were far simpler organisms. The first attempt to separate microorganisms from the plant or animal kingdom came about in 1866 when Ernst Haeckel, a disciple of Darwin's, proposed that all microorganisms be placed in the kingdom *Protista.* Unfortunately, Haeckel's idea did not gain wide acceptance.

PROCARYOTES AND EUCARYOTES

When more refined microscopes became available in the twentieth century, the French scientist, Edouard Chatton (1883–1947) described membrane-bound structures in one-celled organisms. Continuing improvements in microscopes and microscopic techniques allowed cytologists to study the internal components of many types of cells. Some cells lacked membranous structures subsequently called **organelles:** others contained distinct membrane-bound nuclei as well as other membranous structures with specialized functions. The primitive cells with no internal membranes were named **procaryotes;** the more complex cells with internal membrane systems were called **eucaryotes.** All bacterial cells are procaryotes. Cells of protozoa, algae, fungi, plants, and animals are eucaryotes. Further details on these life forms and their structure are found in Chapters 4, 8, and 9.

BACTERIA, ARCHAEA, AND EUCARYA

In the late 1970s, Carl Woese described some unusual microorganisms that resembled bacteria, but which grew in harsh environments incapable of supporting most other forms of life. Although their physical resemblance to bacteria is striking, they also share some properties with the eucaryotes.

The ability of the newly discovered life forms to live under extreme environmental conditions suggests that the organisms may be descendants of early forms of life on Earth. With their discovery, it became apparent that there were three primary domains of living organisms: (1) **bacteria** (formerly eubacteria), (2) **archaea** (formerly archaebacteria), and (3) the cells of larger organisms known as **eucarya.** More information on the differences between bacteria and archaea appears in Chapter 8.

It is believed that bacteria, archaea, and eucarya arose from a common ancestor (Fig. 1–13). Furthermore, archaea appear to be more widely distributed in nature than was originally believed. Most known surviving archaea found on Earth today live in very hot, acidic, or salty environments.

Biologists have now established separate kingdoms for bacteria and archaea (Table 1–1). Most kingdoms are divided into groups known as **phyla** or **divisions** and further subdivided into **classes, orders,** and **families** (Table 1–2). Each category contains organisms with some shared characteristics. There is a decreasing order of inclusiveness beginning with the phyla or division, with families being the least inclusive.

The ninth edition of *Bergey's Manual of Systemic Bacteriology,* an authoritative source for classification of bacteria, places eubacteria (bacteria) and archaebacteria (archaea) in the kingdom Procaryotae. The kingdom is broken down into four divisions, which will be examined in Chapter 8. Classification of the bacteria into further groups is pending.

The advances in technology have made it possible to study genetic relatedness of both unicel-

Table 1–1
THE SIX-KINGDOM CLASSIFICATION

KINGDOM	EXAMPLES
ARCHAEBACTERIA	Thermophiles Acidophiles Methanogens
EUBACTERIA	Cyanobacteria Nitrogen-fixing bacteria Most pathogenic bacteria
PROTISTA	Algae Protozoa
FUNGI	Fungi Slime molds
PLANTAE	Mosses Ferns Seed plants
ANIMALIA	Sponges Jellyfish Worms Arthropods Echinoderms Chordates

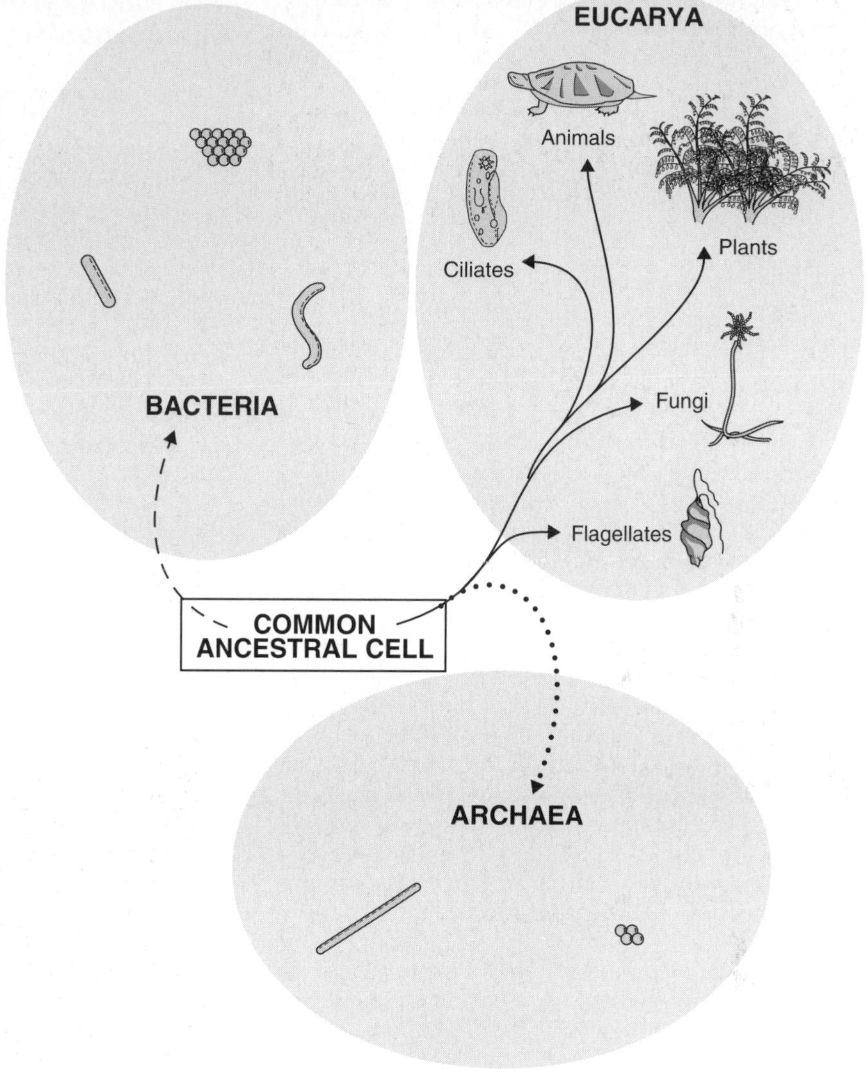

Figure 1–13 ◆ The three domains of cellular life showing proposed relationships between *Archaea, Bacteria,* and *Eucarya* based on rRNA studies. The unbroken arrows indicate relationships between members of the *Eucarya* as derived from a common ancestral cell. The dashed arrow shows the origin of *Bacteria* from the same common ancestral cell. The dotted arrow represents early branching of *Archaea* from the ancestral cell.

Table 1–2
EXAMPLES OF THE CLASSIFICATION OF ORGANISMS IN THREE KINGDOMS

	QUERCUS VIRGINIANA (LIVE OAK)	*FELIS DOMESTICA* (HOUSE CAT)	*TREPONEMA PALLIDUM* (AGENT OF SYPHILIS)
Kingdom	Plantae	Animalia	Procaryotae
Phylum (division)	Angiosperm	Chordata	Gracilicutes
Class	Dicotyledon	Mammalia	Scotobacteria
Order	Fagales	Carnivora	Spirochaetales
Family	Fagaceae	Felidae	Spirochaetaceae

lular and multicellular organisms. The degree of relatedness allows taxonomists to have insight on the time of appearance of particular organisms on Earth.

Classification systems are constantly changing. All systems fall short of perfection, but such systems do provide us with some order to the rapidly expanding knowledge of the microbial world.

THE BINOMIAL SYSTEM OF NOMENCLATURE

The binomial system of naming organisms, first proposed by Carolus Linnaeus (1707–1778), a Swedish botanist, provided an orderly approach for dividing living things into groups **(taxons)** and for naming specific organisms. According to the Linnaean system of binomial nomenclature, each organism is given two names: a generic name (genus, pl. genera) of Latin or Greek derivation, and a specific name (species), consisting of a descriptive adjective pertaining to a source, characteristic, or even discoverer of the organism. Within a species, there may be organisms that differ slightly from the organism originally described (the **prototype**). These differing types are referred to as the **strains** of that particular genus and species. Genus names are always capitalized; species names are lower case. Letters, numbers, or names following the genus and species designation refer to strains. Genus and species names are italicized or underlined in print and writing.

Sometimes a common name is used to refer to individual organisms in the particular same genus. For example, bacteria belonging to the genus *Mycoplasma, Salmonella,* or *Yersinia* may be called mycoplasmas, salmonellas, or yersinias. These common names of bacteria are not italicized or capitalized. Occasionally, other simplified terms are employed for particular bacteria. The terms meningococcus and pneumococcus are descriptive names for *Neisseria meningitidis* and *Streptococcus pneumoniae,* respectively.

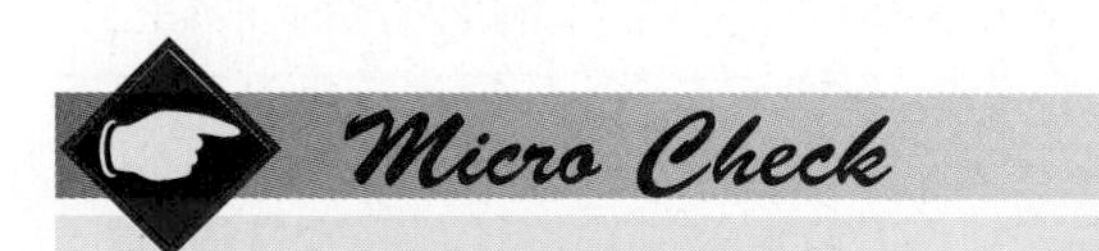

- What purpose do classification systems serve?
- How are microorganisms named?
- What is meant by a strain of a particular genus and species?

The Major Groups of Microorganisms

The major groups of cellular microorganisms are the bacteria, algae, protozoa, and fungi. The members of each group are easily recognizable with the aid of a light microscope used in most laboratories. Acellular particles, known as viruses, viroids, and prions, can be seen only with an electron microscope. These very small forms have often been described as perfect parasites because they find refuge inside cells and use the resources of cells to produce up to 10,000 offspring in as little as seven hours. Viruses are responsible for most of the emerging microbial diseases today. The cells on which they depend are called **host cells.**

ARCHAEA

Archaea are presumed to have evolved before oxygen existed in the atmosphere. The single cells developed some unique pathways to produce energy in the absence of oxygen. Some archaea are found in nutrient-deficient barren environments; others have adapted to extreme temperatures or salinity. Archaea have been found living, though sparsely, in granite far below the Earth's crust. Such tenacity to hang on to life, despite adverse conditions, is not shared by most other microorganisms. The archaea are both structurally and chemically diverse from eubacteria and microbial eucaryotes. They remain of great interest to researchers seeking ways to resolve toxic waste problems on Earth in the belief that some toxins produced by life on the surface of the planet could be food for life of subsurface microbes.

BACTERIA

Bacteria are a structurally diverse and a widely distributed group of unicellular organisms (Fig. 1–14). Most bacteria are capable of living independently under favorable environmental conditions; however, the rickettsias and chlamydias require host cells as sources of energy for metabolic and reproductive activities.

A majority of bacteria produce materials that sustain other forms of life. Some aquatic bacteria contain light-harvesting pigments that permit them to use energy from the sun to make nutrients. The process is called **photosynthesis** and is discussed in greater detail in Chapter 8. Some photosynthetic bacteria, known as cyanobacteria,

FOCAL POINT

Dwellers of the Deep—Some Like it Hot

Once it was conventional wisdom that only the surface of the Earth was inhabited by plants, animals, and microscopic forms of life. Biologists speculate that some microbes escaped from assaults of meteorites and ultraviolet rays from the sun by seeking refuge in subsurface layers. The deep dwellers have been discovered nearly 3 km below the ground where temperatures reach 75°C (167°F) and nutrients are sparse. Colonies of microbes have lived in a state of suspended animation since dinosaurs were thundering overhead 80 to 160 million years ago. The independent heat-loving microbes, like *Bacillus infernans,* are able to convert the barest of inorganic materials of rock into organic molecules. Thomas Gold of Cornell University speculates that the weight of subterranean microbes could be at least equal to that of their microbial counterparts above the surface. Some biologists believe that life could have started in the hot, barren depths of the subsurface layers of the Earth. Life may even be hiding beneath the red dust on the surface of Mars.

Adapted from Science News 151:192–193, 1997

are also capable of converting atmospheric nitrogen into nitrogenous compounds by a method called **nitrogen fixation** (Color Plates 1 to 3). Some species of nonphotosynthetic bacteria fix nitrogen independently, but others require the aid of a leguminous plant, such as alfalfa, clover, or soybean (Fig. 1–15). Large numbers of bacteria degrade carbon-containing compounds in nature and return carbon dioxide to the atmosphere. Certain other bacteria are used in making valuable food products, such as cheeses, yogurt, and vinegar. In recent years bacteria have

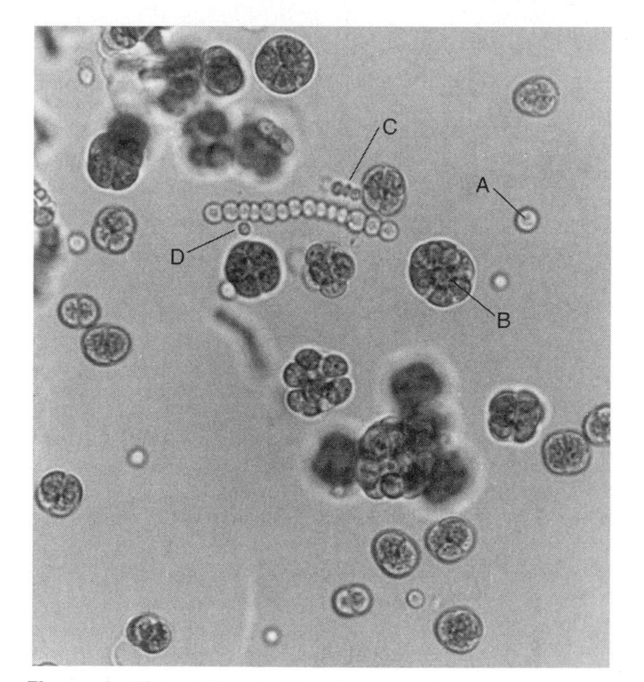

Figure 1–14 ◆ Cells of *Chlorogloea fritschii* illustrating major morphological types of chlorophyll-containing bacteria: single granulated cells (A), colonial aggregates surrounded by a sheath (B), small cells in short filaments (C), and larger cells in long filaments (D).

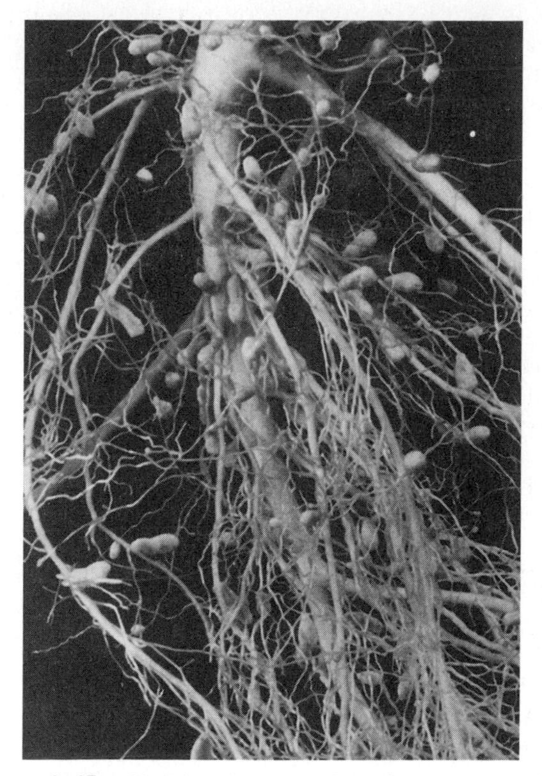

Figure 1–15 ◆ Nodules of nitrogen-fixing bacteria on a crimson clover plant.

been programmed by genetic engineering to produce an increasing number of agricultural, industrial, and biological products.

The importance of bacteria as causes of life-threatening diseases in humans, animals, and plants continues to have a significant influence on world population and on the individual's quality of life. The devastation caused by epidemics of puerperal fever, plague, and yellow fever is now history. We can only speculate on the long-term effects of today's microbial enemies.

MICROBIAL EUCARYA

Like the other eucarya, the microbial eucarya have membrane-bound organelles and share molecular characteristics. On the molecular level the eucarya resemble the many molecules of archaea more than the bacteria. Construction of a universal tree of life is full of pitfalls. Sequences of different molecules yield conflicting results. Among the microbial eucarya are algae, protozoa, and fungi. We shall consider the structural characteristics of these organaisms in Chapter 9.

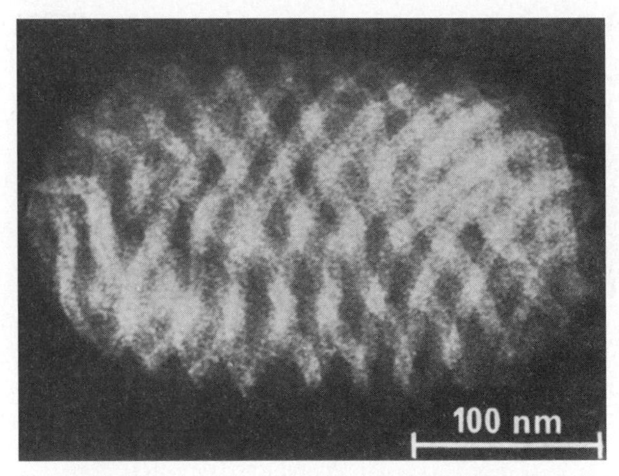

Figure 1–16 ◆ An electron micrograph showing the criss-cross pattern of the Orf virus, which is the cause of pustular dermatitis in animals and humans.

ACELLULAR PARTICLES

The classification schemes we have discussed pertain to cellular organisms. The study of microbiology includes the study of tiny particles lacking cellular organization which depend on bacterial, archeal, or eucaryotic host cells for replication. The largest group of the dependent particles are called **viruses.** Most viruses are visible only with an electron microscope (Fig. 1–16). Some viruses cause mild, often unrecognizable diseases in plants and animals. However, the acellular particles are also responsible for such serious diseases as hepatitis, poliomyelitis, influenza, yellow fever, rabies, and AIDS. Viruses are discussed in more detail in Chapter 10.

Understanding Microbiology

1. Why did it take so long to disprove the theory of spontaneous generation?
2. Why can Koch's postulates not always be met?
3. Why is it so easy to take for granted the contributions of beneficial microorganisms to our biosphere?
4. Describe the roles of vaccinations and chemotherapy in combating infectious disease.
5. Describe two reasons why classification schemes can be expected to change with time.

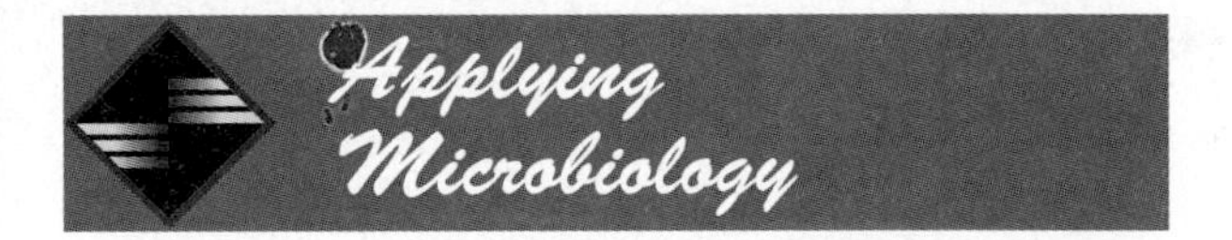

6. Assume the role of Oliver Wendell Holmes or Ignaz Semmelweis and attempt to convince health care workers of the need for handwashing between patients.

Chapter 2 The Chemistry of Life

Chapter Outline

Learning Objectives

After you read this chapter, you should be able to:

1. Name the four major elements found in cells.
2. Define element, atom, compound, molecule, and mixture.
3. Explain how electrons in the outer shell determine the behavior of atoms.
4. Describe three types of chemical bonds.
5. Explain the origin of chemical symbols.
6. Describe two major types of chemical reactions.
7. Name the four major organic molecules found in living things and the elements they contain.

We are all affected by chemistry in our daily lives. The air we breathe, the food we eat, and the availability of a safe supply of water are all related to the quality of human lives. Likewise, other forms of life, including microorganisms, depend on gases in the atmosphere, chemical content of nutrients, and availability of water to sustain life.

A knowledge of the basic principles of chemistry is increasingly important as we attempt to solve the problems created by overcrowding, inadequate food supplies, emissions from automobiles, endangered species, waste disposal, and the appearance of new infectious diseases. How do the emerging microorganisms cause disease? Why do some drugs inhibit growth of certain microorganisms? How do other microorganisms become resistant to drugs?

ELEMENTS AND COMPOUNDS

We can begin to answer these questions by becoming familiar with the language of the

Table 2–1
MAJOR ELEMENTS FOUND IN A BACTERIUM AND IN THE HUMAN BODY

ELEMENT	A TYPICAL BACTERIUM	THE HUMAN BODY
Oxygen	65.0%	69.0%
Carbon	18.0%	15.0%
Hydrogen	10.0%	11.0%
Nitrogen	3.0%	3.0%
Phosphorus	1.0%	1.2%
Sulfur	0.25%	0.3%

Note: Figures represent gross composition of representative cells.

chemists. **Matter** is described as anything that occupies space and has mass. It can exist in gaseous, liquid, or solid states. All living and nonliving matter is composed of basic substances known as elements. An **element** is a substance that cannot be broken down into simpler components. An **atom** is the smallest particle of an element that still retains the characteristics of that element. Atoms are so small that 100 million atoms placed end to end would measure less than one inch.

There are 92 naturally occurring elements, but only four represent the major components of cells: carbon, hydrogen, oxygen, and nitrogen. These elements, along with phosphorus and sulfur, are the major elements found in microbial cells (Table 2–1).

On Earth, elements are found rarely in the free state, but usually exist in combination with other elements, forming compounds or mixtures. A **compound** is created when two or more elements chemically combine in definite proportions. For example, water is the most abundant compound in all cells, making up approximately 70 percent of a cell's contents. Water consists of hydrogen and oxygen in a ratio of 2 to 1. The smallest portion of a compound that can exist is called a **molecule,** and therefore, one molecule of water contains two atoms of hydrogen and one atom of oxygen.

Mixtures contain two or more elements or compounds in varying proportions that have not undergone a chemical reaction to unite them. The ingredients of a mixture retain their own identifying characteristics. Air is an example of a mixture containing such vital substances as oxygen, nitrogen, and carbon dioxide.

Chemical Shorthand

The representation of elements by **symbols** is the basis for a type of chemical shorthand. A list of common elements and their symbols is found in Table 2–2. In chemical shorthand, the symbol for an element represents one atom of that element.

A chemical symbol consists of one or two letters and begins with a capital, based on its name. When several elements have names beginning with the same letter, the most common element has been given the symbol of a single capitalized letter. Symbols of the others begin with the same capital letter but are distinguished by a second letter, which is not capitalized. For example, carbon, calcium, chlorine, and copper all begin with the letter C. The symbol C represents carbon, whereas calcium, chlorine, and copper are represented by Ca, Cl, and Cu, respectively. Some elements were originally given Latin names. For example, the symbol Cu for copper comes from the Latin name *cuprum* and the symbol Na for sodium comes from the Latin name *natrium.*

The chemical shorthand for a compound is called a **formula.** A formula contains the symbols of the atoms that make up the compound. Because atoms do not always combine in equal proportions, it is necessary to use numerical subscripts following symbols when more than one atom is present in a molecule. The well-known chemical formula for water is H_2O, which stands for one molecule of water. To refer to more than one molecule of water, an arabic number is

Table 2–2
ATOMIC NUMBERS AND WEIGHTS OF COMMON ELEMENTS

ELEMENT	SYMBOL	ATOMIC NUMBER	ATOMIC WEIGHT
Hydrogen	H	1	1
Carbon	C	6	12
Nitrogen	N	7	14
Oxygen	O	8	16
Sodium	Na	11	23
Magnesium	Mg	12	24
Phosphorus	P	15	31
Sulfur	S	16	32
Chlorine	Cl	17	35
Potassium	K	19	39
Calcium	Ca	20	40
Iron	Fe	26	56
Iodine	I	53	127

placed in front of the formula. Therefore, $2H_2O$ means two molecules of water in chemical shorthand. Using chemical shorthand saves time and provides us with an international method of communication. Can you think of another international means of communication that does not involve language arts?

Functional Groups

Certain atoms are consistently found in energy relationships with the same types of atoms. The resulting bonding forms groups of atoms known as **functional groups.** The functional groups behave quite differently than the individual atoms of which they are composed. Examples of functional groups are given in Table 2–3. Some molecules contain more than one functional group. The functional groups on a single molecule may be the same or different functional groups. For example, amino acids always contain an amino (NH_2) group and a carboxyl (COOH) group. It is important to recognize functional groups because they are often the sites of action in chemical reactions.

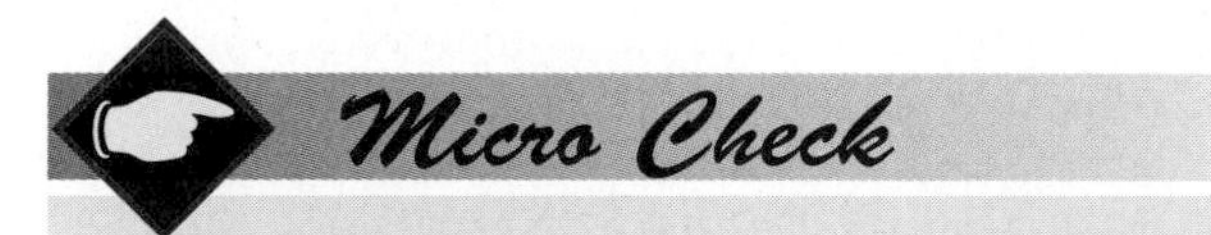

- What are the advantages of using symbols and formulas to express atoms and molecules?
- What does a subscript after the symbol of an atom in a formula indicate?
- Why is it important to be able to recognize functional groups?

Table 2–3
COMMON FUNCTIONAL GROUPS

FUNCTIONAL GROUP	FORMULA
Acetyl	CH_3
Amino	NH_2
Ammonium	NH_4
Bicarbonate	HCO_3
Carbonate	CO_3
Carboxyl	COOH
Ethyl	C_2H_5
Hydroxyl	OH
Nitrate	NO_3
Methyl	CH_3
Phosphate	PO_4
Sulfate	SO_4

The constant interactions of molecules within microbial cells provide the basis for their behavior. What governs the molecular interactions? How are the atoms organized within molecules that makes their behavior predictable? Why are some molecules more active than others? Let us examine the structure of atoms for the answers to these questions.

THE STRUCTURE OF ATOMS

Atoms contain three major types of particles: **protons, neutrons,** and **electrons.** The central portion of an atom, sometimes called the **atomic nucleus,** contains the positively charged (+) protons and the uncharged (neutral) neutrons. Negatively charged (−) electrons revolve around the atomic nucleus in orbits called **shells** (Fig. 2–1). Every electron has a specific amount of energy. Electrons having similar amounts of energy are located in the same shell. The energy level of electrons increases with distance of the shells from the nucleus. The first shell never contains more than two electrons. The second shell may have up to eight electrons. The third shell may contain up to 18 electrons, and the fourth shell can accommodate up to 32 electrons (Fig. 2–2). There are additional shells in some atoms, but they are beyond the scope of this text. Most elements found in living things have only two or three shells. The number of electrons in the outermost shell determines an atom's behavior.

Although the number of protons in atoms does not change, the number of neutrons differs in some atoms of the same element. Elements having variable numbers of neutrons are called

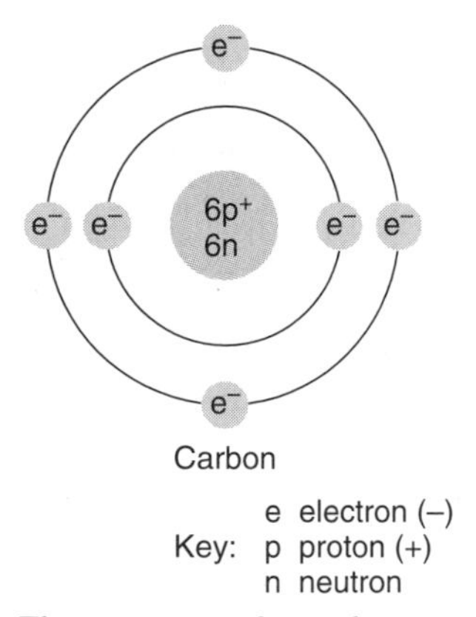

Figure 2–1 ◆ The structure of a carbon atom showing six protons (p^+) and six neutrons (n) in the atomic nucleus and six electrons (e^-) rotating around the nucleus in two shells.

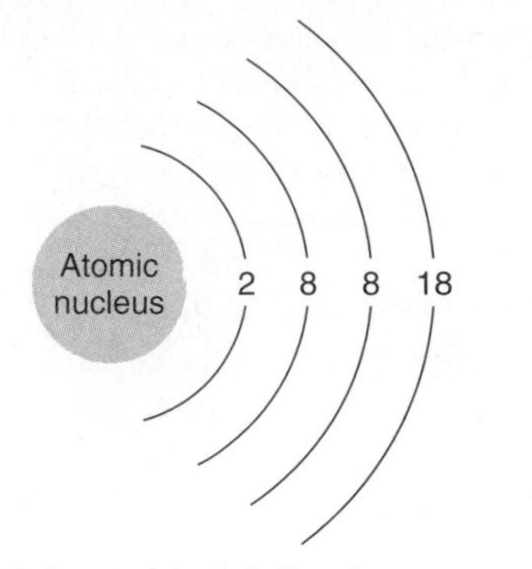

Figure 2–2 ◆ Bohr model of shells of an atom and numbers of electrons of the first four shells. The first shell is spherical, but others may have a more complex pathway.

isotopes. The symbols for isotopes contain a superscript number preceding the symbol of the element. That number indicates the mass of the atom. The number of protons subtracted from the mass number equals the number of neutrons. One isotope of carbon, known as carbon-14 is abbreviated ^{14}C. Because carbon always has six protons, the number of neutrons in this isotope is eight.

Elements having variable numbers of neutrons are unstable and emit subatomic particles and energy. The rate at which such **radioactive** isotopes break down is constant. Therefore, when this rate is known, it is possible to date particular fossils and rock formations by the degree of breakdown of an isotope. It is also possible to use radioactive isotopes, such as ^{14}C, to trace steps in numerous biochemical pathways. Radioactive isotopes are valuable in assessing certain types of anemia, pancreatitis, and thyroid conditions.

Table 2–4
VALENCES OF SOME COMMON ATOMS

ATOM	NUMBER OF ELECTRONS IN OUTER SHELL	IONIC CHARGE OR VALENCE
Calcium	2	+2
Carbon	4	±4
Chlorine	7	−1
Hydrogen	1	+1
Nitrogen	5	−3
Oxygen	6	−2
Potassium	1	+1
Sodium	1	+1

Each atom, beginning with hydrogen, has been assigned an atomic weight, or mass. Every proton and neutron has an atomic mass of 1. The total mass of protons and neutrons is equal to the atomic mass. Because an atom of hydrogen has one proton, no neutrons, and one electron, the atomic mass of hydrogen is 1. The atomic number of an atom equals the number of protons, so the atomic number of hydrogen is also 1. The number of electrons surrounding the atomic nucleus is always equal to the number of protons. Therefore, all uncombined atoms have a net charge of zero.

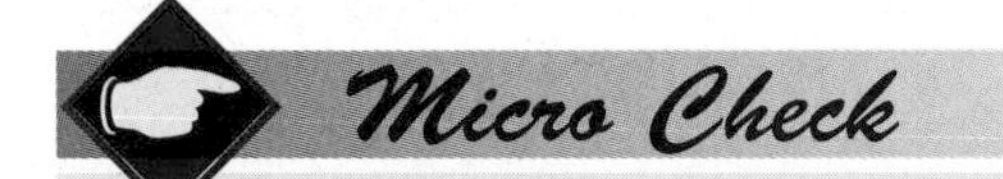

- Name the three types of particles found in atoms.
- How can you explain the net charge of zero exhibited by atoms?
- How have radioactive isotopes contributed to our understanding of the history of life on Earth?

ENERGY RELATIONSHIPS OF ATOMS

Most atoms are not found free in nature. Atoms collide, interact, and form molecules in less than a trillionth of a second. When atoms lose, gain, or share electrons following a collision, an energy relationship known as a **chemical bond** is established between atoms to form compounds. The reactive capacity of atoms is related to the numbers of electrons required to complete their outermost shells to the maximum holding capacity. The electrons in the outermost shells determine the combining power, or **valence,** of atoms (Table 2–4). The behavior of atoms follows the **octet principle,** which states that atoms tend to produce stable arrangements of eight electrons in their outermost orbits by losing, gaining, or sharing electrons. The close energy relationships of atoms provide stability for the participating atoms. The bonds formed during interactions of atoms vary in strength. Some are easily broken; others can withstand considerable stress. Bonds are classified as **ionic, covalent,** or **hydrogen** bonds.

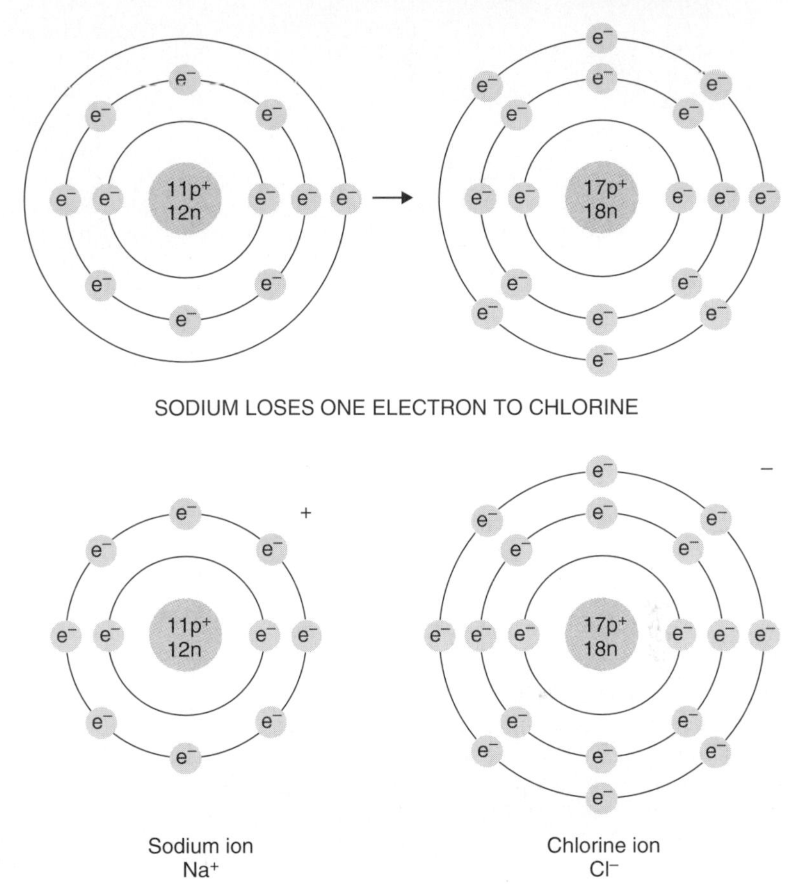

Figure 2–3 ◆ The ionic bond of sodium chloride, which is formed when sodium gives up an electron to chlorine. Sodium acquires a positive charge because it then has one more proton than the number of electrons. Chlorine acquires a negative charge because it then has one more electron than the number of protons.

Ionic Bonds

When electrons of atoms are transferred from the outer shell of one atom to the outer shell of another atom, an **ionic bond** is formed. When sodium, for example, loses the one electron from its outer shell to chlorine, which needs one electron to complete its outer shell, the atom of sodium has one more proton than electron (Fig. 2–3). Therefore, the atom of sodium has a valence of +1. The chlorine atom has one more electron than proton and now has a valence of −1. The charged particles formed by the transfer of one or more electrons to another atom are called **ions.** Negatively charged ions are called **anions;** positively charged ions are called **cations.** The attraction between the oppositely charged atoms causes a stable union; in the case of sodium and chlorine, the resulting compound is sodium chloride, or table salt.

Covalent Bonds

When electrons of atoms are shared, **covalent bonds** are formed. Two atoms of hydrogen, each with a single electron, can share these electrons, completing the outermost shell of each atom to the maximum of two electrons (Fig. 2–4). The resulting molecule of hydrogen is far more stable than the separate hydrogen atoms.

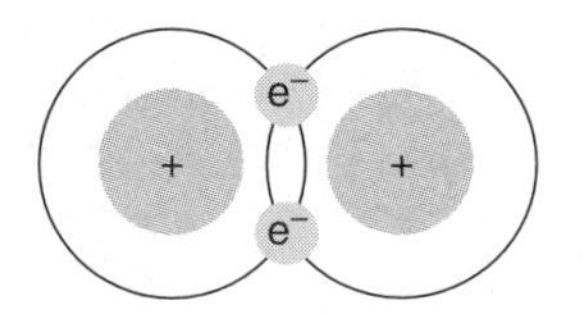

Figure 2–4 ◆ Sharing of electrons in a molecule of hydrogen in which two hydrogen atoms share a pair of electrons, which orbit the two nuclei.

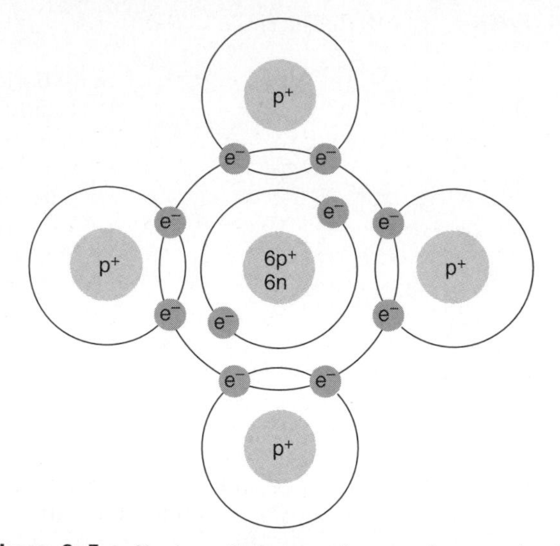

Figure 2–5 ◆ Sharing of electrons in a methane molecule (CH_4). The electrons of four hydrogen atoms are shared with one carbon atom.

Hydrogen atoms can share electrons with other types of atoms as well. In a molecule of methane, for example, the electrons of four hydrogen atoms are shared with one atom of carbon, which requires four electrons to complete its outermost orbit to the maximum of eight (Fig. 2–5). Compounds that contain both carbon and hydrogen are called **organic compounds.** Carbon atoms commonly form covalent bonds with hydrogen, oxygen, nitrogen, sulfur, and phosphorus.

Although an atom of carbon can bond with a maximum of four hydrogen atoms, it may bond with less than four. When that occurs, double or triple covalent bonds are formed between the carbon atoms.

H H
C=C
H H
C_2H_4
Ethylene
H—C≡C—H
C_2H_2
Acetylene

Compounds containing double or triple covalent bonds are described as being **unsaturated,** meaning that the carbon atoms have not bonded with the maximum number of hydrogen atoms. If bonding occurs with the maximum number of hydrogen atoms, the compound is described by the term **saturated.** The butter you may have used on your bread today is an example of a saturated compound. The corn oil used in cooking is an example of an unsaturated compound.

If atoms forming covalent bonds exert a pull of the same magnitude on shared electrons, the bond is called a **nonpolar covalent bond.** The bonding that occurs with shared electrons of two hydrogen atoms is an example. If one atom of a covalent bond exerts a greater pull than another atom, a **polar covalent bond** is formed. When two hydrogen atoms bond with an oxygen atom to form water, the electrons orbit the oxygen's atomic nucleus with greater frequency than the atomic nuclei of hydrogen (Fig. 2–6). This creates an unequal distribution of charges, and therefore, the atom of oxygen is partially negatively charged and the hydrogen atoms are partially positively charged.

Hydrogen Bonds

A third type of bond between molecules having polar covalent bonds is the **hydrogen bond.** A partially negatively charged atom of one molecule attracts a partially positively charged atom of another molecule. Hydrogen bonds form between hydrogen atoms covalently bonded to oxygen or nitrogen and a negatively charged acceptor atom on another molecule. Water molecules exhibit polarity. The unequal sharing of electrons in a molecule of water causes oxygen to be negative enough to attract a partially positively charged atom of hydrogen in an adjacent water molecule. If large numbers of water molecules

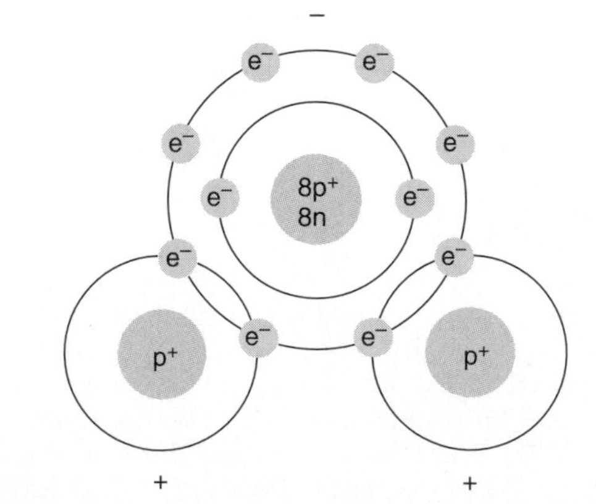

Figure 2–6 ◆ Polar covalent bond in a molecule of water. The shared electrons of hydrogen orbit the atomic nucleus of oxygen with greater frequency than the atomic nuclei of hydrogen, causing the oxygen to have a negative charge. Each of the hydrogen atoms carries a slight positive charge.

are bonded together in this manner, a latticework of water molecules is formed (Fig. 2–7). Hydrogen bonds are much weaker than covalent bonds. However, if they are present in sufficient numbers, hydrogen bonds can hold molecules together. Proteins and nucleic acid molecules contain hundreds of hydrogen bonds.

Energy Content of Bonds

The amounts of energy contained in the three types of bonds has been determined by measuring the amounts of energy required to break them. The energy of bonds is measured in kilocalories (kcal) per gram molecular weight. A **kilocalorie** (a thousand calories) is the amount of energy needed to heat 1000 grams (1 kg) of water from 14.5°C to 15.5°C at standard atmospheric pressure. The gram molecular weight is the sum of the atomic masses of the atoms within a molecule expressed in grams.

The energy content of covalent bonds ranges from 80 to 110 kcal per mole. Both hydrogen and ionic bonds contain less energy. Hydrogen bonds yield 4 to 6 kcal per mole; ionic bonds in cells store about 5 kcal per mole.

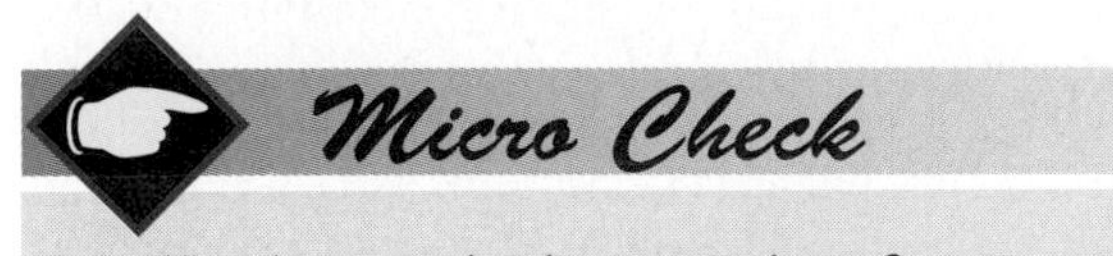

- What is meant by the term valence?
- Which types of bonds release the greatest amounts of energy?
- How are gram molecular weights determined?

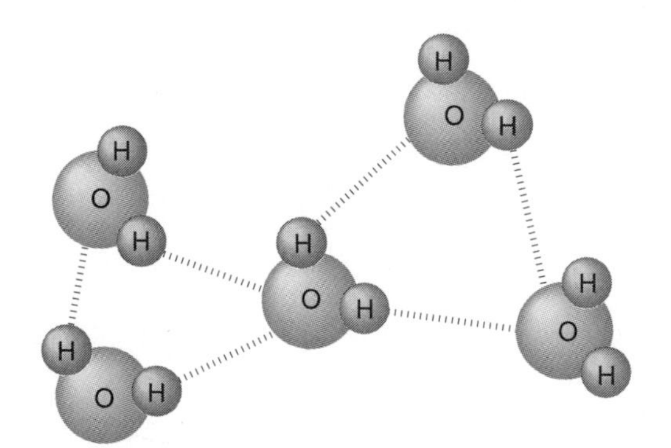

Figure 2–7 ◆ Hydrogen bonding between water molecules. Unequal sharing of electrons between hydrogen and oxygen in a water molecule causes an oxygen atom of one molecule to attract a hydrogen atom of another molecule. The hydrogen bonds between molecules provide water with unique properties.

Types of Chemical Reactions

All chemical reactions build or break bonds between atoms. Energy is required in building chemical bonds of molecules; energy is released in breaking chemical bonds of molecules. The two basic types of reactions may be described as **energy-requiring (endergonic)** reactions and **energy-liberating (exergonic)** reactions. The synthesis of compounds within cells requires energy to form bonds. Synthesis can be expressed quite simply by representing atoms, ions, or molecules with letters of the alphabet.

$$A + B \longrightarrow AB$$

In this reaction the newly synthesized molecule is AB. The degradation of another molecule CD may be expressed as follows:

$$CD \longrightarrow C + D$$

The products C and D may be atoms, ions, or molecules.

Sometimes building or breaking of bonds occurs simultaneously when energy exchanges are made. For example, if the molecules AB and CD make an even exchange of energy, that exchange could be represented as follows:

$$AB + CD \longrightarrow AD + BC$$

Very few chemical reactions occur without the help of external forces. The external forces may be something as simple as exposure to air, light, heat, or water or may be more complex, such as the action of chemicals known as enzymes found in living systems. The role of enzymes in chemical reactions is described in Chapter 6.

Until recently, scientists could readily recognize final products in the birth of molecules, but knew little about intermediate reactions. The molecules formed in the developmental stages exist for very brief periods of time measured in trillionths of a second. With lasers and molecular beams, it has been determined that hydrogen iodide (HI) can collide with carbon dioxide (CO_2) in five trillionths of a second. We actually live in a chemical world in which molecular change is not only constant, but extremely rapid.

Reversibility of Reactions

Theoretically all chemical reactions are reversible under appropriate circumstances. If a chemical reaction is readily reversible, double arrows are used to indicate that the reaction occurs in either direction.

$$A + B \rightleftharpoons AB$$

If molecules are stable and environmental conditions remain unchanged, reversible reactions do not occur. Internal conditions within cells are dynamic rather than static, however, and the time span of many intermediates in biochemical pathways is extremely limited.

A Chemical Accounting System

The chemists also have an accounting system to express chemical reactions. The accounting system consists of **equations** that, like the accountant's debits and credits, must balance. An equation consists of a left side and a right side, showing the reactants (left) and products (right) in a reaction. The numbers and types of atoms on one side of the equation must balance the numbers and types of atoms on the other side of the equation.

Active gaseous elements travel in pairs of atoms, so if the gas is oxygen, it is correctly written O_2. Because both atoms enter into a reaction, it may be necessary to indicate two molecules of a product to balance the equation. For example, it takes two atoms of magnesium (Mg) to react with molecular oxygen (O_2):

$$2Mg + O_2 \longrightarrow 2MgO$$

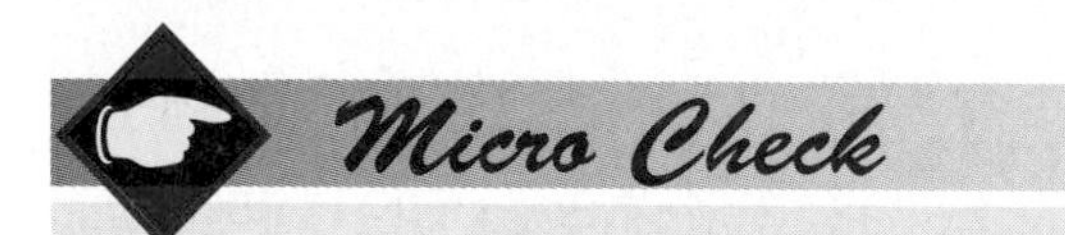

- What are the two basic types of chemical reactions?
- Why is the time span of many molecules in cells extremely limited?
- What do accountants and chemists have in common?

ACIDS, BASES, AND SALTS

Many chemical substances dissociate when dissolved in water. When dissociation occurs, the component parts develop charges and are properly called **ions.** Components releasing hydrogen ions (H^+) upon dissociation are called **acids.** Compounds releasing hydroxyl ions (OH^-) upon dissociation are called **bases.** Neutral solutions contain an equal number of hydrogen ions (H^+) and hydroxyl ions (OH^-). Positively charged ions are called **cations** because they are attracted to the cathode (negative pole) in an electrical field; negatively charged ions are called **anions** because they migrate to the anode (positive pole) in an electrical field. Compounds that dissociate in water producing cations other than H^+ and anions other than OH^- are known as **salts.** Table 2–5 contains a list of common acids, bases, and salts and their products of dissociation. Acids produce hydrogen ions (H^+) in solution; bases release hydroxyl ions (OH^-) in solution. The carbonated beverages, such as the colas, contain CO_2, which forms carbonic acid (H_2CO_3) when it dissolves. Oranges, lemons, and grapefruit contain citric acid. Lactic acid, produced by bacteria, is responsible for the souring of milk. Common bases include drain openers, detergents, window cleaning products, and antacids. The term alkaline is sometimes used to describe bases.

The chemical reactions of all cells are greatly affected by even moderate alterations in acidity or alkalinity. Most microorganisms carry on their activities in neutral or slightly alkaline environments, but exceptions do exist. Yeasts and molds grow best under mild acid conditions. Some sulfur-oxidizing bacteria found in sulfide-rich environments tolerate highly acid conditions.

Measurements of Acidity (pH)

The acidity of a solution (pH) is measured by the concentration of hydrogen ions (H^+) in a solution. Measurements of pH range from 0 to 14, depending on the negative logarithm of the hydrogen ion concentration (Fig. 2–8):

$$pH = \log \frac{1}{(H^+)} \text{ or } -\log(H^+)$$

A change in one unit on the scale represents a tenfold change in hydrogen ion concentration. Pure water in which the concentrations of hydrogen ions (H^+) and hydroxyl (OH^-) ions are equal has a pH of 7 on the scale. Seawater has a somewhat more alkaline pH, ranging from 7.8 to 8.3. What does that tell us about microorganisms that live in marine habitats? How can we recreate and maintain nature's environment to grow microorganisms in the laboratory?

Table 2–5
PRODUCTS OF DISSOCIATED ACIDS, BASES, AND SALTS

	FORMULAS	CATIONS	ANIONS
Acids			
Acetic acid	CH_3COOH	H^+	CH_3COO^-
Hydrochloric	HCl	H^+	Cl^-
Sulfuric	H_2SO_4	H^+	SO_4^{2-}
Nitric	HNO_3	H^+	NO_3^-
Boric acid	H_3BO_3	H^+	BO_3^{3-}
Carbonic acid	H_2CO_3	H^+	CO_3^{2-}
Bases			
Ethyl alcohol	C_2H_5OH	$C_2H_5^+$	OH^-
Sodium hydroxide	$NaOH$	Na^+	OH^-
Potassium hydroxide	KOH	K^+	OH^-
Calcium hydroxide	$Ca(OH)_2$	Ca^{2+}	OH^-
Ammonium hydroxide	NH_4OH	NH_4^-	OH^-
Salts			
Sodium chloride	$NaCl$	Na^+	Cl^-
Copper sulfate	$CuSO_4$	Cu^{2+}	SO_4^-
Silver nitrate	$AgNO_3$	Ag^+	NO_3^-
Zinc chloride	$ZnCl_2$	Zn^+	Cl^-
Mercuric nitrate	$Hg\ (NO_3)_2$	Hg^{2+}	NO_3^-

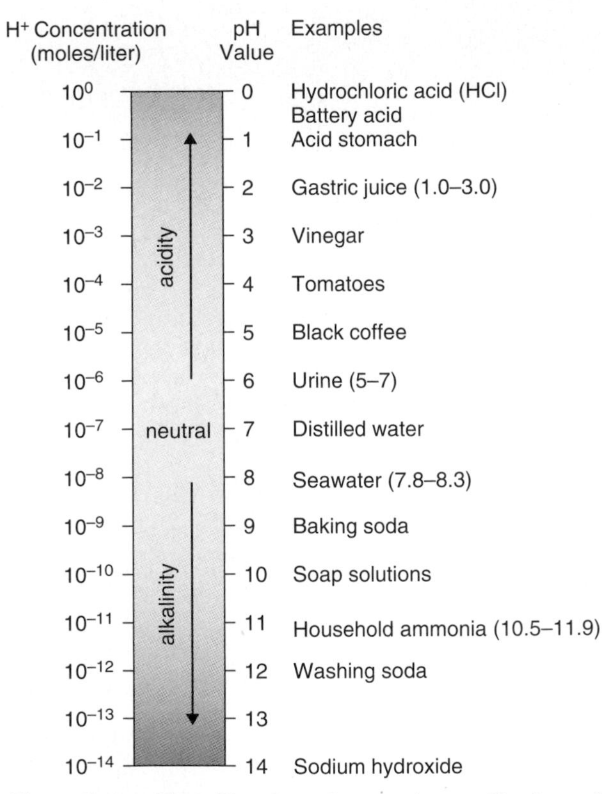

Figure 2–8 ◆ The pH scale and approximate pH values of some common substances.

The Role of Buffers

Certain salts can combine with excess hydrogen (H^+) or hydroxyl (OH^-) ions to produce substances that are less acid or alkaline. Those salts are called **buffers.** One active buffer in cells is bicarbonate:

$$HCO_3^- + H^+ \rightleftharpoons H_2CO_3$$

The reaction is readily reversible so that in the presence of carbonic acid or other buffers, adjustments in pH can be made to sustain the living state.

Populations of large numbers of microorganisms grown in the laboratory can be severely limited, however, by acidic or basic products of metabolism. Nontoxic buffers may be added to nutrient materials to counteract the accumulation of acid or alkaline metabolic products which would interfere with growth. Buffers are discussed in more detail in Chapter 5.

ORGANIC MOLECULES

The major organic (carbon- and hydrogen-containing) molecules found in living things are carbohydrates, proteins, lipids, and nucleic acids. The proteins, nucleic acids, and some carbohydrates are classified as **macromolecules** because of their large size. The organic molecules contain hydrogen (H), oxygen (O), and nitrogen (N) in addition to carbon (C). Sulfur (S) and phosphorus (P) are found with lesser frequency. Most of the carbon (C) atoms are bonded to hydrogen (H) atoms.

Carbohydrates: The Energy-Rich Molecules

Carbohydrates, including sugars and starches, are major sources of energy for all living things. They contain carbon (C), hydrogen (H), and oxygen (O). The atoms are arranged in H—C—OH configurations. The empirical formula for a carbohydrate is expressed as $(CH_2O)_n$ in which n is 3 or greater. The simplest carbohydrates are **trioses** in which n is equal to 3.

Carbohydrates are commonly classified on the basis of the number of simple units or **monomers** making up the molecules. The most abundant monomer in nature is glucose, in which n equals 6.

MONOSACCHARIDES

Simple carbohydrates, containing three to seven carbon atoms (C) and either an aldehyde group (CH=O) or a keto group (C=O) are called **monosaccharides.** The most biologically active monosaccharides are the five-carbon pentoses and the six-carbon hexoses. The monosaccharides having five or more carbon atoms are often represented by linear formulas or closed ring structures known as Haworth formulas.

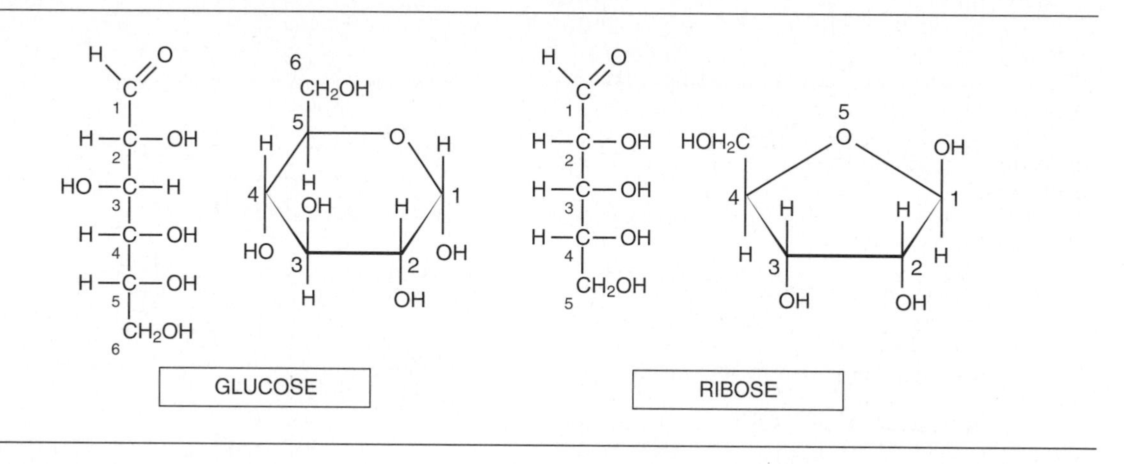

Numbering the carbon atoms of either type of formula is helpful in understanding and describing the bonding between monomers of carbohydrates and chemical reactions occurring with other molecules.

Monosaccharides can exist in either a right-handed (D) configuration or a left-handed (L) configuration. If the C-5 of a hexose or the C-4 of a pentose is isolated from the rest of the structures, it can be observed that the carbon can be bonded on the right or the left side with the hydroxyl group (—OH).

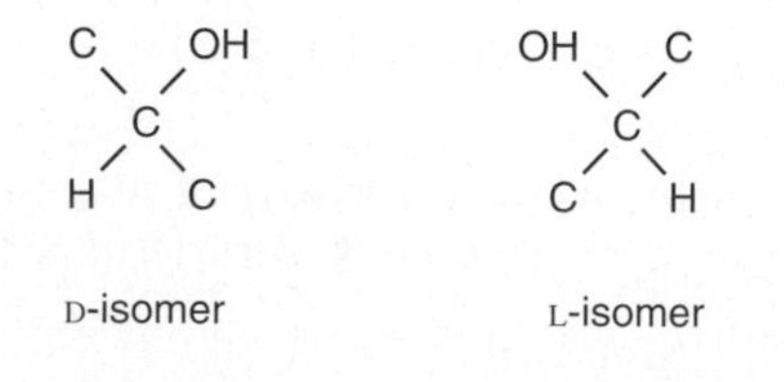

Chemical compounds containing the same numbers and types of atoms in different positions are called **isomers.** D- and L-isomers are mirror images of each other. The D-isomers are more abundant in nature and, therefore, the most significant to microbial life.

Two other types of isomers can be formed when monosaccharides cyclize. If the —OH group of ribose or glucose is positioned below the plane of the ring at C-1, the molecule is called an α-isomer. If the —OH group is attached to the C-1 above the plane of the ring, the molecule is referred to as a β-isomer (see the structures at the top of the next page). On other monosaccharides the —OH group alternates positions above or below C-2, C-3, or C-4. In this chapter, simple modified structural formulas will be used as much as possible to show positioning of bonds between molecules or alterations in molecules.

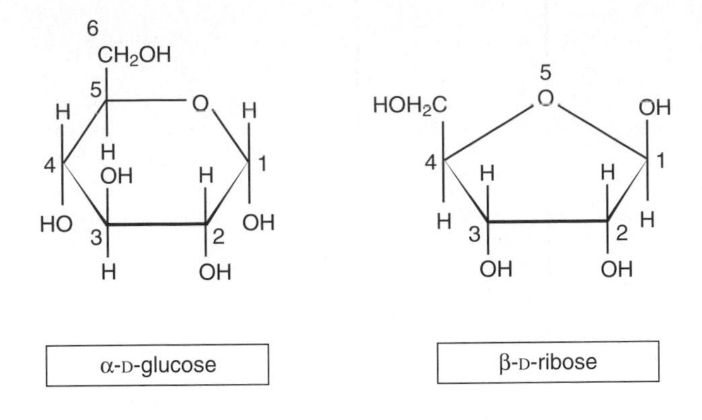

DISACCHARIDES

Combinations of two molecules of monosaccharides with the loss of one molecule of water at the bonding site forms disaccharides. The monomers of disaccharides may be similar or dissimilar. When water is lost as a result of the union of two monosaccharides, a **glycosidic bond** between the monomers is formed at the site of the water loss.

Maltose is a disaccharide that contains two monomers of glucose linked in the C-1 and C-4 positions.

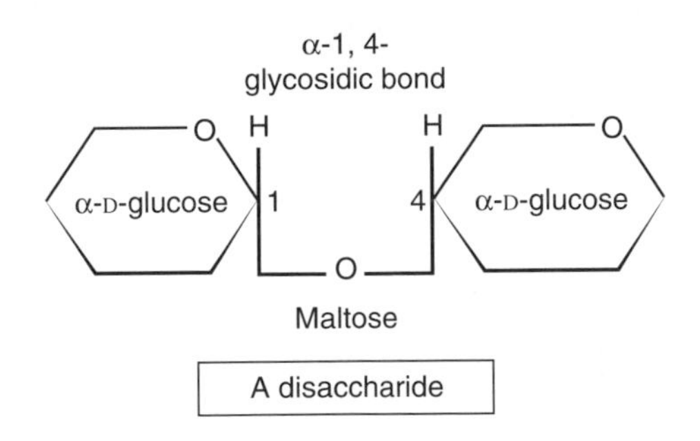

Sucrose is a disaccharide that contains a monomer of glucose and a monomer of fructose. In the combined form fructose exists as a five-membered structure instead of the usual six-membered ring.

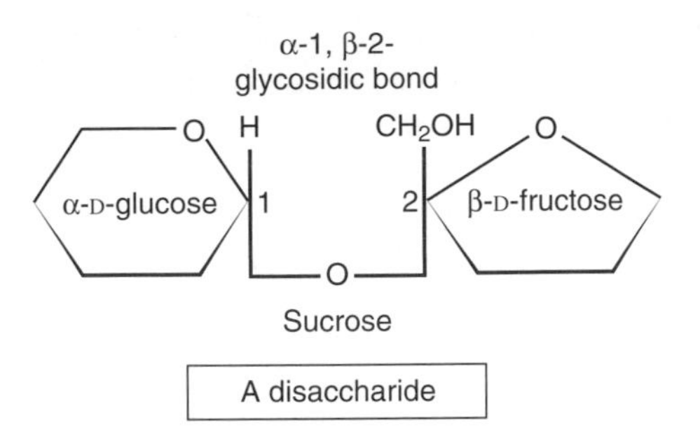

Lactose contains a molecule of glucose and a molecule of galactose in a 1,4-glycosidic bond. Both monomers exist as six-membered rings.

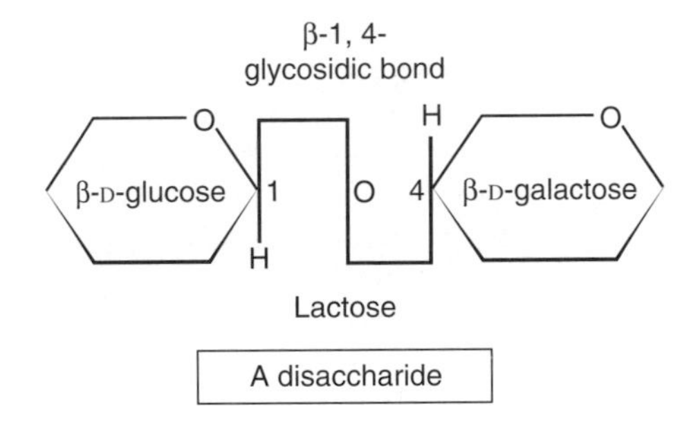

POLYSACCHARIDES

The polysaccharides consist of multiple hexoses or pentoses with numerous glycosidic bonds. Starch, the form in which carbohydrates are

FOCAL POINT

Lesser Known Sugar Rescues Children from Middle Ear Infections

Xylitol, a sugar found naturally in birch trees, has the potential to rescue the 50 percent of children one to three years of age destined to have a middle ear infection annually. The infection is caused by invasions of bacteria into the cavity of the middle ear. In a study conducted in Finland, preschoolers receiving 10 grams of xylitol five times a day came down with fewer middle ear infections over three months than a similar group receiving gum sweetened with sucrose. Furthermore, the birch sugar inhibited the growth of *Streptococcus pneumoniae,* the major bacterial culprit in the ear infections. It seems to prevent attachment of the bacterium to the mucous membranes of the mouth and throat.

Adapted from Science News 154(18):287, 1998

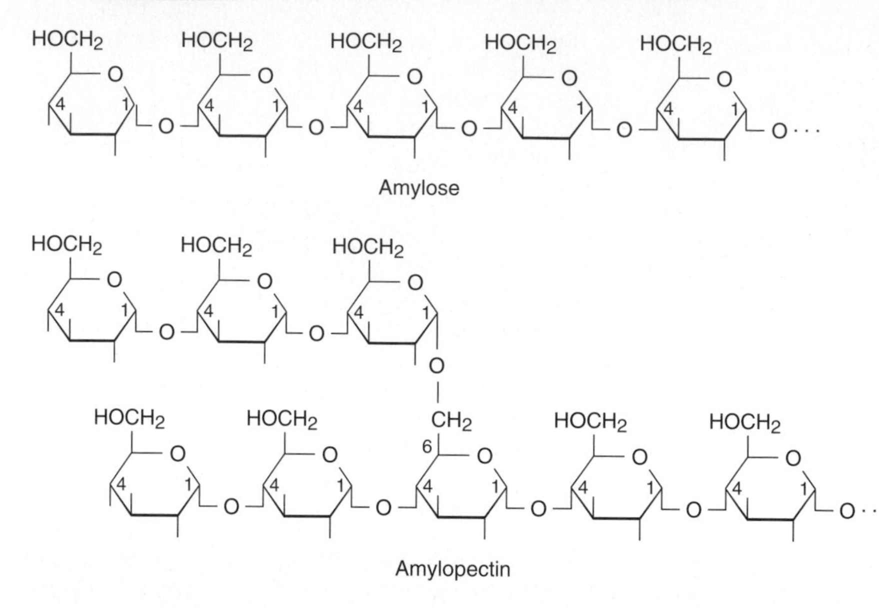

Figure 2–9 ◆ The amylase and amylopectin components of a starch molecule showing 1,4- and 1,6-glycosidic bonds.

stored in plants, contains an **amylose** and an **amylopectin component.** The amylose unit is composed of glucose monomers connected linearly by 1,4-glycosidic bonds; the molecular weight is variable. Amylose constitutes 15 to 25 percent starch. Amylopectin is a branched molecule containing several thousand glucose units with 1,4- and 1,6-glycosidic bonds (Fig. 2–9).

Cellulose is the most abundant polysaccharide in nature; it is a major constituent of the cell walls of plants, fungi, and most algae. It consists of long chains of glucose units connected by 1,4-glycosidic bonds. It differs from amylose in that the bonding is arranged differently and the chains are longer.

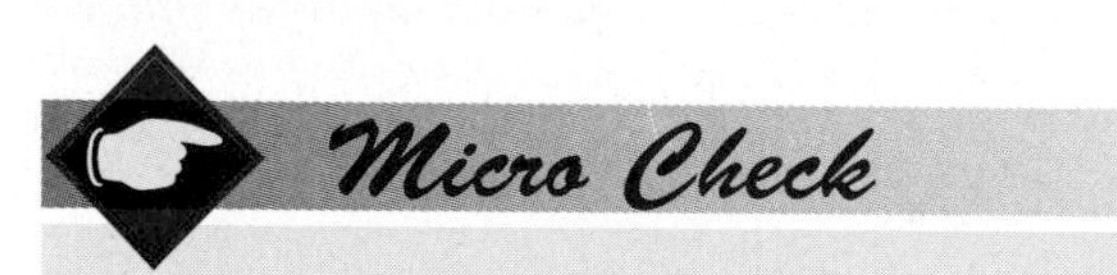

- ◆ Why are carbohydrates needed to sustain life?
- ◆ How can you recognize the formula of a carbohydrate?
- ◆ What is the purpose of numbering carbon positions in closed ring structures?

Proteins: The Determinants of Diversity

The proteins are macromolecules containing carbon (C), hydrogen (H), oxygen (O), and sometimes iron (Fe) or sulfur (S). The monomers of proteins consist of subunits known as **amino acids.** All amino acids have an amino (NH_2) group, a carboxyl (COOH) group, and a side chain which is designated by R. Amino acids, like the monosaccharides, can exist as D- or L-isomers.

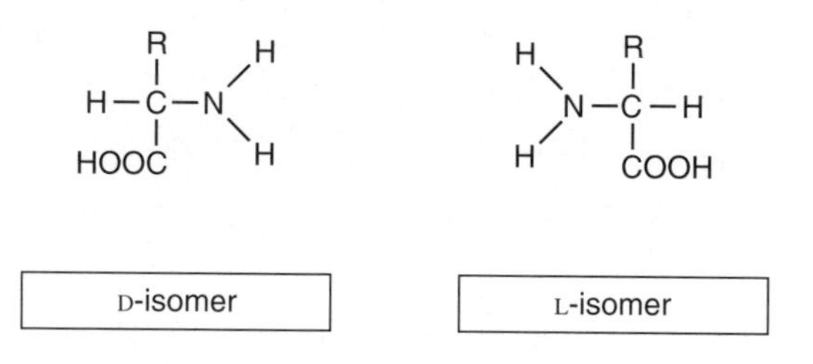

Proteins constitute about 50 percent of all living things (Fig. 2–10). An elephant, a mouse, a giant sequoia, and even the smallest microbes are dependent on structural proteins that make up their component parts. Proteins of our cell membranes make us all unique as individuals unless we have an identical twin. Other proteins speed up, or catalyze, chemical reactions in cells. Proteins often contain 100 to 10,000 amino acids, but it is the sequence of their appearance and the folding of their chains that determines their function. The configuration of protein molecules is best understood by consideration of the four sequential arrangements designated as primary, secondary, tertiary, and quaternary structures occurring in the synthesis of proteins.

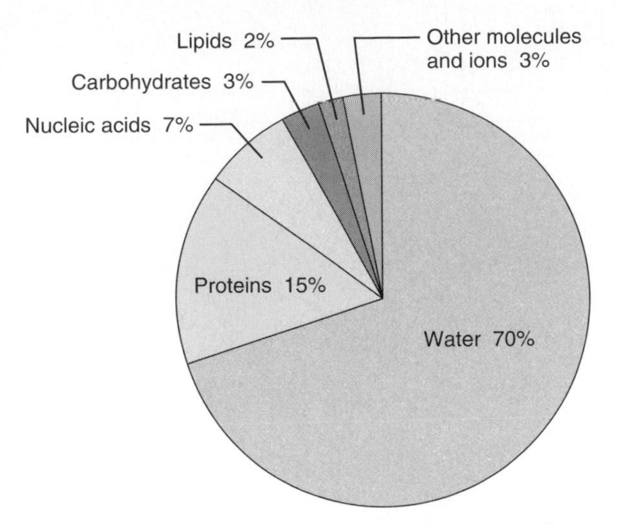

Figure 2–10 ◆ Percentages of major molecules found in a typical bacterial cell. Proteins are the most abundant organic constituents.

PRIMARY STRUCTURE

Amino acids are connected by **peptide bonds,** which join a carboxyl group (COOH) of one amino acid with an amino group (NH_2) of another; one molecule of water is lost by a single peptide bond, as in glycosidic bonding.

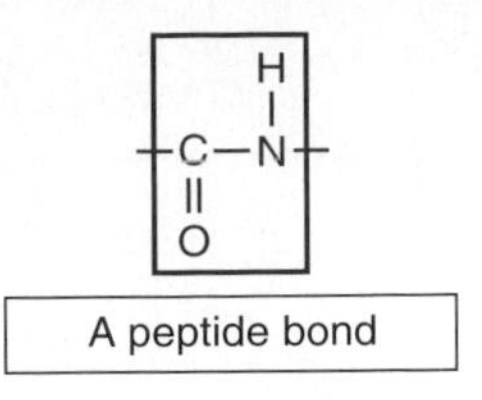

Two amino acids joined by a peptide bond are called **dipeptides;** three amino acids bonded similarly are **tripeptides;** a chain of 10 or more amino acids constitutes a **polypeptide.** One molecule each of alanine (Ala), cysteine (Cys), and glycine (Gly) make up a tripeptide (Fig. 2–11). However, five other possible combinations of the three amino acids could exist. If we use Ala, Cys, and Gly to represent the amino acids, six tripeptides could be formed, depending on the arrangements of the molecules:

Ala Cys Gly Cys Gly Ala Gly Ala Cys
Ala Gly Cys Cys Ala Gly Gly Cys Ala

There are 20 commonly occurring amino acids in nature (Table 2–6). If 20 amino acids are used, almost an infinite variety of combinations and chain lengths of amino acids can be envisioned. The variety of polypeptides made possible by combinations of amino acids is responsible for the diversity of both structure and function among living things.

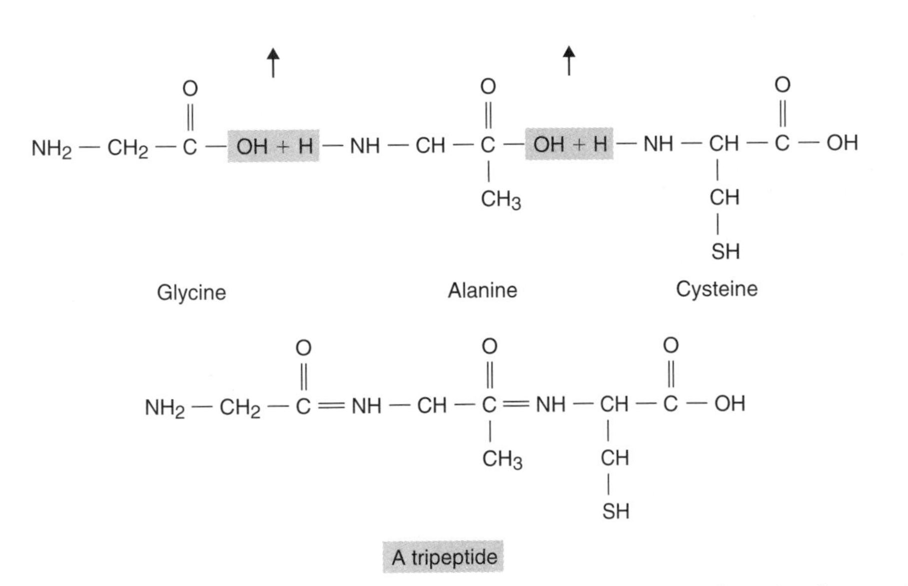

Figure 2–11 ◆ Structure of a tripeptide. One molecule each of glycine, alanine, and cysteine form a tripeptide. Carbon and nitrogen atoms are joined by double bonds when water is lost in each peptide bond.

Table 2–6

TWENTY COMMONLY OCCURRING AMINO ACIDS

AMINO ACID	ABBREVIATION	FORMULA
Alanine	Ala	$CH_3-CH(NH_3)-COOH$
Arginine	Arg	$H_2N-C(=NH_2)-NH-CH_2-CH_2-CH_2-CH(NH_3)-COOH$
Asparagine	Asn	$NH_2(O=)C-CH_2-CH(NH_3)-COOH$
Aspartic Acid	Asp	$^{-}O(O=)C-CH_2-CH(NH_3)-COOH$
Cysteine	Cys	$HS-CH_2-CH(NH_3)-COOH$
Glutamic Acid	Glu	$^{-}O(O=)C-CH_2-CH_2-CH(NH_3)-COOH$
Glutamine	Gln	$NH_2(O=)C-CH_2-CH_2-CH(NH_3)-COOH$
Glycine	Gly	$H-CH(NH_3)-COOH$

Table 2–6
TWENTY COMMONLY OCCURRING AMINO ACIDS *Continued*

AMINO ACID	ABBREVIATION	FORMULA
Histidine	His	$HC{=}C{-}CH_2{-}CH(NH_3){-}COOH$; ring: $HC{=}C$, HN^{+}, NH, $C{-}H$ (imidazole: $HC{=}C{-}NH{-}CH{=}N^{+}H{-}$)
Isoleucine	Ile	$CH_3{-}CH_2{-}CH(CH_3){-}CH(NH_3){-}COOH$
Leucine	Leu	$(CH_3)_2CH{-}CH_2{-}CH(NH_3){-}COOH$
Lysine	Lys	$H_3N{-}CH_2{-}CH_2{-}CH_2{-}CH_2{-}CH(NH_3){-}COOH$
Methionine	Met	$CH_3{-}S{-}CH_2{-}CH_2{-}CH(NH_3){-}COOH$
Phenylalanine	Phe	$C_6H_5{-}CH_2{-}CH(NH_3){-}COOH$
Proline	Pro	ring H_2C, H_2C, H_2C, $N{-}H$, $C(H){-}COOH$
Serine	Ser	$HO{-}CH_2{-}CH(NH_3){-}COOH$

Table continued on following page

Table 2–6
TWENTY COMMONLY OCCURRING AMINO ACIDS *Continued*

AMINO ACID	ABBREVIATION	FORMULA
Threonine	Thr	$CH_3-C(OH)(H)-C(H)(NH_3)-COOH$
Tryptophan	Trp	$C_6H_4(NH-CH=C)-CH_2-C(H)(NH_3)-COOH$
Tyrosine	Tyr	$HO-C_6H_4-CH_2-C(H)(NH_3)-COOH$
Valine	Val	$(CH_3)_2CH-C(H)(NH_3)-COOH$

SECONDARY STRUCTURE

Long chains of polypeptides tend to form a helix or to occur in a pleated sheet arrangement. Much of the coiling and pleating is maintained by hydrogen bonds in which the hydrogen (H) of an amino group (NH_2) of one amino acid bonds with one oxygen (O) of a carbonyl group (C═O) of another amino acid.

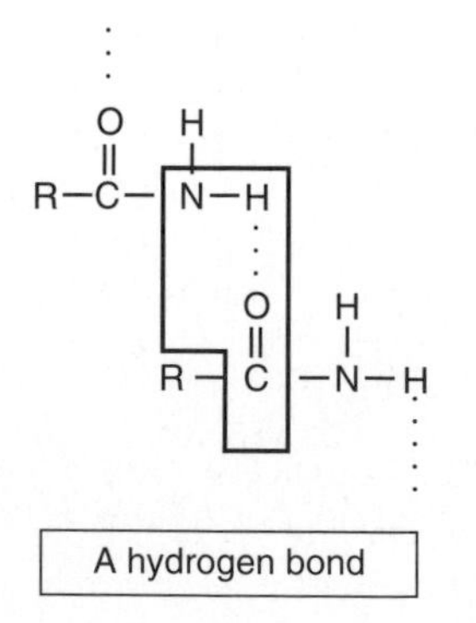

A hydrogen bond

Although a single hydrogen bond is weak, many hundred such bonds collectively provide structural integrity for proteins. Helical proteins include the keratins, myosin, and collagen. Fibroin, a protein found in silk, has a pleated sheet arrangement.

TERTIARY STRUCTURE

The helices or pleated sheets of polypeptides may undergo additional coiling and folding to become globular in shape. The tertiary structure formed in this manner is stabilized by the formation of additional hydrogen, ionic, and disulfide bonds.

Ionic bonds form between the $—COO^-$ of the side chains of acidic amino acids and the $—NH_3^+$ of the side chains of basic amino acids.

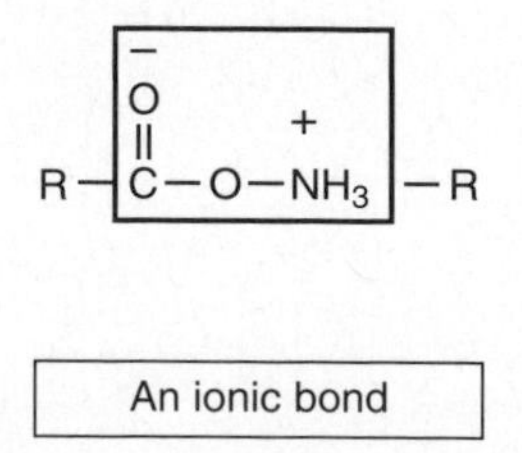

An ionic bond

The sulfur-containing amino acid cysteine plays an important role in linking polypeptide chains. Disulfide bonds form between sulfur atoms of two cysteine side chains.

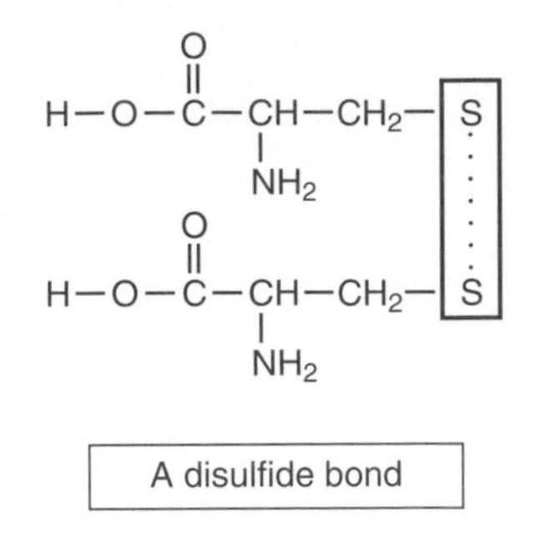

A disulfide bond

A fourth factor contributing to the higher order structure of proteins is the position of polar and nonpolar chains of side chains of amino acids. **Hydrophobic** (water-hating) nonpolar side chains are positioned on the inside of the protein molecule. **Hydrophilic** (water-loving) polar chains are on the outside of the protein molecule. The positioning of side chains in this manner favors hydrogen bonding between amino acids. The ease with which hydrogen bonds are formed and broken accounts for the dynamic state of proteins in cell membranes.

QUATERNARY STRUCTURE

Proteins that contain more than one polypeptide chain demonstrate a fourth level of organization called a **quaternary structure.** The same noncovalent forces promoting the formation of tertiary structures are responsible for binding of polypeptide chains. All four levels of organization can be seen in Figure 2–12.

CONJUGATED PROTEINS

A protein combined with a nonprotein, either an inorganic or organic compound, is called a **conjugated protein.** Proteins may be conjugated with carbohydrates (glycoproteins), lipids (lipoproteins), nucleic acids (nucleoproteins), phosphorus (phosphoproteins), or pigments.

DENATURATION OF PROTEINS

The unfolding or uncoiling of a protein by destruction of bonds is called **denaturation.** Heat, acids, bases, radiation, salts of heavy metals, and organic solvents can denature proteins. The proteins lose their shapes and are no longer biologically active. Beating of egg whites causes albumin molecules to unfold. If you used a stove or a microwave oven to cook your food today, you broke hydrogen bonds of proteins. Like the fallen Humpty Dumpty, who could not be put together again, denaturation is not reversible.

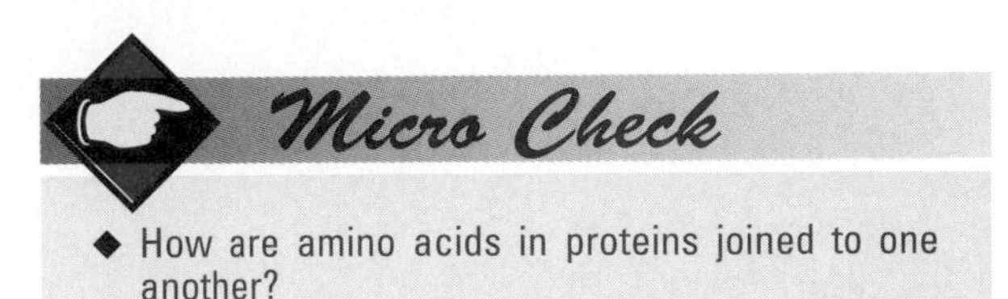

- How are amino acids in proteins joined to one another?
- What factors contribute to the stability of tertiary and quaternary structures of proteins?
- What happens when proteins are denatured?

Lipids: The Distant Cousins

The lipids of microorganisms consist of a heterogeneous group of compounds containing carbon (C), hydrogen (H), oxygen (O), and sometimes phosphorus (P) and nitrogen (N). All are sparingly soluble in water, but are readily soluble in organic solvents such as ether, acetone, chloroform, benzene, or the alcohols. The structures of lipids are diverse, and often, like distant cousins, it is difficult to identify members of the same family. Lipids are major constituents of plasma membranes of cellular organisms. The dissimilarity of lipids makes any classification somewhat arbitrary.

SIMPLE LIPIDS

Fats, oils, and waxes consist of fatty acids and glycerol or other alcohols. Fatty acids, are straight, unbranched hydrocarbon compounds usually containing a terminal methyl group (CH_3), a long hydrocarbon chain with a varying number of units of CH_2, and a terminal carboxyl group (COOH). Subscripts are often used to indicate the number of CH_2 units.

$$CH_3(CH_2)_{16}COOH$$

Stearic acid

A saturated fatty acid

Fatty acids may possess one to four carbon-to-carbon double bonds (C=C) or only single bonds between carbon atoms. Each carbon atom linked to another carbon atom by a double bond

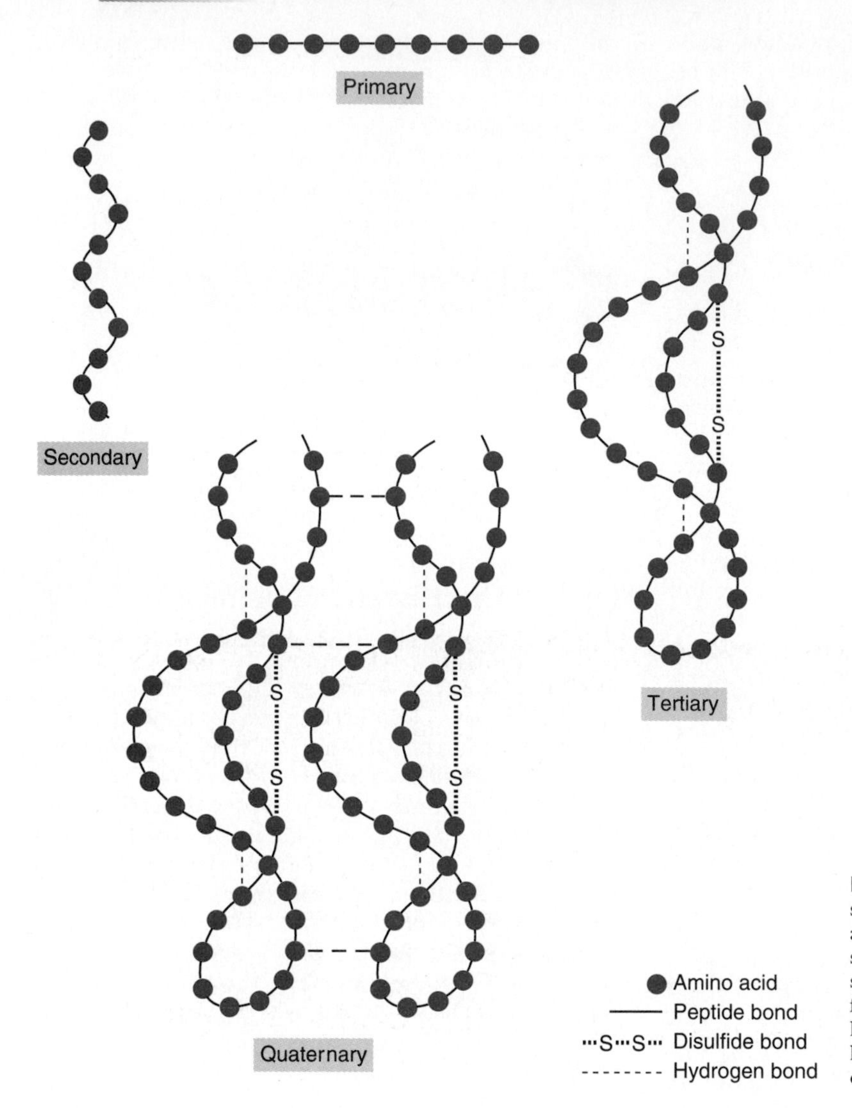

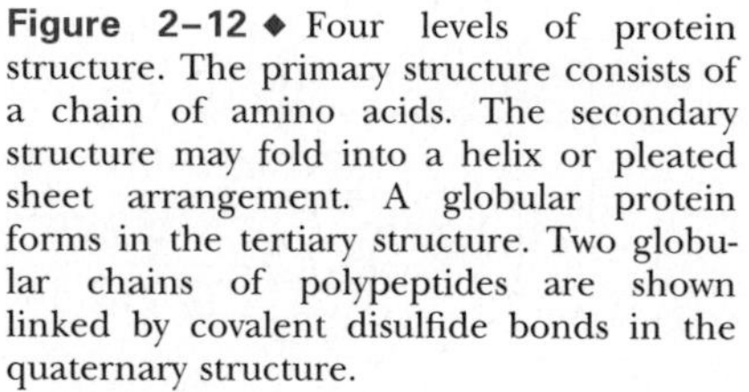

Figure 2–12 ◆ Four levels of protein structure. The primary structure consists of a chain of amino acids. The secondary structure may fold into a helix or pleated sheet arrangement. A globular protein forms in the tertiary structure. Two globular chains of polypeptides are shown linked by covalent disulfide bonds in the quaternary structure.

binds one less hydrogen atom than carbon atoms joined by a single bond. Therefore, fatty acids that contain double bonds are called **unsaturated fatty acids.** The unsaturated fatty acids are liquid at room temperature. Unsaturated fatty acids include oleic, linoleic, linolenic, and arachidonic acids. The most widely distributed fatty acid in nature is oleic acid.

$$CH_3(CH_2)_7CH = CH(CH_2)_7COOH$$

Oleic acid

An unsaturated fatty acid

Fatty acids having no carbon-to-carbon double bonds possess the maximal number of atoms of hydrogen at carbon-bonding sites and therefore are called **saturated fatty acids.** The most important saturated fatty acids are lauric, myristic, palmitic, and stearic acids. Saturated fatty acids with less than 10 carbon atoms are liquids at room temperature; saturated fatty acids with chains of more than 12 to 14 carbon atoms are solids.

The true fats contain fatty acids and glycerol, a trihydroxyl alcohol derived from a triose. They may alternately be called **glycerides.** The bonding between the hydroxyl group (OH) of glycerol and the carboxyl group (COOH) of a fatty acid with the loss of a water molecule is called an **ester bond.**

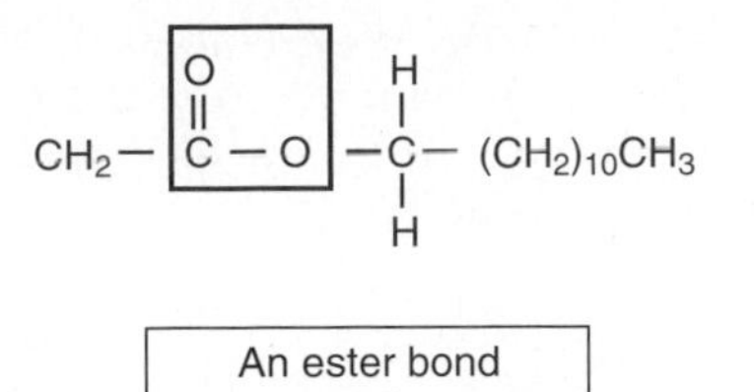

An ester bond

If a single ester bond is formed, the compound is a **monoglyceride;** two ester bonds with the same or different fatty acids form a **diglyceride;** three ester bonds with similar or dissimilar fatty acids form a **triglyceride.** Triglycerides containing mixed fatty acids are more common in nature; they are sometimes called **neutral fats** (Fig. 2–13). Waxes are formed when fatty acids combine with long-chain alcohols; they have high melting points and are more stable than true fats.

COMPOUND LIPIDS

The most important compound lipids of microorganisms are **phospholipids, glycolipids,** and **steroids.** The phospholipids are derivatives of glycerol phosphate. Some have a nitrogen-containing group. The nitrogen-containing portion may be choline, ethanolamine, or L-serine.

$HO-CH_2-CH_2-N\equiv(CH_3)_3$	Choline
$HO-CH_2-CH_2-NH_2$	Ethanolamine
$HO-CH_2-CH(COOH)-NH_2$	L-Serine

The glycolipids contain fatty acids and a sugar linked to sphingosine, a nitrogen-containing compound with no glycerol.

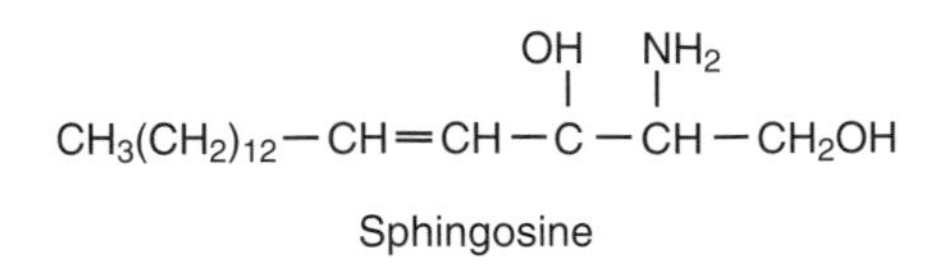

Sphingosine

Steroids are a group of structurally complex compounds which have diverse physiological roles in mammalian cells. They have a polycyclic carbon skeleton and contain an alcohol group. Hence, steroids may be called **sterols.** The most common sterol is cholesterol. Cholesterol is classified as a lipid because it is insoluble in water.

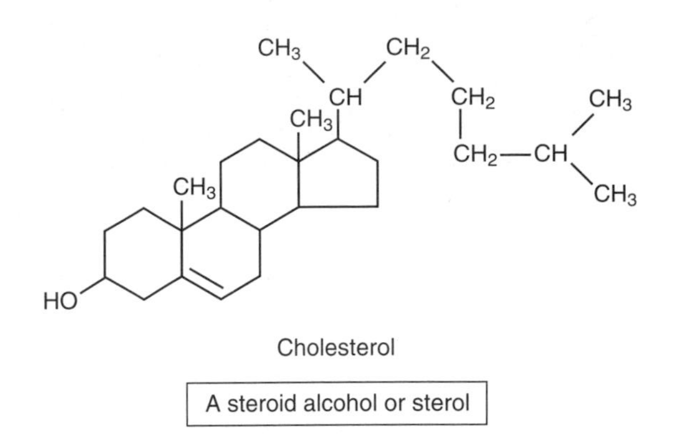

Cholesterol

A steroid alcohol or sterol

Micro Check

- What are the structural components of glycerides?
- How does a saturated fatty acid differ from an unsaturated fatty acid?
- Why is cholesterol classified as a lipid?

Nucleic Acids: The Informational Molecules

The nucleic acids are macromolecules containing carbon (C), hydrogen (H), oxygen (O), nitrogen (N), and phosphorus (P). The names are derived from the type of sugar contained within the molecules. Ribose, a pentose, is associated with RNA (ribonucleic acid). The sugar in DNA

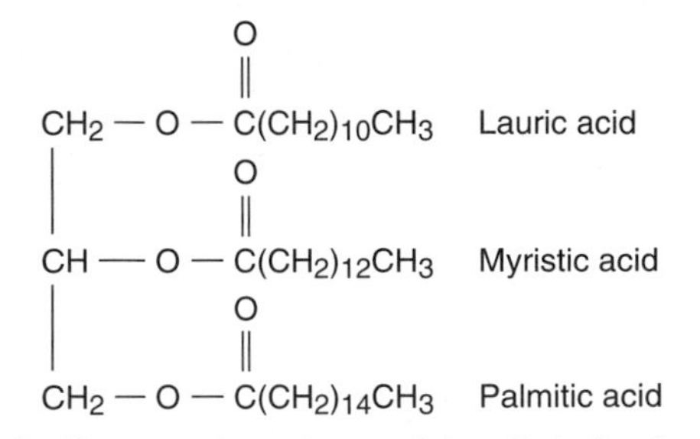

Figure 2–13 ◆ A triglyceride containing dissimilar fatty acids.

(deoxyribonucleic acid) has one oxygen atom missing, making it deoxyribose.

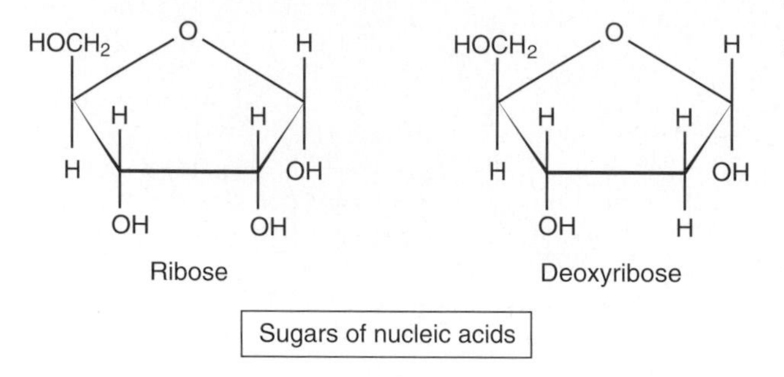

Sugars of nucleic acids

DNA is responsible for inherited characteristics, growth, and reproduction of cells. This macromolecule determines such things as our skin, eye, and hair color, height, and blood type and is the source of nearly 4000 human disorders, including some types of cancer. DNA is found in nucleated and nonnucleated cells and is a major component of one group of viruses. Other viruses contain RNA instead of DNA. DNA molecules store the information necessary for making proteins in most organisms. The viruses containing RNA are the only examples in nature of RNA being the repository of stored information. In cellular organisms, instructions supplied by DNA are passed on to molecules of RNA. Three types of RNA are needed to make proteins as specified by DNA. Only in viruses containing RNA does the process differ. The specific roles of DNA and RNA in cellular microorganisms are discussed in greater detail in Chapter 7. The functions of the nucleic acids in viral replication are explained in Chapter 10.

NUCLEOSIDES AND NUCLEOTIDES

The nitrogen-containing portions of nucleic acids are mixtures of basic substances known as **purines** and **pyrimidines.** The major pyrimidines in nucleic acids are **uracil** (U), **thymine** (T), and **cytosine** (C); they are six-membered ring structures with minor variations in the numbers of atoms.

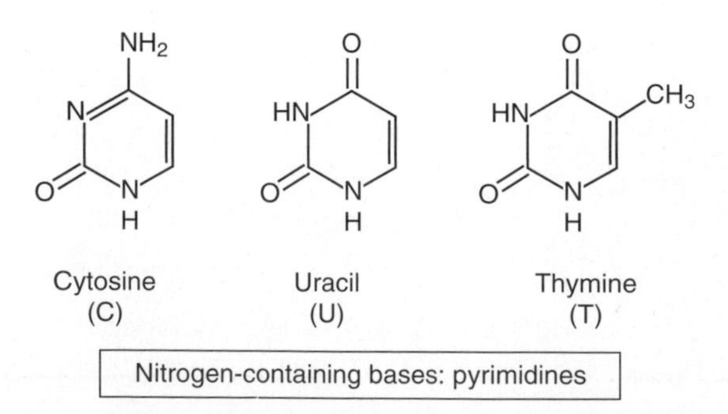

Nitrogen-containing bases: pyrimidines

The purines are six-membered pyrimidine rings fused to a five-membered imidazole ring. The principal purines in nucleic acids are **adenine** (A) and **guanine** (G).

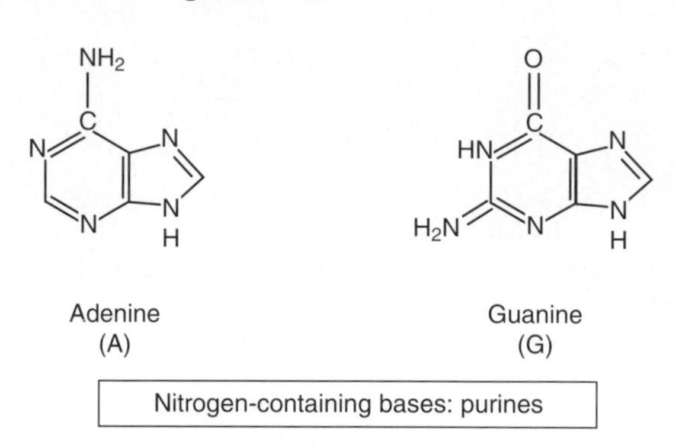

Nitrogen-containing bases: purines

The positions of the carbon atoms (C) in the cyclic structures can be numbered in much the same manner as they are numbered for carbohydrates.

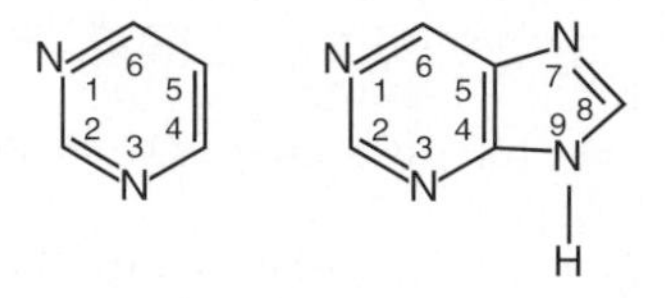

This is often helpful in understanding reactions between the pyrimidine or purine portions of the nucleic acids.

The subunits of nucleic acids, formed when a purine or pyrimidine is linked to ribose or deoxyribose, are called **nucleosides** (Table 2–7). In order to differentiate the positions of the carbon (C) atoms of the sugars from those of the nitrogenous bases, a prime (′) is used to identify the carbon positions of the sugars. The addition of phosphate (PO_4) to ribose in an ester bond at position 2′, 3′, or 5′ or to deoxyribose at position 3′ or 5′ forms a **nucleotide.** Nucleotides are considered the building blocks of nucleic acids.

DEOXYRIBONUCLEIC ACID

Pyrimidines and purines of double-stranded DNA are joined by hydrogen bonds. DNA molecules occur as helices with purines appearing opposite pyrimidines. The purine adenine (A) always pairs with thymine (T), the pyrimidine; the purine guanine (G) always pairs with the pyrimidine cytosine (C) (Fig. 2–14). The A-T base pairs are joined by two hydrogen bonds. The C-G base pairs are connected by three hydrogen bonds. This precise pairing of pyrimidines and purines is known as **complementarity.** Nitrogen bases occurring opposite one another in those positions are said to be complementary to one another.

RIBONUCLEIC ACID

Ribonucleic acid (RNA) is distinguished from DNA by the (1) presence of the pyrimidine uracil (U) instead of thymine (T), (2) the substitution of ribose for deoxyribose, (3) its location within the cell, and (4) its specialized functions in the synthesis of proteins. All three types of RNA originate from the instructions supplied by DNA. The strands of RNA are complementary to the DNA strands in the same manner that a new strand of DNA is complementary to an unwound strand of DNA, except for the replacement of uracil (U) for thymine (T).

The genetic information copied from DNA is contained in three types of RNA. Most of the RNA of cells is associated with structures known as **ribosomes,** the protein factories of cells (see Table 2–7). This type is called **ribosomal** RNA (rRNA). The rRNA is a major structural component of ribosomes. **Messenger** RNA (mRNA) contains the information that codes for the sequence of amino acids in proteins. Triplets of bases, known as **codons,** direct the position of specific amino acids in polypeptide chains. A third type of low-molecular-weight RNA, called **transfer**

Table 2–7
SUBUNITS OF RNA AND DNA MOLECULES

BASE FORMULA	BASE	NUCLEOSIDE	NUCLEOTIDE
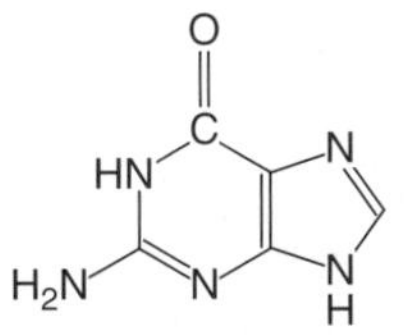 O, C, HN, N, N, H₂N, N, H	Adenine A	Adenosine A	Adenosine monophosphate AMP
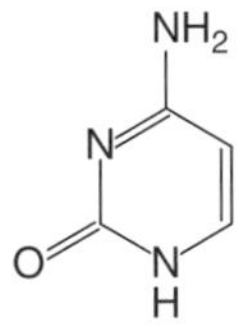 NH_2, N, O, N, H	Cytosine C	Cytidine C	Cytidine monophosphate CMP
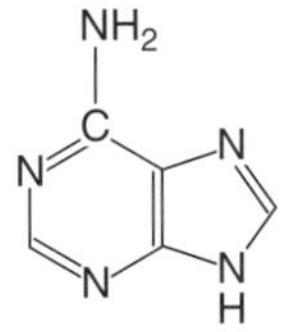 NH_2, C, N, N, N, N, H	Guanine G	Guanosine G	Guanosine monophosphate GMP
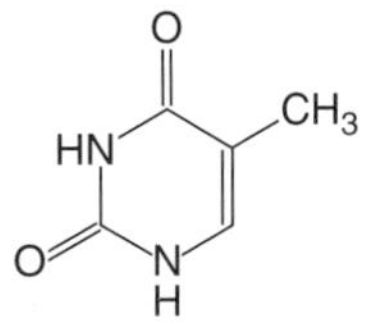 O, HN, CH_3, O, N, H	Thymine T	Thymidine T	Thymidine monophosphate TMP
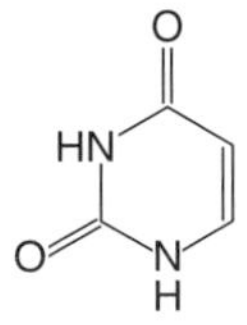 O, HN, O, N, H	Uracil U	Uridine U	Uridine monophosphate UMP

RNA (tRNA), occurs in part as a cloverleaf configuration with paired bases (Fig. 2–15). The lower loop of the cloverleaf contains a triplet of unpaired nitrogen bases known as an **anticodon.** The bases of anticodons are complementary to the bases present on codons for each of the 20 amino acids. A detailed discussion of protein synthesis is presented in Chapter 7.

Micro Check

- What is the difference between a nucleoside and a nucleotide?
- What is the difference in chemical composition of DNA and RNA?
- How are nucleotides held together in nucleic acids?

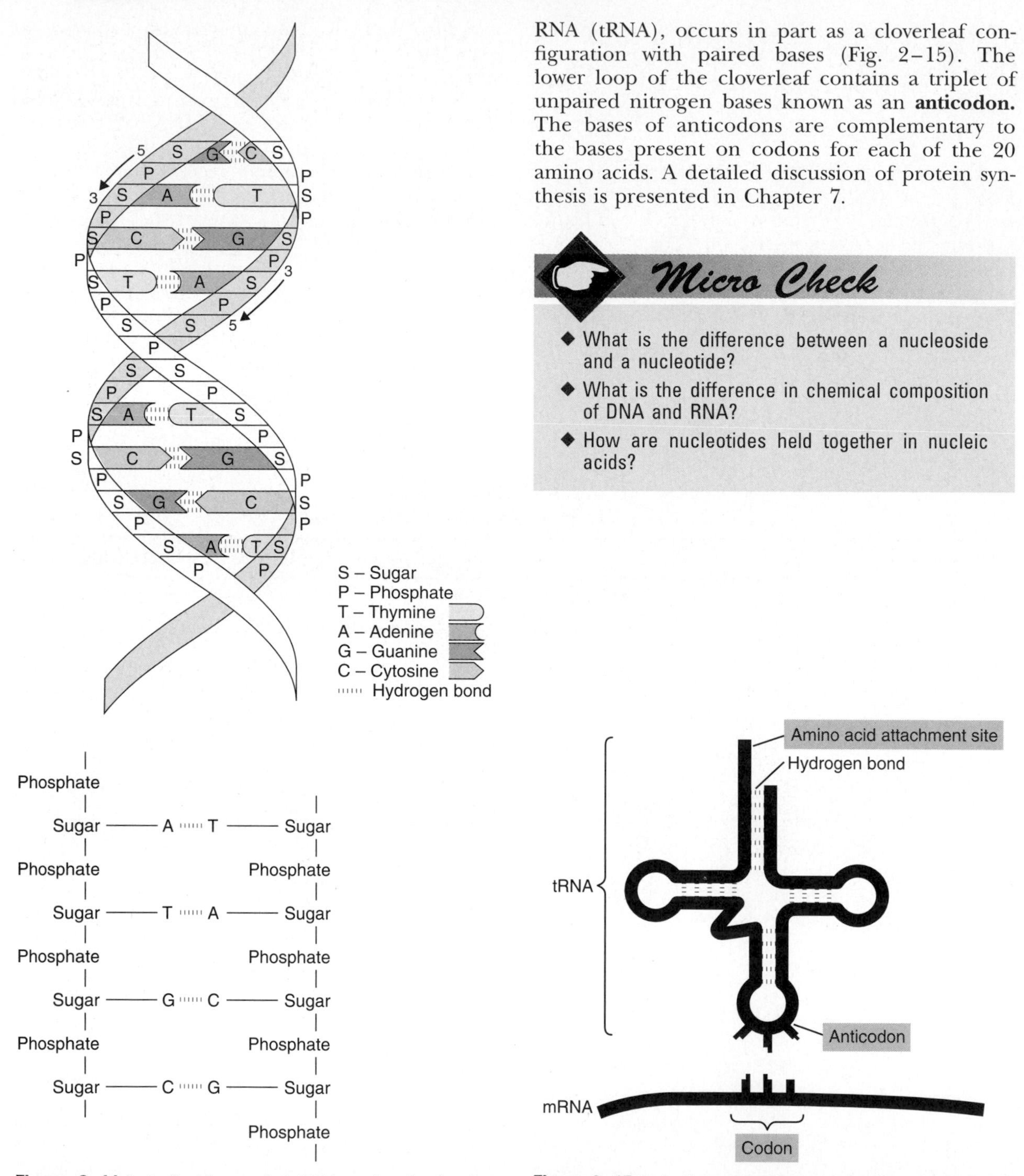

Figure 2–14 ◆ A double-stranded DNA molecule showing complementarity. Adenine (A) pairs with thymine (T) and cytosine (C) pairs with guanine (G).

Figure 2–15 ◆ A diagrammatic representation of one tRNA. The triplet of bases (anticodon) in the bottom loop is complementary to a triplet of bases (codon) on mRNA.

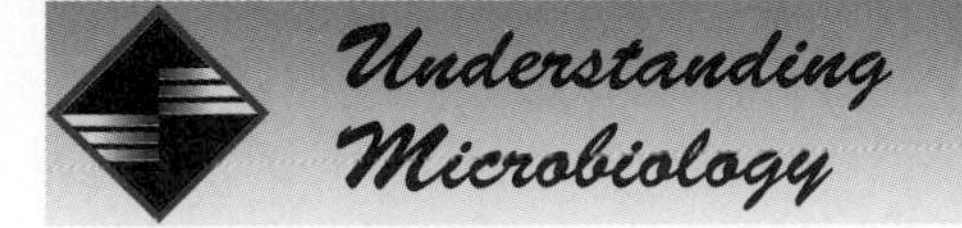

1. Why is air classified as a mixture rather than a compound?
2. How is the atomic number of an element determined?
3. How are molecular weights of compounds determined?
4. Name and describe three types of chemical bonds.
5. Why are proteins considered the determinants of diversity?

Applying Microbiology

6. If a segment of DNA contained the following triplets of bases, construct the mRNA with its appropriate codons and the complementary strand of tRNA with its appropriate anticodons.

TAC CAT TAG GAG CCC ATT

Chapter 3

Observation of Microorganisms

Chapter Outline

- **TYPES OF MICROSCOPES**
  - The Bright-Field Microscope
  - The Dark-Field Microscope
  - The Phase-Contrast Microscope
  - The Differential Interference Contrast Microscope
  - The Fluorescence Microscope
  - The Transmission Electron Microscope
  - The Scanning Electron Microscope
- **PREPARATION OF MATERIALS FOR BRIGHT-FIELD MICROSCOPIC EXAMINATION**
  - Wet and Hanging-Drop Wet Mounts
  - Fixed Stained Smears
  - Simple Stains
  - Differential Stains
  - Special Stains
  - Negative Stains

Learning Objectives

After you have read this chapter, you should be able to:

1. Describe seven types of microscopes and one specific use for each of them.
2. Differentiate between the magnifying and resolving power of a microscope.
3. Explain how the magnification of the light microscope is determined.
4. Compare the image obtained with a transmission electron microscope with that obtained with a scanning electron microscope.
5. Explain the need for a variety of staining techniques.

Microscopes have been used to study microorganisms since the seventeenth century, but microscopes were in existence for at least a half century before van Leeuwenhoek made his first one. Microscopes remain invaluable instruments and are found in every microbiology laboratory. Technological advances since the time of van Leeuwenhoek have provided us with a variety of microscopes and methods for examining microorganisms. The magnification of van Leeuwenhoek's microscope was only 300, but with today's electron microscopes, magnifications of 100,000 or greater make it possible to see minute details of microbial structure.

TYPES OF MICROSCOPES

Bright-field, dark-field, and phase-contrast microscopy use visible light as a source of illumination. Fluorescent microscopy employs ultraviolet radiation and special stains that cause microorganisms to glow. Electron microscopy uses electrons, directed by electromagnets under a vacuum, to obtain pictures on a screen or images that may be stored magnetically. Preparation of materials for electron microscopy is more complex and time consuming than methods required by other types of microscopy.

The choice of a microscope depends on the purpose for which it is to be used. Most microbiology laboratories have several types of microscopes, but the bright-field microscope is the most popular instrument for examination of stained smears of microorganisms. The phase-contrast microscope is used to observe detailed structures of living unstained microorganisms.

The Bright-Field Microscope

The first bright-field microscopes were single-lensed or **simple** microscopes. As primitive as simple microscopes seem to us today, these instruments did revolutionize thinking about the world in which we live. Simple microscopes introduced the concept of the cell as a basic structural unit and demonstrated phenomena such as brownian movement, cytoplasmic streaming, and phagocytosis. For the first time, it was possible to see and study a whole gamut of microorganisms not known to exist.

Most bright-field microscopes made today contain two sets of lenses for magnification and are, therefore, called **compound** microscopes (Fig. 3–1). The lens closer to the eye when viewing an object is called the **ocular lens;** the lens closer to the object being viewed is called the **objective lens.**

Magnification of a compound microscope is a product of the enlarging powers of the individual lenses. The ocular lens commonly has a magnifying power of 10, although lenses with a power of 5 or 15 are also used. The usual laboratory microscope has at least three objective lenses mounted on a revolving nosepiece so that they can be rotated according to need. The total magnification is determined by multiplying the power of the ocular lens by the power of the objective lens. The low-power objective lens has a magnifying power of 10, making a total magnification of 100× possible.

Magnifications of 400× or more are obtainable with high-power lenses of 40×. The lens of a third or oil-immersion objective usually magnifies 100 times; it requires a drop of immersion oil to be placed between the specimen and the objective lens. Oil is applied to increase the amount of light diffracted by the sample. If an image remains in view as the lenses are rotated into position, the microscope is **parfocal.**

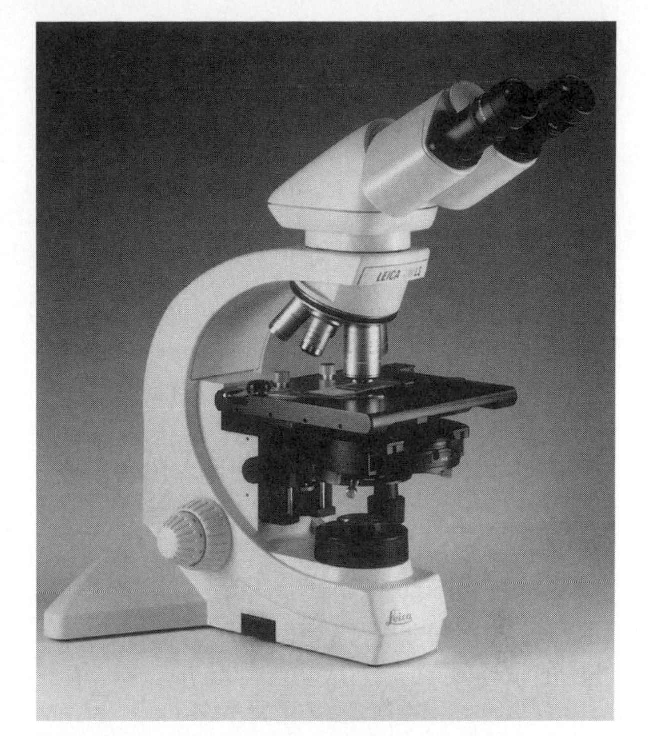

Figure 3–1 ◆ A binocular compound bright-field microscope.

The resolving power of a microscope is the minimal distance at which two points can be seen as separate objects. The resolving power of bright-field microscopes under oil is 0.2 μm. The factors limiting resolution are the wavelength of visible light and the aperture of the lens system. Wavelengths of visible light range from 400 to 700 nm. The shorter wavelengths produce better resolution. The numerical aperture (NA) is a mathematical expression of the light-gathering ability of a lens. It is derived from the refractive index of the lens and the angle of the cone of light entering the lens (Fig. 3–2). The focal length is the distance between the point at which light rays from an outside source converge and a focal point in the center of the lens.

The magnification, numerical aperture, and equivalent focal length of objective lenses are usually engraved on the sides of objectives (Fig. 3–3). The working distances are the amounts of space between the objective lenses and the slide needed to bring an object into sharp focus. Objectives containing lenses with numerical apertures of 0.5 or more generally need a substage condenser to concentrate the light rays. A shut-

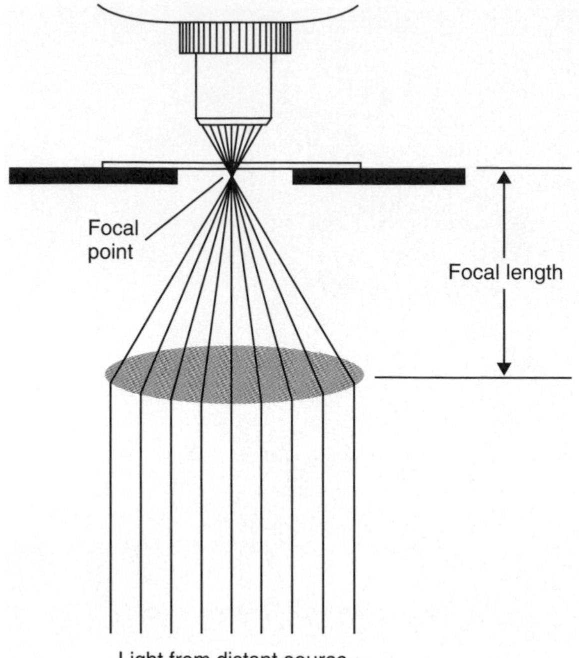

Figure 3–2 ◆ A beam of light is converged to a focal point from the center of a lens. The distance between the two is the focal length of an objective.

ter, known as an iris diaphragm, regulates the amount of light reaching the microscopic field. The depth of field or thickness of a specimen observable at one time decreases as the numerical aperture and magnification increase. The depth of field diminishes somewhat with lesser ability of an observer's eye to adjust for distance. With age the lens of the human eye gradually loses elasticity required for accommodation.

The size of a microscopic field diminishes as magnification is increased. Optical parameters for three common objectives are given in Table 3–1.

In general, the greater the power of the lens, the more light is required for detailed observations of an object under the microscope. Proper illumination is best obtained by a substage lamp and adjustment of the condenser and diaphragm to regulate the amount of light (Fig. 3–4).

For best visualization, an object should be placed in the center of the field. The coarse and fine adjustment knobs are used to obtain a sharp image. A good microscopist constantly adjusts both light and focal distance for optimal viewing. Careful interpretations based on bright-field microscopy take both time and patience as well as familiarity with a particular microscope.

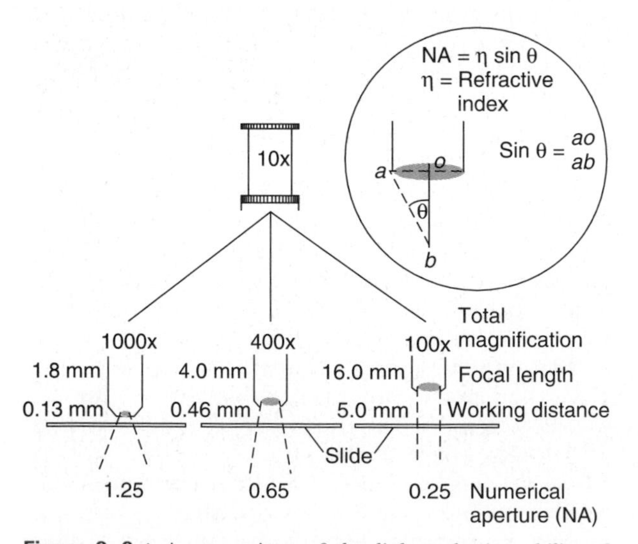

Figure 3–3 ◆ A comparison of the light-gathering ability of three objective lenses. The lens with the largest numerical aperture has the greatest ability to gather light.

The Dark-Field Microscope

A dark-field microscope has one or more special condensers that block out the central rays of light and cause the peripheral rays to hit the object from the side (Fig. 3–5). Under dark-field illumination microorganisms appear light against a black background. Some bright-field microscopes are constructed in such a way that the light-field condenser can easily be replaced by a dark-field condenser. Bacteria that are difficult to stain, such as spirochetes, are best seen with a dark-field microscope. The dark-field technique is frequently used to observe living spirochetes that cause syphilis or to visualize capsules of microorganisms (Fig. 3–6). Capsules are protective layers that surround the cell walls of some bacteria and yeasts. Because no special staining is necessary, there is little or no distortion in shape or size of

Table 3–1
OPTICAL PARAMETERS FOR COMMON OBJECTIVES

OBJECTIVE	DIAMETER OF FIELD	DEPTH OF FIELD	RESOLVING POWER
10×	1500 μm	7.0 μm	2.00 μm
40×	375 μm	1.3 μm	0.45 μm
100×	150 μm	0.5 μm	0.20 μm

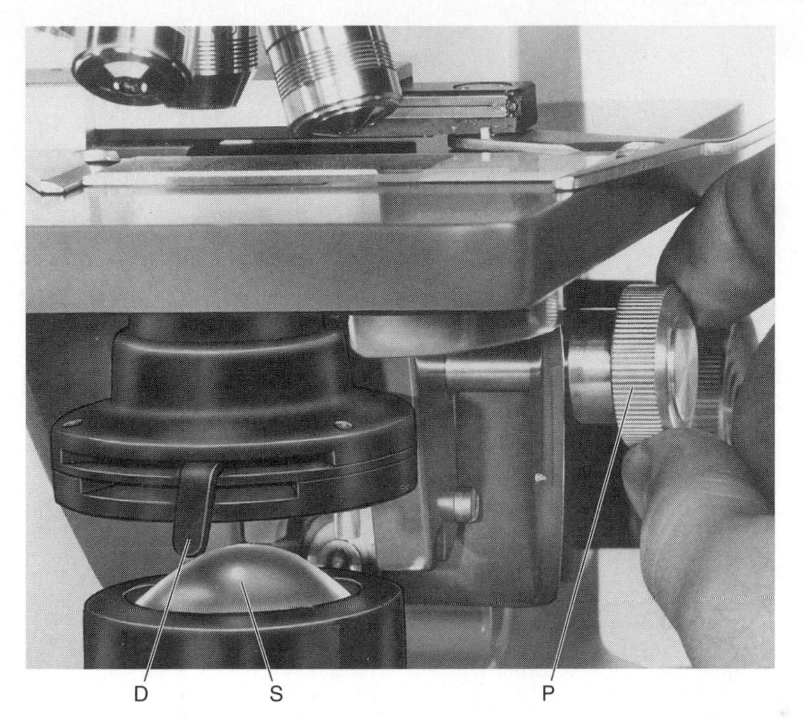

Figure 3–4 ◆ Mechanism for adjusting condenser and diaphragm to obtain proper illumination. S, substage lamp; D, diaphragm; P, pinion knob to raise and lower condenser.

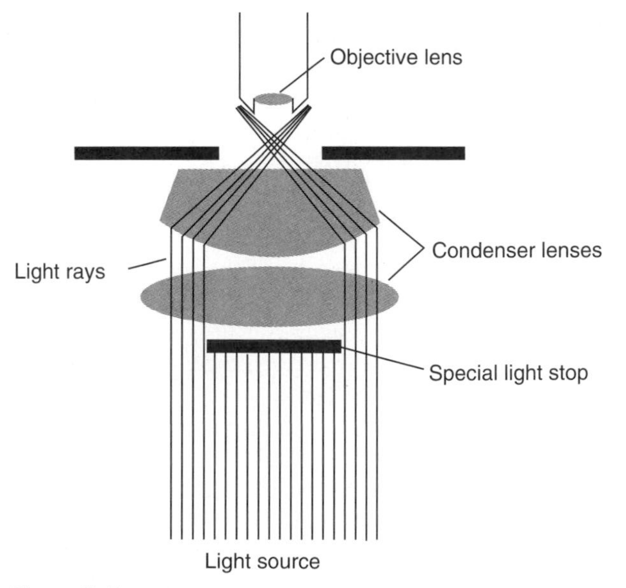

Figure 3–5 ◆ The dark-field microscope. A special condenser blocks central rays of light and directs peripheral rays to a focal point. The small portion of light reflected through the specimen causes objects to appear light against a black background.

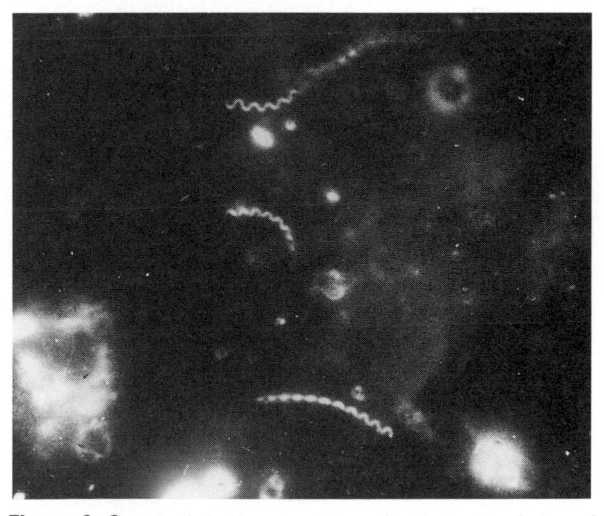

Figure 3–6 ◆ Dark-field preparation showing spirochetes of *Treponema pallidum* in scrapings from a chancre of a patient with syphilis.

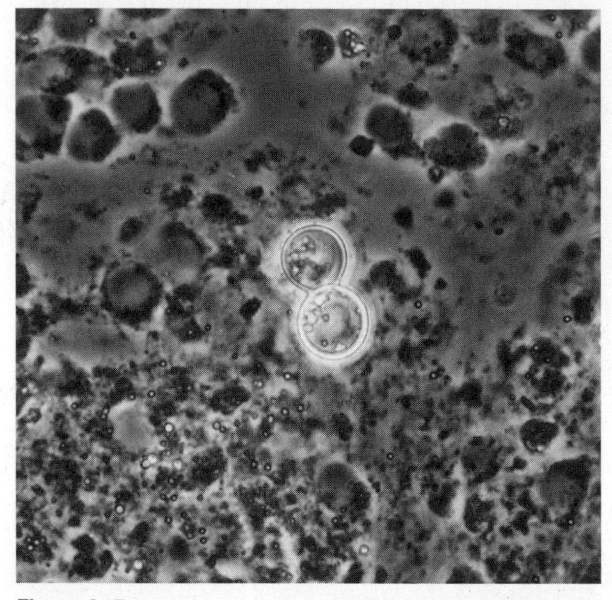

Figure 3–7 ◆ A phase-contrast micrograph of a budding cell of the yeast *Blastomyces dermatitidis*. The contrast between the background and the yeast cell is accomplished with a special condenser and a special objective.

microorganisms observed with a dark-field microscope.

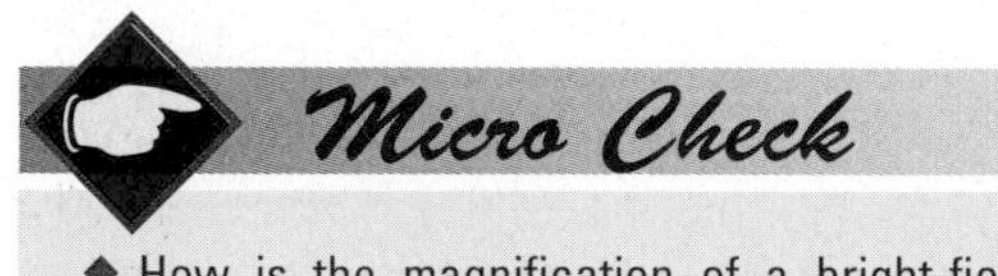

- ◆ How is the magnification of a bright-field microscope determined?
- ◆ Differentiate between magnification and resolving power of a microscope.
- ◆ For what purpose is dark-field microscopy used?

The Phase-Contrast Microscope

More detailed observation of living cells is possible with a phase-contrast microscope. The microscope contains a special condenser and a special lens objective assembly that accentuates differences in density of cell structures. Light waves are diverted so that structures with varying densities are out of phase with one another. When the light waves are recombined, alterations in the magnitude of light waves are seen as differences in light intensity (Fig. 3–7). No greater magnification or resolution is obtainable with phase-contrast microscopy, but the greater clarification of detail makes it an especially useful tool in studying intracellular structures of cells.

Phase-contrast microscopy is also valuable in demonstrating motility, cytoplasmic streaming, and the dynamic states of organelles. The application of cinema micrography and video microscopy to phase-contrast microscopic studies has recorded vividly such processes as mitosis, binary fission, budding, fragmentation, and phagocytosis.

The Differential Interference Contrast Microscope

The differential interference contrast (DIC) microscope contains a polarizing filter to split a light beam and a prism analyzer to recombine light refracted by a specimen. The microscope can be used to produce three-dimensional images and to accentuate phase-contrast differences of unstained cells (Fig. 3–8). The Nomarski interference contrast microscope has a resolution greater than the phase-contrast microscope, but

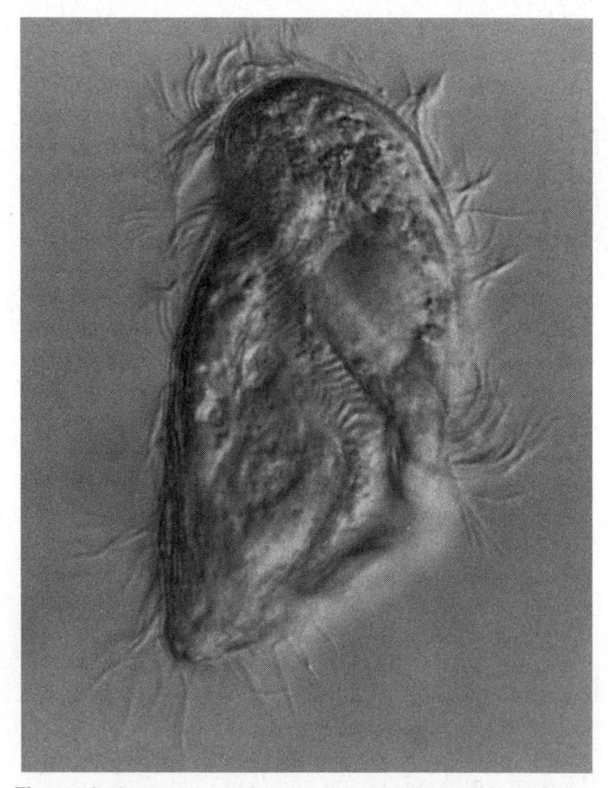

Figure 3–8 ◆ View of the protozoan *Metopus pulcher* with a differential interference contrast (DIC) microscope.

lesser depth of focus at a set point. The lesser focal depth makes it possible to observe sharply defined images.

The Fluorescence Microscope

Another type of microscope, important as a tool in the diagnosis of infectious diseases, is the fluorescence microscope. The use of fluorescence to accentuate objects is based on the principle that fluorescent materials emit a light of a different color when illuminated by ultraviolet radiation. A barrier filter allows only light that has been taken up by a specimen to be transmitted through the optical system. Fluorescence microscopy is employed to visualize objects which fluoresce naturally or those stained with fluorescent dyes such as fluorescein, auramine, or rhodamine B. Special filters limit the wavelength to that required for fluorescence.

There are many applications of fluorescent techniques in microbiology, including those employed for the identification of some bacteria, fungi, and viruses in clinical specimens. Fluorescent techniques are also used to identify specific **antibodies.** Antibodies are proteins produced by humans and some other animals in response to the presence of "nonself" substances on microorganisms. The "nonself" substances are called **antigens.** Antigens combine with specific antibodies to form complexes sometimes seen with difficulty under a bright-field microscope. If fluorescent dyes are attached to the protein molecules to produce **labeled antibodies,** the complexes are more easily identified under a fluorescent microscope.

The Transmission Electron Microscope

The most valuable tool of microbial cytologists and virologists is the transmission electron microscope (TEM) (Fig. 3–9). Transmission electron microscopy employs a stream of fast-moving electrons with a very short wavelength. Magnetic fields rather than optical lenses are used to focus electron beams and project an image on a fluorescent screen or film plate (Fig. 3–10). The picture captured on film is called an **electron micrograph.** Magnification 100 times greater than can be obtained with the bright-field microscope is possible. The resolving power of the TEM is 0.002 μm. If photographs are taken and enlarged, magnifications of 1 million or more can be obtained.

Drawbacks of the TEM are the expense of the equipment, elaborate and time-consuming procedures necessary to prepare specimens, and requirement of specially trained personnel for its operation.

Despite cumbersome procedures and the inability to examine living microorganisms, the TEM is needed for ultrastructural analysis of structures which are beyond the resolving power of light microscopes. Microbiologists are completely dependent on TEM for observing viruses.

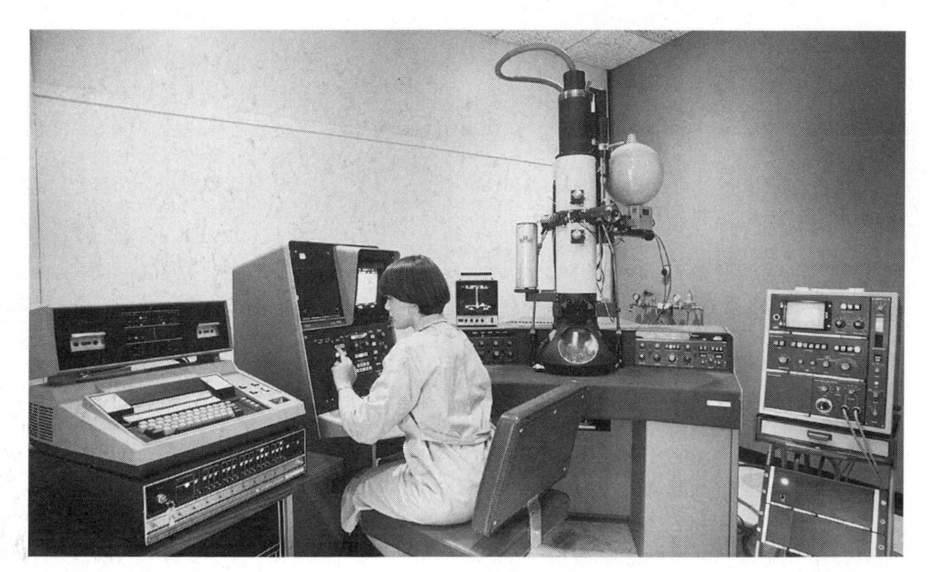

Figure 3–9 ◆ One of many electron microscopes available to cytologists and virologists.

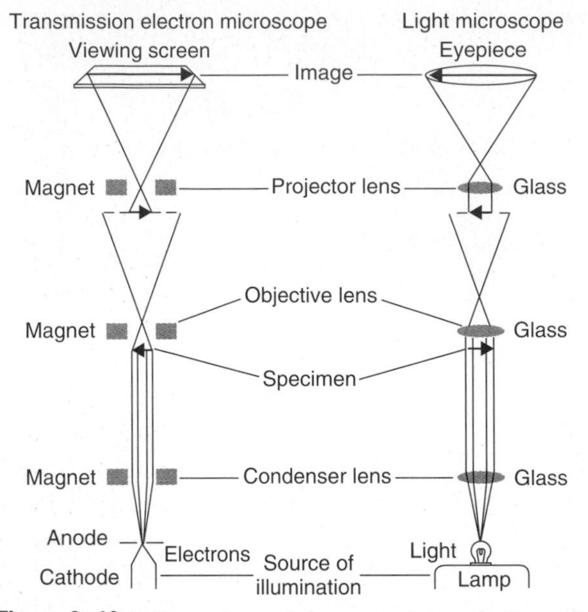

Figure 3–10 ◆ Comparison of the transmission electron microscope (TEM) and a light microscope.

Observation of morphological characteristics of viruses on electron micrographs has enabled virologists to classify the tiny particles according to size, shape, and symmetry (Fig. 3–11).

The freeze-etching technique may be used to prepare material for transmission electron microscopy. Cell specimens are frozen and thin sections are chipped off and coated with a fine layer of carbon. This technique has two major advantages over chemical fixation. First, it eliminates many changes in appearance produced by the fixation process. Second, it gives the images a new dimension; electron photomicrographs can reveal the topography or surface appearance of specimens (Fig. 3–12).

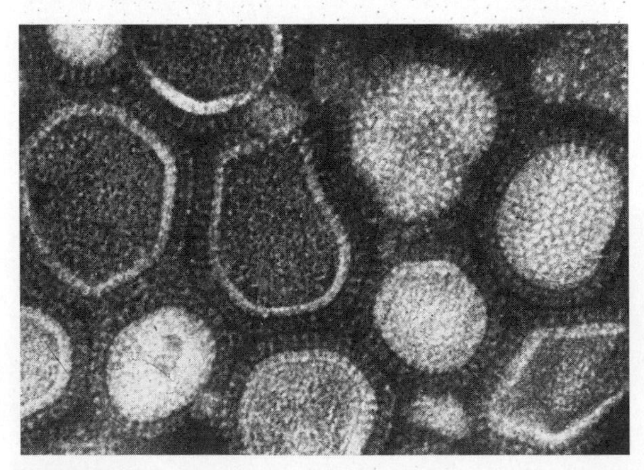

Figure 3–11 ◆ An electron micrograph of the influenza virus. The viral particles vary in size from 80 to 120 nm.

The Scanning Electron Microscope

A modification of electron microscopy is the scanning electron microscope (SEM), which provides three-dimensional images with limited resolution. The images show realistic contours of specimens rather than the two-dimensional representations of the conventional electron microscope (Fig. 3–13). The surface images obtained

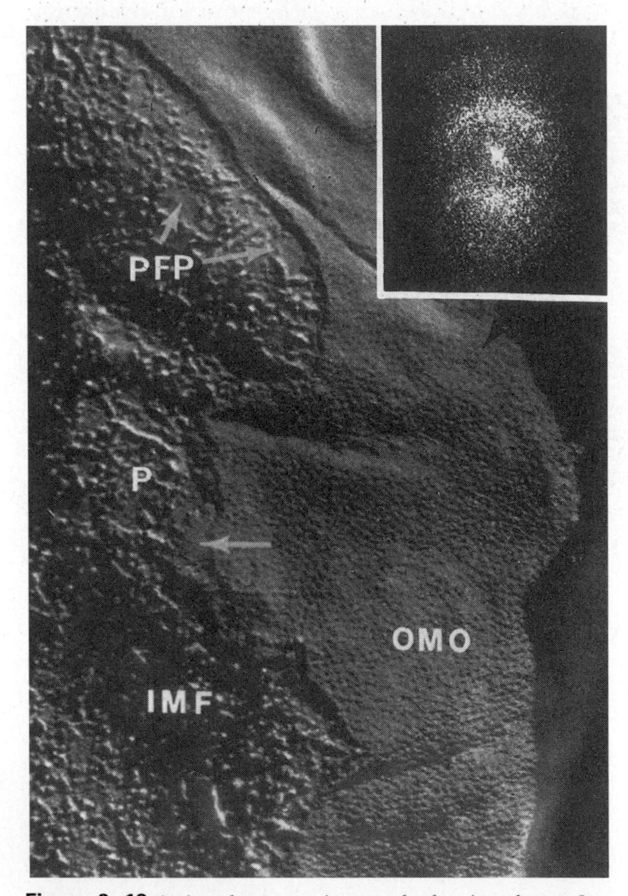

Figure 3–12 ◆ An electron micrograph showing the surface of the bacterium *Escherichia coli,* prepared by freeze-etching. A concave and a convex surface can be discerned. IMF, inner membrane fracture plane; OMO, outer face of outer membrane; P, particle within fracture plane; PFP, particle-free patches, as shown by arrows. The insert is a diffractogram of central pitted area showing a random arrangement of pits.

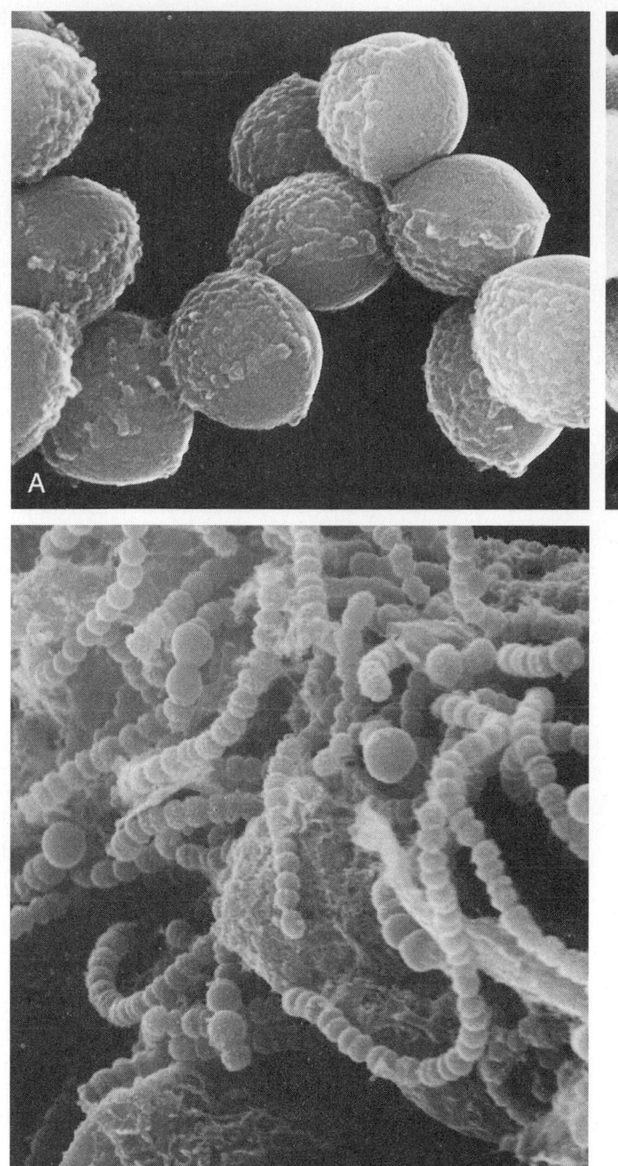

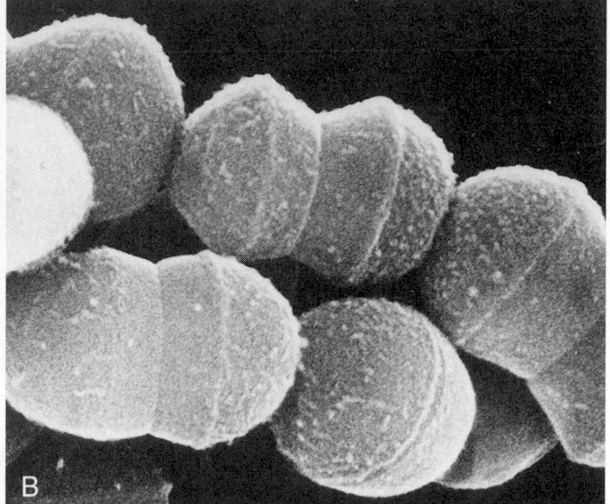

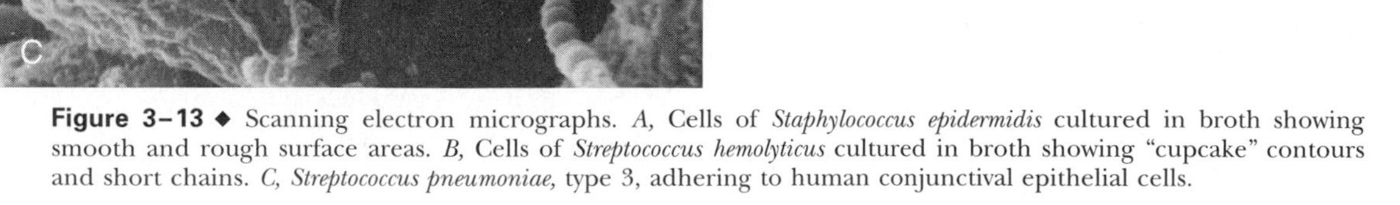
Figure 3–13 ◆ Scanning electron micrographs. *A,* Cells of *Staphylococcus epidermidis* cultured in broth showing smooth and rough surface areas. *B,* Cells of *Streptococcus hemolyticus* cultured in broth showing "cupcake" contours and short chains. *C, Streptococcus pneumoniae,* type 3, adhering to human conjunctival epithelial cells.

by SEM are startlingly realistic, but resolving power and magnification are much less than those of a TEM. The SEM has a resolving power of 0.01 to 0.02 μm and a magnification up to 100,000×.

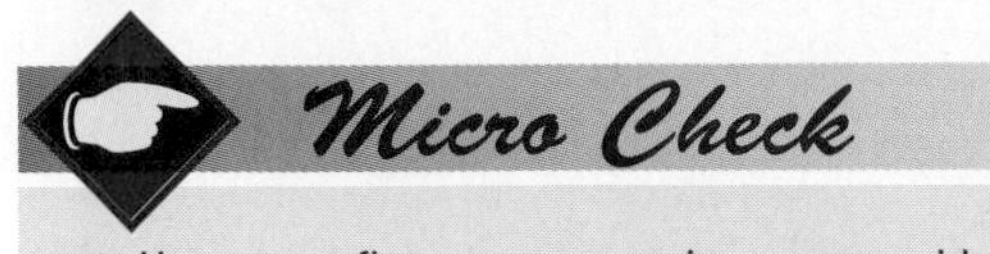

- How can fluorescence microscopy aid in the diagnosis of infectious diseases?
- What advantages does phase-contrast microscopy have over bright-field microscopy?
- How is an electron micrograph obtained?

Most of today's diagnostic laboratories are equipped with several types of light microscopes. The need for electron microscopes is usually limited to those laboratories engaging in basic research on viruses or ultrastructure of other microorganisms. The primary uses of the various types of microscopes are summarized in Table 3–2. Whatever microscope is used, there is no substitute for the knowledge and skills of a microbiologist in unraveling the mysteries revealed by microscopy.

PREPARATION OF MATERIALS FOR BRIGHT-FIELD MICROSCOPIC EXAMINATION

The preparation of materials for microscopic examination varies with the type of microscope and the type of specimen. Specimens to be examined may be living microorganisms suspended in a liquid, but more often are dead microorganisms to which chemical fixatives and stains have been applied. Only fixed and dried specimens can be examined with an electron microscope because life is not compatible with the vacuum required to prevent scattering of the electron beam. Because the bright-field microscope remains the basic tool of most microbiology laboratories, only methods used to prepare materials for examination with that microscope are presented.

Wet And Hanging-Drop Wet Mounts

A simple wet mount of a microbial suspension can be used to study living microorganisms. It is made by putting a drop of the suspension on a clean glass slide and placing a coverslip over the material (Fig. 3–14). Low power is frequently ad-

Table 3–2
COMPARISON OF TYPES OF MICROSCOPES

TYPE	USUAL MAGNIFICATION	RESOLVING POWER	PRIMARY USE
Bright-field	1000×	0.2 μm	Examination of stained and unstained microorganisms
Dark-field	1000×	0.2 μm	Visualization of organisms or structures that stain with difficulty
Fluorescence	1000×	0.2 μm	Demonstration of microorganisms and antibodies in diagnostic procedures
Phase contrast	1000×	0.2 μm	Demonstration of living microorganisms or their activities
Differential interference	1000×	0.2 μm	Visualization of organisms in three dimensions
Transmission electron	500,000 to 1,000,000×	0.002 μm	Visualization of viruses and ultrastructure of microorganisms
Scanning electron	10,000 to 100,000×	0.01 to 0.02 μm	Production of three-dimensional images and examination of details of surface structures of microorganisms

FOCAL POINT

Robot Microscopes to the Rescue

Final diagnosis of many diseases often requires laborious hours of scanning microscopic slides looking for microorganisms, stages of multicellular parasites, or cancer cells. Sometimes a second opinion is sought from another microbiologist or pathologist who is not necessarily on the premises. Valuable time is spent sending slides or tissue samples to other experts. Now the development of robotically controlled microscopes may make shuttling of specimens unnecessary. Corabi Telemetrics, located in Alexandria, VA, employs the robot microscope, computers, custom software, and high definition television (HDTV) cameras, and monitors to transmit images on fiberoptic cables. Recipients use keypads to focus and to control illumination for projection on a high-resolution screen. Nikon built the computer-controlled microscope for Corabi. After two years of testing, the elaborate system was first installed in 1990 at Emory University Hospital and at Grady Memorial Hospital in Atlanta, Ga. Future installation will allow a unique networking of hospitals in remote geographic areas. Corabi has not been the first to commercialize "telemedicine." A precedent was made a few years earlier in radiology. However, the technological requirements to produce accurate colors, high resolution, and flexibility of both magnification and illumination were quite different for microscopy. The implications of computer-controlled microscopes are far reaching. Interactive networks employing the new technology will be able to diagnose diseases and provide a basis for appropriate treatment faster than ever before. As an educational tool, robot microscopes would permit large numbers of students to observe the same fields without the time-consuming, often frustrating, experience of individual searching and focusing on appropriate fields for study. The partnership between microscopes and computers appears destined for success of the most extraordinary kind with potential benefits for us all.

equate to observe the general form and structure of larger organisms. High power will reveal additional details. Small bacteria are often difficult to see, and reduced illumination or contrast microscopy may be required.

Although motility may be discernible on a simple wet mount, a hanging-drop wet mount is often more reliable. To prepare this mount, a small quantity of petroleum jelly is applied to the corners of one surface of a cover slip. A drop of liquid is placed on the cover slip and a special slide, with a depression, is inverted and positioned so that the petroleum jelly touches and adheres to the slide. The slide is carefully turned right side up so that the drop of liquid is suspended from the cover slip into the depression. (Fig. 3–15). The specimen is viewed under the high-power or oil-immersion objective.

True motility must be differentiated from **brownian movement,** a type of movement exhibited by both living and nonliving small particles in aqueous suspensions. Brownian movement is caused by forces created by bombardment of water molecules. A particle exhibiting brownian movement moves in a haphazard fashion. A motile bacterium progresses in a definite direction

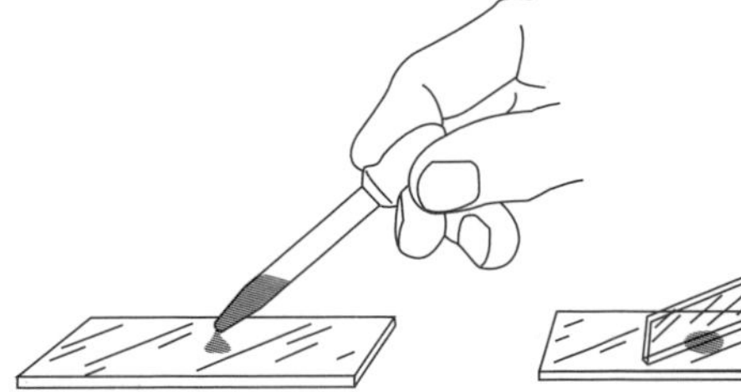
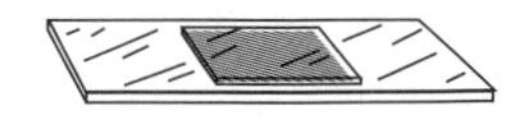

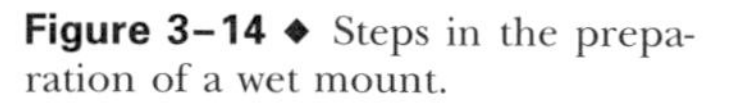
Figure 3–14 ◆ Steps in the preparation of a wet mount.

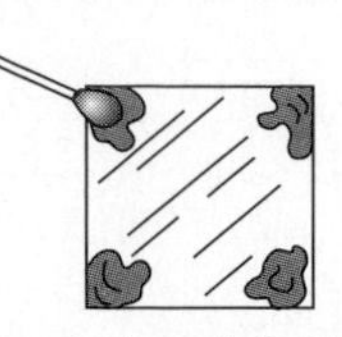

(1) Apply petroleum jelly to the corners of one surface of a cover slip.

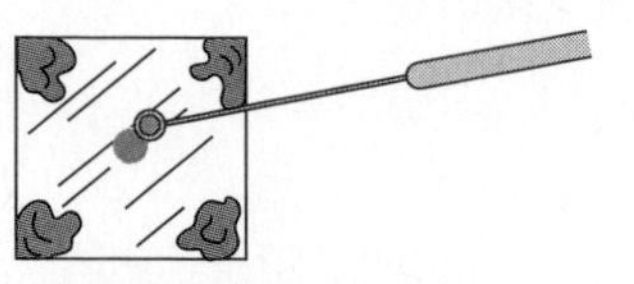

(2) Place a loopful of culture material on the center of the cover slip.

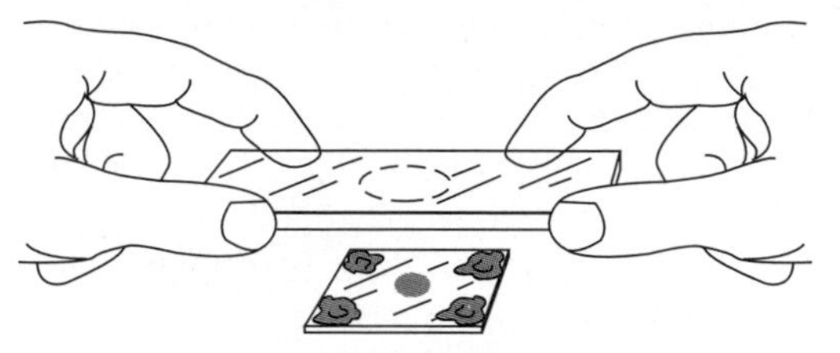

(3) Invert the hanging-drop slide so the depression is over the drop and lower it until it touches the cover slip.

Cover glass

Petroleum jelly

Hanging drop

(4) Invert the hanging-drop slide.

Figure 3–15 ◆ Steps in the preparation of a hanging-drop wet mount.

and may often be observed turning end-to-end as well.

Microscopic examination is a time-consuming method for detecting motility on the large numbers of bacterial isolates in diagnostic laboratories. A cultural method, which employs a semisolid medium, is a reliable alternative for demonstrating motility.

Fixed Stained Smears

Materials that have been dried on glass slides are most useful for detecting the presence of microorganisms or for studying their sizes and shapes. The preparations are called **smears.** The dried smears are **fixed** or fastened to the slide by treatment with chemicals or heat before staining. Unstained bacteria are difficult to distinguish from their surroundings. Staining provides the means for obtaining contrast between bacteria and background material.

Solutions of a number of organic dyes may be applied for staining smears. An organic dye is classified chemically as a salt because it contains positively and negatively charged ions. A **basic dye** contains the staining component in the positive (cationic) portion of the molecule; an **acidic dye** has the staining component associated with the negative (anionic) portion of the molecule. Some stains are called polychromatic because they produce a variety of colors.

Bacteria have an affinity for basic aniline dyes, such as crystal violet, safranin, and methylene blue, because of the negative charges on cell walls. Acidic dyes, such as acid fuchsin, eosin, and nigrosin, are repelled by the negative charges of bacteria. Polychromatic stains are valuable for staining blood, tissue, and fecal smears or any materials suspected of containing eucaryotic cells. Negative charges of nucleic acid are confined to nuclei which take up basic components of dyes. The basic charges of the eucaryotic cytoplasm have an affinity for acid stains. The contrast, provided by mixtures of dyes in polychromatic stains, makes it possible to differentiate the types of eucaryotic cells from one another. Such differentiation can be very important in mixed infections and for observing white blood cells in peripheral blood.

Rarely can bacteria be identified by microscopic examination alone for there are too many "look-alikes." However, careful examination of stained smears can provide information on staining characteristics, shape, size, and groupings of bacteria. Microorganisms must be differentiated from other cells and debris on smears prepared from specimens obtained from infected individuals.

The fact that microorganisms cannot be seen upon microscopic examination of a smear does not necessarily mean that no organisms are present. The organisms may not be present in sufficient numbers to be observable in the limited sampling of the specimen placed on the slide. For this reason, cultures are more reliable for detecting the presence of infectious agents. When culturing is not feasible, multiple smears should be prepared from repeated samplings of specimens.

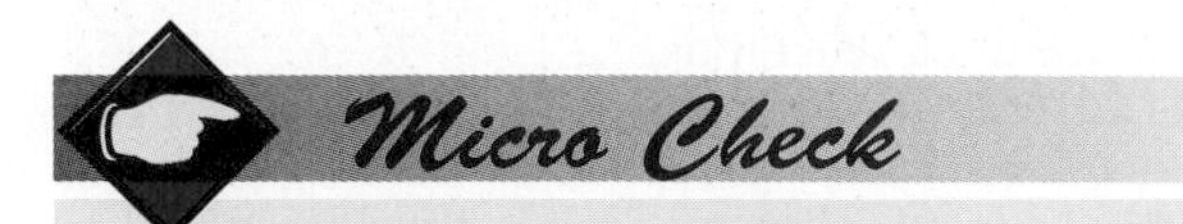

- What is brownian movement?
- Why do bacteria stain with basic dyes?
- Why is microscopic examination insufficient to identify bacteria?
- Why are cultures more reliable than microscopic examinations in establishing the presence of an infection?

Simple Stains

Simple staining is the application of a single stain to a fixed smear. Methylene blue, crystal violet, safranin, or another stain is allowed to react with bacteria on a heat-fixed smear for 30 to 60 seconds. The smear is then washed with water and blotted dry.

The simple-stain technique will allow the shape, size, and groupings of bacteria to be discerned using the oil-immersion objective. Sometimes the presence of inclusions or resistant stages, known as endospores, can also be detected. Most inclusions have a greater affinity for basic dyes than the surrounding protoplasm and stain darker than the rest of the cell. Endospores do not take up dyes readily and appear colorless unless special procedures are used for staining.

FOCAL POINT

A Giant Among Microbial Dwarfs

UNITS OF LENGTH

Kilometer	km	1000 m	10^3 m
Meter	m	m	m
Decimeter	dm	0.1 m	10^{-1} m
Centimeter	cm	0.01 m	10^{-2} m
Millimeter	mm	0.001 m	10^{-3} m
Micrometer	μm	0.000001 m	10^{-6} m
Nanometer	nm	0.000000001 m	10^{-9} m
Angstrom	Å	0.0000000001 m	10^{-10} m

Microorganisms are usually measured in microscopic units known as micrometers (μm) or nanometers (nm). For example, the bacterium that causes tuberculosis is only 0.5 to 4.0 μm in length. The virus that causes AIDS measures a mere 100 nm in diameter. Some ciliated protozoa may attain lengths up to 180 μm. One bacterium, *Epulopiscium fishelsoni,* has gained fame as a giant microorganism because of its size. The organism, found in the intestines of the surgeonfish, is about 1 million times larger than its bacterial relatives and appears to be related to members of the genus *Clostridium* (klos-TREH-dee-um) on the basis of rRNA sequences of nucleotides. Some of the giant-sized bacteria grow to be longer than 0.5 mm, making them visible to the naked eye. The clostridia are gram-positive spore-forming bacilli found in soil and intestinal tracts of humans and animals. It is not known if there are other giant bacteria in undiscovered habitats. The discovery of such huge microorganisms, which resemble bacteria in every other way except size, provides us with additional evidence for the continuum of life forms.

From ASM News 59(10):519, 1993.

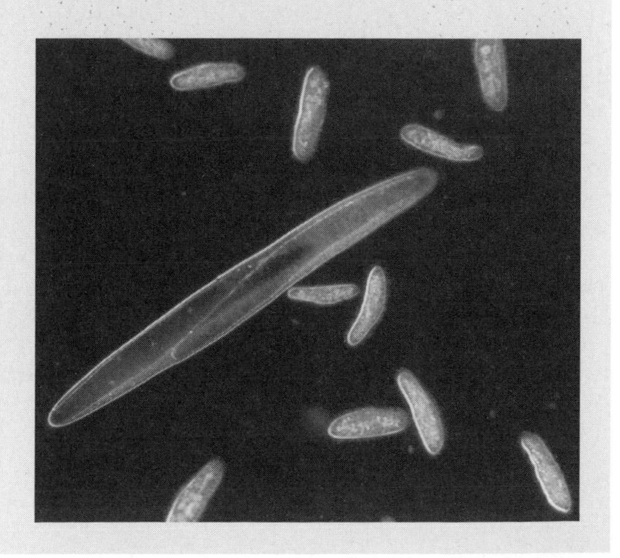

Table 3–3
THE GRAM STAIN PROCEDURE

1. Cover the smear with crystal violet for one minute and rinse in tap water.
2. Cover the smear with Gram's iodine for one minute and rinse in tap water.
3. Decolorize by adding 95 percent ethyl alcohol drop by drop to the slide in a tilted position until the primary stain fails to wash from the smear, but *no longer*. Rinse in tap water.
4. Cover the smear with safranin for 30 seconds. Wash in tap water and blot dry.

Differential Stains

Differential staining is the application of more than one stain to a fixed smear. The procedure is used to demonstrate different staining characteristics of cells. A number of differential staining techniques are used in microbiology, but the most widely used is the Gram stain (Table 3–3).

GRAM STAIN

Hans Christian Gram, a Danish bacteriologist, developed a four-step staining process for separating bacteria into two groups in 1884. Gram staining requires the sequential use of a crystal violet dye, an iodine solution, an alcohol solution, and a safranin dye.

Crystal violet is allowed to react with bacteria on a heat-fixed smear for one minute, and then the smear is rinsed in tap water. Gram's iodine, a mordant, is applied and allowed to react for an additional minute before the smear is rinsed in tap water. A **mordant** is a chemical used to promote or fix the staining reaction. Gram's iodine reacts specifically with the crystal violet to form intracellular complexes. At this point in the procedure all bacteria are stained purple (Fig. 3–16). The smear is next subjected to decolorization by applying a mixture of acetone and ethyl alcohol or 95 percent ethyl alcohol, drop by drop, until the primary stain of crystal violet fails to wash from the smear. The smear is rinsed once again in tap water. In the final step the smear is flooded with a counterstain of safranin for 30 seconds before rinsing in tap water for the last time.

The most critical step in successful Gram staining is the decolorizing procedure. Bacteria retaining the primary stain of crystal violet are designated as **gram-positive;** bacteria taking on the red color of the counterstain safranin are described as **gram-negative.**

The Gram reaction is not an all-or-none phenomenon. The crystal violet–iodine complex forms in both types of cells, but application of the decolorizer alters the permeability of cell walls. Variation in retention of the dye-iodine complex has been attributed to differences in physical and chemical structures of cell walls. The thicker walls of gram-positive cells are dehydrated by the application of the decolorizer, causing pores to diminish in size. The thin-walled gram-negative bacteria have outer membranes of lipopolysaccharide which surround the cell walls (see Chapter 4). The outer membranes are destroyed by alcohol-treatment, and the walls are

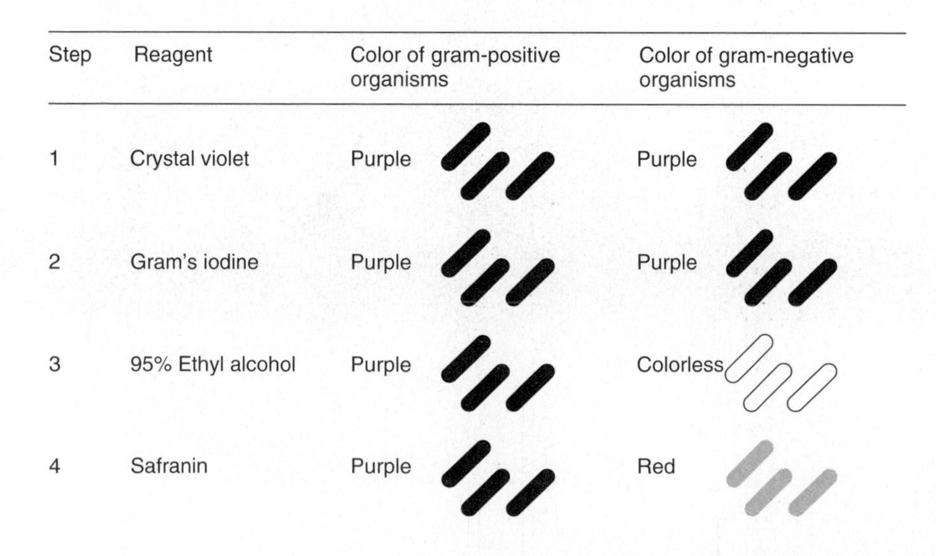

Figure 3–16 ◆ A comparison of gram-positive and gram-negative bacteria during steps of Gram staining.

Table 3–4
THE ZIEHL-NEELSEN ACID-FAST STAIN PROCEDURE

1. Cover the smear with basic carbolfuchsin and heat slowly to the steaming point.
2. Steam gently for 5 to 10 minutes replacing stain as necessary.
3. Allow slide to cool and wash in tap water.
4. Decolorize by adding acid alcohol drop by drop to the slide in a tilted position until the primary stain fails to wash from the smear. Wash in tap water.
5. Cover the smear with methylene blue for 30 seconds. Wash in tap water and blot dry.

too thin to retain crystal violet–iodine complexes. The counterstain of safranin must be applied to the decolorized cells so they can be seen and differentiated from the purple cells.

Gram stains performed on young cultures are the most reliable. Some gram-positive bacteria lose their ability to retain the crystal violet–iodine precipitate with age. Gram-positive bacteria from old cultures may appear red or purple. Some bacteria demonstrate variability in Gram staining. Nevertheless, the Gram stain technique has no parallel for dividing bacteria into two major groups. The implications of differences in staining go beyond mere differences in the physical and chemical characteristics of cell walls, however. The Gram reactivity is of significance in the choice of other procedures needed for identification of bacterial species. Furthermore, a physician can sometimes make a presumptive diagnosis on the basis of a Gram stain and begin appropriate antimicrobial therapy.

ACID-FAST STAIN

Another differential staining technique is the **acid-fast stain,** which is employed primarily in the diagnosis of tuberculosis, nocardiosis, bacterial diseases, and a protozoan disease known as cryptosporidiosis. Acid-fast bacilli can be demonstrated in sputum or gastric washings of individuals having tuberculosis. Acid-fast developmental stages of protozoan oocysts are found in stool specimens of persons having cryptosporidiosis, an infection commonly found in AIDS patients.

In the acid-fast staining procedures, basic carbolfuchsin is used as the primary stain; methylene blue is employed for counterstaining (Table 3–4). Acid alcohol is used as a decolorizer. It contains 3 percent hydrochloric acid (HCl) in 95 percent ethyl alcohol and is a much more potent decolorizer than that used in the Gram stain technique. Acid-fast bacteria appear red against a blue background. The organisms are called **acid-fast** because they retain the primary stain despite decolorization with acid alcohol. Other bacteria or background material take up the counterstain.

The Ziehl-Neelsen acid-fast staining procedure requires heat to permit basic carbolfuchsin to permeate the walls of bacterial cells or developmental stages of cryptosporidia. The decolorizer and counterstain are applied to cooled cells. The Kinyoun acid-fast staining technique is an alternative procedure that does not require heat. The lipid-rich walls of acid-fast organisms make them resistant not only to dyes, but also to the action of some antimicrobial agents and disinfectants.

OTHER DIFFERENTIAL STAINS

A number of differential staining techniques are also used for the demonstration of protozoa and fungi. Many protozoan staining procedures employ mixtures of dyes. With the trichrome staining procedure, it is possible to obtain several colors for differentiation of cell types and structures. The cytoplasm of cysts and trophozoites appears blue-green with tinges of purple, whereas nuclei and bacteria stain red.

Wright's or Giemsa's stain is used to examine some spirochetes, intracellular bacteria, and some infective forms of protozoa. Both stains are compound stains containing eosin and methylene blue. The most important blood organisms detected by these stains are the protozoa causing malaria (Fig. 3–17).

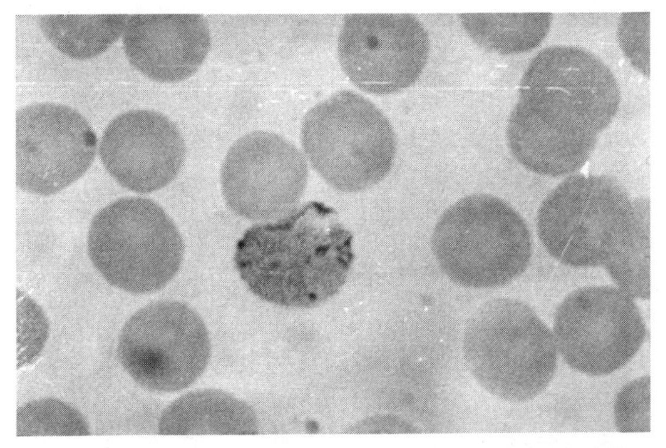

Figure 3–17 ◆ A Giemsa-stained blood smear showing Schüffner's granules of a malarial parasite in a red blood cell.

Special Stains

Special staining techniques are used to demonstrate flagella, capsules, and endospores of bacteria. Flagella are threadlike appendages of locomotion found on some bacteria. Their diameter is beyond the resolution of light microscopes. Flagella must be coated with tannic acid and basic fuchsin to increase their diameters sufficiently to make them visible. The location and numbers of flagella on motile bacteria are crucial to the identification of some organisms.

Some bacteria and yeasts contain protective layers known as capsules which surround cells. Capsules do not stain well with most stains. Although they can sometimes be seen as clear halos around the cells, their presence can often be detected more easily if smears, stained with crystal violet, are rinsed with 20 percent aqueous copper sulfate. Capsules appear as blue halos surrounding purple cells.

Certain bacteria form stages, known as endospores, during their life cycles. Endospores are spherical or oval structures which may be seen within cells or as free entities. They resist staining so are seen as clear spaces on Gram stains. Endospores will stain, however, if a 5 percent aqueous solution of malachite green, a weak basic dye, and heat are applied to smears. Rinsing in water removes malachite green from other portions of cells. A counterstain with safranin makes it easy to distinguish endospores from the rest of the cells.

More than one special stain may be necessary to demonstrate fungi in tissue. Nonviable fungi do not stain readily and may be difficult to distinguish from other tissue elements. A silver nitrate stain is preferred for screening purposes. Fungi

FOCAL POINT

A New Generation of Microscopes

A new generation of microscopes has revived the hope of one day visualizing DNA and other smaller molecules in atomic dimension. A scanning-probe instrument, such as the scanning tunneling microscope (STM), makes it possible to examine naked DNA without heavy metal coatings. The instrument contains a needlelike probe that is scanned back and forth over a specimen within a few angstroms of the surface. Vertical movement of the probe is monitored and adjusted to maintain either a constant signal or a constant distance from the surface. By plotting vertical versus translational movement in a series of scans a detailed three-dimensional map of surface properties can be constructed. Not surprisingly, DNA was one of the first specimens to be examined. Other molecules that have been examined include RNA, phosphorylase kinase, catalase, and ferritin. Reliable measurements of helical pitch, half-pitch, groove width, and center-to-center packing distance have been obtained by STM. Even small molecules, such as carbon monoxide and benzene, can be imaged by STM. Progress is being made in imaging proteins and protein–nucleic acid complexes. It is hoped that STM will ultimately supply answers to some very old problems. Although individual double-ring structures of adenine and atoms of phosphate can be visualized, the pathway of electron transport through DNA has not been determined. The STM has already given us a much closer look at nucleic acids and proteins than methods used previously. No doubt other secrets of nature, long shrouded in shadows or by stains, remain to be discovered by STM.

ASM News, 56(3):136, 1990

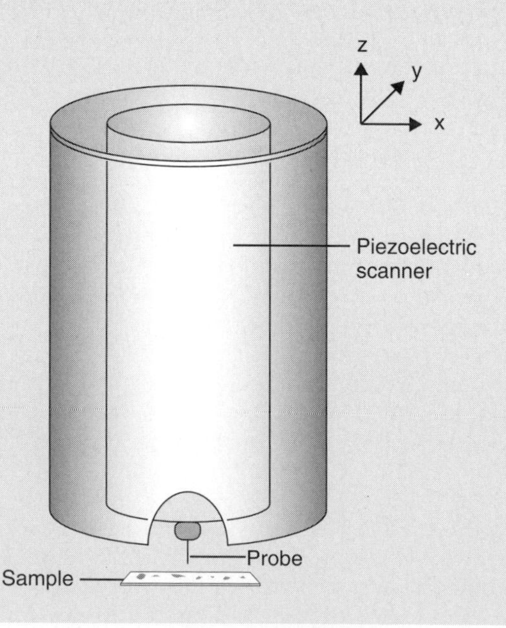

impregnated with silver nitrate appear black-brown against a yellow background.

Negative Stains

The application of acidic stains, such as India ink or nigrosin, to microorganisms produces a dark background against which unstained bacteria can be observed. The cells do not stain because the negatively charged dyes are repelled by the negatively charged bacteria. The appearance of the organisms is somewhat analogous to their appearance in dark-field microscopy. Little distortion of microorganisms occurs with negative stains since no fixing is required. Furthermore, only a bright-field microscope is required. Negative staining techniques are particularly valuable for demonstrating some spirochetes and capsules of some bacteria and yeasts. Capsules appear as clear halos surrounding cells. Flagella, capsules, and endospores are described in greater detail in Chapter 4.

Micro Check

- What is the role of the cell wall as a determinant of Gram reactivity?
- For what purposes is the acid-fast stain used?
- Why is it necessary to employ different staining techniques for eucaryotic cells than for procaryotic cells?

Understanding Microbiology

1. Why is proper illumination so important in making accurate microscopic observations?
2. What is meant by the term parfocal in referring to a microscope?
3. What factors account for Gram reactivity of bacteria?
4. What is the most critical step in the Gram stain?
5. Name two advantages associated with the use of negative stains.

Applying Microbiology

6. If one student obtained gram-negative bacilli and another obtained gram-positive bacilli from the same culture, how can you explain the results?

Chapter 4

Structure of Microbial Cells

Chapter Outline

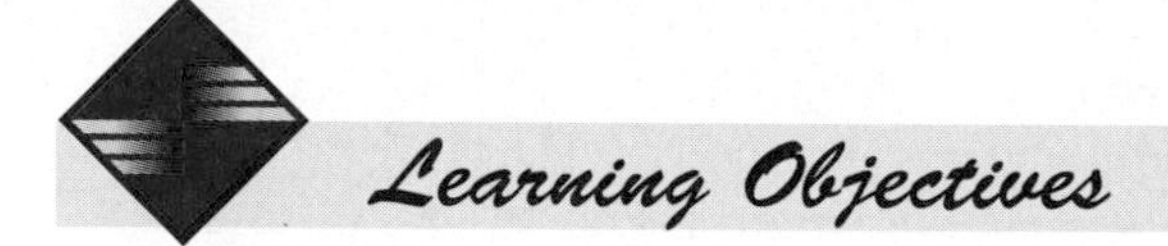

Learning Objectives

After you have read this chapter, you should be able to:

1. Describe the major differences between procaryotes and eucaryotes.
2. Differentiate between the cell walls of gram-positive and gram-negative bacteria.
3. Describe the significance of the outer membrane of gram-negative bacteria.
4. Explain passive and active transport of molecules across plasma membranes.
5. Explain the significance of bacterial endospores.
6. List the membranous organelles of eucaryotes.

Biological cells look somewhat like the small rooms for which they were named by Robert Hooke in 1665. Hooke, a curator of instruments for the Royal Society of London, looked at thin pieces of cork through a microscope. The barren compartments resembled the cells that monks occupied in the monasteries of that time. Hooke was the first to use the term "cells" to describe these microscopic units. We now know that cells are far from the barren compartments that Hooke saw through a primitive microscope.

It soon became apparent that there were differences between plant and animal cells. Viewing those differences and those of the single-celled microorganisms continues to fascinate students today. At first, bacteria did not seem to fit early descriptions of the cell because no nucleus was observed in the unicellular organisms. Later it was discovered that nuclear material did exist in bacteria but that it was not bounded by a membrane. The bacteria are the smallest life forms that can exist as independent organisms.

Today's microscopes allow us to see structures of cells in great detail. Success in combating infections is based on knowledge obtained from examining the chemistry and architectural design of microbial cells. Searches for mechanisms of pathogenesis (ability to cause disease), identifica-

Table 4–1
COMPARISON OF PROCARYOTIC AND EUCARYOTIC CELLS

CHARACTERISTIC	PROCARYOTES	EUCARYOTES
Size	0.2–60.0 μm	5–100 μm
Nuclear membrane	None	Present
Chromosome	One	Multiple
Cytoplasmic streaming	Not detectable	Detectable
Sterols in cytoplasmic membrane	Usually absent	Present
Internal membranes	Absent or simple	Complex
Membranous organelles	Absent	Abundant
Site of photosynthesis	Membrane	Chloroplast
Site of respiration	Membrane	Mitochondria
Mode of reproduction	Asexual	Asexual and sexual
Mitotic apparatus	None	Microtubular spindles
Ribosomes	70S particles	80S particles
Appendages	Flagella, pili, and prosthecae	Flagella and cilia

tion procedures, effective treatments, and preventive measures all require detailed information about cell structure and function.

Cellular microorganisms are divided into **procaryotes** and **eucaryotes** based on their patterns of organization. Table 4–1 summarizes the major differences between procaryotes and eucaryotes.

PROCARYOTES

Procaryotes can be distinguished from eucaryotes by the lack of membrane-bound organelles (Fig. 4–1). The nuclei of eucaryotic cells are readily observable as dense, dark-staining structures under a bright-field microscope. Detailed structure of both the cytoplasm and the nucleus can be seen with an electron microscope. A few bacteria are so small that they are difficult to see under a bright-field microscope. Other bacteria, the mycoplasmas, are smaller than some viruses and can be observed only with an electron microscope.

Shapes, Sizes, and Arrangements of Procaryotic Cells

Bacteria vary in shape, size, and arrangements of cells. Most bacteria may be classified according to shape as (1) rod-shaped (**bacilli**), (2) spherical

FOCAL POINT

The Mighty Midgets of The Planet Earth

Bacteria are able to carry out all activities necessary to sustain life despite their small size. Like eucaryotic cells of microorganisms and multicellular organisms, these small cells must take in nutrients from the environment and dispel waste products. The rate at which these materials pass in and out of cells is inversely proportional to cell size. Most bacteria are at least ten times smaller than eucaryotic microorganisms. The cell surface area is determined by the amount of plasma membrane available for exchanges of materials between the cell and the environment. The resulting increase in cell volume is always greater than the increase in cell surface. Bacteria and other microorganisms make up the single largest mass of life on Earth. The bacteria are the major inhabitants in open oceans. The activities of these mighty midgets sustain all other forms of life on the planet, and thus, our lives are irrevocably intertwined with theirs.

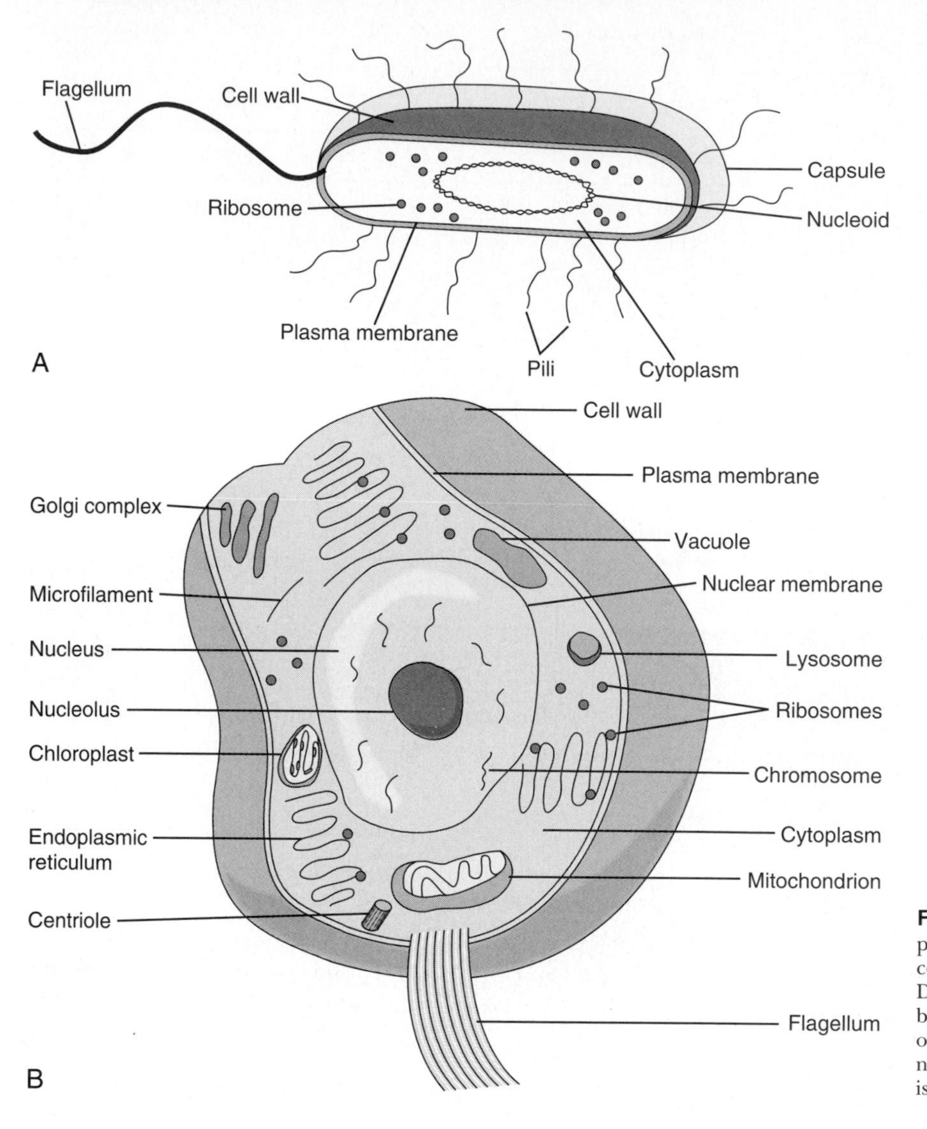

Figure 4–1 ◆ *A,* Composite of a procaryotic cell showing structures commonly associated with bacteria. DNA is not enclosed in a membrane. *B,* Composite of a eucaryotic cell showing membrane-bound nucleus and other organelles. DNA is contained in chromosomes.

(**cocci**), or (3) spiral (**spirilla**) (Fig. 4–2, Color Plate 4). Some bacteria, however, have quite different shapes. **Vibrios** are short, slightly curved rods. **Spirochetes** are flexible, helical cells capable of rapid movement. Elongated coccal forms are sometimes called **coccobacilli.** Bacilli that occur in long threads are described as **filamentous** bacilli; those with tapered ends are known as **fusiform** bacilli. Square bacteria have been observed in recent years, but they appear to be a rarity in nature. The majority of bacteria range from 0.2 to 1.5 μm in diameter and are 1.0 to 6.0 μm long. The spirilla are an exception; some attain lengths of 500 μm. Most bacteria exhibit some variation in size and shape depending on environmental conditions. This variation in morphologic appearance is called **pleomorphism.**

Bacteria sometimes occur in groups rather than singly. Cell division takes place along a single axis in bacilli, so sometimes they are seen in **pairs, chains,** or a steplike arrangement called a **palisade.** Cocci divide along one or more planes producing cells in pairs (**diplococci**), cells in chains (**streptococci**), cells in packets (**sarcinae**), or cells in clusters (**staphylococci**) (Fig. 4–3). The size, shape, and arrangements of cells are often the first clues in the identification of a bacterium. Because there are many "look-alikes," methods other than microscopy must be used to determine the genus and species of an organism.

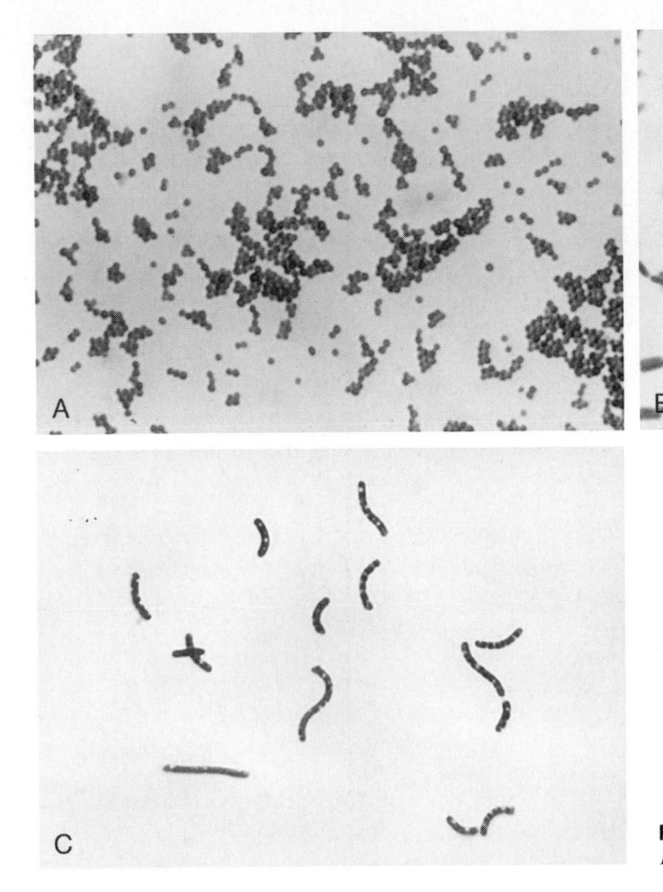

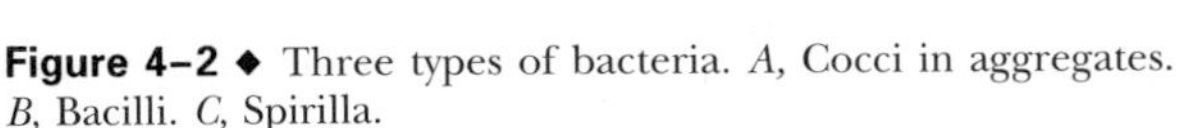

Figure 4–2 ◆ Three types of bacteria. *A,* Cocci in aggregates. *B,* Bacilli. *C,* Spirilla.

Cell Surface Structures

All bacteria, except mycoplasmas, are enclosed in rigid, porous cell walls. The cell walls provide support and protection necessary to maintain shape. The cytoplasm of all cells is surrounded by a plasma membrane that permits certain molecules to enter and leave cells.

GLYCOCALYX

Some bacteria have an additional layer outside the cell wall. This extracellular structure is called a **glycocalyx.** If the covering consists of polysaccharides and is firmly attached to the cell wall, the structure is a **capsule** (see Fig. 4–1*A*). If the surface layer consists of a mass of glycoproteins loosely associated with the cell wall, it is a **slime layer.** Capsules adhere to solid surfaces and to nutrients in the environment. The adhesive power of capsules is a major determinant in the initiation of some bacterial diseases. Capsules allow certain pathogens to avoid phagocytosis. The ingestion and destruction of microorganisms by white blood cells, known as **phagocytes,** was first described by Metchnikoff in 1882. More details on phagocytosis are discussed in Chapter 13.

The encapsulated strains of *Streptococcus pneumoniae, Haemophilus influenzae,* and *Neisseria meningitidis* cause life-threatening infections. It takes 10 or fewer encapsulated cells of *S. pneumoniae* to kill a mouse. Fortunately, vaccines made from capsular polysaccharides are available to protect human populations against diseases caused by these pathogens.

Slime layers also cause bacteria to adhere to solid surfaces and to adhere to one another. The slime layer of *Streptococcus mutans* allows that organism to accumulate in great numbers on tooth enamel. Other bacteria in the mouth become trapped in the slime to form **plaque.** Many organisms, including *S. mutans,* break down dietary sugars to lactic acid, which destroys enamel. Thus, bacterial slime contributes to dental caries, the commonest of all infections in the Western World.

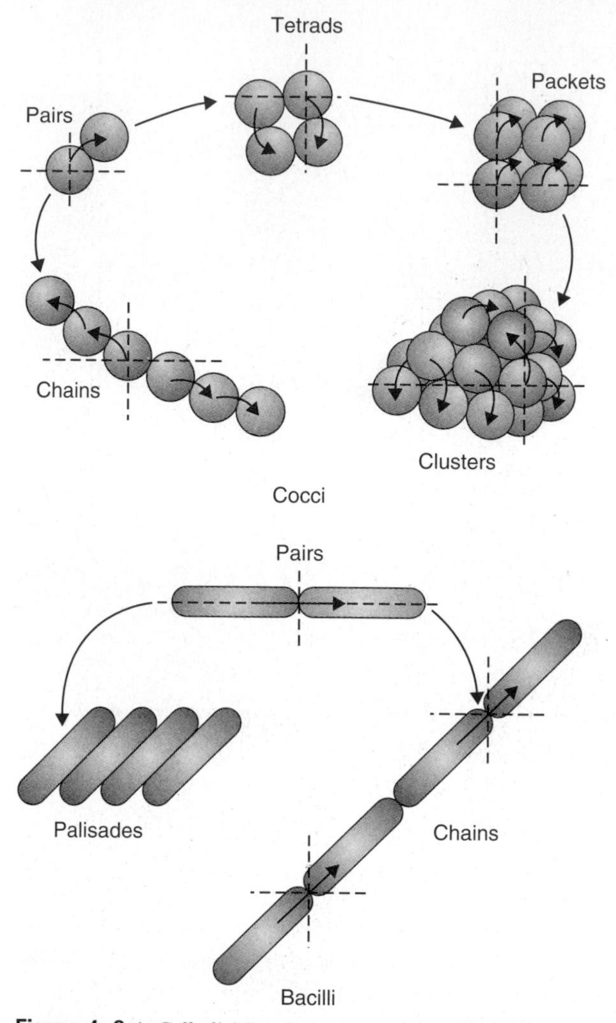

Figure 4–3 ◆ Cell division in cocci and bacilli. Division occurs along more than one axis in cocci, but bacilli divide across their short axes.

CELL WALL

The cell walls of bacteria surround the plasma membranes. The rigid shapes of the organisms are maintained as long as cell walls are intact. If all or part of a cell wall is destroyed, environmental stress produces bizarre shapes, and death will ensue.

The strength of the cell wall can be attributed to the presence of a component known as a **peptidoglycan.** The backbone of peptidoglycan molecules is composed of two derivatives of glucose, *N*-acetylglucosamine (NAG) and *N*-acetylmuramic acid (NAM), alternately connected by glycosidic bonds (Fig. 4–4). Some of the carbohydrate derivatives are attached to tetrapeptides (chains of four amino acids). The amino acids in the side chains are often D-isomers rather than the L-isomers more commonly found in nature. The D- and L-isomers of amino acids are mirror images of each other, having the same chemical composition but a reverse arrangement of the the atoms. These amino acids include D-alanine, L-alanine, D-glutamic acid, and L-lysine or **diaminopimelic acid (DAP).** DAP is not known to exist elsewhere in nature.

The tetrapeptides are connected by larger interpeptide bridges of five amino acids. The number of interpeptide bridges are fewer in gram-negative bacteria than in gram-positive bacteria. The widely used penicillins and cephalosporins interfere with linking of the interpeptides. Cell walls without the cross links are structurally weak and disintegrate when the cells divide. Microorganisms that do not contain peptidoglycan are not susceptible to the action of those drugs. Penicillins and cephalosporins can be used to treat many bacterial infections because the wall-less eucaryotic cells of humans are exempt from attack. Other differences between cell walls of gram-positive and gram-negative bacteria are summarized in Table 4–2.

The Cell Wall of Gram-Positive Bacteria. Peptidoglycan makes up as much as 90 percent of the thick, compact cell wall in gram-positive bacteria (Fig. 4–5). Some species of gram-positive bacteria possess small amounts of polysaccharides

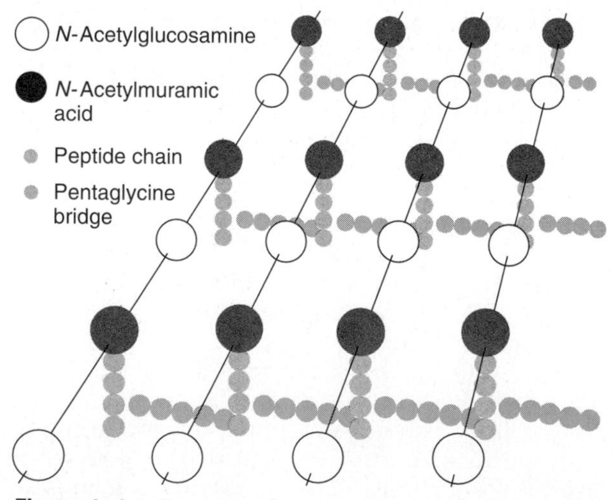

Figure 4–4 ◆ Structure of the peptidoglycan of a gram-positive cell wall. A continuum of sugar derivatives (*N*-acetylglucosamine and *N*-acetylmuramic acid) is wound around the cell. Reinforcement is supplied by cross linkages with chains and bridges of amino acids.

Table 4–2
MAJOR DIFFERENCES BETWEEN GRAM-POSITIVE AND GRAM-NEGATIVE BACTERIA

CHARACTERISTICS	GRAM-POSITIVE	GRAM-NEGATIVE
Thickness of peptidoglycan wall	200–800 Å	140–155 Å
Amino acids of peptidoglycan	Limited types	Variety of types
Teichoic acids	Present	Absent
Outer membranous wall	Absent	Present
Periplasmic space	Absent	Present
Flagellar structure	Two rings	Four rings
Pili	Rare	Abundant
Endospore formation	Common in some genera	Absent
Susceptibility to penicillin	Greater	Lesser
Ability to evade phagocytosis	Lesser	Greater

or lipids in their walls. Cell walls of some gram-positive cocci contain ribitol or glycerol derivatives called **teichoic acids.** Teichoic acids appear to stabilize cell walls by binding magnesium. Lipids called **mycolic acids** are abundant in cell walls of *Mycobacterium tuberculosis.*

The Cell Wall of Gram-Negative Bacteria. The walls of gram-negative bacteria are more complex in chemical composition, thinner, and less compact. Peptidoglycan constitutes only 5 to 20 percent of the cell wall in typical gram-negative bacteria. The peptidoglycan is not the outermost layer, but occupies a space between the plasma membrane and an **outer membrane.** Short pieces of peptidoglycan are cross-linked together into a gel. The outer membrane is similar to the plasma membrane in that it contains proteins and phospholipids. It differs because the arrangement of the molecules is not symmetrical and demonstrates less selective permeability. The inner layer contains phospholipids, but the outer portion is composed of lipopolysaccharides. Outer membranes are directly in contact with the environment unless gram-negative bacteria have capsules or slime layers. The space between the cell wall and the plasma membrane is called the **periplasm.** The periplasm processes and controls molecular traffic entering or leaving the cell. The peptidoglycan molecules are not as accessible to the action of antibiotics that interfere with synthesis of peptidoglycan as those in gram-positive bacteria. The lipopolysaccharide (LPS) layer of outer membranes is a harmful substance classified as an **endotoxin.** Endotoxins are discussed in further detail in Chapter 12.

The Cell Wall in Cell Division. The cell wall has a primary role in cell growth and in cell division. Growth of a cell causes changes in the contour of surface layers as the volume of a cell increases. During cell division there is an infolding of the cell wall at a point midway between opposite ends of the cell. A cross wall is formed as newly synthesized cell wall material is deposited, forming a partition between dividing cells. Cell division is complete when separation occurs.

SURFACE APPENDAGES

Some procaryotes have distinct appendages that enable them to move about or to adhere to solid surfaces. They consist of delicate strands of proteins, which require special staining tech-

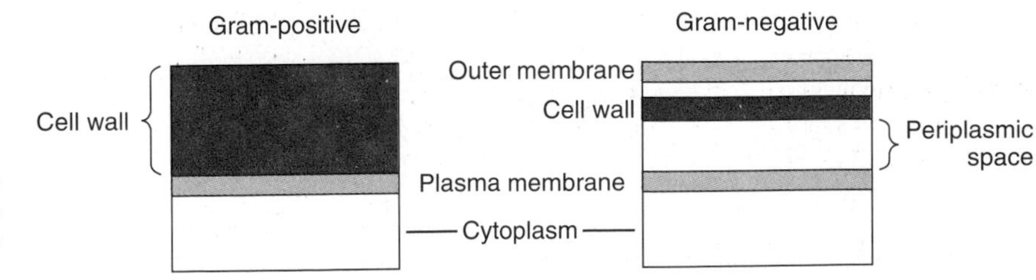

Figure 4–5 ◆ Comparison of the wall and membranes of a gram-positive cell (left) and a gram-negative cell (right).

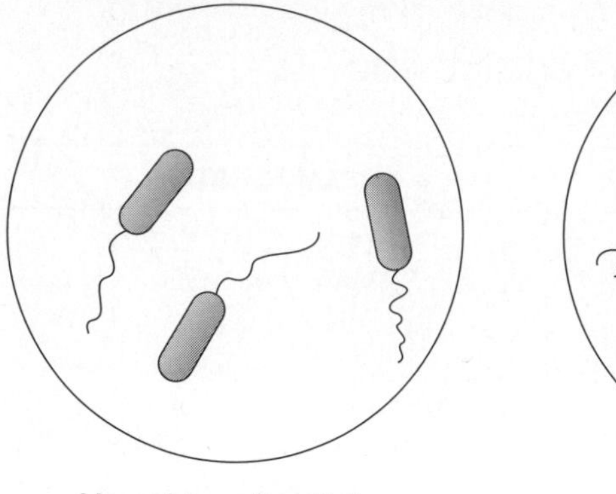

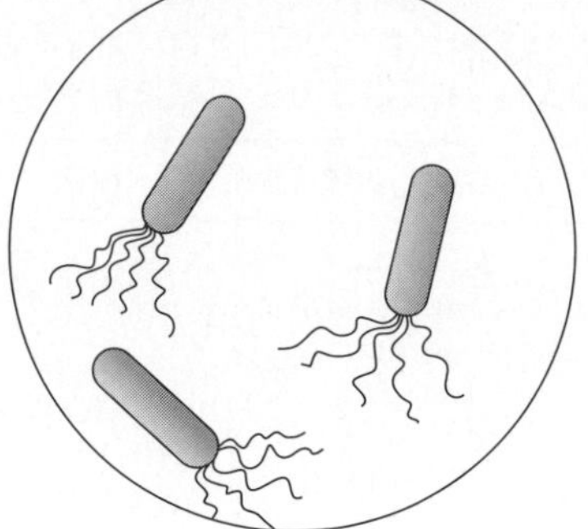

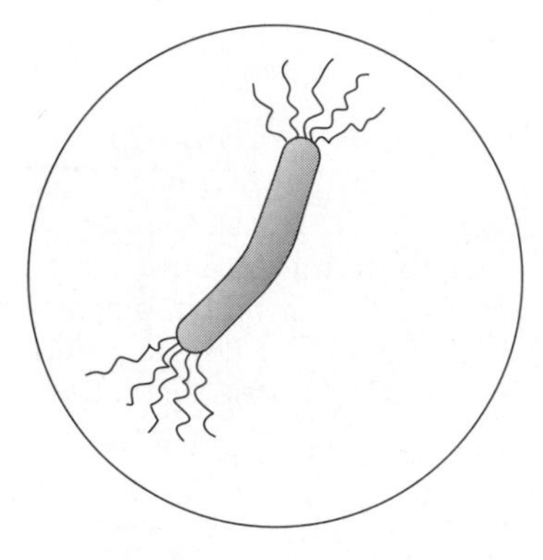

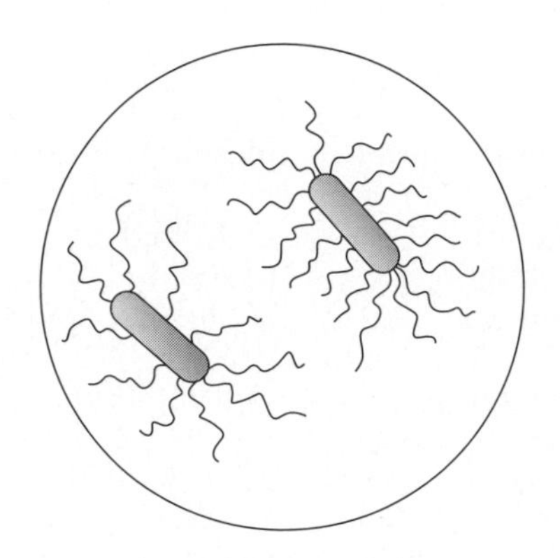

Figure 4–6 ◆ Arrangements of flagella in bacteria. Flagella may be polar or surround an entire cell.

niques for observation under a bright-field microscope. The presence of appendages provides some procaryotes with a survival advantage.

Flagella. Long, thin extensions, known as **flagella,** permit some bacteria to move about freely in aqueous environments. Flagella are usually longer than the organism on which they are located. Polar flagella may be present at one or both ends of a bacterium. Polar types of flagellation include (1) **monotrichous** (a single flagellum at one end), (2) **amphitrichous** (a single flagellum at each end), and (3) **lophotrichous** (a tuft of flagella at one or both ends) (Fig. 4–6). If flagella are present at multiple sites on the surface of a bacterium, the type of flagellation is called **peritrichous.** The arrangement of flagella is constant for a particular species.

Flagella consist of stacked, barbell-shaped proteins known as **flagellins.** Each filament of flagellins is attached to the bacterial cell by a flexible hook and a basal body. The basal body consists of one or more sets of rings anchored in the cell wall or plasma membrane (Fig. 4–7). The inner rings (M and S) are associated with the plasma membrane. Gram-negative bacteria also have two outer rings (L and P) embedded in the peptidoglycan of the cell wall. A flagellated bacterium is

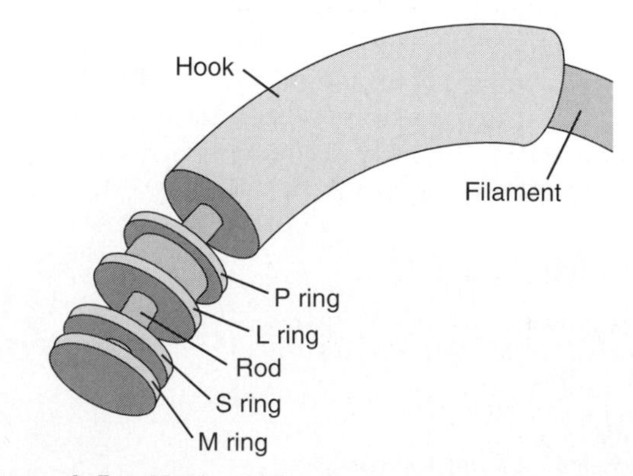

Figure 4–7 ◆ Hook and basal structures of a flagellum of a gram-negative bacterium. The S and M rings are attached to the plasma membrane.

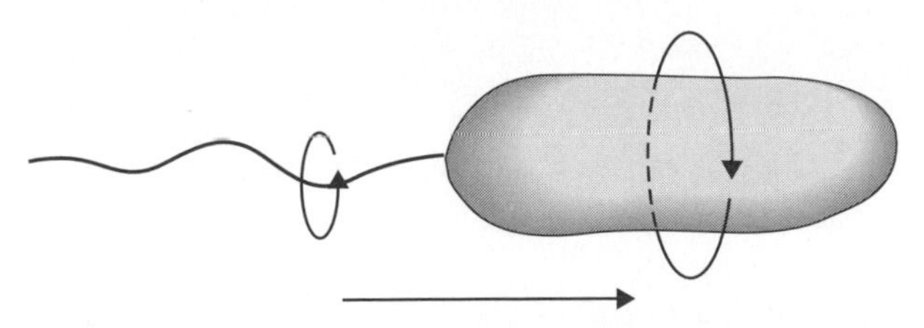

Figure 4–8 ◆ A bacterium showing clockwise rotary movement of the body as a flagellum completes one counterclockwise rotation.

propelled forward when energy from ATP causes rotation of the rings. A complete counterclockwise rotation is necessary to propel a bacterium a small fraction of its length (Fig. 4–8).

The direction of movement caused by the molecular motors of the flagella often appear to be random, but can be influenced by chemicals, wavelengths of light, and magnetic fields. Movement toward a nutrient or away from a harmful chemical is called **chemotaxis.** The progress in any direction is interrupted by short tumbles or **twiddles** (Fig. 4–9). The presence of an unfavorable environment causes more tumbling than one rich in nutrients.

Axial Filaments. The molecular motors of spirochetes are packaged quite differently. The structures, known as **axial filaments** or endoflagella, lie between an outer sheath of the organisms and the outermost layer of cytoplasm (Fig. 4–10). Axial filaments wind around organisms

FOCAL POINT

The Intrigue of Molecular Motors

Inside a black concrete building belonging to Stanley Electric Company, in Tsukuba, Japan, automobile engineers have been sharing space with some unlikely benchmates. While the engineers have been working on the next generation of automobile parts for the highly successful Japanese automobile industry, a team of biophysicists have been studying bacterial flagella of some common bacteria belonging to the genus *Salmonella.* The whiplike flagella are one of nature's smallest mechanical devices. The speeds, attained by the organisms as they propel themselves in a fluid environment, reach about 15,000 revolutions per minute. The biophysicists have discovered that the S-ring is part of a very large folded protein that makes up ten types of stacked, barbell proteins in the flagellar motor structure. A computer model of a flagellar filament has been developed, and the researchers are attempting to clone the genes in the rotor structure. The stators which the rotator pushes against have yet to be identified. The stators have been difficult to analyze because they are embedded in the plasma membrane. The efficiency of the motor mechanism in bacteria is unparalleled. Scientists estimate that perfection of molecular machines may take 20 to 30 years. The molecular-scale motors may one day be used to deliver drugs to specific organs in the body. Understanding the molecular and physical basis of flagellar movement could lead to more energy efficient automobiles. Nature's secrets have but to be unlocked.

Scientific American 265(3):168–169, 1991

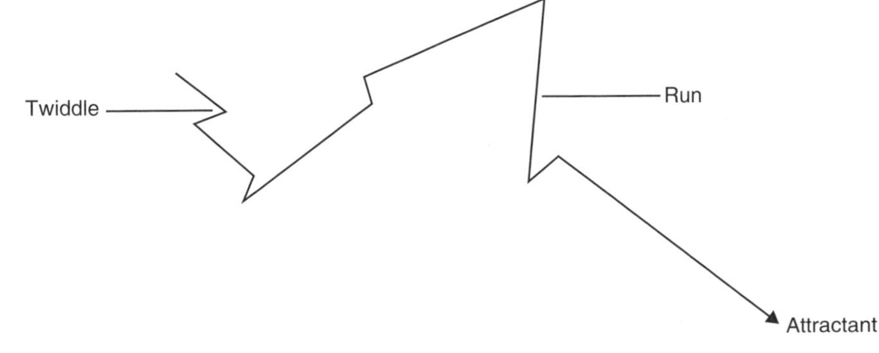

Figure 4–9 ◆ Tracking record of movement by a bacterium toward an attractant. Efficiency of movement in the direction of the attractant is interrupted by bizarre movements known as twiddles. Probability of twiddles decreases as movement is directed in runs of increasing length.

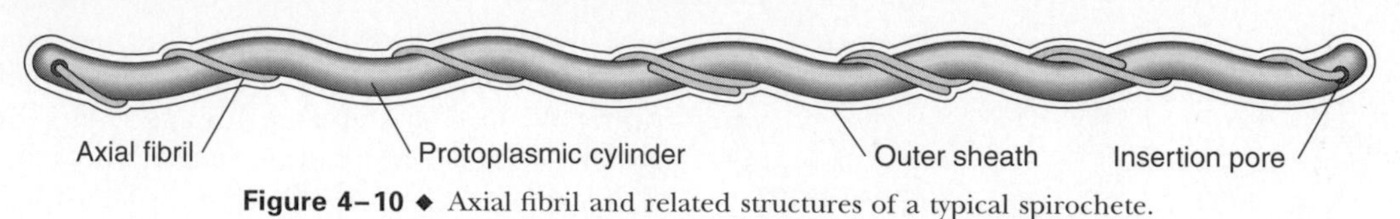

Figure 4–10 ◆ Axial fibril and related structures of a typical spirochete.

with some overlapping in the middle. Flexible hooks and paired rings are found at insertion points, but each filament is surrounded by a flexible sheath. Movement occurs in wavelike succession and is rapid. The vigorous motility of *Treponema pallidum,* the spirochete that causes syphilis, is attributed to an axial filament. It allows the spirochete to move well in highly viscous (syrupy) fluids.

Pili (Fimbriae). A number of gram-negative bacteria have shorter, finer appendages that surround the cells (see Fig. 4–1*A*). The hairlike filamentous structures are called **pili** (singular, pilus) or **fimbriae** (singular, fimbria) but have no role in motility. They permit bacteria to adhere to solid surfaces. Pili are responsible for the attraction of some organisms to epithelial surfaces during an initial encounter and throughout an infection. *Escherichia coli, Neisseria gonorrhoeae,* and *Bordetella pertussis* all have pili that promote colonization on epithelial tissue. Particular pili, designated as sex pili, have a role in cell contact required in transfer of DNA from one bacterium to another.

PLASMA (CYTOPLASMIC) MEMBRANE

Procaryotic cells are surrounded by a continuous layer of a lipid-protein "mosaic" called the **plasma** or **cytoplasmic membrane.** The membrane is composed of proteins embedded in two layers of phospholipids (a lipid bilayer) (Fig. 4–11). The phospholipid molecules are oriented in such a manner that the **hydrophilic** (water-loving) head ends are directed outward and the **hydrophobic** (water-hating) tail ends are directed inward toward each other. The hydrophilic nature of some proteins keeps them on the surface of membranes. Most proteins are hydrophobic and are buried within the lipid matrix.

Some surface proteins are constructed so that pores are formed in the membrane. Other proteins are linked to polysaccharides to form glycoproteins. The protein and phospholipids are constantly moving while maintaining a mosaic pattern. The unique construction and fluidity is often described as a **fluid mosaic model.**

The Plasma Membrane As a Barrier. The primary function of the plasma membrane is to regulate the movement of molecules entering or leaving the cell. Not all molecules can be transported across the plasma membrane. Limitations include size, solubility in membrane lipids, availability of carrier molecules, and sufficient quantities of stored energy. The size of the pores, formed by protein molecules of the membrane, allow water, water-soluble sugars, and small ions to move freely across the membrane. Uncharged particles and lipid-soluble substances enter cells through lipids of the membrane. Most large mol-

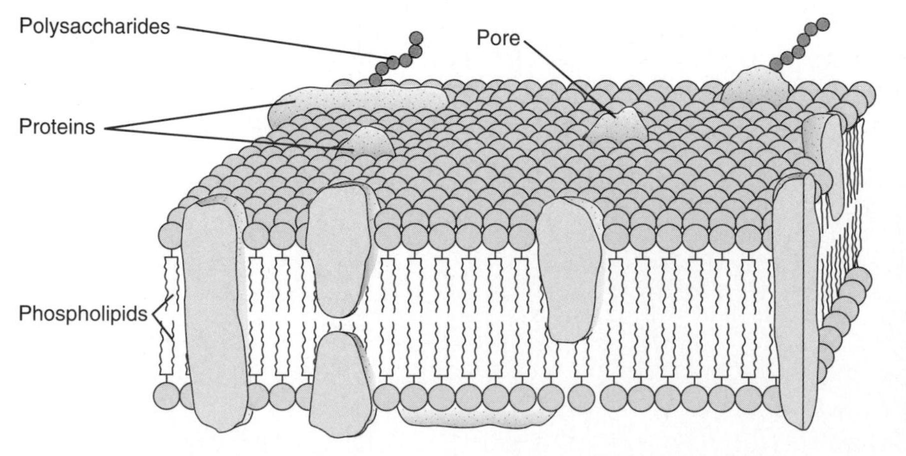

Figure 4–11 ◆ Plasma membrane of a procaryote showing distribution of polysaccharides and the lipid-protein "mosaic." Most proteins are embedded in the lipid matrix. Some surface proteins form pores through which molecules can pass.

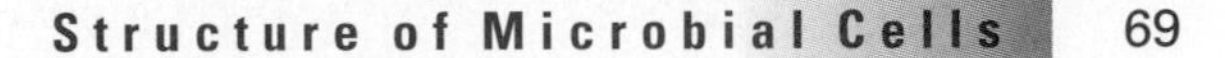

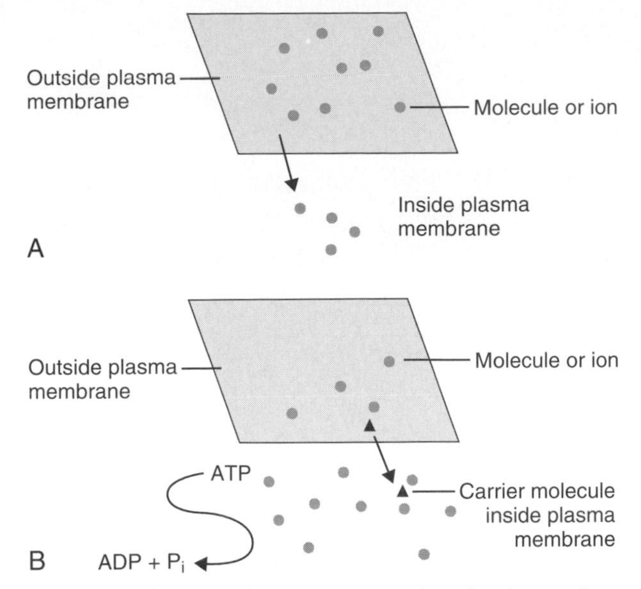

Figure 4–12 ◆ *A,* Passive transport of molecules or ions across the plasma membrane in the presence of a concentration gradient. Molecules move from an area of greater concentration to an area of lesser concentration. *B,* Active transport with expenditure of ATP in the absence of a concentration gradient. Carrier molecules are required to move molecules against a concentration gradient.

ecules cannot enter cells in the absence of help from a carrier molecule. The restrictions imposed by chemical constituents and arrangement of membrane molecules are responsible for **selective permeability** of the membrane.

Movement of molecules across the plasma membrane requires energy in some form. If no energy sources of the cell are expended, movement is by **passive transport** (Fig. 4–12*A*). In **simple diffusion,** molecules of a substance move from an area of greater concentration to an area of lesser concentration. The driving force is the inherent energy of molecules, which keeps them in motion. The driving force is proportional to the difference in concentrations of the molecules. The differences in concentrations are referred to as a **concentration gradient.** Molecules move freely across the plasma membrane in the presence of a concentration gradient if the particles are small enough to pass through the pores.

The **rate of diffusion** depends on the concentration gradient, the molecular size, and the temperature of the environment. The greater the concentration gradient, the more rapid is the diffusion of molecules. Small molecules move faster than larger molecules at a constant temperature. A rise in temperature causes molecules to move more rapidly. Diffusion continues until a point of equilibrium is reached. At that point, there is a uniform distribution of molecules on both sides of the membrane.

Some enzymes, known as permeases, assist in diffusion of molecules across the plasma membrane. The enzymes act as carrier molecules, but movement of molecules occurs only in the presence of a concentration gradient. The process is called **facilitated diffusion.** Specific molecules move across membranes more rapidly if diffusion is facilitated by carrier molecules. Some permeases assist in the transport of a wide variety of substances; others are highly specific in their facilitating ability. Many permeases are synthesized only in response to the presence of particular substrates in the environment.

Diffusion of water molecules across the plasma membrane is called **osmosis.** The difference in concentrations of water molecules, separated by a membrane, generates a driving force known as **osmotic pressure** (Fig. 4–13). The environment of a cell may contain amounts of dissolved substances, or **solutes,** that are equal to, less than, or greater than those found within a cell. An **isotonic** solution is one containing a concentration of solutes equal to that found within a cell.

A **hypotonic** solution is one containing fewer solutes than those found within a cell. The concentration of water molecules is greater than that found inside the cell. Water molecules enter cells, causing them to swell. Cells without walls rupture quickly, releasing cytoplasmic contents into the environment when placed in a hypotonic solution. Cells with walls can withstand more pressure before bursting but will eventually succumb from osmotic shock.

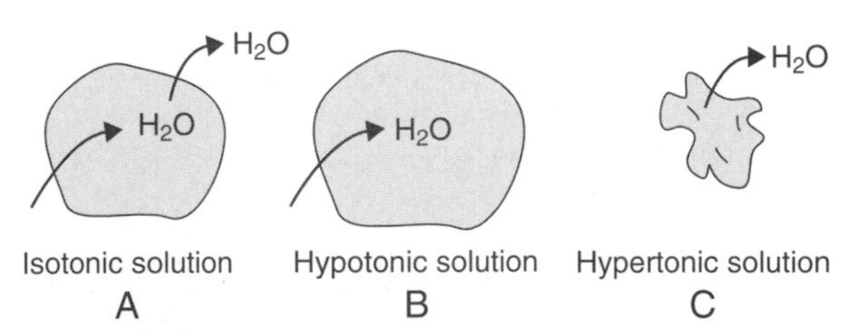

Figure 4–13 ◆ Effect of differences in concentrations of water in the external and internal environments of red blood cells. *A,* Red blood cells remain the same size in an isotonic solution because there is no change in concentrations of dissolved salts on either side of the plasma membrane. *B,* Water molecules move into cells in a hypotonic solution causing them to swell. *C,* Water molecules leave cells in a hypertonic solution causing them to shrink. The driving force for the movement of water molecules is osmotic pressure.

A hypertonic solution is one containing more solutes than those found within a cell. The concentration of water molecules is greater inside the cell than that found in the environment. Water molecules leave cells, causing them to shrink. Cells without walls shrink readily in hypertonic environments. Most cells with walls can survive in moderately hypertonic surroundings, but ultimately, the osmotic pressure causes a loss of water.

The number and type of molecules transported passively across membranes could not sustain microbial life. Most molecules move across plasma membranes by **active transport.** The process is analogous to a pump in which energy is used to move water uphill. The types of active transport are classified according to the source of energy used to drive molecules across membranes.

In **ATP-driven active transport,** energy is derived from adenosine triphosphate (ATP) to drive substances across plasma membranes with the aid of carrier molecules (see Fig. 4–12*B*). Solutes are bound to carrier proteins located on the membrane or in the periplasm. The reaction is coupled with the breakdown of ATP to adenosine diphosphate (ADP). The energy-linked reaction lowers the affinity of the carrier for the solute so that separation occurs within the cell. The ATP molecules are quickly restored as energy from fermentation, respiration, or the sun is trapped again in phosphate bonds.

In **group translocation,** nutrients enter cells only after modification of the molecules by the addition of chemical groups. In the phosphotransferase system (PTS) of bacteria, entering molecules are phosphorylated during transport. For example, glucose is converted to glucose 6-phosphate when a high-energy phosphate bond is given up by phosphoenolpyruvate (PEP). Movement of the phosphate group requires four special proteins (Fig. 4–14). Group translocation is far more complex than the other forms of transport, but requires less energy than does ATP-driven active transport.

The Membrane and Chemical Activity. The plasma membrane has a number of roles. It is the portal of entry or exit for large numbers of molecules. The enzyme-rich membranes carry on the ATP-liberating reactions of photosynthesis and respiration. Pigments that trap energy from the sun in photosynthetic bacteria are abundant in the plasma membrane. The membrane is also the site where structural components of membranes, cell walls, and glycocalyces are synthesized.

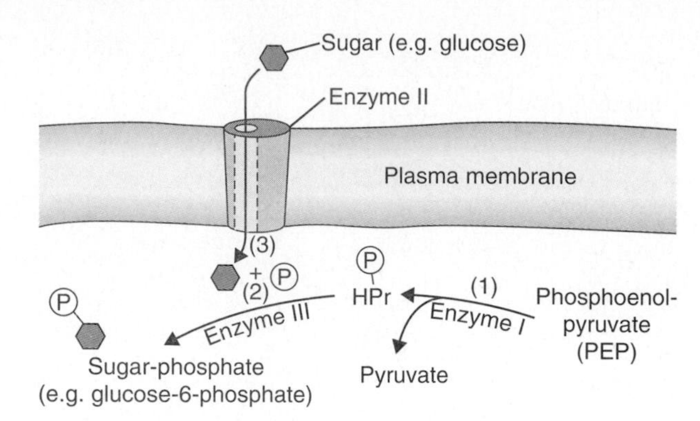

Figure 4–14 ◆ Mechanism of group translocation showing roles of three enzymes and a heat-stable protein (HPr) of phosphoenolpyruvate (PEP) in the transport of a sugar across the plasma membrane.

The Plasma Membrane in Secretion. A number of products necessary for the survival of organisms are secreted through plasma membranes. Those products include hydrolytic enzymes, potent toxins, and proteases that can interfere with protective factors known as **antibodies.**

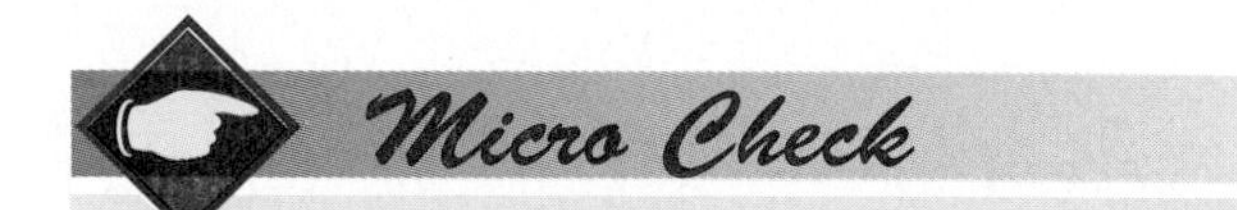

- Describe three basic shapes of bacteria.
- How do cell walls of gram-positive and gram-negative bacteria differ?
- What is meant when plasma membranes are described as selectively permeable?

Cytoplasm

The cytoplasm of procaryotic cells consists of a mixture of water, carbohydrates, proteins, lipids, and inorganic salts. Electron microscopy reveals the presence of internal membranes in many procaryotes. The internal membranes are diverse in structure and function, but have the same chemical composition as the plasma membrane.

GRANULES

The lipid, poly-β-hydroxybutyric (PBH) acid is one of the most common energy reserve products stored in granules of procaryotes. Other reserve materials found in granules include glycogen, sulfur, and inorganic phosphates, which

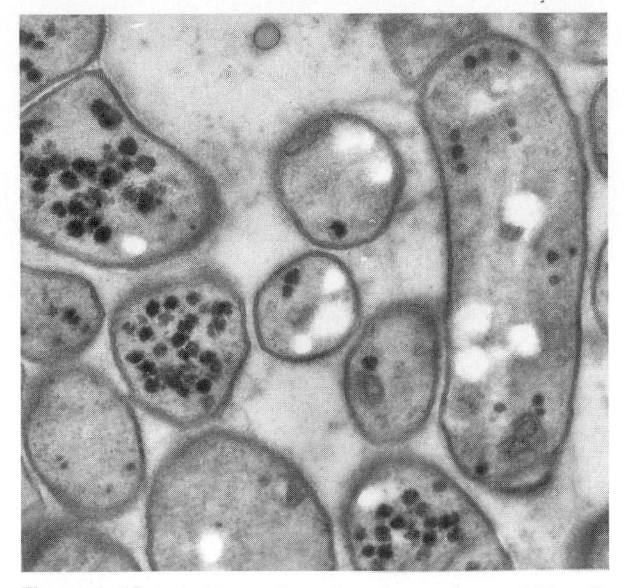

Figure 4–15 ◆ A thin section of a young culture of *Nocardia asteroides* showing dark-staining glycogen granules and clear, lipid-containing vacuoles.

make up the volutin granules (Fig. 4–15). The volutin granules appear **metachromatic** (changing in color) when they are stained with basic blue dyes. The stored materials enable bacteria to survive in environments depleted in carbon and energy sources.

RIBOSOMES

Ribosomes are small, numerous particles distributed throughout the cytoplasm or attached to the plasma membranes of procaryotes. The ribosomes are made up of one type of RNA and proteins. Each procaryotic ribosome is composed of two particles whose sizes are expressed in Svedberg (S) units. S units represent sedimentation constants obtained by a procedure that separates the particles in a high-velocity ultracentrifuge. A 30S subunit and a 50S subunit are obtained from ribosomes of procaryotic cells. Intact ribosomes have an S value of 70. There are 10,000 or more ribosomes in a metabolically active bacterium. They are beyond the resolution of a bright-field microscope, but can be observed readily by electron microscopy (Fig. 4–16). Ribosomes are the sites of protein synthesis. Most of the energy of the cell is consumed in making proteins. The synthesis of proteins is discussed in Chapter 7.

The S values of bacterial ribosomes are smaller than those of human ribosomes. Streptomycin, chloramphenicol, and erythromycin are used to treat bacterial infections because they act selectively on 70S ribosomes. The inhibition of protein synthesis eventually leads to death of the bacteria. The antibacterial drugs have no effect on the 80S component of human ribosomes.

NUCLEOID

DNA is found in distinct regions of procaryotes known as the **nucleoid.** The DNA is not separated from the cytoplasm by membranes. Nucleoid regions can be differentiated from the more dense cytoplasm on electron micrographs (Fig. 4–17).

A single double-stranded circular molecule of DNA makes up the nucleoid of a procaryote (see Fig. 4–1*A*). The molecule of DNA is tightly coiled, but if stretched end to end, the molecule would be a thousand or more times longer than a bacterial cell. The DNA of procaryotic cells constitutes a single chromosome even though it is not packaged as a rodlike structure. The DNA of that chromosome contains all the genetic information required to sustain life.

PLASMIDS

Some bacteria contain small segments of double-stranded, circular DNA that exist as separate

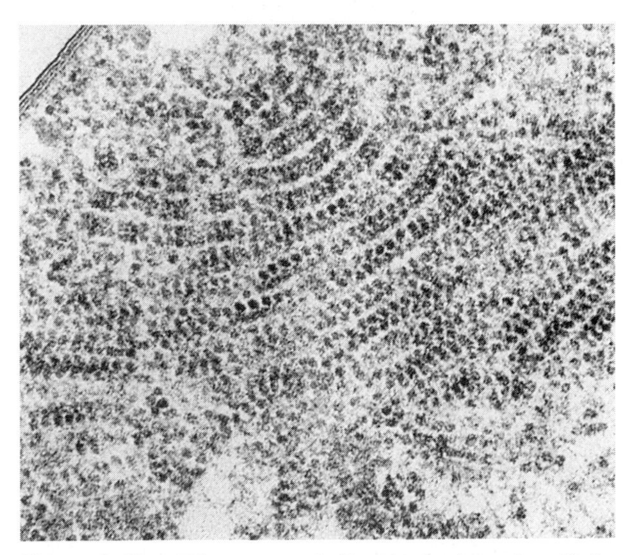

Figure 4–16 ◆ Ribosomes as helices in the bacterium *Escherichia coli.*

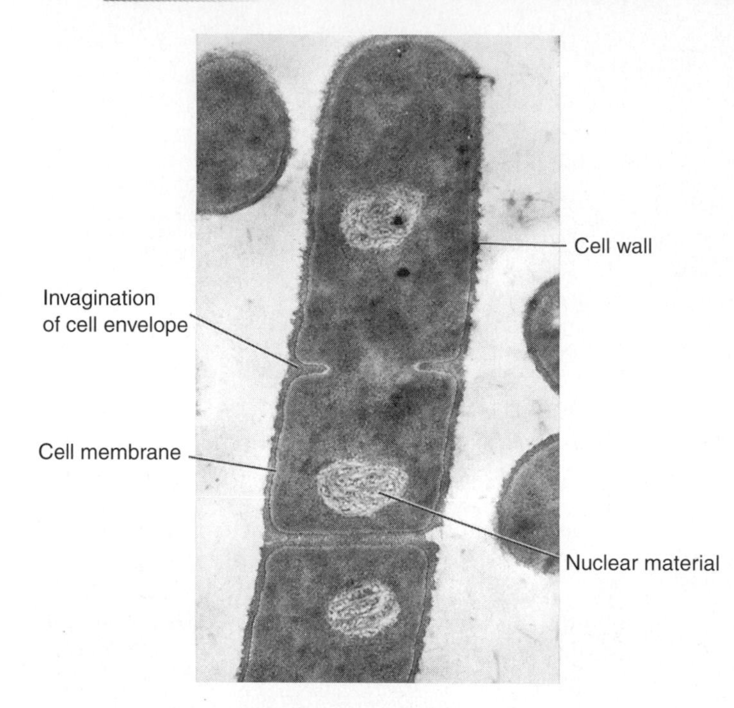

Figure 4–17 ◆ A cell of *Bacillus subtilis* showing nuclear material in regions making up the nucleoid.

entities in the cytoplasm. The fragments of DNA are called **plasmids.** Plasmids are not essential for the usual life-sustaining activities of the cell, but may be the difference between life and death in a hostile environment. The DNA of plasmids functions in an analogous manner to that of chromosomal DNA, but is exempt from chromosomal control unless it becomes chromosome-associated. Among the plasmids of special interest are those responsible for production of antibiotic resistance factors, toxins, and antimicrobial substances.

Endospores

A distinctive characteristic of some procaryotes is the ability to produce resting structures known as **endospores.** The dormant structures are frequently multilayered and are metabolically inactive. Endospores often travel long distances in the air and can survive for years in nutritionally deficient environments. Cells that are metabolically active are called **vegetative** cells to differentiate them from resting structures.

Only certain bacteria, usually bacilli and only rarely cocci and vibrios, form endospores. Frequently, these structures are simply called spores. The most important spore-formers are members of the genera *Bacillus* and *Clostridium.* Sporulation begins when an infolding of the plasma membrane separates a portion of DNA and cytoplasm from the rest of the cell. Several protective layers are deposited around a spherical or oval **forespore** (Fig. 4–18). The forespore is surrounded by a layer of peptides known as the **cortex.** The next outermost layer is composed principally of peptidoglycan differing from that of vegetative cells. It makes up the **spore coat.** Additional water-impermeable peptides may surround the spore coat to make up an **exosporium.**

Spores are the heat-stable forms of bacteria first described by Tyndall, discussed in Chapter 1. The dormant structures are remarkably resistant to heat, drying, radiation, dyes, and disinfectants. Heat resistance appears to be related to the presence of dipicolinic acid (DPA) and calcium in the core of spores. DPA is not found in vegetative cells. A return to the vegetative state is triggered by an environmental factor such as heat. The process is called **spore germination.** Once the spore coat is broken, **outgrowth** occurs. The process proceeds in an orderly manner if the environment can support vegetative cell growth. Emergence of the developing cell is followed by elongation until it is freed from the confines of its temporary imprisonment (Fig. 4–19). The time required for germination and outgrowth to take place is only a few minutes.

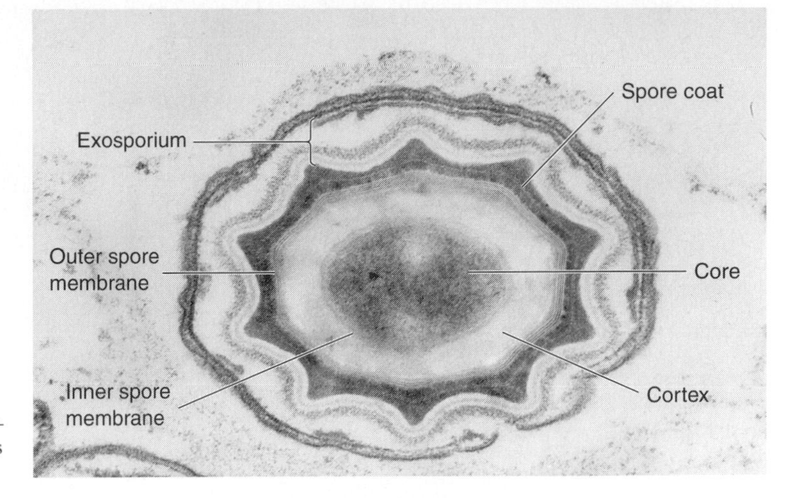

Figure 4–18 ◆ A mature spore of *Bacillus macerans* in cross section showing protective layers and core.

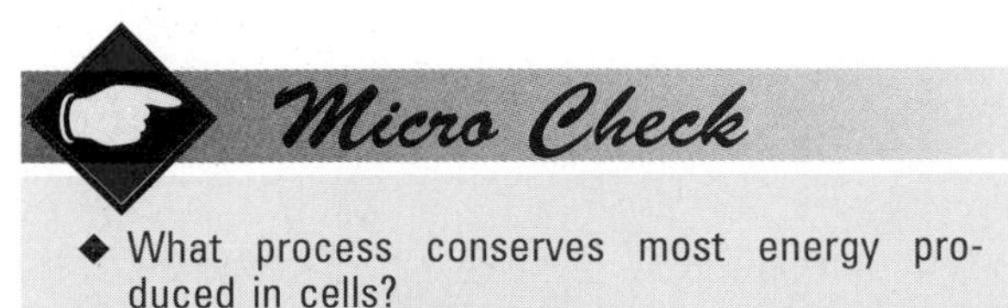

- ◆ What process conserves most energy produced in cells?
- ◆ Of what significance are plasmids to bacteria?
- ◆ How are some bacteria able to survive under unfavorable environmental conditions?

EUCARYOTES

The microbial eucaryotes consist of a diverse group of unicellular and multicellular organisms whose cells have membrane-bound nuclei and specialized membrane-bound structures known as **organelles,** which perform life-sustaining activities (see Fig. 4–1*B*). They include the photosynthetic algae and nonphotosynthetic protozoa and fungi and are found in a variety of terrestrial and aquatic habitats. The algae and fungi have cell walls; the protozoa are bounded only by plasma membranes. Algae are the principal site of photosynthesis on Earth, but rarely cause disease. Although the numbers of protozoa and fungi causing disease are fewer than numbers of bacteria producing illness, the diseases they cause can be life-threatening.

Shapes, Sizes, and Arrangements of Eucaryotic Cells

The cells of the eucaryotic microorganisms are spherical, cylindrical, or elongated and, sometimes, form long chains of connected cells or aggregate into colonies of cells. Some very small unicellular eucaryotes may not be bigger than 1.0 μm in diameter, but some protozoa like *Pelomyxa carolinensis,* measure 600 μm or more. The fungi comprise unicellular spherical, elliptical, or elongated forms, known as yeasts, and the multicellular molds containing tubular filaments (hyphae) of varying lengths, measuring 5 to 10 μm in width. More details on algae, protozoa, and fungi are found in Chapter 9.

Cell Surface Structures

Algae and fungi have cell walls, but the cytoplasm of protozoa is enclosed only in a plasma membrane in most species. A few marine protozoa produce shells containing small pores through which nutrients and wastes can pass. The famous White Cliffs of Dover are actually deposits of calcium carbonate derived from residues of protozoan shells that at one time inhabited the coastal waters. The cell walls of eucaryotes are largely protective but also provide these cells with their characteristic shapes.

CELL WALL

Many algae and a few fungi have cell walls composed of cellulose. The walls of most fungi contain **chitin,** a polymer of *N*-acetylglucosamine, which is also present in the exoskeletons of crustaceans and some insects. Some algae have walls of silica, polysaccharides, and proteins that form interesting geometric patterns (Fig. 4–20).

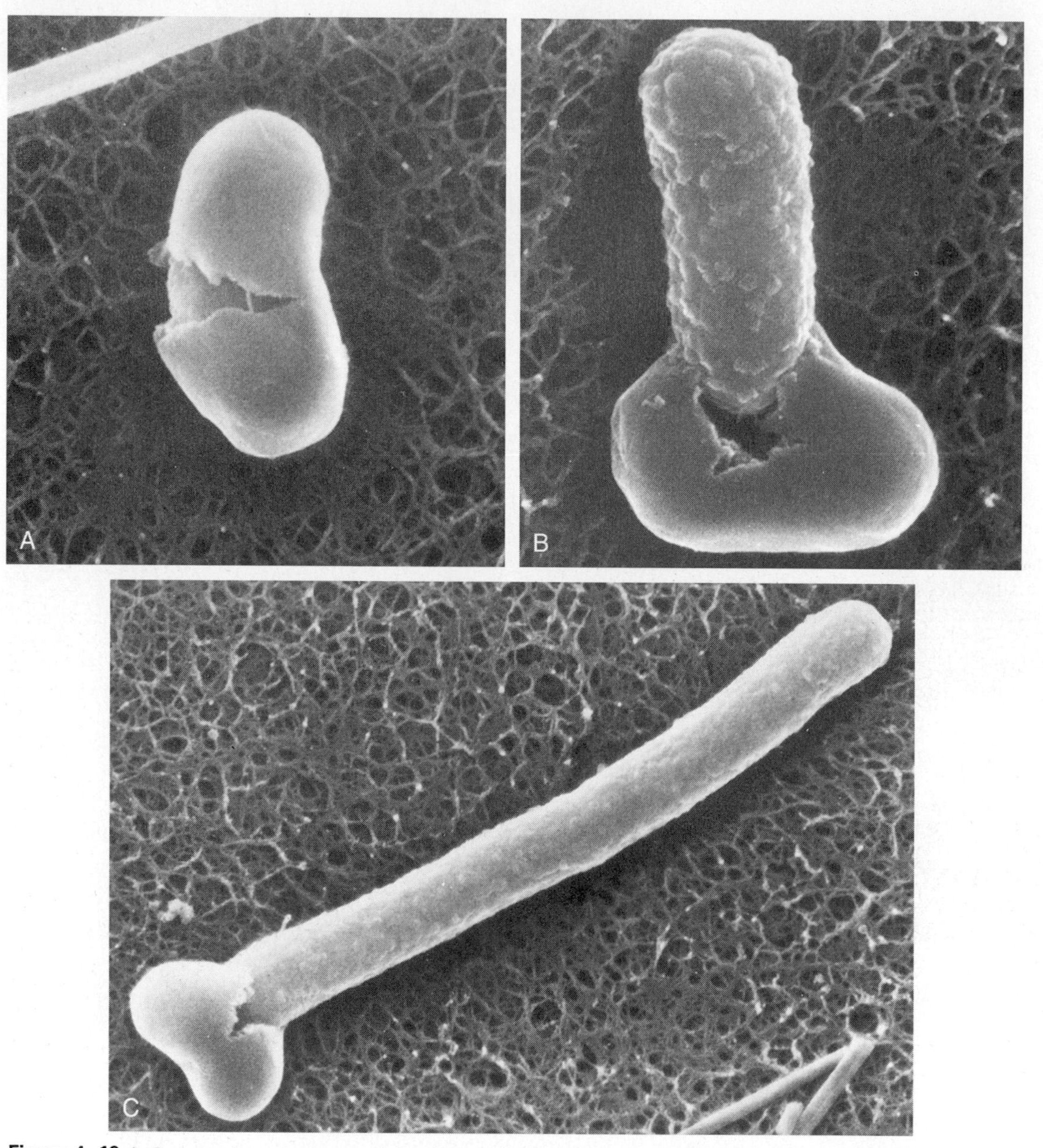

Figure 4–19 ◆ Germination of a spore of *Bacillus subtilis* after triggering by heat at 60°C and growth at 37°C on thin layer agar. *A,* Disruption of spore wall and emergence of spore at 60 minutes. *B,* Initial stage of outgrowth at 120 minutes. *C,* Terminal stage of outgrowth at 150 minutes.

Cell walls of eucaryotes contain no peptidoglycan. Fungi are not susceptible, therefore, to antibiotics, such as penicillin, that interfere with the synthesis of peptidoglycan. The drug of choice for the treatment of infections caused by microorganisms is dependent on several factors, but the chemical composition of cell walls, if they are present, is a prime consideration.

SURFACE APPENDAGES

Most protozoa and some algae are motile during at least one stage of their development. Some protozoa move quite slowly by extending temporary projections of the cytoplasm called **pseudopodia** (false feet), but other protozoa have true appendages that propel them in aqueous environments.

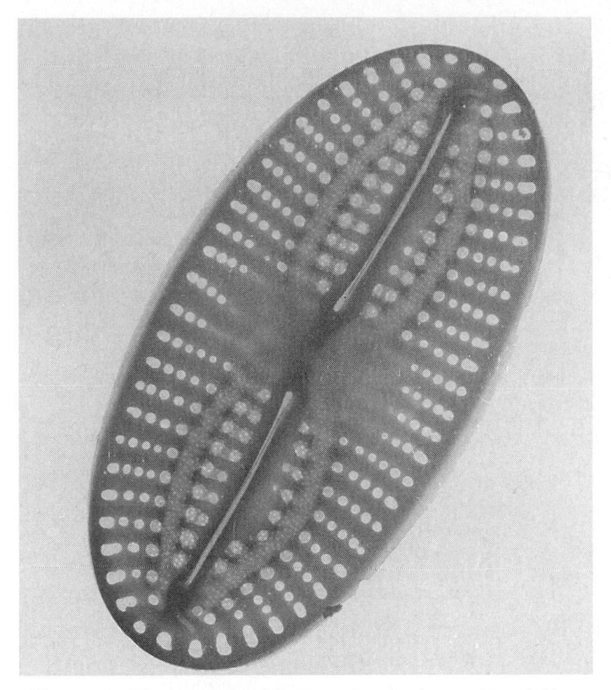

Figure 4–20 ◆ A cell wall of an alga having walls of silica.

Flagella. Some protozoa and algae move by means of flagella. Eucaryotic flagella are large enough to be seen readily with a bright-field microscope. Eucaryotic cells usually have one or two polar flagella, but may have up to eight flagella. Each flagellum contains a peripheral ring of nine double hollow filaments called **microtubules** surrounding two central microtubules (Fig. 4–21). The microtubules are made up of subunits of a protein known as **tubulin.** The outer microtubules are connected to the central microtubules and to each other by thin microfilaments of protein in a spokelike arrangement. Each flagellum is enclosed by a continuation of the plasma membrane. The appendages are anchored in a basal body located in the cytoplasm. Coordinated sliding movements of the microtubules enable some protozoa to attain speeds of 30 to 250 μm per second. The energy for movement is supplied by ATP.

Cilia. One group of protozoa move by means of shorter and more numerous hairlike appendages known as **cilia.** The cilia may surround the entire cell or occur in an area near a food-gathering structure known as an **oral groove.** The structure of cilia consists of the same "9 + 2 pattern" of microtubules in eucaryotic flagella. The coordinated movements of multiple cilia produce a wavelike motion that permits some organisms to move at ten times or more the speed of flagellated eucaryotes.

PLASMA (CYTOPLASMIC) MEMBRANE

The plasma membrane of eucaryotic cells is similar in structure and function to the membrane of procaryotic cells. One notable exception, however, is the universal presence of **sterols** in the eucaryotic plasma membrane. Only the procaryotic mycoplasmas have sterols in their membranes. The protein and carbohydrate constituents of eucaryotic plasma membranes differ from those found in procaryotes but permit movement of molecules across membranes by both passive and active transport mechanisms. In addition, protozoa are able to take in or to expel solutes or particles that are too large to pass through the plasma membrane. That movement is made possible by active transport mechanisms known as **endocytosis** and **exocytosis** (Fig. 4–22).

Entering materials become trapped within an indented portion of the membrane. As more membrane material is synthesized, a vesicle is formed that moves into the cytoplasm.

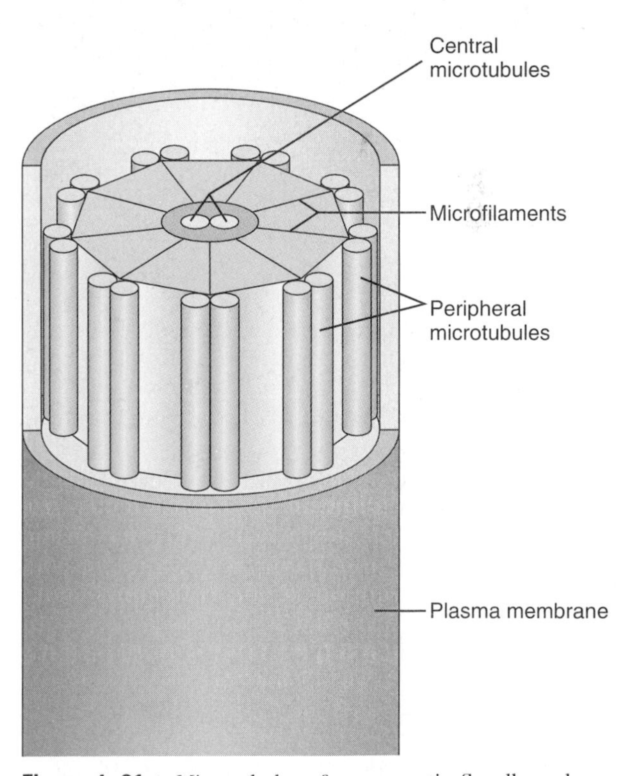

Figure 4–21 ◆ Microtubules of a eucaryotic flagellum showing an arrangement called the "9 + 2 array." There are nine pairs of peripheral tubules and two central tubules.

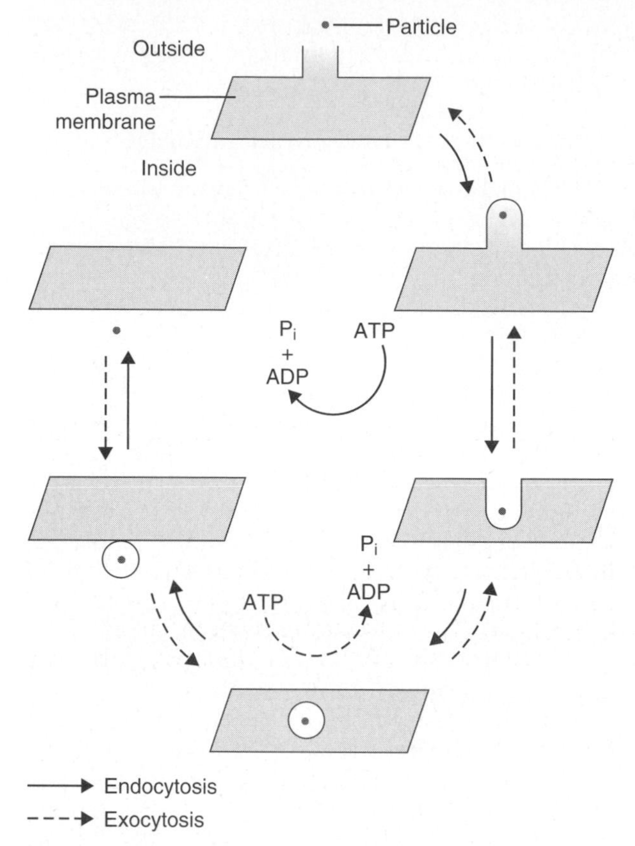

Figure 4–22 ◆ In endocytosis a particle is surrounded by extensions of the plasma membrane. The extensions fuse to form a vesicle from which the particle is ultimately released into the cytoplasm. In exocytosis a vesicle containing a waste product is formed from extensions of the plasma membrane. It is carried to the outside of the cell and released into the environment. Both methods of transport require ATP.

Exocytosis is the release of materials from cells by reverse endocytosis. Cytoplasmic vesicles containing waste products move to the cell surface. Vesicles fuse with the plasma membrane allowing liquids or particles to be discharged. Undigested food and debris taken in by the processes of endocytosis are returned to the environment by exocytosis.

Bacteria and small eucaryotes are often ingested and destroyed by phagocytic protozoa. Sometimes bacteria can survive in the cytoplasm of their protozoan predators and interact with their hosts. The association leads to a partnership called **endosymbiosis.** If both partners benefit from the association, it can be classified as **mutualism.** If one organism benefits and the other is unaffected, it is described as **commensalism.** If one partner benefits and the other is harmed, the term **parasitism** is applied to the association. Mutualistic endosymbiosis often provides a survival advantage to both microorganisms.

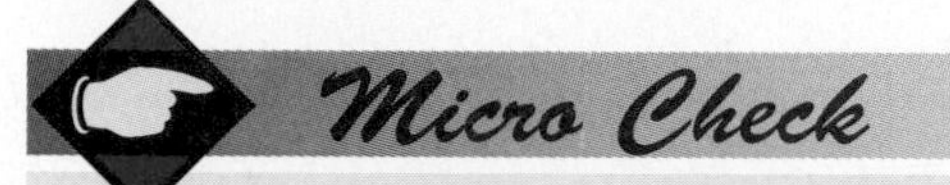

- Name three groups of microorganisms classified as eucaryotes.
- How do cell walls of eucaryotes differ chemically from those of procaryotes?
- Differentiate between endocytosis and exocytosis.

Cytoplasm

The cytoplasm of eucaryotic cells, like that of procaryotes, is a mixture of organic and inorganic materials. The cytoplasm is constantly in motion. The continuous movement is an efficient transportation system for the distribution of molecules throughout the cell. The flowing movement, known as **cytoplasmic streaming,** also allows organelles to interact with one another. The higher viscosity of procaryotic cytoplasm limits the interactions of cell contents. Accumulations of nutrients or cellular products are frequently stored in **granules** or in the membranous **vacuoles** or **vesicles.**

INTERNAL MEMBRANES

The cytoplasm of eucaryotes contains a system of internal membranes known as the **endoplasmic reticulum** (ER) (Fig. 4–23). The membranes are extensions of the plasma and nuclear membranes. The network of fluid-filled channels is a transport system for products synthesized by a cell. The association of ribosomes with the ER give it a rough appearance. ER that lacks ribosomal attachments appears smooth. Membranes of both rough and smooth ER synthesize phospholipids.

GRANULES

Granules of eucaryotic cells contain polysaccharides and several kinds of energy-rich lipids. Algin, a polysaccharide produced and stored by some algae, is used widely as a stabilizer in the food and dairy industries. Agar, another polysaccharide used as a solidifying agent in culture media, is produced by some red marine algae.

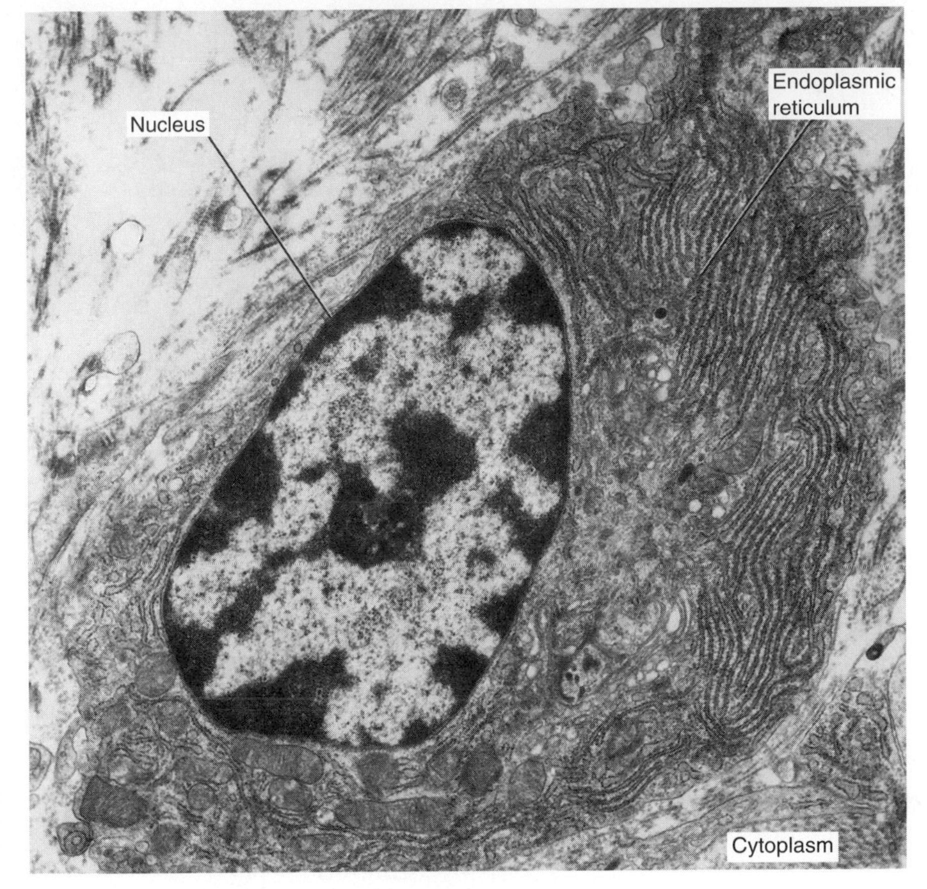

Figure 4–23 ◆ An electron micrograph of a typical eucaryotic cell showing a distinct nucleus and distinct channels of endoplasmic reticulum.

VACUOLES

The vacuoles of eucaryotic cells appear to be empty sacs, but looks can be deceiving. The vacuoles contain a variety of fluids, soluble materials, and ingested particles. Some vacuoles are critical to the survival of certain protozoa. Many freshwater protozoa would be destroyed by the influx of water molecules if it were not for their ability to expel water into the environment by **contractile vacuoles.** Other specialized vacuoles have a role in food gathering.

VESICLES

The infoldings of the plasma membrane that occur in endocytosis or exocytosis are called **vesicles.** A vesicle is typically smaller than 1.0 μm. The vesicles, formed while taking in or discharging materials, are of a transitory nature. The fluid nature of the plasma membrane is responsible for the ability to form vesicles.

RIBOSOMES

The ribosomes of eucaryotic cells are larger than those found in procaryotes. The subunits consist of a 60S and a 40S particle. Intact ribosomes of eucaryotes make up 80S particles. Smaller ribosomes, similar to those of procaryotes, are located in highly specialized organelles known as **mitochondria** and **chloroplasts.** The ribosomes function, as in procaryotes, in the synthesis of proteins.

MITOCHONDRIA

Mitochondria are the sites of respiration and fatty acid synthesis in eucaryotic cells. The oval or rod-shaped mitochondria are often called the "power houses of the cell" because energy is released from nutrients in the mitochondria during respiration. The chemical reactions of respiration are discussed in Chapter 6. Mitochondria are enclosed by a two-layered membrane and contain

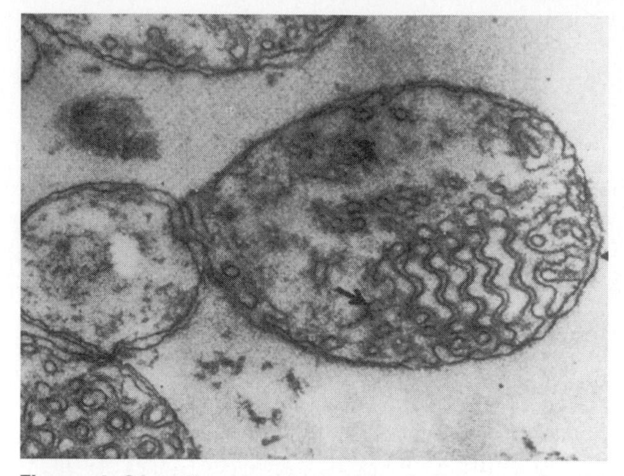

Figure 4–24 ◆ Electron micrograph of a section through part of an ameba *(Pelomyxa carolinensis)* showing a mitochondrion formed by infoldings of the inner membrane. Arrow indicates fibrous inclusions in the matrix space.

inner membranes called **cristae** (Fig. 4–24). Mitochondria vary in size, depending on the species, but most are 1.0 to 2.0 μm long and 0.3 to 0.7 μm wide. Some cells have as many as a thousand mitochondria, but a few types of cells have one very large mitochondrion with connecting branches. Replication of mitochondria can proceed independently of nuclear DNA replication, but the organelles are not completely autonomous.

The membranes of mitochondria resemble plasma membranes of procaryotes in that sterols are not present. Their ribosomes are consistent in size with those found in bacteria. Their resemblance to procaryotes has caused speculation that mitochondria may have evolved from bacterial endosymbionts. However, mitochondrial DNA has sequences differing from chromosomal DNA of procaryotes. Furthermore, the protein-synthesizing systems of mitochondria are unlike those found in ribosomes of procaryotes or eucaryotes. The unique organelles are not merely domesticated procaryotes or ancient relics of eucaryotes. Mitochondria have been able to develop and maintain individuality in the competitive environment of eucaryotic cells.

CHLOROPLASTS

Photosynthesis occurs in algae within distinct pigment-containing, membranous organelles known as **chloroplasts** (Fig. 4–25). Like mitochondria, chloroplasts have double-layered outer and inner membranes. The inner membranes or **thylakoids** are often stacked in parallel arrangements. There are usually many chloroplasts in a single cell. Chloroplasts are spherical or oval bodies measuring 3.0 to 8.0 μm in diameter. The thylakoids possess pigments, like chlorophyll, and enzymes required for photosynthesis. The chemi-

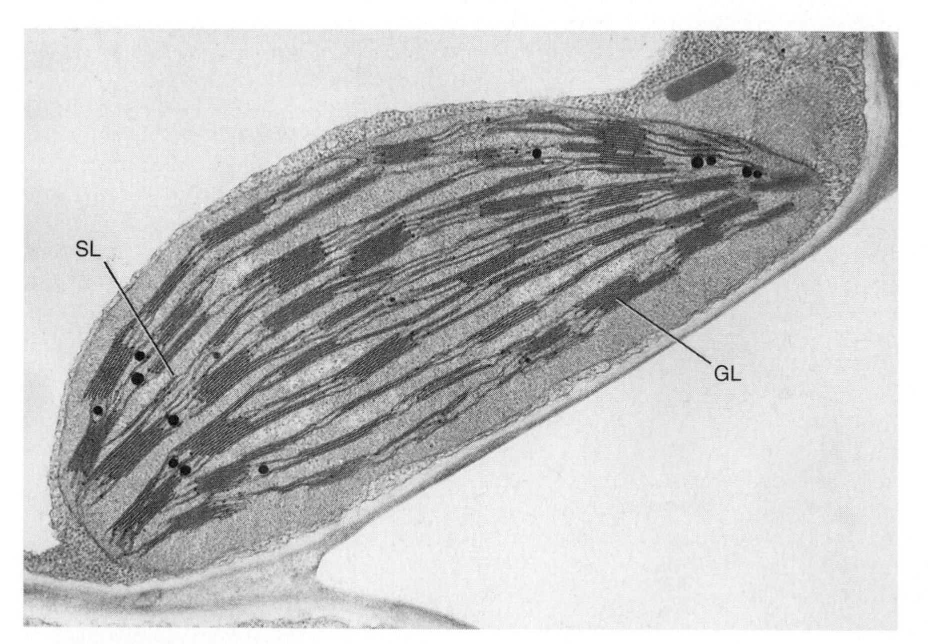

Figure 4–25 ◆ Mature chloroplast containing well-developed internal membrane system consisting of grana lamellae (GL) and stroma lamellae (SL).

cal reactions of photosynthesis are discussed in Chapter 6.

Chloroplasts possess their own DNA and ribosomes that have S values similar to those for procaryotic ribosomes. The susceptibility of chloroplast and bacterial ribosomes to antibiotics is almost identical. Like mitochondria, chloroplasts are self-replicating units, but they do require some proteins coded for by chromosomal DNA. Some scientists trace the origin of chloroplasts to early procaryotes, but if, like the mitochondria, they were derived from endosymbionts, modifications have occurred over the years from living in a protected environment.

THE GOLGI COMPLEX

The **Golgi complex** consists of narrowly stacked membranes, known as **cisternae,** surrounded by vesicles. The membranes are connected to the ER and usually located near the nucleus (Fig. 4–26). The Golgi complex is responsible for modifying and packaging of lipids, proteins, and carbohydrates into more complex structural components. The final products are carried by vesicles to the surfaces of cells, storage depots, or other membranous organelles. Eucaryotic cells depend on the efficient assembly and packaging of molecules in the Golgi complex to maintain the integrity of their parts.

LYSOSOMES

The lysosomes are membranous sacs produced by the Golgi complex which contain large quantities of digestive enzymes (Fig. 4–27). The small sacs, often below the lower limit of resolution of the bright-field microscope, release enzymes when lysosomes fuse with vacuoles or vesicles formed during endocytosis. The confinement of the potent enzymes within enzyme-bound organelles in the cell is advantageous because the enzymes can dissolve (lyse) the cell itself if they escape into the surrounding cytoplasm. Rupture of lysosomal membranes, and subsequent digestion of cell constituents, does occur when a cell dies. Sometimes lysosomes of seemingly healthy cells release their enzymes and cause cell death; for this reason lysosomes are called "suicide bags." The granules of some white blood cells are lysosomes that release enzymes and destroy engulfed pathogens.

CYTOSKELETON

Eucaryotic cells contain a network of microtubules and microfilaments that make up a framework known as the **cytoskeleton.** The tubules and filaments are located throughout the cytoplasm, but are more visible along the margin of the plasma membrane. They anchor organelles, maintain the shape of wall-less cells, and permit some cells to move. Microtubules are made up of an unusual protein called **tubulin.** The tubulin alternates between assembled and disassembled states in different stages of the cell cycle. The presence of the contractile protein **actin** in microfilaments provides those structures with flexibility exhibited by intracellular movements. The dynamic nature of the cytoskeleton can be observed during cell division when the spindle fibers aid the movement of chromosomes to opposite ends of the cell.

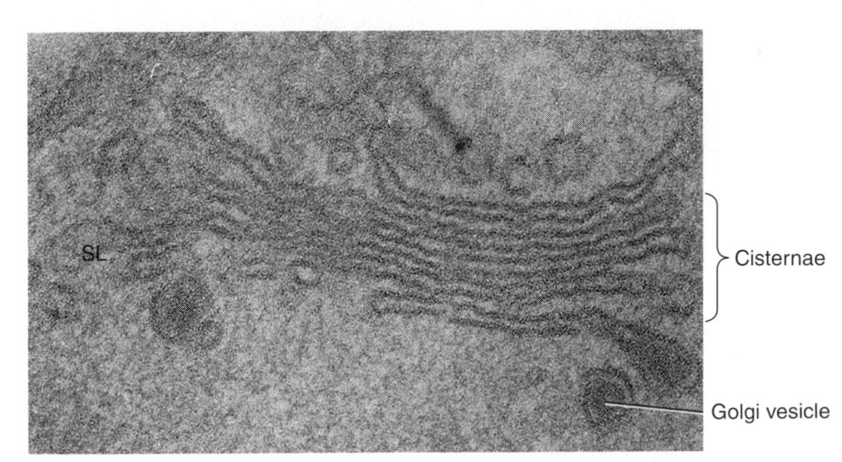

Figure 4–26 ◆ A Golgi complex in the aquatic fungus *Chytridiomyces.*

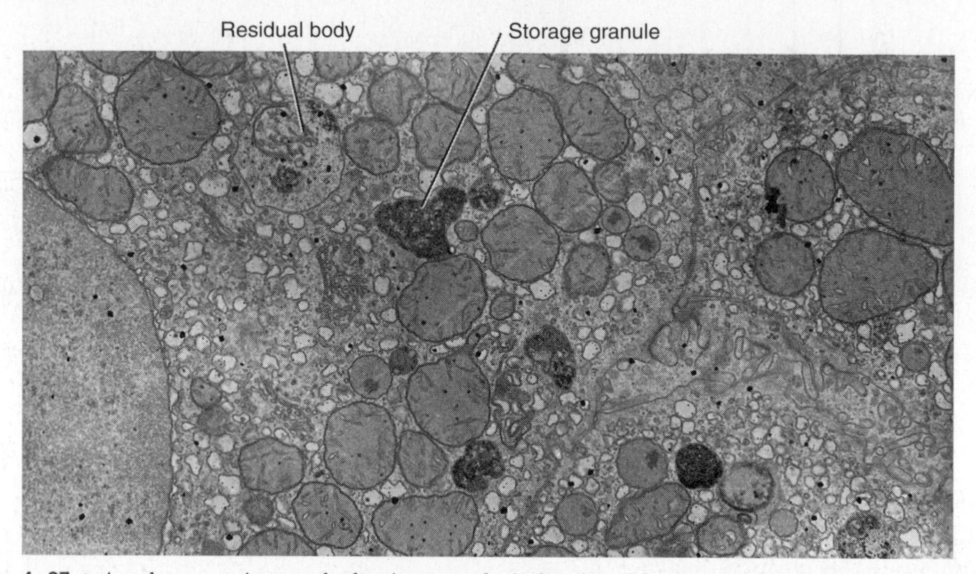

Figure 4–27 ◆ An electron micrograph showing two physical states of lysosomes in a rat kidney cell. The dark irregularly shaped structures are storage granules. The spherical structures are residual bodies.

NUCLEUS

The genetic material of eucaryotic cells is housed in a dense membrane-bound organelle known as the **nucleus.** The nucleus is by far the largest of the organelles and is easily recognized under the low power of a bright-field microscope. Distinct pores in the double-layered nuclear membrane permit large molecules to enter or leave the nucleus (Fig. 4–28). The quantity of DNA is greater in eucaryotic cells than in procaryotes. A yeast cell contains three times as much DNA as do most bacterial cells. The DNA is packaged in units called **chromosomes.**

As one or more small, darker staining areas within the nucleus, **nucleoli** can be observed in some cells. The nucleoli are aggregates of one type of RNA necessary for protein synthesis in ribosomes. Nucleoli, sometimes called karyosomes in nuclei of some trophozoites or cysts of protozoa, are important identifying characteristics.

Some nuclear DNA is complexed with proteins called **histones.** Histones neutralize negative

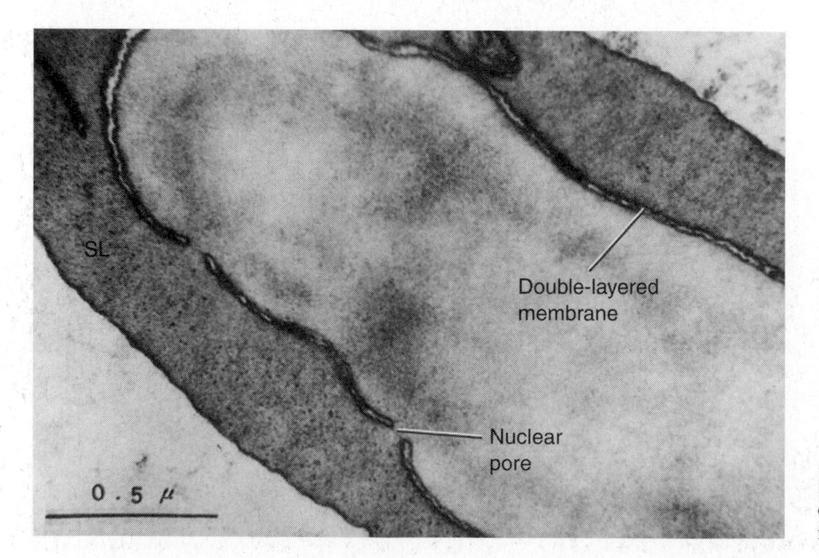

Figure 4–28 ◆ Electron micrograph of a typical eucaryotic cell showing the double-layered nuclear membrane and nuclear pores.

charges on DNA molecules and appear to have a role in condensation of chromatin into chromosomes during cell division. The association of the macromolecules causes spherical subunits, the **nucleosomes,** to form. The nucleosomes are connected by thin strands of naked DNA. The nucleosomes look much like beads spaced at regular intervals on a string. The strands of molecular beads make up the **chromatin** of the nucleus.

PLASMIDS

Small segments of circular DNA are contained in **plasmids** of some fungi. The expression of the extrachromosomal DNA is sometimes independent of chromosomal control. In other instances, the plasmid DNA is subject to regulation by chromosomal DNA. Although bacteria are more commonly used to house genes from plants or animals, yeast cells are also hosts of choice for some genetically engineered products. Genetic engineering techniques are discussed in Chapter 7.

Cysts

Some protozoa form dormant, nonmotile stages known as **cysts** in the presence of unfavorable environmental conditions. Cysts are usually spherical or oval walled structures with one or more nuclei (Fig. 4–29). Unlike endospores of bacteria, cysts are quite susceptible to drying and heat, but will withstand freezing temperatures. Cysts are the infective stages of several protozoa that cause intestinal disease in humans. The cysts are transmitted by contaminated water or food. When the cell wall of a cyst disintegrates, the emerging cells are the motile, feeding trophozoites. The ability to produce cysts is responsible for survival of some protozoa outside the humans or animals they parasitize.

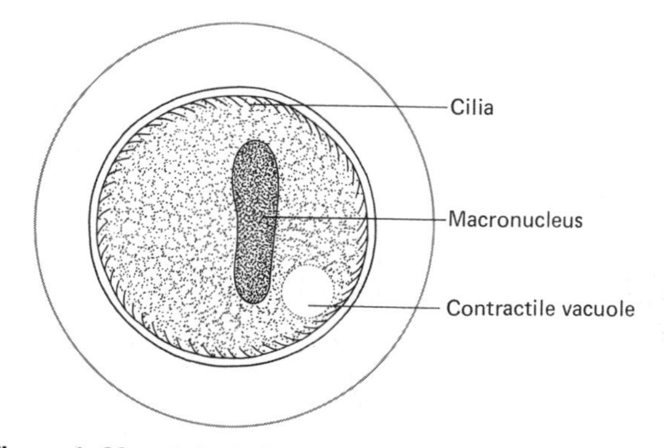

Figure 4–29 ◆ Spherical cyst of the ciliated protozoan *Balantidium coli.* The cyst is responsible for transmission of an intestinal infection.

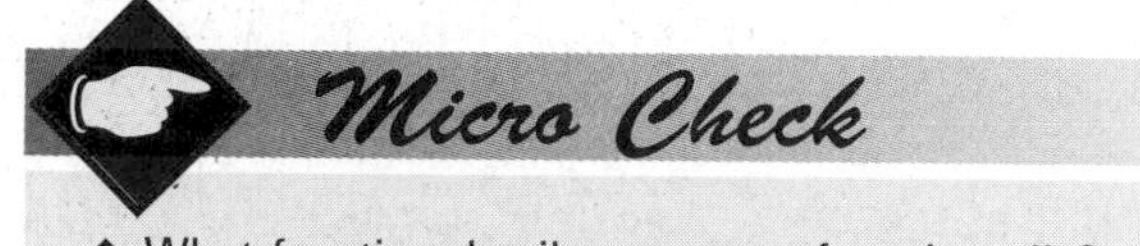

- What function do ribosomes perform in cells?
- Why are mitochondria called "power houses?"
- Explain the difference between a nucleus and a nucleoid.

Understanding Microbiology

1. How do cell walls of gram-negative bacteria differ from those of gram-positive bacteria?
2. Explain how molecules can move across a plasma membrane against a concentration gradient?
3. How do ribosomes of procaryotes differ from those of eucaryotes?
4. What characteristics do mitochondria and chloroplasts have in common?
5. How do some bacilli survive in nutritionally deficient environments?

Applying Microbiology

6. How would you go about telling procaryotes from eucaryotes in a hay infusion under a bright-field microscope?

Unit 2

Growth, Metabolism, and Variation

Chapter 5

Microbial Growth

Chapter Outline

- **THE POPULATION GROWTH CURVE**
  - The Lag Phase
  - The Logarithmic or Exponential Phase
  - The Stationary Phase
  - The Death Phase
  - Significance of a Population-Growth Curve
- **FACTORS INFLUENCING MICROBIAL GROWTH**
  - Temperature
  - Water
  - Osmotic Pressure
  - Salinity
  - Hydrostatic Pressure
  - Atmospheric Conditions
  - pH
  - Light Intensity
  - Nutritional Requirements
- **CULTIVATION OF MICROORGANISMS IN THE LABORATORY**
  - Liquid, Semisolid, and Solid Media
  - Selective and Differential Media
  - Pure Culture Techniques
  - Special Culture Techniques
  - Animal Inoculation
- **CONTINUOUS AND SYNCHRONIZED CULTURES**
  - Continuous Cultures
  - Synchronized Cultures
- **METHODS OF MEASURING GROWTH**
  - Measurements of Cell Mass
  - Measurement of Cell Number

Learning Objectives

After you have read this chapter, you should be able to:

1. Define generation time.
2. Identify the phases of growth on a population-growth curve.
3. Explain why logarithmic growth is rarely encountered in nature.
4. Classify microorganisms according to energy and carbon source.
5. Describe conditions that must be met in the laboratory in order to culture microorganisms.
6. Describe three methods for obtaining isolated colonies of bacteria.
7. Contrast the advantages or disadvantages of direct and indirect estimations of bacterial numbers.

Microbial growth consists of a uniform increase in components of the cell culminating in reproduction. Reproduction occurs when sufficient amounts of biomolecules are available to provide structural and metabolic requirements of two cells. A metabolically active organism capable of reproduction is considered to be **viable.** The time required for growth and reproduction is known as the doubling or **generation time.** Generation time is a function of the rate of growth. The short generation times of some microorganisms account for both beneficial and harmful effects of microorganisms. The rapid generation times of some microorganisms make them ideal

Table 5–1
GENERATION TIMES OF SOME BACTERIA AND FUNGI UNDER OPTIMAL CONDITIONS

ORGANISM	GROWTH TEMPERATURE (°C)	GENERATION TIME (MIN)
Bacillus mycoides	37	28
Escherichia coli	37	12.5
Mycobacterium tuberculosis	37	792–932
Staphylococcus aureus	37	27–30
Treponema pallidum	37	1,980

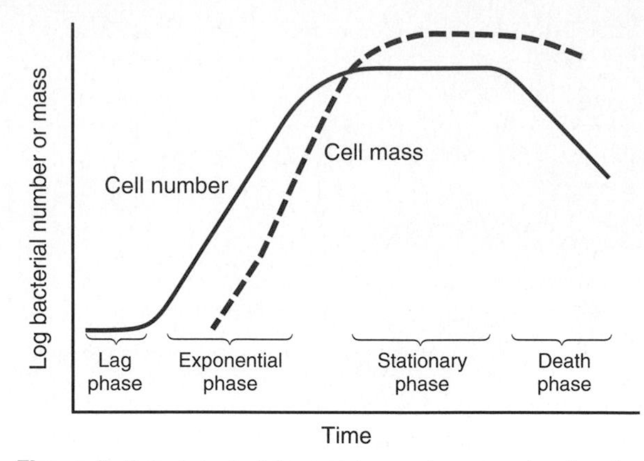

Figure 5–1 ◆ A typical bacterial growth curve showing four phases.

agents to make a variety of useful products by the process of fermentation. Maximal recoveries of products are made possible by supplying optimal conditions for growth. Animal, plant, and human hosts often provide environments that are ideal for growth of microorganisms.

The generation times of procaryotes are usually shorter than those of eucaryotes, but even procaryotes demonstrate wide variation in generation times. *Mycobacterium tuberculosis* and *Treponema pallidum* have exceptionally long generation times, which are responsible for the chronic nature of those diseases. The variations in generation times can be demonstrated in the laboratory by supplying cultures of single species with optimal conditions for growth of cells (Table 5–1).

THE POPULATION GROWTH CURVE

The term growth is usually applied to populations of microorganisms rather than to individual organisms in much the same manner as one refers to the growth in population of a particular geographic area. In the laboratory, four phases of a bacterial growth curve can be demonstrated: (1) lag, 2) logarithmic or exponential, (3) stationary, and (4) death.

The Lag Phase

An identifiable **lag phase** occurs when bacteria are transferred to a fresh culture medium (Fig. 5–1). During the lag phase, bacteria are adjusting to a new environment and the number of cells does not increase appreciably. However, the cells are metabolically active, synthesizing the biomolecules in preparation for cell division. Cells divide at different rates because concentrations of enzymes and coenzymes vary. Therefore, a very gradual increase in cell population occurs.

The Logarithmic or Exponential Phase

The lag phase is followed by the **logarithmic** or **exponential phase** when the rate of growth increases with time. Each bacterium placed in a supporting medium divides by binary fission into two cells. When those two cells each divide, there are four cells. Each time binary fission occurs, there is a doubling in numbers of bacteria under favorable growth conditions (Table 5–2). If a

Table 5–2
INCREASE IN CELL COUNT AS A RESULT OF BINARY FISSION

GENERATION NUMBER	CELL COUNT
0	1
1	2
2	4
3	8
4	16
5	32
6	64
7	128
8	256
9	512
10	1,024
20	1,048,576

culture medium is inoculated with 10^6 cells, only 20 generations would produce a staggering number of cells.

Very large populations of microorganisms are needed to produce observable results in laboratory tests. These large populations necessitate that a logarithmic, rather than an arithmetic, scale be used to represent populations during growth phases. A logarithm is an algebraic shorthand using small numbers and exponents for expressing huge numbers, as found in these populations. Logarithmic growth can be observed with pure cultures in the laboratory, but such growth rarely is encountered in nature. This is because most microorganisms do not experience pure culture conditions in nature, and therefore, optimal growth conditions are not sustained over long periods of time.

The Stationary Phase

A number of factors limit population growth. An essential nutrient may be depleted, or products of metabolism may accumulate. Ultimately, a **stationary phase** occurs in which the total number of viable cells remains constant. A depletion of nutrients causes cells to be smaller. Toxic metabolic products limit cell division. The stationary phase may last for a few hours to several days.

The Death Phase

The death phase begins when growth stops and the number of dead cells outnumber the viable cells. Death is caused primarily by the hostile environment created by toxic waste products. The death phase continues until most, if not all, microorganisms die. The rate of the death phase does not always occur exponentially. Some species of bacteria, particularly spore-formers, demonstrate remarkable resistance to the cumulative factors limiting growth and will survive if transferred to a new culture medium.

Significance of a Population Growth Curve

Information obtained from growth curves of particular bacteria under controlled conditions provides essential information to microbiologists. Microorganisms are most active metabolically during the logarithmic phase. Because identification of species requires the use of a variety of substrates and determination of end products, microorganisms ideally should be transferred during the logarithmic phase. Moreover, if industrial fermentation processes are to yield maximal amounts of end products, nutritional requirements and growth rates of microorganisms must be understood.

Micro Check

- What is the advantage of expressing numbers as logarithms?
- Which growth phase of bacteria is constant with time?
- What factors limit bacterial growth?

FACTORS INFLUENCING MICROBIAL GROWTH

The natural habitats of microorganisms reveal a great diversity in environmental conditions. Microbial populations are a reflection of physical and chemical parameters of the immediate surroundings of microorganisms. An environmental factor required by one microorganism may limit the growth of another one. For example, some microorganisms can tolerate extremes of temperature, high osmotic pressure, and a wide range of other atmospheric conditions. Others have a very limited range in which they can grow and reproduce.

Changing environmental conditions and competition for nutrients prevent the expansion of microbial populations in nature. In medical laboratories and industrial fermentation plants, efforts are made to create ideal environmental conditions for particular organisms. Competition is eliminated permitting sufficient growth to identify disease-producing microorganisms or to recover specific products.

Temperature

Almost all microorganisms grow over a broad range of temperatures, but optimal growth is obtained over a relatively narrow range. The lowest temperature supporting growth of an organism is the **minimal growth temperature;** the highest temperature supporting growth is the **maximal growth temperature.**

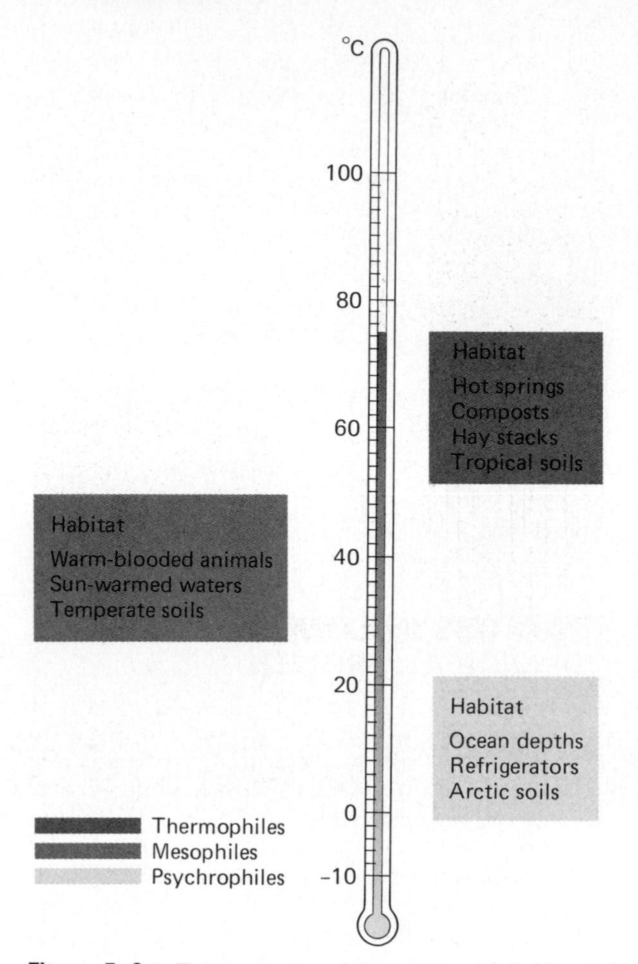

Figure 5–2 ◆ Temperature growth ranges and habitats of psychrophiles, mesophiles, and thermophiles.

MESOPHILES

The **optimal growth temperature** for most medically important bacteria ranges between 20° and 45°C (Fig. 5–2). These organisms are called **mesophiles.** Disease-producing microorganisms often grow best at temperatures optimal for growth of the cells of their hosts. In medical laboratories, human pathogens are usually grown in incubators having thermostats which maintain temperatures at 37°C. Some fungi grow better at 30°C.

THERMOPHILES

Microorganisms that grow best at temperatures of 45°C or above are called **thermophiles** (heat-loving). Thermophiles occur in many natural environments such as hot springs, deep-sea hydrothermal vents, tropical soil composts, and haystacks. The spontaneous combustion of stacked hay is caused, in part, by thermophilic action producing temperatures as high as 75°C. Bacteria even occur in boiling-water environments, where many reproduce quite well. Members of the genus *Pyrodictium* found in a thermal vent off the coast of Italy are able to grow at temperatures up to 110°C. The growth of most photosynthetic procaryotes is limited by temperatures of 70° to 73°C. Most eucaryotic microorganisms cannot tolerate a temperature above 60°C.

The optimal temperature limits have been determined for a number of thermophiles. Thermophiles may play a significant role in the biotechnology of the future. The efficiency of many fermentative processes could be increased immeasurably if thermophiles could be used instead of the usual heat-sensitive mesophiles.

PSYCHROPHILES

Microorganisms that can grow at 0°C or lower and have an optimal growth temperature of about 15°C are called **psychrophiles** or **cryophiles** (cold-loving). These organisms are found at great depths in the oceans or in the soil in areas with cold climates. Representative examples of psychrophiles may be found among the algae, fungi,

Table 5–3
CLASSIFICATION OF BACTERIA BY SOURCES OF ENERGY AND CARBON

NUTRITIONAL TYPE	ENERGY SOURCE	CARBON SOURCE	REPRESENTATIVE GENERA
Photoautotroph	Light	CO_2	*Chromatium, Thiospirillum*
Photoheterotroph	Light	Organic molecules	*Rhodomicrobium, Rhodospirillum*
Chemoautotroph	Inorganic molecules	CO_2	*Sphaerotilus, Nitrosomonas*
Chemoheterotroph	Organic molecules	Organic molecules	*Escherichia, Pseudomonas*

and bacteria. The pink snow that can be observed at high altitudes in many parts of the world is caused by growth of the red alga *Chlamydomonas nivalis.* Psychrophiles are difficult to study because they are often killed by even brief exposure to higher temperatures.

True psychrophiles must not be confused with **psychrotrophs,** which grow very slowly at 0°C, but have an optimal growth temperature range of 25° to 30°C. These organisms are abundant in nature and can cause food spoilage at refrigerator temperatures.

Water

The most abundant molecule in all forms of life is water. Microorganisms contain at least 70 percent water. Water participates in most chemical reactions of cells. It is lost in condensation reactions when a hydrogen ion (H^+) from one functional group on a monomer and a hydroxyl ion (OH^-) from another monomer combine. Conversely, water is required to break down polymers by **hydrolysis.**

Water also participates in the formation of hydrogen bonds when hydrogen and oxygen atoms from different molecules are attracted to one another. Hydrogen bonding is responsible for shape and chemical characteristics of large molecules, such as proteins and nucleic acids.

Water is capable of dissolving many different substances. Chemical compounds having the ability to store dissolved substances in solution are called **solvents.** The dissolved substances are called **solutes.** Solutes are transported across plasma membranes with water molecules.

Water is an essential component of all natural and artificial media. The hydrogen bonds of water molecules insulate microorganisms from sudden changes in temperature.

The availability of water in the environment is expressed as A_W or water activity. As less water is available, growth rates decrease (Fig. 5–3).

The amount of water necessary to support metabolic activities varies among microorganisms. Some can survive for long periods of time; others are very sensitive to the lack of an available source of water. This is cause for concern in transporting swabs taken from certain body sites in the isolation of *Neisseria gonorrhoeae.* A transport medium is frequently inoculated immediately at the collection site prior to being sent to the laboratory. The special medium minimizes drying of specimens on swabs.

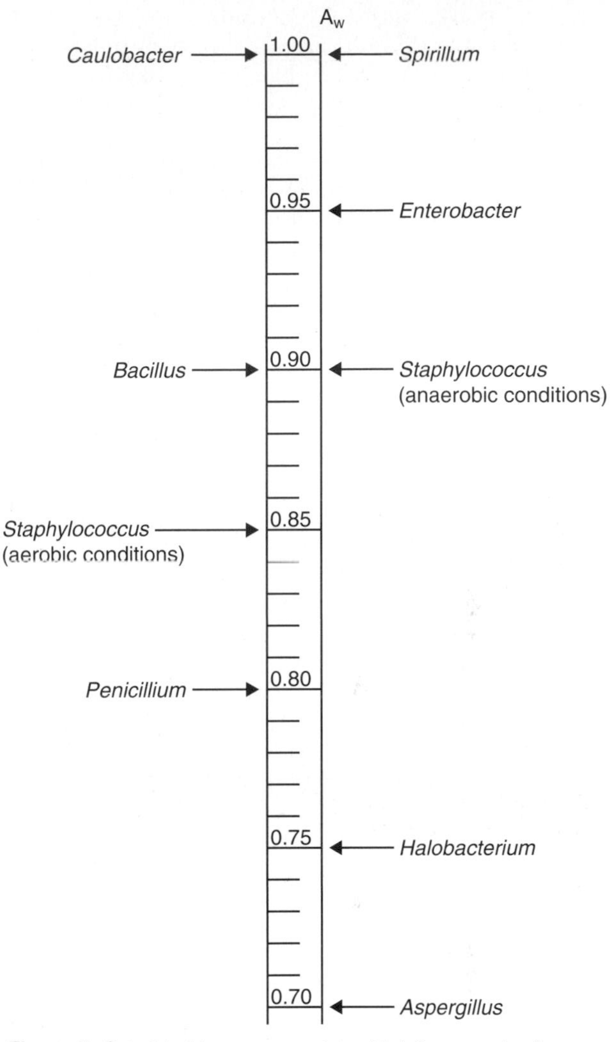

Figure 5–3 ◆ Limiting water activity (A_w) for growth of some bacteria and fungi.

Osmotic Pressure

Most microorganisms do not tolerate an environment in which the concentration of solutes exceeds by far that in the cells. Although most microorganisms with cell walls can tolerate solute concentrations of 1 to 2 percent, optimal growth is obtained when solute concentrations in cells and the environment are the same (isotonic).

A higher solute concentration in cells than in the environment facilitates the movement of water molecules into cells. A lower solute concentration in cells than in the environment causes water molecules to leave the cell. A solute concentration which is greater than that contained in cells constitutes a **hypertonic** environment. A solute concentration of the environment surrounding cells which is less than that found in cells is described as **hypotonic.** Sufficient uptake or loss of water results in cell destruction (see Chap. 4). The force with which water molecules move through the plasma membrane is known as **osmotic pressure.** Microorganisms that can grow in the presence of excess solutes are called **osmotolerant.** Other microorganisms, known as **osmophiles,** require high solute concentrations for optimal growth.

Salinity

Although most microorganisms cannot tolerate hypertonic concentrations of sodium chloride (NaCl) in the environment, some require it for optimal growth. Others do not need a high level of salinity, but can tolerate relatively high concentrations of NaCl. The **obligate halophiles** (salt-requiring) bacteria include archaea belonging to the genera *Halobacterium* and *Halococcus* found in saline lakes and basins where levels of NaCl approximate the saturation level. Other obligate halophiles, which grow optimally at concentrations of about 3.5 percent NaCl, are found in the oceans of the world. The **facultative halophiles** (salt-tolerating) bacteria can live in concentrations of NaCl up to 10 percent. Facultative halophiles include *Staphylococcus aureus,* the cause of many skin infections, and *Enterococcus fecalis,* a normal inhabitant of the intestinal tract.

The high salt tolerance of staphylococci and enterococci explains their ability to survive on skin surfaces despite the concentration of salt in sweat. It also explains the availability of staphylococci to enter even small breaks in the skin and cause serious infections.

The ability of bacteria to tolerate high NaCl concentrations is the basis of some selective culturing procedures. An interesting relationship exists between temperatures and salt requirements in some lactic acid bacteria. In general, optimal temperatures are higher as concentrations of NaCl in the environment are increased.

Hydrostatic Pressure

Another type of environmental pressure exerted on aquatic microorganisms is **hydrostatic pressure** from the weight of water. Most microorganisms are inhibited by hydrostatic pressures of 200 to 600 atmospheres (atm), which would be equivalent to a depth of 2000 to 4000 meters of ocean. Those than can survive under conditions of increased hydrostatic pressure are called **barotolerant.** Microorganisms that grow best at high hydrostatic pressures are true **barophiles.** True barophiles are found only in the deepest parts of oceans.

Atmospheric Conditions

Many microorganisms require molecular oxygen (O_2) to carry on metabolic activities. Other microorganisms generate energy by biochemical pathways in which O_2 is not involved. **Obligate aerobes** grow only in the presence of O_2. **Obligate anaerobes** grow only in the absence of O_2. The presence of O_2 not only inhibits growth but is highly toxic to some obligate anaerobes.

The reason for the extreme O_2 sensitivity of some bacteria is not well understood, but is believed to be related to the anaerobe's inability to destroy toxic forms of O_2, produced as metabolic waste products. The alternate forms of oxygen, are superoxide (O_2^-) and hydrogen peroxide (H_2O_2). The destruction of these toxic products requires the enzymes superoxide dismutase and catalase. One or both enzymes are found in aerotolerant organisms. The breakdown of O_2 to singlet oxygen (O_2^-) occurs in two steps:

$$20_2^- + H_2 \xrightarrow[\text{dismutase}]{\text{superoxide}} H_2O_2 + O_2\uparrow$$

$$2H_2O_2 \xrightarrow{\text{catalase}} 2H_2O + O_2\uparrow$$

Facultative bacteria grow in the presence or absence of oxygen. Many yeast and enteric bacteria have both aerobic and anaerobic pathways. In nature the facultative anaerobes have great survival capacity because they can shift "metabolic gears" in response to atmospheric conditions.

Microaerophilic bacteria require O_2 in quantities less than that found in the atmosphere. Capneic bacteria need carbon dioxide (CO_2) in amounts greater than that found under ordinary atmospheric conditions. Growth of many pathogens is stimulated by increased concentrations of CO_2. Moreover, CO_2 is an important reactant in some biosynthetic pathways.

Knowledge of atmospheric requirements for particular types of microorganisms must be considered in obtaining, transporting, and culturing materials suspected of containing certain microorganisms.

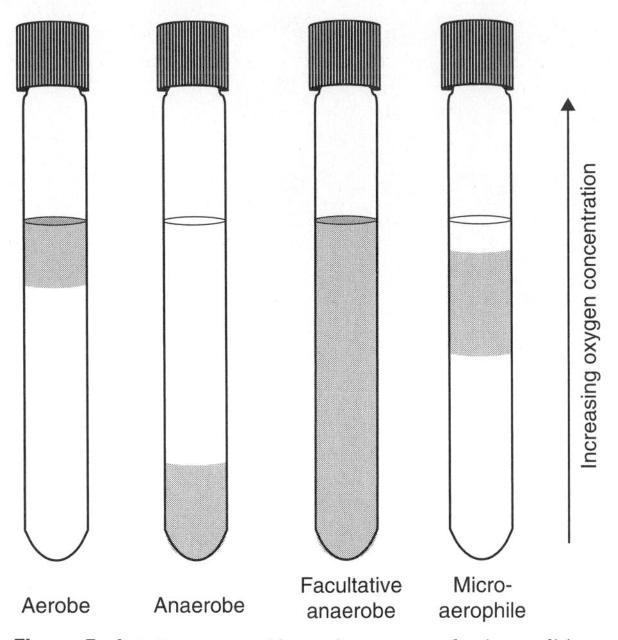

Figure 5–4 ◆ Response of bacteria to atmospheric conditions in thioglycolate broth.

A reducing agent, such as sodium thioglycolate, can also create degrees of anaerobiosis when it is added to a liquid containing essential nutrients. The sodium thioglycolate binds to any O_2 which diffuses into the medium from the atmosphere. If a tube of the broth is boiled to remove as much O_2 as possible before it is inoculated, obligate aerobes grow near the surface and obligate anaerobes grow in the bottom (Fig. 5–4). Microaerophilic organisms grow in an intermediate zone where O_2 tension is reduced, and facultative anaerobes grow throughout the tube.

Anaerobes may also be isolated by using a sealed jar containing a pack that generates H_2 and CO_2 in the presence of a platinum catalyst (Fig. 5–5). Atmospheric oxygen is eliminated in the sealed jar when it combines with hydrogen to form water. Some laboratories employ anaerobic growth chambers, which maintain an O_2-free atmosphere for inoculating specimens suspected of containing anaerobes (Fig. 5–6). Capneic organisms are often grown in a CO_2 incubator where atmospheric concentration is controlled by a gauge connected to a tank of CO_2.

pH

Almost all microorganisms grow best at a pH approximating neutrality, but will tolerate mild acidic or alkaline environments (Table 5–4). Some species of *Thiobacillus* are remarkable bacteria because optimal growth is obtained at a pH of about 2.0. Such bacteria have developed adaptive mechanisms for dealing with a high hydrogen ion (H^+) concentration.

A vibrio, *Helicobacter pylori,* thrives on gastric epithelium despite the acidity of the stomach and is believed to be the cause of peptic ulcers. The ability of the organism to survive in such a hostile environment has been attributed to ammonia released by the action of the enzyme urease.

Several groups of archaea are thermoacidophiles that grow at high temperatures and a low pH. The three major groups of archaea are discussed in Chapter 8. A few bacteria, such as the vibrio that causes cholera, grow at a pH of 8.5 or greater. Fungi are more acid tolerant than bacteria and many grow best at a pH of 5.0 to 6.0. Differing requirements for pH can be used in selecting for growth of particular microorganisms.

The pH of culture media is controlled by the addition of substances known as buffers, which resist changes in pH. The buffers stabilize pH by combining either with hydrogen ions (H^+) of

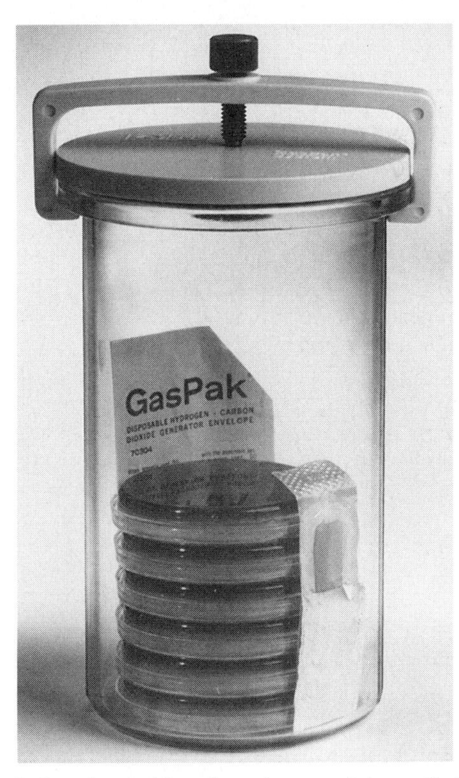

Figure 5–5 ◆ Anaerobic culture jar containing a GasPak envelope for generating H_2 and CO_2.

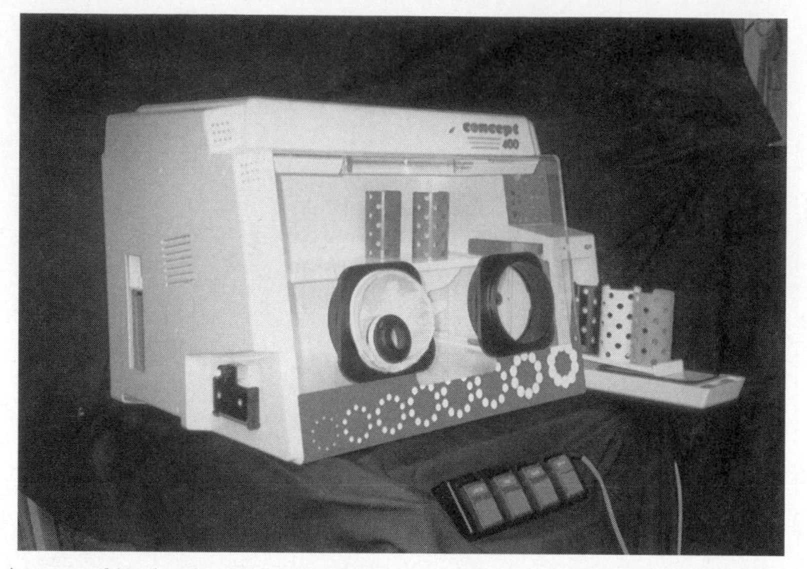

Figure 5–6 ◆ An anaerobic chamber which maintains an oxygen-free atmosphere. Hands and arms are placed through glove ports to inoculate media.

strong acids to produce weak acids or with hydroxyl ions (OH^-) of strong bases to form weak acids and water:

$$H^+ + HPO_4^{2-} \longrightarrow H_2PO_4^-$$

$$OH^- + H_2PO_4^- \longrightarrow HPO_4^{2-} + HOH$$

Disodium phosphate (Na_2HPO_4) and monosodium phosphate (NaH_2PO_4) are often used in combination to obtain a final pH of 7.0 in culture media. Depletion of buffers allows acid or alkaline metabolites to accumulate and limits growth.

Light Intensity

Although photosynthetic microorganisms require light to carry out life-sustaining activities, high intensities of ultraviolet (UV) and visible light are harmful to other microorganisms. Both proteins and nucleic acid absorb UV, but nucleic acids mutate easily when exposed to light. The effect of UV on DNA is discussed in Chapter 21. Large quantities of visible light activate cytochromes and flavins of nonphotosynthetic microorganisms. However, instead of the energy being diverted to an energy-requiring reaction, it is dissipated to produce potentially lethal free radicals. The free radicals can damage proteins or nucleic acids, causing cell death. Pigmented bacteria can tolerate higher intensities of light than nonpig-

Table 5–4
EXAMPLES OF ENRICHMENT MEDIA

MEDIUM	ENRICHMENT	RECOMMENDED USE
Blood agar	Sheep blood	Good general purpose medium for isolation of pathogens
Charcoal yeast extract	Yeast extract	Isolation of *Legionella* species
Chocolate agar	Hemoglobin, yeast extract	Isolation of *Neisseria* and *Haemophilus* species
Nagler agar	Egg yolk	Isolation of *Clostridium* species
Mueller-Hinton agar	Starch	Antimicrobial susceptibility tests

mented forms because the pigments absorb light rays preventing susceptible molecules from being damaged.

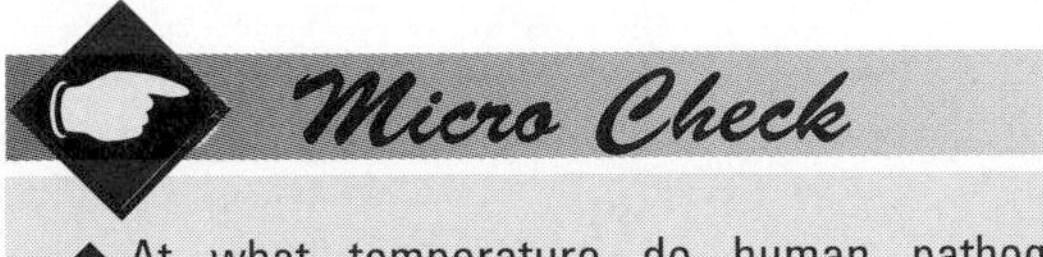

- At what temperature do human pathogens grow best?
- Where are true barophiles found?
- How can the sensitivity of microorganisms to light be explained?

Nutritional Requirements

The nutritional requirements of particular microorganisms differ even more substantially than their physical needs. Microorganisms absorb energy from the sun or release energy from nutrients. Organisms that derive energy from the sun are called **phototrophs,** whereas those which obtain energy from chemical compounds are known as **chemotrophs.** The pathways for the generation of energy by photosynthesis, fermentation, and respiration are discussed in Chapter 6. Specific atoms of nutrients are necessary for microbial growth.

CARBON

Carbon atoms are essential constituents of the molecules of life. Some microorganisms obtain carbon from atmospheric carbon dioxide. They are called **autotrophs** to distinguish them from **heterotrophs,** which depend on organic compounds for carbon. Microorganisms may be classified according to their energy and carbon sources as **photoautotrophs, chemoautotrophs, photoheterotrophs,** and **chemoheterotrophs** (see Table 5–3). The prefixes "photo-" (light) and "chemo-" (chemical compound) indicate the source of energy. "Hetero-" refers to sources of carbon other than or different from carbon dioxide used by autotrophs.

The versatility of microorganisms can be seen in the types of organic compounds that serve as carbon and energy sources. Many chemoheterotrophs derive their carbon and energy sources from the same organic compounds. For example,

FOCAL POINT

The Chemoautotrophic Way of Life

The Russian Sergei Winogradsky (1856–1953) and the Dutchman Martinus Beijerninck (1851–1931) first described the chemoautotrophic way of life. The significance of their findings was somewhat eclipsed by the interest in microorganisms emerging as agents of infectious disease. Eventually the role of microorganisms as geochemical agents responsible for large-scale chemical transformations in nature was recognized largely because of the painstaking efforts of Winogradsky and Beijerninck.

In order to study microorganisms that could grow in an environment devoid of organic sources of energy and carbon, these two men used an **enrichment-culture** technique with media of defined inorganic chemical composition. The technique permitted a single metabolic type to predominate in media inoculated with soil. In 1887 Winogradsky described a large bacterium, *Beggiatoa,* which did not require organic material for growth but which thrived in an environment rich in hydrogen sulfide (H_2S). The filamentous bacterium was able to oxidize H_2S as a source of energy with the formation of intracellular elemental sulfur deposits and use carbon dioxide (CO_2) as a source of carbon. The sulfur was further oxidized to sulfates. Later Winogradsky studied iron bacteria which grew if supplied with a high content of reduced iron salts. By using a medium devoid of combined nitrogen, but containing other requirements, Winogradsky was also able to demonstrate an anaerobic nitrifying spore-forming soil bacterium, which he named *Clostridium pasteurianum* after Pasteur. Beijerninck altered atmospheric conditions to provide an aerobic environment to demonstrate bacterial nitrifiers belonging to the genus *Azotobacter* in soil.

The great metabolic versatility of microorganisms enables them to live in some extreme habitats in which most plants and animals cannot exist. In recent years, the chemoautotrophic way of life has taken on increased significance with the discovery of the ability of bacteria of hydrothermal vents to support complete ecosystems in the deepest parts of the sea.

some species of *Pseudomonas* can use over 90 organic compounds as sources of carbon and energy. *Pseudomonas* organisms can be particularly troublesome in the hospital environment. Their ability to use so many carbon sources enables them to grow in liquid soap dispensers and some respiratory therapy equipment. Many of the metabolic genes in those organisms are plasmid encoded.

NITROGEN

All life forms require nitrogen (N). Many bacteria make enzymes that degrade proteins to amino acids. Other bacteria obtain nitrogen from inorganic sources, such as nitrites (NO_2^-), nitrates (NO_3^-), and ammonium (NH_4^+) compounds. A fewer number are able to reduce atmospheric nitrogen independently or in association with plants known as legumes in a process known as **nitrogen fixation** (see Chap. 23). Nitrogen is an essential component of proteins.

SULFUR AND PHOSPHORUS

Sulfur (S) and phosphorus (P) requirements of microorganisms can be met by organic or inorganic compounds. Inorganic salts of sulfates (SO_4^{3-}), sulfides (S^{2-}), and thiosulfates (SH^-) are common sources of sulfur. The need for S in a reduced form can be met. by supplying microorganisms with the sulfur-containing amino acids, cysteine, or methionine. The requirement for P may be met by inorganic salts of phosphates (PO_4^{3-}) and less frequently by phosphorus-containing organic molecules. The lack of availability of soluble PO_4^{3-} salts is often a limiting factor for growth of microorganisms in nature.

OTHER MINERALS

Microorganisms require other minerals, such as potassium (K^+), magnesium (Mg^{2+}), calcium (Ca^{2+}), molybdenum (Mo^{2+}), manganese (Mn^{2+}), divalent iron (Fe^{2+}), trivalent iron (Fe^{3+}), and zinc (Zn^{2+}), in trace amounts. Many enzymes are activated only in the presence of these elements. Potassium (K^+) and manganese (Mg^{2+}) are important in the synthesis of proteins. Divalent iron (Fe^{2+}) and trivalent iron (Fe^{3+}) are needed for synthesis of cytochromes and the enzymes catalase and peroxidase. Zinc (Zn^{2+}) and manganese (Mn^{2+}) activate certain hydrolytic enzymes. Calcium (Ca^{2+}) is an important component of bacterial spores. Cobalt (Co^{2+}) and molybdenum (Mo^{2+}) are required for vitamin B_{12} synthesis and nitrogen reduction, respectively.

GROWTH FACTORS

Growth factors are small organic compounds that include vitamins, amino acids, purines, pyrimidines, and porphyrins. If they are not synthesized in sufficient amounts by microorganisms to support growth, they must be supplied in the environment. The lactic acid bacteria, such as *Lactobacillus* and *Streptococcus* species, depend on an environmental source for some amino acids and vitamins. Some members of the genus *Haemophilus* grow only in the presence of hemin (X factor) and NAD (V factor). Other *Haemophilus* species require only one of the growth factors.

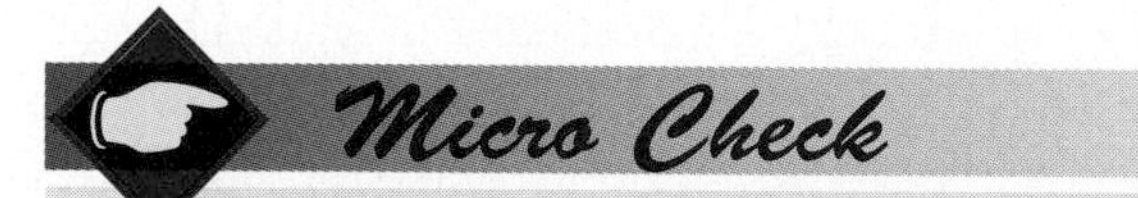

- Where do obligate chemoautotrophs obtain carbon?
- From what inorganic sources do microorganisms obtain nitrogen?
- Of what importance are minerals in microbial nutrition?

CULTIVATION OF MICROORGANISMS IN THE LABORATORY

The successful cultivation of microorganisms depends on the availability of appropriate nutrients and environmental conditions. Substances that support the growth of microorganisms are called **media.** Some microorganisms grow well on simple media containing glucose and minimal salts; others require special growth factors. A few will not grow on any nonliving material.

Mixtures in which all components are known are called **defined media**. All defined culture media must contain available sources of energy, carbon, nitrogen, water, and inorganic salts. **Complex media** may consist of ill-defined mixtures of ingredients that supply essential nutrients. The ingredients of a culture medium and atmospheric conditions can be adjusted to meet growth requirements of particular organisms.

One can provide requirements for a specific metabolic type by enrichment with particular growth factors. Media that contain specific growth factors or ingredients are called **enriched media.** Atmospheric conditions can be adjusted to provide necessary aerobic or anaerobic environments. Media used to cultivate human pathogens are often enriched with materials, such as yeast extract or sheep blood, known to be good sources of nutrients (Table 5–4). Some microorganisms grow poorly or not at all under laboratory conditions because it is impossible to duplicate conditions of nature or the human host.

Various defined culture media are available commercially in dehydrated form. Water is added to carefully weighed amounts of the powdered products. Frequently, heat must be applied to solubilize ingredients before dispensing them in suitable tubes, bottles, or Petri plates. Media must be free of microbial contamination if organisms are to be grown in pure culture. Sterilization is accomplished by autoclaving, by exposure to flowing steam for intermittent periods, or by filtration processes described in Chapter 21.

Many laboratories find it more convenient to purchase sterile media ready for use. Commercially prepared media are subjected to rigid quality control procedures to ensure reliability and reproducibility of test results.

Liquid, Semisolid, and Solid Media

Components of culture media may be supplied in tubes or bottles as **liquid media,** called broths. The consistency of a liquid medium may be modified by the addition of a solidifying agent, such as agar or gelatin, to change it to a **semisolid** or a **solid medium.** Liquid and semisolid media are usually dispensed in tubes, but solid media are dispensed in Petri plates or slanted in tubes or bottles to provide maximal surfaces for growing bacteria or fungi.

Enriched broths are used to grow bacteria which may be few in number in specimens obtained from patients. Semisolid media is valuable in establishing patterns of growth or motility. Solid media is used to obtain pure colonies of any organisms present.

Selective and Differential Media

Media that inhibit the growth of unwanted organisms and allow the growth of others are called **selective media** (Table 5–5). Dyes, salts, or antimicrobial agents can be added to media to inhibit the growth of particular organisms. For example, cycloheximide and chloramphenicol are sometimes added to media designed to culture pathogenic fungi to prevent growth of contaminating fungi and bacteria. Selective media are useful in isolating bacteria or fungi from specimens containing more than one organism.

Media designed to separate organisms based on type of growth or end products of metabolic reactions are called **differential media.** Differential media contain particular substrates, dyes, salts, or pH indicators that make it possible to divide organisms into two or more groups. For example, if a pH indicator such as phenol red, is added to lactose broth, fermentation of lactose can be detected by a color change of red to yellow.

Enriched and selective media may be classified as differential media as well if they make it possible to differentiate between two or more groups of organisms. For example, blood agar, containing 5 to 10 percent sheep blood, permits the

Table 5–5
EXAMPLES OF SELECTIVE MEDIA

MEDIUM	INHIBITORY AGENTS	SELECTIVITY*
Columbia colistin-nalidixic (CNA) agar	Colistin, nalidixic acid	Aerobic and facultative gram-positive bacteria
Eosin methylene blue (EMB) agar	Eosin, methylene blue	Enteric gram-negative bacilli
MacConkey's (MAC) agar	Crystal violet, bile salts	Enteric gram-negative bacilli
Mannitol-salt (MS) agar	7.5% sodium chloride	Salt-tolerant staphylococci
Sabouraud's agar	Acid pH, glucose	Fungi
Thayer-Martin agar	Vancomycin, colistin, nystatin	*Neisseria* species

*These microorganisms will grow on the medium.

more fastidious organisms to grow, but also differentiates organisms based on the amount of hemolysis (destruction of red blood cells) produced surrounding colonies. A green zone of discoloration around colonies indicates partial destruction of red blood cells and is called **alpha hemolysis.** A clear zone around colonies indicates complete destruction of red blood cells and is called **beta hemolysis.**

Mannitol salt agar is an example of a medium selective for growing staphylococci. The high salt concentration inhibits the growth of most other bacteria. In a medium called eosin methylene blue (EMB) agar, the dyes eosin and methylene blue are used to inhibit the growth of gram-positive bacteria. If lactose is added to EMB agar, the medium will differentiate lactose-fermenting from nonlactose-fermenting gram-negative bacteria. The lactose fermenters produce colored colonies on EMB agar.

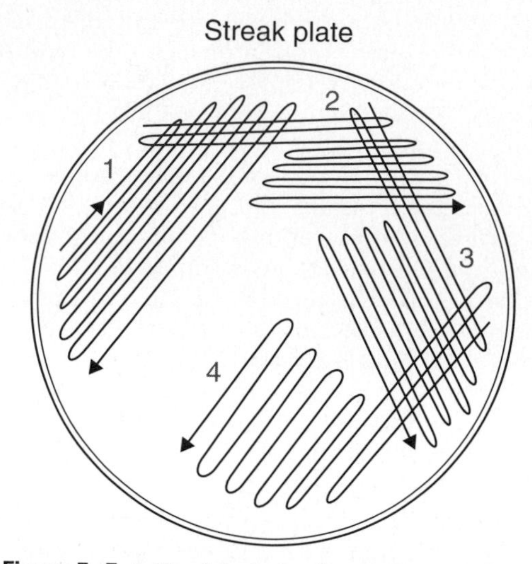

Figure 5–7 ◆ The "clock-plate" method of streaking.

Pure Culture Techniques

The identification of bacteria depends on isolating colonies containing a single species of an organism. Isolation of bacteria can be accomplished by use of three techniques: (1) a streak plate, (2) a pour plate, or (3) a spread plate.

The **streak-plate** technique uses an inoculating loop for isolating bacteria on the surface of agar in a process called streaking. Patterns of streaking vary, but the purpose is to disperse the original inoculum so that pure colonies of organisms are obtained (Fig. 5–7). It is necessary to have pure colonies to identify bacteria and perform antibiotic susceptibility tests.

In the **pour-plate** technique, bacteria are inoculated into a tube of melted agar cooled to a temperature of 45° to 47°C, mixed, and poured into a sterile Petri plate (Fig. 5–8). An alternative procedure is sometimes used in which dilutions of milk water, food, or soil samples are placed directly into sterile Petri plates before adding melted and cooled sterile nutrient agar.

The **spread-plate** technique requires that surfaces of plates be well dried before inoculation. A small amount of a liquid inoculum is placed in the center of an agar medium in a plate and spread over the surface with a bent sterile glass rod (Fig. 5–9). Plates must be allowed to dry an hour or two before inverting them for incubation.

It is important that all inoculated plates be incubated in an inverted position with the bottom agar-containing part of the Petri plate on top. Positioning plates in this manner prevents condensed moisture on the lid from dripping onto the surface of the agar. Any excess moisture on the surface of agar prevents the isolation of

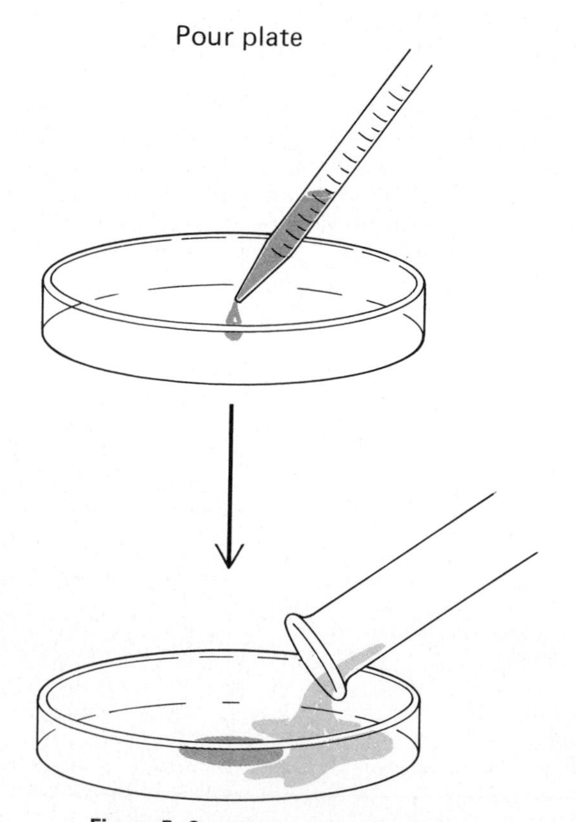

Figure 5–8 ◆ The pour-plate technique.

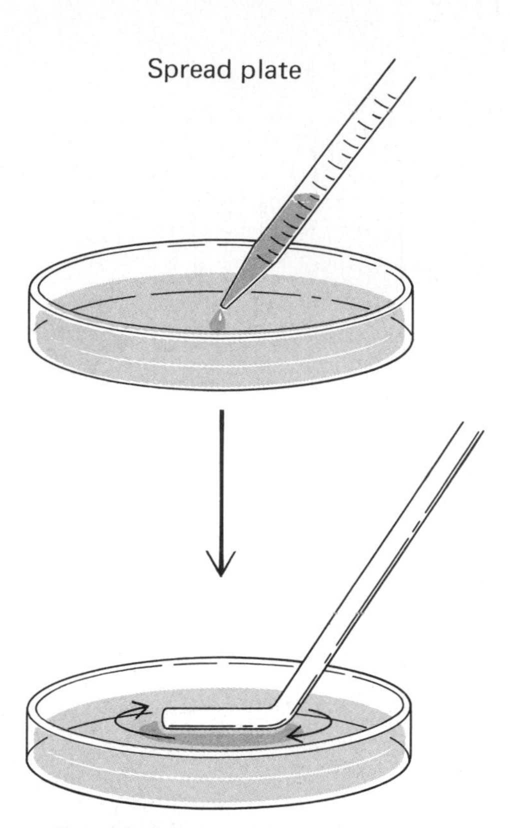

Figure 5–9 ◆ The spread-plate technique.

distinct colonies, causing them to develop instead as a single mass of growth.

Incubated pour plates contain both surface and subsurface colonies; streak and spread plates, if inoculated properly, contain only surface colonies (Fig. 5–10). Colonies obtained by any of these techniques may be examined for colony morphology and used to prepare smears for Gram staining. Only pure colonies should be used to subculture for purposes of identification.

Special Culture Techniques

Sometimes it is necessary to use special culture techniques in growing microorganisms in the laboratory. Viruses and certain bacteria, known as rickettsias and chlamydias, do not grow on artificial culture media. The organisms must be grown in embryonated eggs or in tissue cultures. Growth media for tissue cultures consist of balanced salt solutions enriched with sera, amniotic fluid, tissue extracts, or products of protein digestion.

Cells used as host cells for culturing viruses, rickettsias, or chlamydias are allowed to grow until a single layer of cells, known as a **monolayer,** is obtained before specimens are added. Cultures require replacement of media and rinsing at periodic intervals to maintain optimal growth conditions. Specific changes in cells, known as cytopathic effects (CPE) caused by microorganisms in host cells can be seen with a bright-field microscope. Specific viruses cause a CPE which is typical. CPEs are discussed in Chapter 10. Tissues also may be stained or be allowed to react with antibodies labeled with special stains for examination by fluorescent microscopy.

Cultivation of protozoa is time-consuming and requires both special materials and equipment. It is not practical for most laboratories to attempt

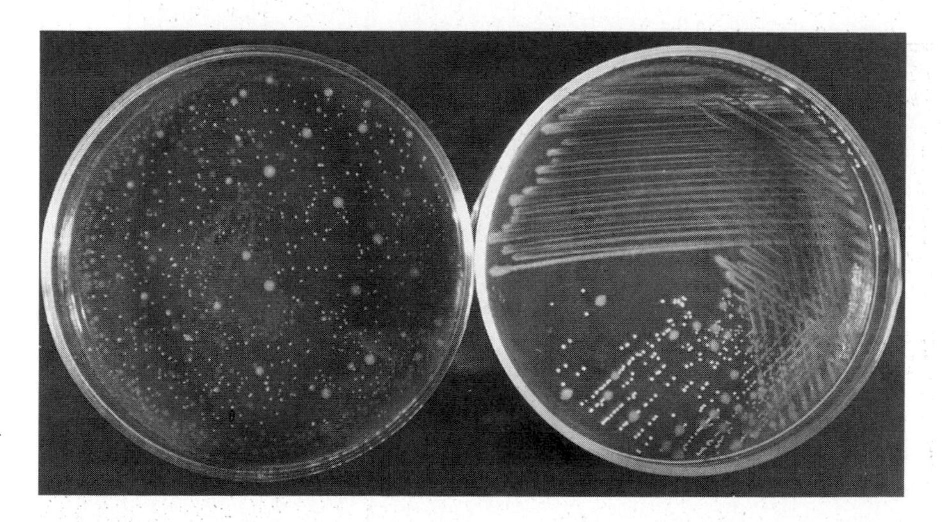

Figure 5–10 ◆ Appearance of colonies on a pour plate (left) and on a streak plate (right).

to grow the parasites. The only cultural methods in general use are those used for the isolation of amebas and a few flagellates.

Animal Inoculation

When microbiology was developing as a science, animals were used to confirm the pathogenicity of bacteria isolated from cases of human infections. Animal inoculations are not used very often in the average diagnostic laboratory. Occasionally, mice or hamsters are injected intraperitoneally with exudates, fluids, or suspensions of tissues from some patients with suspected viral, fungal or protozoal infections. Mice or guinea pigs are used to demonstrate the presence of specific toxins, such as those produced by the etiological agents of botulism and diphtheria.

Very few pathogens will not grow on some form of artificial media. Notable exceptions are bacteria that cause leprosy and syphilis. *Mycobacterium leprae* can be cultured only in the footpads of mice or in the nine-banded armadillo. *Treponema pallidum* does not grow well, if at all, on artificial laboratory media. Fortunately, the acid-fast *M. leprae* usually can be visualized in skin scrapings. Antibodies to *T. pallidum* can be detected in serum of patients with syphilis.

CONTINUOUS AND SYNCHRONIZED CULTURES

Overnight cultures are employed in most hospital and public health laboratories, but continuous culture techniques are used in industrial and research laboratories. Not only can large numbers of microorganisms be obtained, but high yields of products can be recovered. Sometimes it is necessary to synchronize growth in studying details of particular cell cycles so that populations can be studied at the same stages of their life cycles.

Continuous Cultures

Provision for continuous culture can be made in a growth chamber known as a **chemostat** (Fig. 5–11). Fresh nutrients are supplied and used medium is removed at a constant rate. Under carefully controlled conditions, cells in the open system remain in the logarithmic phase of growth for a long period (see Fig. 5–1). The increase in cell population is described as **steady-state growth.** During steady-state growth cell mass and cell number are proportional.

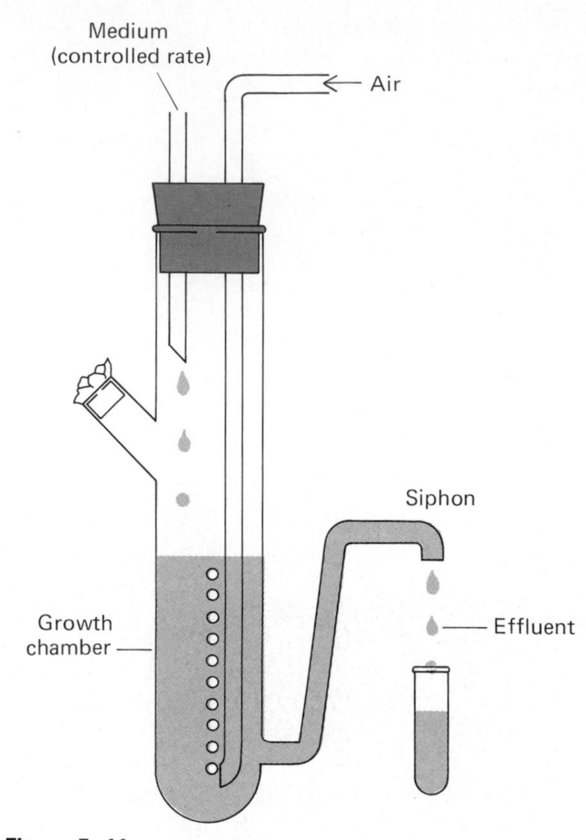

Figure 5–11 ◆ A simplified version of a chemostat. Bacteria in the growth chamber remain in the logarithmic phase of growth.

Synchronized Cultures

There are advantages to having all cells of a culture dividing at the same time. Such cultures are said to be **synchronized.** Most of us are familiar with synchronizing the time of our watches if we are to meet someone at a specified time. Synchronizing the cells of a culture of microbial cells in different growth phases is more difficult.

Synchronized growth can be obtained by physiological or mechanical selection procedures. The process of physiological selection to start synchronized growth is based on control of specific requirements for growth. DNA replication can be inhibited by a reduction in temperature or deprivation of an essential nutrient such as thymine. Growth will start again when the temperature is increased or when the missing nutrient is made available. Growth is synchronized by controlled restoration of the medium and removal of waste products in a chemostat.

Mechanical selection, by employing filter paper, permits only the smallest cells to pass through the filter. The young cells can be transferred to a fresh culture medium where cells will be dividing at the same time.

Yields of metabolic products are maximal during the time cells are in synchrony. Cells become asynchronous after three or four generations, presumably because of individual differences in partition of cytoplasm during cell division (Fig. 5–12). Synchronized cultures are used to study the dynamics of cell growth in research and to obtain high density of cells in the logarithmic phase in industry.

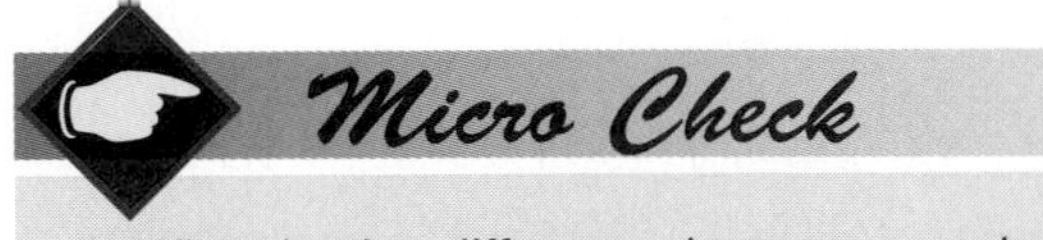

- What is the difference between a selective and a differential medium?
- What methods are used to obtain pure cultures?
- Why is it necessary to use special techniques to grow viruses and certain bacteria?

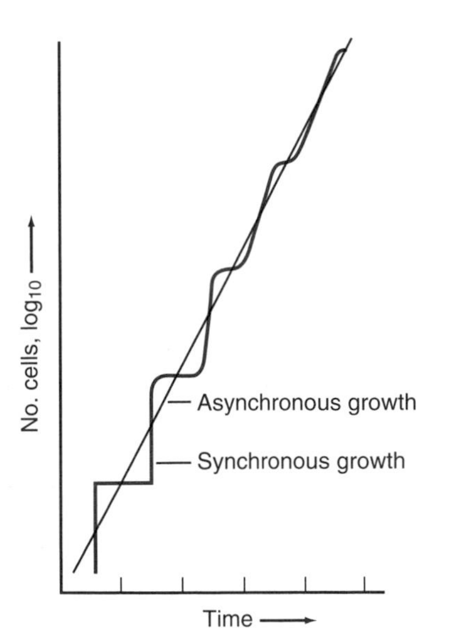

Figure 5–12 ◆ Synchronous and asynchronous growth compared. Cells become asynchronous after three or four generations.

METHODS OF MEASURING GROWTH

It is often pertinent to ascertain numbers as well as types of microorganisms present in milk, food, water, soil, or even urine in cases of bladder or kidney infections. Growth can be measured as an increase in cell mass or cell numbers.

Measurements of Cell Mass

Cell mass can be determined directly by measuring weight or indirectly by measuring turbidity in a liquid medium or a cellular component. The choice of a method depends on the anticipated range of the population size and the availability of required equipment. All methods have some limitations. No method differentiates between living and dead cells.

MEASUREMENT OF CELL WEIGHT

Cell mass can be determined by dry or wet weight after harvesting cells. Dry weight measurements are more time-consuming but allow a more accurate estimation of cell masses because amounts of water in cells may not be directly related to protoplasmic content. Cells must be washed thoroughly and subsequently dried before cells can be weighed. Dry weight of cells is about 20 to 25 percent of the wet weight of cells. Average weights can be obtained by dividing the weight of a population of cells by the total number of cells. Measurement of cell weight is not practical unless one is dealing with massive populations of cells.

TURBIDIMETRIC MEASUREMENT

Microbial growth in a liquid medium causes visible turbidity (cloudiness), which can be measured in a spectrophotometer. The turbidity is measured in optical density (O.D.) units (Fig. 5–13). The O.D. is the logarithm of the ratio of intensity of light striking the suspension to that amount which is transmitted. The greater the cell mass present, the less light will pass through the instrument. The O.D. is proportional to cell mass between 0.01 mg and 0.5 mg dry weight. Measurement of very large populations requires dilution in order to obtain accurate estimates of cell mass.

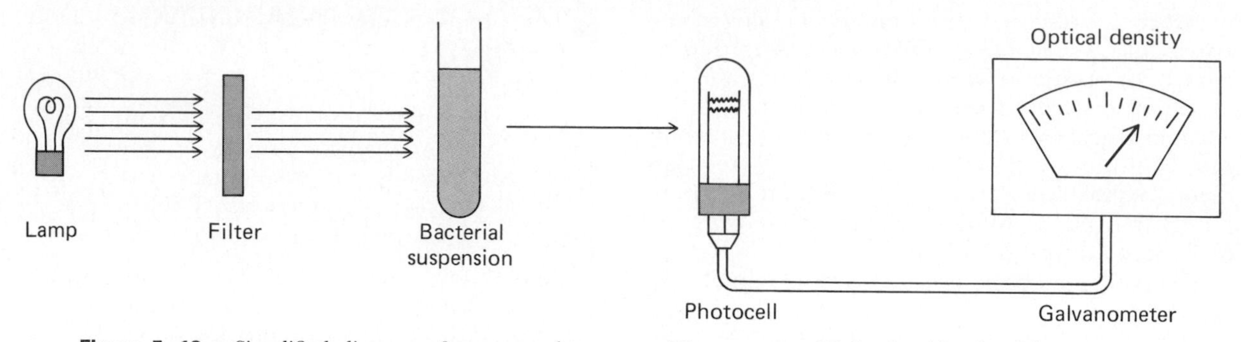

Figure 5–13 ◆ Simplified diagram of a spectrophotometer. The amount of light that hits the galvanometer is inversely proportional to the mass of cells in the bacterial suspension.

CHEMICAL ANALYSIS

The amount of a particular cellular component of a microbial population is proportional to cell mass. For example, the total nitrogen content is frequently measured to assess biomass. Determining total nitrogen is complex and time-consuming. Cells must be washed repeatedly to remove extraneous material and digested prior to chemical analysis for nitrogen. This procedure is largely used in research laboratories.

Measurement of Cell Number

Numbers of cells in a microbial population can be estimated directly by microscopy or electronic devices. Viable cell counts are determined by a culture technique. Indirect methods which measure a particular end product or amount of dye reduction can sometimes provide quantitative or semiquantitative information.

DIRECT CELL COUNTS

The number of cells in a suspension can be counted microscopically in counting chambers known as **Petroff-Hauser chambers.** The Petroff-Hauser counting chamber consists of a slide etched with a grid of 25 small squares within one square millimeter (1 mm^2) and a cover slip (Fig. 5–14). The space occupied by the sample is 1/50 mm. A bacterial suspension, contained in 0.001 ml, is added carefully so that it covers the grid completely, but does not overflow the chamber. Several squares are counted and the average is used to calculate the number of cells per milliliter.

$$N = \text{average cells} \times 25 \times 50 \times 10^3$$

Cells may also be counted by a stained-smear technique if the population is large enough. Usually 0.01 ml of a well-mixed bacterial suspension is spread over one square centimeter on an ordinary glass slide, dried, stained, and counted. Several randomly selected fields are usually counted. The number of fields in 1 cm^2 can be ascertained by using a stage micrometer. The number of fields multiplied by the average number of cells per field times the dilution factor of 100 equals the number of cells per milliliter of sample. Both the counting chamber and stained-smear techniques are subject to many technical errors.

Estimation of total cells by an electronic counter eliminates some of the human error and gives more rapid results. A small volume of a dilute bacterial suspension is allowed to flow past a pair of electrodes. Interruption in the current by the cells is recorded as a pulse on an electronic device.

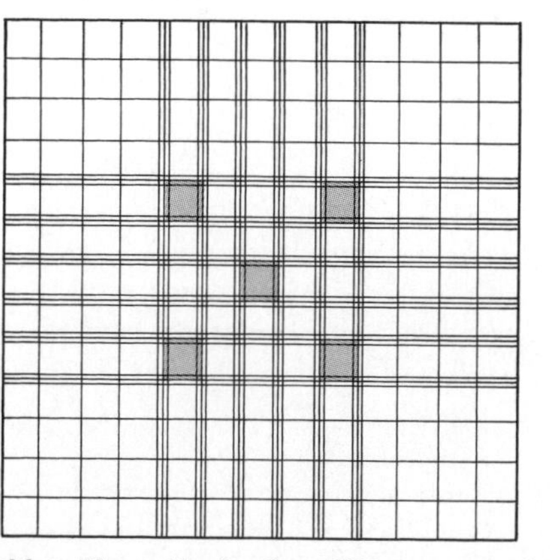

Figure 5–14 ◆ The grid of a Petroff-Hauser counting chamber. Several small squares are counted, averaged, and multiplied by a dilution factor to calculate the number of cells in a milliliter of sample.

Direct microscopic and electronic counts have many limitations. They do not differentiate between living and dead cells. In addition, if two cells adhere to each other, they are recorded as a single cell by electronic counters. Furthermore, microbial cells cannot always be differentiated from debris.

VIABLE CELL COUNTS

The number of viable bacteria is important in evaluating the quality of water, milk, other foods, and soil. Uniform procedures are essential in such assessments because minor variations in techniques can cause significant changes in results.

Standard Plate Count. One of the most practical methods for determining numbers of viable bacteria is the **standard plate count** (SPC), which uses small volumes of a series of 10-fold (10^{-1}) or 100-fold (10^{-2}) dilutions of samples (Fig. 5–15). Measured amounts of each dilution are added to each of two sterile Petri plates. Fifteen to 20 ml of appropriate melted and cooled agar medium are added to each plate. The contents of each plate are mixed by gentle swirling. The technique is based on the premise that single organisms will give rise to colonies after incubation at an appropriate temperature.

Duplicate plates of the same dilution of samples having 30 to 300 colonies after incubation are selected for counting. Petri plates are placed directly on an illuminated instrument called a Quebec colony counter. The counter has a magnifying lens which permits one to see and count colonies. An electronic colony counter can also be used to save time when large numbers of counts are performed (Fig. 5–16). The electronic device contains a video camera that scans and counts the colonies. The count appears on a viewing monitor.

The average number of colonies on duplicate plates of the same dilution of sample is multiplied by the dilution factor to obtain the number of **colony-forming units** (CFU) per milliliter. If two plates of a 10^{-2} dilution were found to have 230 and 220 CFU, respectively, the average is multiplied by 10^2.

$$225 \times 10^2 = 22{,}500 \text{ CFU/ml}$$

Membrane-Filter Counts. A modification of a standard plate count uses a membrane filter to trap bacteria as samples of water or other liquids are passed through it (Fig. 5–17). The membrane filter is then placed in a sterile Petri plate containing a pad saturated with an appropriate medium. The medium diffuses into the membrane filter, causing trapped bacteria to develop into colonies after incubation.

Membrane colony counts are determined by counting numbers of colonies detected on a Quebec or an electronic colony counter and re-

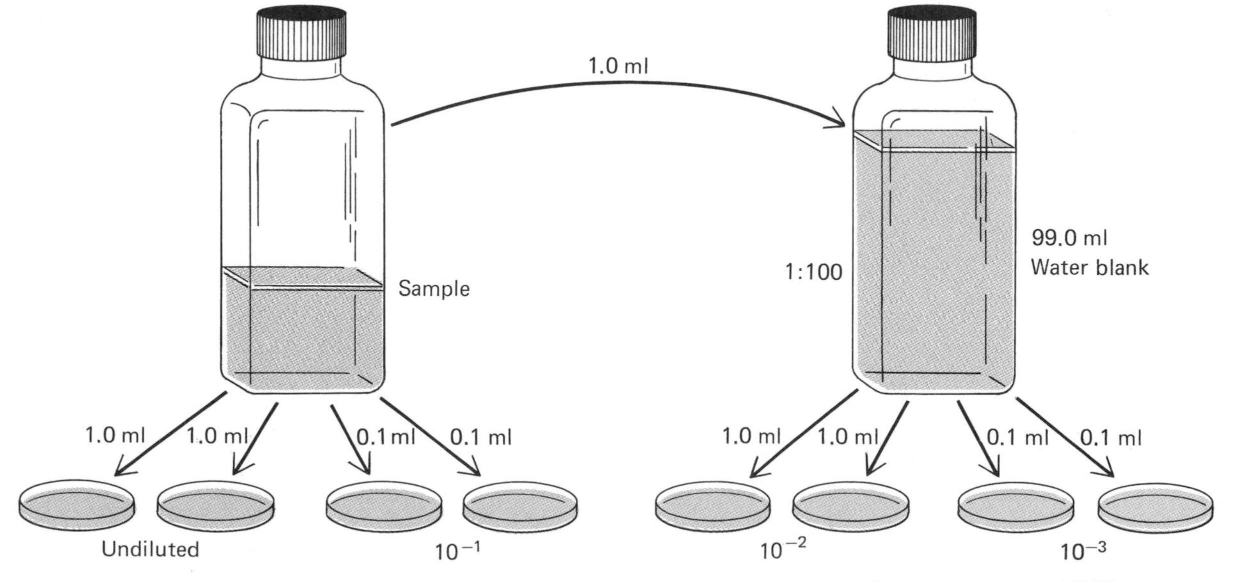

Figure 5–15 ◆ The technique employed in the standard plate count to obtain colony-forming units (CFU) per milliliter. Plates of each dilution are prepared in duplicate.

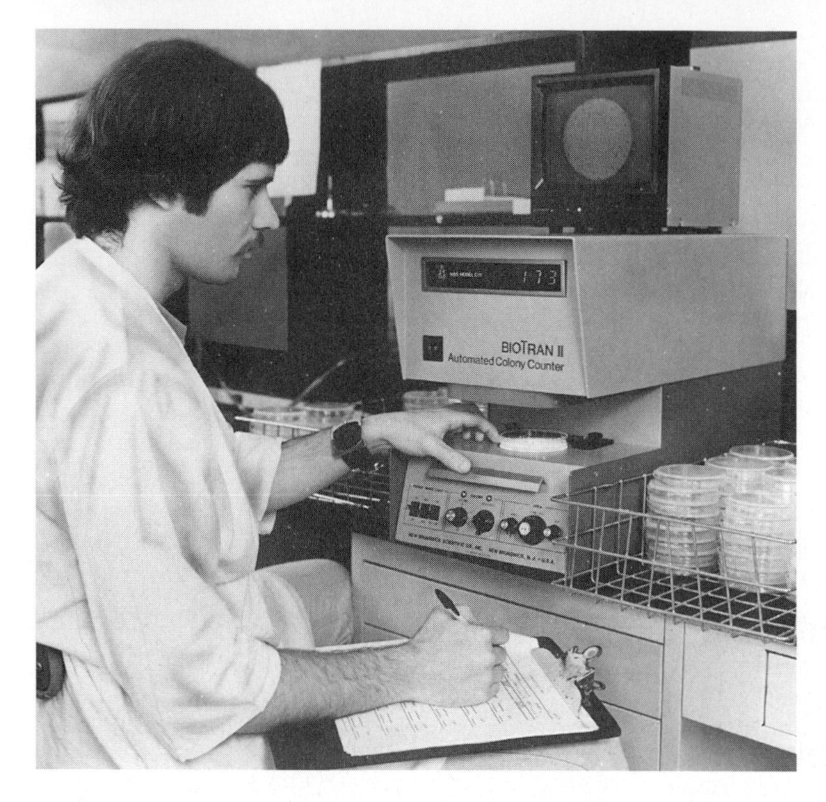

Figure 5–16 ◆ An electronic colony counter and viewing monitor. An integrated video camera scans the culture plate, and the colony count appears on a digital readout.

ported per volume of sample filtered. In the analysis of water, 100 ml volumes are used. If 67 CFUs were counted on the membrane filter, it would be reported as 67 CFU per 100 ml of the sample.

Membrane-filter counts have the same limitations as SPCs, because a single plating medium will not support the growth of all bacteria. Membrane-filter counts can be used only when a limited number of bacteria are present. However, both techniques permit the isolation of colonies, which can be identified by additional tests.

INDIRECT MEASUREMENTS

Indirect methods for estimating numbers of a bacterial population depend on the ability of bacteria to reduce dyes or to produce a measurable end product from particular substrates. In the methylene blue reduction test, a change in color of the dye from blue (the oxidized state) to a colorless compound (the reduced state) is the basis for determining relative numbers of bacteria. The test is limited in that reduction of methylene blue by mixed population may represent varying degrees of metabolic activity, but it is generally considered a reliable, semiquantitative method for grading milk. The test is described in Chapter 24.

Under carefully controlled conditions, the amount of an end product yielded by a specific metabolic reaction is proportional to the density of a bacterial population. Quantitative determinations of end products, such as ammonia, reducing sugars, or acids, are usually reserved for studies on pure cultures. Bacteria in mixed cultures differ in growth rates, so yields of products would no longer be proportional to numbers of organisms.

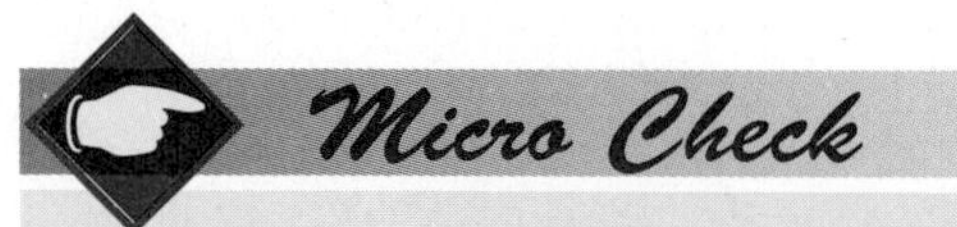

- What is the major limitation of direct or electronic cell counts?
- What is the major advantage of determining numbers of bacteria by standard plate counts?
- Why are quantitative determinations for particular end products usually reserved for studies on pure cultures?

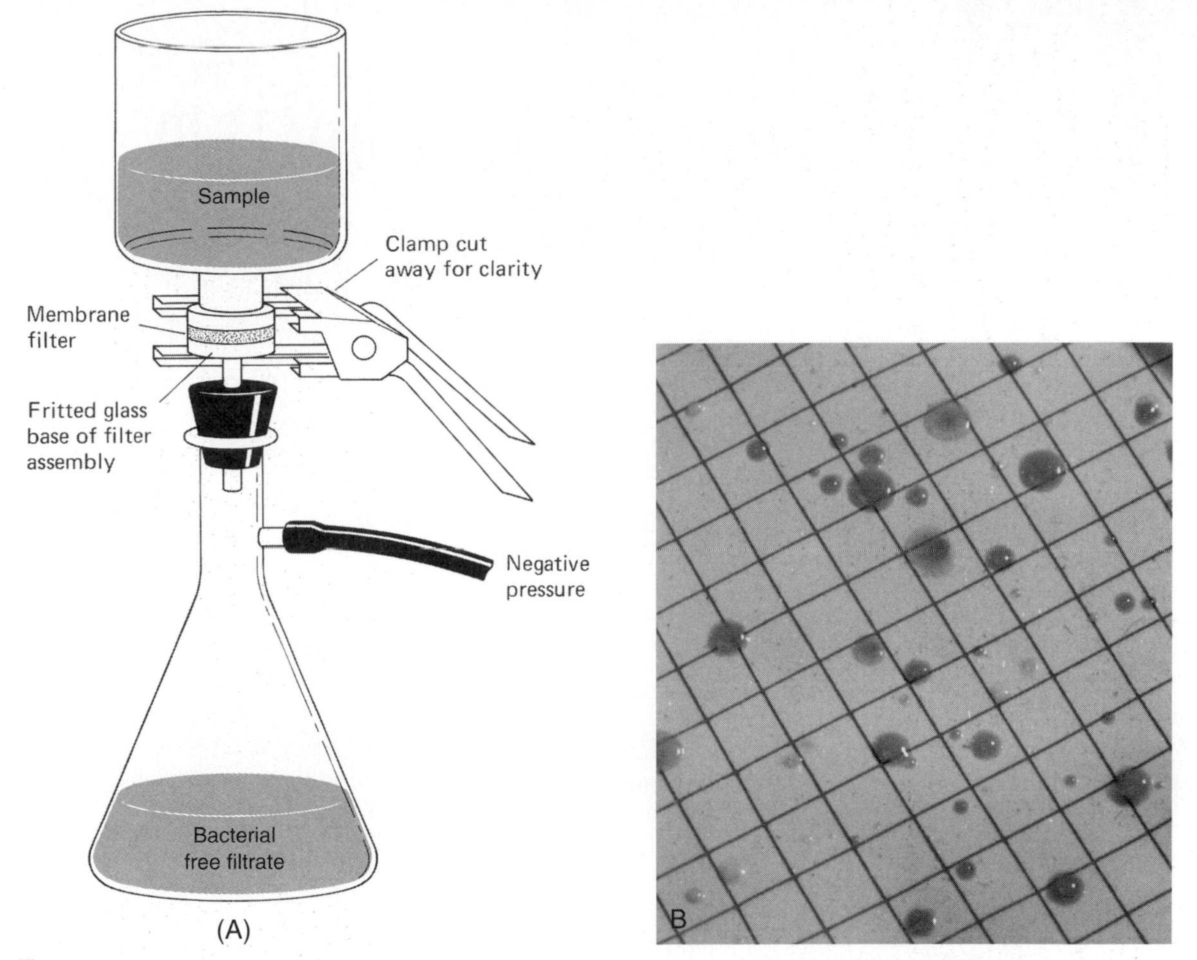

Figure 5–17 ◆ Membrane-filter technique. *A,* Bacteria are trapped on membrane filter when negative pressure is applied. *B,* Bacteria develop into colonies after saturation in medium and an overnight incubation period.

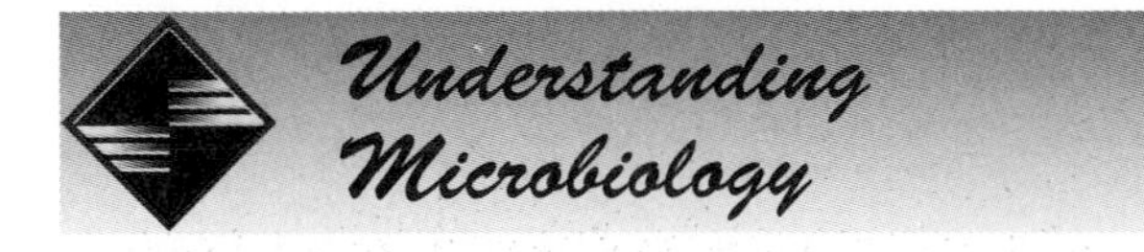

1. Name four phases of a microbial population growth curve.
2. How can the detrimental effect of acidic or basic products resulting from microbial metabolism be controlled in artificial culture media?
3. Explain why facultative anaerobes have a survival advantage over obligate anaerobes.
4. Explain how it is possible for a medium to be both selective and differential.
5. What are the limitations of viable cell counts?

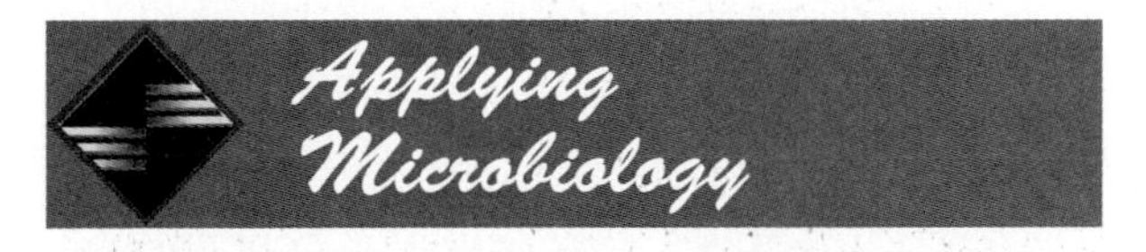

6. If a bacterium has an average doubling time of 30 minutes and you use an inoculum of 3×10^3 cells/ml, what would the final population be at the end of eight hours of incubation under optimal conditions for growth?

Chapter 6

Microbial Metabolism and Regulation

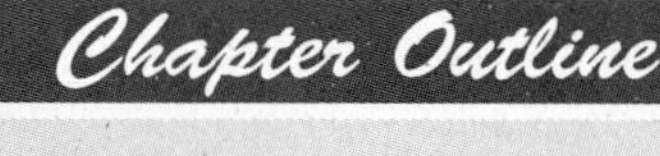

Chapter Outline

- **ENERGY RESOURCES**
  - Role of Enzymes
  - Classification of Enzymes
  - Naming of Enzymes
  - Coenzymes and Essential Ions
- **FACTORS INFLUENCING THE RATE OF ENZYME REACTIONS**
  - pH
  - Temperature
  - Substrate Concentration
  - Enzyme Concentration
  - Product Concentration
  - Inhibiting Substances
- **CATABOLISM: ENERGY-GENERATING REACTIONS**
  - Respiration
  - Fermentation
  - Metabolism of Other Carbohydrates, Lipids, and Proteins
  - Photosynthesis
- **ANABOLISM: ENERGY-REQUIRING REACTIONS**
  - Synthesis of Carbohydrates
  - Synthesis of Proteins
  - Synthesis of Lipids
- **INTEGRATION OF CATABOLISM AND ANABOLISM**
- **CONTROL MECHANISMS FOR METABOLISM**
  - Allosteric Modulation
  - Covalent Modification
  - Regulated and Constitutive Enzymes
  - Catabolite Repression

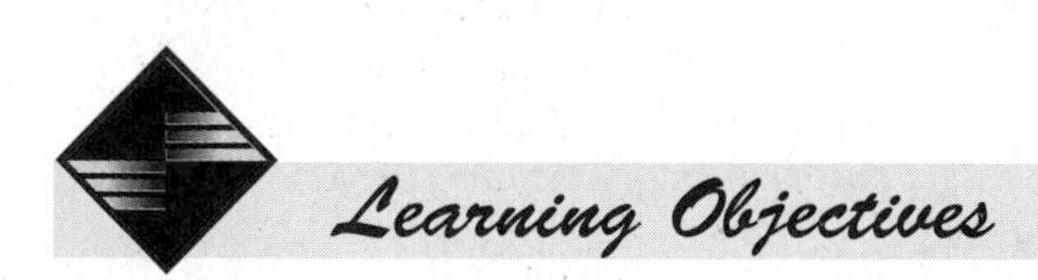

Learning Objectives

After you have read this chapter, you should be able to:

1. Differentiate between catabolic and anabolic reactions.
2. Recognize the six types of enzyme-catalyzed reactions.
3. Identify the three major pathways in aerobic respiration and their roles in generating ATP.
4. Contrast the efficiency of aerobic respiration, fermentation, and anaerobic respiration in metabolism.
5. List the final electron acceptors of aerobes and anaerobes.
6. Identify one or more roles of ATP in metabolism.
7. Describe four mechanisms that control microbial metabolism.

All microorganisms require energy and depend on chemical reactions to be able to sustain life and interact in an increasingly complex environment. Some chemical reactions within microbial cells release energy from nutrients; other reactions require energy to build needed molecules. The energy stored in nutrient molecules is released in **exergonic** reactions, such as those involved in the degradation, or **catabolism,** of glucose. Reactions requiring energy to build molecules such as proteins are called **endergonic** and are examples of **anabolism.** The total of all the reactions of catabolism and anabolism in a cell is known as **metabolism.** Energy released in catabolism is captured in high-energy bonds of **adenosine triphosphate (ATP)** molecules. Some microorganisms require light energy in order to carry out metabolism; these are the **photosynthetic** microorganisms. Not all reactions occur at every moment in the life of a cell. Internal control processes conserve energy by slowing or stopping some reactions or even ceasing the production of some enzymes.

ENERGY RESOURCES

The energy required to generate ATP for **chemotrophs** is supplied by nutrients. Energy is released gradually as the chemical bonds of nutrient molecules are broken. Sunlight energy is the source of energy for **phototrophs.** Phototrophs convert light energy into chemical energy by a process known as **photosynthesis,** which involves the production of glucose from carbon dioxide and water (Fig. 6–1).

Microorganisms, like other forms of life, are dependent on energy conversions. An example is the conversion of energy stored in the bonds of glucose molecules into carbon dioxide, water, and high-energy bonds of ATP by many aerobic bacteria. You will recall from Chapter 2 that the glucose molecule is a closed ring structure containing six carbon atoms with attached hydrogen and oxygen atoms. Glucose is degraded into six molecules of carbon dioxide gas and six molecules of water, some heat energy, and many molecules of energy-rich adenosine triphosphate (ATP). In chemical shorthand, the overall reaction for the catabolism of glucose ($C_6H_{12}O_6$) may be written as:

$$C_6H_{12}O_6 + 6O_2 \longrightarrow 6CO_2 + 6H_2O + \text{energy}$$

More than half of the energy from glucose escapes as heat energy. The remaining energy is used to form the energy-rich chemical bonds of ATP.

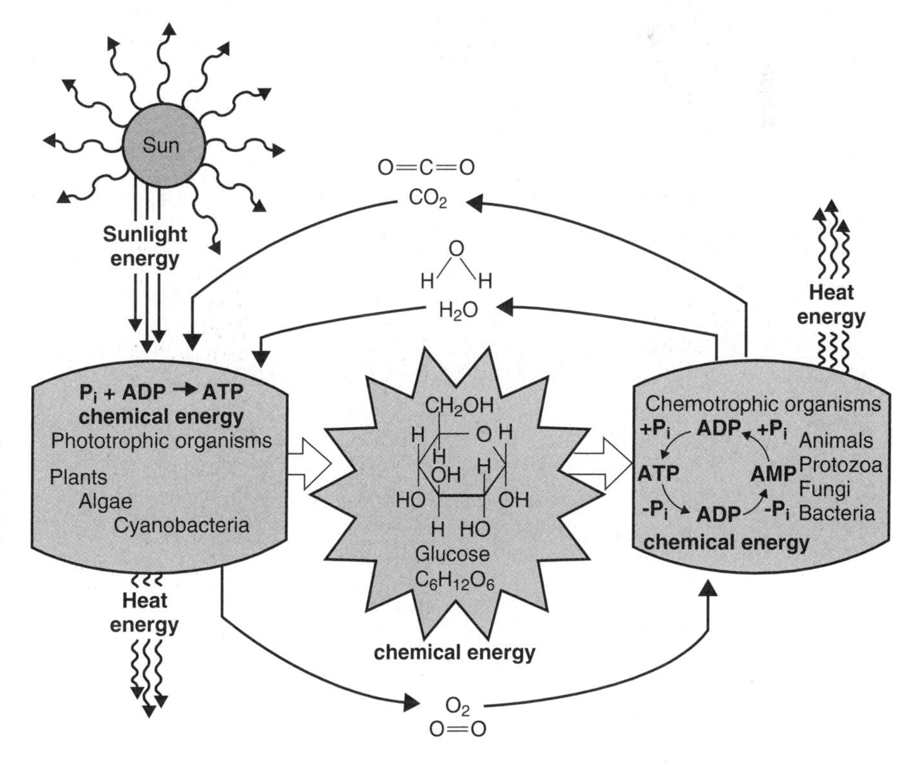

Figure 6–1 ◆ Interrelationships between chemotrophic and phototrophic organisms. Sunlight energy powers the phototrophic organisms to produce glucose and other organic molecules. Some chemotrophic organisms may use CO_2, but others use organic molecules, such as glucose, to supply energy and carbon atoms. Carbon dioxide released by chemotrophs is fixed by phototrophs to produce glucose.

Approximately 7 kcal of energy are stored when a high-energy phosphate bond is added to **adenosine diphosphate (ADP)** to form ATP. In metabolism, ATP is a very important molecule because it is the major source of energy for endergonic reactions. When energy is released from the nutrient molecules, large amounts of energy are used to attach a phosphate group of atoms (PO_4) to ADP to form ATP. The conversion of ADP to ATP is the most common means of transferring energy from one molecule to another (Fig. 6–2).

Energy is neither created nor destroyed by conversions from one form to another. That relationship between matter and energy is true under all known circumstances and constitutes the **First Law of Thermodynamics,** which states that the total energy of a system and its surroundings is constant. The **Second Law of Thermodynamics** tells us that some energy is released as heat energy during conversions. Transformations of energy are not 100 percent efficient. All living organisms require energy just to maintain body structure and to repair damaged or worn-out parts. Cells also need energy for active transport of ions and molecules across plasma membranes, for cell division, and for motility.

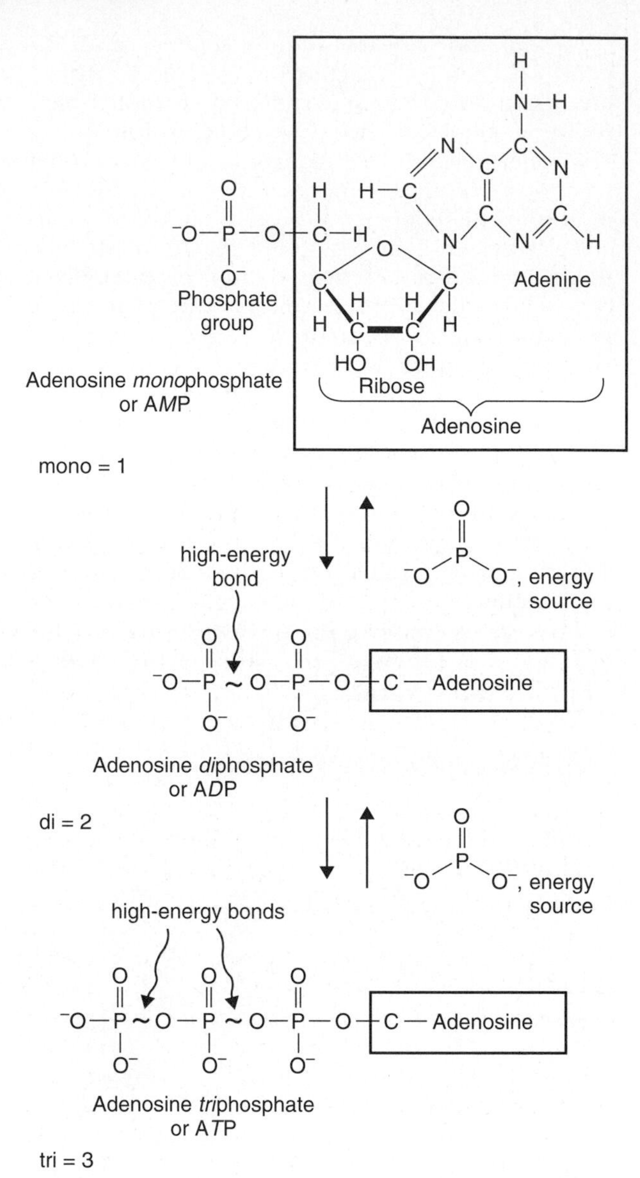

Figure 6–2 ◆ Energy flow in microbial metabolism. Energy is released from nutrients and captured to form energy-rich phosphate bonds on ADP and ATP. Energy requirements for certain enzymes may be supplied by a high-energy phosphate group released from ATP to form ADP (or AMP if two high-energy phosphate groups are removed).

Micro Check

- From what sources do microorganisms obtain energy?
- Why is ATP considered the universal currency of energy exchange?
- Explain the significance of the transfer of a phosphate group to ADP.

Role of Enzymes

An **enzyme** is a protein molecule that **catalyzes** one specific type of reaction and essentially no others. The chemical acted on by the enzyme is called the **substrate.** The enzyme promotes a chemical reaction, but remains unchanged, so it is called a **catalyst.** Without enzymes, cellular metabolism would occur either too slowly to support life or not at all. Enzymes catalyze reactions in cells by binding temporarily with their substrates. The location on the enzyme where the substrate binds is called the **active** or **catalytic site.**

Enzyme-substrate (E-S) binding promotes the formation of reversible covalent bonds. A susceptible bond on the substrate (S) is broken during the catalytic cycle to yield one product (P) or two products (P_1 and P_2):

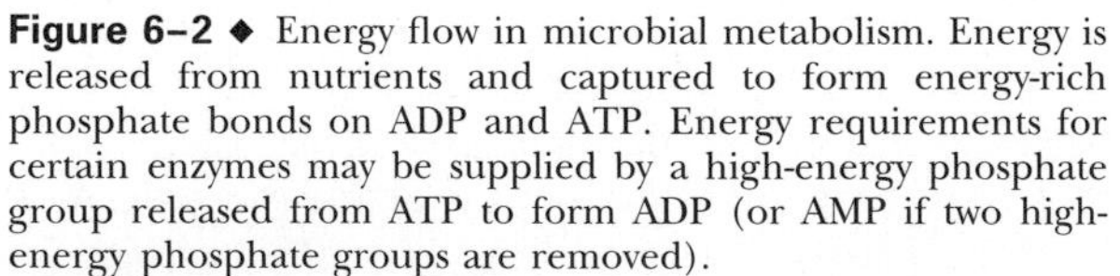

$$E + S \longrightarrow \{E\sim S\} \longrightarrow E + P$$

OR

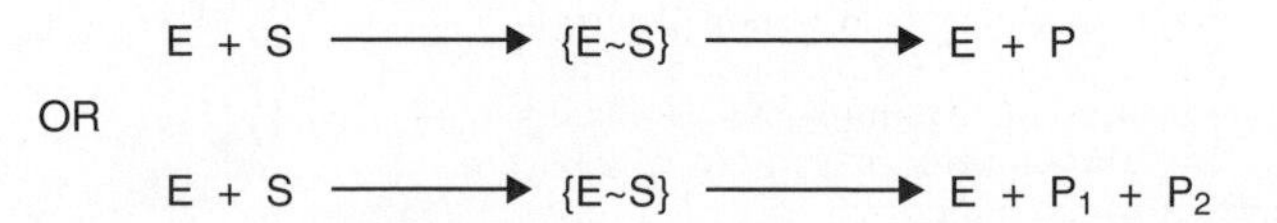

$$E + S \longrightarrow \{E\sim S\} \longrightarrow E + P_1 + P_2$$

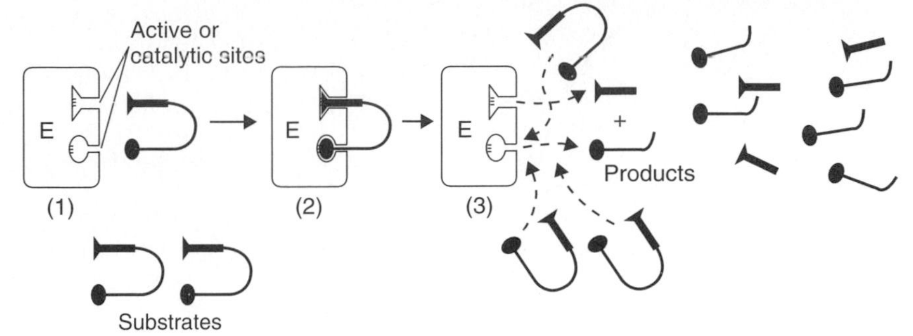

Figure 6–3 ◆ The "lock and key" interaction between an enzyme (E) and a substrate. Opposite electrical charges and spatial configuration between active site and substrate are involved in the attraction between enzyme and substrate (2). The substrate is changed (3) to the product(s) of the enzyme's catalysis; the enzyme and product(s) separate so the enzyme is free to interact with another substrate molecule.

A conformational change of the enzyme occurs during the chemical reaction. After the products are released from the active site, the enzyme is restored to its original shape and can bind to more substrate molecules. The speed with which enzyme-substrate reactions occurs is sometimes difficult to appreciate; most enzymes catalyze about 10,000 reactions a second.

The attraction between an enzyme and its substrate(s) can be explained by (1) differences in charge on the molecules, (2) formation of weak bonds, and (3) the attraction occurring between closely spaced atoms (van der Waals forces). Most enzymes are proteins with a globular shape. The folding of an enzyme molecule produces a three-dimensional configuration that is complementary to the shape of a substrate(s).

An early model devised by Fischer to explain the enzyme-substrate binding is called the "lock and key" theory. Just as a hand guides a key into position in a lock, the attraction of opposite charges on enzyme and substrate help to position and bind a specific substrate molecule(s) on the enzyme (Fig. 6–3). The "lock and key" model is useful, but it implies that the molecules involved are not flexible.

A general "induced fit" model developed by Koshland takes the flexibility of proteins and substrate molecules into consideration. In this model, the substrate induces a three-dimensional shape change in the enzyme for binding, catalytic action, or both (Fig. 6–4). The unique shape of the binding sites place chemical units on the enzyme with particular chemical units on the substrate. This relationship between an enzyme, its substrate, and the reaction catalyzed is termed **specificity.** The changed substrate constitutes the **product** or **products** that are released from the active site.

The amount of energy needed to trigger a chemical reaction is known as the **energy of activation.** Enzymes provide an alternate pathway, a transition-state, identified as (E-S), for the chemical reaction to occur. In the transition state, the energy required to activate a reaction on the substrate is lower (Fig. 6–5). The enzyme protein flexes to bring atoms of the substrate close together within the active site, allowing the reaction to take place at a lower energy of activation.

Classification of Enzymes

Enzymes are classified on the basis of the type of reaction catalyzed. Every metabolic reaction is catalyzed by one of six classes of enzymes. Familiarity with these six classes of enzymes and the reactions catalyzed is helpful for understanding

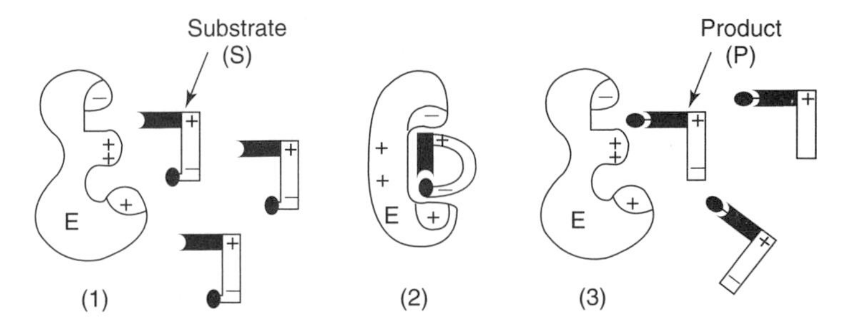

Figure 6–4 ◆ "Induced fit" model for enzyme action. Binding of the enzyme (E) and substrate (S) produces particular changes in the enzyme's conformation (three-dimensional) structure (1). This structural change brings specific parts of the substrate(s) close enough to react in the {E-S} transition state (2). Completion of the reaction results in an enzyme-product complex and subsequent release of product molecules (3).

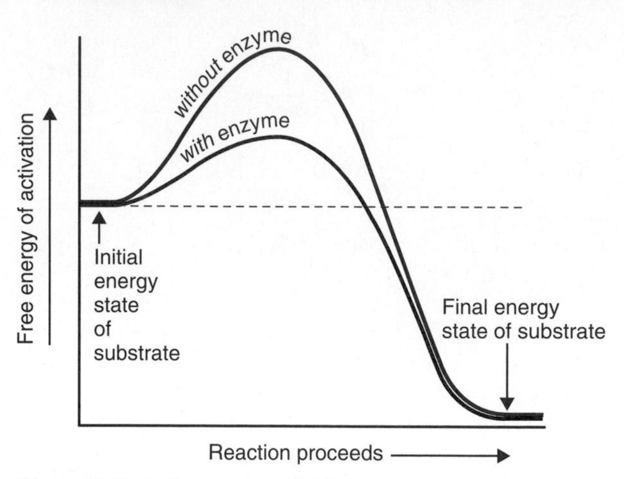

Figure 6–5 ◆ The "energy hill." Energy is required to activate a substrate molecule. This activation energy is lowered by the interaction of substrate with an enzyme.

bioenergetics of microbial metabolism (Table 6–1). Theoretically, all enzyme reactions are reversible, but in cells, conditions do not always exist to drive the reactions in reverse.

OXIDOREDUCTASES

Oxidation is the most common type of reaction in the production of cellular energy. The loss of electrons is called **oxidation;** the gain of electrons is called **reduction.** The enzymes catalyzing transfers of electrons are **oxidoreductases.** The most active oxidoreductases in biological systems are **dehydrogenases,** which catalyze the reactions involved in the transport of hydrogen from one molecule, A, to another molecule, B.

$$AH_2 + B \rightleftharpoons A + BH_2$$

As electrons travel from atoms of greater electronegativity to those of lesser electronegativity, energy is released. One reactant (AH_2) is oxidized to A, while the other reactant (B) is reduced, forming BH_2. Oxidation and reduction operate as **coupled** or **redox reactions.**

TRANSFERASES

During degradation and synthesis of compounds in cells, **functional groups** of atoms are frequently transferred from one substrate to another. The groups transferred include amino (NH_2), carboxyl (COOH), methyl (CH_3), and sulfur- (S) or phosphorus- (P) containing groups. The functional group is identified by the letter R in the following general equation:

$$AR + B \rightleftharpoons BR + A$$

Transferase enzymes are important in metabolism because they modify molecules and transfer energy-rich bonds.

HYDROLASES

The breaking of chemical bonds in the presence of water to release energy is called **hydrolysis.** The enzymes catalyzing hydrolytic reactions are called **hydrolases.** Water, represented by H_2O, can be split to form an H^+ ion and a hydroxyl (OH^-) functional group of atoms:

$$AB + H_2O \rightleftharpoons AOH + BH$$

Some microbial hydrolases, such as cellulase, which breaks down cellulose in plant material,

Table 6–1
SIX CLASSES OF ENZYMES

CLASS	EXAMPLE OF ENZYME	EXAMPLE OF ENZYME ACTION
Oxidoreductases	Oxidases	Redox reactions
	Dehydrogenases	Transfers electrons and hydrogens
Transferases	Deaminases	Transfers amino (NH_2) group between molecules
Hydrolases	Cellulase	Splits cellulose by adding water between sugar molecules
Lyases	Phosphorylase	Removes or adds a phosphate group
Isomerases	Phosphoglucoisomerase	Rearranges atoms in glucose 6-phosphate to make fructose 6-phosphate
Ligases	DNA ligase	Forms bonds between nucleotides to connect the ends of a DNA strand

are liberated into the environment while others remain inside cells.

LYASES

The removal of functional groups (R) from a substrate without adding water or the addition of groups to a double bond are accomplished with the aid of **lyases.**

$$AR \rightleftharpoons A + R$$

Carboxylation, the primary reaction in light-requiring reactions, is catalyzed by a lyase, which adds a carboxyl group (COOH) to a pentose. **Deamination,** the removal of an amino group (NH_2) and **decarboxylation,** the removal of a carboxyl group (COOH) are important reactions for transferring energy.

ISOMERASES

The rearrangement of atoms within a molecule causing a change in the configuration of atoms in a molecule is called **isomerization.** If AB is a molecule, then BA is a change in its structure:

$$AB \rightleftharpoons BA$$

In general, **isomerases** change the geometrical (spatial) arrangement of the atoms in a molecule. The isomerases may be further divided into **epimerases** and **racemases.** If only the specific configuration around a single carbon atom is changed, the enzyme is called an epimerase. If the light rotation properties of a molecule are altered, such as the conversion of an L-isomer to a D-isomer, the enzyme is called a racemase.

LIGASES

The formation of bonds in **polymers,** large molecules produced by linking smaller molecules, involves the action of **ligases** (sometimes still called synthetases). The ligases linking the individual building block units (monomers) of the polymers are also known as polymerases. All endergonic reactions, such as those used to produce proteins from amino acid molecules, require energy derived from ATP:

$$A + B + ATP \rightleftharpoons AB + ADP + P_i$$

Cellular growth occurs as the complex compounds, such as proteins, DNA, or RNA, are synthesized from smaller molecules.

EXOENZYMES AND ENDOENZYMES

Enzymes may also be classified according to the site of their activity. **Exoenzymes** are secreted into the environment and break large molecules into smaller molecules that can enter the cell. For example, a microorganism hydrolyzes starch into sugar units of glucose, maltose, and dextrins if it produces amylase, an exoenzyme. The smaller sugars can be transported across the plasma membrane.

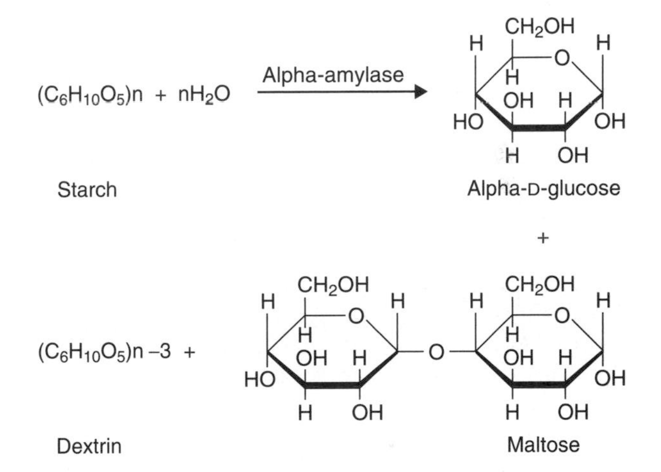

Other examples of exoenzymes include cellulase, which degrades cellulose; caseinase, which breaks down the milk protein, casein; lipases, which act on fats; and nucleotidases, which convert nucleic acids to nucleosides. The products formed by exoenzyme activity may enter catabolic or anabolic pathways.

Endoenzymes carry on their activities within the plasma membrane. Examples of endoenzymes include the enzymes of respiration and ligases, which will be discussed later in this chapter.

Naming of Enzymes

Enzymes are named according to three main criteria: (1) type of reaction catalyzed, (2) the name of the substrate acted upon, and (3) using the suffix **-ase.** A dehydrogenase, for example, is an oxidoreductase that transfers electrons of hydrogen or hydrogen ions from one substrate to another. For example, a lactic acid dehydrogenase acts upon the substrate lactic acid, removing electrons and hydrogen. A polymerase is a ligase catalyzing the combination of monomers into macromolecules. The name DNA polymerase indicates that the molecule synthesized is DNA.

When referring to groups of enzymes that operate on a small class of molecules, the suffix -ase is often added to the class of substrates. For example, enzymes that degrade carbohydrates may be called carbohydrases. Likewise, proteases, lipases, or nucleases are enzyme groups that operate on proteins, lipids, or nucleic acids, respectively.

Coenzymes and Essential Ions

Many enzymes require other molecules or ions in order to catalyze a reaction. The protein portion of an enzyme is known as the **apoenzyme.** The nonprotein portion is an essential ion or an organic molecule called a **coenzyme.** Most coenzymes are bound to their enzymes by noncovalent forces. Those coenzymes which form covalent bonds with enzymes are called **prosthetic groups.** Inorganic ions, such as Mg^{2+}, Fe^{3+}, Zn^{2+}, and Mn^{2+}, often serve as **essential ions** for certain enzyme reactions.

Coenzymes are usually relatively small molecules, but their names are often so long that initials are used regularly to designate them (Table 6–2). Most coenzymes are derived from vitamins. Coenzymes act as carrier molecules to transport electrons, atoms, or functional groups. Three of the most important coenzymes are nicotinamide adenine dinucleotide (NAD^+), nicotinamide adenine dinucleotide phosphate ($NADP^+$), and flavin adenine dinucleotide (FAD^+). NAD^+ and $NADP^+$ are derived from the vitamin niacin. FAD^+ is derived from the vitamin riboflavin.

NAD^+ molecules accept hydrogen ions and electrons from the substrate. The net result is that the substrate loses electrons to become oxidized while NAD^+ gains hydrogen ions and electrons to become reduced ($NADH + H^+$).

In other enzyme reactions, reduced NAD is used to donate its hydrogen ions and electrons to the substrate molecule. Such a reaction results in oxidized NAD molecules. Later in this chapter we shall discuss the role of electron carrier molecules in generating ATP molecules in glucose catabolism.

The important energy exchange molecule, adenosine triphosphate (ATP), is used by some enzymes as a donor molecule of a high-energy phosphate group (PO_4) of atoms (see Table 6–2). When ATP donates one of its phosphate groups, it is changed to adenosine diphosphate (ADP). Occasionally, ADP donates one of its phosphate groups in other enzyme reactions where energy is required. The ADP becomes adenosine monophosphate (AMP). The ADP and AMP molecules can receive phosphate groups from certain substrate molecules, resulting in the formation of high-energy phosphate bonds. When AMP and ADP accept a phosphate group, they are converted to ADP and ATP respectively. In this way, these very important coenzymes are readily available for reactions catalyzing phosphate transfers.

More than 25 percent of all enzymes have tightly bound metal ions or require them for cat-

Table 6–2
SOME COENZYME CARRIER MOLECULES

CARRIER MOLECULE	VITAMIN COMPONENT	PASSENGER ATOMS OR GROUPS
Adenosine triphosphate (ATP)	None	PO_4
Biotin	Biotin	COOH
Coenzyme A (CoA)	Pantothenic acid	CH_3CO
Flavin adenine dinucleotide (FAD)	Riboflavin (B_2)	H
Flavin mononucleotide (FMN)	Riboflavin (B_2)	H_2O
Nicotinamide adenine dinucleotide (NAD)	Niacin	H^+
Nicotinamide adenine dinucleotide phosphate (NADP)	Niacin	H^+
Pyridoxyl phosphate pyridoxamine	Pyridoxine (B_6)	NH_2, COOH
Tetrahydrofolic acid	Folic acid	CHO
Thiamine pyrophosphate (ThPP)	Thiamine (B_1)	COOH

alytic action. The most common ions essential for catalysis are magnesium (Mg^{2+}), manganese (Mn^{2+}), calcium (Ca^{2+}), molybdenum (Mo^{2+}), and zinc (Zn^{2+}). Certain phosphatases and peptidases require specific metallic ions for activity. The metallic ions link the enzyme and substrate with each other. Sometimes, the metal ions share an electron pair or provide an electron.

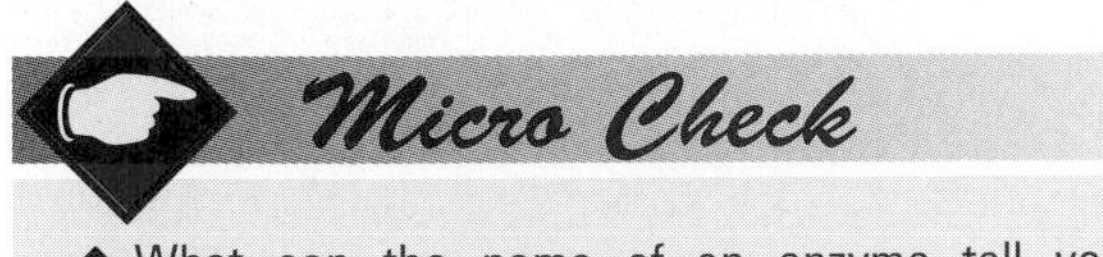

- What can the name of an enzyme tell you about the reaction it catalyzes?
- What effect does the binding of enzyme and substrate have on the chemical bonds of the substrate?
- What "passengers" are carried by coenzymes to the sites of chemical reactions?

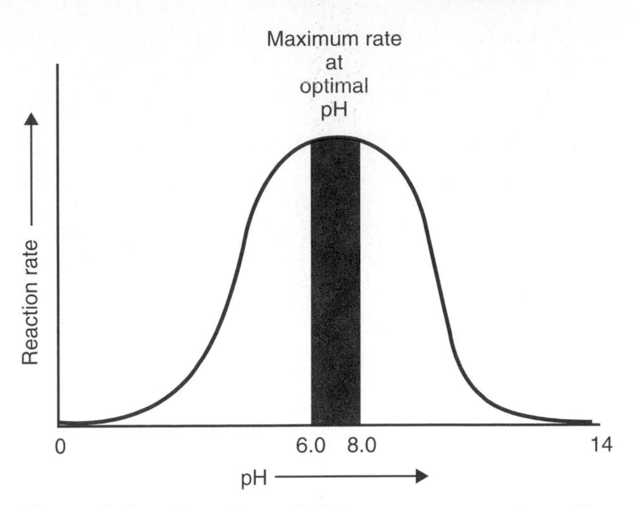

Figure 6–6 ◆ The effect of pH on enzyme reactions. The optimal pH for the microbial enzymes measured for this graph is close to 7.0.

FACTORS INFLUENCING THE RATE OF ENZYME REACTIONS

The rate at which enzyme reactions proceed is influenced by a number of environmental factors including pH, temperature, and the concentrations of substrate, enzyme, and product. Certain ions or other molecules act also to stimulate or inhibit the rate of action of some enzymes. Individual enzymes respond differently to these influences.

pH

The hydrogen ion concentration (pH) of the environment can be a rate-limiting factor. The pH of the cellular environment profoundly affects the electrical charges of enzymes, and may influence the affinities of enzymes for their substrates. Whereas the reactions may proceed over a wide range of pH values, the reaction rate is most rapid at an optimal pH (Fig. 6–6). A majority of microbial enzymes are most active near pH 7.0 (neutrality).

Temperature

The rate of most chemical reactions is increased at higher temperatures unless the temperature is so high that it destroys the integrity of the enzymes. Enzymes are deactivated by exposure to excessive heat or cold (Fig. 6–7). Excessive heat inactivates enzymes by breaking covalent bonds maintaining the three-dimensional configuration of the molecules in a process called **denaturation.** Cold temperatures slow down or in-

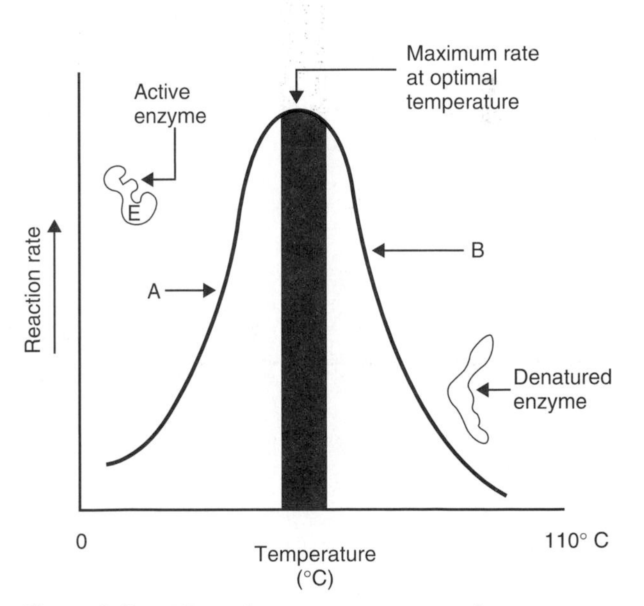

Figure 6–7 ◆ Effect of temperature on rate of enzyme reactions. The rate of a reaction increases (A) as temperature rises to an optimal temperature for the enzyme. As the temperature continues to increase beyond this point, the rate of the reaction decreases (B), with the eventual thermal denaturation of the enzyme.

hibit enzyme activity, but do not change the structure of the enzyme.

Substrate Concentration

Increasing the concentration of substrate in a substrate-enzyme system that has a fixed amount of enzyme will generally increase the velocity or rate of the reaction until the active sites on the enzyme molecules are saturated. The Michaelis-Menten constant expresses the concentration of the substrate which produces one-half of the maximum velocity (Fig. 6–8). The lowest concentration of substrate to yield one-half maximum velocities is the most efficient for conserving cell energy.

Enzyme Concentration

Increased concentrations of an enzyme in a substrate-enzyme system, with a fixed amount of substrate, cause a rapid rise in reaction rate, which levels off as all the available substrate is bound to active sites on the enzyme (Fig. 6–9).

Product Concentration

Many enzymes promote reactions in the forward direction as well as in the reverse direction. If the product(s) of an enzyme reaction accumulate, a reversal of the reaction may occur. However, if these products are then used as substrates in other reactions, the direction of the first reaction remains forward. A state of equilibrium occurs when there is no net change in quantities of substrates or products.

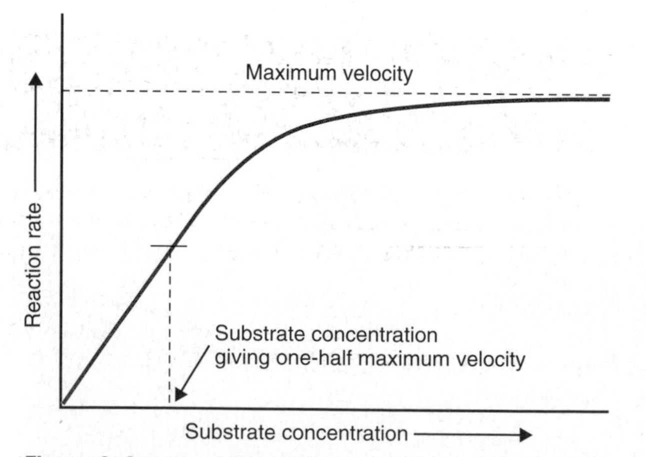

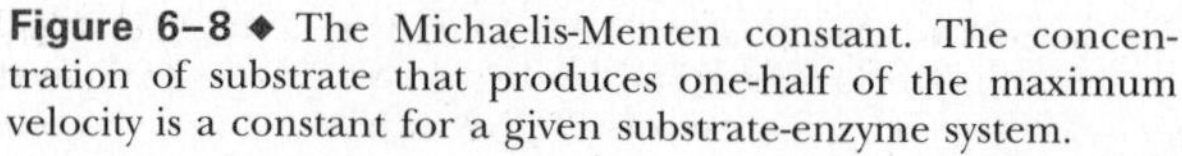

Figure 6–8 ◆ The Michaelis-Menten constant. The concentration of substrate that produces one-half of the maximum velocity is a constant for a given substrate-enzyme system.

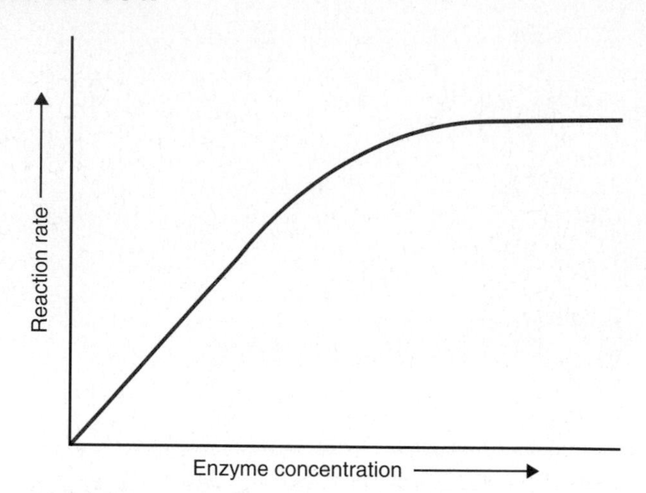

Figure 6–9 ◆ Effect of enzyme concentration on enzyme reactions. With a fixed amount of substrate, the reaction rate increases as more enzyme action is added until all substrate is gone.

Inhibiting Substances

A variety of substances can inhibit the rate of enzyme reactions. The effectiveness of an inhibitor depends upon its ability to bind in a reversible or an irreversible manner with the enzyme. In **competitive inhibition,** the inhibitor molecule competes with a structurally similar substrate for a position on an active site of the enzyme molecule. The degree of inhibition is dependent on the relative concentrations of the substrate and the inhibitor. The inhibition is reversible if the substrate level is increased.

One of the most potent of such inhibitors is malonic acid, which competes effectively with succinic acid for active sites on molecules of succinic acid dehydrogenase (Fig. 6–10). When the ratio of malonic acid to substrate is only 1:50, the dehydrogenase enzyme is inhibited by 50 percent.

Competitive inhibition is the basis for some forms of treatment for infectious diseases. The sulfa drugs, for example, compete with para-aminobenzoic acid (PABA), a raw material used in the synthesis of folic acid. Folic acid is important in the synthesis of a variety of compounds required for the growth of bacteria. A glance at the structures of sulfanilamide and PABA reveals their structural similarity:

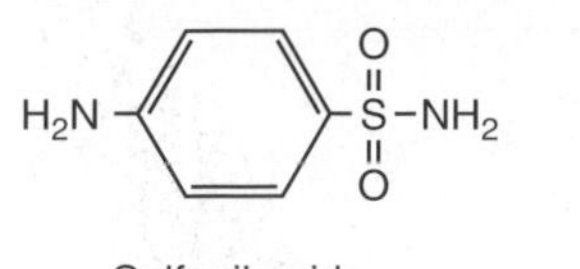

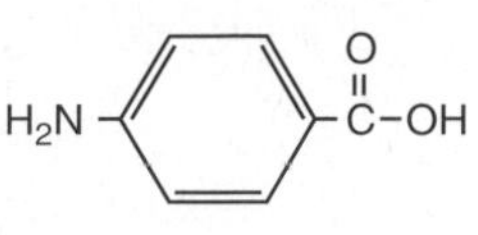

Because humans do not synthesize folic acid, sulfanilamide is useful in treating infections caused by those organisms requiring PABA. Drugs that interfere with metabolism, such as sulfanilamide, are known as **antimetabolites.** Antimetabolites constitute a valuable arsenal of weapons for treating infectious diseases and some types of cancer.

In **noncompetitive inhibition,** the rate of reaction of certain enzymes may be limited by a small molecule combining at an alternate position, called the **allosteric site,** on the enzyme. Enzymes subject to noncompetitive inhibition are called **allosteric enzymes.** Binding of the inhibitor to the allosteric site causes a conformational change in the enzyme that interferes with the binding of the normal substrate at the active site (Fig. 6–11).

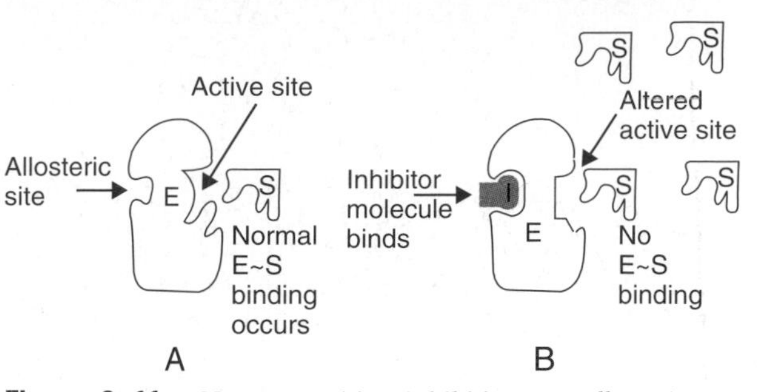

Figure 6–11 ◆ Noncompetitive inhibition on allosteric enzymes. *A,* Normal enzyme (E) with active site reacting with its substrate (S). *B,* Inhibitor (I) binding to the allosteric site causes a change in the conformation of the enzyme so that the normal substrate cannot bind.

The degree of interference in noncompetitive inhibition depends only on the concentration of the inhibitor. Noncompetitive inhibition cannot be reversed by adding additional substrate. Many of the heavy metals, such as mercury (Hg^{2+}) and silver (Ag^{2+}), act as noncompetitive inhibitors of enzymes. Chemical agents containing these metals therefore make good disinfectants.

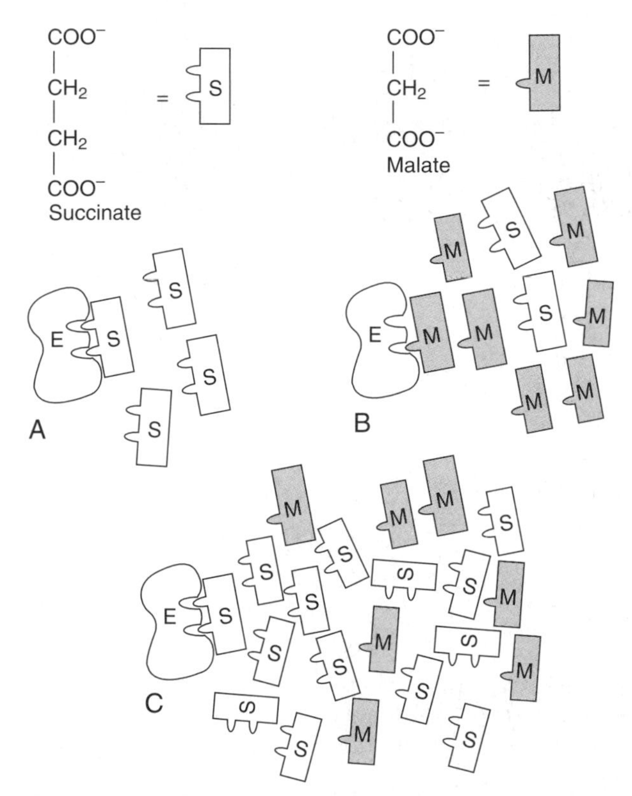

Figure 6–10 ◆ Competitive inhibition of enzyme action. *A,* Normal enzyme-substrate binding between the enzyme (E) succinate dehydrogenase and the substrate molecule (S) succinate. *B,* Malonate (M) competes with succinate for binding sites on the enzyme to block binding of succinate. *C,* If more succinate is added, succinate competes more successfully for binding to the enzyme.

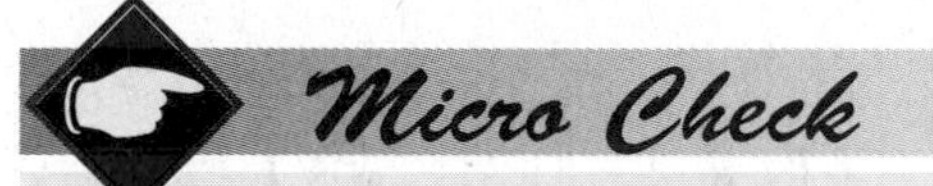

- ◆ What is meant by denaturation of enzymes?
- ◆ How is growth of microorganisms affected by small changes in temperature?
- ◆ Explain the differences between competitive and noncompetitive inhibition.

CATABOLISM: ENERGY-GENERATING REACTIONS

Microbial cells metabolize nutrients to generate ATP by (1) respiration, (2) fermentation, and (3) photosynthesis. Often more than one process is used by microorganisms for producing ATP. Respiration and fermentation generate ATP when chemical energy is released from nutrient molecules. Respiration reactions release more of the total energy available in nutrient molecules than is released during fermentation of the same molecules. Thus, respiration yields more ATP molecules, which are valuable in reactions to synthesize important molecules such as proteins and nucleic acids.

FOCAL POINT

Discovering Phosphorylase

If you could pick one molecule in metabolism to study, what would be your choice? Glucose? In the process, you may become a pioneer in enzyme research discovering the role of enzymes in disease and in energy metabolism. That's what happened for Carl and Gerty Cori, husband and wife, who spent most of their professional lives conducting medical research.

The Coris wanted to understand diseases related to glucose metabolism. Their discovery of the enzyme phosphorylase launched their career. They discovered the cyclic nature of liver and muscle enzymes in glucose metabolism, and their name was attached to the pathway, which became known as the Cori cycle. They also revealed how hormones affected the Cori cycle. Ultimately, they identified four hereditary diseases resulting from defects in carbohydrate metabolism.

Their groundbreaking work showed how phosphorylase breaks down stored glycogen to glucose 1-phosphate, beginning a process that provides energy to the working muscle. With insufficient oxygen, the working muscle accumulates lactate, which is transported to the liver. The Cori cycle is completed as the lactate is metabolized to glucose. Arda Green, a researcher in the Cori laboratories, crystallized the protein phosphorylase. After much successful work, the Coris, in 1947, shared a Nobel Prize in Physiology and Medicine with an Argentinian researcher, Bernardo A. Houssay.

Advanced researchers flocked to Washington University School of Medicine in St. Louis, Missouri, to study their methods. Many enzymes of classic biochemistry were discovered and crystallized by people using techniques often first developed in Gerty Teresa Cori's laboratories. Nobel Prizes were later awarded to eight of these researchers, including Edwin G. Krebs and Arthur Kornberg of the United States, and Severo Ochoa of Spain.

In photosynthesis, energy from light excites electrons of special photopigments. The fast-moving electrons are transported to a series of carrier molecules generating ATP. Carbohydrates, proteins, lipids, and photopigments, like chlorophyll, are excellent sources of energy because they contain so many hydrogen atoms. The atoms of hydrogen contain small packets of energy, the electrons.

Respiration

In the process of respiration, electrons are transferred from a molecule by a series of oxidation-reduction reactions to a final electron acceptor. During the reactions, energy is released and stored in high-energy bonds. Oxygen is the final electron acceptor in **aerobic respiration.** Many microorganisms depend on environmental oxygen as the final electron acceptor. For some microorganisms, oxygen is toxic, and respiration is conducted with other inorganic molecules acting as the final electron acceptors in a process known as **anaerobic respiration.** Often, organisms are able to utilize either aerobic or anaerobic respiration depending on the enzymes in the organism and on the availability of oxygen.

AEROBIC RESPIRATION

We shall begin our catabolic journey with a single molecule of glucose ($C_6H_{12}O_6$) and six molecules of oxygen gas (O_2). At the end of aerobic respiration, the glucose will be degraded to six molecules of carbon dioxide gas (CO_2) and six molecules of water (H_2O) and will release enough energy to form 38 ATP molecules. The overall reaction for the aerobic respiration of glucose is:

$$C_6H_{12}O_6 + 6O_2 \longrightarrow 6CO_2 + 6H_2O + \text{energy}$$

Energy is used to generate ATP in three pathways of aerobic respiration: (1) glycolysis, (2) the citric acid cycle or Krebs cycle, and (3) electron transport.

Glycolysis

The first pathway, glycolysis, involves 10 enzyme reactions and produces a net yield of two molecules of **pyruvic acid** and two molecules of ATP from one molecule of glucose (Fig. 6–12). No oxygen is required for glycolysis to occur. This reaction series also produces two molecules of reduced NAD (designated NADH or $NADH_2$), which is oxidized in later reactions by donating

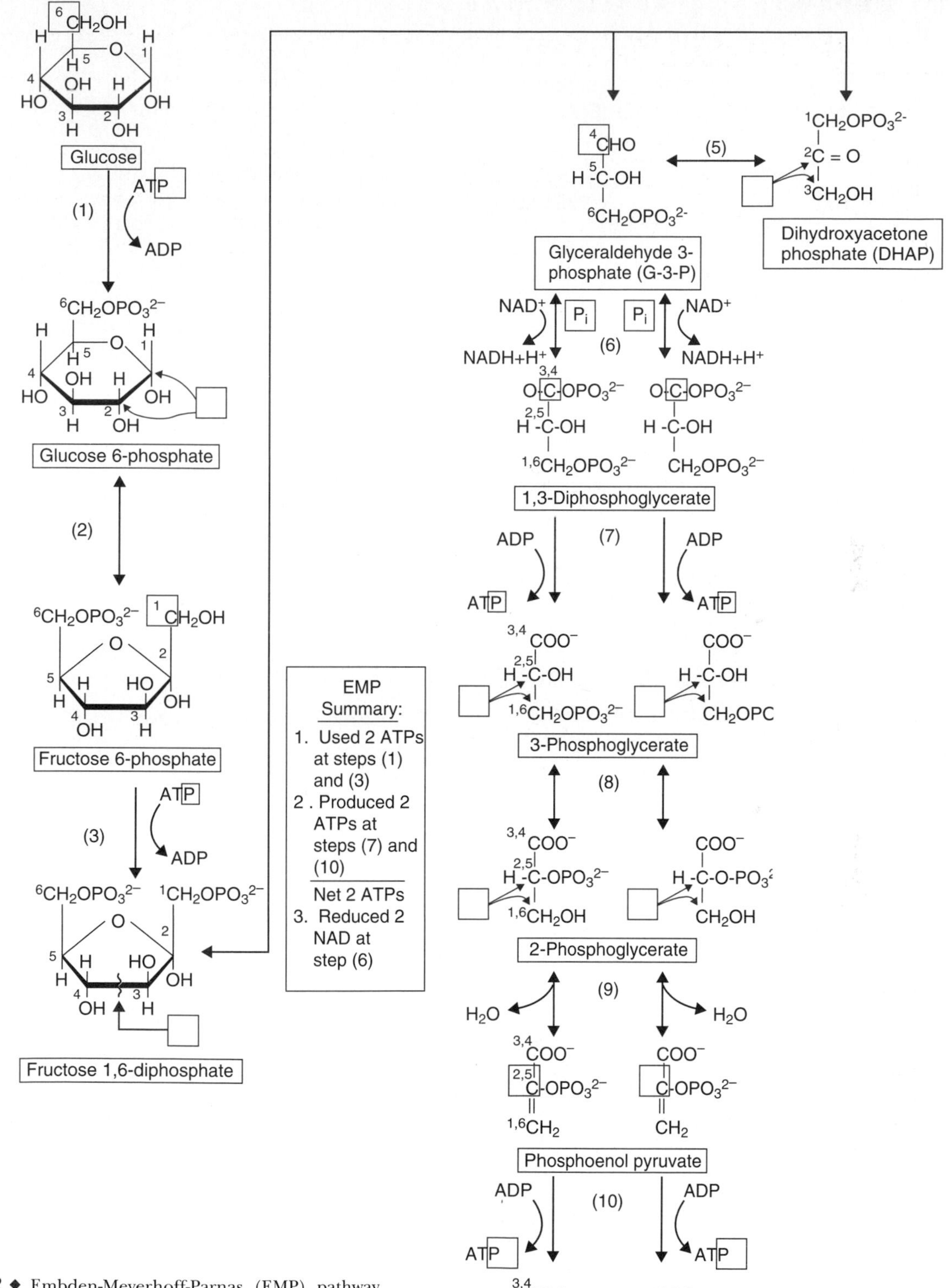

Figure 6–12 ◆ Embden-Meyerhoff-Parnas (EMP) pathway. Degradation of glucose to the key intermediate pyruvic acid (pyruvate) by glycolysis releases enough energy to form two molecules of ATP. Colored squares highlight where the next change will take place. Numbers on the carbon atoms show where the carbon atoms of glucose are found in subsequent reactions.

Table 6–3
ENZYMES OF THE EMBDEN-MEYERHOF-PARNAS (EMP) PATHWAY

STEP	ENZYME	ATP USED (−) OR PRODUCED (+)
1	Hexokinase	−1
2	Phosphoglucoisomerase	0
3	Phosphofructokinase	−1
4	Aldolase	0
5	Triose phosphate isomerase	0
6	Glyceraldehyde phosphate dehydrogenase	0
7	Phosphoglycerate kinase	+1*
8	Phosphoglycerate mutase	0
9	Enolase	0
10	Pyruvate kinase	+1*

*ATP values from reactions 7 and 10 are given per molecule of substrate at these steps. Because reaction 4 splits the six-carbon molecule into two three-carbon molecules, the number of ATP molecules produced at reactions 7 and 10 is doubled.

its hydrogen ions and electrons to other molecules.

$$C_6H_{12}O_6 + 2ADP + 2P_i \longrightarrow 2CH_3COCOOH + 2ATP$$

Glucose → Pyruvic acid

The series of reactions involved in glycolysis is known as the **Embden-Meyerhof-Parnas (EMP) pathway** to recognize the principal investigators of this pathway. The carbon atoms of glucose are numbered on the molecule to make it easier to understand the location of an enzyme's action and the name of the molecules (see Fig. 6–12). Each EMP reaction is catalyzed by a different enzyme (Table 6–3). In the first stage of the EMP pathway two molecules of ATP are required. The four reactions in this stage lead to breaking the glucose chain into two molecules with three carbons each. In the second stage of the EMP pathway, energy is released twice to generate four ATP molecules.

The first stage of glycolysis consists of steps 1 through 5. The energy to initiate the glycolytic pathway is supplied by a molecule of ATP in step 1 and a second ATP molecule in step 3. Steps 6 through 10 constitute the second stage of glycolysis. Two molecules of ATP are generated in step 7 and two more in step 10. A net yield of two ATP molecules results from one glucose entering the EMP pathway.

Two molecules of reduced NAD are also produced in the EMP pathway. To continue metabolizing glucose, these NADH molecules must be oxidized to NAD^+ in other reactions. The fate of reduced NAD is considered in the subsequent sections on fermentation and electron transport

Table 6–4
ENZYMES OF THE "BRIDGE REACTION" AND THE CITRIC ACID CYCLE

REACTION	ENZYME	ENZYME ACTION(S)
Bridge reaction:		
Pyruvate to acetyl-CoA and CO_2	Pyruvate dehydrogenase	Remove H^+ Produce CO_2 Add CoA
Citric acid cycle		
Acetyl-CoA and oxaloacetate to citrate	Citrate synthase	Condensation to citric acid
Citrate to isocitrate	Aconitase	Isomerization
Isocitrate to alpha-ketoglutarate	Isocitrate dehydrogenase	Remove H^+ Produce CO_2
Alpha-ketoglutarate to succinyl-CoA	Alpha-ketoglutarate dehydrogenase	Remove H^+ Add CoA Produce CO_2
Succinyl-CoA to succinate	Succinate thiokinase	Remove CoA Form high-energy phosphate bond on GDP
Succinate to fumarate	Succinate dehydrogenase	Remove H^+
Fumarate to malate	Fumarase	Add H_2O
Malate to oxaloacetate	Malate dehydrogenase	Remove H^+

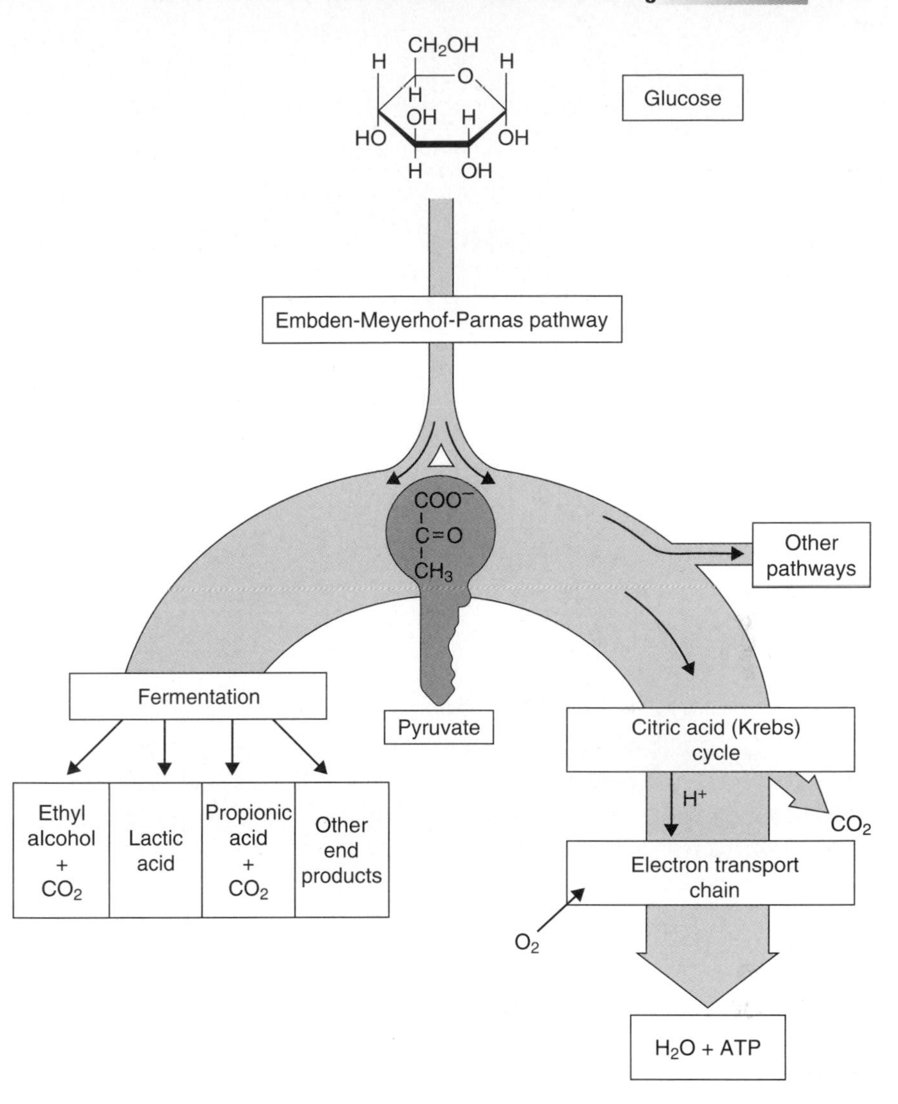

Figure 6–13 ◆ Pyruvate acts as a "bridge" to other pathways. Glycolytic enzymes produce pyruvate, which may be further metabolized by the citric acid cycle, fermentation, or in other pathways.

in this chapter. The end product of glycolysis, pyruvate or pyruvic acid, is considered a key metabolite because it participates in so many chemical reactions in cells (Fig. 6–13).

The Metabolic Bridge

We are all familiar with bridges that link highways to one another. The chemical pathways in cells are often connected by reactions that can be considered metabolic bridges. Molecular traffic is directed to one or more biochemical pathways. In aerobic respiration, pyruvate connects glycolysis to the citric acid cycle by an enzyme converting the pyruvate to **acetyl-coenzyme A (acetyl-CoA)** and carbon dioxide (CO_2) while transferring two hydrogen ions to NAD^+ (Table 6–4).

The two electrons and hydrogen ions accepted by NAD^+ reduce this molecule to $NADH + H^+$. The fate of the reduced NAD molecules is discussed in the section describing the electron transport chain.

$$\underset{\text{Pyruvic acid}}{CH_3COCOOH} + \underset{\text{Coenzyme A}}{CoA{-}SH} + NAD^+ \longrightarrow \underset{\text{Acetyl-CoA}}{CH_3CO{-}S{-}CoA} + CO_2 + \underset{\text{Reduced NAD}}{NADH_2}$$

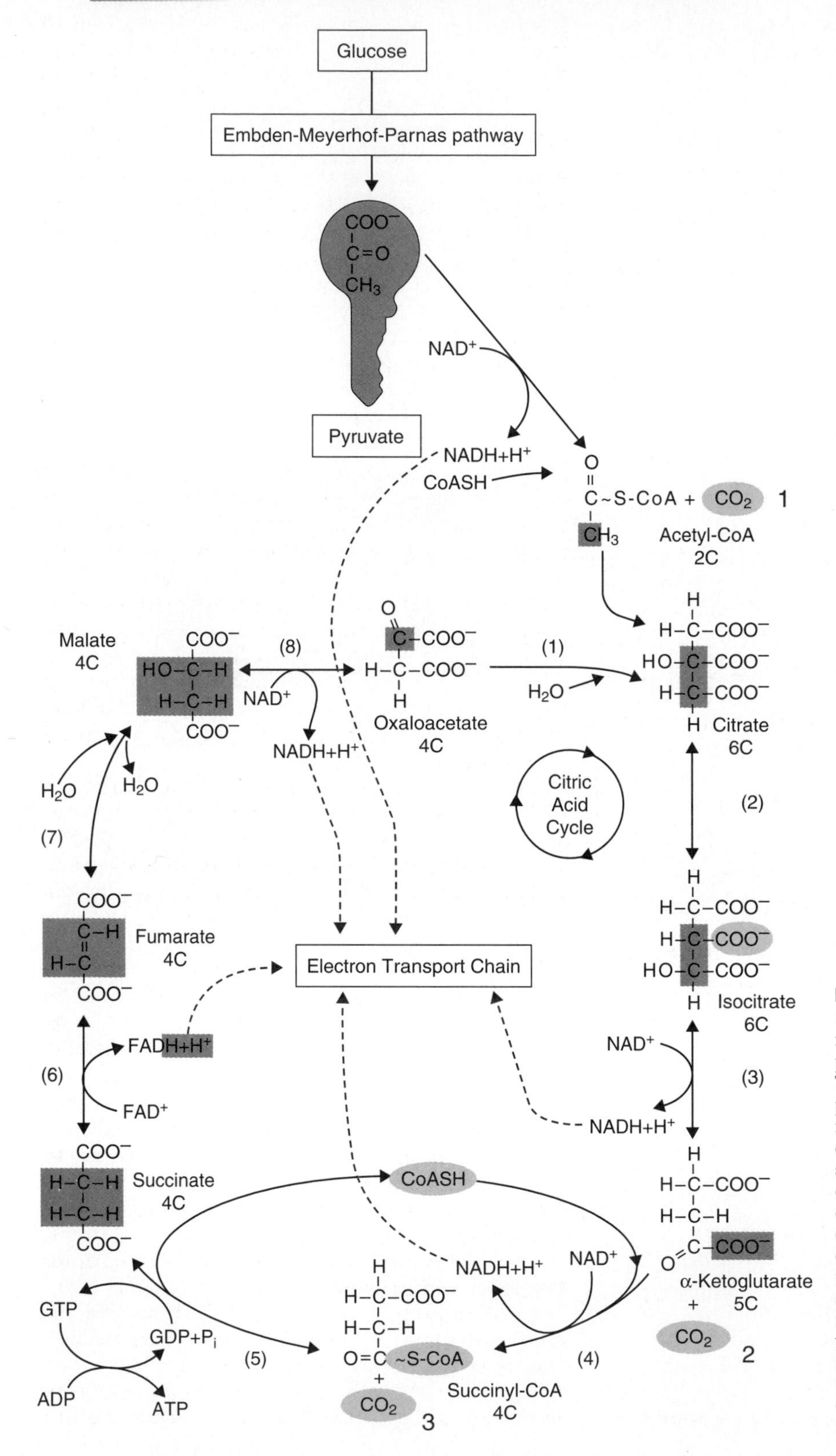

Figure 6–14 ◆ The citric acid (Krebs) cycle showing intermediate metabolites and the reactions that produce reduced NAD and FAD. The pink dashed arrows show the path of these reduced coenzyme molecules to the electron transport chain where they are oxidized. The shaded pink ovals show the three decarboxylation reactions to produce CO_2. The shaded pink ovals of coenzyme A (CoASH) show it is cycled from reaction (4) to reaction (5) where it is released to react again. The colored squares and rectangles indicate which atoms will participate in the next reaction. Finally, the cycle ends with the same molecule it started with, oxaloacetate, which reacts with acetyl-CoA for another cycle.

Coenzyme A (CoA) is a sulfur-containing (S) carrier molecule that transports the acetyl group (CH_3CO—) to the citric acid cycle.

The Citric Acid Cycle

The second pathway in aerobic respiration, the **citric acid cycle** has eight steps that end with the molecules needed to restart the cycle (Fig. 6–14). The cycle is also known by two other names: (1) the **tricarboxylic acid cycle** because citric acid has three carboxyl groups in its structure and (2) the **Krebs cycle** to honor the major researcher of this cycle, Hans Krebs. The relationship between the pathways by which glucose is catabolized aerobically by EMP, citric acid cycle, and the electron transport chain is indicated in Figure 6–14. Enzymes of the citric acid cycle are found on the plasma membrane in procaryotes and within the matrix of mitochondria in eucaryotes (see Table 6–4).

During one turn of the citric acid cycle, three molecules of NADH, one molecule of FADH, and one molecule of an energy-rich guanosine triphosphate (GTP) are generated. Because two molecules of acetyl-CoA are derived from one molecule of glucose, the cycle operates twice for each molecule of glucose oxidized. For two turns of the cycle, the figures for NADH, FADH, and GTP are multiplied by two to represent the yield from one molecule of glucose: 6 NADH, 2 FADH, 2 GTP.

The phosphate group of GTP is transferred to ADP to form one molecule of ATP in a side reaction. At steps 3 and 4, CO_2 is released. Small amounts of CO_2 produced during the citric acid cycle are used in endergonic pathways. Excess CO_2 is excreted as a gas into the environment. The citric acid cycle makes one turn and ends with oxaloacetate. Oxaloacetate reacts with a second acetyl-CoA to form citrate or citric acid, thus beginning a second turn of the cycle for each glucose utilized.

Molecules of NAD^+ and FAD^+ are essential in the glycolysis pathway and the citric acid cycle to pick up hydrogens and electrons. The reduced forms of these molecules are oxidized in the electron transport chain, a series of reduction-oxidation (redox) reactions to regenerate these coenzymes while producing ATP, O_2, and H_2O.

The Electron Transport Chain

To regenerate NAD^+ and FAD^+, electrons and hydrogen ions are transferred from reduced NAD and FAD molecules to carrier molecules in the electron transport or **respiratory chain** (Fig. 6–15). The last carrier transfers the electrons to oxygen, which is the final electron acceptor in aerobic respiration. The carrier molecules vary in different organisms and even in a single species, depending on growth conditions. In certain reactions, the carrier molecules release sufficient quantities of energy to result in the formation of high-energy phosphate bonds on ADP to produce ATP. Three molecules of ATP are produced by electron transport per each molecule of reduced NAD. Two molecules of ATP are produced by electron transport per each molecule of reduced FAD.

The power of the electron transport chain lies in the stepwise release of energy from hydrogen ions and electrons to make a large number of ATP molecules per glucose molecule. The energy requirements for cellular growth, division, locomotion, and many other functions are supplied by ATP.

In eucaryotic organisms, most of the electron carriers are contained within the inner membranes of mitochondria (Fig. 6–16*D*). A few carriers are located in the external membranes of mitochondria. The electron transport chain in procaryotes is associated with the plasma membrane (Fig. 6–16*A*).

The electrons travel from carrier molecules with low redox potentials to carriers with increasingly higher redox potentials (see Fig. 6–15). The electron carriers include **flavoproteins** (such as flavin mononucleotide, FMN), **iron-sulfur enzymes** (Fe/S), nonprotein quinones such as **coenzyme Q (CoQ),** and a few **cytochromes** (proteins containing an iron group). As the hydrogen ions and electrons are transferred from NADH to the chain of carriers, energy is released and captured by phosphorylating ADP to generate ATP. Further energy-yielding reactions (exergonic) occur to these electrons and hydrogen ions as they pass through the chain of carrier molecules.

The exergonic reactions provide a force to move protons or hydrogen ions (H^+) from the inner surface of a membrane to the outer surface of the membrane. While the protons travel through the membrane, electrons move down the chain of carrier molecules.

As more protons are pumped to the outside of the membrane, an electrical and concentration difference, or **proton gradient,** develops. The area outside the membrane becomes more positive (more H^+) and more acid. The protons

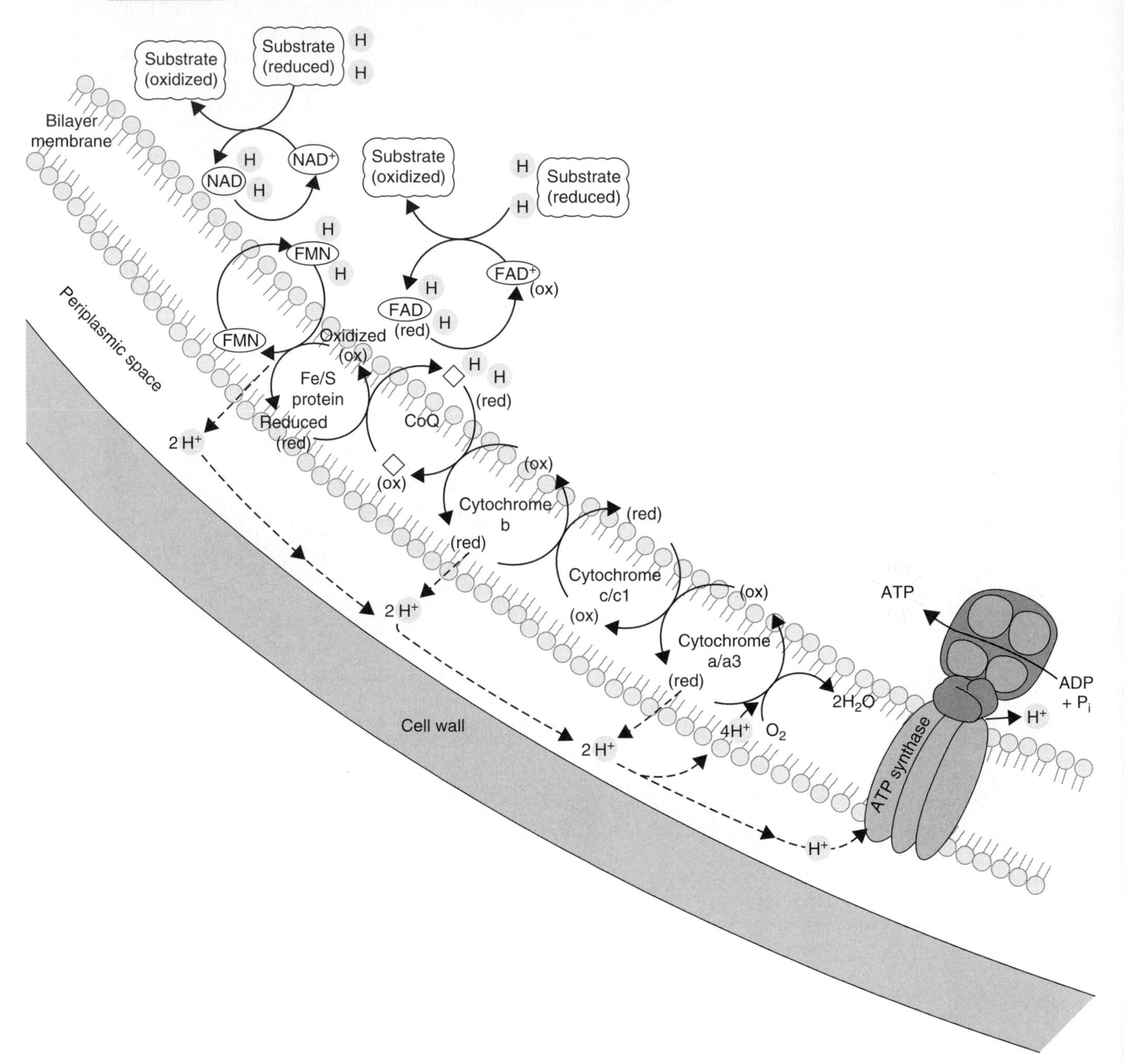

Figure 6–15 ◆ One model of an electron transport chain. Electrons proceed from $NADH^+$ and $FADH^+$ to other electron carriers in a chain of molecules located in membranes. Oxygen is a final electron acceptor in aerobic metabolism. As hydrogen ions (H^+) are released, they move to the outer side of the membrane. Accumulation of H^+ on the outer side of the membrane creates a proton motive force to drive the H^+ ions back to the inner side through the pores of ATP synthase. The proton motive force releases energy to generate ATP as the H^+ ions (protons) travel through the ATP synthase complex.

move from the region of high proton concentration to the inner surface of the membrane where protons are in low concentration in a process termed **chemiosmosis.** The return movement of protons occurs through a specific enzyme complex located in the membrane, ATP synthase (see Figs. 6–15 and 6–16*D*). Transporting H^+ through ATP synthase energizes the enzyme com-

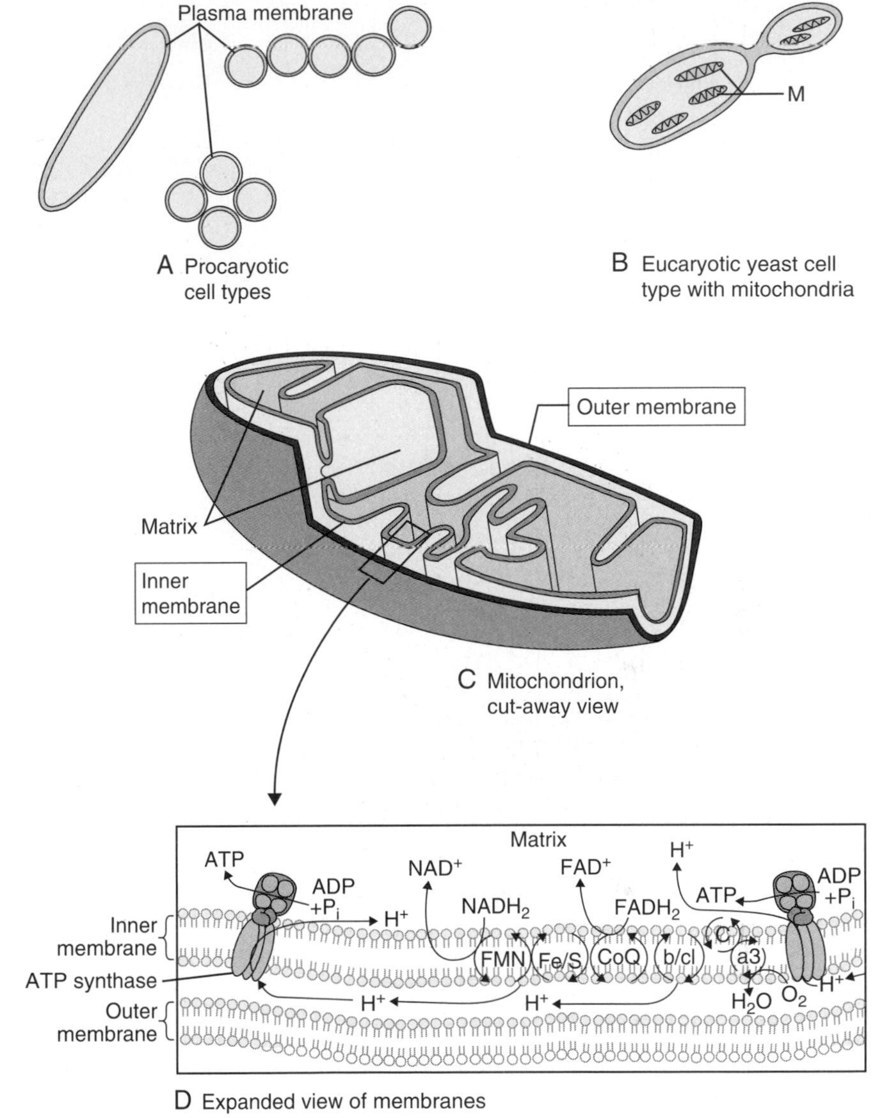

Figure 6–16 ◆ Electron transport chain locations. *A,* In procaryotes, the chain is found on the plasma cell membrane. *B,* In eucaryotes such as yeast cells, the chain is found on the inner membrane of the mitochondrion. *C,* A mitochondrion is shown in a cut-away view, which reveals the matrix and the inner and outer membranes. *D,* An expanded view of the mitochondrial membranes shows the association of electron carriers and ATP synthase with the inner membrane. As H^+ ions (protons) accumulate in the space between membranes, a proton motive force (PMF) develops to push the protons back across the membrane through the pore of ATP synthase. The energy released by PMF is captured by ATP synthase to produce ATP.

plex to form ATP while releasing the protons to the inside of the membrane (see Figs. 6–15 and 6–16*D*). This mechanism is responsible for most of the ATP in cells.

Phosphorylation, occurring in the electron transport chain, is called **oxidative phosphorylation** because it is always coupled with oxidation of carrier molecules. Some chemical inhibitors of electron transport, such as cyanide, uncouple oxidative phosphorylation and limit the generation of ATP. This uncoupling, ultimately, causes a critical energy shortage, which often leads to death.

Tallying the Score of Energy Yields

Now we can make a tally of the number of molecules of ATP and reduced NAD and FAD molecules in glycolysis and the citric acid cycle (Table 6–5). Glycolysis resulted in a net production of two molecules of ATP by a **substrate phosphorylation** reaction. In aerobic respiration with a membrane system of electron transport, the two molecules of reduced NAD (step 6 of glycolysis) yield six molecules of ATP.

In the “bridge” reaction, in which pyruvate is decarboxylated to acetyl-CoA, reduced NAD is formed. Because two molecules of pyruvate are

Table 6–5
TALLY OF MOLECULAR YIELD FROM ONE MOLECULE OF GLUCOSE IN AEROBIC RESPIRATION

PATHWAY	NADH	FADH	ATP
Glycolysis	2	0	2
Metabolic bridge	2		
Citric acid cycle	6	2	2*
Electron transport system	0	0	34
Totals	10†	2‡	38

*ATP is produced when one PO_4 is transferred from GTP to form ATP.

†Three molecules of ATP are produced during electron transport from each molecule of NADH.

‡Two molecules of ATP are produced during electron transport from each molecule of FADH.

produced per glucose, two molecules of reduced NAD are produced. If we assume all the reduced NAD molecules are oxidized by the electron transport chain, then six molecules of ATP are produced by oxidative phosphorylation.

In the citric acid cycle, two molecules of ATP are produced by substrate phosphorylation at step 5. The six molecules of reduced NAD will generate 18 molecules of ATP by oxidative phosphorylation. The two molecules of reduced FAD will generate four molecules of ATP. The net number of ATP molecules generated as glucose is broken down aerobically is 38 (Table 6–5).

Aerobic respiration in some eucaryotes yields 36 ATP molecules. One explanation for this difference may be that ATP energy is used to transport two pyruvate molecules from the cytoplasm across the mitochondrial membrane. In eucaryotes, glycolysis occurs in the cytoplasm while reactions of the citric acid cycle and electron transport chain occur in the mitochondria. In procaryotes, the reactions of glycolysis, citric acid cycle, and electron transport occur in the cytoplasm and plasma membrane of the cell.

Recent studies indicate that the number of molecules of ATP generated by oxidative phosphorylation vary from the numbers generally reported in introductory textbooks. Some studies suggest that 2.5 molecules of ATP are generated per molecule of reduced NAD, and 1.5 molecules of ATP per molecule of reduced FAD. For our purposes, we find it convenient to continue using the generally acceptable values given in this section.

Micro Check

- In which pathway are most reduced NAD molecules formed?
- Where do the reactions of the citric acid cycle take place in procaryotes? In eucaryotes?
- What is the effect of uncoupling (inhibiting) oxidative phosphorylation?

ANAEROBIC RESPIRATION

Some bacteria utilize anaerobic respiration for generating energy. In this process, the final electron acceptor in electron transport is an inorganic electron acceptor, but not oxygen. Obligate anaerobes lack the enzymes necessary to release the total potential energy from glucose and are extremely sensitive to the presence of atmospheric oxygen. Oxygen is so toxic to strict anaerobes that even brief exposure to an air atmosphere kills most of the population. Facultatively anaerobic bacteria, such as *Escherichia coli,* may use anaerobic respiration when oxygen is limited or absent.

Depending on the species of anaerobic bacteria, the final electron acceptor may be either CO_2, the sulfate ion (SO_4^{2-}), or the nitrate ion (NO_3^-).

$$CO_2 + 4H_2 \longrightarrow CH_4 + 2H_2O \quad \text{(Type 1)}$$

$$Na_2SO_4 + H_2 \longrightarrow Na_2SO_3 + H_2O \quad \text{(Type 2)}$$

$$NaNO_3 + H_2 \longrightarrow NaNO_2 + H_2O \quad \text{(Type 3)}$$

The methane (CH_4) producers (Type 1) and the sulfate-reducing bacteria (Type 2) such as *Desulfovibrio* are obligate anaerobes, which are widely distributed in polluted waters, swamps, and marshes. The denitrifiers (Type 3) include bacteria in the genera *Pseudomonas, Bacillus,* and *Escherichia.* These bacteria are essential to the natural cycling of nitrogen and sulfur in soil and water.

Fermentation

When electrons are transferred to organic molecules in the final step of electron transport, the process is known as **fermentation.** Organic molecules serve as electron donors and acceptors in fermentation. Fermentation usually begins with the EMP pathway but varies with the end products that are produced.

Each species of fermenting bacteria and yeast has specific enzymes by which the key metabolite, pyruvic acid, is metabolized further to make the final products (Fig. 6–17). In all the pathways by which pyruvate is metabolized, reduced NAD is oxidized by an organic molecule accepting electrons and hydrogens. In this way, step 6 of the EMP pathway continues, so the cell continues to catabolize sugars. However, fermentation is not as efficient as aerobic respiration in gaining energy from the sugar. In most fermentations, the net yield is two molecules of ATP.

Fermentation is used industrially to make a number of useful products, including alcoholic beverages, bread, and fermented milk products, such as cheese and yogurt. In the making of wine or beer, special strains of yeasts are used to ferment sugars in the starting material. Industrial fermentations are discussed in Chapter 24.

The overall reaction for glucose in an alcoholic fermentation is as follows:

$$\underset{\text{Glucose}}{C_6H_{12}O_6} + 2ADP + 2P_i \longrightarrow \underset{\text{Ethyl alcohol}}{2C_2H_5OH} + 2CO_2 + 2ATP$$

Ethyl alcohol and CO_2 are the primary end products. Because only partial oxidation of glucose occurs, the energy released by fermentation is much less than that which accompanies complete oxidation of a glucose molecule to six CO_2 molecules.

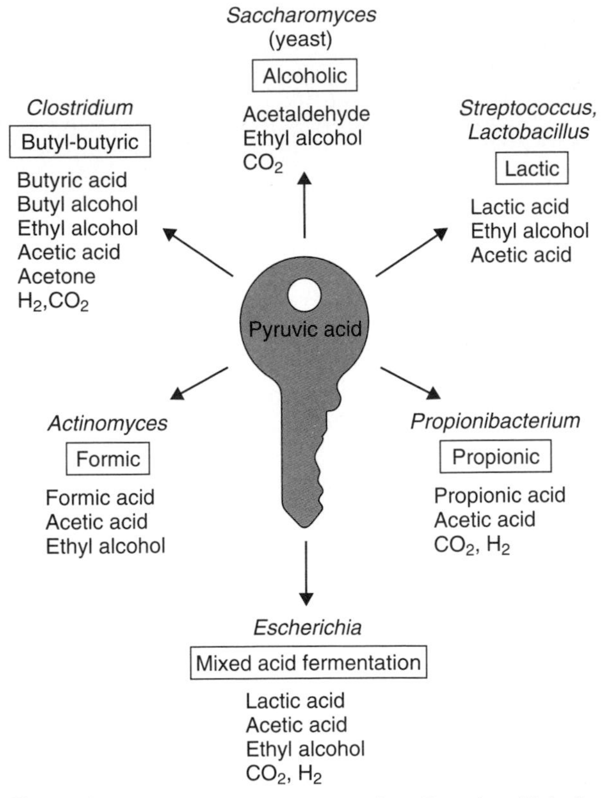

Figure 6–17 ◆ Products of fermentation. Pyruvic acid is the key intermediate metabolite, which is converted by different species to a variety of end products. The lactic acid fermentations are extremely useful in the commercial production of bread, wine, beer, and fermented dairy and vegetable products.

Among the lactic acid bacteria, fermentation of lactose may produce lactic acid, acetic acid, ethanol, and some gases. If lactic acid is the primary end product of fermentation, the microorganisms are said to be **homofermentative.** The homofermentative lactic acid bacteria such as *Streptococcus thermophilus* and *Lactobacillus bulgaricus* are important in the commercial production of yogurt. An overall reaction for the homofermentation of glucose in milk follows:

$$\underset{\text{Glucose}}{C_6H_{12}O_6} + 2ADP + 2P_i \longrightarrow \underset{\text{Lactic acid}}{2C_3H_6O_3} + 2ATP$$

A **heterofermentative** microorganism produces a mixture of acids, alcohols, and gases as the end products of fermentation. The commercial fermentation of cabbage to sauerkraut involves heterofermentative bacterial species such as *Leuconostoc mesenteroides.*

Although fermentation is not an efficient energy-yielding process for microorganisms, it does provide an alternative metabolic pathway for facultative anaerobes in the absence of oxygen. Microbiologists use a variety of fermentation tests as aids in the identification of organisms.

Metabolism of Other Carbohydrates, Lipids, and Proteins

Glucose represents only one carbohydrate source of energy for microorganisms. Sucrose, fructose, lactose, galactose, mannose, xylose, mannitol, and sorbitol are a few other sugars used as an energy source.

Microorganisms degrade a wide variety of other carbon-containing compounds. Before a large polymeric molecule can be used by cells, it must be broken down to its smaller monomer units. The monomers can enter catabolic pathways at various points (Fig. 6–18). For example, polysaccharide molecules such as starch and cellulose are degraded to their component sugars, such as glucose. Fatty acids and glycerol are the breakdown products of fats and lipids, which act as energy sources for catabolism in the respiration pathways. Proteins are broken down into amino acid units or short chains of amino acids known as peptides. These amino acids are produced from and used in respiration pathways.

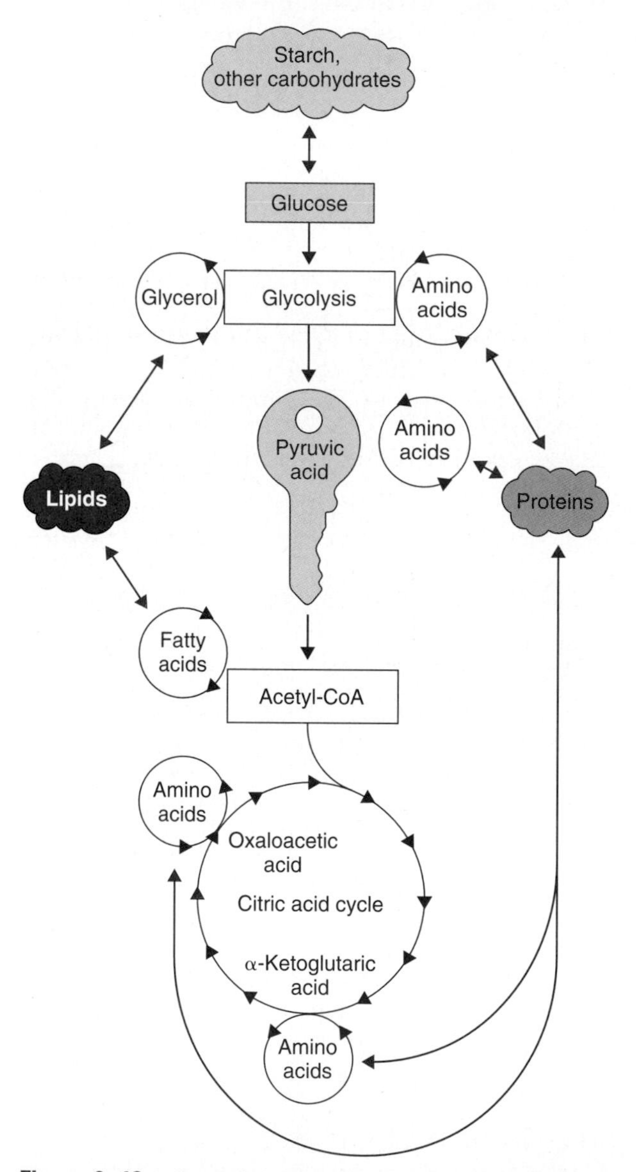

Figure 6–18 ◆ Interrelationships in the degradation of carbohydrates, lipids, and proteins. In catabolic reactions, fats, proteins, and carbohydrates are degraded to smaller molecules, which are metabolized by way of the Embden-Meyerhof-Parnas pathway or the citric acid cycle. These same metabolic pathways may operate in the opposite direction to construct or synthesize proteins, fats, and carbohydrates as needed.

Photosynthesis

Most algae, plants, cyanobacteria, and some other phototrophic bacteria have the ability to convert light energy into chemical energy, such as ATP, by the process of **photosynthesis.** The photosynthetic process in cyanobacteria, algae, and plants employs water as a source of hydrogen and produces oxygen gas in a process called **oxygenic photosynthesis** (Fig. 6–19).

Photosynthesis in a different group of bacteria, the phototrophic green sulfur and purple sulfur bacteria, takes place only under anaerobic conditions and is described as **anoxygenic photosynthesis.** Instead of water, sulfur (S), hydrogen sulfide (H_2S) or hydrogen gas (H_2) serves as a source of hydrogen to reduce carbon dioxide. An overall general reaction for photosynthesis may be expressed as follows:

$$CO_2 + 2H_2X \xrightarrow{\text{light}} (CH_2O) + 2X + H_2O$$

The H_2X symbolizes H_20 in cyanobacteria, algae, and plants and symbolizes H_2S in the photosynthetic sulfur bacteria. To initiate photosynthesis, light wavelengths of 700 nm or less are necessary in chlorophyll-containing eucaryotic cells. Wavelengths between 725 and 1035 nm are useful in procaryotic cells, which have different chlorophylls called bacteriochlorophylls.

The reactions of photosynthesis are often divided into reactions that require light and those which are light-independent and can take place in the light or dark. The light reactions start when a molecule of a photopigment, such as chlorophyll a, absorbs light energy. The absorbed light is transferred very rapidly to other molecules of pigment until it reaches a special molecule of chlorophyll located in a reaction center. Electron flow is generated from the light excitation of these photopigments.

The pattern of electron flow differs in oxygenic and anoxygenic photosynthesis, but carrier

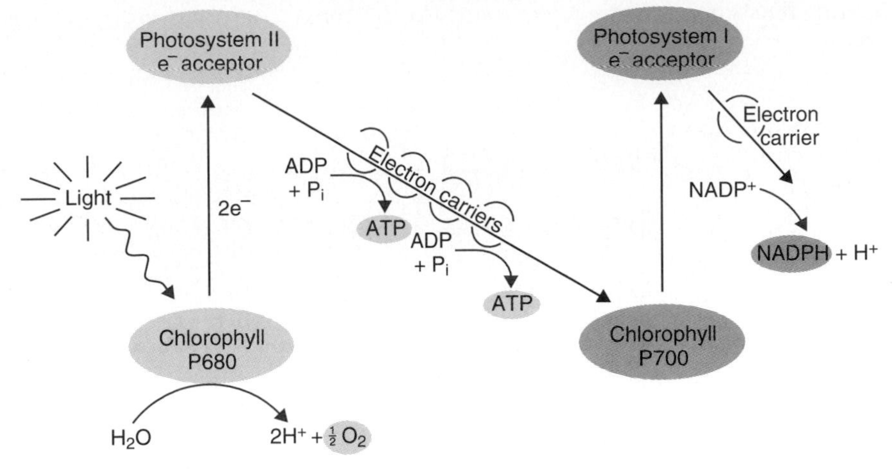

Figure 6–19 ◆ Noncyclic photophosphorylation. The electron released from chlorophyll is carried eventually to $NADP^+$. ATP and $NADPH_2$ are generated in this process. The hydrolysis of water generates the electron for another passage through the photosystems. Oxygen gas (O_2) is released from two molecules of water.

molecules are similar to those found in the electron transport chain. ATP is generated as a proton gradient and is established across the intracellular membranes of phototrophic bacteria or the thylakoid membranes of eucaryotic chloroplasts. The role of proton gradients (proton motive force, PMF) in membrane transport and generation of ATP was discussed earlier in this chapter. The generation of ATP from light energy is called **photophosphorylation.**

The fixation (reduction) of CO_2 occurs in a cyclic series of chemical reactions that do not require light (Fig. 6–20), known as the **Calvin-Benson cycle.** Although fixation of CO_2 was first studied in algae, the same reactions occur in most autotrophs. In those reactions, CO_2 is reduced or fixed to produce a series of intermediate compounds which enter biosynthetic pathways at particular points. Because an input of ATP is needed to initiate the cycle, de-

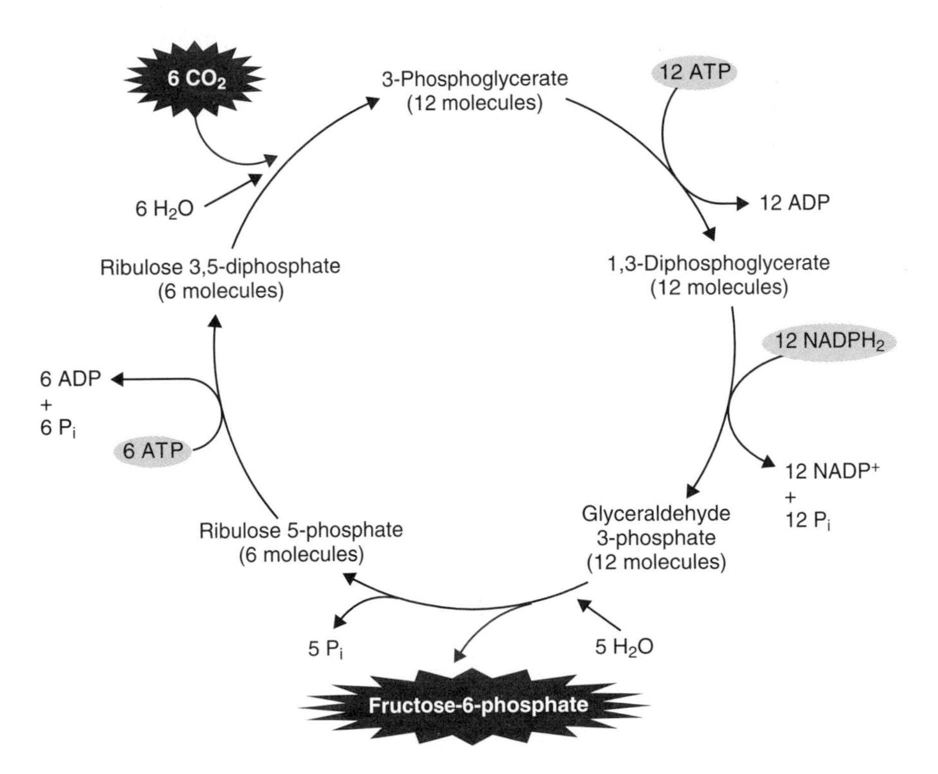

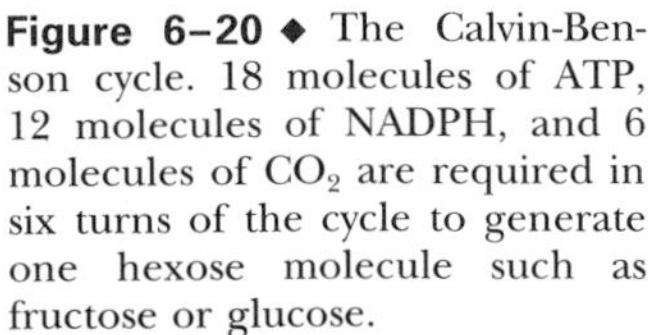

Figure 6–20 ◆ The Calvin-Benson cycle. 18 molecules of ATP, 12 molecules of NADPH, and 6 molecules of CO_2 are required in six turns of the cycle to generate one hexose molecule such as fructose or glucose.

tailed reactions will be discussed in the next section.

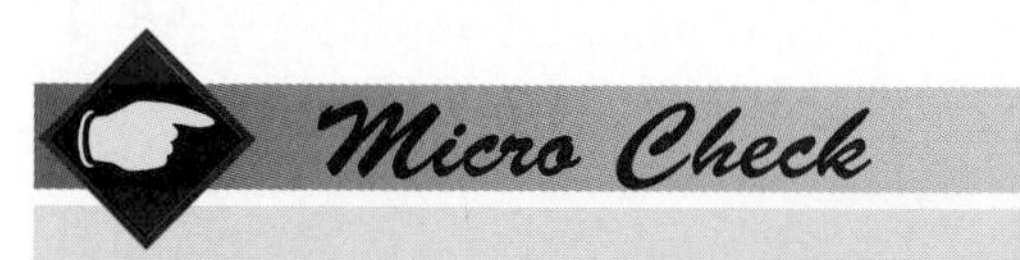

- What gas is produced in oxygenic photosynthesis?
- What cycle is involved in fixing carbon dioxide gas to produce sugar?
- What is the relationship between humans and other animals and photosynthetic organisms?

ANABOLISM: ENERGY-REQUIRING REACTIONS

Energy released by catabolism is used to synthesize important cellular molecules in anabolic reactions. Some microorganisms are able to synthesize organic compounds from inorganic molecules. Other microorganisms use intermediate products formed by a series of degradation reactions for the synthesis of carbohydrates, proteins, lipids, and nucleic acids. For example, **autotrophs** use CO_2 as a sole source of carbon to produce complex organic molecules. Other bacteria known as **heterotrophs** depend on organic molecules primarily. They use ATP and intermediate products of catabolism for synthezing carbohydrates, proteins, lipids, and nucleic acids. The energy requirements for CO_2 fixation are derived from photosynthesis, fermentation, or respiration. The major products of CO_2 fixation are carbohydrates.

Synthesis of Carbohydrates

Carbohydrate molecules are a diverse group of molecules including simple sugars like glucose, disaccharides (two sugars joined to each other by a glycosidic bond) such as sucrose, and polysaccharides containing multiple glycosidic bonds such as starch and cellulose. Their synthesis involves ATP energy and carbon-containing molecules, the simplest of which is CO_2. See Chapter 2 for a discussion of carbohydrates and glycosidic bonds.

The major product of CO_2 fixation in autotrophs is 3-phosphoglycerate. When CO_2 reacts with ribulose 1,5-diphosphate, two molecules of 3-phosphoglycerate are formed. Six turns of the Calvin-Benson cycle provided by six molecules of CO_2 produce one hexose, fructose 6-phosphate (see Fig. 6–20). A constant supply of ribulose is generated in the cycle. The molecules of ATP and reduced NADP are provided by the light reactions of photosynthesis. Intermediates of the cycle enter other synthetic pathways to form polysaccharides or to enter the EMP pathway.

A number of hexoses (sugars with six carbons) are derived from the glucose 6-phosphate formed in glycolysis. Many pathways involve uridine diphosphate glucose (UDPG), an intermediate nucleoside molecule containing glucose. Other nucleosides participate in the synthesis of sugars like those found in peptidoglycan of bacterial cell walls. Nucleosides are discussed in Chapter 2.

In the synthesis of polysaccharides, a primer, often consisting of a small polysaccharide fragment, is required (Fig. 6–21). The primer acts as a material on which subsequent chemical reactions can bind, much as applying a primer (base)

FOCAL POINT

Ribozymes: Discovery of a Catalytic Role for RNA

The 1989 Nobel Prize in Chemistry went to Sidney Altman of Yale University and Thomas Cech of the University of Colorado for their independent discoveries that RNA molecules can act as enzymes. Until that time, enzymatic catalysis was thought to be the exclusive domain of proteins. Cech found that pre-ribosomal RNA was capable of removing nonessential sequences from a large molecule of RNA and then splicing the ends of the remaining RNA.

Altman demonstrated that the catalytic activity of a ribonuclease was in the RNA subunit. Cech's work was done with an eucaryotic microorganism called *Tetrahymena.* The mechanism is now known to occur universally in mitochondria. Some scientists hypothesize that life on early Earth was an "RNA world" where RNA carried out the necessary activities of life without the help of either proteins or DNA.

Adapted from Science 246:325, 1989

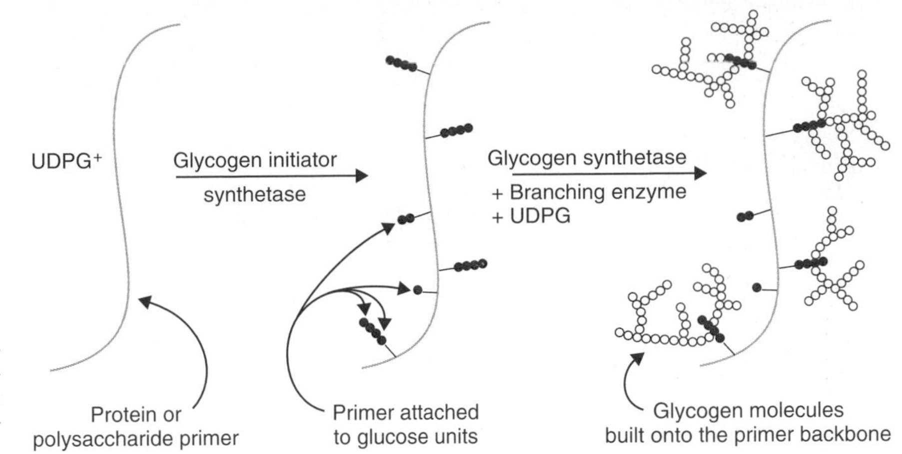

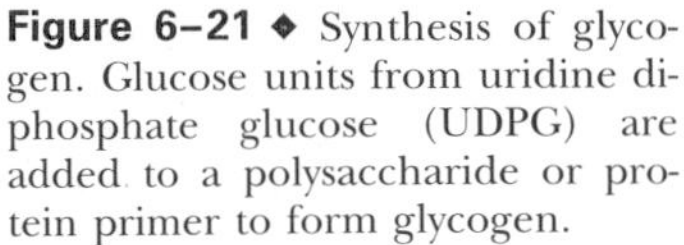
Figure 6–21 ◆ Synthesis of glycogen. Glucose units from uridine diphosphate glucose (UDPG) are added to a polysaccharide or protein primer to form glycogen.

coat of paint to a new surface helps bind the top coat of paint. For example, the synthesis of cellulose and starch is initiated by dextrins as primers. Dextrins are branching chains of glucose and maltose sugars. Glucose units are added to the primer with energy supplied by a nucleoside such as uridine diphosphoglucose (UDPG). The glucose units are connected by glycosidic linkages as water molecules are lost.

Synthesis of Proteins

The synthesis of proteins is dependent on the availability of amino acids in the cytoplasm. The carbon skeletons of most of the amino acids are derived from organic acid intermediates in the glycolysis and citric acid cycle pathways (Fig. 6–22). Many microorganisms also possess enzymes for making amino acids if they are not present in adequate amounts in the environment.

The properties of proteins are determined by their amino acid composition and the sequence of amino acids in the protein chain. Linkage of amino acids by peptide bonds to form proteins is described in Chapter 2. A more detailed description of protein synthesis and the roles of nucleic acids in that process is found in Chapter 7.

Synthesis of Lipids

Microorganisms incorporate fatty acids of the environment into phospholipids of plasma membranes and other membranes. If fatty acids are absent in the growth medium, they are synthesized from acetyl-CoA by a CO_2-biotin–dependent mechanism (Fig. 6–23). Two carbon fragments of acetyl-CoA become linked to an acetyl carrier protein (ACP) producing malonyl-ACP. The fatty acid chain is added to certain groups in the ACP. When butryl-ACP is formed by a reduction reaction from acetoacetyl-ACP, the product is spiraled within the ACP complex to react with another molecule on ACP to become two carbons longer. The spiraling of product continues on ACP, adding two-carbon units to build a fatty acid such as palmitic acid. When fatty acid synthesis is complete, ACP separates from the fatty acid.

Ethanolamine is another major constituent of many bacterial phospholipids derived from activated glycerol. It contains two ester linkages between fatty acids (Fig. 6–24). The synthesis of phosphatidyl ethanolamine proceeds in 15 steps; seven high-energy bonds of ATP are required to complete a single molecule of the phospholipid.

Activated glycerol, formed during glycolysis, combines with three fatty acids to form **triglycerides,** which are important reserve energy sources for fungi (Fig. 6–25). Bacteria do not store triglycerides, but instead accumulate **poly-β-hydroxybutyric acid (PHB)** as a major energy reserve. PHB can be synthesized either from butyryl-ACP in the fatty acid synthetic pathway or from the fermentation of pyruvic acid.

Some microbial lipids are polymers of the five-carbon molecule, isoprene:

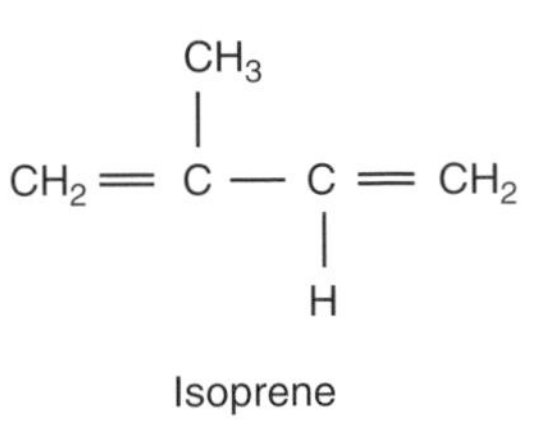

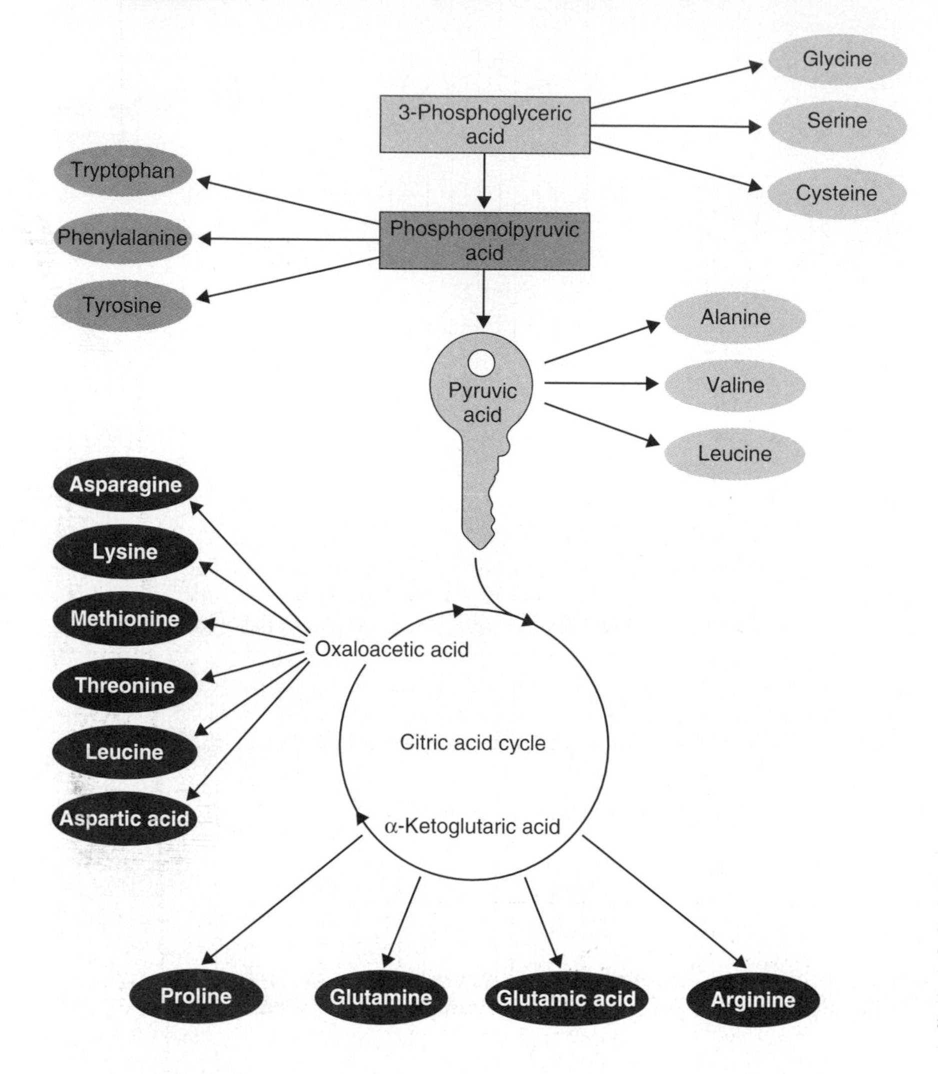

Figure 6–22 ◆ Precursors of amino acids. Intermediate molecules in glycolysis and the citric acid cycle serve as precursor molecules to form amino acids. By attaching one or more amino groups to an organic acid such as pyruvic acid an amino acid is formed.

Chlorophyll, carotenoids, bactoprenols, coenzyme Q, and cholesterol are all derived from isoprene subunits. The synthetic pathway begins with acetyl-CoA and proceeds by way of an important intermediate product known as mevalonic acid.

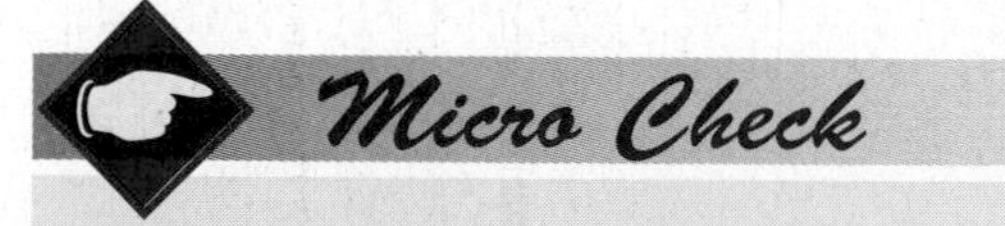

- Why are anabolic pathways not merely the reverse of catabolic pathways?
- What happens to excess products of anabolic pathways?
- What are the advantages of the variety of anabolic capabilities of microorganisms?

INTEGRATION OF CATABOLISM AND ANABOLISM

For the most part, catabolic and anabolic pathways are distinct from one another. However, the two types of pathways are linked by means of certain key metabolites that, at particular junctions, can either be degraded further or be used as building materials. Biochemical pathways that participate in catabolic and anabolic reactions are called **amphibolic pathways** and are indicated by double-headed arrows on Figure 6–18. The ATP-ADP system links energy-generating and energy-requiring reactions. That system shuttles phosphate (PO_4) groups back and forth with incredible speed.

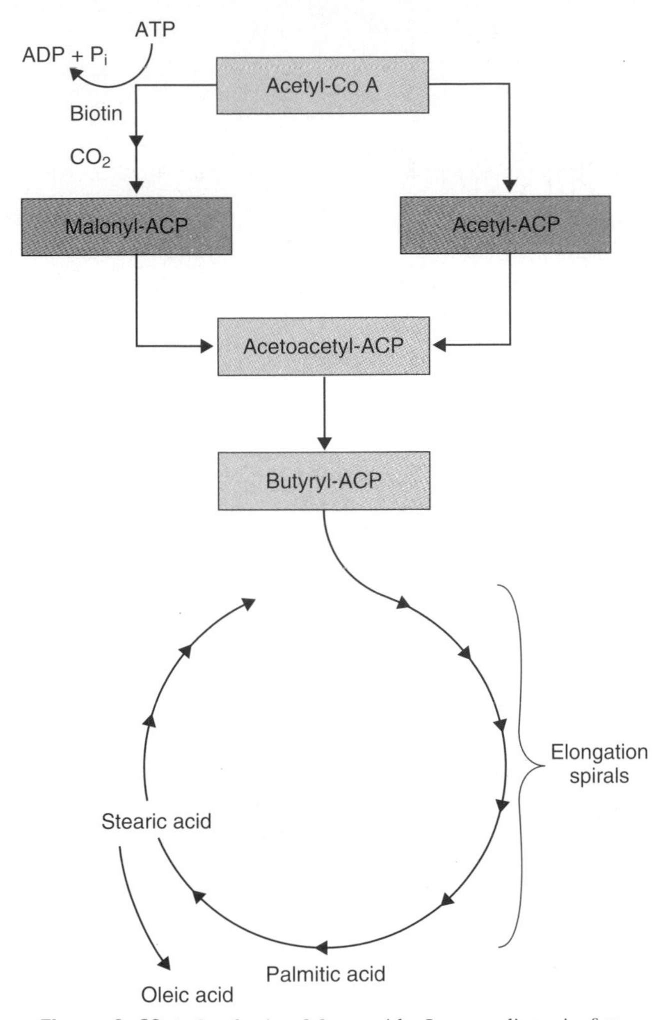

Figure 6–23 ◆ Synthesis of fatty acids. Intermediates in fatty acid synthesis are linked to an acyl carrier protein (ACP). Formation of malonyl—ACP involves fixation of CO_2 activated by biotin. Fatty acid chains increase in length in the elongation spirals as acetyl groups are added to the growing chain on ACP.

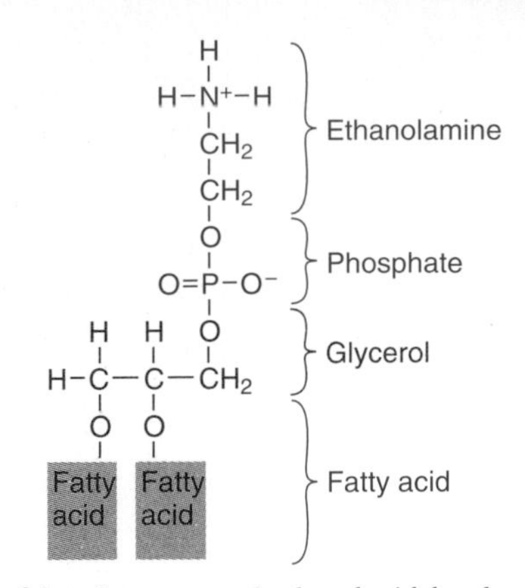

Figure 6–24 ◆ Structure of phosphatidyl ethanolamine, a phospholipid found in cell membranes. The phosphoglyceride is a derivative of activated glycerol.

CONTROL MECHANISMS FOR METABOLISM

The degree of chemical activity in a typical bacterium, such as *Escherichia coli,* can be appreciated when we realize there are probably at least a thousand interdependent reactions carried out in a single cell. Moreover, those reactions are subject to change with alterations in the immediate environment. If the movement of a thousand cars on city streets were not controlled by traffic signals, traffic could not flow in an orderly manner. Molecular traffic likewise could not move efficiently within cells without molecular traffic signals.

A number of control mechanisms exist for molecular traffic in cells. Eucaryotic cells have specific activities confined to different types of organelles as one means of regulation. Because biochemical pathways of procaryotic cells are not confined to organelles, they are subject to different regulatory mechanisms.

Allosteric Modulation

The most responsive control mechanism affecting enzyme activity is **allosteric modulation.** Allosteric enzymes are discussed earlier in the chapter. End products often act as allosteric inhibitors in synthetic pathways, but it is possible that a change in an active site can also give it a greater affinity for the substrate. A simple **feedback inhibition** occurs if the first enzyme of a pathway is

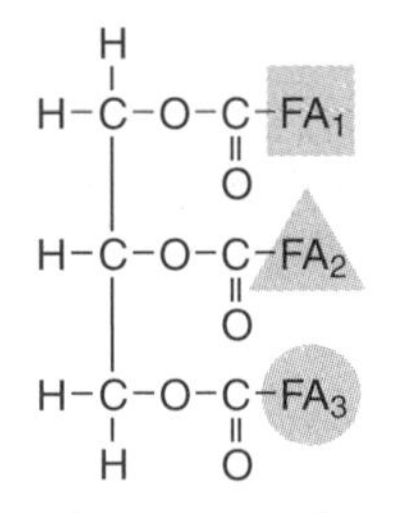

Figure 6–25 ◆ General structure of a triglyceride, showing the three fatty acids (FA_1, FA_2, FA_3). The three fatty acids may be identical or different. Variations in fatty acids accounts for different triglyceride molecules.

inhibited by the end product. In the following example, letters A through E represent the different molecules in the pathway, ending with molecule E; the arrows indicate a reaction by an enzyme. The arrow from the end product E to the enzyme between A and B identifies E as a molecule that inhibits the first enzyme in the pathway:

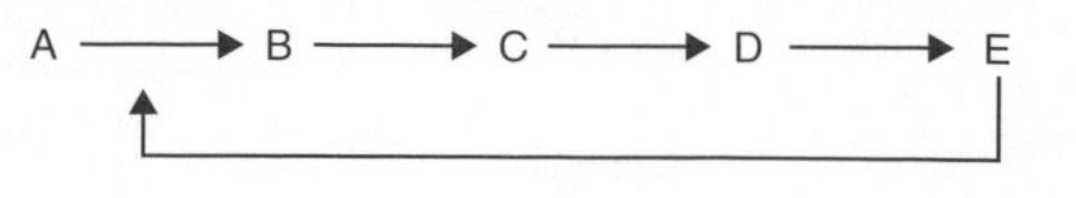

Sometimes more than one enzyme of a pathway is affected by an allosteric modulator. Multiple allosteric modulations take place in branched pathways:

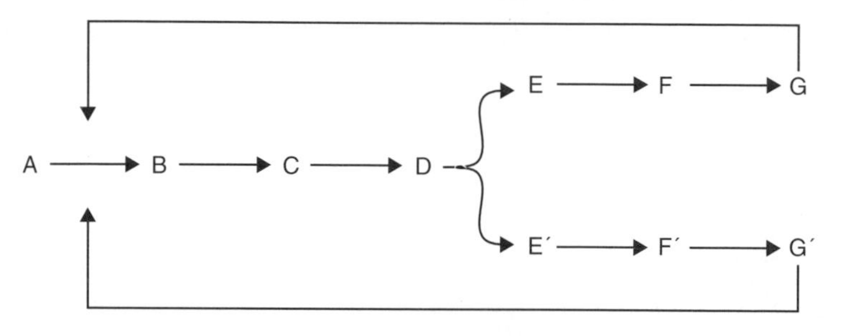

Covalent Modification

The activity of some enzymes in eucaryotic cells is further altered by forming covalent bonds with modifying groups. The activity of the enzyme may be enhanced or diminished. For example, the activity of glycogen synthetase is inhibited by the addition of a phosphate (PO_4) group to the molecule. Phosphorylation of glycogen phosphorylase enhances its activity. Glycogen synthetase is usually inactive when glycogen phosphorylase is active. There are fewer examples of covalent modification in procaryotic cells.

Regulated and Constitutive Enzymes

Another level of metabolic control occurs by regulating the amount of certain enzymes. Some enzymes are synthesized only when their substrates are available. These regulated enzymes are classified as **inducible** enzymes. The presence of controls at the genetic level for the regulated enzymes of certain metabolic pathways conserves cellular energy. The cell does not produce certain enzymes unless a particular substrate is available. The regulated enzymes will be discussed in Chapter 7.

Enzymes which do not respond to the presence or concentrations of substrates or products are called **constitutive** enzymes. Enzymes of glycolysis and the citric acid cycle are examples of constitutive enzymes since they are always present in cells.

Catabolite Repression

A less specific type of repression affects a number of inducible enzymes. Certain inducible enzymes are not produced if glucose is available. Constitutive enzymes release energy from glucose and are preferentially used in the presence of glucose. When glucose is depleted and other nutrients are available, the required enzymes are synthesized.

Glucose is often referred to as a **global repressor** because of its far-reaching repression of other enzymes. As cells produce lots of ATP from metabolizing glucose, the concentration of **cyclic AMP** is lowered. Molecules of cyclic AMP serve as regulator molecules to induce the synthesis of lactose-degrading enzymes.

When glucose and lactose are both supplied in a culture medium inoculated with *Escherichia coli,* a **diauxic** growth curve is obtained (Fig. 6–26). Glucose is metabolized, producing an initial peak of growth. Much of the AMP molecules are phosphorylated to ATP. When the concentration of glucose becomes very low, ATP is converted to AMP by various pathways. Some AMP molecules become cyclic and act as inducers of the lactose enzymes producing a second growth peak.

Catabolic repression represents another form of energy conservation because the bacterium does not synthesize molecules of lactose-degrading enzymes until glucose is depleted. The mechanism is sometimes called the **glucose effect.** If an organism cannot use glucose as a source of energy, there is no glucose effect.

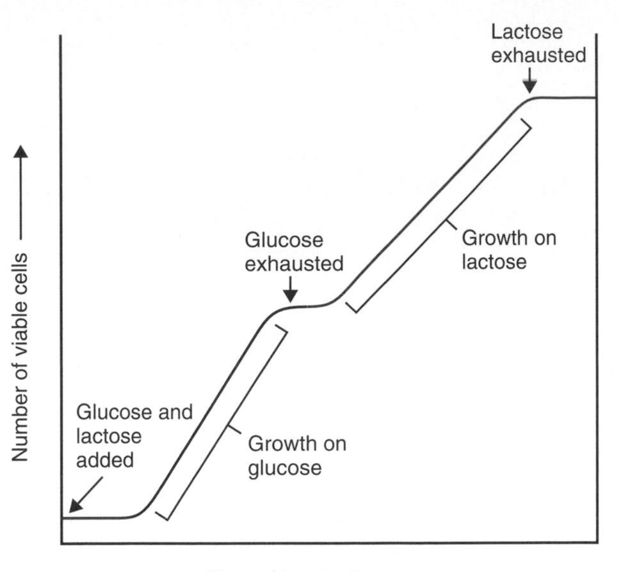

Figure 6–26 ◆ A diauxic growth curve of *Escherichia coli* growing in a broth containing both glucose and lactose. Only when the supply of glucose is depleted does the bacterium begin to use lactose.

Micro Check

- ◆ What is the difference between allosteric and covalent modification?
- ◆ How does regulation of inducible enzyme synthesis conserve energy of cells?
- ◆ What is one role of cyclic AMP?

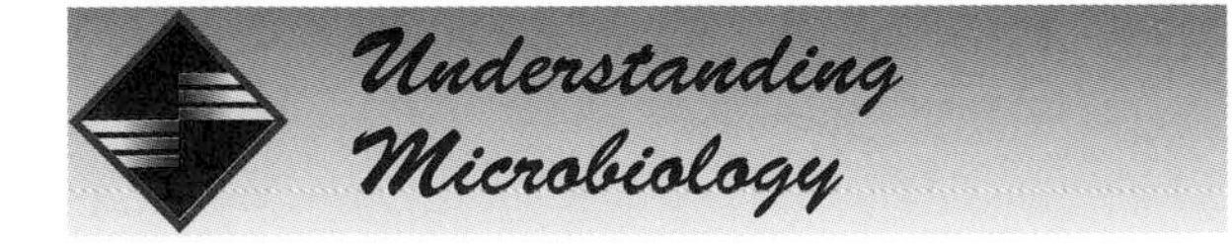

Understanding Microbiology

1. What is the difference between catabolic and anabolic reactions?
2. Name three sources of energy used by microbial cells.
3. What is the function of enzymes in cells?
4. Name the type of enzyme involved in each of the following representative reactions.

(a) $AB + H_2O \rightleftharpoons AOH + BH$

(b) $AR \rightleftharpoons A + R$

(c) $A + B + ATP \rightleftharpoons AB + ADP + P_i$

(d) $AB \rightleftharpoons BA$

(e) $AH_2 + B \rightleftharpoons A + BH_2$

5. Name six factors that influence the rate of enzyme reactions.

Applying Microbiology

6. On your next shopping trip to the grocery store or supermarket visit the bread aisle, the canned food aisle, the beer and wine section, and the dairy section to find fermented foods and beverages. Make a list of 10 to 15 different fermented foods. Identify the type of fermentation that occurred in that food: alcoholic, heterofermentative lactic acid, homofermentative lactic acid, and propionic acid. Do you enjoy fermented foods? Are there other fermented foods found in your market?

Chapter 7

Microbial Genetics

Chapter Outline

- GENOTYPE VS. PHENOTYPE
- REPLICATION AND EXPRESSION OF DNA
  - Replication
  - Transcription
  - Translation
- MUTATIONS
  - The Parameters of Mutation
  - Types of Mutations
- THE MOLECULAR BASIS OF MUTATION
  - Classification of Mutations
  - Detection of Mutants
  - Detection of Chemical Mutagens
- GENETIC TRANSFER IN PROCARYOTIC CELLS
  - Transformation
  - Transduction
  - Conjugation
- REGULATION OF GENE EXPRESSION IN PROCARYOTES
- RECOMBINATION IN EUCARYOTES
- RECOMBINANT DNA TECHNOLOGY
  - Gene Cloning Systems
  - Selection of Recombinant DNA Hosts
  - Gene Amplification
- THE ETHICS OF BIOCHEMICAL ENGINEERING

Learning Objectives

After you have read this chapter, you should be able to:

1. Differentiate between genotype and phenotype.
2. Describe the process of replication.
3. Differentiate between transcription and translation.
4. Differentiate between an auxotroph and a prototroph.
5. Describe three methods of genetic transfer in procaryotes.
6. Discuss the role of transposons in genetic expression.
7. Describe one mechanism each for repression and induction.
8. Describe the basis of recombinant DNA technology.

Classical genetics began in the middle of the nineteenth century when Gregor Mendel, an Austrian monk, studied characteristics of pea plants. Mendel introduced the concept of structural units called **genes** as the agents responsible for heredity. The contributions of Mendel have been invaluable in the understanding of inheritable variance in multicellular plants and animals. Until 1944, some geneticists believed that genes were composed of proteins. In that year, Oswald Avery, Colin MacLeod, and Maclyn McCarty demonstrated that genetic specificity resides within DNA molecules. James Watson and Sir Francis Crick deciphered the structure for DNA in 1953. Their work depended on the x-ray crystallography research on DNA conducted in Wendell Wilkins' laboratory by Rosalind Franklin. Watson, Crick, and Wilkins received the Nobel Prize in 1962 for their discovery of the double helix of DNA, which provided the foundation for molecular genetics.

Research in microbial genetics during the past several decades has revealed universal genetic principles. A gene is now recognized as a unit of

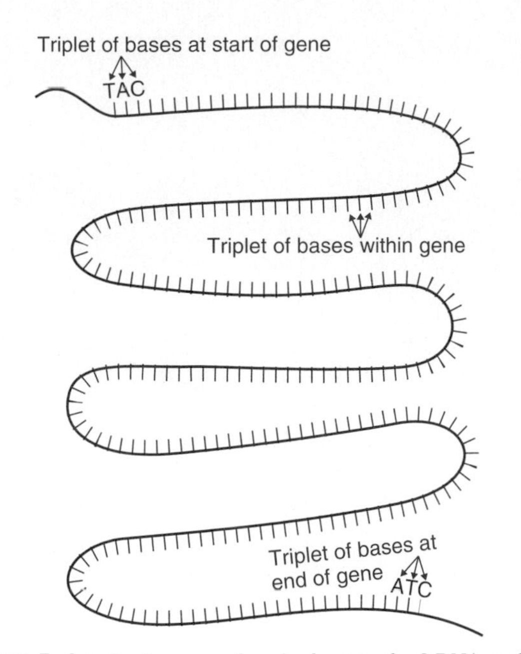

Figure 7–1 ◆ A diagram of a single strand of DNA coding for one gene. The set of three letters represents the nitrogen bases for a "start" code (TAC) at the beginning of the gene and "stop" code (ATC) at the end of the gene.

structure and function on a segment of DNA (Fig. 7–1). A **chromosome** contains many genes. All the genes of an organism constitute its **genome,** its inherited properties or characteristics. The functions of genes are to direct the synthesis of DNA and the three types of RNA necessary to make proteins.

Most bacteria contain one circular chromosome, but some also contain smaller circular segments of DNA known as **plasmids.** Plasmid DNA is self-replicating; it may code for synthesis of fertility pili, substances that destroy antibiotics, enzymes, or other properties. Eucaryotic chromosomes are more complex, involving DNA with attached proteins and special methods for cell division, such as mitosis and meiosis.

GENOTYPE VS. PHENOTYPE

The sum total of genetic information contained in an individual member of a species is called its **genotype.** The genes determine all characteristics or traits of an organism, but not all genes are expressed all the time. For example, most *Escherichia coli* strains have genes for the production of lactose-fermenting enzymes (genotype), but these genes are not expressed until lactose is in the environment. If we examine the enzymes in *E. coli* cells when no lactose is present in the culture medium, no lactose-fermenting enzymes are detectable. If we transfer the *E. coli* cells to a lactose broth, within a short time, the cells produce lactose-fermenting enzymes. This phenomenon of enzyme induction is discussed later in this chapter. The genes that are expressed and can be measured constitute the **phenotype** of an organism.

Changes in genotype, known as **mutations,** occur either as a result of a sudden, inheritable change in a gene or by **genetic transfer,** a process that introduces foreign DNA into a cell under special conditions.

Genetic transfer in procaryotes can occur spontaneously, but it is rare. **Recombination,** the process whereby transferred or donor DNA combines with the DNA of a recipient cell, is observed in many medically important bacterial species. Antibiotic-resistance genes are often transferred between cells of the same or related species, resulting in serious diseases that are difficult to treat. In eucaryotes, the process of recombination is more complex and occurs during asexual or sexual reproduction.

Changes in phenotype may be induced environmentally without changing an organism's genotype. Environmental variations in temperature, available nutrients, pH, and physical state of a culture medium may influence the phenotypes of some bacteria, fungi, and other microorganisms. Environmentally induced changes in phenotype affect all exposed cells in a population; genotypic changes affect only those cells that undergo a mutation.

One example of phenotypic variation is in the bacterium *Serratia marcescens,* which produces a bright red colony when grown at 25°C (see Color Plate 17). This bacterial species produces a brick-red pigment known as **prodigiosin.** When *S. marcescens* is grown at 37°C, the colony is pale pink or colorless. The pigment is not produced at 37°C probably because at least one of the enzymes needed for pigment production is not active at the higher temperature.

An example in fungi demonstrates how temperature changes affects phenotype. For example, *Sporothrix schenckii* produces a yeastlike colony at 37°C and a moldlike colony at room temperatures of 20°–25°C (Fig. 7–2). This ability to grow either as a yeast or mold depending on the temperature is known as **dimorphism.**

Some strains of actively motile bacteria belonging to the genus *Proteus* "swarm" or spread over the surface of a moist agar plate. The "swarming" cells produce a series of waves on the agar sur-

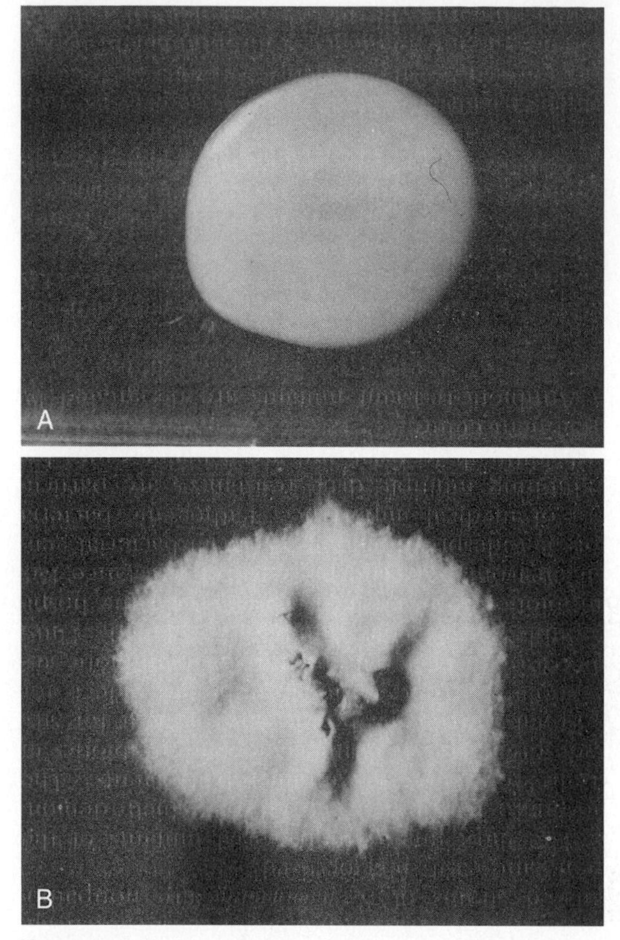

Figure 7–2 ◆ Dimorphism expressed by a fungus, *Sporothrix schenckii*, at two temperatures. *A,* A typical yeast colony at 37°C. *B,* A typical mold colony at 20° to 25°C.

face (Fig. 7–3). If the medium contains bile salts, swarming is inhibited. In these examples, the genotype remains the same, but the phenotype is influenced by the environment.

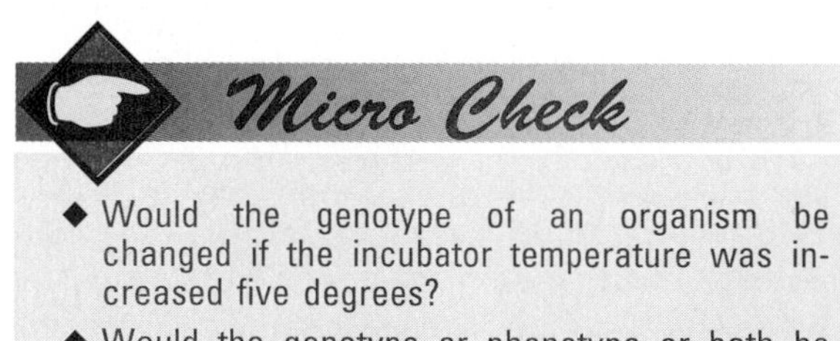

- Would the genotype of an organism be changed if the incubator temperature was increased five degrees?
- Would the genotype or phenotype or both be altered if an organism was exposed to a mutagen?
- Does genetic transfer of DNA between two cells alter the recipient's genotype or the donor's genotype?

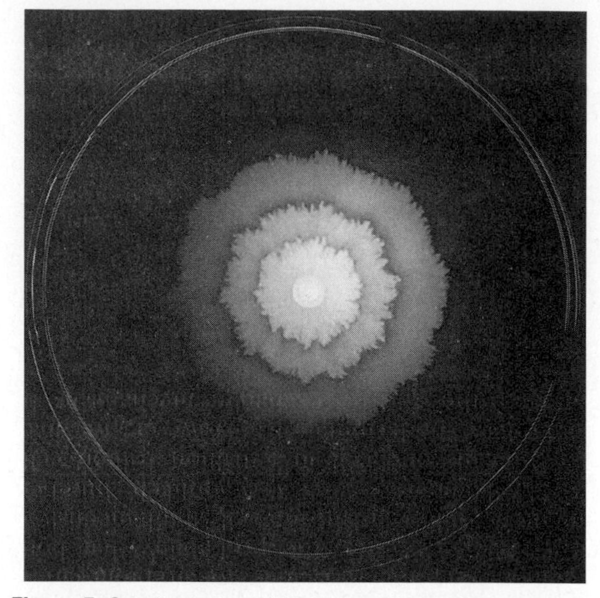

Figure 7–3 ◆ Swarming of *Proteus* on the surface of a nutrient agar plate. The spreading pattern of growth occurs in successive waves during overnight incubation at 37°C.

REPLICATION AND EXPRESSION OF DNA

DNA consists of two chains of complementary **nucleotides** wound around each other to form a double helix. The nucleotides consist of three elements: a phosphate unit, a **deoxyribose** sugar molecule and one of four nitrogen bases. Because the sugar element is deoxyribose, the nucleotides are known as **deoxyribonucleotides.** The four bases in DNA are adenine (A), cytosine (C), guanine (G), and thymine (T). The base adenine (A) always pairs with its **complementary base,** thymine (T) forming an A-T **base pair,** and cytosine (C) always pairs with its complement, guanine (G), forming a G-C base pair. Two hydrogen bonds join the A-T base pairs and three hydrogen bonds link G-C base pairs. The structure of nucleotides and their bases are discussed in Chapter 2.

Replication

As cells prepare to divide, DNA is duplicated so that each cell, after division, has an exact copy of the original DNA. The process of duplicating cellular DNA is called **replication.** A helicase enzyme begins replication by unwinding and separating the two strands of DNA. The site of sepa-

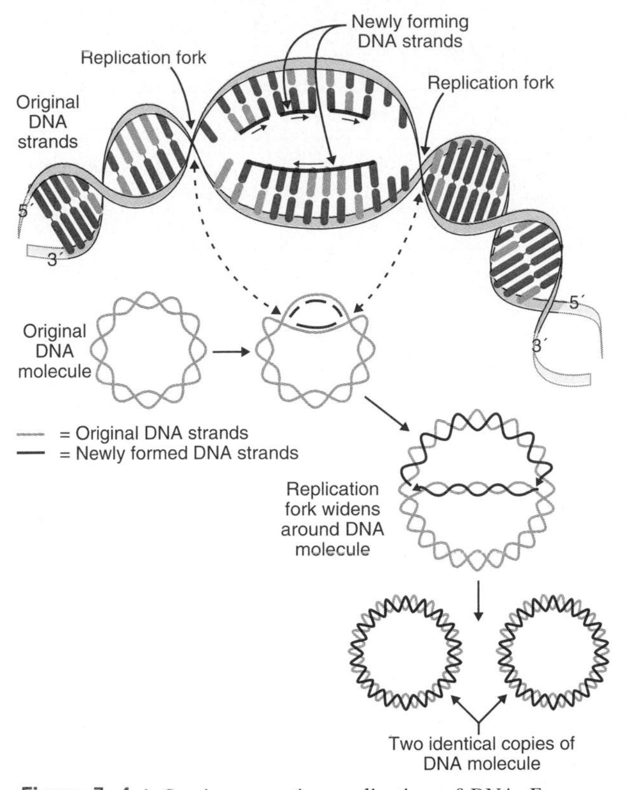

Figure 7–4 ◆ Semiconservative replication of DNA. Enzymes cause separation of the two strands at an origin position. The new strands complement the base sequence on the original strand, resulting in two identical DNA molecules, each having one original and one new strand.

ration is called the **replication fork** (Fig. 7–4). Synthesis of new DNA is initiated by the temporary binding of short, complementary strands of RNA, called **primer RNA,** to each parent strand of DNA (Fig. 7–5). The primer RNA serves as an attachment point for another enzyme that builds a DNA chain complementary to the parent DNA. After the DNA chain lengthens, another enzyme removes the primer RNA, replacing it with DNA.

Once complementary nucleotides are positioned opposite each of the nucleotides on the parent strand, covalent bonds are formed between the sugar and phosphate groups of adjacent deoxyribonucleotides on the new chain. Hydrogen bonds join the complementary base pairs between the parent DNA and new DNA. Covalent and hydrogen bonds have been described in Chapter 2. The new strands are constructed in fragments of about 1000 nucleotides on one chain. These fragments are then joined by another enzyme, **DNA ligase.** Replication proceeds until the entire chromosome has been duplicated, forming two identical DNA molecules. The process is called **semiconservative replication** because each of the double-stranded molecules of DNA retains or conserves one of the original strands of DNA.

Transcription

DNA also serves as the template for the synthesis of three types of RNA in a process known as **transcription.** These RNA types include messenger RNA (mRNA), transfer RNA (tRNA), and ribosomal RNA (rRNA) (Table 7–1). All three RNA molecules are essential for protein synthesis.

The basic building block of DNA and RNA molecules is the nucleotide. The nucleotides in RNA contain three elements: a phosphate group,

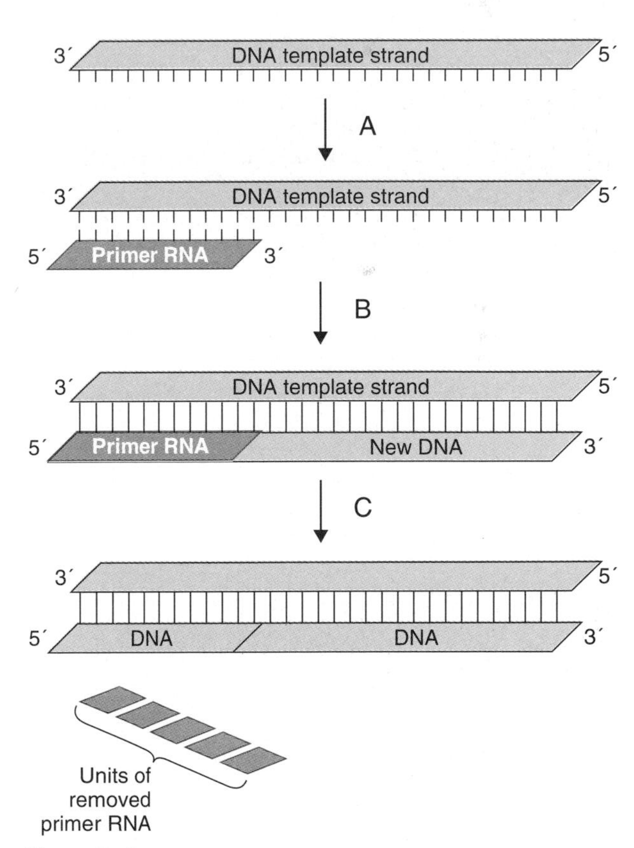

Figure 7–5 ◆ Initiation of DNA synthesis. At A, a short complementary fragment of primer RNA is synthesized on the DNA template. At B, new DNA is synthesized using the primer RNA fragment as a start point. At C, the RNA fragment is removed by another enzyme that replaces the ribonucleotides by deoxyribonucleotides.

Table 7–1
TYPES OF RNA MOLECULES

TYPE	ABBREVIATION	APPROXIMATE AMOUNT	FUNCTION
Ribosomal RNA	rRNA	80%	Structural component of ribosomes
Messenger RNA	mRNA	5%	Directs the synthesis of polypeptides
Transfer RNA	tRNA	15%	Transports amino acids to ribosomes

a ribose sugar, and one of four nitrogen bases. Because the sugar is ribose, these nucleotides are called **ribonucleotides.** The base in a ribonucleotide is either adenine (A), cytosine (C), guanine (G), or uracil (U). The structure of uracil resembles thymine. In replication and other processes in which RNA molecules form base pairs with DNA or RNA, uracil acts like thymine and forms hydrogen bonds with adenine.

Most RNA molecules are single-stranded except for those found in some viruses. However, almost every RNA molecule folds back on itself, producing hairpin loops with double-helical structures. The proportion of helical regions varies in the three types of RNA. The configuration of tRNA resembles a cloverleaf, which is formed when about half of the ribonucleotides containing complementary nitrogen bases are joined by hydrogen bonds at specific points (Fig. 7–6).

Transcription of RNA proceeds in three steps: (1) **initiation,** (2) **elongation,** and (3) **termination** (Fig. 7–7). In the first step, an RNA polymerase binds to a **promoter site** on DNA to open the double strands. In the second step, RNA polymerase synthesizes a chain of ribonucleotides complementary to the DNA strand with the gene to be transcribed, the **sense strand.** In the third step, elongation stops when a terminator region on the gene is reached. The RNA molecule releases from the DNA molecule, then forms its active configuration, either as a linear or a folded molecule. Synthesis of more RNA molecules continues as long as the gene remains in an "open" state. When the gene "closes," the two DNA strands bind together. Regulation of DNA expression will be discussed later in this chapter.

Translation

The synthesis of polypeptides, or protein chains, occurs on the ribosomes. The process, under the direction of a mRNA molecule, is called **translation.** The sequence of nitrogen bases of mRNA are complementary to the base sequence on a gene. At the ribosome, these bases are translated in groups of three, called **codons.** Each codon on mRNA directs the exact placement of one amino acid in a polypeptide chain. When all combinations of the four bases are arranged in patterns of three, 64 groups of three are possible. However, only 20 amino acids are found in the proteins of living things. Therefore, most amino acids are specified by more than one codon. The **genetic code** consists of the mRNA codons and their associated amino acid (Table 7–2). The specification of the same amino acid by two or more codons is known as **degeneracy.** This property of degeneracy allows for some degree of resistance to mutations, especially if a mutation occurs in the third base in the codon. Do you see groups of codons in Table 7–2 that

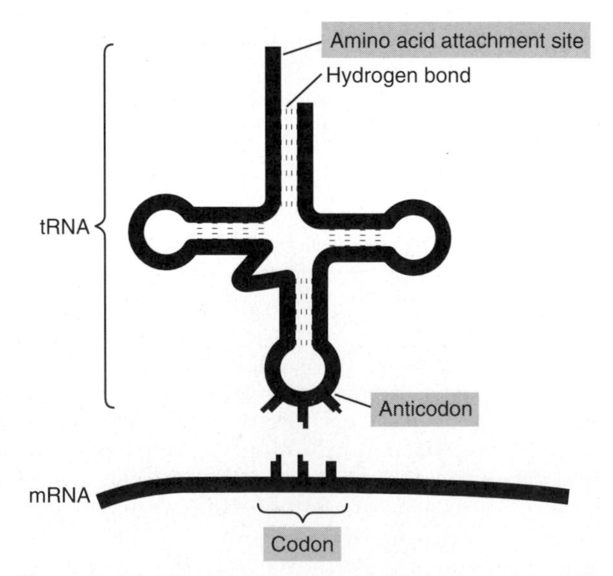

Figure 7–6 ◆ The three-dimensional tRNA places the triplet bases of the anticodon opposite the complementary triplet base codon on mRNA during translation at the ribosome. The tRNA carries a specific amino acid at its amino acid attachment site.

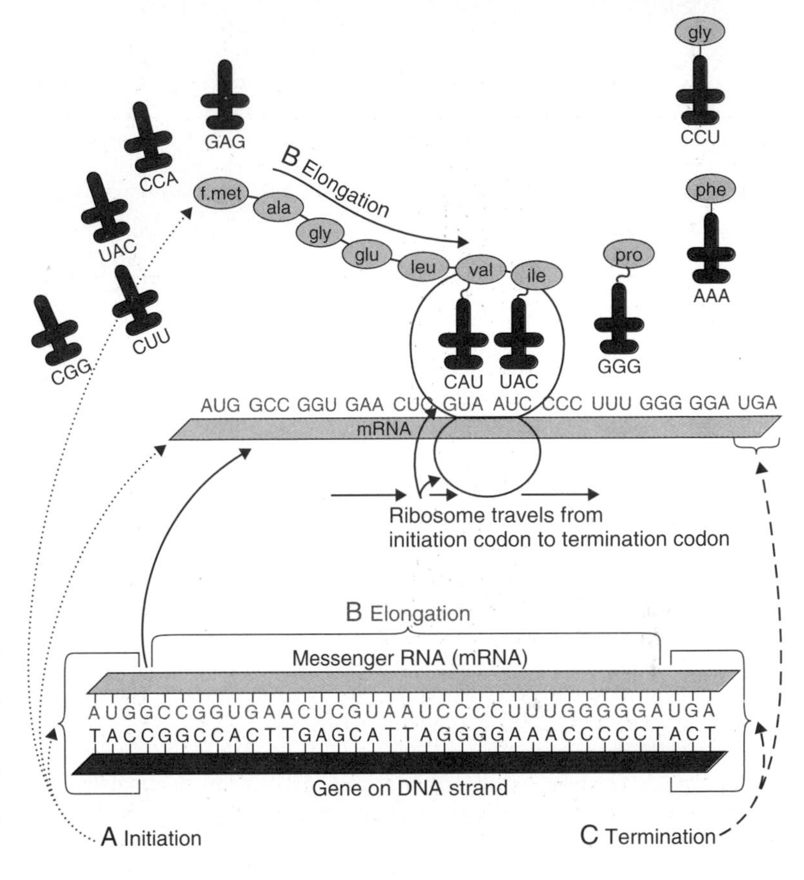

Figure 7–7 ◆ The three stages of polypeptide synthesis in procaryotic cells. *Initiation* (A) begins at the codon, AUG, for the amino acid *N*-formylmethionine (f-met). *Elongation* (B) of the chain of amino acids proceeds as tRNA molecules carry amino acids to the ribosome for correct placement on mRNA. *Termination* (C) happens at a STOP codon, such as UGA, signaling the release of the completed polypeptide chain.

Table 7–2
CODONS ON mRNA FOR THE AMINO ACIDS

FIRST POSITION	SECOND POSITION U		C		A		G		THIRD POSITION
U	UUU	Phe	UCU	Ser	UAU	Tyr	UGU	Cys	U
	UUC	Phe	UCC	Ser	UAC	Tyr	UGC	Cys	C
	UUA	Leu	UCA	Ser	UAA	STOP	UGA	STOP	A
	UUG	Leu	UCG	Ser	UAG	STOP	UGG	Trp	G
C	CUU	Leu	CCU	Pro	CAU	His	CGU	Arg	U
	CUC	Leu	CCC	Pro	CAC	His	CGC	Arg	C
	CUA	Leu	CCA	Pro	CAA	Gln	CGA	Arg	A
	CUG	Leu	CCG	Pro	CAG	Gln	CGG	Arg	G
A	AUU	Ile	ACU	Thr	AAU	Asn	AGU	Ser	U
	AUC	Ile	ACC	Thr	AAC	Asn	AGC	Ser	C
	AUA	Ile	ACA	Thr	AAA	Lys	AGA	Arg	A
	AUG	Met START	ACG	Thr	AAG	Lys	AGG	Arg	G
G	GUU	Val	GCU	Ala	GAU	Asp	GGU	Gly	U
	GUC	Val	GCC	Ala	GAC	Asp	GGC	Gly	C
	GUA	Val	GCA	Ala	GAA	Glu	GGA	Gly	A
	GUG	Val	GCG	Ala	GAG	Glu	GGG	Gly	G

specify the same amino acid? Notice the only difference for many of these groups is the third base in the codon.

The synthesis of polypeptides, or proteins, is also divided into three stages with the same names as used in the transcription of RNA: (1) initiation, (2) elongation, and (3) termination (see Fig. 7–7). In the first stage, one codon, AUG, serves as the "start" codon to specify the amino acid, formylmethionine (f-met), initiating translation. In the second stage, each codon, following AUG, specifies a particular amino acid in the polypeptide chain. Ribosomes bind to the "start" end of the mRNA to begin protein synthesis. The amino acids needed to elongate the amino acid chain are delivered by tRNA molecules.

In procaryotes, there are between 50 and 70 different types of tRNA molecules. The tRNA molecule has two distinct sections, the **amino acid binding site** and the **anticodon site** (see Fig. 7–6). The anticodon site has three bases. A tRNA molecule carrying a specific amino acid attached to its amino acid binding site is activated to deliver the amino acid to the ribosome. The activated-tRNA molecule attaches to the mRNA molecule as it is positioned on the ribosome. Complementary base pairing occurs between the codon and anticodon sites.

Ribosomes contain two subunits, one large and one small subunit. Each subunit contains rRNA molecules and proteins. The structure of ribosomes is discussed in Chapter 4. The ribosome forms a unit with the mRNA molecule at the "start" codon only, allowing the message contained in the mRNA molecule to be translated from beginning to end. The ribosome has two binding sites to which tRNA molecules can attach. As translation proceeds, the mRNA molecule is moved along the ribosome to bring the next codon into position for another activated-tRNA molecule.

Two amino acids positioned next to each other on the ribosome are linked by peptide bonds. Peptide bonds are described in Chapter 2. Then the tRNA occupying the first position leaves the ribosome and moves to the cytoplasm to attach to another molecule of the same amino acid. The mRNA molecule moves across the ribosome, bringing the next codon into second position. Another tRNA molecule with the correct anticodon binds to this codon, bringing the next amino acid. Enzymes in the ribosome form a peptide bond between the amino acids in first position and the new amino acid. The tRNA molecule in first position leaves, and the elongation process continues, positioning the next codon on the ribosome. When one of the "stop" codons (UAA, UAG, UGA) on mRNA reaches the ribosome, the process is complete. The polypeptide and the mRNA are released from the ribosome. The mRNA moves to other ribosomes where additional molecules of the same polypeptide are synthesized. If the concentration of protein molecules reaches a suitable level for the cellular needs, the mRNA molecules for making the protein are degraded into ribonucleotides. These ribonucleotides are used to build another mRNA molecule.

The energy required for transcription and translation is supplied by high-energy phosphate bonds usually supplied by ATP. Energy is required for many stages of protein synthesis: (1) to bind an amino acid to tRNA, (2) to bind an activated-tRNA to a codon, (3) to form a peptide bond, and (4) in other steps in protein synthesis.

Replication, transcription, and translation are highly ordered processes dependent on the controlling function of DNA molecules. Cells expend most of their energy for protein synthesis. The relationships of DNA, RNA, and proteins are critical in their influence on cellular activities.

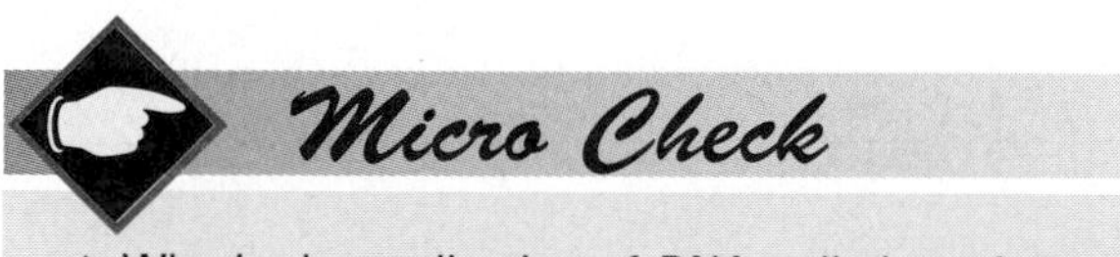

- Why is the replication of DNA called semiconservative?
- Which nitrogen base on RNA is complementary to adenine on DNA in transcription?
- What roles do rRNA, mRNA, and tRNA play in polypeptide synthesis?

MUTATIONS

Mutations are inherited changes in the DNA molecule. **Spontaneous mutations** occur naturally with no known cause, but they rarely affect more than one cell in a population of 10^6 to 10^{10} cells. Genetic changes produced in the laboratory are called **induced mutations.** Induced mutations also occur in nature when cells are exposed to radiation or gene-altering chemicals. Gene-altering physical, chemical, or biological agents are **mutagens** or **mutagenic agents.**

The disaster in Chernobyl is a real example of exposure of living organisms to the mutagenic effects of radioactive dust. The explosion of the nuclear power plant in the city of Chernobyl, Russia, discharged radioactive particles across the continent and to other parts of the world by air currents. The potential mutagenic consequences of this event are difficult to measure.

The **mutation rate** is a measure of the rate of genetic change. The rate can be increased in the laboratory or in nature by exposing cells to mutagens. Certain chemicals or radiation such as ultraviolet radiation, x-rays, or gamma rays can increase the number of cells with altered genotypes to approximately one cell in a population of 10^3 to 10^5 cells.

Mutant strains usually lose one or more traits present in the parent strain, often weakening the mutant strain. Lethal mutations cause death of the cell or organism when severe damage occurs. Some nucleotide sequences are highly mutable, but the reasons for such "hot spots" is unclear. Mutations occurring over millions of years are responsible in part for the great diversity of characteristics in all life forms.

The Parameters of Mutation

Mutation is a random and an unpredictable event. The parameters of mutations can be expressed in terms of a mutation rate, which is constant for a particular type of mutation, and **mutant frequency,** which varies with the mutation rate and the rate of selection for a specific type of mutant. The mutation rate is the probability that a certain average number of mutations will occur per cell per generation. A mutation rate of 10^{-6} would mean that when 1×10^6 cells divided to generate 2×10^6 cells, one mutant cell occurred.

The probability that two mutations will occur simultaneously in the same cell is equal to the product of the individual probabilities. Much of the information on multiple mutation rates comes from studying drug-resistant mutants. If a bacterium has a mutation rate for resistance to chloramphenicol of 10^{-8}/cell/generation and the mutation rate for resistance to streptomycin is 10^{-10}/cell/generation, the probability that both mutations will occur in one cell simultaneously is 10^{-18}/cell/generation. A very unlikely number, 10^{-18}, means one cell in a trillion trillion cells would have both mutations. However, we shall see later the genetic exchange mechanisms by which bacterial strains with resistance to two, four, or more drugs develop.

The mutant frequency is the number of a particular mutant type in a population of cells. A mutant frequency of 10^{-5} means that there is one mutant in a population of 100,000 cells.

Types of Mutations

Any characteristic of an organism can be altered by a spontaneous or an induced mutation. Bacterial mutants requiring specific amino acids, vitamins, purines, or pyrimidines for growth are common. Nutritional mutants are called **auxotrophs** because they require added amino acids or vitamins to grow. The parents or "wild types," from which they are derived, are called **prototrophs;** they do not require specific added nutrients. Auxotrophs have lost the ability to produce important growth factors. To designate a mutation, mutants lacking the ability to produce the amino acid, histidine, for example, are designated by his$^-$. A mutant strain lacking the ability to produce two amino acids such as histidine and proline are designated as his$^-$ pro$^-$. Alternately, a mutant may lose the ability to digest a particular substrate, such as lactose. A lac$^-$ strain cannot ferment lactose.

Mutants may exhibit alterations in composition of structural proteins or polysaccharides that alter the virulence or host-range of microorganisms. Encapsulated strains of *Streptococcus pneumoniae,* for example, are highly virulent because they resist phagocytosis. The capsule layer around the cell protects the cell from phagocytosis by the body's defensive white blood cells. Nonencapsulated strains of *S. pneumoniae* are nonpathogenic and easily phagocytized.

The most important bacterial mutants of the hospital environment are those which demonstrate resistance to antimicrobial agents. The widespread use of disinfectants and antibiotics in hospitals provides a hostile environment for susceptible microorganisms. Antibiotics select for the resistant bacterial mutants since antibiotic-susceptible bacteria are inhibited or killed. Thus, antibiotic use is a selective pressure in the hospital environment. The presence of resistance factors is widespread among nearly all bacterial genera of medical importance. Pathogenic bacteria exhibiting multiple drug resistances are particularly difficult to treat and are a major cause for treatment failure.

Antibiotic-resistant mutants are designated by

the first three letters of the antibiotic followed by a superscript letter r. Antibiotic-susceptible mutants are identified with the superscript letter s to the right of the three-letter abbreviation for the antibiotic. Thus, a streptomycin-resistant mutant is designated as str^r, and a streptomycin-susceptible strain is designated as str^s.

Certain mutations are expressed only under particular environmental conditions. Examples of such conditionally dependent mutants are those which are temperature-sensitive or osmotically sensitive such as to a decreased solute concentration in the environment. In these mutations, the restricting environment blocks the function or synthesis of either a gene product or a tRNA.

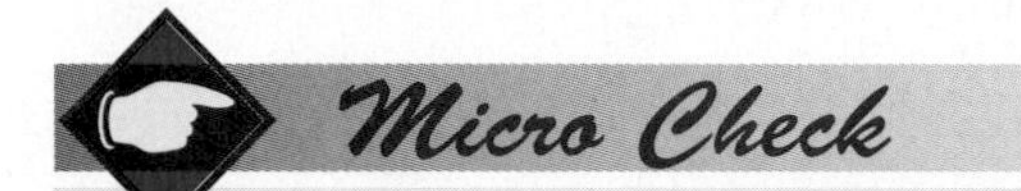

- What does a spontaneous mutation rate of 10^{-6} mean?
- What would be the probability of four mutations occurring simultaneously in one cell if each mutation had an individual rate of 10^{-5}?
- Using abbreviations, how might one designate the mutations in a bacterium that is histidine-requiring, lactose-negative, and ampicillin-susceptible?

THE MOLECULAR BASIS OF MUTATION

DNA was described by Watson and Crick as a double-helical structure with two chains of nucleotides coiled around each other and held together by hydrogen bonds. The amount of coiling can be appreciated when one considers that the estimated length of DNA in *E. coli* is approximately 1000 times as long as the length of the bacterial cell. Continuing studies on the DNA of microorganisms over the last several decades revealed that DNA is not always double-stranded; the DNA genome of some DNA viruses is single-stranded.

Many procaryotes also contain small circular molecules of DNA called plasmids. Plasmids replicate independent of chromosomal DNA and have genes that encode for a variety of products. Among the phenotypes encoded by plasmids are (1) production of pigments, toxins, and antibiotics; (2) resistance to antimicrobial agents; (3) ability to degrade particular carbon sources; (4) ability to invade or colonize certain tissue; (5) sensitivity to **bacteriophage** (viruses that attack bacteria); and (6) ability to transfer genetic material between cells of the same or closely related species. Conjugation, transduction, and transformation methods for transferring plasmids between related cells will be discussed in a later section of this chapter.

Because a gene codes for a specific amino acid sequence in its polypeptide, alterations in DNA are usually reflected in a changed amino acid at the corresponding position on the polypeptide chain (Fig. 7–8).

Classification of Mutations

The consequences of exposure to a mutagen may be classified according to the extent of damage done to a DNA molecule. If only a single

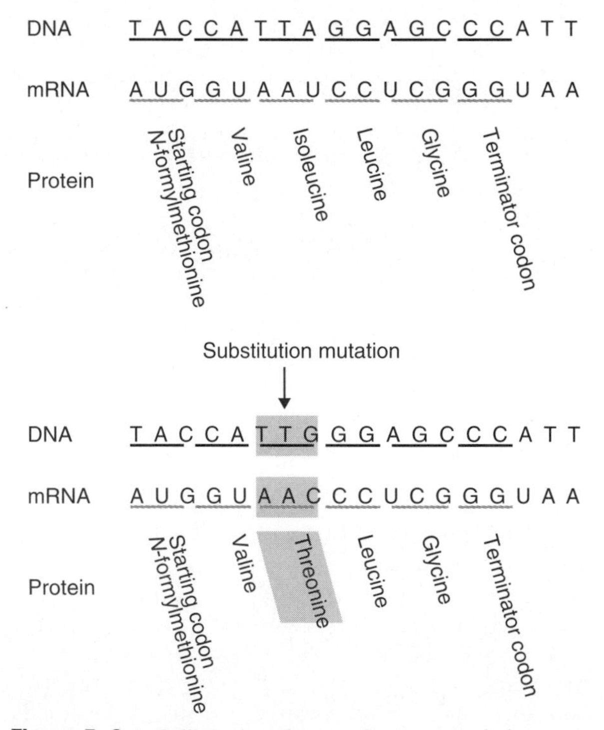

Figure 7–8 ◆ Collinearity of part of a gene and the amino acids of the protein molecule for which it codes. A base substitution in DNA such as G replacing A produces a change on mRNA. Cytosine (C) replaces uracil (U), resulting in the amino acid threonine replacing isoleucine in the polypeptide chain.

Table 7–3
CLASSIFICATION OF MUTATIONS ACCORDING TO TYPES OF LESIONS PRODUCED

Microlesions involve base substitution of the normal base by a different base:
- Point mutations
  - Transitions
  - Transversions

Macrolesions involve removal or addition of one or several nucleotides causing frame-shift mutations:
- Deletions
- Insertions
- Inversions
- Transposons

base pair is altered, the injury is described as a **microlesion.** If a number of base pairs or several genes are affected, the impairment is called a **macrolesion** (Table 7–3).

POINT MUTATIONS

A **point mutation** involves a change in a single base of a nucleotide. One base replaced by another base is the most frequent type of mutation and is known as **base substitution.** When a purine base replaces another purine or a pyrimidine base replaces another pyrimidine, the substitution is called a **transition** (Fig. 7–9). When a purine is replaced by a pyrimidine or the reverse

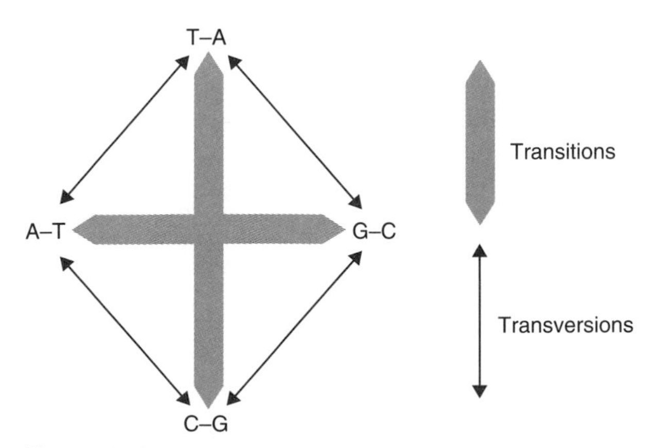

Figure 7–9 ◆ Possible alterations in a single nucleotide. Transitions are the replacement of a purine with another purine or a pyrimidine with another pyrimidine. Transversions are the substitution of a purine for a pyrimidine or a pyrimidine for a purine.

occurs, the substitution is called a **transversion.** Purine and pyrimidine bases are discussed in Chapter 2.

Transitions may be produced by **base analogs,** which are nitrogen bases that resemble the usual bases in DNA, except for their distribution of hydrogen atoms. Hydrogen atoms are responsible for base pair formation. Base analogs, such as 5-bromouracil (5-BU), which resembles thymine, or 2-aminopurine (2-AP), which resembles adenine, are incorporated into a DNA molecule in place of the normal base and alter the normal base pairing.

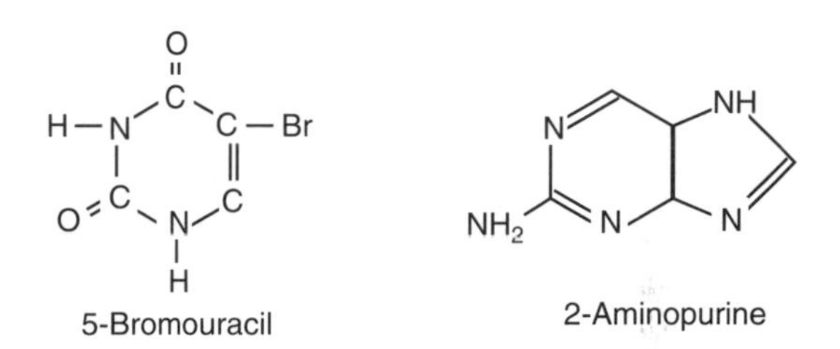

If the bonding properties are altered, the consequence will be a transition from an A-T base pair to a C-G pair or a G-C to A-T transition.

Base analogs are useful for designing antiviral drug treatments. Viral replication is either stopped, or the synthesis or function of important proteins is blocked. The best-known base analog is azidothymidine (AZT), which has an important use in treating AIDS.

Some chemical mutagens, chiefly nitrous acid, promote transitions by acting upon resting DNA. Nitrous acid removes amino groups (NH_2) from adenine, guanine, and cytosine. The deaminated products do not pair with the purines or pyrimidines that are complementary to the original bases.

Alkylating agents are chemicals that change the bases of DNA by adding short chains of carbon atoms. Chemical agents such as the nitrogen mustards and ethylene oxide, are powerful mutagens causing changes in base pairing. These chemical agents are known to cause both transitions and transversions. For example, alkylation of a guanine on DNA may cause it to pair with thymine instead of cytosine. This example is one method for development of a point mutation.

When a codon is changed by the substitution of one base for another, the codon could still contain instructions for the same amino acid. In that event, the protein molecule would remain unchanged by the substitution. Such mutations

	Amino acid sequence							
	1	2	3	4	5	6	7	8
Hemoglobin A (normal)	val	his	leu	thr	pro	glu	glu	lys ...
Hemoglobin S	val	his	leu	thr	pro	val	glu	lys ...

Figure 7–10 ◆ A single base substitution on the gene for the hemoglobin A molecule results in a change in the amino acid on position 6 of the β-globin chain. Hemoglobin A, which has normal oxygen-carrying capacity, is converted to hemoglobin S. Hemoglobin S has diminished oxygen-carrying capacity and is responsible for sickle cell anemia.

are called **silent mutations** because the gene product has not changed.

A single base substitution can code for a different amino acid. Depending on how the substitution affects the final form and function of the protein, the consequence may be negligible, harmful, or even lethal. Such substitutions can alter the properties of a protein significantly or not at all. An example with serious health consequences involves the protein of the hemoglobin molecule in red blood cells. The hemoglobin A gene is changed to a hemoglobin S gene by a transversion. The hemoglobin molecules of persons with sickle cell anemia contain the amino acid valine in place of glutamic acid in normal hemoglobin (Fig. 7–10). This single amino acid change produces a hemoglobin variant with a lower affinity for oxygen and causes disease.

If a functionally inactive protein is synthesized from a mutant gene, the result may be lethal for an organism. If a nonsense codon is formed by a point mutation, no amino acid is specified, and polypeptide synthesis is terminated.

FRAMESHIFT MUTATIONS

The **deletion** or **insertion** of one or several bases or the insertion of certain dyes can cause a **frameshift mutation.** This type of mutation causes a misreading, or shift in the reading, of the genetic code. The mRNA molecule produced from such altered DNA may have a large number of different codons with the subsequent production of nonfunctional proteins.

An analogy using words is often helpful to visualize the effect of a frameshift mutation. If we substitute three-letter words for six codons, and assume the deletion of a single letter (base), then nonsense words having no meaning occur. In the example below, the e in "The" is deleted, and the remaining letters are read in groups of three, resulting in a nonsense message.

The cat ate the fat rat.
Thc ata tet hef atr at.

Deletions and insertions cause frameshift mutations because they involve changes in one or more bases. They are classified as macrolesions. Small deletions may appear spontaneously, but loss of extended segments of DNA results from exposure to mutagenic agents, such as radiation and chemical mutagens.

Ultraviolet radiation promotes the formation of thymine dimers between two adjacent thymines on a strand of DNA. Thymine dimers have the effect of deleting the thymines from the base sequence message of the gene. The dimers distort DNA and prevent replication and transcription (Fig. 7–11). Most bacteria have enzyme repair systems that undo the damage on the DNA molecule if special conditions are available. These mechanisms are discussed in Chapter 21.

Radiation such as x-rays and gamma rays cause chains of large molecules to break, leaving smaller molecules that are electrically charged, or ionized. These types of radiation are termed **ionizing radiation.** Proteins and nucleic acid molecules are especially susceptible to ionizing radiation. If the dose of radiation is high or sustained for a long period, the chemistry of the cells is

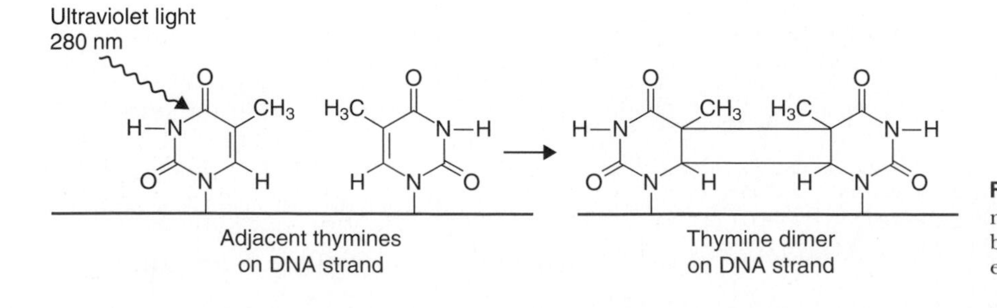

Figure 7–11 ◆ Formation of thymine dimers. Adjacent thymine bases on DNA form a dimer when exposed to ultraviolet radiation.

altered drastically. If the cell dies as a consequence, the radiation dose is said to produce a **lethal mutation.**

Mutations resulting from the removal of nucleotides on a portion of a DNA strand are known as **deletions.** Known mutagenic agents that operate in this way include hydrogen peroxide, organic peroxides, *N*-methyl-*N*-nitrosoguanidine (NTG), and manganous chloride. NTG is an extremely efficient mutagen. In populations of cells subjected to NTG, mutation rates may exceed 10 percent.

A seemingly small deletion can have rather dramatic effects on the organism suffering the loss. In the human disease of cystic fibrosis (CF), a gene deletion of only three nucleotides coding for the amino acid phenylalanine in position 508 of the protein was found. In North America, 70 percent of CF patients have this deletion, involving only three bases in the 250,000 base pairs of the normal CF gene. The removed bases and a few others alter the activity of the protein product. The protein product of the normal CF gene regulates normal transport of chloride and sodium ions across cell membranes. In CF patients, ion transport is disrupted, causing retention of water, a build-up of mucus, and lung damage.

Mutations resulting from the addition of one or several bases are insertions. **Intercalating agents** are mutagenic chemicals that insert (intercalate) between bases in the DNA strands. The base pairs that would be next to each other normally are separated by the molecules of mutagen. When DNA is replicated, additional bases are inserted into the space, changing the base sequence. Ethidium bromide is an intercalating agent; it carries a warning to handle with care because it is a **carcinogen** (cancer-causing agent).

INVERSIONS

Inversions are classified as macrolesions because long sequences of bases may be altered. When a segment of DNA is inverted, the change in the sequence of bases promotes nonsense codons. With an inversion, there is a high probability of the loss of gene function.

TRANSPOSONS

Some genes have gained a reputation as frequent travelers within the genome of eucaryotic and procaryotic cells. The genes that move from one segment of DNA to another on chromosomes, on plasmids, or within viruses are called **transposons (Tns)**. They are sometimes also called "jumping genes" (Fig. 7–12). Transposons are segments of DNA that contain inverted repeat (IR) segments of bases on the ends and a transposase gene. The simplest version is the **insertion sequence (IS) element.** They may also contain other genes such as drug resistance genes in the middle.

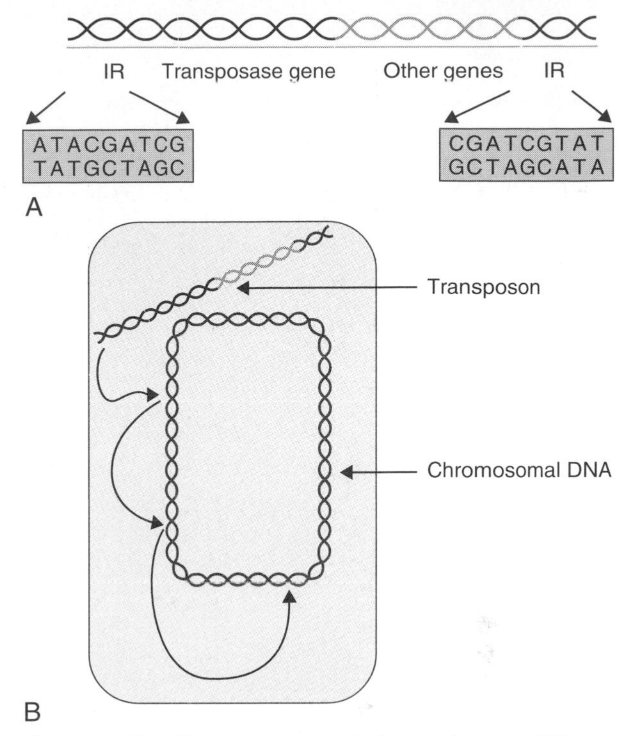

Figure 7–12 ◆ Transposons contain inverted repeat (IR) segments of bases on the ends, a transposase gene, and other genes such as drug resistance genes (*A*). The transposon can insert and "jump" from one location to another in the chromosome (*B*).

Within a cell, the transposon can insert itself into the chromosomal DNA of a cell for a time. The transposon may "jump" from one location to another in the chromosome, interrupting gene sequences. All transposons are potential mutagens because they alter the DNA sequence as they integrate into a new position. The transposon may prevent expression of a gene or a cluster of genes into which it has integrated. Transposons provide yet another mechanism to explain diversity of phenotypes.

FOCAL POINT

Barbara McClintock's Amazing Maize

In 1951, Barbara McClintock, a plant geneticist working with Indian corn, or maize, observed a great variation in the color of their kernels. She suggested a revolutionary explanation for the color variation in corn kernels: *jumping genes.* Certain DNA segments she called transposons move from one location to another, causing interrupted expression of genes encoding pigment production. Her peers took a dim view of genes that could relocate, or transpose. With time, the techniques of molecular biology improved so that many more scientists identified transposable elements in other organisms, including bacteria.

The phenomenon of transposons implicates them as agents for genetic change in bacteria, plants, the fruit fly, and perhaps even humans. Not only did Barbara McClintock win the Nobel Prize in Medicine or Physiology in 1983, she was given an annual $80,000 lifetime grant from the MacArthur Foundation and six other awards. Unlike winning a prize for a display of the sweetest or largest ears of corn at the annual state fair, Barbara McClintock waited over 30 years for her prize. Her amazing maize brought her the belated recognition she so richly deserved, making her a member of the prestigious Nobel Prize laureates.

REVERSIONS

Some mutants can revert to wild-type phenotypes in a process known as **back mutation** or **reversion.** The restoration in phenotype can occur by a variety of mechanisms. The base sequence can be changed back to the original sequence by the action of mutagens.

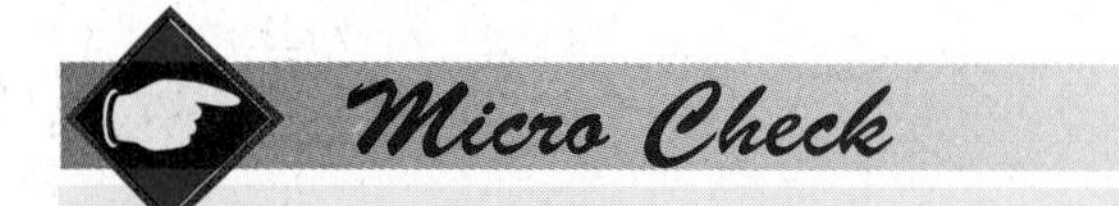

- How is it possible for a variation in phenotype to be environmentally induced?
- What is the difference between mutation rate and mutation frequency?
- What is meant by transposon?

Detection of Mutants

Because mutation rates are so low, it is to be expected that mutants are difficult to detect. Under ordinary cultural techniques, mutants may go unnoticed—just one in a crowd in a population of a million or more cells. Therefore, it is necessary to use special cultural techniques designed to select for the mutants.

ENRICHMENT OF MUTANT CELLS

When culturing microorganisms, adding a non-nutrient chemical or virus to the culture medium allows the researcher to discover, or select mutant cells. For example, mutants having resistance to an antimicrobial agent can be observed in a culture medium with the agent added. Only colonies of resistant mutant cells will grow in the presence of the antibiotic or toxic chemical. To detect bacterial cells within a population that are resistant to attack by bacterial viruses, known as bacteriophages (or **phages,** for short), direct enrichment is used by adding phages to which they are susceptible to the culture medium. When a mixed population of bacteria is grown on plates containing a specific phage, only colonies of phage-resistant mutants grow, while phage-sensitive cells are destroyed.

An alternate enrichment technique detects mutants with additional nutritional requirements, that is, auxotrophs, from a mixed cell population of both prototrophic (parent or "wild"-type cells) and auxotrophic cells. A selective agent, such as a lethal concentration of penicillin, is added to a **minimal broth,** a broth designed to cultivate only prototrophic cells. After inoculating this broth with the mixed cell population, the penicillin destroys the growing prototrophs. Auxotrophs survive because they cannot grow, and penicillin does not affect nongrowing cells. The remaining auxotrophic cells must be transferred to a minimal agar containing glucose, mineral salts, and the essential nutrient or growth factor for the desired mutant (Fig. 7–13). This is a simple method for isolating the mutant strain from the mixed population.

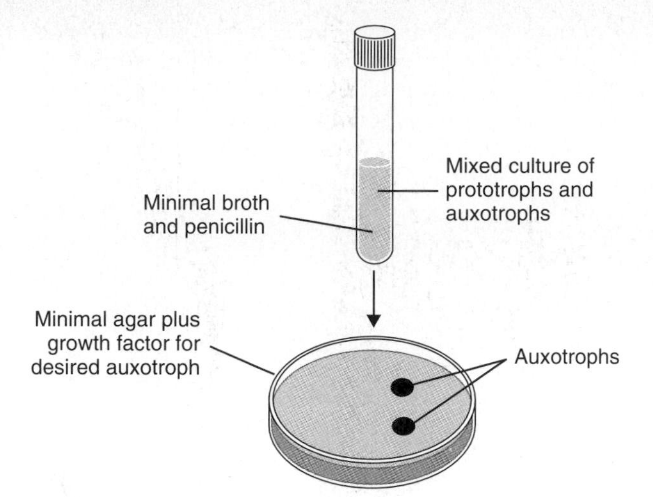

Figure 7–13 ◆ Penicillin-enrichment technique for selecting auxotrophic mutants in a mixed population. Penicillin kills prototrophs growing in minimal broth. Auxotrophs survive the exposure to penicillin and later grow on an agar with complete nutrients for its growth.

SELECTION FOR MUTANT CELLS

A technique known as **replica plating** is very efficient for separating nutritionally deficient mutants from mixed populations of cells. Colonies on a master plate of a nutritionally complete agar medium are transferred to other plates by means of a velveteen "stamp." Sterile velveteen is wrapped tightly around a support block. By pressing the velveteen fabric gently onto the master plate, cells from the colonies are transferred to the velveteen fibers. These fibers act like thousands of inoculating needles. The velveteen block is then "stamped" onto: (1) a sterile minimal agar plate that supports growth of prototrophs only and (2) a sterile nutritionally complete agar plate that supports growth of both prototrophs and auxotrophs (Fig. 7–14).

An arrow marked on the stamping block and on the plates ensures that the position of each colony on the master plate can be compared to the transfer plates. Colonies unable to grow on the minimal agar represent auxotrophs. To determine which nutrient is required by auxotrophic mutants of different types, several plates of minimal agar containing a different growth factor are made. The replica-plating technique is used to inoculate the colonies. The auxotrophic colonies will grow only on the plate with the needed growth factor. Ten or more replica plates can be made from a single imprint on a velveteen "stamp."

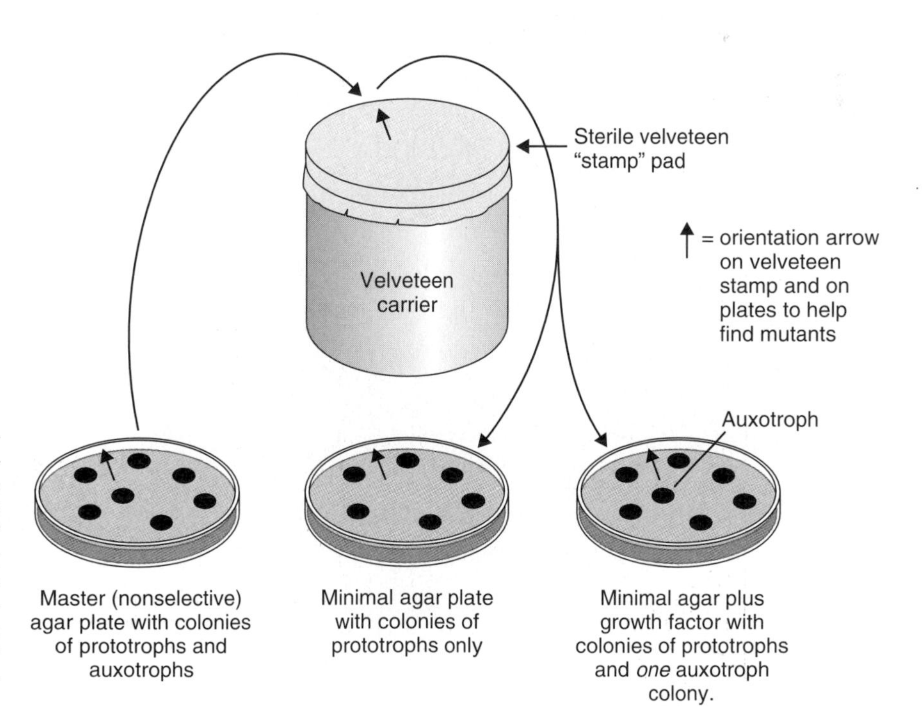

Figure 7–14 ◆ Replica-plating technique. Sterile velveteen on a cylindrical support picks up cells from each colony on a master plate. The velveteen is imprinted, or "stamped," onto the surface of a minimal agar plate and minimal agar plates with an added growth factor. After incubation, auxotrophs grow only on the medium with the growth factor that meets their nutritional requirements.

Detection of Chemical Mutagens

Mutant strains of many microorganisms are valuable for understanding metabolic pathways, host susceptibility, and antibiotic resistance. A histidine-negative mutant of *Salmonella typhimurium* is especially useful for detecting chemical mutagens in a testing procedure developed by Bruce Ames. Because many chemical mutagens are also carcinogenic, the Ames test is valuable for screening potential carcinogens. This in vitro system for detecting potential carcinogens is more economical than large-scale animal studies. If the test chemical is a mutagen, the bacterial mutant will be genetically altered, and some cells will revert back to the original phenotype for histidine production, or be histidine-positive (his^+).

In the Ames test, rat liver homogenates are added to histidine-deficient agar seeded with an *S. typhimurium* his^- strain. Discs containing suspected mutagenic chemicals are placed on the surface of the agar. In the presence of a mutagen and rat liver homogenates, the DNA of the mutant bacterial strain is repaired by a reverse mutation to restore the original phenotype. Rat liver homogenates activate mutagens and allow the bacterial system to simulate a mammalian system. Colonies of histidine-positive (his^+) bacteria grow in the immediate areas surrounding the discs (Fig. 7–15). The number of colonies is related to the degree of mutagenicity of the chemical.

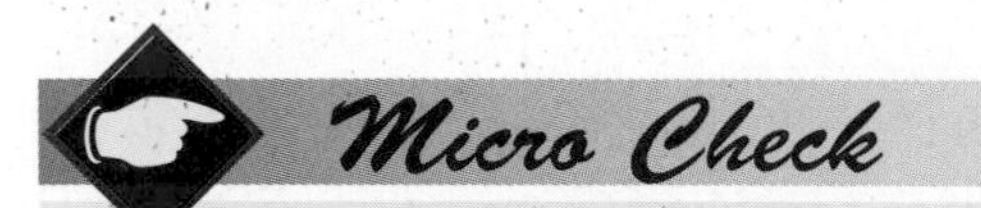

- Why are special techniques required to detect mutants?
- How can the replica-plating technique be used to detect nutritional mutants?
- What advantages does the Ames test have over animal tests in detection of possible carcinogens?

GENETIC TRANSFER IN PROCARYOTIC CELLS

Procaryotes can acquire new genetic material from another closely related organism by three naturally occurring gene transfer processes: **transformation, transduction,** and **conjugation.** In all instances, cells that transfer DNA are called **do-**

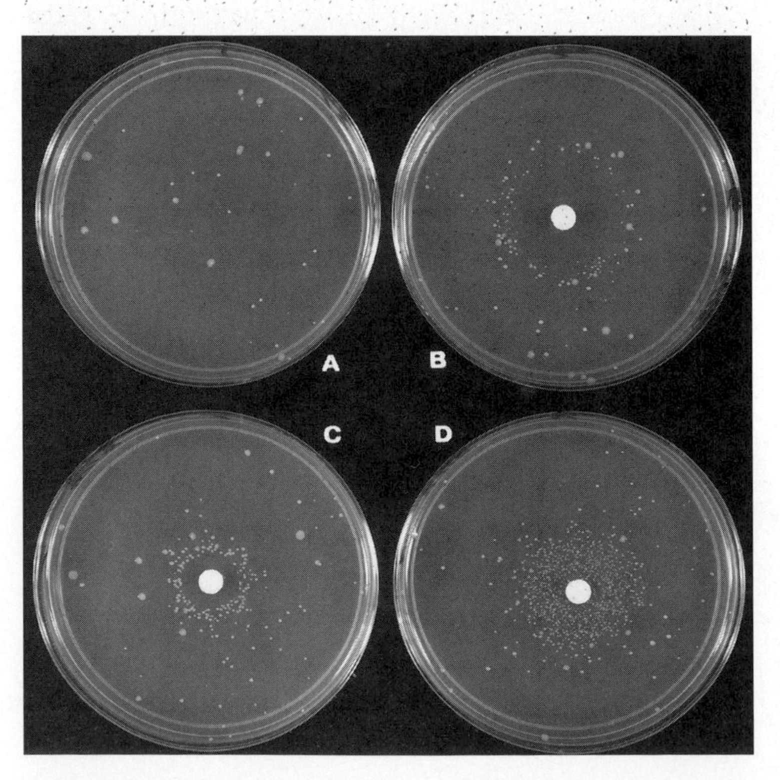

Figure 7–15 ◆ The Ames spot test. Each plate contains a histidine-negative (his^-) strain of *Salmonella typhimurium;* plates C and D contain rat liver homogenate. Spontaneous revertants appear on plate A. Colonies of induced revertants surround furylfuramide, AF-2 (1 μg) on plate B; aflatoxin (1 μg) on plate C; and 2-aminoflurorente (10 μg) on plate D.

nors and cells in which new DNA is introduced are known as **recipients.**

Transformation is the transfer of free (naked) DNA from one cell to another cell. Transduction is the transfer of DNA from a bacteriophage containing bacterial DNA to another cell. Conjugation requires cell-to-cell contact to initiate transfer of DNA from one cell to another. These genetic transfer methods provide a mechanism for genetic diversity in microorganisms that lack the ability to reproduce sexually.

Transformation

The process of transformation was first observed and named by the British bacteriologist Frederick Griffith in 1928 (Fig. 7–16). He was studying *Streptococcus pneumoniae,* known by the common name, pneumococcus. The encapsulated form of this bacterium causes pneumonia in humans. The virulent strain produces a capsule around its cells. The avirulent mutant strain of pneumococcus has no capsule-producing gene.

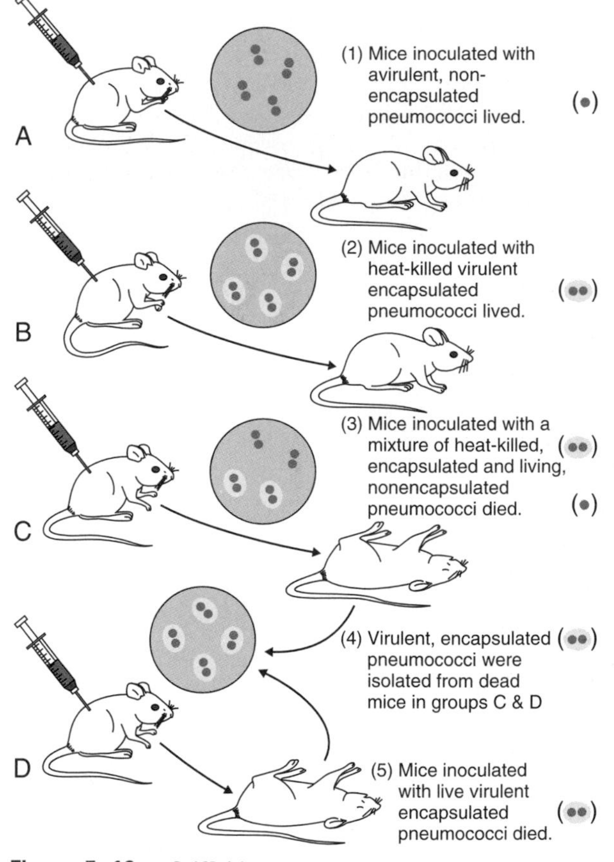

Figure 7–16 ◆ Griffith's experiment in which the "naked" DNA released from killed cells of virulent pneumococcus "transformed" the avirulent pneumococci into disease-producing organisms (group C). The other three experimental groups serve as control groups.

In his experiments, Griffith inoculated one group of mice with the mutant nonencapsulated strain of *S. pneumoniae.* The nonencapsulated strain of the organism did not cause pneumonia in the mice. He inoculated a second group of mice with heat-killed cells of the encapsulated strain of the organism. This group of mice did not contract pneumonia. In a third group of mice he injected a mixture of heat-killed encapsulated and living nonencapsulated organisms. The mice receiving this mixture of the two strains died from pneumonia. In a fourth group of mice, he injected live encapsulated pneumococcal cells. These mice developed pneumonia and died. The virulent strain of pneumococcus was isolated from the dead animals in the third and fourth groups.

From his results, Griffith concluded that in some manner, the harmless, nonencapsulated bacteria in the mixture used in the third group of mice had been "transformed" into virulent, encapsulated organisms. He called the responsible agent a "transforming principle" and the process transformation. When Griffith conducted these experiments, the exact nature of the hereditary molecules was still unknown.

In 1944, Oswald Avery, Colin MacLeod, and Maclyn McCarty identified the "transforming" substance as DNA. These researchers and Fred Griffith received the Nobel Prize for their contributions to understanding the chemical nature of heredity. Transformation occurs naturally in many species of procaryotes. In the laboratory, the process is a powerful tool for manipulating the genetic makeup of bacterial cells. A number of factors influence the uptake of DNA by "competent" cells, those cells able to transport a DNA segment into the cell interior. These factors include environmental conditions, density of cell population, and DNA size, concentration, and strandedness.

Transduction

The process of transduction was discovered by accident in 1951 when Joshua and Esther Lederberg worked with a talented graduate student, Norton Zinder, to conduct conjugation experiments with mutants of *Salmonella typhimurium.*

During the course of their studies, a transfer of genetic material occurred when a culture of one mutant was exposed to a cell-free extract of another mutant. At first, it was thought that transformation had occurred. Later, cells were grown in a specially constructed U-shaped tube fitted with a filter at the bottom of the U-tube. Cells could not pass through the filter. The enzyme, DNAse, was added to the liquid culture medium to break down any free DNA, thus preventing transformation.

Two auxotrophic strains were inoculated into the U-tube, each strain separated by the filter, thus preventing cell contact and conjugation. During incubation, one of the strains showed a degree of recombination of genes that came from the other strain. The transfer agent was discovered to be a bacteriophage that was infecting one of the bacterial strains. This phage is now known as P22. The phage was small enough to pass through the filter carrying DNA from its host bacterium in its virus coat to the second bacterial host on the other side of the filter. The process was called transduction and the bacteriophages transferring the genetic material were named **transducing particles** (Fig. 7–17).

During the development of some bacteriophages about one particle in 10^5 to 10^7 particles incorporates a small fragment of host DNA. Because it does not contain sufficient viral DNA to code for the manufacture of a new virus in another cell, this particle is also known as defective. Once released from the host, viral particles may infect a new host cell. Transduced DNA fragments from the dead host may recombine with recipient cell DNA, perhaps introducing new genes. Some phage DNA may be degraded or may persist in the host as nonreplicating units.

Some phages transfer a restricted set of genes at relatively high frequency. The transfer of a limited number of specific genes is called **specialized transduction.** Conversely, if a transducing particle transfers any segment of donor DNA, it is known as **generalized transduction.** A small number of transducing particles are capable of promoting both types of transduction.

Conjugation

Conjugation involves a transfer of some genetic material during cell-to-cell contact. The cells are of two different mating types within a species or between closely related species. Mating types include a donor and a recipient cell. The donor cell carries a specialized pilus, called the **sex pilus** or **F pilus** (F meaning fertility), to establish contact between cells. The recipient cell has no F pilus. The process was first demonstrated by Joshua Lederberg and Edward Tatum in 1946, when they studied specific mutants of *E. coli* K-12. It is now known that gram-negative bacteria and some gram-positive bacteria are capable of conjugation.

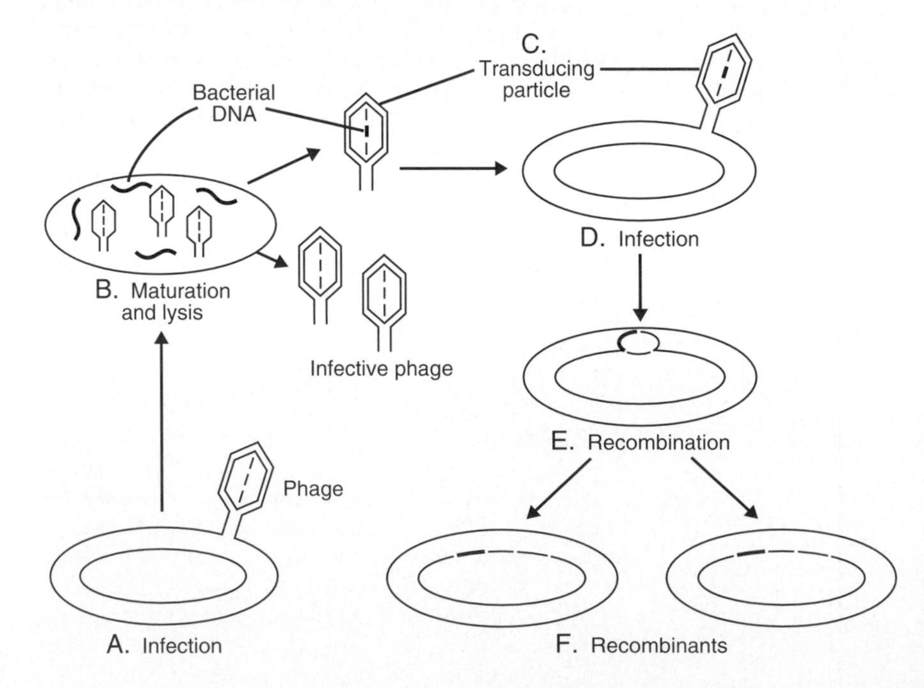

Figure 7–17 ◆ Generalized transduction. When a phage enters a bacterium, a lytic cycle is established (A and B). If bacterial DNA is accidentally packaged into a phage (C), it becomes a transducing particle. When the bacterial DNA of a transducing particle enters another bacterium (D), recombination can occur (E). The offspring cells carrying the new transduced gene(s) are also called recombinants (F).

Lederberg and Tatum found that in a mixed population of mutants, the transfer of genetic material always proceeded in a single direction from one population of mutants to another during contact between cells (Fig. 7–18). Later, it was discovered that donor strains contained an **F plasmid (F^+)** with genes for self-replication and formation of a mating pilus. Recipient strains lacked the F plasmid (F^-). Only F^+ cells, therefore, can be donors. In nature, F^- strains are more prevalent than F^+ strains because the plasmid is quite sensitive to temperatures above 42°C. Transfer of the F plasmid in crosses between F^+ and F^- strains approaches 100 percent. Chromosomal DNA is rarely transferred in an $F^+ \times F^-$ mating.

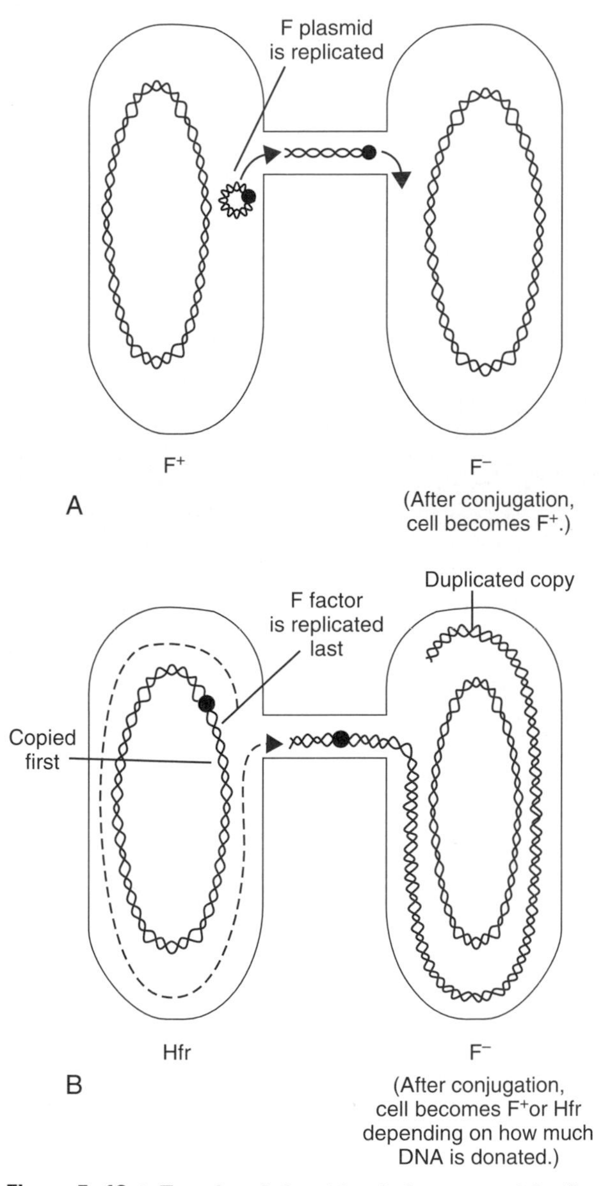

Figure 7–18 ◆ Transfer of plasmid and chromosomal fertility factor (F). *A,* In a cross between F^+ and F^- cells, a copy of the F factor is transferred independent of chromosomal transfer. *B,* In a cross between Hfr and F^- cells, a copy of the integrated F factor is transferred only after chromosomal transfer.

When the F plasmid integrates into the chromosome of recipient cells, the new donor cells are designated as Hfr (high frequency of recombination). Hfr indicates their ability to transfer chromosomal DNA with greater efficiency. Hfr cells mate with F^- cells transferring genes from the chromosome. Because the F factor is transferred after all the chromosomal genes, F^- cells may remain F^- if the cell contact time is short. Recombinants can be demonstrated in approximately 1 percent of cells after a cross between F^- and Hfr mating types.

By periodic interruptions in matings, François Jacob and Elie Wollman demonstrated in 1955 that Hfr cells transfer genetic material to recipient F^- cells in a specific orientation. The sequence of genes entering the recipient cell is also the order of their arrangement on the donor chromosome. The entire chromosome of *E. coli* enters a recipient cell in 90 minutes, if mating is not interrupted. Because cells rarely remain in contact that long, the transfer of an entire chromosome including the F plasmid is rare.

Conjugation experiments have revealed much about the nature of the bacterial chromosome. The circular conformation of the bacterial chromosome was first established by conjugation experiments. Conjugation has made it possible to locate or map positions of genes on bacterial chromosomes, producing **linkage maps.**

Bacteria containing new DNA often have survival advantages. Newly acquired traits are frequently protective or provide organisms with the ability to use a greater variety of carbon or energy sources.

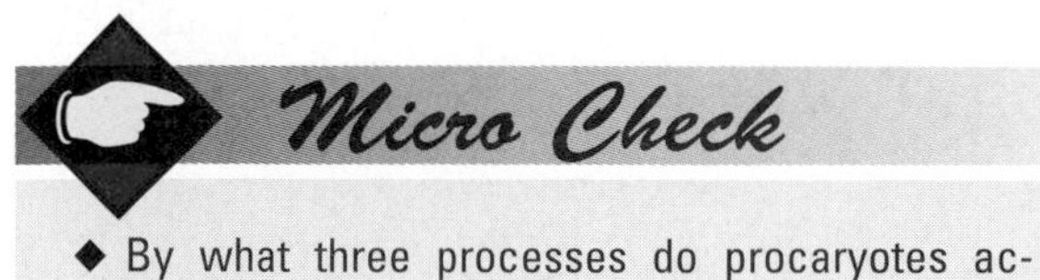

- By what three processes do procaryotes acquire genetic material from other procaryotes?
- What determines the amount of DNA transferred in conjugation?
- Of what importance is genetic transfer to survival of bacterial species?

REGULATION OF GENE EXPRESSION IN PROCARYOTES

Regulation of the synthesis of some enzymes occurs at the genetic level. Transcription of genes for regulated enzymes is controlled by either **negative** or **positive** (sometimes both) **control mechanisms**. Negative control involves a **regulatory protein** binding to DNA to block transcription of a genetic unit. Positive control permits transcription when a regulatory protein binds to DNA.

Operons are distinct genetic units on the bacterial chromosome controlled by regulatory proteins. A trait such as lactose fermentation or tryptophan synthesis is controlled by a single operon. An operon includes structural genes for producing enzymes and some genes for controlling transcription of structural genes.

The main regions of an operon are (1) a **regulator gene,** (2) a **promoter,** (3) an **operator,** and (4) **structural genes** (Fig. 7–19). The regulator gene codes for a regulatory protein. The promoter (P) binds RNA polymerase to initiate transcription. The operator (O) is next to the promoter and may overlap it. The operator acts as an "on-off" switch for transcription of the structural genes. The regulatory protein binds to the operator to turn it on (positive control) or off (negative control).

Operons that have negative control mechanisms in *E. coli* include the **lactose operon (lac operon)** and **tryptophan operon (trp operon).** The lac operon codes for lactose degrading en-

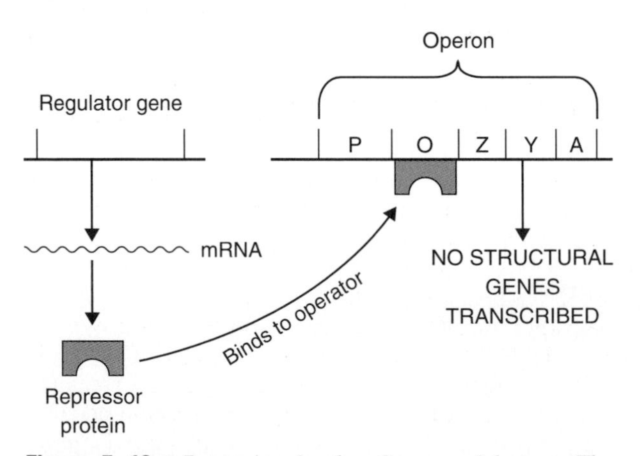

Figure 7–19 ◆ Repression in the absence of lactose. The operon is in the "off" position in the absence of lactose. A lac repressor protein attaches to the operator gene (O), preventing transcription of structural genes Z, Y, and A.

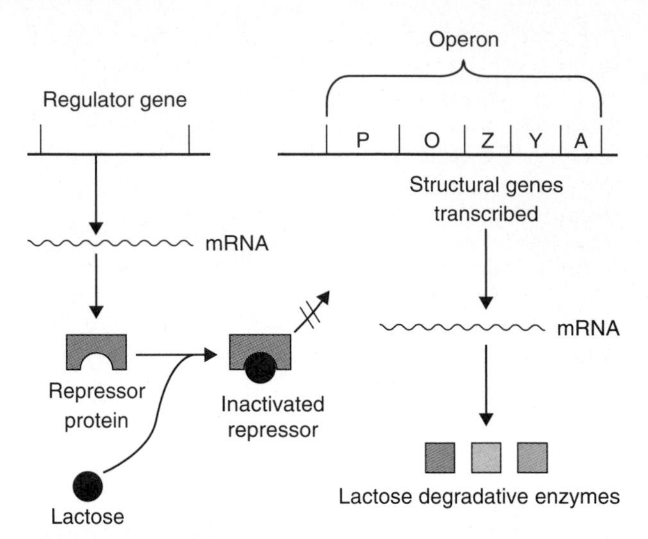

Figure 7–20 ◆ Induction. The operon is in the "on" position in the presence of lactose. The lactose (inducer) inactivates the lac repressor molecule, releasing the operator gene. Transcription of the structural genes Z, Y, and A proceeds.

zymes. The operon is essentially "off," or not transcribed significantly, when lactose is not available. In this way, the bacterial cell does not synthesize unnecessary enzymes. The regulatory protein is a **repressor protein** that actively binds to the operator when lactose is absent and blocks transcription. When lactose is available, a form of lactose known as allolactose binds to the repressor protein (Fig. 7–20). This binding alters the shape of the repressor causing it to leave the operator, thus turning "on" the operon.

The three structural genes, Z, Y, and A, code for three enzymes: β-galactosidase breaks lactose into its two component sugars; a galactoside permease transports lactose into the cell; and a galactoside transacetylase, which has an unknown function. Because these genes are transcribed when their substrate lactose acts as an "inducer," their products are called **inducible enzymes.**

The trp operon codes for five enzymes that produce tryptophan. The end product of the metabolic pathway, tryptophan, is involved in turning "off," or repressing, the operon. This type of control is called **end product repression.** When tryptophan is produced in excess, some molecules bind to inactive trp repressor proteins activating them. Activated repressors attach to the operator of the trp operon and block transcription. When tryptophan is absent, the trp repressor is inactive and the operon is "on."

An additional regulatory mechanism called **attenuation** complements the action of the operator in the synthesis of some amino acids. Attenuation together with the operator provides a finer control on gene expression. In the trp operon exists an additional DNA region called the leader between the operator and the first structural gene. This region has a length of DNA that contains two codons for tryptophan and a stop signal called the **attenuator.**

In bacteria, transcription produces an mRNA molecule that is translated almost simultaneously. If tryptophan is in excess, translation proceeds quickly through the two trp codons in the leader transcript of the mRNA. This rapid translation results in the formation of a double-stranded fold on the mRNA called a **terminator hairpin.** This hairpin loop exposes the attenuator causing RNA polymerase to stop transcription. If tryptophan is in low supply, however, translation of the leader transcript is stalled, the mRNA folds into a different antiterminator loop that does not expose the attenuator and RNA polymerase transcribes all the structural genes. Translation of the mRNA results in enzymes to synthesize tryptophan.

Operons for fermenting the sugars arabinose and maltose are examples of positive control. The substrate, arabinose or maltose, activates a regulatory substance that in turn binds to the operator to initiate transcription of the structural genes. In the absence of substrate molecules, these operons remain turned "off."

One example of a positive regulator for several operons including the lac operon is **catabolite activator protein (CAP),** an allosteric protein. CAP becomes active when cyclic AMP(cAMP) binds to it. The CAP-cAMP complex binds to the lac operator to initiate transcription by RNA polymerase. An example of this type of control is catabolite repression described in Chapter 6. When the supply of glucose is depleted, cAMP becomes available to bind to CAP. If lactose is available, the CAP-cAMP complex turns on the lac operon. The lac operon is an example of dual control by both positive and negative control mechanisms.

RECOMBINATION IN EUCARYOTES

Sexual reproduction provides the means for genetic recombination to occur in most eucaryotes. The process is more complex than in procaryotes because eucaryotic cells have more than one chromosome (Table 7–4). The chromosome number is reduced by one-half during formation of gametes (sex cells) by a process of reduction-division known as **meiosis** (Fig. 7–21). Prior to meiosis, DNA replication occurs, producing duplicate strands of DNA called **chromatids.** Two identical chromosomes have a tetrad (set of four) of chromatids. Segments of like chromatids become attached to one another at some points. Crossing-over of fragments of chromatids may occur, causing genes to be moved from one location to another. These new linkage associations or recombinations are important for their implication in causing mutations (Fig. 7–22).

The tetrads separate and undergo cell division, resulting in four cells in the haploid state, each having half the number of chromosomes as the original cell. In animals, these haploid cells in a male are four gametes that mature into **sperm** cells; in the female, the gametes produce an **ovum.** Cell fusion, which occurs when a sperm fertilizes an ovum, restores the diploid number of chromosomes.

Table 7–4
DIPLOID CHROMOSOME NUMBERS OF COMMON EUCARYOTES

COMMON NAME	SCIENTIFIC NAME	CHROMOSOME NUMBER
Mold	*Aspergillus nidulans*	8
Yeast	*Saccharomyces cerevisiae*	8
Corn	*Zea mays*	20
Potato	*Solanum tuberosum*	48
Fly	*Musca domestica*	12
Cat	*Felis catus*	38
Dog	*Canis familiaris*	78
Human	*Homo sapiens*	46

RECOMBINANT DNA TECHNOLOGY

The ability to program cells to make particular products is known as **recombinant DNA technology** or **genetic engineering. Biotechnology** is a discipline that encompasses natural sciences, engineering, and computer sciences to produce valuable products from recombinant DNA research. DNA of microbial, plant, or animal origin can be transferred to some bacterial or yeast cells. Recipient cells, known as **recombinant cells,** transcribe and translate the transferred genes along with their own genes. The recombinant cells become cell "factories," producing large quantities of important proteins, or other prod-

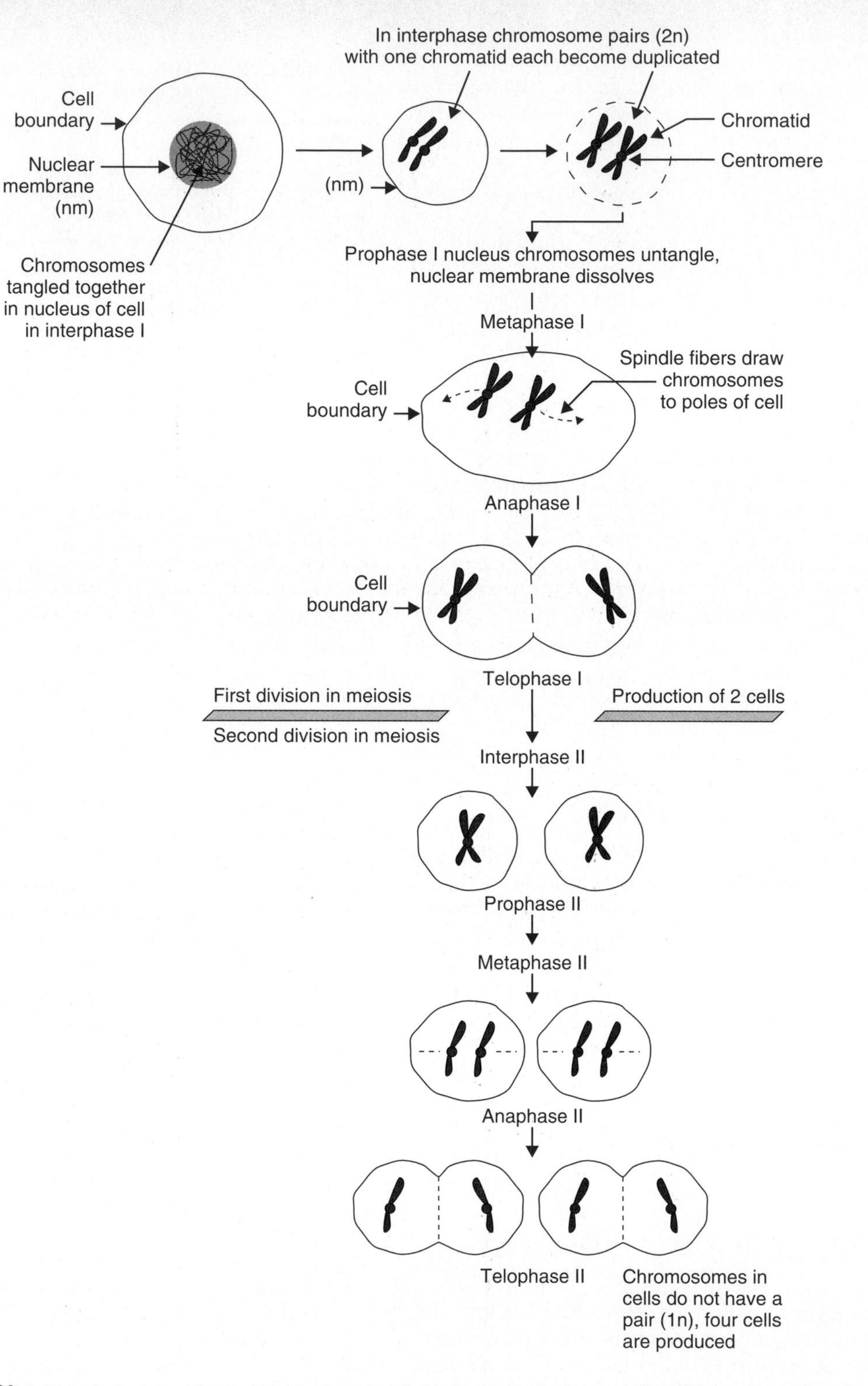

Figure 7–21 ◆ Meiosis in sex cells. Only a single pair of chromosomes is shown within the nucleus. Metaphase has been omitted from the diagram. The daughter cells formed during the first meiotic division are diploid, but the daughter cells formed during second meiotic division are haploid.

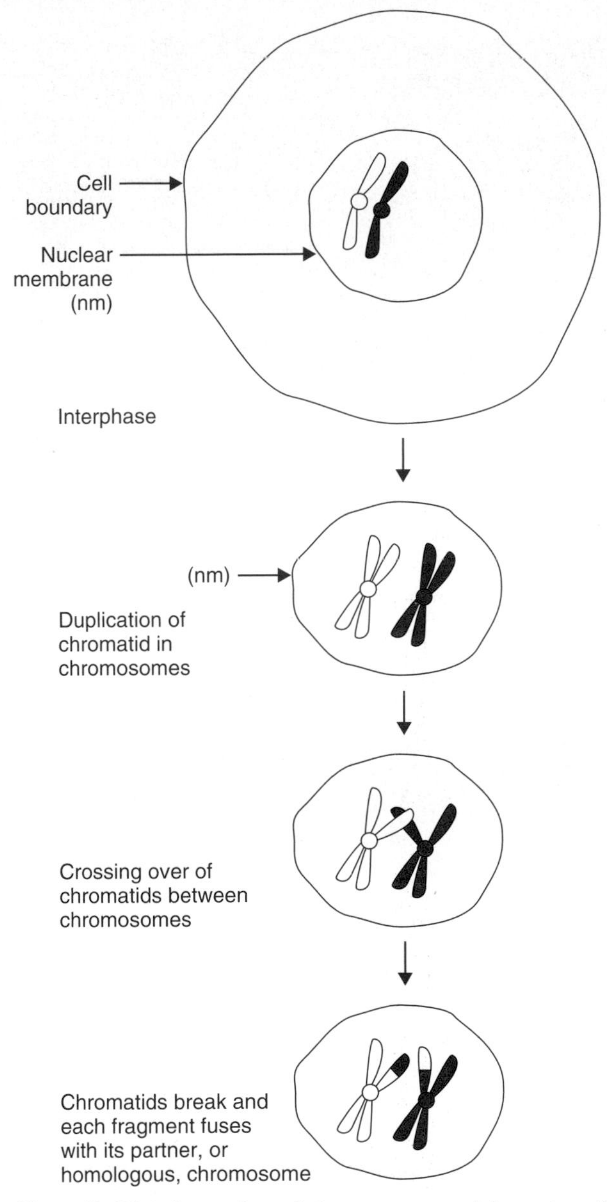

Figure 7–22 ◆ Separation of chromosomes and formation of new linkages between chromatids during crossover.

ucts. **Gene cloning** involves cultivating recombinant cells to increase the number of cells with copies of the recombined gene of interest. A population of such cells is called a **clone.**

Biotechnology makes possible the industrial synthesis of medically useful products such as hormones, vaccines, monoclonal antibodies, immune modulators, and others (Table 7–5). In agricultural science, recombinant DNA technology introduces desirable genes into plants. Gross sales of genetically engineered products account for billions of dollars of income each year, and biotechnology industries can be expected to increase over the next several decades.

Gene Cloning Systems

Methods for preparing to clone a gene may include (1) isolation of a fragment of DNA of interest, (2) synthesis of **complementary DNA (cDNA)** from an mRNA template, or (3) construction of a recombinant plasmid carrying a gene of interest.

For the isolation of a DNA of interest, **restriction enzymes** that cut DNA at specific sites are required. The enzymes, sometimes known as "molecular scissors," typically recognize short sequences of bases that are identical if read either from one direction or the other. Such sequences are called palindromes. The words "Otto" and "toot" are examples of palindromes. Examples of palindromes in DNA sequences include the following:

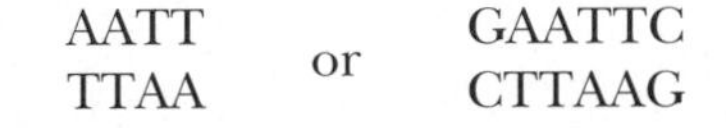

A restriction enzyme may break bonds between the adenines in the AATT sequence on both strands. This creates a break in the DNA molecule where the ends of each strand have a sequence of complementary bases, or "sticky ends."

By using the same restriction enzyme on DNA molecules from two or more different sources, the same "sticky ends" are produced on each DNA fragment. After mixing the DNA fragments together, some recombinant DNA molecules will form as their "sticky ends" form hydrogen bonds between complementary bases. In this way, recombinant DNA fragments are constructed. Recombinant DNA carrying *E. coli* DNA and the human insulin gene as well as other types of combinations have been produced in this way.

Complementary DNA (cDNA) is produced from mRNA when **reverse transcriptase** synthesizes DNA from the RNA template. This method is especially valuable for genes that have noncoding sequences of nucleotides. Many DNA molecules of eucaryotes and a very few procaryotes have coding and noncoding regions within a gene. The coding gene is called an **exon,** for expressed gene. The noncoding segments within the exon are called **introns,** meaning intervening sequences. The value of the unusual genetic

Table 7–5
GENETICALLY ENGINEERED PRODUCTS MANUFACTURED BY RECOMBINANT MICROORGANISMS

PRODUCT	FUNCTION
Epidermal growth factor	Regulates calcium levels, stimulates growth of epidermal cells
Erythropoietin	Stimulates production of red blood cells
Granulocyte stimulating factor	Stimulates production of white blood cells
Human growth hormone	Regulates growth of human body
Insulin	Regulates blood sugar levels
Interferon alpha	Interfere with replication of viral pathogens, anti-tumor, anti-inflammatory effects
Interferon beta	
Interferon gamma	
Interleukin 2	Stimulates antigen-activated CD4+ helper cells
Tissue plasminogen activator	Dissolves blood clots
Tumor necrosis factor	Destroys tumor cells
Hepatitis B vaccine	Protects against hepatitis B infection
Monoclonal antibody specific for hormone, human chorionic gonadotropin	Pregnancy testing

structure is unknown. The introns may be warehouses for extra genetic material. For exons with one or more introns, an mRNA template is more useful in genetic engineering to replicate a desired gene minus its intron segments.

Donor fragments of DNA are incorporated into a small self-replicating **vector,** a DNA molecule used to transfer foreign DNA into a cell or organism. That vector may be a plasmid, phage, or a phage-hybrid plasmid, known as a **cosmid.** Ligases covalently link vector and donor DNA fragments into a self-replicating unit of recombinant DNA (Fig. 7–23).

Selection of Recombinant DNA Hosts

The recombinant DNA can be introduced into a microbial host by transformation, transduction, or by a process known as **protoplast fusion** after cell walls are removed. Actual fusion, and therefore, the opportunity to transfer genes, can be increased by treatment with polyethylene glycol (PEG) or exposure to an electric current. Sometimes additional techniques must be employed to promote expression of a gene by the foreign host cell.

E coli, Bacillus subtilis, and the yeast *Saccharomyces cerevisiae* have been used extensively as host cells for clone vectors. Genetic information has been transferred from one plant to another by using a plant-cloning vector, the tumor-inducing (T_i) plasmid of *Agrobacterium tumefaciens.*

Detection of Clones. Special procedures must be used to select for a clone of interest among a large population of organisms. One approach is to look for the gene product if it is being expressed. Another technique employs nucleic acid hybridization to detect the presence of a specific gene.

Demonstration of New Products. New products of recombinant hosts may be detected by the use of selective media or product-specific antibodies. Often the product of a recombinant organism is an enzyme whose activity can be measured by a color reaction. In other instances, nonrecombinants may grow only in the presence of specific nutrients, whereas recombinants will grow even in the absence of a specific nutrient. It is necessary to have a reliable method to detect the recombinants producing the desired products.

Nucleic Acid Hybridization. If a newly acquired gene of a recombinant is not expressed, its protein products are not detectable in the

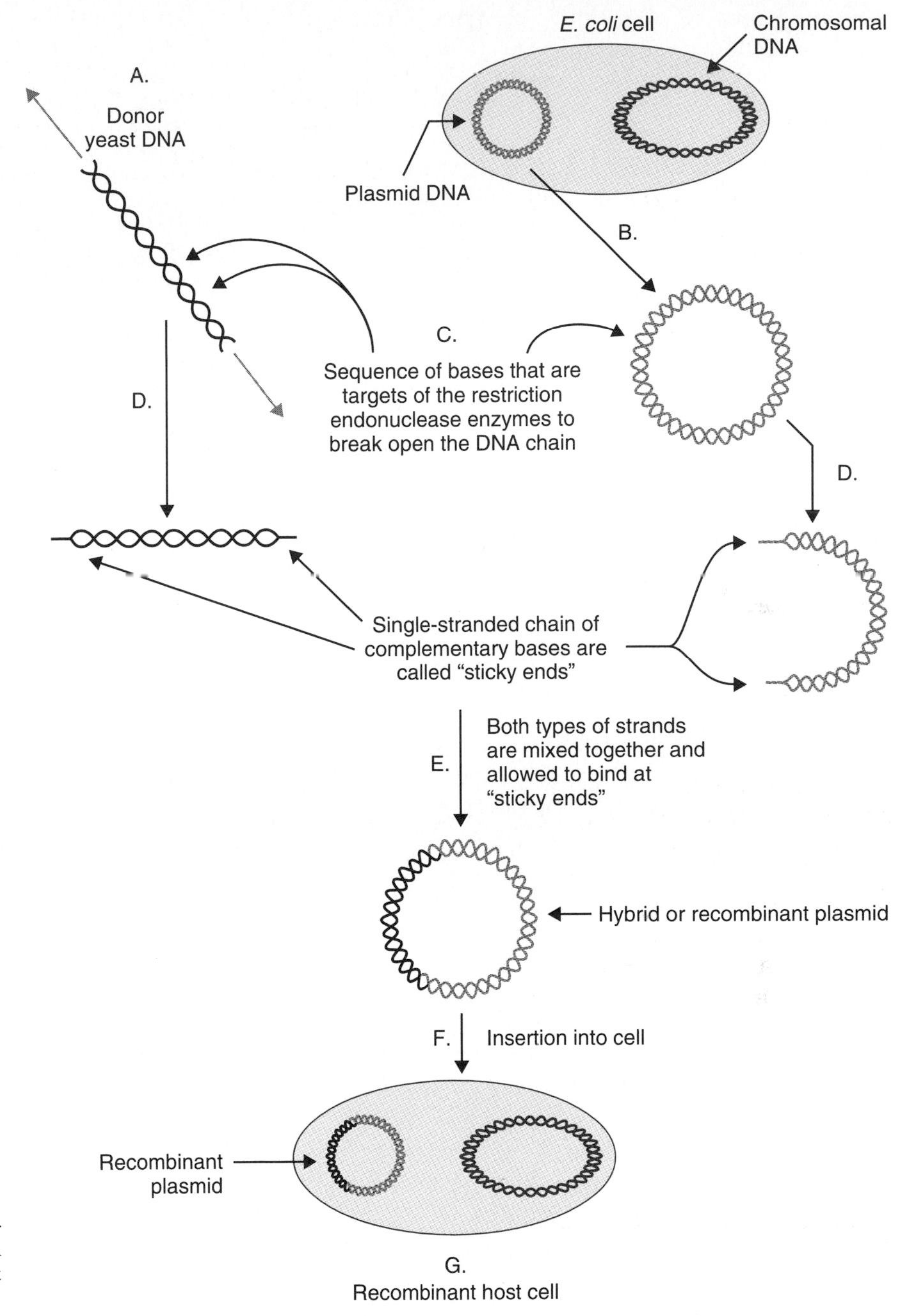

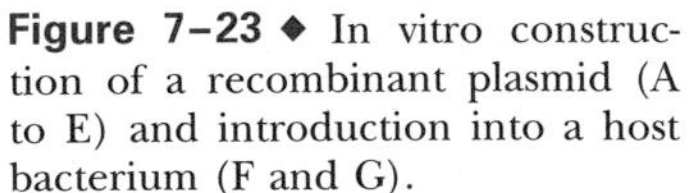
Figure 7–23 ◆ In vitro construction of a recombinant plasmid (A to E) and introduction into a host bacterium (F and G).

cells. Nucleic acid hybridization may be used to detect the DNA of interest in these bacteria. In this technique, a radioactively labeled short, single strand of DNA or RNA, called a **probe,** is synthesized. The probe has a base sequence complementary to a portion of the gene of interest. A mixed cell population with recombinant and nonrecombinant cells is cultured on a plate. The colonies are then replicated onto a nitrocellulose filter and dissolved, and their DNA molecules are treated to produce single strands. The radioactive probe is added to the filter. The probe will form base pairs with DNA sequences that are complementary; these base pairs are from the recombinant colonies. Exposing the filter to x-ray film will produce an image of the radioactivity and identify the recombinant colonies on the master plate.

Gene Amplification

The DNA of a single gene can be stimulated to replicate rapidly by a process known as gene amplification. The technique, known as a **polymerase chain reaction (PCR),** starts with a single fragment of DNA and produces billions of copies in a few hours (Fig. 7–24). The original fragment of DNA must first be heated to separate the two strands of DNA. The synthesis of new DNA proceeds in the presence of an ample supply of deoxyribonucleotides, a heat-stable DNA polymerase, and short segments of DNA needed to prime the reaction. The two strands of the original DNA act as templates for the new strands of DNA. As the temperature is lowered, the primer binds to the DNA and replication begins on each strand to form two DNA molecules. At the end of the replication cycle, heat is applied to separate the two strands of newly synthesized DNA to prepare for another replication cycle. When the temperature is lowered, the primers attach to the DNA and begin the process again. The heating-cooling cycle continues automatically in PCR to produce a massive quantity of identical DNA molecules.

Application of PCR has made it possible to develop tests for the diagnosis of carriers of human genetic diseases. For many infectious diseases, diagnosis can be made in retrospect if tissue samples are available. The technique is especially valuable for identifying organisms, such as *Mycobacterium tuberculosis,* which grow slowly in the laboratory.

The ability to amplify the DNA in minute samples of blood or even in a single hair at a crime scene has introduced to forensic (legal) medicine a powerful technology for identifying people. This **DNA "fingerprinting"** technique, or DNA typing, is based on detecting unique short repetitive sequences in DNA, called **variable number of tandem repeats (VNTRs),** found in blood or other body fluids (Fig. 7–25). Although the same sequences may appear in other people, the num-

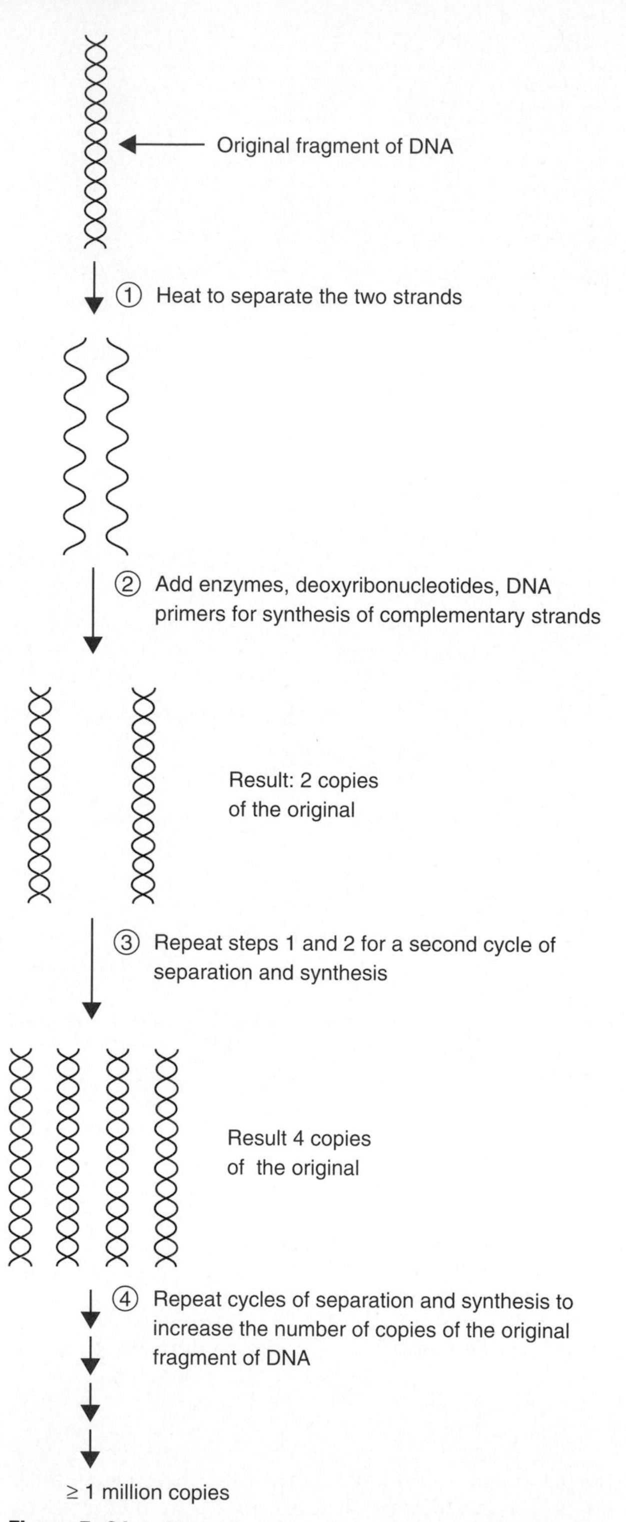

Figure 7–24 ◆ The polymerase chain reaction (PCR). An exponential increase in fragments of DNA occurs in a temperature-cycling instrument.

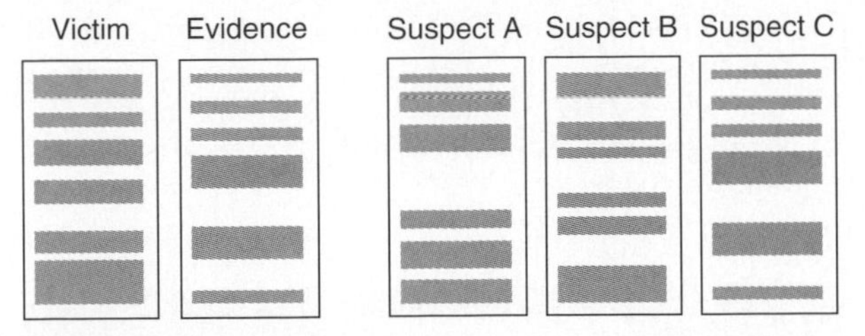

Figure 7–25 ◆ Diagram of DNA fingerprints. The DNA fingerprint of Suspect C matches the blood obtained from the scene of the crime.

bers of times they appear in any one individual differ. The banding patterns of DNA sequences are compared between the victim, evidence, and any suspects to find a match. Some courts have allowed DNA fingerprints to be introduced into evidence against a defendant since 1987; other courts have been slow to accept the new technology.

More than 25 countries use DNA fingerprinting for forensics and paternity testing. The highly publicized trial of O. J. Simpson increased the awareness of the general public to the power of DNA fingerprinting. Conservation groups use DNA fingerprinting to detect illegal slaughter of whales or other protected animals. Unlabeled meat sold in Japanese markets was identified as coming from two protected species, the humpback and fin whales.

THE ETHICS OF BIOCHEMICAL ENGINEERING

The potential for altering the evolutionary process by using in vitro recombinant DNA has aroused both enthusiasm and apprehension among scientists. The fear that genetically altered microorganisms could destroy entire populations in biological warfare is very real. Some countries prohibit or require authorization for certain experiments. The risk factors must be carefully weighed. Supporters of genetic engineering believe that commitment to responsible experimentation can improve the quality of life for millions. Human genome mapping is sure to generate new diagnostic tests, and the research has the potential to lead to cures for many diseases.

Opponents contend that the potential for misuse of information obtained by DNA technology could cause employers or insurance companies to demand genetic screening. How much do we need to know? If a fatal illness, for which there is no cure, is diagnosed before signs or symptoms appear, what are the legal implications? Can the temptation to tinker with reproductive cells be avoided? Who will have access to our DNA fingerprints? Is the search for biology's "Holy Grail," the mapping of the human genome, justified? Only time can resolve these ethical issues.

FOCAL POINT

Simpson Trial Spurred Action To Conserve Microbe

An unusual bacterium, found in a hot spring in Yellowstone National Park, has entered the crowded field of notables in the O.J. Simpson murder case. The heat-loving microbe, *Thermus aquaticus,* is the source of a thermostable polymerase used in the DNA fingerprinting technique. The role of the enzyme in the polymerase chain reaction (PCR) is crucial in the diagnosis of many infectious diseases and to the field of criminology. Because heat is required to synthesize additional fragments of DNA, the polymerase used must be heat-stable.

Environmentalists have seized the opportunity of the publicity surrounding the Simpson case to raise public consciousness of the need for preserving the habitats of *T. aquaticus.* Continued protection becomes more expensive as visitors to Yellowstone National Park continue to increase each year. There is no money in the park's annual budget to protect the geysers, hot springs, and steam vents from the ravages of human carelessness. In addition, *T. aquaticus* and other microbial inhabitants of the hot springs provide scientists with clues as to the nature of early life forms. Conservationists feel that well drilling on land adjacent to Yellowstone might alter geothermal activities in the park. The question remains as to whether the newfound fame of *T. aquaticus* can save the unique environment that permits it and other heat-tolerant microbes to survive.

Los Angeles Times, August 31, 1994.

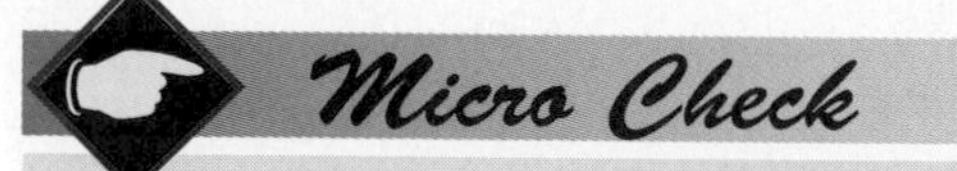

- What vectors are used in gene cloning?
- How are the vectors transferred to appropriate hosts?
- What risks are associated with DNA technology?

Understanding Microbiology

1. Give three examples of the influence of environmental conditions on phenotype.
2. What is the significance of drug-resistant mutant bacterial strains in a hospital?
3. How can plasmids influence expression of phenotypes?
4. What is the significance of "jumping genes"?
5. Why is genetic engineering a controversial technology?

Applying Microbiology

6. Formulate an argument for presentation before a congressional committee to convince them of the need for supporting basic research on mutagens in air, water, and food. Anticipate at least five questions members of Congress may ask, and provide definitive answers to them.

Unit 3

Major Groups of Microorganisms

Chapter 8

Procaryotes: Bacteria and Archaea

Chapter Outline

- **THE CONCEPT OF SPECIES**
- **HOW GENUS AND SPECIES ARE NAMED**
- **RANKING THE BACTERIA**
- **CRITERIA FOR CLASSIFYING BACTERIA**
  - Chemotaxonomy
  - Nucleic Acid Relatedness
  - Genetic Recombination
  - Numerical Taxonomy
- **THE BACTERIA**
  - The Spirochetes
  - Aerobic/Microaerophilic Helical Vibrioid Gram-Negative Bacteria
  - Gram-Negative Rods and Cocci
  - Facultatively Anaerobic Gram-Negative Rods
  - Anaerobic Gram-Negative Rods
  - Anaerobic Gram-Negative Cocci
  - The Rickettsias and Chlamydias
  - Mycoplasmas
  - Gram-Positive Cocci
  - Endospore-Forming Gram-Positive Rods and Cocci
  - Regular Nonsporing Gram-Positive Rods
  - Irregular Nonsporing Gram-Positive Rods
  - Mycobacteria
  - Nocardioforms
  - Streptomycetes and Their Allies
- **THE ARCHAEA**
  - The Methanogens
  - The Extreme Thermophiles
  - The Extreme Halophiles

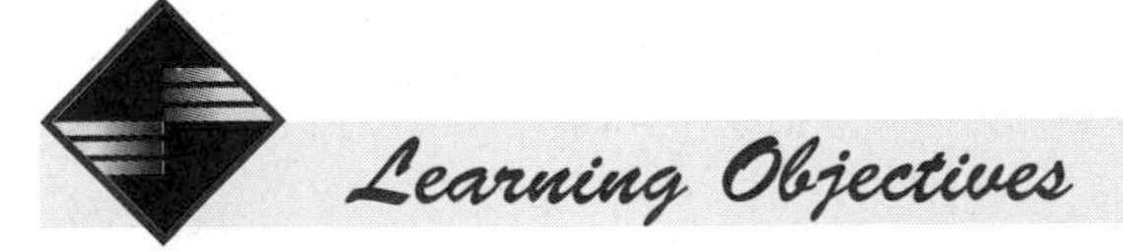

Learning Objectives

After you have read this chapter, you should be able to:

1. Explain the concept of species.
2. Describe the derivation of genus and species names.
3. List the major criteria used in classifying bacteria and archaea.
4. Explain the significance of chemotaxonomy, nucleic acid relatedness, and genetic recombination in phylogeny of the procaryotes.
5. Name the four divisions to which bacteria and archaea belong.
6. Explain why no classification scheme for procaryotes can be considered complete.

All one-celled microorganisms lacking nuclear membranes are procaryotes despite differences in structure, chemistry, and habitat. The procaryotes are divided into two groups: *bacteria* and *archaea.* For reasons not understood, the procaryotes never evolved beyond the microbial stage, whereas the microscopic eucaryotes evolved into more complex organisms.

There is an abundance of information about bacteria. Less is known about the archaea for understandable reasons. The archaea tend to live in less accessible habitats and therefore are less involved in our everyday lives. By comparison, the bacteria, particularly the bacterial pathogens, have received more attention over to the years. It is beyond the scope of this chapter to make the reader familiar with all groups of bacteria and archaea that have been described. Only the most prominent members of certain groups will be examined.

THE CONCEPT OF SPECIES

We shall be referring to particular "species" of bacteria throughout this text; therefore, it is essential to understand how bacteria are assigned to a species. The assignment of a bacterium to a species cannot be based on the same principles that govern such placements in the plant and animal kingdoms. A bacterial species is not the result of an interbreeding population. Bacteria reproduce by binary or multiple fission and, therefore, cannot be classified by means of breeding groups. Each of the offspring may evolve in a different direction by mutation or the mechanisms of gene transfer coupled with selective environmental pressures.

It is difficult to assess the contribution of gene movement from one organism to another because the frequencies with which they occur in nature are unknown. Mutations are rare, but their sudden and random nature makes it impossible to define a species in terms of a limited number of characteristics. There is not a battery of stable characteristics upon which we can depend with certainty. Instead, a bacterial species is defined as a group of bacteria that share a large number of similar characteristics. A bacterium, as originally described, is known as the **prototype.** It is deposited in one of several hundred culture collections in the world for safekeeping. The American Type Culture Collection (ATCC) is located in Rockville, MD. If a subsequently isolated bacterium is found to differ only slightly from the prototype, it is called a **strain** of that species.

HOW GENUS AND SPECIES ARE NAMED

Bacteria are named by using the **binomial system of nomenclature** first proposed by the Swedish botanist, Carolus Linnaeus. The first name, which is always capitalized, indicates the genus of the organism. *Staphylococcus, Escherichia,* and *Bacillus* are examples of genus names. The second name, which is not capitalized, refers to a specific member of a genus—hence the name species. Although genus names, or genera, are often used without a species name, a species name is never used without the accompanying genus name or its initial. Thus, *Escherichia coli* may be referred to as *E. coli* and *Staphylococcus aureus* may be written simply *S. aureus* if the genus name has already appeared so that no confusion exists as to the meaning of the abbreviation. Both genus and species names are italicized or underlined in print and writing.

The endings of genus names are "latinized" and may be feminine, masculine, or neuter in gender. *Salmonella, Shigella,* and *Legionella* end in "a," which is a feminine singular ending. Occasionally, the plural ending "ae" is assigned to an uncapitalized genus name when less formality is required. An English plural form may be used as an alternative. Therefore, both the terms salmonellae and salmonellas constitute acceptable usage. *Proteus, Haemophilus,* and *Bacillus* take a masculine singular ending (us). The letter "i" replaces "us" if individual names are used collectively and are not capitalized. The uncapitalized plural forms of *Proteus* and *Haemophilus* are seldom used, but a plural form is used for members of the genus *Bacillus* if it is established that members of that genus are being discussed. However, the term bacilli (uncapitalized) more commonly refers to shape of bacteria. *Clostridium, Corynebacterium,* and *Propionibacterium* end in "ium," which is a singular neuter ending. The ending "ia" is used in the plural uncapitalized names. For example, it is acceptable to refer to members of the genus *Clostridium* as clostridia. It is usually considered appropriate to use the casual, plural, uncapitalized forms in publications of general interest or in lengthy discussions of a genus.

Sometimes a genus name indicates a shape or even a shape and grouping of an organism. For example, all members of the genus *Bacillus* are bacilli. Likewise, members of the genus *Streptococcus* are cocci in chains. The name *Streptococcus* is derived from the Greek words "streptos," meaning twisted, and "kokkos," meaning berry. Other times, a genus is named for its discoverer. The genus name *Neisseria* was named for Albert Neisser, who discovered the bacterium that causes gonorrhea in 1879. Part of a genus name may be derived from a habitat of the organism. Archaea belonging to the genus *Thermoplasma* can tolerate temperatures up to 65°C.

Species names are often more descriptive than genus names, but may also be derived from the names of their discoverer. The names are either adjectives or nouns. The endings may agree with the gender of the genus name, or if adjectives are used as a past participle of verbs, the species names have a common ending for all genders.

When nouns in the genitive (possessive) are used, the species names do not necessarily agree in gender or number. Examples are *Salmonella pullorum* (*Salmonella* of chicks), *Mycoplasma hominis* (*Mycoplasma* of man), and *Streptococcus lactis* (*Streptococcus* of milk). A less common method of naming species is the use of explanatory nouns. They also do not necessarily agree with the gender of the genus name. Examples are *Salmonella dublin* (*Salmonella* of Dublin), *Enterobacter aerogenes* (*Enterobacter* of air), and *Yersinia pestis* (*Yersinia* of plague).

Genus and species names often change when new information becomes available. All changes must be approved by the International Committee on Systematic Bacteriology. Because new information accumulates more rapidly than ever before with today's array of laboratory methods, one of the challenges that microbiologists face is keeping up with name changes. The names contained in the four volumes of *Bergey's Manual of Systematic Bacteriology* are accepted internationally. This manual classifies procaryotes according to genetic relatedness as revealed by the techniques of molecular biology. The goal of the manual is to indicate relatedness only; it is not meant to aid in identification of bacteria. Practical aids for identifying bacteria are contained in *Bergey's Manual of Determinative Bacteriology*. The bacteria are divided into 35 groups.

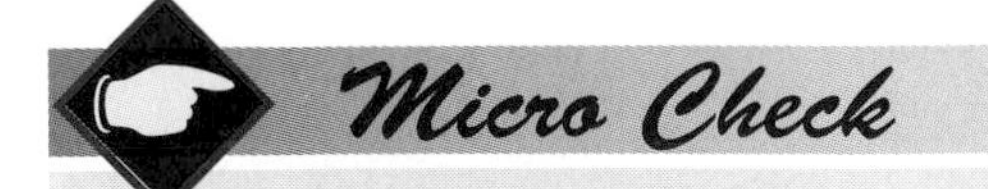

- Why is it not possible to define a species of bacteria by only a few characteristics?
- How do strains of species originate?

RANKING THE BACTERIA

Bacteria may be placed in particular ranks, or **taxons,** based on similarities of observed characteristics or evolutionary relatedness. Those taxons include domains or kingdoms, divisions, classes, orders, families, and genera. Early attempts at assigning bacteria to taxons relied primarily on morphological and physiological characteristics. Classification schemes based solely on phenotype are really artificial, but are quite practical (Table 8–1).

Classification systems for plants and animals are based on evolutionary data obtained from fossil records or dating procedures using radioactive carbon. Until rather recently, no fossil records of microorganisms in sedimentary rock had been uncovered. Evidence reveals that bacteria existed at least 3.5 billion years ago on Earth, but fossil records tell us almost nothing about the phylogeny or evolution of procaryotes.

Advances in biotechnology in the last decade have increased our knowledge of phylogenetic relationships of bacteria, but the information is far from complete. Because of incomplete information, the placement of organisms, in particular taxons, is still based on some phenotypic characteristics.

Criteria used to divide bacteria into four divisions described in *Bergey's Manual of Systematic Bacteriology* are (1) the presence or absence of cell walls and (2) the chemical composition of the cell walls. Bacteria have been assigned to the following four divisions:

1. *Gracilicutes.* The bacteria are gram-negative and have thin cell walls containing peptidoglycan. They include the photosynthetic bacteria and cyanobacteria.
2. *Firmicutes.* The bacteria are usually gram-positive and have thick, rigid cell walls containing peptidoglycan. Members of the division include the filamentous bacteria.
3. *Tenericutes.* The bacteria are gram-negative and have no cell walls.

Table 8–1
THE FORMAL RANKS OF A REPRESENTATIVE BACTERIUM

RANK	EXAMPLE	TAXON ENDING
Kingdom or domain	Procaryotae or Bacteria	-a, -ae
Division	Gracilicutes	-utes
Class	Scotobacteria	-ia
Order	Pseudomonadales	-ales
Family	Pseudomonadaceae	-aceae
Genus	*Ralstonia*	*Variable*
Species	*pickettii*	Variable

4. *Mendosicutes.* The bacteria may be gram-positive or gram-negative and have nonpeptidoglycan-containing cell walls. The archaea are the only members of the division.

Additional characteristics of the first three divisions appear in Table 8–2.

The contributors to *Bergey's Manual of Systematic Bacteriology* are quick to point out that the classification system presented in the four volumes of that book is not the "official classification" for bacteria. No official classification for bacteria exists. The listings merely represent an attempt to find order in an ever-accumulating body of information.

Taxonomists can be divided into "lumpers" and "splitters." Lumpers tend to ignore small differences and place emphasis on a limited number of characteristics. Splitters divide organisms into larger numbers of groups and attach more importance to minor differences. Just as there is no official classification for bacteria, there are no correct or incorrect taxons if the system is based on scientific evidence. Lumpers and splitters have contributed equally to classification schemes. It is well to remember that classification schemes are valid only if they serve a purpose for microbiologists.

CRITERIA FOR CLASSIFYING BACTERIA

Whereas morphologic features of plants and animals are reliable characteristics for classifying those organisms, the large number of "look-alikes" among microorganisms presents different

Table 8–2
CHARACTERISTICS OF GRACILICUTES, FIRMICUTES, AND TENERICUTES

PROPERTY	GRACILICUTES	FIRMICUTES	TENERICUTES
Appendages	Can produce several types of appendages—pili and fimbriae, prosthecae, and stalks	Usually lack appendages (may have spores on hyphae)	Lack appendages
Cell shape	Spheres, ovals, straight or curved rods, helices or filaments; some have sheaths or capsules	Spheres, rods, or filaments; may show true branching	Pleomorphic in shape; may be filamentous and branching
Cell wall	Gram-negative type wall with inner 2–10 nm peptidoglycan layer and outer membrane (8–10 nm thick) of lipid, protein, and lipopolysaccharide	Gram-positive type wall with a thick cell wall (20–80 nm) composed mainly of peptidoglycan; other polysaccharides and teichoic acids may be present	Lack a cell wall; enclosed by a plasma membrane
Endospores	No endospores	Some groups have endospores	No endospores
Metabolism	Phototrophic, chemoautotrophic, or chemoheterotrophic	Usually chemoheterotrophic	Chemoheterotrophic; most require cholesterol and long-chain fatty acids for growth
Motility	Motile or nonmotile; flagellation—polar, amphitrichous, lophotrichous, or peritrichous; motility may also result from the use of axial filaments (spirochetes) or gliding motility	Most often nonmotile; have peritrichous flagellation when motile	Usually nonmotile
Reproduction	Binary fission, sometimes budding	Binary fission	Budding, fragmentation, and/or binary fission

problems. Differential staining techniques are quite valuable in separating bacteria of medical importance. A Gram stain, for example, often provides the first clue to the cause of an infection. Growth characteristics provide additional information, but chemical profiles based on enzymatic activities most often permit the identification of genus and species. Serological techniques are dependable for demonstrating antigens specific for a particular species or strain, but closely related organisms may contain some of the same antigens.

Analyses, such as chemotaxonomy, nucleic acid relatedness, genetic recombination, and numerical taxonomy, have made it possible to deduce some of the most probable phylogenetic relationships. The technology is rapidly being improved, but the following methods were used as a basis for grouping bacteria and archaea in *Bergey's Manual of Systematic Bacteriology*.

Chemotaxonomy

Chemotaxonomy classifies bacteria on the basis of chemical composition of whole cells or parts of cells. Cell wall composition, plasma membrane components, **cytochrome** variables, amino acid sequencing, and protein profiles are among the criteria that can be used to divide bacteria into groups.

Cell Wall Composition. Peptidoglycan was described in Chapter 4 as the major chemical of procaryotic cell walls of bacteria. The amino acid composition of peptidoglycan is nearly the same as in gram-negative bacteria, but the amino acid and carbohydrate contents differ substantially among the gram-positive bacteria. The amino acids of cell walls are now included in generic descriptions of bacteria in *Bergey's Manual of Systematic Bacteriology*. The archaea contain walls, plasma membranes, ribosomes, and RNA sequences that set them apart from bacteria; some archaea have no cell walls.

Plasma Membrane Components. Lipids are present in the plasma membranes of bacteria and as storage depots in some cells. The fatty acid content is influenced by environmental factors, including the chemical composition of the medium. Mycolic acids are exceptions; their presence is environmentally independent. Mycolic acids are found in the cell walls of only a limited number of genera, such as *Mycobacterium* and *Nocardia*. Other lipids of chemotaxonomic significance are phospholipids, glycolipids, and carotenoids.

Cytochrome Variables. Cytochromes were described in Chapter 5 as special proteins that could be alternately reduced and oxidized in electron transport. Cytochromes such as a, a_1, b, c, c_1, and d may be found in bacteria. The distribution of cytochromes differs more in procaryotes than in eucaryotes. Some lactic acid bacteria contain only cytochrome b. Species of *Clostridium* lack all cytochromes. Cytochrome d is found in many gram-negative bacteria. If cytochrome variables are to be used for taxonomic purposes, growth conditions must be standardized.

Amino Acid Sequences. Closely related bacteria share many amino acid sequences in common. Proteins that have been analyzed for amino acid content are ferredoxins, flavodoxins, azurins, and cytochrome c. Sometimes some startling results are obtained by amino acid sequencing. The amino acid content of a limited sequence of cytochrome c of two organisms is seen in Table 8–3. The constancy of residues of cytochrome c in both procaryotes and eucaryotes is attributed to the three-dimensional structure of the molecule.

Protein Profiles. Protein profiles of bacteria can be obtained by polyacrylamide gel electrophoresis (PAGE). The bands of migrated proteins when stained are often called "fingerprints." Molecular weights can be assigned to bands by comparing them with molecular weight standards

Table 8–3
AMINO ACID SEQUENCES FOR A SEGMENT OF CYTOCHROME C FROM TWO BACTERIA

POSITION	*Pseudomonas aeruginosa*	*Azotobacter vinelandii*
15	Cysteine	Cysteine
16	Valine	Threonine*
17	Alanine	Valine*
18	Cysteine	Cysteine
19	Histidine	Histidine
20	Alanine	Alanine
21	Isoleucine	Isoleucine
22	Asparagine	Asparagine
23	Threonine	Serine*

*Differences are seen in the 16, 17, and 23 positions.

Source: Dickerson RE: Cytochrome c and the evolution of energy metabolism. Sci Am *242*(3):137, 1980.

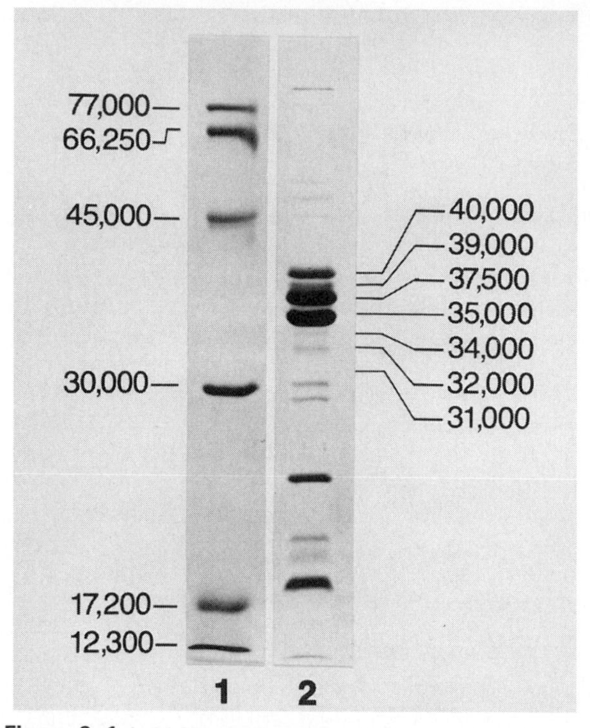

Figure 8–1 ◆ PAGE profiles. Lane 2 shows stains of outer layer membrane proteins of *Citrobacter diversus.* Protein standards are shown in lane 1. Determination of PAGE profiles is useful in epidemiological studies.

of known proteins (Fig. 8–1). Protein profiles are often of value in epidemiological investigations of particular diseases. Fingerprints of outer membrane proteins have been useful in studying some outbreaks of meningitis.

Nucleic Acid Relatedness

Methods for determining nucleic acid content are very reliable for determining relatedness of bacteria. The nitrogen bases of DNA and RNA are less subject to frequent changes. Nucleic acid studies have become increasingly important over the past three decades. Nucleic acid techniques can be expected to replace long-standing tests based on phenotypic characteristics.

DNA Base Composition. Early studies on the DNA base composition revealed that percent guanine (G) + cytosine (C) values for bacteria range from about 25 to 75. The percent of the bases varies little for a particular species. The ranges for some common species are found in Table 8–

Table 8–4
DNA BASE COMPOSITION OF SELECTED BACTERIA

PERCENT GUANINE + CYTOSINE	ORGANISM
30–32	*Clostridium perfringens*
38–40	*Haemophilus influenzae*
42–44	*Bacillus subtilis*
46–48	*Vibrio cholerae*
50–52	*Escherichia coli*
52–54	*Corynebacterium diphtheriae*
60–62	*Pseudomonas fluorescens*
66–68	*Mycobacterium tuberculosis*
70–80	*Sarcina lutea*

Source: Modified from Marmur RJ, Falkow S, Mandel M: New approaches to bacterial taxonomy. Ann Rev Microbiol *17*:329, 1963.

4. However, organisms with similar ranges of percent G + C are not necessarily related. Bacteria presumed at one time to be closely related on the basis of their phenotypic characteristics have been found to be merely distant cousins.

One method for determining percent G + C is called **thermal denaturation.** Heating causes disruption of hydrogen bonds between base pairs of double-stranded DNA and an increase in absorbance. The temperature at the midpoint of a curve obtained by plotting temperature against absorbance is the melting temperature, or T_m (Fig. 8–2). DNA molecules with greater numbers of G-C base pairs have higher T_m values than those with more A-T (adenosine-thymine) base

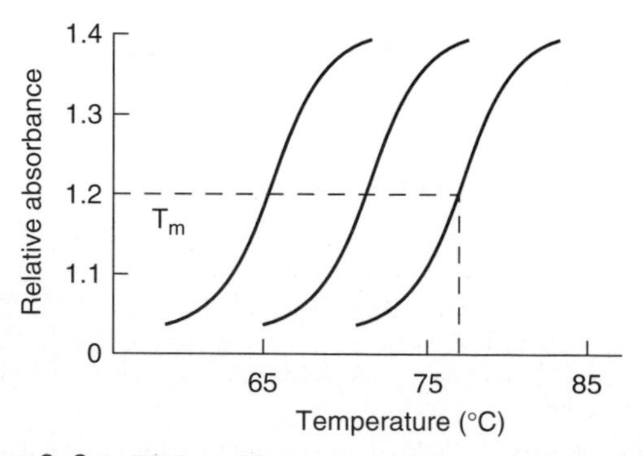

Figure 8–2 ◆ DNA melting curves of three organisms. Heat separates double-stranded DNA by disrupting hydrogen bonds. The melting point (T_m) is the temperature at midpoint determined by plotting temperature against absorbance.

pairs. G-C base pairs are more stable because they are linked by three hydrogen bonds. A-T base pairs are held in place by two hydrogen bonds.

A limitation of determining base composition by thermal denaturation is that the order of the nucleotides is not revealed. Percent G + C values have not been determined for all species described in *Bergey's Manual of Systematic Bacteriology*, so other surprises may be in store for taxonomists.

Nucleic Acid Hybridization. The degree of genetic relatedness between organisms can be determined also by hybridization between common sequences of their DNAs. Double strands of DNA from two organisms can be separated by treatment with heat. If the single strands of DNA from the organisms are mixed, double-stranded sequences or *duplexes* will form between complementary single-stranded sequences by a process called **annealing.** Hydrogen bonding occurs between adenine (A) and thymine (T) and guanine (G) and cytosine (C). The duplexes of double-stranded DNA are called **hybrids.** The degree of hybridization is proportional to the degree of relatedness (Fig. 8–3).

Nucleic Acid Sequences. DNA and RNA sequencing is a valuable determinant of bacterial relatedness. The 16S component of the 30S subunit and the 5S component of the 50S subunit of ribosomal RNA (rRNA) are universally present in procaryotes. The sequences of the bases can be studied in these components after treatment with ribonuclease. Some sequences are constant; others demonstrate a degree of variability. The sequences of ribosomal RNA of bacteria indicate relatedness with each other, but are substantially different from the 5S and 16S components isolated from archaea. Those differences constitute one of the major forms of evidence for separate lineages for bacteria and archaea.

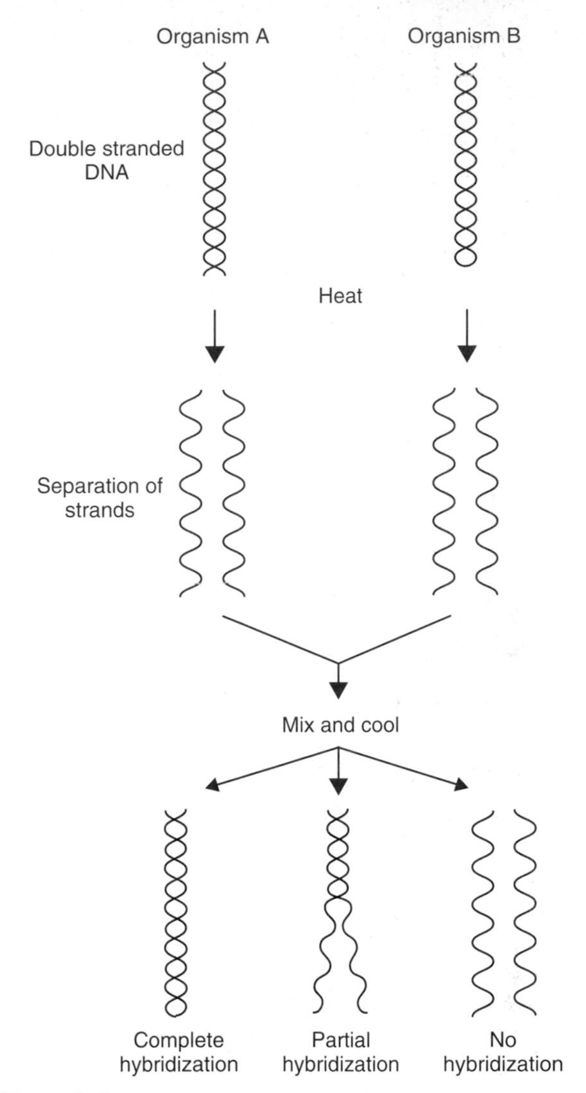

Figure 8–3 ◆ Genetic relatedness by DNA hybridization studies. Double-stranded DNA from two organisms is heated to separate DNA into single strands. After mixing and cooling, the amount of hybridization is proportional to the genetic relatedness.

Genetic Recombination

The availability of laboratory-induced techniques for genetic transfer has provided important information on bacterial relatedness. The three processes of gene transfer are described in Chapter 7. Such studies have proved to be valuable in establishing evolutionary relationships.

Some kinds of gene transfer occur between different species of the same genus and less often between two genera of bacteria. Chromosomal or extrachromosomal DNA may be transferred. It is well established that transferred genes contribute to bacterial phenotypic diversity. Antibiotic resistance is conferred by newly acquired genetic material in certain enteric pathogens; toxin production is dependent on integration of genes from bacterial viruses in *Corynebacterium diphtheriae*, *Streptococcus pyogenes*, and *Clostridium botulinum*. Lysogeny refers to a relationship between a bacterial host and the viral DNA. The process is described in detail in Chapter 10.

Numerical Taxonomy

Numerical taxonomy is a computer-based method for classifying bacteria for which a large number of characteristics are known. The technique is especially applicable for assessing similarities or differences in phenotype or genotype. It is used less frequently for analyzing ancestral origin.

The groups of interest to numerical taxonomists are usually strains, but can be species or genera. The taxons are called **operational taxonomic units** (OTUs). The number of strains analyzed must be substantive and should include both recently isolated and worldwide strains. It is generally agreed that the number of characteristics studied must be a minimum of 50. It is not practical or possible to assess all characteristics of strains. Most numerical taxonomy methods divulge only 10 to 20 percent of the total genetic potential of a strain. Each characteristic is given equal weight.

Percentage of similarity (%S) for any two strains can be expressed as follows:

$$\%S = \frac{NS}{NS + ND}$$

where NS is the number of similar characteristics and ND is the number of different characteristics.

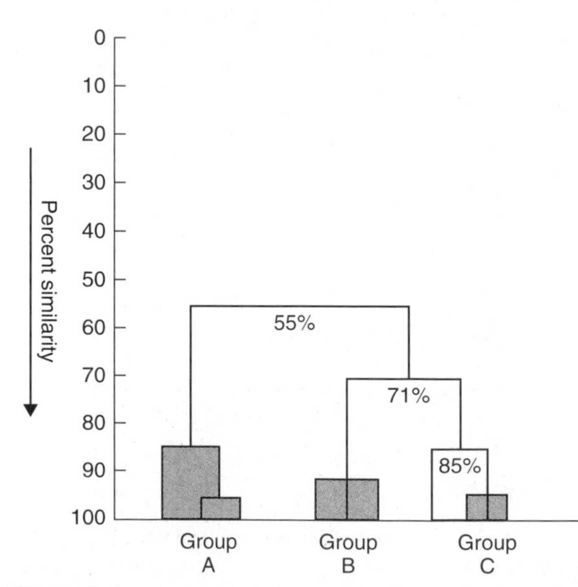

Figure 8–4 ◆ A hypothetical example of a dendrogram showing similarities of three groups of bacteria.

Percentage of similarity can be determined by assigning a value of 1 to a positive test and a zero to a negative test. A computer is used to compare characteristics of each organism with other organisms. A **dendrogram** can be made to express relatedness by placing bacteria with similar characteristics into groups (Fig. 8–4). At least a 90 percent similarity is obtained with organisms of the same OTU. In rapid identification schemes, varying weights are assigned to particular characteristics, depending on the demonstrated stability of each characteristic. Patient care demands quick answers to select appropriate antibiotic therapy. Computer-based analyses of large numbers of strains of species provide clinical laboratories with invaluable tools.

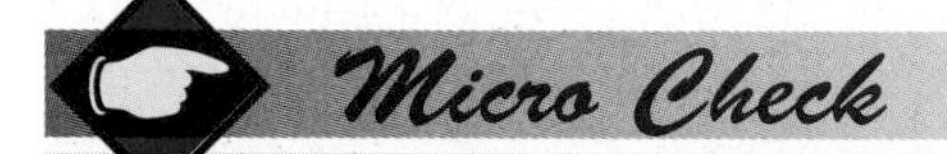

- ◆ What is meant by a phylogenetic classification scheme?
- ◆ How can chemical analyses be used to determine relatedness of bacteria?
- ◆ What is the role of computers in numerical taxonomy?

THE BACTERIA

The presence or absence of a cell wall and the nature of that wall, if present, are of primary importance in classifying bacteria. All bacteria with walls containing peptidoglycan belong to the divisions Gracilicutes or Firmicutes. Those lacking rigid cell walls are members of the division Tenericutes.

Procaryotes are described in 33 sections of the four volumes of *Bergey's Manual of Systematic Bacteriology*. All groups are not of medical significance, but all contribute to the diverse activities of the microbial world. Only brief descriptions of major groups of bacteria can be included in this chapter, but even a brief encounter with certain bacteria can be memorable. Each group exemplifies the diversity of morphology, chemical activities, and habitats.

The Spirochetes

The spirochetes are helical, motile bacteria that sometimes attain lengths up to 250 μm. They demonstrate a unique flexibility due to the

FOCAL POINT

Metabolic "Breathprints" of Microorganisms

A novel approach to bacterial identification has been proposed by a biologist in Hayward, California. The new approach employs the redox dye, tetrazolium violet, to detect oxidation of 95 carbon sources. Cell suspensions are added to wells containing the dye, appropriate nutrients, and the test carbon source. After incubation for four to 24 hours, the reduced product, a purple formazan, occurs in wells if the test organism can oxidize the carbon source.

For identification, the metabolic "breathprint" is analyzed on a computer against a database of at least several thousand strains. The gram-negative test battery has been extensively developed. One advantage of this technology is that it detects oxidation of carbon substrates that do not produce enough acid to produce a change in pH sufficient to alter a typical pH indicator dye. The breathprint method is also more rapid than the much used pH indicator tests. The final step of dye reduction is irreversible. In methods based on pH, products formed from metabolic activity are often unstable and reversions can occur.

Strains of particular gram-negative bacteria rarely differ by more than five of the 95 tests. Although initial testing was on pathogens, information using metabolic "breathprints" of environmental nonpathogens is rapidly increasing. The technique is applicable to demonstrating microbial ecology in bodies of water where mixed microbial populations degrade organic wastes. The redox method can likewise be used to study catalytic capabilities of bioremedial microorganisms. The time required to set up a battery of 95 tests is no longer than that required to streak onc Petri plate.

ASM News 55(10), 1989.

twisting motions of their axial fibrils. The axial fibrils, a type of endocellular flagella, are wound around their cell bodies. Free-living spirochetes are found in a variety of aqueous environments or in association with human or animal hosts (Fig. 8–5). Three notorious pathogens, which are spirochetes, are (1) *Treponema pallidum,* the cause of syphilis, (2) *Borrelia burgdorferi,* which is responsible for Lyme disease, and (3) *Leptospira interrogans,* a pathogen of both animals and humans. Some spirochetes only grow with difficulty in the laboratory, and the pathogenic treponemes do not grow on artificial culture media or in tissue cultures.

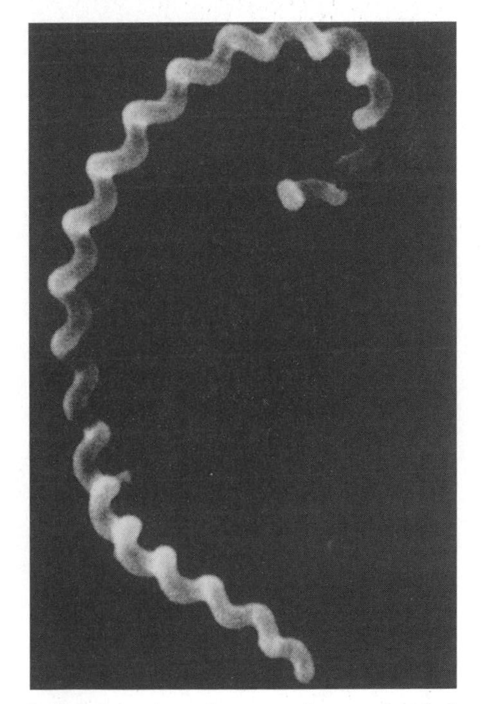

Figure 8–5 ◆ Scanning electron micrograph of the spirochete *Leptospira interrogans,* which causes disease in animals and humans.

Aerobic/Microaerophilic Helical Vibrioid Gram-Negative Bacteria

The helical/vibrioid (comma-shaped) gram-negative bacteria may be slightly curved or possess multiple helical turns. All are motile by flagella. Many live in fresh or coastal water, and a few are capable of producing animal or human diseases. Various species of microaerophilic *Campylobacter* cause infections of the gastrointestinal tract or blood in humans. *Helicobacter pylori* has been associated with peptic and duodenal ulcers. Other vibrios, such as members of the genera

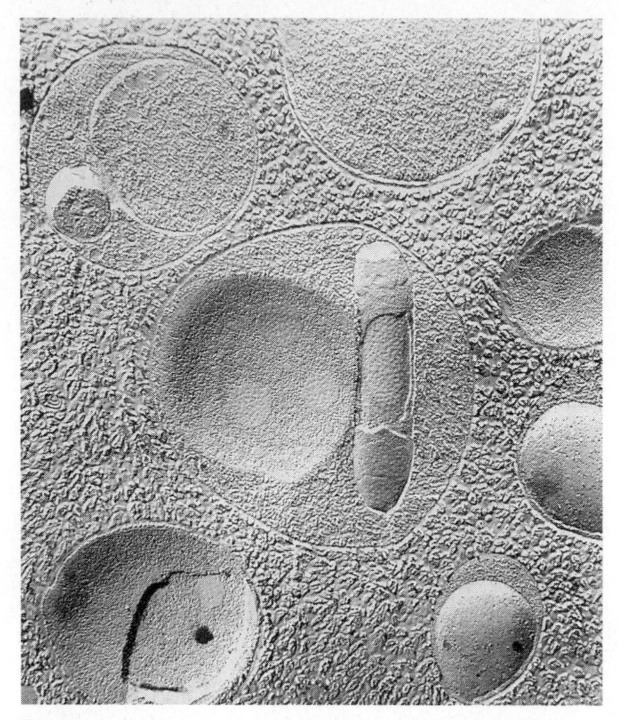

Figure 8–6 ◆ Electron micrograph of a *Bdellovibrio* cell in the periplasmic space of host *Escherichia coli.* The vibrio loses its flagellum during the penetration process.

Bdellovibrio and *Vampirovibrio,* are bacterial or algal predators (Fig. 8–6). Isolation of some vibrios in the laboratory requires an atmosphere containing 5 percent O_2, 10 percent CO_2, and 85 percent N_2.

Gram-Negative Aerobic Rods and Cocci

The gram-negative aerobic rods and cocci include a diverse group of bacteria that have been studied extensively. Their metabolism is respiratory—never fermentative. Both the rods and cocci are widely distributed in nature, and many are human and animal pathogens. *Rhizobium* species are of particular interest because they are able to fix atmospheric nitrogen (convert it to a nongaseous form) when growing in nodules on roots of certain leguminous plants (Fig. 8–7). All plants require fixed nitrogen. **Legumes** include such plants as sweet peas, clover, beans, peanuts, and alfalfa. Another large group, the pseudomonads, are important as decomposers of organic debris in the soil. The bacterium *Legionella pneumophila,* which caused the mysterious legionnaires' disease (legionellosis) in 1976 in Philadelphia, is a member of this group. Other human pathogens in this group include *Neisseria gonorrhoeae,* the cause of gonorrhea, *Bordetella pertussis,* the cause of whooping cough, and *Franciscella tularensis,* the cause of a febrile disease called tularemia.

Facultatively Anaerobic Gram-Negative Rods

The facultatively anaerobic gram-negative rods constitute a very large group of bacteria with rel-

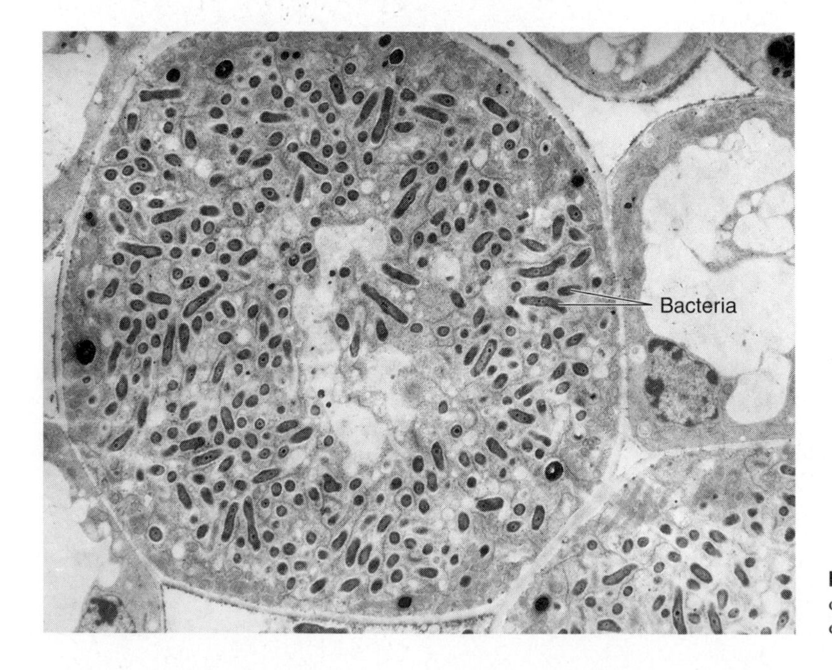

Figure 8–7 ◆ Appearance of a nodule cell containing nitrogen-fixing bacteria under the electron microscope.

atively simple nutritional requirements. If motile, all have peritrichous flagella except for members of the genus *Tatumella* (Fig. 8–8). The bacilli are widely distributed in nature and are found in soil, water, and intestinal tracts of animals and humans. Those found in the intestinal tract of animals and humans are known as the *enteric* bacteria. Members of the genera *Escherichia, Salmonella, Shigella, Enterobacter, Proteus,* and *Providencia* are among the enteric bacteria. *Escherichia coli* is by far the best-known enteric bacterium. It has been invaluable in recombinant DNA technology. *E. coli* and other inhabitants of the intestinal tracts of humans and warm-blooded animals are called **coliforms.** The presence of coliforms in drinking water is indicative of fecal pollution by public health standards in the United States and many other countries.

Anaerobic Gram-Negative Rods

The anaerobic gram-negative rods may be straight, curved, or helical and are motile or nonmotile. They are found in the intestinal tracts of animals and humans. Most can be isolated from sewage if appropriate growth conditions are supplied. *Leptospira buccalis* can be isolated from plaque near the gum line on most tooth surfaces. The spindle-shaped *Fusobacterium* species also frequently live along the gingival margin. The best known pathogens of the group belong to the genus *Bacteroides.* They are common causes of anaerobic bacteremia, rectal abscesses, and postsurgical wounds.

Anaerobic Gram-Negative Cocci

The anaerobic gram-negative cocci frequently occur in pairs. The most important of the strict anaerobes belong to the genus *Veillonella.* The organisms are found in the mouth, the intestines, and the vagina. Their role in disease is uncertain.

Micro Check

- Why are classification schemes subject to change?
- What distinguishes *Bdellovibrio* and *Vampirovibrio* from other vibrios?
- What is the significance of coliforms in water?

The Rickettsias and Chlamydias

The rickettsias and chlamydias are very small, gram-negative bacteria, most of which require host cells for replication. They are usually rod-shaped, but may also appear coccoidal (Fig. 8–9). Many of the host-dependent organisms cause diseases of humans and animals. Rickettsias require both a vertebrate and an arthropod host. The best studied rickettsia is *Rickettsia prowazekii,* the cause of epidemic typhus.

The chlamydias have a complex developmental cycle but do not infect invertebrates. They do cause disease in some birds and mammals. Chlamydias are responsible for the human disease

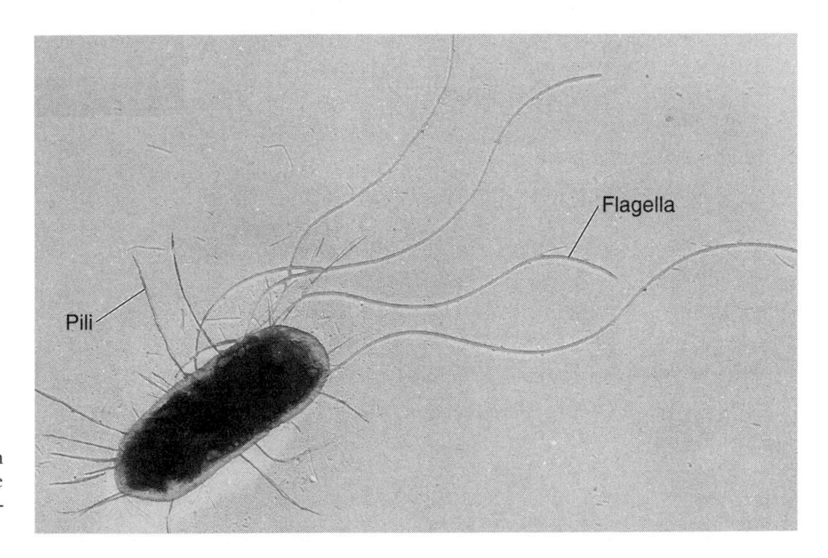

Figure 8–8 ◆ Appendages of the bacterium *Escherichia coli.* The longer appendages are flagella, which may be longer than the organism.

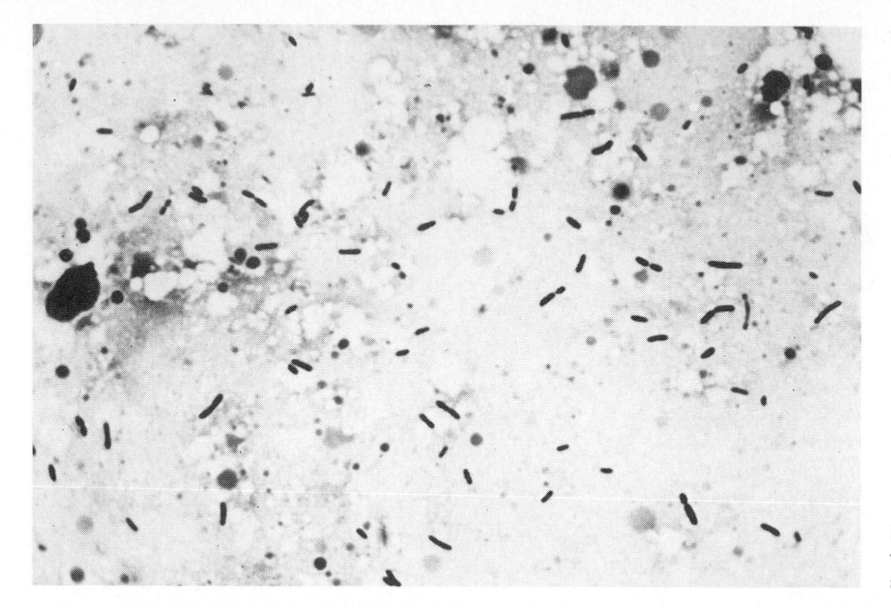

Figure 8–9 ◆ *Rickettsia rickettsii* as viewed under the bright-field microscope in an egg yolk sac.

known as trachoma, a leading cause of blindness in the world, and for at least two sexually transmitted diseases (STDs) of humans.

Mycoplasmas

The mycoplasmas are the smallest of the free-living bacteria. These organisms have no cell walls and therefore are highly pleomorphic. They vary from spherical or pear-shaped cells, measuring 0.3 to 0.8 μm in diameter, to branched or helical filaments (Fig. 8–10).

The mycoplasmas have special growth requirements that can be supplied by incorporating yeast and beef extracts into media. The wall-less bacteria should not be confused with L-phase variants of other bacteria. The wall-defective L-forms are induced by some types of antibiotic therapy. Unlike mycoplasmas, L-phase variants can revert to the parent wall–containing bacteria by serially subculturing in the absence of antibiotics.

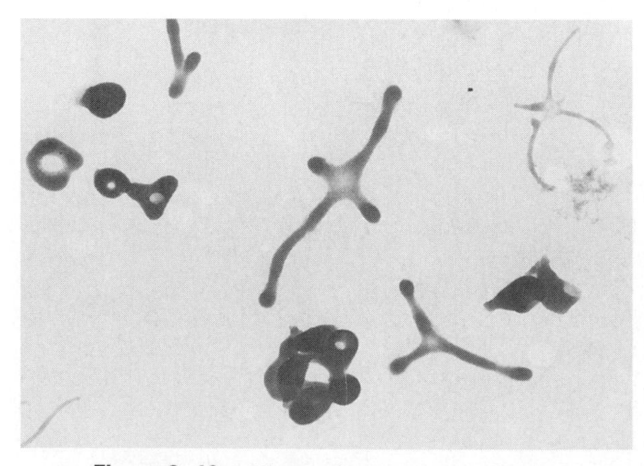

Figure 8–10 ◆ Bizarre shapes of mycoplasmas.

Most pathogenic mycoplasmas are host-specific, causing disease in animals, plants, and humans. The best-known pathogen, *Mycoplasma pneumoniae,* causes primary atypical pneumonia in humans. Another mycoplasma, *Spiroplasma citri,* is pathogenic for citrus plants and certain insects.

Gram-Positive Cocci

The gram-positive cocci consist of both aerobic and anaerobic spherical cells that range from free-living, harmless organisms to some highly virulent forms. They are differentiated by their atmospheric requirements, by their tendency to show particular groupings, and by the presence or absence of catalase.

The micrococci include aerobic members of the genus *Micrococcus* and facultative anaerobes belonging to the genus *Staphylococcus. Micrococcus* species are not associated with disease, but *Staphylococcus aureus* and *Staphylococcus epidermidis* continue to cause new and serious diseases. Some pathogenic strains of *S. aureus* produce as many as 18 extracellular products with the ability to harm human or animal hosts. *S. epidermidis* is a skin resident that is isolated with increasing frequency from postsurgical wounds, urinary tract infections, and cases of subacute bacterial endocarditis.

The streptococci are a diverse group of microaerophilic or facultatively anaerobic organisms that produce lactic acid. They are classified by the ability of their colonies to demonstrate hemolysis (dissolution of red blood cells) on blood agar and by the presence of certain antigens on their cell surfaces. Alpha streptococci produce a green area surrounding colonies, and beta streptococci cause complete lysis of red blood cells around colonies resulting in clear areas. A third group of streptococci produce no hemolysis on blood agar. Among the important human pathogens are *Streptococcus pneumoniae,* a cause of lobar pneumonia, and *Streptococcus pyogenes,* the primary isolate in bacterial pharyngitis.

The peptococci are obligate anaerobes that frequently colonize the mucous membranes of the respiratory, urogenital, and digestive tracts. The cocci promote serious infections when they gain access to devitalized tissue. Members of the two genera *Peptococcus* and *Peptostreptococcus* are difficult to distinguish from one another without extensive laboratory tests.

Endospore-Forming Gram-Positive Rods and Cocci

The endospore-forming rods and cocci are important because of the resistance of their spores to heat and disinfectants. Members of the genera *Bacillus* and *Clostridium* are important in the food industry and in medicine (Fig. 8–11). *Bacillus* species are obligate aerobes or facultative anaerobes; all *Clostridium* organisms are obligate anaerobes. Members of both genera are widespread in the soil. Thermophilic species of *Bacillus* are common food spoilage organisms in the canning industry. Some species of *Bacillus* are insect pathogens. *B. anthracis* is the cause of anthrax, and *B. cereus* is associated with one type of food poisoning. Clostridia are etiologic agents of botulism, tetanus, gas gangrene, and perfringens food poisoning.

Regular Nonsporing Gram-Positive Rods

The regular nonsporing gram-positive rods are obligate or facultative anaerobes that have complex nutritional requirements. Some lactobacilli are common inhabitants of the mouth, intestinal tract, and vagina. Others are invaluable in the production of fermented food products and beverages. Their role in making yogurt, pickles, and sauerkraut is discussed in Chapter 24.

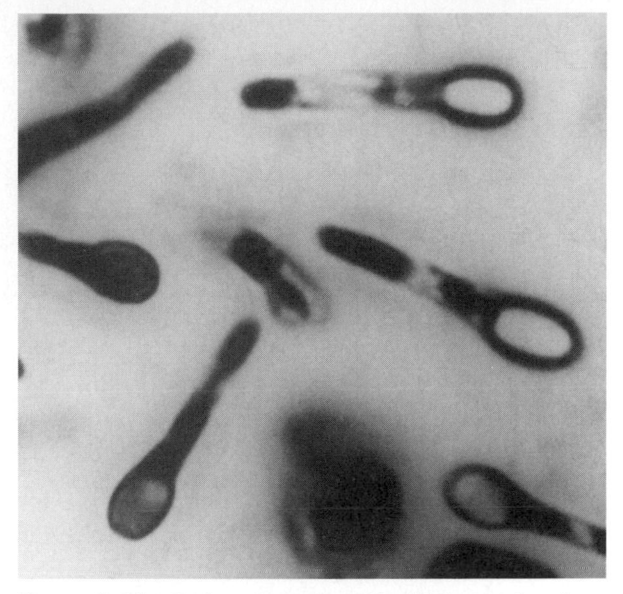

Figure 8–11 ◆ Endospores of a clostridial organism in a stained, wet-mount preparation.

Among the human pathogens in this group is *Listeria monocytogenes,* the cause of an inflammatory disease of the brain and meninges. The organism has the unusual ability to multiply both at high (45°C) and low (4°C) temperatures. Its tolerance for a variable pH and a high salt concentration permits it to grow in soft cheeses, raw meat, seafood, and vegetables. The organism is considered an environmental contaminant that most likely gains entrance to food products during processing.

Irregular Nonsporing Gram-Positive Rods

The irregular nonsporing gram-positive rods have unusual shapes which are often clublike. The pleomorphic bacteria are mostly facultative anaerobes; a few are obligate aerobes. The genus *Corynebacterium* contains organisms called **diphtheroids,** which reside on mucous membranes of the respiratory tract. The bacilli have an interesting type of binary fission known as **snapping division.** After division, bacteria remain partially attached. The attached cells, sometimes described as resembling Chinese characters, are unmistakable. The most important pathogen in this group is *Corynebacterium diphtheriae,* which is the cause of diphtheria and stains irregularly (Fig. 8–12)

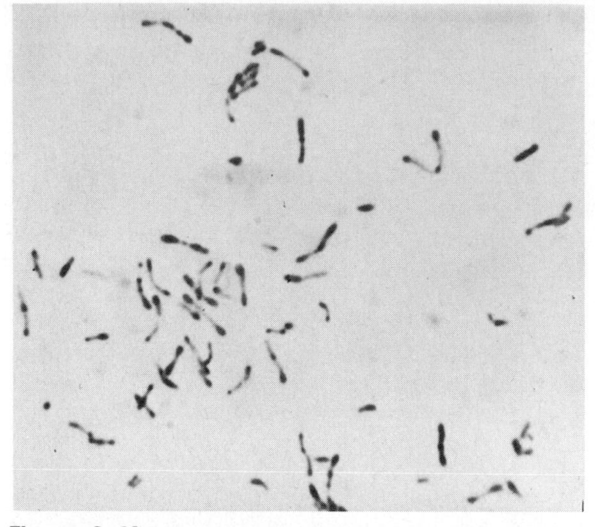

Figure 8–12 ◆ Micrograph of *Corynebacterium diphtheriae* showing irregular staining of some bacteria after division.

The anaerobic propionibacteria are also members of this group. *Propionibacterium acnes* is a common skin resident and is frequently the cause of acne. Another species, *P. shermanii,* is used to make Swiss cheese. The large amount of carbon dioxide produced during fermentation is responsible for the holes in the cheese.

Members of the genus *Actinomyces* consist of bacteria that produce aerial hyphae (Fig. 8–13). They are either obligate or facultative anaerobes and are abundant in the soil. Some are found on the mucous membranes of the respiratory and gastrointestinal tracts of humans and animals. The most important pathogen, *Actinomyces israelii,* is sometimes isolated from periodontal abscesses or infections of the lung.

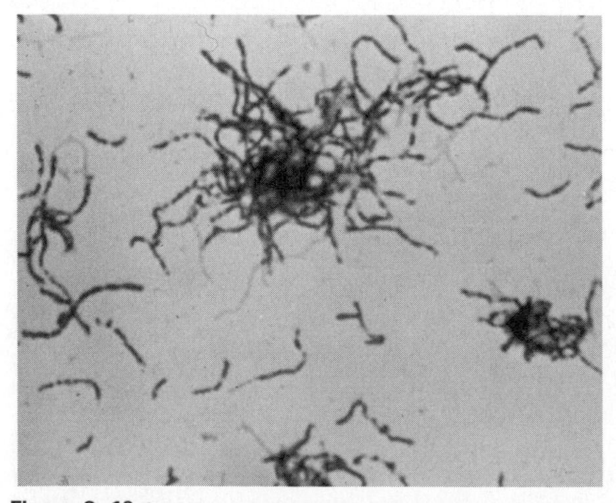

Figure 8–13 ◆ Gram stain from a colony of an *Actinomyces* species showing filamentous, gram-positive bacilli.

Mycobacteria

The mycobacteria are a group of aerobic, acid-fast rods with a tendency to form filaments. The filaments, unlike those of the *Actinomyces,* are unstable and break up easily into rods. Their acid-fast quality (ability to retain the dye, basic carbolfuchsin, despite treatment with acid alcohol) is due to a high lipid content in the cell walls. Many soil mycobacteria are **saprophytes** and grow readily on laboratory media. The causative agents of tuberculosis and leprosy (Hansen's disease) are mycobacteria. *Mycobacterium tuberculosis* is slow-growing and requires complex media. *M. leprae* does not grow on artificial culture media.

Nocardioforms

Species of *Nocardia* are aerobic, gram-positive, hyphae-producing bacteria. They are only partially acid-fast and grow readily in the laboratory. The nocardias are occasionally the cause of lung or skin infections.

Streptomycetes and Their Allies

The streptomycetes are soil inhabitants that resemble the filamentous *Actinomyces* except for being aerobic. The streptomycetes produce aerial hyphae and spores. None are pathogens, but many species of *Streptomyces* are important sources of antibiotics. Among the antimicrobial agents derived from the soil organisms are streptomycin, cycloheximide, and tetracycline.

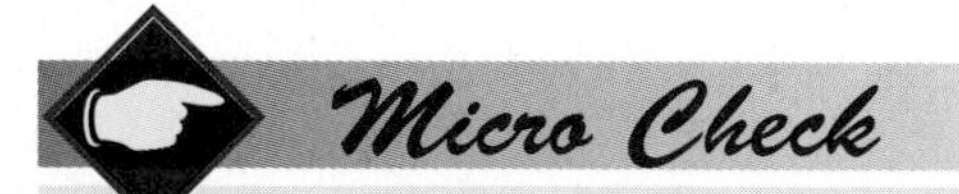

- How do rickettsias and chlamydias differ from other bacteria?
- How do mycoplasmas differ from L-forms?
- Of what significance is the ability of bacteria to form endospores?

THE ARCHAEA

Members of the domain Archaea and the division Mendosicutes represent a group of bacteria that have features uniquely distinct from Eucarya or Bacteria. All have unusual cell walls, with the exception of the **thermoacidophiles,** which are found in hot acid springs. Cell walls of the other archaea do not contain peptidoglycan. Lipids in archaea contain isoprenyl units instead of fatty acids linked to glycerol. Differing sequences of nucleotides on rRNA distinguish archaea from both eucarya and bacteria. The archaea are found often in unusual or extreme habitats.

The organisms are divided into three major groups based on their habitats: (1) **methanogens,** (2) **thermophiles,** and (3) **halophiles.** The environments in which each group is found differ profoundly in chemical and physical characteristics. Their ability to survive in extreme environments has piqued the curiosity of many microbiologists.

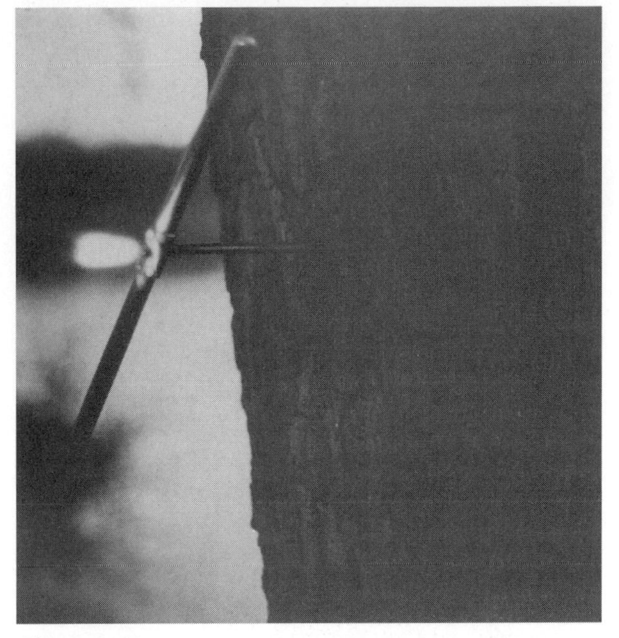

Figure 8–14 ◆ Microbial origin of methane in a living tree.

The Methanogens

The methanogens grow in anaerobic environments, such as swamps, marshes, marine sediments, sludge, and hydrothermal vents. Some are endosymbionts in anaerobic protozoa. **Endosymbiosis** is a unique relationship in which one organism is housed by another organism, with each deriving benefits from the association. There are at least 14 genera differing in morphology, cell wall composition, and substrates utilized. All generate methane as a consequence of their metabolic activities (Fig. 8–14).

The Extreme Thermophiles

The thermophilic archaea differ from the bacterial thermophiles by thriving in extremes of heat (Fig. 8–15). Some can grow at temperatures up to 150°C under enormous hydrostatic pressure in deep ocean springs. Many archaeal thermophiles also grow in highly acid environments

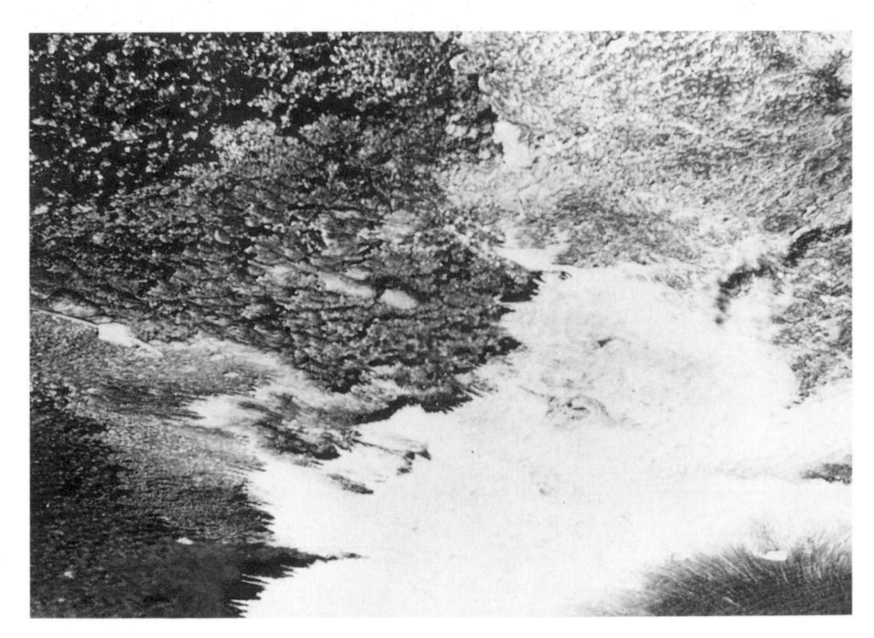

Figure 8–15 ◆ A hot-spring habitat where temperatures may reach 85°C or more, and where the presence of sulfur acts as an energy source for thermophilic archaea.

and require sulfur. Studies suggest that the early ocean environments were oxygen-free and had temperatures as high as 200°C. The microorganisms appearing on Earth during the first 2 billion years must have been thermophiles.

The Extreme Halophiles

The archaeal halophiles are unusual in that they require high concentrations of sodium chloride. These aerobic organisms live in salt lakes, salt-evaporating ponds, and brines used to preserve meat or fish. Extreme halophiles need at least 8.8 percent sodium chloride for growth, but will also grow in an environment with a salinity as high as 32 percent. Despite the frequency of extreme halophiles in brines, used for food preservation in some parts of the world, no foodborne illness due to the salt-tolerant organisms has been described.

Micro Check

- What atmosphere do swamps and marshes supply that is required by methanogens?
- Why is it likely that extreme thermophiles were early inhabitants on Earth?
- Where are the extreme thermophiles found?

Understanding Microbiology

1. Why is it impossible to define species of bacteria with a limited number of characteristics?
2. Why are classification schemes for bacteria phenotypic rather than phylogenetic?
3. Name and briefly describe the four divisions of bacteria.
4. How are streptococci differentiated from one another?
5. What characteristics of archaea make them uniquely different from eucarya and bacteria?

Applying Microbiology

6. If the following results on percent guanine + cytosine were found in three unknown organisms, what conclusion would you reach on relatedness? What other tests on nucleic acids would you recommend for clarification?

ORGANISM	PERCENT GUANINE + CYTOSINE
A	62–65
B	31–36
C	59–64

Chapter 9

Eucaryotes: Algae, Protozoa, and Fungi

Chapter Outline

- **ALGAE**
  - Ranking the Algae
  - Green Algae (Chlorophyta)
  - Euglenoids (Euglenophyta)
  - Diatoms, Yellow-Green, and Golden Brown Algae (Chrysophyta)
  - Brown Algae (Phaeophyta)
  - Dinoflagellates (Pyrrophyta)
  - Red Algae (Rhodophyta)
- **PROTOZOA**
  - Ranking the Protozoa
  - Pseudopods (Sarcodina)
  - Flagellates (Mastigophora)
  - Ciliates (Ciliata)
  - Sporozoans (Sporozoa)
- **FUNGI**
  - Ranking the Fungi
  - Water Molds (Zygomycota)
  - Sac Fungi (Ascomycota)
  - Club Fungi (Basidiomycota)
  - Imperfect Fungi (Deuteromycota)
  - Slime Molds

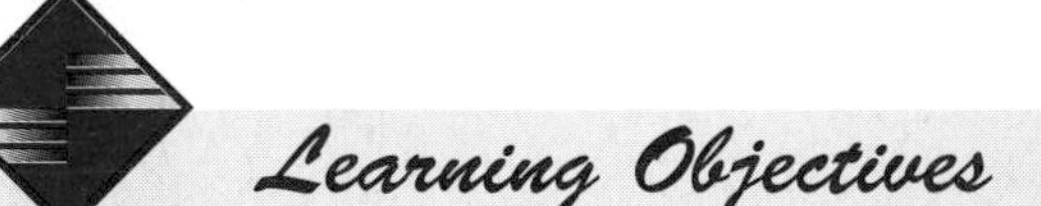

After you have read this chapter, you should be able to:

1. Describe the major characteristics of algae, protozoa, and fungi.
2. Explain what advantage colonization has for algae.
3. Describe the basis used for classifying algae into the major divisions.
4. Describe the basis for classifying fungi.
5. Differentiate between acellular and cellular slime molds.

The eucaryotic microorganisms are unicellular or multicellular organisms whose cells have membrane-bound nuclei. The cells of eucaryotes are more complex in structure than procaryotic cells. The differences in these two patterns of cellular organization are discussed in Chapter 4. Microbial eucaryotes include the photosynthetic **algae,** the nonphotosynthetic **protozoa** belonging to the kingdom Protista, and the nonphotosynthetic yeasts and molds belonging to the kingdom Fungi (Table 9–1). The larger, multicellular brown and red algae have been placed in the kingdom Plantae. The microscopic protozoa and algae make up **plankton,** the primary food source for aquatic animals. Fungi are major decomposers of organic components in the soil.

ALGAE

The algae consist of microscopic unicellular or multicellular organisms as well as macroscopic or-

Table 9–1
DIFFERENTIAL CHARACTERISTICS OF ALGAE, PROTOZOA, AND FUNGI

CHARACTERISTIC	MICROSCOPIC ALGAE	MACROSCOPIC ALGAE	PROTOZOA	FUNGI
Cellularity	Unicellular or multicellular	Multicellular	Unicellular	Unicellular or multicellular
Photopigments	Present	Present	Absent	Absent
Cell walls	Present	Present	Absent	Present
Motility	Flagella (if motile)	None	Pseudopodia, flagella, cilia	None
Kingdom	Protista	Plantae	Protista	Fungi

ganisms, such as the seaweed kelp (Fig. 9–1). All algae contain chlorophyll a and either chlorophyll b, c, or d. Some algae produce accessory pigments, known as **phycobilins,** which cause them to appear yellow-green, brown, or red. Motile algae have one or more anterior or posterior flagella. Algae reproduce asexually or sexually. Sexual reproduction involves the formation of sex cells known as **gametes,** which originate from the same or different algal organisms.

Algae are found in abundance in both freshwater and marine habitats (Fig. 9–2). Despite a wide variation in size and shape, algae share the typical membrane-bound nuclei and cytoplasmic organelles. It is the similarity of algae to protozoa and fungi and their role in photosynthesis that provide the basis for our interest in the algae. Most algae do not produce human disease.

Ranking the Algae

The diversity of size and structural characteristics among the algae has led to much confusion in classification over the years. It now appears from ultrastructural and molecular studies that algae and protozoa are not separate protistan groups. The names "algae" and "protozoa" should not be used in a classfication scheme that purports to express genetic relatedness. We shall

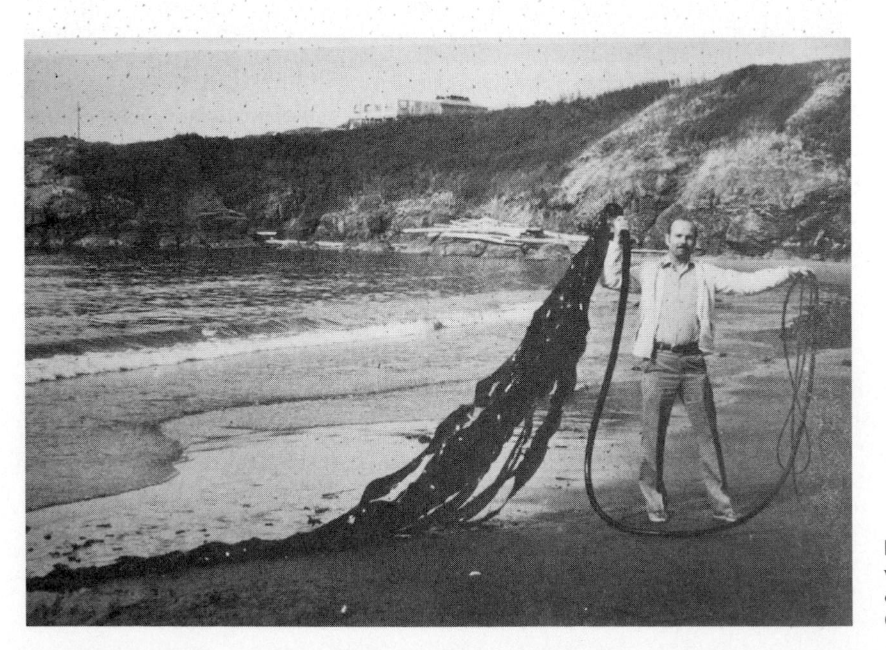

Figure 9–1 ◆ *Neurocystis luetkeana* washed up on shore on the Pacific coast. The kelp may reach a length of 60 m.

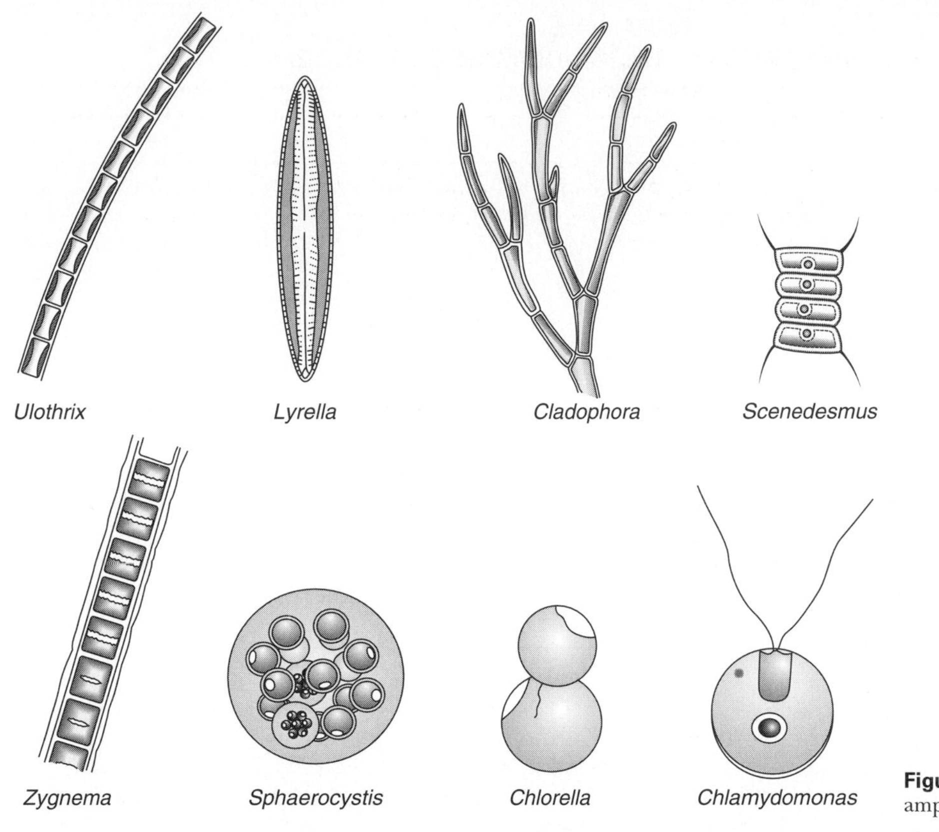

Figure 9–2 ◆ Representative examples of algae found in nature.

maintain the use of these terms as a matter of convenience in grouping algae and protozoa based on certain shared expressed characteristics. Algae may be classified into divisions based on the type of photopigments, chemical nature of cell walls, methods of reproduction, and kinds of materials stored as reserves (Table 9–2). Only the major divisions and a few examples of algae belonging to the divisions appear below.

Green Algae (Chlorophyta)

The green algae contain chlorophylls a and c and carotenes. Some members of the division are unicellular; most are multicellular (see Color Plates 13 to 15). They reproduce asexually by mitosis, but also produce mating strains that fuse to produce zygotes (Fig. 9–3). When zygotes undergo meiosis, actively motile cells are formed. Because zygotes contain two copies of each chromosome, the term **diploid** (2N) is used to describe them. The mating strains are described by the term **haploid** (N) because they contain a single copy of each chromosome. All the green algae are haploid for most of their lives, forming zygotes and the subsequent zygospores only in stressful environments. Among the best known green algae are species of unicellular *Chlamydomonas* and *Chlorella* and the multicellular species of *Spirogyra* and *Volvox.*

The flagellated *Chlamydomonas* organisms are among the most studied algal cells. Each cell has two anterior flagella and a single chloroplast. The chloroplast is the site of photosynthesis, but it also is the storage depot for starch, the major energy reserve produced by all green algae. A **stigma** (red eyespot) guides the organism toward light.

Chlorella is representative of nonmotile unicellular green algae (see Fig. 9–2). It has a very small nucleus and no eyespot. The tiny cells of *Chlorella* gained fame when they were used by Melvin Calvin to uncover the dark reactions of photosynthesis.

Several species of nonchlorophyll-containing mutants of *Chlorella,* found in soil, cause disease in animals and humans. The algal mutants,

Table 9–2
CHARACTERISTICS OF MAJOR DIVISIONS OF ALGAE

DIVISION	COMMON NAME	CELL WALL MATERIAL	MAJOR PIGMENTS	RESERVE PRODUCT
Chlorophyta	Green algae	Cellulose, pectin	Chlorophylls a and b, carotenes	Starch
Euglenophyta	Euglenoids	No true wall	Chlorophylls a and b, carotenes	Carbohydrates, oils
Chrysophyta	Yellow-green algae, golden brown algae, diatoms	Pectin, silica	Chlorophylls a and c, carotenes	Oils
Phaeophyta	Brown algae	Algin, cellulose, pectin	Chlorophylls a and c, beta-carotene, fucoxanthin, xanthophylls	Carbohydrates, oils
Pyrrophyta	Dinoflagellates	Cellulose, silica	Chlorophylls a and c, beta-carotene, xanthophylls	Starch, oils
Rhodophyta	Red algae	Cellulose, pectin	Chlorophylls a and d, phycoerythrin, phycocyanin	Starch

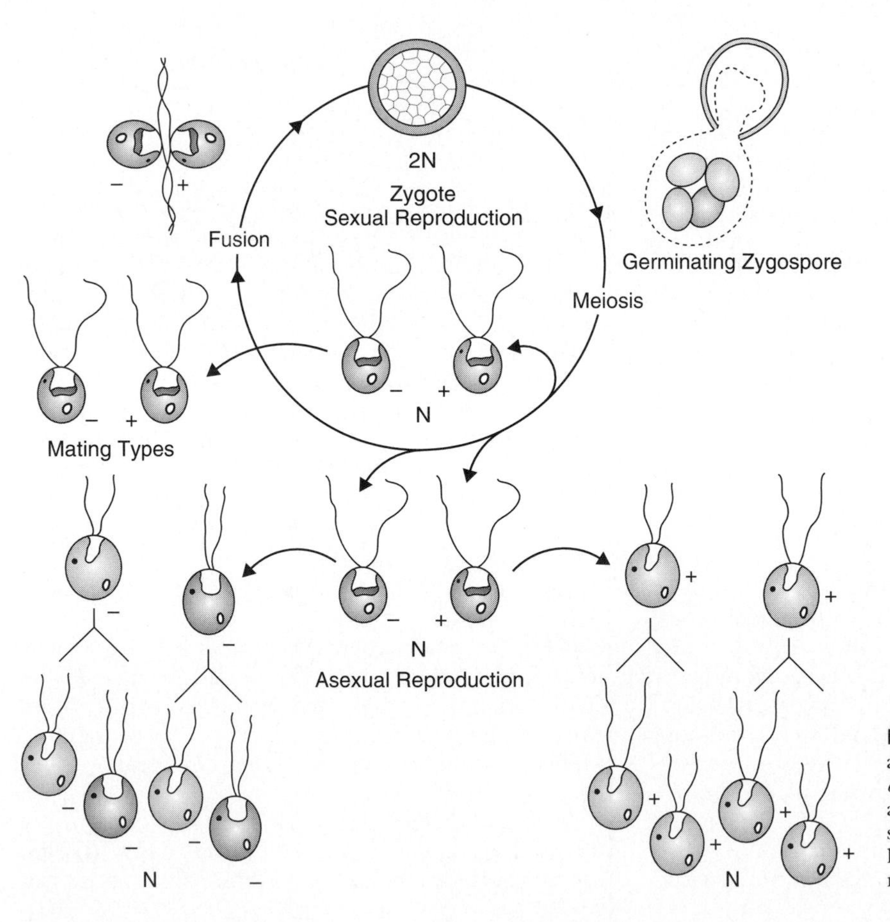

Figure 9–3 ◆ A summary of sexual and asexual reproduction in *Chlamydomonas.* Mating types fuse to form a zygospore. The germinating zygospore divides by meiosis to produce haploid cells, which more commonly multiply asexually.

which belong to the genus *Prototheca,* adapt with ease to a heterotrophic mode of nutrition. The algae have been isolated with some frequency from skin lesions in severely immunosuppressed patients.

The multicellular *Spirogyra* forms long filaments consisting of single cells joined end to end. The chloroplasts are arranged in ribbonlike spirals within individual cells. The cells reproduce by a sexual form of reproduction known as conjugation (Fig. 9–4). Two filaments line up next to one another during conjugation. The contents of one cell of a filament are transferred to an adjacent cell of another filament. Sometime later the recipient cell undergoes meiosis to produce new filaments. Filaments of *Spirogyra* accumulate in large numbers in scum on the surfaces of ponds and lakes.

Spherical colonies of *Volvox* are made up of individual flagellated cells in a gel-like sheath (Fig. 9–5). Coordinated movements of the flagella of individual cells causes the spheres to rotate in aquatic environments. Sometimes daughter colonies can be seen within parent colonies. Eventually the daughter colonies leave to establish an independent existence.

Euglenoids (Euglenophyta)

The euglenoids are unicellular, motile organisms that have no cell walls. They contain a flexible outer layer, called a **pellicle,** chlorophylls a and b, carotene, and two anterior flagella. The longer flagella is responsible for cell movement. Storage products are oils and carbohydrates. Like the green algae, euglenoids possess a stigma that directs them to a light source. Euglenoids reproduce asexually by binary fission. Some of the most studied euglenoids belong to the genus *Euglena* (Fig. 9–6; Color Plate 16).

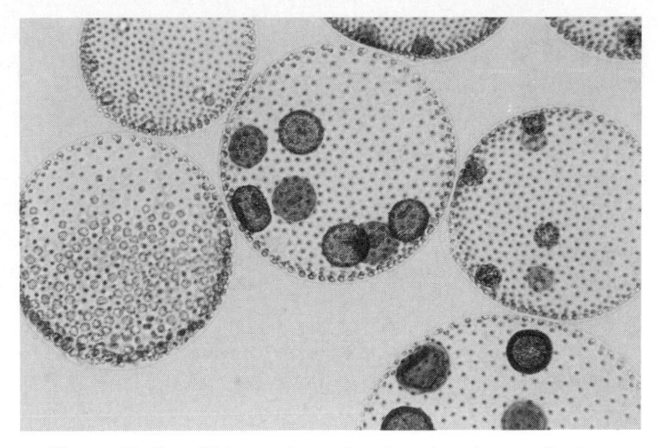

Figure 9–5 ◆ *Volvox* colony showing daughter colonies.

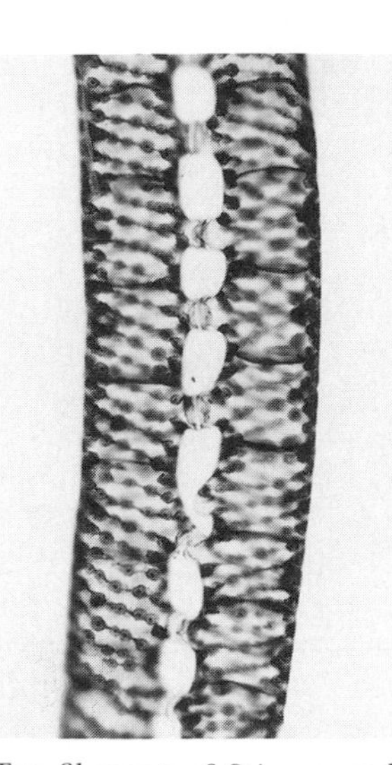

Figure 9–4 ◆ Two filaments of *Spirogyra* undergoing conjugation. Tubular outgrowths develop and fuse to form zygotes.

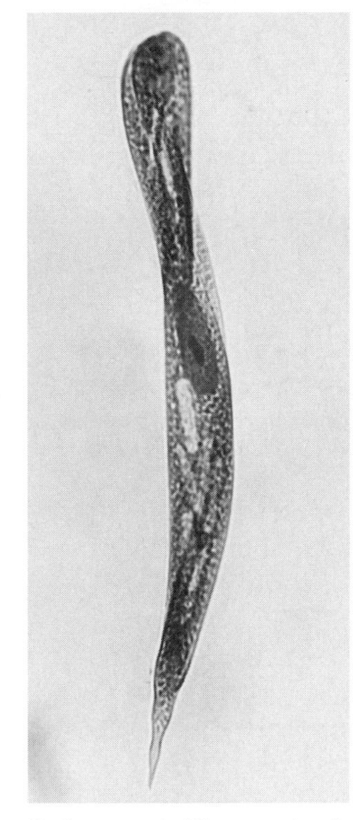

Figure 9–6 ◆ *Euglena oxyuris.* The organism has distinct chloroplasts and lacks a cell wall.

Some biologists consider euglenoids to be protozoa because of the missing cell walls. They do resemble protozoa except for the distinct chloroplasts located throughout the cytoplasm. The fact that euglenoids have characteristics of both algae and protozoa reminds us that the continuum of life forms often makes it difficult to place all organisms in distinct groups without detailed molecular studies.

Diatoms, Yellow-Green, and Golden Brown Algae (Chrysophyta)

Most of the chrysophytes are unicellular organisms that possess an abundance of carotenes as well as chlorophylls a and c. The carotenes are responsible for the golden brown color of some members of the division. Diatoms are capable of only limited mobility. These organisms secrete a mucoid material that enables them to glide on solid surfaces.

Diatoms have two-part overlapping cell walls called **frustules.** The patterns of the frustules are unique in nature, and their beautiful and intricate formations have been termed the "jewelry of nature" (Fig. 9–7; Color Plate 17). The walls contain cellulose, pectin, and silica. Holes in walls permit the nutrients to enter and waste products to exit. Reproduction by mitosis produces smaller diatoms with each division until the size of offspring are only about one third of the original size. Sexual reproduction restores them to their former size. Oils are the major storage materials. Diatoms are especially abundant in cool ocean waters.

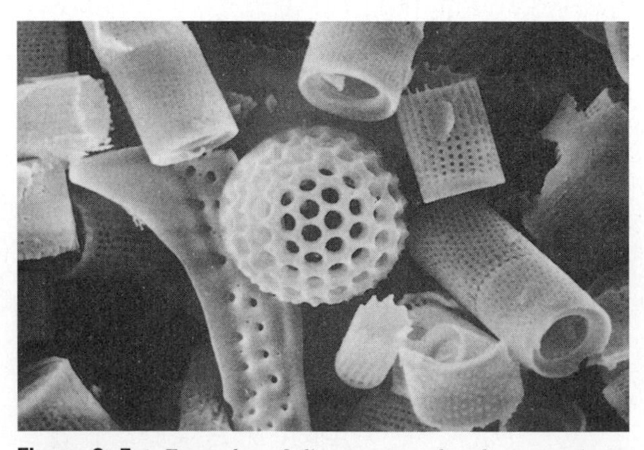

Figure 9–7 ◆ Examples of diatoms seen by electron microscopy showing intricate patterns of frustules.

When diatoms die, the residual silica, which is deposited on the ocean floor, forms what is known as *diatomaceous earth.* The broken bits of one-time cell walls, also known as fuller's earth, are added to cosmetics, paints, polishes, and insulation materials.

Brown Algae (Phaeophyta)

The brown algae are complex, multicellular organisms that superficially resemble plants. Their distinctive coloring is due to the presence of **fucoxanthin.** The organisms also contain chlorophylls a and c, carotenes, and other xanthophylls. Brown algae grow along the shore line of marine environments. They are often anchored by primitive organs known as **holdfasts.** Brown algae attain lengths up to 100 m and are able to reproduce sexually and asexually. The storage products are carbohydrates and oils.

Cell walls of brown algae contain algin, a commercially useful product. Algin is widely employed as a stabilizer in milk products, salad dressings, and chewing gum. It is sometimes added to processed beverages to prevent foaming.

Dinoflagellates (Pyrrophyta)

The dinoflagellates are primarily unicellular marine forms. Most dinoflagellates contain chlorophylls a and c, carotenes, and xanthophylls; some emit light in a phenomenon known as **bioluminescence.** As their flagella beat, dinoflagellates move rapidly through a liquid.

The two-plate cell walls of dinoflagellates are composed of cellulose and silica in ornate patterns. The organisms have the ability to use an organic energy source in the absence of light. Storage depots contain starch and oils. Most dinoflagellates reproduce asexually by longitudinal fission.

Dinoflagellates are responsible for "red tides" that commonly occur in coastal waters of the United States and Canada in summer and early autumn (see Color Plate 18). The populations, often called **blooms,** produce a potent neurotoxin that accumulates in shellfish and kills thousands of other fish along the coasts. Ingestion of shellfish containing the neurotoxin causes a human disease known as paralytic shellfish poisoning. The disease can be fatal if respiratory muscles are affected.

Red Algae (Rhodophyta)

The red algae are nonmotile unicellular or multicellular filamentous organisms. Their bright color is due to **phycoerythrin.** The organism also contains phycocyanin and chlorophylls a and d. The variety of photopigments enables red algae to carry on photosynthesis in coastal waters of the oceans or in depths up to 1 m. The accessory photopigments are destroyed by light so algae may appear green or brown in surface waters. The red algae have complex reproductive cycles involving asexual and sexual reproduction.

The agar used as a solidifying agent in microbiological culture media comes from red algae belonging to the genera *Gelidium* and *Gracilaria.* Agar is also added to ice cream, jellies, jams, and some drugs. Carrageenans, extracted from walls of other red algae, are used as stabilizers in milk products and some cosmetics.

Micro Check

- What is the major role of algae in nature?
- How do algae differ from plants?
- What is the source of diatomaceous earth?

PROTOZOA

Protozoa consist of a large group of unicellular organisms as diverse as unicellular algae (Fig. 9–8). There are no multicellular forms. Some spherical forms are only 1.0 μm in diameter; elongated cells attain lengths of 100 μm or more. The protozoa typically do not contain photopigments or cell walls.

Protozoa are found in fresh water, marine habitats, and moist soil. Their diet includes bacteria, small algae, and other protozoa. Food particles are engulfed by the plasma membrane or enter through a primitive mouth. The feeding stages of protozoa are called **trophozoites.** The survival of protozoa despite unfavorable environmental conditions is attributed to (1) the variety of methods of reproduction and (2) the ability of certain protozoa to form resting stages called **cysts** (Fig. 9–9). Asexual reproduction occurs by binary or multiple fission involving a series of nuclear changes associated with mitosis. During the process, protozoa assume a variety of shapes. Members of the genus *Plasmodium* reproduce both asexually and sexually. The life cycle of *Plasmodium* species is discussed in Chapter 20.

Some protozoa can remain viable as cysts for long periods of time outside their hosts. The

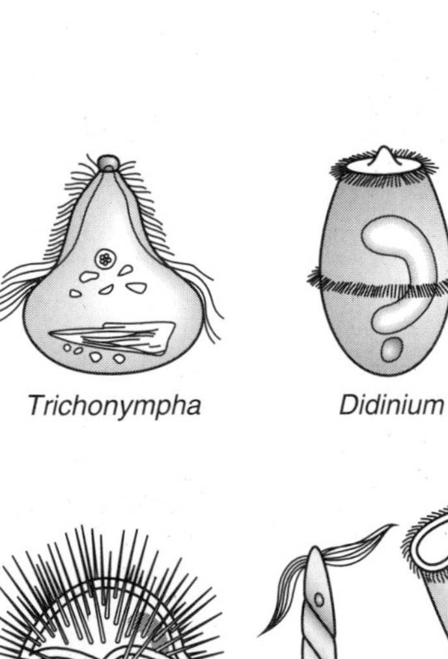

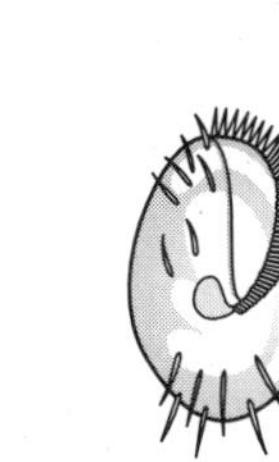

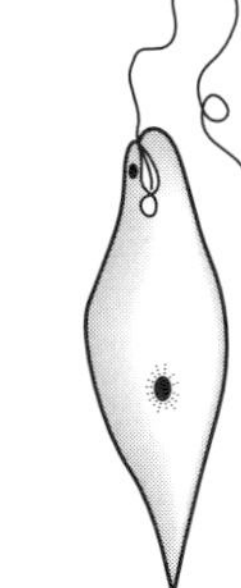

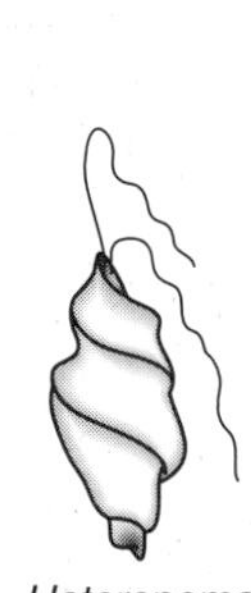

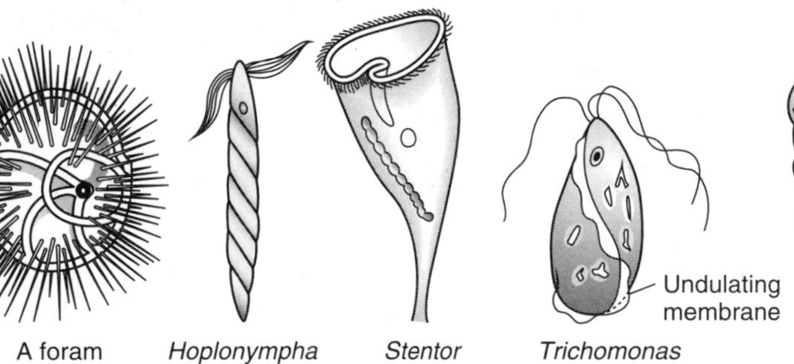

Figure 9–8 ◆ Representative examples of protozoa found in nature.

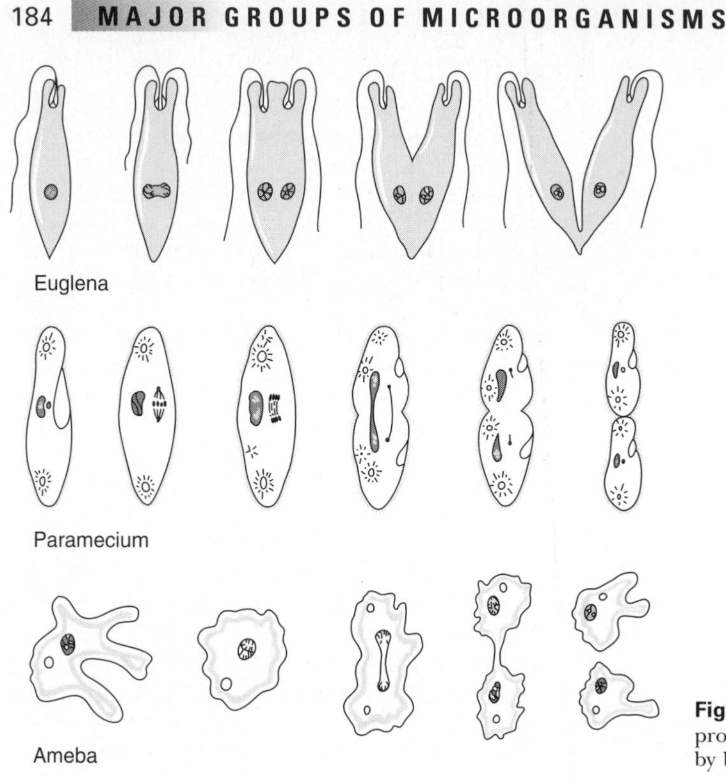

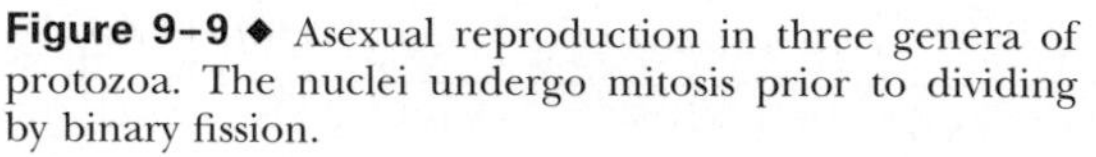
Figure 9–9 ◆ Asexual reproduction in three genera of protozoa. The nuclei undergo mitosis prior to dividing by binary fission.

thick walls of the cysts make them resistant to drying. Certain species reproduce in the encysted stage. The newly formed trophozoites are released when walls of cysts are disrupted by host enzymes.

Protozoa, like algae, are food sources for aquatic animals. Some play a role in degradative processes that return carbon dioxide (CO_2) to the atmosphere. A majority of protozoa do not cause disease, but some live in vertebrate hosts and do damage while living in that protected environment. A small number of protozoa are responsible for intestinal infections of humans; others invade the blood, lungs, liver, or brain.

Ranking the Protozoa

Protozoa are classified on the basis of mode of motility and cell structure (Table 9–3). Some protozoa have complex life cycles and are nonmotile as adults. The photosynthetic euglenoids and dinoflagellates may be classified as algae or protozoa because they share characteristics with

Table 9–3
CHARACTERISTICS OF THE MAJOR CLASSES OF PROTOZOA

CLASS	PRIMARY MODE OF MOTILITY	TYPE OF REPRODUCTION
Sarcodina	Pseudopodia	Binary fission
Mastigophora	Flagella	Longitudinal fission
Ciliata	Cilia	Transverse fission, conjugation
Sporozoa	Adults—nonmotile; immature forms and gametes—flagella	Multiple fission, syngamy

both major groups. All classes of protozoa contain some pathogens.

Pseudopods (Sarcodina)

Members of the class Sarcodina move by means of pseudopodia, or false feet. Members of this class include free-living and parasitic amebas (see Color Plate 19). The ameboids are the slowest moving of the protozoa as they seek food and react to both physical and chemical stimuli.

Certain pseudopods survive by forming cysts in hostile environments. Amebas divide by binary fission, but division of nuclei also occurs in cysts. At least six species of amebas are common parasites of humans. A few free-living amebas are able to cause human infections. The best known parasitic ameba is *Entamoeba histolytica,* which causes a type of dysentery (Fig. 9–10). The ameba can migrate to extraintestinal sites or cause recurrent debilitating enteric disease. It must be differentiated from nonpathogenic amebas, which occasionally inhabit intestinal tracts of humans without causing harm.

Flagellates (Mastigophora)

The flagellates belong to the class Mastigophora. They contain one or more flagella, located most often on the anterior end. The intestinal flagellates have internal structures, such as undulating membranes, axostyles, or sucking disks, which provide them with enough flexibility to withstand peristaltic action. Most flagellates encyst under unfavorable conditions. Trophozoites reproduce asexually by longitudinal binary fission. Division of encysted flagellates produces at least two daughter cells.

Flagellates that cause human infections are *Giardia lamblia,* an intestinal parasite, *Trichomonas vaginalis,* a cause of genitourinary disease, and the trypanosomes associated with sleeping sickness in parts of Africa (Fig. 9–11). A lesser known flagellate, carried by sandflies, is the cause of the skin disease leishmaniasis. At least 200 participants of the Gulf War in 1992 developed the cutaneous lesions of one type of leishmaniasis when returning to the United States. More information on intestinal and blood flagellates is found in Chapters 17 and 20.

Ciliates (Ciliata)

The ciliates are a large group of protozoa that move by means of short, hairlike appendages surrounding the plasma membrane or extending from only part of the cell (see Color Plate 20). The appendages, known as *cilia* also help to procure food by creating waves that propel food morsels into a primitive mouth. Ciliates have at least one macronucleus and one or more micronuclei.

The paramecia are representative examples of ciliates with macro- and micronuclei. They are often found in abundance in fresh water containing aquatic plants and decaying organic material. The cilia can reverse the path of rotation, making them versatile in a hostile environment. The only ciliate that is pathogenic to humans is the

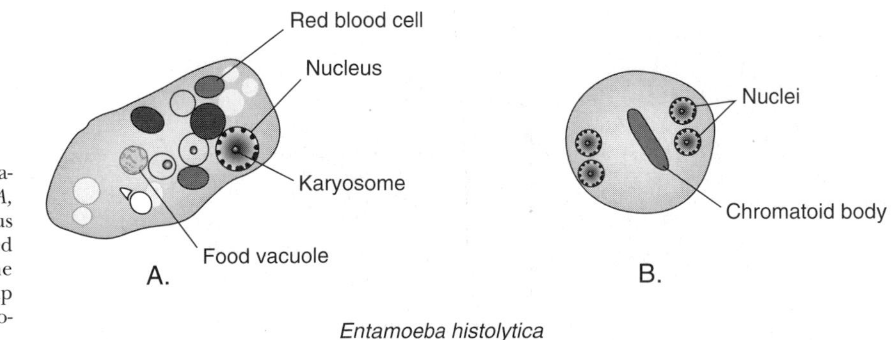

Figure 9–10 ◆ Stages of the parasitic ameba *Entamoeba histolytica. A,* The trophozoite has a single nucleus with a distinct karyosome. Ingested red blood cells are present in the cytoplasm. *B,* The cyst can have up to four nuclei and often has a chromatoid body.

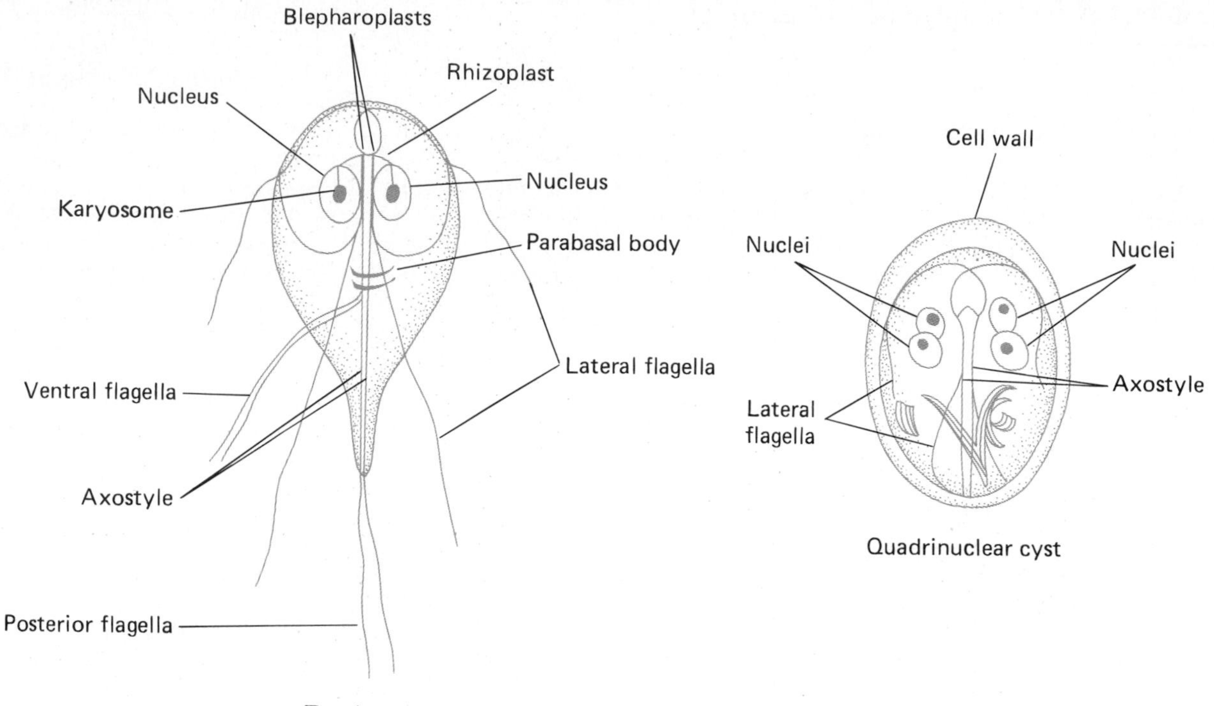

Figure 9–11 ◆ Stages of the parasitic flagellate *Giardia lamblia.* The trophozoite has two nuclei, prominent karyosomes, and flagella, which are often difficult to see. The cyst has four nuclei and no flagella.

saclike *Balantidium coli,* which can penetrate the intestinal mucosa (Fig. 9–12).

Sporozoans (Sporozoa)

The sporozoans have complex life cycles and are nonmotile upon reaching maturity. All members of the class cause infections in one or more hosts. The malarial parasites, belonging to the genus *Plasmodium,* require a vertebrate host and a mosquito to complete their life cycles. Their life cycles include both sexual and asexual forms of reproduction. Asexual cycles occur in red blood cells of vertebrate hosts; sexual cycles take place in certain female mosquitos. Various stages in the asexual cycle can be seen in red blood cells of infected vertebrates. More information on the sexual and asexual cycles of plasmodia is presented in Chapter 20.

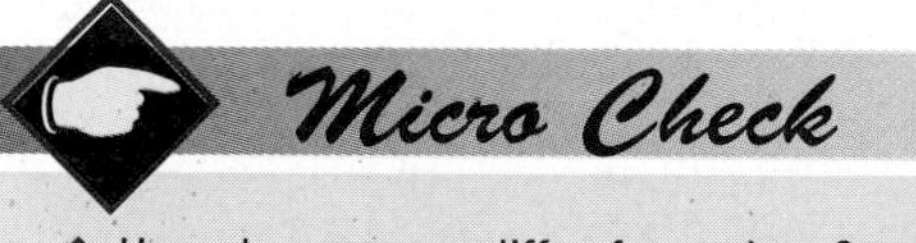

- How do protozoa differ from algae?
- On what basis are protozoa classified?
- Why are flagellates not propelled along with contents of the intestine during peristalsis?

FUNGI

The fungi include both microscopic organisms and larger organisms, such as mushrooms and toadstools. The microscopic fungi consist of unicellular spherical, oval, or elongated **yeast** cells and multicellular organisms called **molds** (Fig. 9–13). Some dimorphic fungi are capable of growing as yeasts or molds, depending on environ-

FOCAL POINT

Pneumocystis carinii: A Protozoan-like Fungus?

Pneumocystis carinii, once known as the cause of a rare disease in mostly premature infants, has emerged to be a major cause of death in AIDS patients. Probably everyone in the United States has been exposed to the organism by the age of 40. Immune mechanisms in a healthy person allow the organism to exist in a dormant state. Suppression of cell immunity, characteristic of AIDS, allows the organism to multiply in the spaces between the air sacs. It appears that the trophozoite multiplies or forms a thin-walled cyst containing eight sporozoites. Once thought to be a protozoan, *P. carinii* is now thought to be a fungus, even though the terms trophozoite and cyst are still used to describe stages of its life cycle.

P. carinii is difficult to grow in the laboratory, and appropriate animal models do not exist. The basis for classifying the organism as a fungus comes from analysis of RNA sequences showing a greater degree of relatedness to fungi than to protozoa. *P. carinii* pneumonia (PCP) can be treated with a variety of drugs, but causes recurrent life-threatening infections in immunosuppressed patients. The primary challenge is in preventing the infection by use of prophylactic drugs. Perhaps one day it shall be possible to establish beyond doubt its taxonomic position.

mental conditions. The dimorphic fungi more commonly grow as yeasts at temperatures above 30°C, but as molds at room temperature or below. The basic structural unit of molds is a tubular filament called a **hypha** (see Color Plate 21). The hyphae may have cross walls **(septa)** or consist of a single elongated, nucleated cell. A hypha with no cross walls is described as a nonseptate or **coenocytic** hypha (Fig. 9–14). A mass of intertwined hyphae is known as a **mycelium.** You have probably seen these fuzzlike structures on old bread or on rotting fruit.

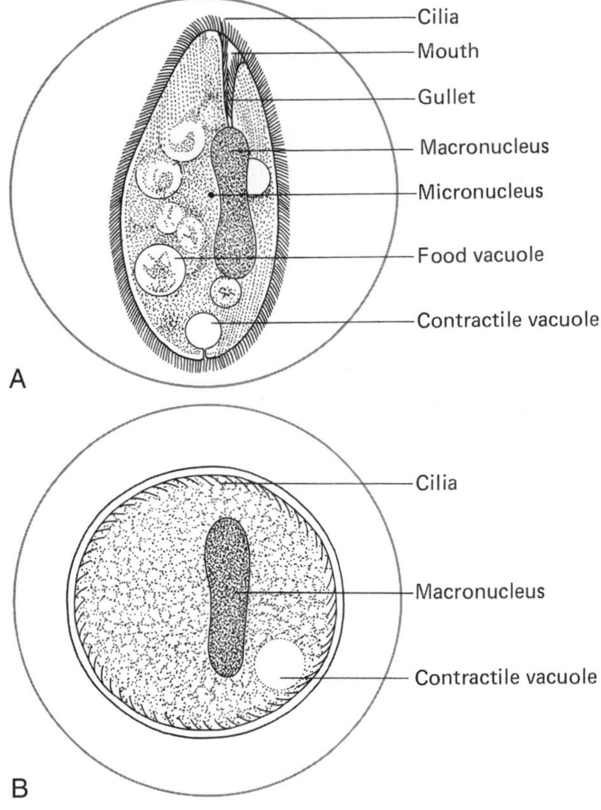

Figure 9–12 ◆ Stages of the parasitic ciliate *Balantidium coli. A,* The ovoid trophozoite has a kidney bean–shaped macronucleus, a small spherical micronucleus, and a primitive gullet and mouth. *B,* The cyst is more spherical and retains both nuclei although the micronucleus may not be visible.

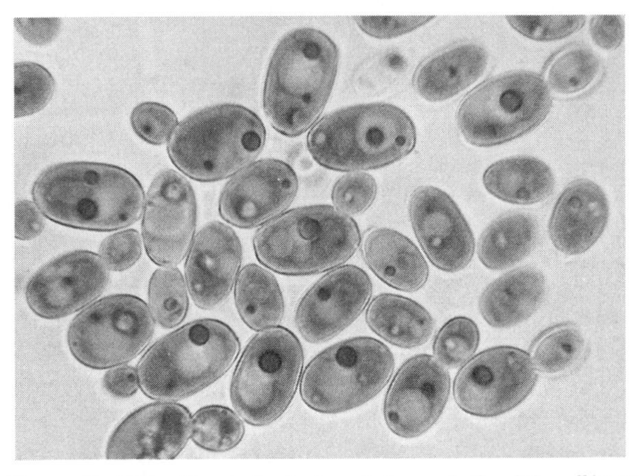

Figure 9–13 ◆ Morphological variation of *Candida albicans* yeast cells.

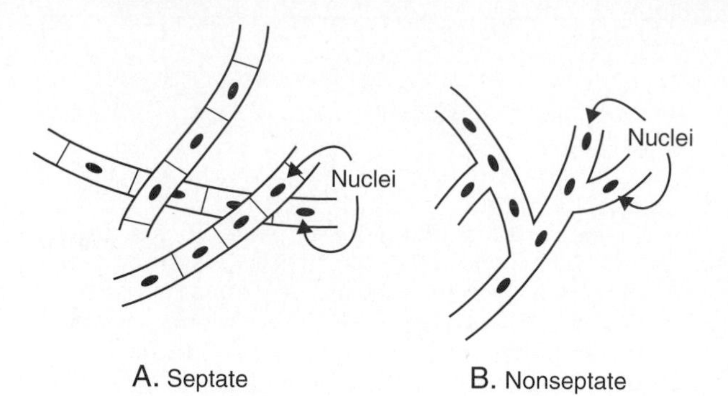

Figure 9–14 ◆ Types of hyphae *A,* Septate hyphae with cross walls between cells. *B,* Nonseptate hyphae with no cross walls separating individual cells.

All fungi lack photopigments; most have rigid cell walls composed of chitin and other carbohydrates. Fungi are major decomposers of organic material in soil, but there are some aquatic fungi. The optimal pH for most fungi ranges between 5.0 and 5.5. Most are aerobic; a few yeasts are facultatively anaerobic. Fungi grow well at temperatures ranging from 20° to 30°C.

A majority of fungi obtain their nutrients from dead organic matter, but some are attracted to living tissue of plants, humans, and other animals. Destructive fungal diseases of plants have completely annihilated some crops and have had devastating effects on the world economy. Late blight potato disease, caused by a fungus, caused a famine in Ireland in 1845 and led to the migration of over 1.5 million Irish people to the United States. Without the destructive capacity of a single fungus, Americans might have never experienced the "wearing of the green" on Saint Patrick's Day—a day we all celebrate with Irish Americans.

The number of fungi causing disease in animals, including humans, is relatively small, but the superficial or generalized infections they cause are often difficult to treat. The human **mycoses** (infections caused by fungi) are discussed in several subsequent chapters.

Ranking the Fungi

Methods of classifying fungi are constantly being updated as new information becomes available. Microbiologists are primarily interested in four classes of the division Amastigomycota (Table 9–4). Fungi are classified by their type of hyphae, modes of reproduction, and kinds of reproductive structures. Asexual structures are called asexual spores or **conidia.** Those produced sexually are referred to as sexual **spores** or simply spores.

The five types of asexual spores are (1) arthroconidia, (2) blastoconidia, (3) chlamydoconidia, (4) conidia, and (5) sporangioconidia (Fig. 9–15). The conidia are classified according to size as macroconidia or microconidia. Small spherical or elliptical microconidia are unicellular. The club- or spindle-shaped macroconidia are multicellular with visible cell walls. Some fungi produce more than one type of asexual spore, although one type may be more characteristic of a particular species. Sexual spores are not produced under the usual laboratory conditions. The formation of sexual spores occurs in nature under adverse environmental conditions. Many fungi bear sexual spores on tips of hyphae, in sacs called asci, or on clublike structures known as basidia. The large number of asexual spores produced by all four classes of fungi ensures survival of most species, since some of the spores are bound to land or be carried to places suitable for germination and growth.

Table 9–4
DIFFERENTIAL CHARACTERISTICS OF FUNGI

CLASS	TYPE OF HYPHAE	TYPE OF CONIDIA	TYPE OF SPORES
Zycomycota	Nonseptate	Sporangioconidia, conidioconidia	Zygospores
Ascomycota	Septate	Blastoconidia, conidia	Ascospores
Basidiomycota	Septate	Usually absent	Basidiospores
Deuteromycota	Septate	Arthroconidia, conidia	Absent

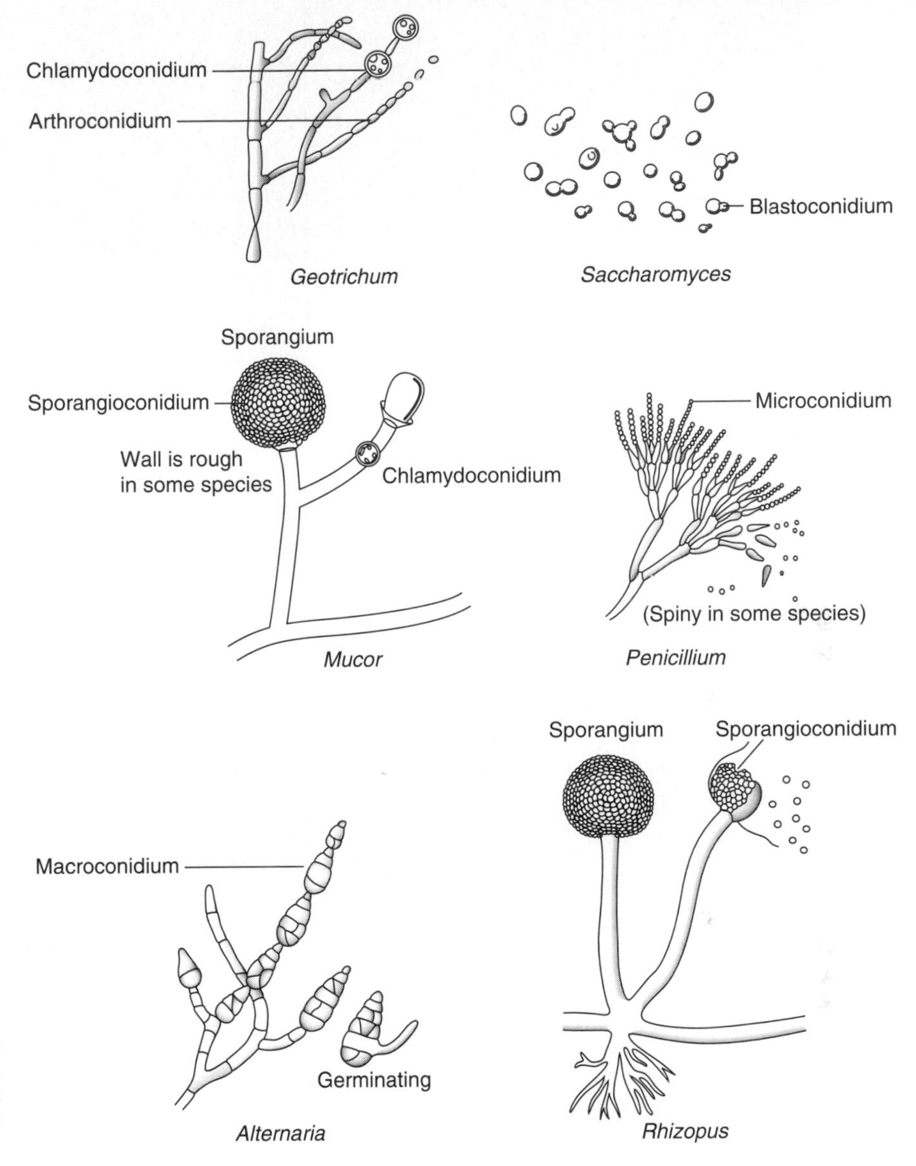

Figure 9–15 ◆ Asexual reproductive structures of common molds. Most are borne externally except for sporangioconidia, which are produced within enlarged cells.

Water Molds (Zygomycota)

The water molds and some related fungi do not live exclusively in water despite their name. Many are soil residents. They have nonseptate hyphae and produce sporangioconidia, chlamydoconidia, and conidia. Sexual reproduction involves the formation of **zygospores** when sex cells fuse (Fig. 9–16).

The common bread mold, *Rhizopus stolonifer,* is an example of a water mold (Fig. 9–17). Some species of **Zygomycota** cause opportunistic infections in patients compromised by burns or immunodeficiency disease.

Sac Fungi (Ascomycota)

The sac fungi consist of yeasts and some molds having septate hyphae. The yeasts reproduce asexually by forming **blastoconidia;** the molds typically produce **microconidia.** The sexual spores or **ascospores** are contained in sacs called **asci.**

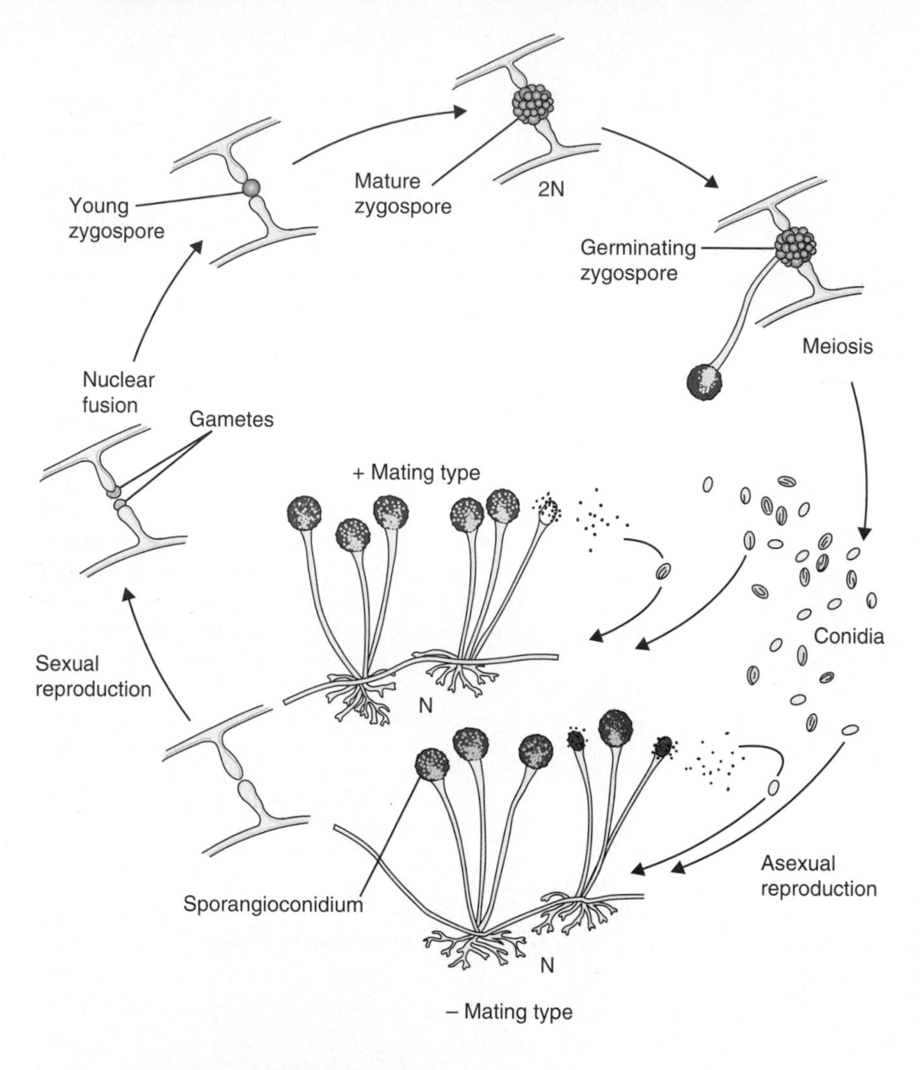

Figure 9–16 ◆ A summary of sexual and asexual reproduction in *Rhizopus*. Mating types fuse to form a zygospore. The germinating zygospore undergoes meiosis to produce haploid cells, which can reproduce asexually.

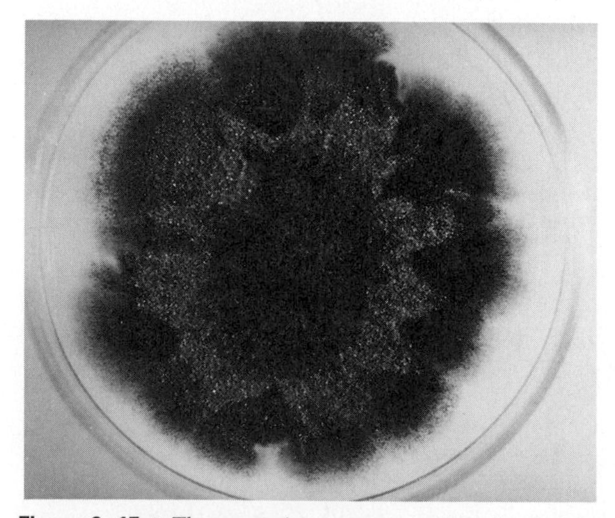

Figure 9–17 ◆ The vegetative structure or mycelium of the common bread mold, *Rhizopus stolonifer,* growing on a culture medium in the laboratory.

The yeasts used in making bread, beer, and wine are sac fungi. Although most members of the class are nonpathogens, a few are particularly aggressive in causing diseases of plants and animals. Chestnut blight, Dutch elm disease, and ergot, a disease of rye and other grasses, are caused by sac fungi. If the toxin of *Claviceps purpurea,* the agent of ergot, is ingested by animals, including humans, it promotes delusions, nerve spasms, and convulsions, sometimes resulting in death (Fig. 9–18).

Club Fungi (Basidiomycota)

The club fungi include rusts, smuts, mushrooms, and toadstools. The structure we know as a mushroom starts with branching hyphae in the soil (Fig. 9–19). The fungus reproduces asexually

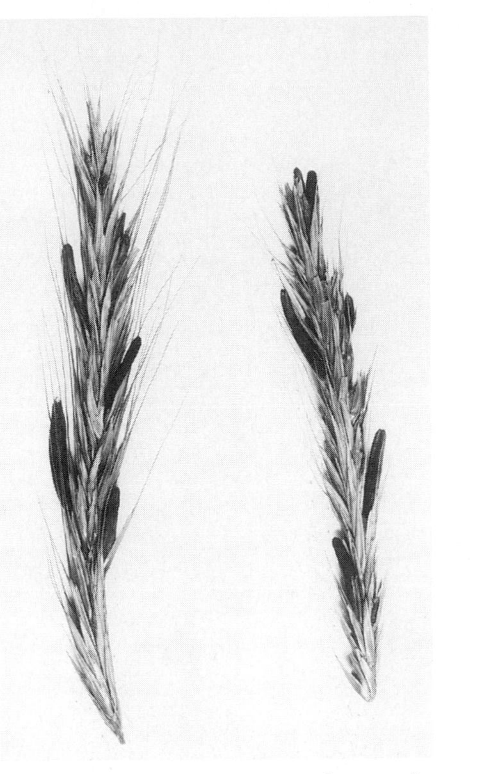

Figure 9–18 ◆ *Claviceps purpurea,* a pathogen of rye, transforms the seeds to large spurs (sclerotia).

in soil by means of blastoconidia and microconidia but also reproduces sexually by producing a large fruiting body called a **basidiocarp.** The fruiting body begins to form underground. It continues developing with the formation of a cap above the soil revealing gills and special spore-bearing structures called **basidia.** The sexual spores or **basidiospores** land on the ground where they start new mycelia if conditions are favorable.

Mushrooms are eaten and enjoyed by people all over the world. However, some mushrooms, such as *Amanita phalloides,* produce toxins that cause gastrointestinal or hallucinogenic symptoms. Coma and death are not uncommon. Because there are no simple tests to differentiate toxic from edible mushrooms, it is best to obtain mushrooms from reliable sources.

Cryptococcus neoformans, a cause of pulmonary disease and meningitis, is the only human pathogen of this class. The most virulent strains are found in sites contaminated with pigeon droppings.

Imperfect Fungi (Deuteromycota)

The imperfect fungi are not known to reproduce sexually. It is a class of "leftovers" for fungi that have either lost their ability to produce sexual spores or have not found a need to develop sexual spores in order to survive. Many fungi, once considered imperfect fungi, have been assigned to one of the other three classes upon the discovery of a sexual form of reproduction. Many of the imperfect fungi are dimorphic and most produce more than one type of asexual spore. The majority are nonpathogenic or parasitize plants; a few cause important diseases of humans and other animals.

A few imperfect fungi, such as *Aspergillus flavus,* which grows readily on stored cereal and nuts, produce potent toxins called **aflatoxins.** The toxins have been implicated in liver cancer in animals. More information on aflatoxins as health hazards is found in Chapter 17. Diseases caused by fungi are discussed in subsequent chapters.

Some species of *Penicillium* produce substances with antimicrobial properties; others give unique flavors to cheeses. Chapter 24 contains more information on the uses of fungi in beverage and food production.

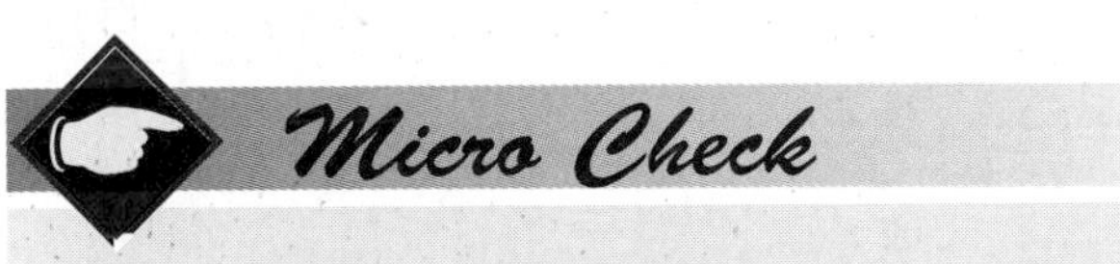

- How do the imperfect fungi differ from the three other classes of fungi?
- How do yeasts differ from molds?
- What is a dimorphic fungus?

Slime Molds

Slime molds have piqued the curiosity of biologists for years because they resemble both protozoa and fungi (see Color Plate 22). Taxonomists classify them as protozoa because at one stage of development they resemble amebas. Their ability to produce distinct fruiting bodies and spores causes them to resemble molds. There are both acellular and cellular slime molds.

ACELLULAR SLIME MOLDS

The acellular slime molds consist of masses of cytoplasm with many nuclei. The streaming mass of cytoplasm, devoid of cell boundaries, is called

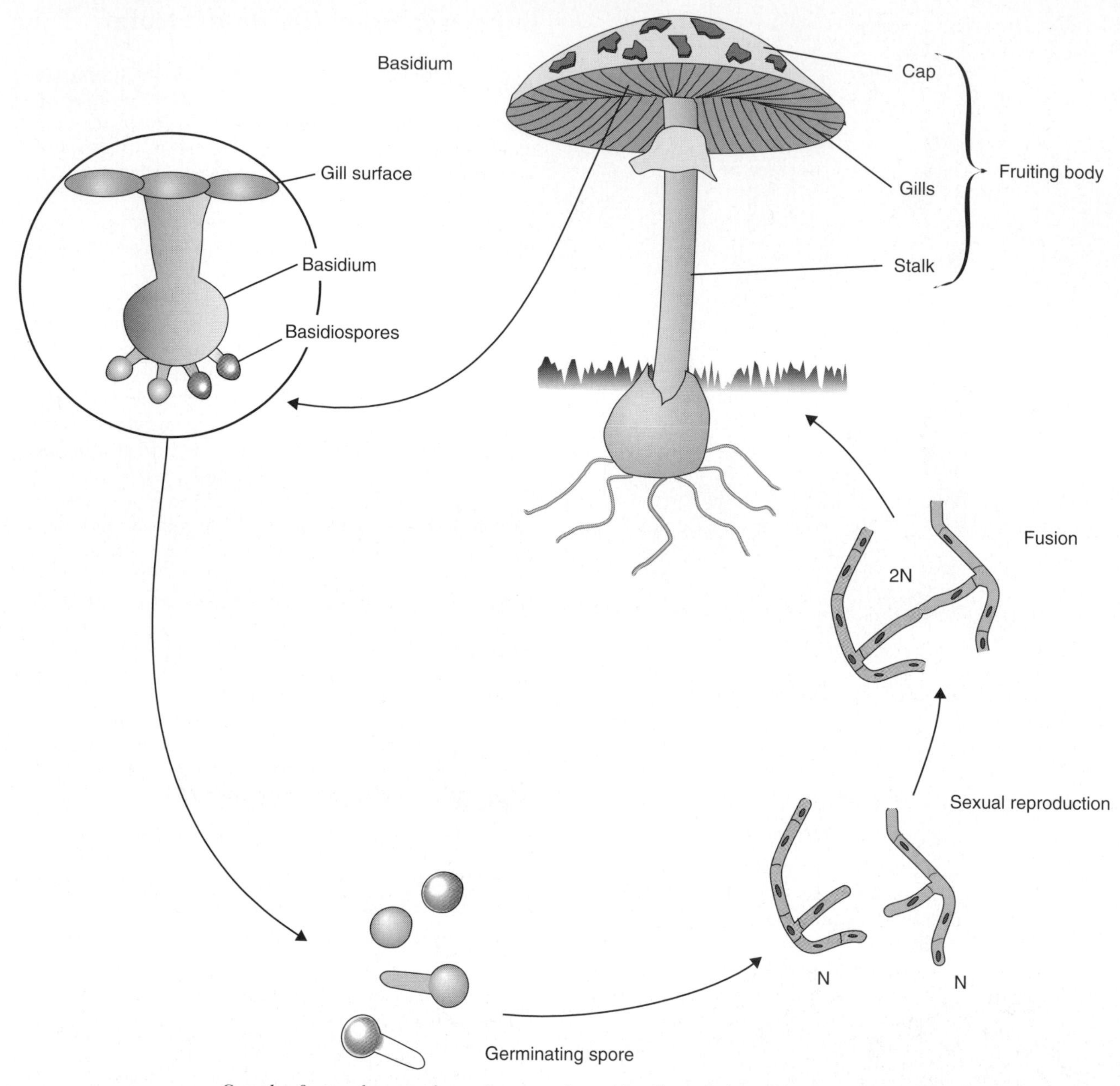

Growth of a mushroom above the ground resulting from fusion of hyphae of two mating types. Diploid basidiospores are produced on basidia in the gills under the cap. Favorable environmental conditions permit germination of spores.

a **plasmodium.** The amorphous mass of cytoplasm creeps along on moist surfaces, taking in morsels of food as it moves. The nuclei undergo division as the plasmodium grows. Growth stops if there is insufficient food or moisture, and fruiting bodies appear on the tops of stalks. The fruiting bodies are often multicolored, ornate structures, which release spores into the environment. The life cycle continues as spores germinate and form a new plasmodium.

FOCAL POINT

Discovery of a Mammoth and Ancient Fungus

Biologists throughout the world were stunned by the discovery of a giant and very old fungus in 1992. The fungus, found in a forest near Crystal Falls, Michigan, weighs about 100 tons and occupies more than 30 acres. The mushroom, *Armillaria bulbosa,* which dwarfs the much admired sequoia trees and even blue whales, challenges the supremacy of the dinosaurs as the largest organisms ever existing on the Earth. The new heavyweight champion could be from 1500 to 10,000 years old. It may have been growing since the end of the last Ice Age. DNA analysis confirms that all tendrils of the organism are genetically uniform. The discovery serves to emphasize that, given favorable conditions, including moisture and nutrients, and lack of competition, growth for some forms of life may be indeterminant. Scientists believe that the fungus has attained its maximum size because of encroaching fungi at one or more of its current borders. The possibility that expansive patches of giant fungi or other organisms may exist in remote parts of the world challenges some of the basic premises of biology in which organisms have been defined in terms of size.

Nature 256:428–431, 1992.

CELLULAR SLIME MOLDS

Cellular slime molds resemble amebas with membrane-bound nuclei. They feed on smaller microorganisms and reproduce asexually under favorable conditions. If food supplies are inadequate, cellular slime molds form a loose association of cells called **pseudoplasmodium.** The enclosed communities of cells move as units on logs, the bark of trees, or organic debris, leaving behind a trail of slime. Entire pseudoplasmodia are sometimes called **slugs.** Individual ameboid cells migrate within the pseudoplasmodia and, ultimately, form spore-bearing fruiting bodies. Fruiting bodies release mature spores into the environment where germination occurs to start new life cycles (Fig. 9–20).

Slime molds are important models for studying cell differentiation. They have important roles in the food chain, feeding on other microorganisms and serving as food for larger organisms. Some cellular slime molds even prey on other cellular slime molds, eliminating their competitors by a type of cannibalization.

FOCAL POINT

Why The English Drink Tea

Until the middle of the nineteenth century, the English consumed about the same amount of coffee as they did tea. At the beginning of that century, there were 500 coffee houses in London alone. The coffee houses were places where political views could be exchanged in a comfortable, stimulating atmosphere. The insurance institution Lloyds of London was an outgrowth of a coffee house.

All coffee was purchased from Ceylon (now known as Sri Lanka), Java, India, and Malaya (now a part of Malaysia). Those countries were a part of the British Empire. A disease, known as coffee rust, appeared on a coffee plantation in Ceylon about 1867. It was caused by a fungus, *Hemileia vastatrix,* which grows primarily on the leaves of the coffee plant. The fungus produces an abundance of spores, which were easily spread by wind and rain to adjacent coffee fields. By 1871 the coffee grown in Ceylon was less than half of the former production. Exports of coffee dropped to less than 7 percent of former shipments by 1893. The British had no desire to buy coffee from Brazil, which was fast becoming the major coffee-producing country of the world. Instead, the British turned to tea, which had originally been brought to Europe by the Dutch in the seventeenth century. By the twentieth century, tea drinkers outnumbered coffee drinkers in England six to one. England imports at least 500 million pounds of tea annually. It is estimated that the average English person consumes about 2000 cups of tea a year.

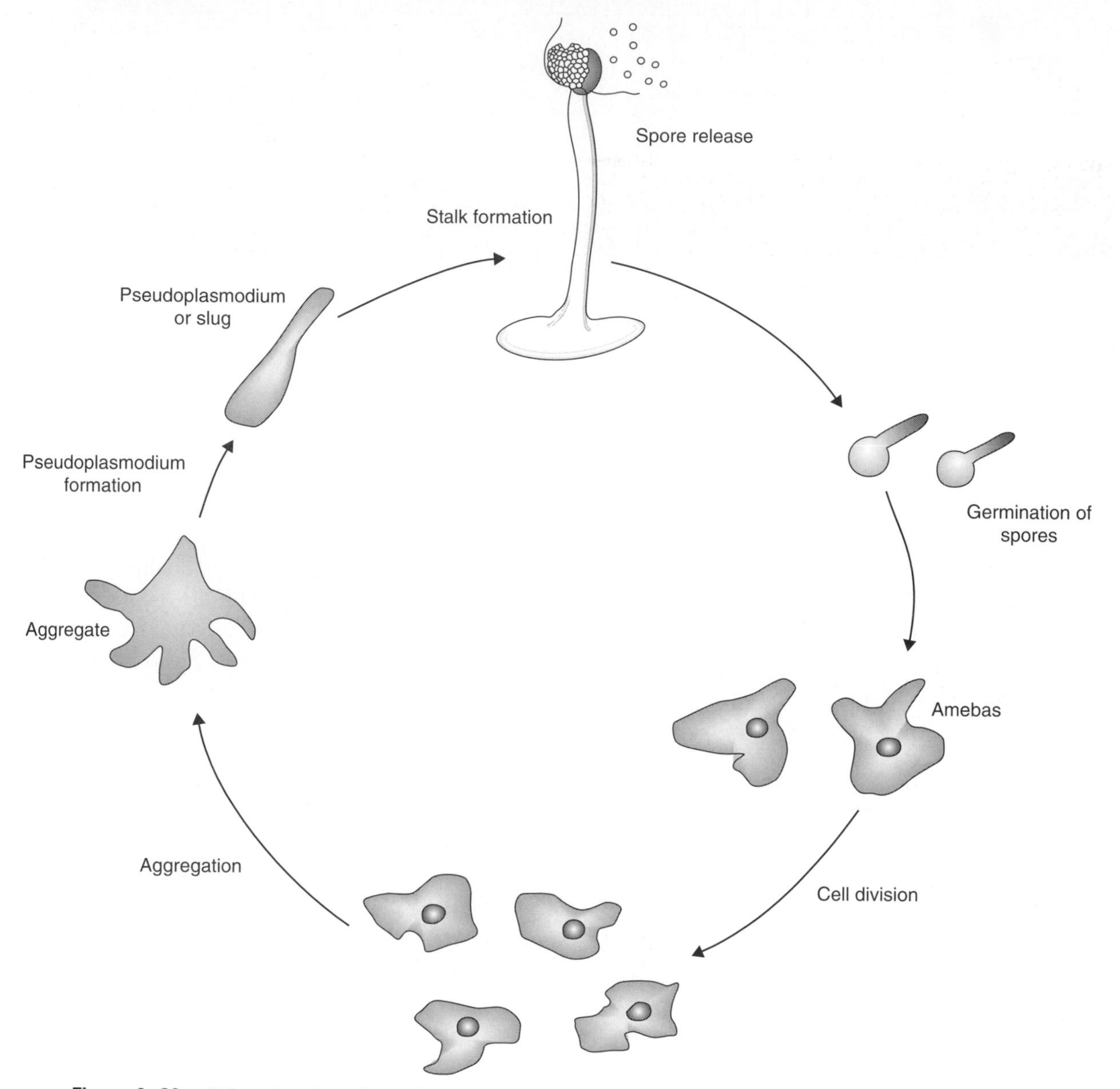

Figure 9–20 ◆ Life cycle of a cellular slime mold. Spores, released from fruiting bodies, germinate to produce amebas. Aggregated amebas form a migrating stage known as a slug, which ultimately differentiates into a stalk.

Micro Check

- ◆ How do slime molds differ from other molds?
- ◆ How do cellular slime molds resemble amebas?
- ◆ Why are slime molds important?

Understanding Microbiology

1. To what kingdoms do the microbial eucaryotes belong?
2. Why are pseudopodia not considered true appendages of locomotion?

3. Name four classes of protozoa.
4. Why are some fungi considered to be imperfect?
5. What makes slime molds difficult to classify?

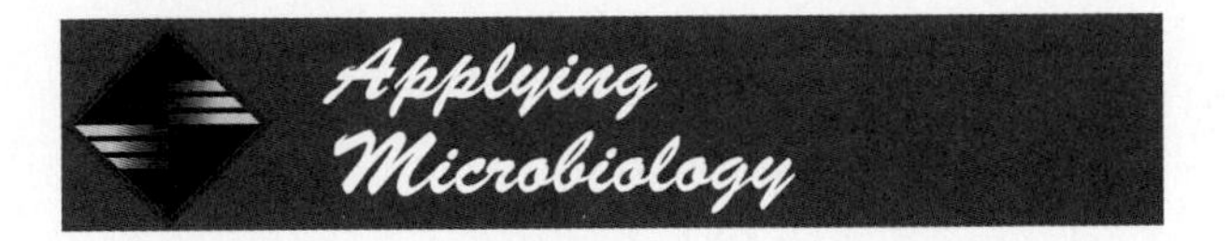

6. Assume you have been given a sample of pond water and asked to count the types of algae and protozoa seen. Name the criteria you would use in differentiating algae from protozoa. How would you be sure you were counting a particular type of organism only once?

Chapter

10 Viruses

Chapter Outline

Learning Objectives

After you have read this chapter, you should be able to:

1. Define capsid, capsomere, virion, nucleocapsid, and envelope.
2. Explain the basis for classification of viruses into two major groups.
3. Describe three major morphological types of viruses.
4. Describe the sequence of events occurring in the replicative cycle of viruses.
5. List three in vitro methods of cultivating viruses.
6. Explain the significance of the 50 percent infectious dose (ID_{50}).
7. Explain the difference between a lytic cycle and lysogeny.
8. Describe the role of reverse transcriptase in cells infected with retroviruses.

The first to recognize that viruses were different from other forms of life was the Dutch botanist and microbiologist Martinus Beijerinck (1851–1931). He was the first to propose the existence of a noncellular form of life in 1899. More than 35 years later, W. M. Stanley (1904–1971) concluded that the tobacco mosaic virus was protein in nature. It was not until 1952 that the core of a virus was found to contain a nucleic acid. We now know that viruses are ultramicroscopic biological entities containing either DNA or RNA surrounded by a protein coat. The tiny particles only exhibit properties associated with life within host cells because they lack the ability to generate energy to support independent living. Infectious disease specialists view viruses as the causes of some serious diseases, but molecular biologists consider them resources for the diversity of the gene pools in many organisms.

THE STRUCTURE AND SPECIFICITY OF VIRUSES

Viruses are not merely particles of ill-defined shape or detail, but they actually consist of almost perfect geometric designs. In the extracellular phase, viruses exist as inert particles known as **virions.** Virions have an inner core of nucleic

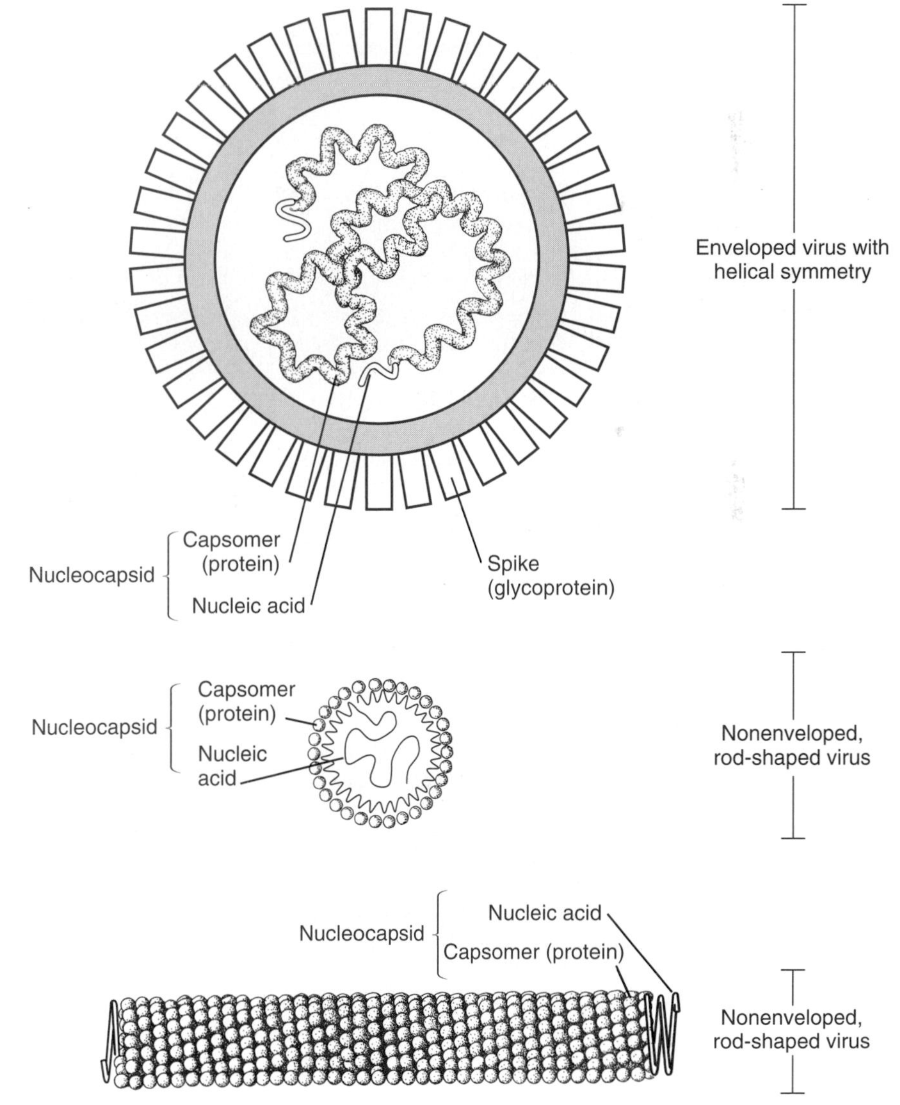

Figure 10–1 ◆ Morphology of viruses. Representations of three forms of viruses: enveloped with helical symmetry; nonenveloped, spheroidal; and nonenveloped, rod-shaped.

acid surrounded by proteins, which make up the **capsid.** Aggregates of the structural units of the protein, which can be seen by electron microscopy, are called **capsomeres.** The nucleic acid and the capsid make up the **nucleocapsid.**

Shape and Size

Most nucleocapsids demonstrate helical or polyhedral symmetry (Fig. 10–1). The tobacco mosaic virus is a good example of a helical virus. The inner core of RNA is surrounded by a capsid made up of about 2000 capsomeres (Fig. 10–2). Many of the nucleocapsids are geometric figures with 12 corners, 20 triangular faces, and 30 edges. The multifaced structures are known as **icosahedrons.** The herpes simplex virus is an example of a virus with icosahedral symmetry (Fig. 10–3). It contains 12 five-sided capsomeres and 150 six-sided capsomeres.

Some nucleocapsids are enclosed in an envelope of host-cell membrane or viral origin; others are nonenveloped. The nonenveloped viruses are often described as naked. Some envelopes have surface projections, called **spikes,** which are made up of glycoproteins. Most virions range in size from 20 to 300 nm.

Bacteriophages (viruses that infect bacterial cells) have **heads** with icosahedral symmetry and distinct appendages, known as **tails,** with helical symmetry. The T-even phages of *Escherichia coli* are typical of the tailed bacterial viruses (Fig. 10–4). The heads of bacteriophages contain nucleic acid surrounded by protein; tails contain several proteins. The tail is used like a syringe to inject viral nucleic acid after attachment to the cell. The outer core of protein is surrounded by a contractile sheath and is attached to an end plate and tail fibers.

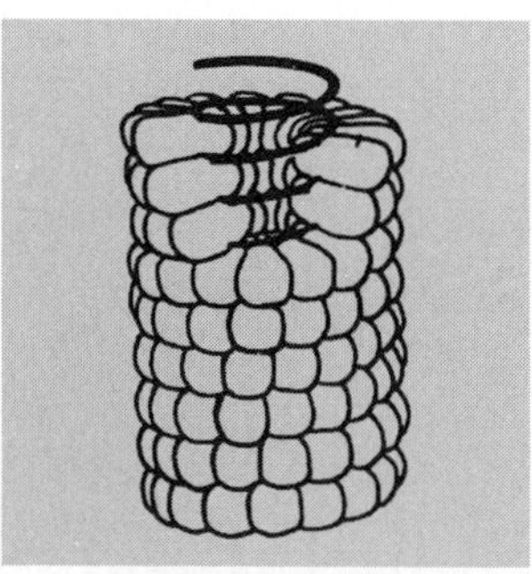

Figure 10–2 ◆ Tobacco mosaic virus showing helical symmetry. The RNA is embedded in the protein.

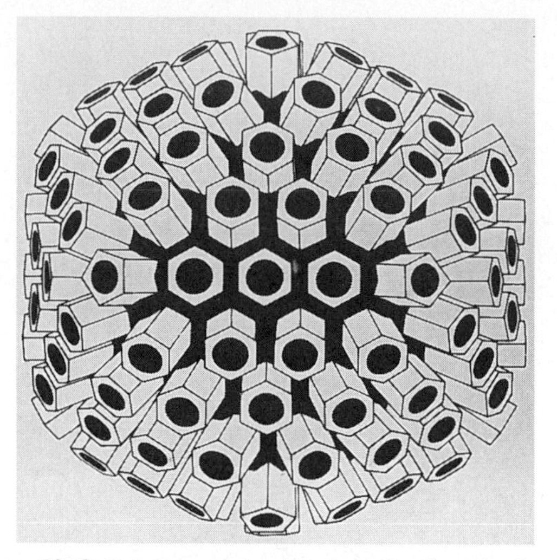

Figure 10–3 ◆ A herpes simplex virus showing the icosahedral symmetry of the virus.

The poxviruses are even more complex in structure. Many of the virions are brick-shaped, with the nucleic acid arranged as a tubular structure in a crisscross pattern. The orf virus, which causes infectious pustular dermatitis, mainly in sheep, is a virus showing this crisscross structure (Fig. 10–5).

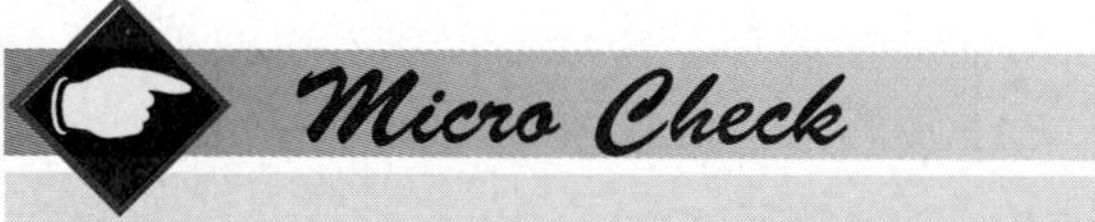

- Why are viruses unable to replicate independently of host cells?
- How do viruses differ from their host cells?
- Why do molecular biologists view viruses as important resources on Earth?

Host Range and Specificity

Viruses outnumber their host cells, and numerous specific viruses can infect a single type of cell. The ability of viruses to become incorporated into the nucleic acid of host cells makes it impossible to take an accurate census of their numbers.

The specificity of viruses for particular cell types is an indication of the ability of those cells to support their replication. Some viruses demonstrate a high degree of specificity. HIV, for example, infects cells known as $CD4^+$ cells, whereas

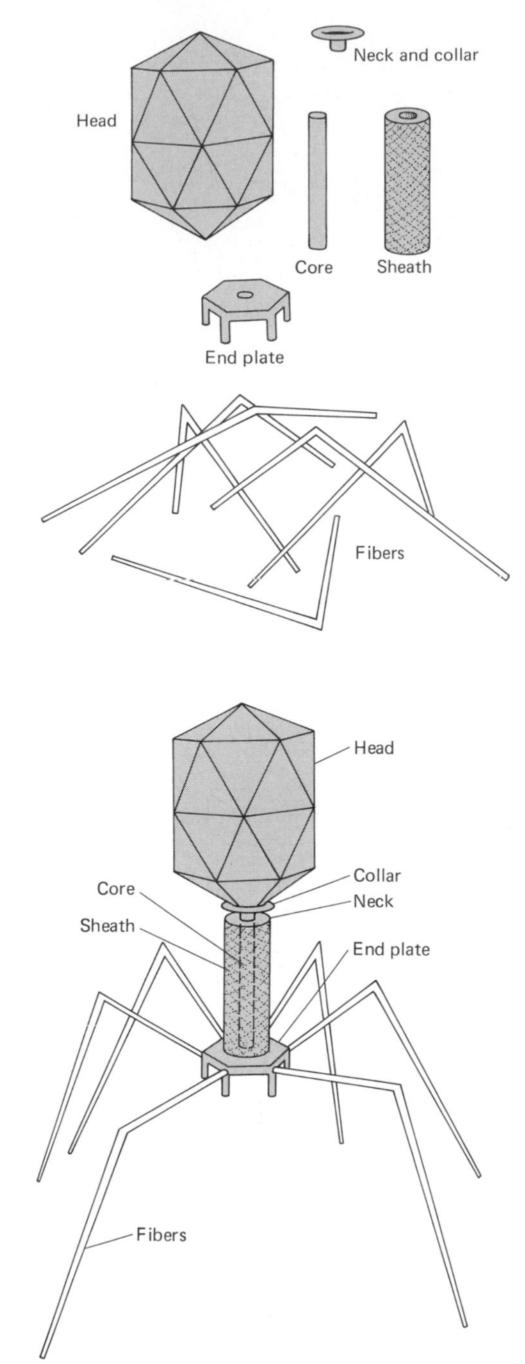

Figure 10–4 ◆ T-even phage. The component parts and the assembled phage are shown.

the hepatitis viruses infect only liver cells. Some other viruses are able to cause multiorgan disease because cells of more than one organ support their replication. The mumps virus is best known for the facial distortion caused by the presence of the virus in the salivary glands. However, the thyroid, pancreas, testicles, ovaries, and meninges are not uncommon sites of mumps infection.

Unfortunately, some viruses can cross the placenta and infect the fetus. Less than one fourth of HIV-infected mothers pass the infection on to their infants by placental transfer. Cytomegalovirus (CMV) infection during pregnancy is a major cause of mental retardation, blindness, and impaired hearing in children.

Binding of viruses to particular cells is dependent on the presence of receptors specific for those viruses on plasma membranes. Antigens on envelopes or capsids bind to the specific receptors when viruses and potential host cells collide. Infection is initiated when viruses enter the cells.

Classification of Viruses

Viruses are divided into two major groups on the basis of the type of nucleic acid contained within the particles. A virus contains either DNA or RNA in the core. Additional characteristics, such as molecular weight of nucleic acid strands, size and shape of virions, nucleocapsid symmetry, and strategy of replication, are used to categorize viruses. Some single-stranded RNA viruses bind directly to ribosomes of host cells. The DNA viruses and double-stranded RNA viruses are transcribed to mRNA directly or indirectly by replicative intermediates (RIs) (intervening compounds necessary for duplication). Transcription is described in Chapter 7.

A strand of RNA that acts as mRNA in the synthesis of proteins is called a **positive sense RNA.** A strand of RNA that must be transcribed to form a complementary strand of mRNA is called a **negative sense RNA.** Positive or negative

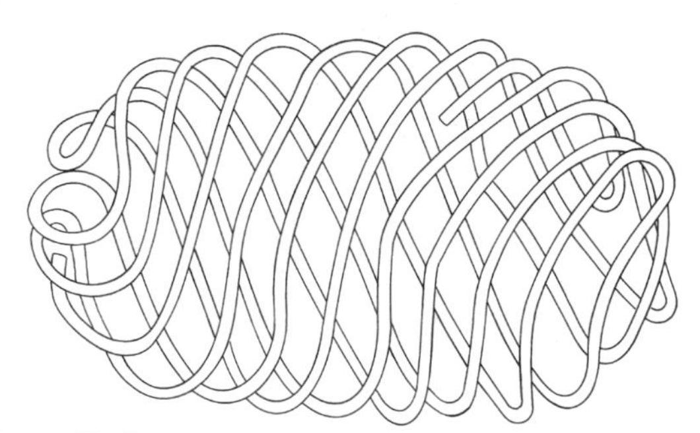

Figure 10–5 ◆ Orf virus with complex winding of the viral DNA.

Table 10–1
PROPERTIES OF MAJOR DNA VIRUSES OF VERTEBRATES

GROUP	NUMBER OF STRANDS	SIZE OF VIRION	SHAPE OF VIRION	NUCLEOCAPSID	ENVELOPE
Parvovirus	1	18–24 nm	Cubical	Icosahedral	−
Hepadnavirus	1.5	42–47 nm	Usually spherical	Icosahedral	+
Papovavirus	2	40–55 nm	Cubical	Icosahedral	−
Adenovirus	2	70–80 nm	Cubical	Icosahedral	−
Herpesvirus	2	180–200 nm	Pleomorphic	Icosahedral	+
Poxvirus	2	230–300 nm	Brick-shaped	Complex	−

sense strands of DNA also exist, but single strands are always converted to double-stranded molecules before mRNA is transcribed. Antisense DNA or RNA has application in blocking the flow of genetic expression in the synthesis of undesired products.

Some RNA viruses, containing negative sense sequences, code for the enzyme **reverse transcriptase.** The enzyme is responsible for making a copy of DNA from RNA in a process of reverse transcription.

Family names, ending in "idae," are used in classifying viruses, but the simplified group names have remained popular. All viruses in a group share common characteristics, but may differ in host-cell specificity. The subdivision of families into genera has gained some acceptance, but medical microbiologists rarely use generic names. They still refer to them by the disease they cause. The properties of the major viruses causing disease in vertebrates, including humans, are listed in Tables 10–1 and 10–2.

REPLICATION OF VIRUSES

The host-parasite relationship between cells and viruses is unique in that resources of host cells are used for viral replication. An orderly series of events occurring during the synthesis of viruses within cells constitutes the infectious process. The sequence of events includes attachment, penetration, uncoating, multiplication, assembly, and release. The events caused by virulent viruses is called a **lytic cycle** (Fig. 10–6). Bacterial cells infected with virulent bacteriophages are destroyed when new infective particles are released.

Attachment

The initial contact between viruses and susceptible cells is a random event. After collision, the virus particles bind to receptor sites on host cells.

Table 10–2
PROPERTIES OF MAJOR RNA VIRUSES OF VERTEBRATES

GROUP	NUMBER OF STRANDS	SIZE OF VIRION	SHAPE OF VIRION	NUCLEOCAPSID SYMMETRY	ENVELOPE
Reovirus	2	54–75 nm	Cubical	Icosahedral	−
Calicivirus	1	27–30 nm	Cubical	Icosahedral	−
Picornavirus	1	18–30 nm	Cubical	Icosahedral	−
Togavirus	1	60–70 nm	Cubical	Icosahedral	+
Flavivirus	1	40–50 nm	Spherical	Icosahedral	+
Orthomyxovirus	1	80–120 nm	Roughly spherical	Helical	+
Paramyxovirus	1	100–300 nm	Pleomorphic	Helical	+
Rhabdovirus	1	60–225 nm	Bullet-shaped	Helical	+
Bunyavirus	1	90–100 nm	Roughly spherical	Helical	+
Retrovirus	1	100 nm	Roughly spherical	Icosahedral	+

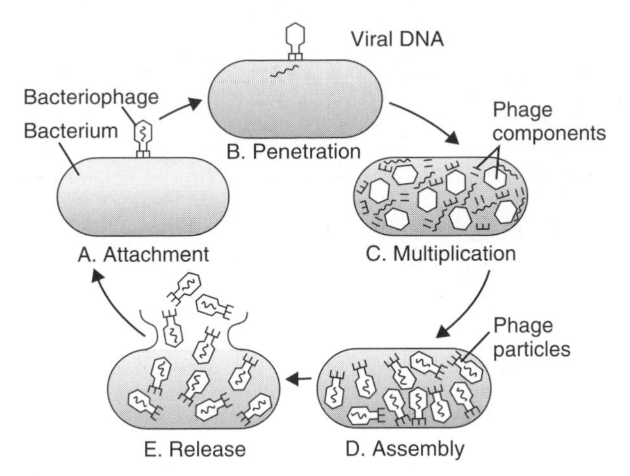

Figure 10–6 ◆ Lytic cycle of a typical bacteriophage showing the sequence of events in replication.

The tail fibers of bacteriophages and the spikes of enveloped viruses are well adapted for attachment. The receptors are often proteins that are located on particular types of cells. It is the lack of specific receptors on cells that restricts most viruses from having a wide host-cell range.

Penetration

Viruses may play an active or a passive role in the penetration process that follows attachment. The T_2 bacteriophage of *Escherichia coli* injects only the nucleic acid portion of the virus particle through the bacterial cell wall. Transfer of other viruses across plasma membranes requires no viral activity. Some viruses appear to be engulfed by cells in a process called **viropexis** (Fig. 10–7). A fusion of the plasma membrane and the virus facilitates entry of the virus.

Uncoating

Penetration and uncoating of the nucleic acid of viruses are sometimes coupled steps, occurring during or before completion of penetration. Capsids of bacteriophages never enter host cells. Other capsids are destroyed after entry of whole virions by cellular or viral-coded enzymes. A few viruses retain small amounts of protein.

Multiplication

Multiplication of specific viruses usually takes place only in the cytoplasm or the nucleus of cells (Fig. 10–8). Both the cytoplasm and the nucleus of a few host cells support replication. The steps involved in the production of more infective particles parallel very closely the synthetic processes in cells except that viral nucleic acid supplies the genetic information. Transcription of RNA from host DNA ceases almost immediately after penetration. The complete resources of host cells are committed to the synthesis of viral nucleic acid and proteins.

Assembly

The assembly of newly synthesized nucleic acids and proteins sometimes requires special enzymes made by virus-directed synthetic processes. Assembly of the components of a few viruses has been accomplished in vitro, but the exact mechanism for packaging viral nucleic acid into a preconstructed capsid is not well understood. The period from the entry of a virus into a host cell and the appearance of infectious progeny is called the **eclipse period** (Fig. 10–9). The eclipse period ranges from 5 to 20 hours for DNA viruses and from 2 to 10 hours for RNA viruses.

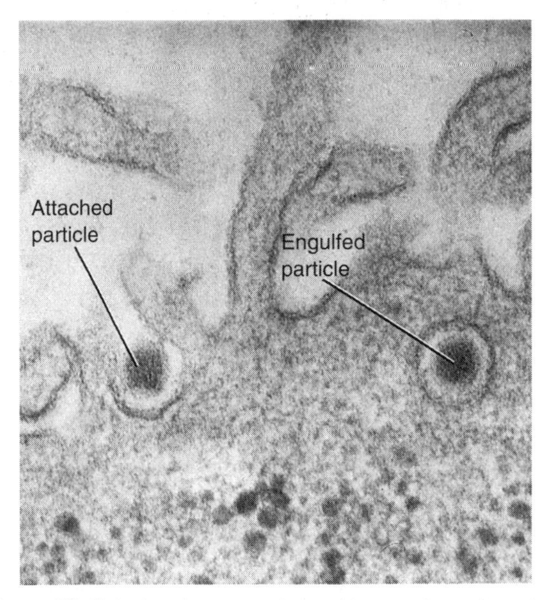

Figure 10–7 ◆ Attachment and engulfment of an adenovirus. One particle is attached to the surface of a cell; the second has been engulfed by the process of viropexis.

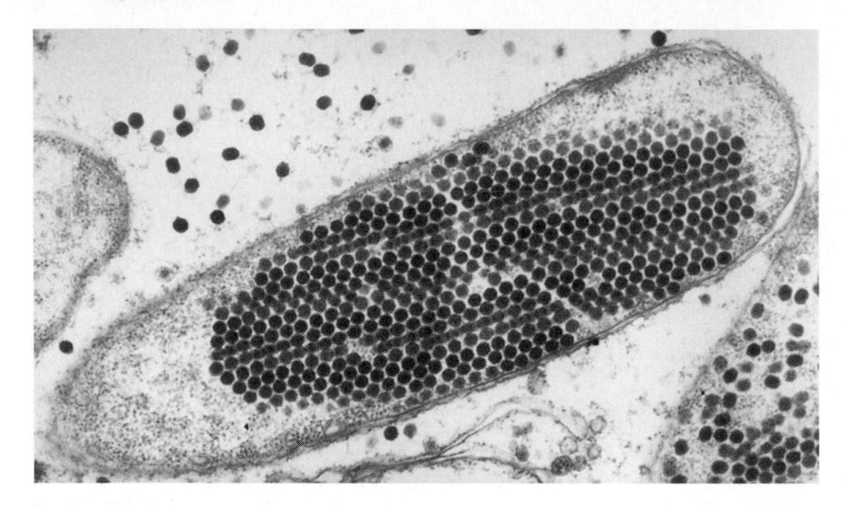

Figure 10–8 ◆ Electron micrograph of ultrathin section of T_2-infected *Escherichia coli*. The polyhedral bodies represent condensates and intact phage particles.

Release

Mature progeny of bacteriophages are liberated from their bacterial hosts when a viral-coded enzyme promotes cell lysis (dissolution). Infective particles of some animal viruses form at the cell surface and are released by a budding process (Fig. 10–10). Budding is initiated when a viral glycoprotein is inserted into the plasma membrane. With movement of assembled virions, cellular proteins are displaced and incorporated into viral capsids or envelopes. The yield of infective particles varies with the host-virus system. A bacterium produces 200 or more infective particles; a human cell frequently makes as many as 10^5 to 10^6 infective particles.

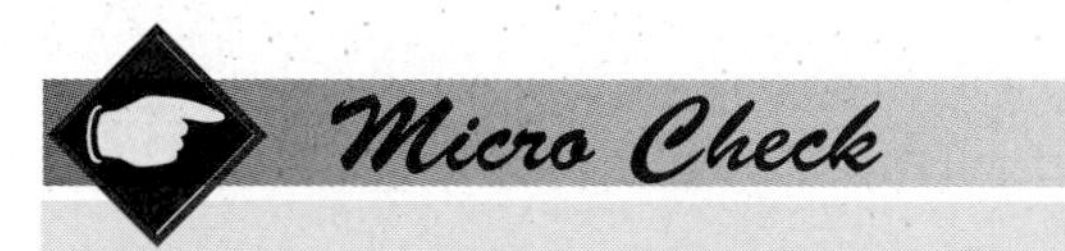

- What is meant by positive and negative sense nucleic acids?
- What is the major criterion used to classify viruses?
- What is an eclipse period?

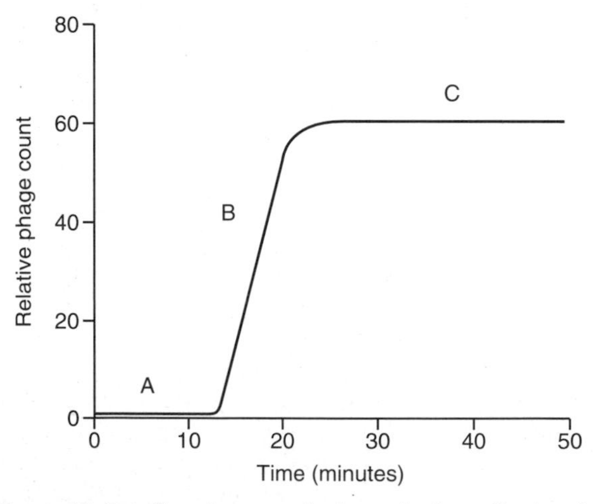

Figure 10–9 ◆ Growth curve of a bacteriophage. During the eclipse period (A) no intact viruses can be recovered from cultures. In the rise period (B) phages are released when cells lyse. The yield is maximal (C) when all bacterial cells have been destroyed.

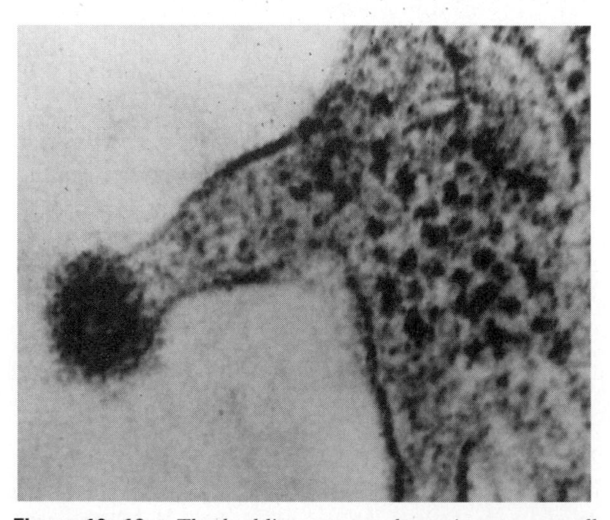

Figure 10–10 ◆ The budding process shown in a tumor cell of a mouse. Completed particles can infect other susceptible cells.

HIDDEN VIRUSES

Some of the most fascinating relationships exist between viruses and their host cells. Long known for their ability to destroy infected cells, some viruses establish a stable carrier state within infected cells by becoming integrated into host chromosomes. Sometimes, integrated genes are transcribed along with those of host cells; other times they alter expression of some of the host's genes. We are just beginning to discover the ramifications of intimate, but often hidden, relationships of viral and host genes, which have been evolving over hundreds of years.

Lysogeny

When DNA of viral origin is integrated into genetic material of a host bacterium, the phage loses its ability to produce a lytic cycle. The integrated DNA forms a relationship with its host cell known as lysogeny (Fig. 10–11). The phage is called a **prophage.** Bacteriophages capable of integrating into host-cell DNA are called **temperate** phages. During the association, bacterial cells are immune to infection by a phage of the same type. If part of the prophage is transcribed, it confers new properties to the host bacterium. The expression of one or more new characteristics of a bacterium containing a prophage is known as **lysogenic conversion.**

The ability of bacteria, such as *Corynebacterium diphtheriae, Streptococcus pyogenes,* and *Clostridium botulinum,* to produce potent exotoxins is derived from lysogenic conversions. Lysogeny occurs frequently in nature, but rarely in bacteria grown in the laboratory. The traits acquired by lysogenic conversion often are protective or permit the host bacterium to use a greater variety of energy sources.

A prophage can revert to a lytic phage spontaneously or in response to an environmental factor. Ultraviolet light, alkylating agents, and some carcinogens are known to induce the reversion. The return to the lytic phage is called **zygotic induction.**

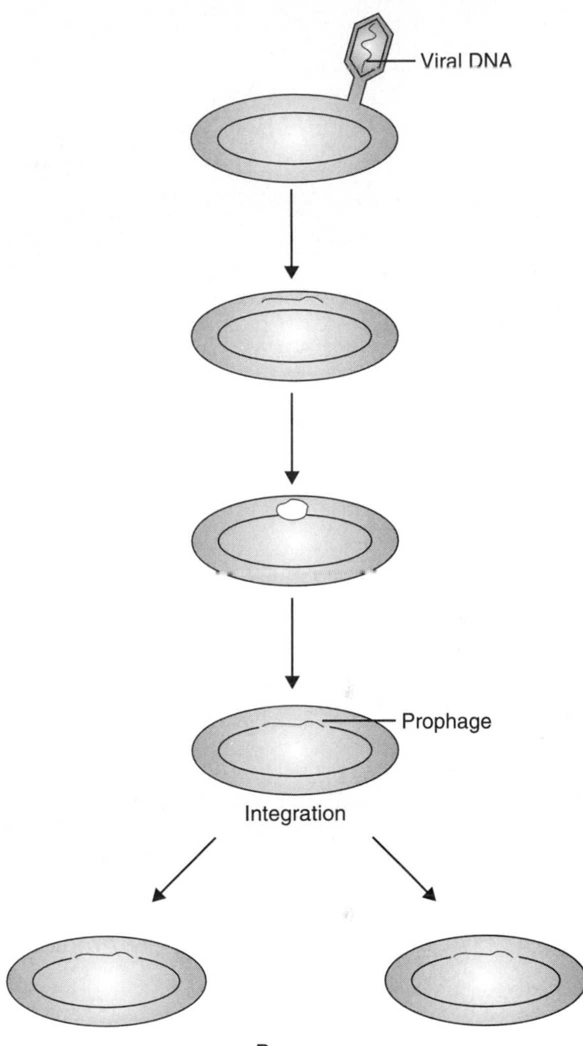

Figure 10–11 ◆ Lysogeny. Viral DNA becomes integrated into DNA of a host bacterium, producing a prophage.

Latency

Some viruses establish a latent (dormant) state in host cells. The viral nucleic acid becomes integrated into the nucleic acid of a host cell. The hidden viral DNA is known as a **provirus.** A latent virus can be reactivated in the future and produce infective viral particles followed by signs and symptoms of the infectious state in a host. Factors known to trigger activation of latent viruses include stress, another viral infection, and exposure to ultraviolet light. Among the human viruses that exhibit latency are those that cause fever blisters, chickenpox, and HIV infection. A major problem caused by latency is the unpredictability of its duration. Latent periods for HIV have not been much over two years in some individuals. Other persons having an HIV infection have experienced prolonged periods of HIV latency and remained in good health for several years.

CULTIVATION OF VIRUSES

Because viruses need the resources of living cells for replication, the techniques for cultivating them are more complex than those required for growing bacteria. The propagation of type-specific bacteriophages can be accomplished by adding infectious phage particles to a culture of susceptible bacteria. Within a few hours, lysis of cells occurs and phage particles can be harvested.

Animals or plants were employed in the earliest attempts to cultivate viruses affecting those organisms, but only limited information on host cell-virus relationships could be obtained. It became feasible to cultivate cells in vitro when plant or animal cells could be freed from tissue by the enzyme trypsin and when antibiotics became available for preventing contamination of cultures. The three most common methods for culturing animal viruses employ (1) embryonated eggs, (2) cell cultures, and (3) animals.

Embryonated Eggs

The developing chicken embryo is a suitable medium for growing a variety of viruses including those of influenza, rabies, canine distemper, and mumps. It takes 21 days for a fertilized ovum to develop into a chick. During the first week after fertilization, the extraembryonic membranes and cavities are formed. Viruses show some selectivity for particular embryonic structures. The age of the embryo required and the route of inoculation depend on the virus to be grown (Fig. 10–12). Some grow best in the allantoic or amniotic cavities; others multiply more readily on the chorioallantoic membrane, in the yolk sac, or less frequently, in the developing embryo.

A candling device, which exposes embryonated eggs to a concentrated beam of light, identifies the vascular structure of the chorioallantois prior to inoculation. Eggs are marked on the shell at a point of inoculation that avoids large blood vessels. Shells are disinfected and punctured, and viruses are injected into the appropriate structure of the eggs. Eggs are examined for evidence of virus infection after a week or more of incubation at 35° to 37°C. Some viruses produce distinct lesions, known as pocks, on the chorioallantoic membrane (Fig. 10–13). Sometimes growth of the embryo is only stunted; other times the embryo dies. The presence of viruses in embryonic fluids is detected by animal inoculation or hemagglutination activity (clumping of red blood cells). Viruses causing vaccinia (cowpox), mumps,

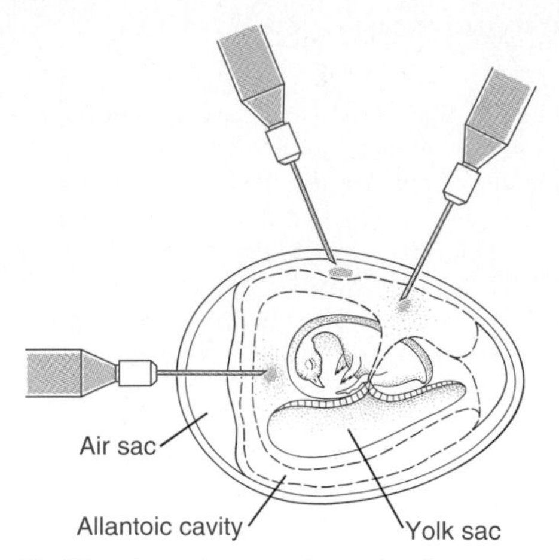

Figure 10–12 ◆ An embryonated egg showing routes of inoculation. The virus grows on cells of membranes lining cavities.

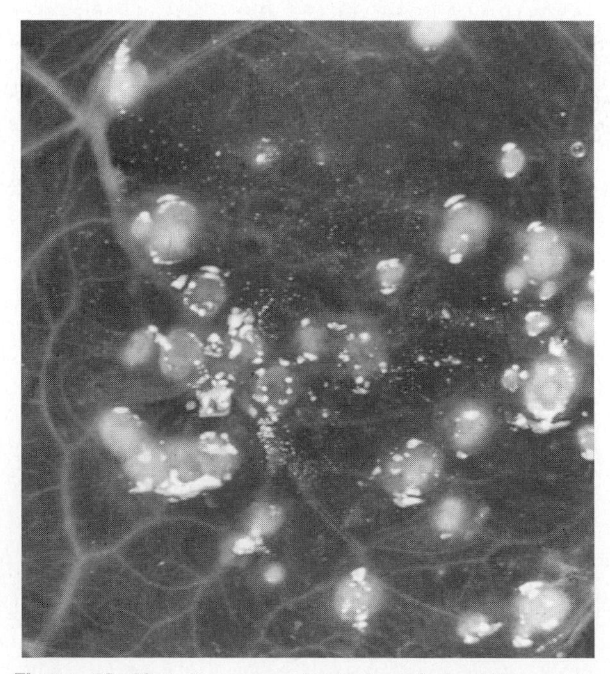

Figure 10–13 ◆ Pox on a chorioallantoic membrane of a chicken embryo infected with vaccinia virus.

and influenza bind to receptors on some red blood cells, producing visible agglutination.

Cell Cultures

Cell cultures are the most desirable method for studying host cell-virus relationships. Viruses may be grown in **primary** cell cultures, which have limited capacities for subculture, or in **continuous** cell lines, which can be transferred an indefinite number of times in media containing essential nutrients. Primary cells usually can be successfully grown for only one to three months. They retain the diploid number of chromosomes of the parent tissue, but may undergo other alterations with serial culturing.

Continuous cell lines have adapted to an in vitro environment, but no longer resemble the host cells. The chromosome number usually increases, causing a condition known as **polyploidy.** Other changes may occur so that continuous cell lines actually consist of **cancerous cells.** Examples of continuous cell lines include monkey kidney cells, human fibroblasts, and human neoplastic (abnormally growing) cells.

Viruses may destroy cells of primary or continuous lines, change their appearance, or have no apparent effect on them. Infected cells often become round and more refractile than uninfected cells (Fig. 10–14). A more distinct morphological change, known as a **cytopathic effect** (CPE) may occur. The CPE is generally characteristic of a particular host cell-virus system. For example, multinucleated giant cells can be observed in tissue cultures infected with measles virus (Fig. 10–15). The CPE produced by some other viruses takes the form of inclusion bodies. The inclusion bodies appear at the site of viral replication and may consist of actual viral particles, their components, or remnants of viral particles.

Virus-infected cells may show no visible changes, but may have alterations in plasma membranes or metabolic activities. For example, the plasma membranes of some virus-infected cells have an affinity for red blood cells and will adsorb them (Fig. 10–16). Cells infected with adenoviruses sometimes agglutinate because plasma membranes are attracted to the red blood cells. Infected cells often bring about a change in the pH of the surrounding medium. With some host cell-virus systems, injury is associated with increases in pH; other viruses cause cells to produce acidic end products.

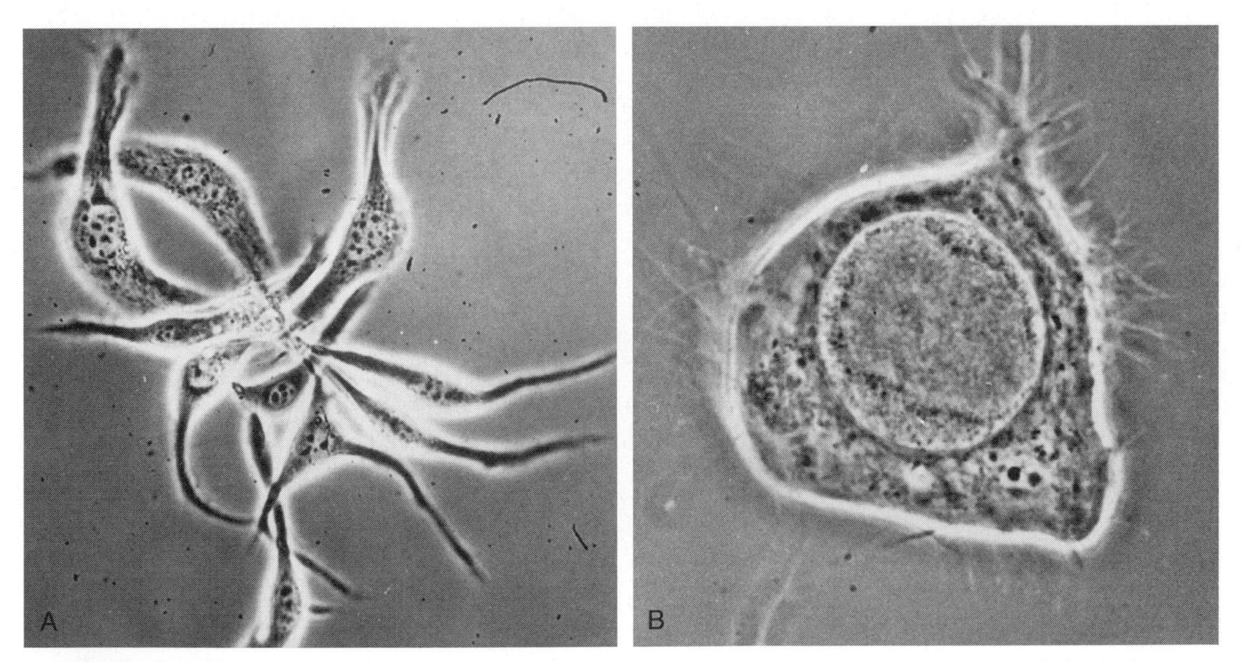

Figure 10–14 ◆ Effects of virus infection on cells. *A,* Uninfected ovarian cells. *B,* Early stage of a viral infection showing rounding of a cell.

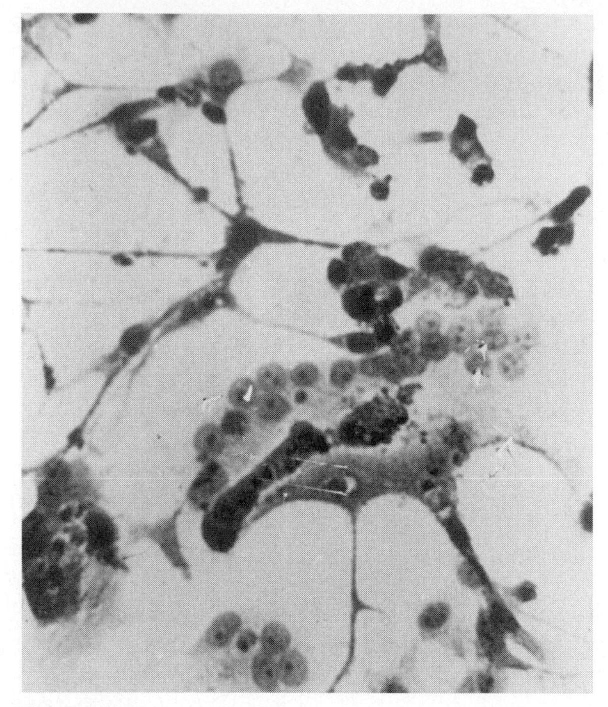

Figure 10–15 ◆ Human amnion cells infected with measles virus. Changes include formation of multinuclear giant cells.

Animals

Animals are still used for the isolation and identification of some viruses. For example, mice are employed for demonstration of the causative agents of encephalitis and rabies. In addition, chickens, mice, hamsters, guinea pigs, and rats are valuable in studying the viruses that induce tumors. Animals may be inoculated intracerebrally, intraperitoneally, intravenously, intranasally, intratracheally, or intradermally with nasal or throat washings, urine, or other body fluids. When mice are inoculated with rabies virus, the animals exhibit muscle incoordination and paralysis within a week or more after injection. Sections of brain may demonstrate cytoplasmic inclusions, known as Negri bodies. Viruses on brain-impression smears react with fluorescein-tagged antibodies. It is sometimes necessary with other viruses to mince tissue to free viruses for serological testing.

ENUMERATION OF VIRUSES

The small size of viruses and the complex methods required for cultivation prevent the use of bacteriological assay techniques for enumeration of virus particles. A count of physical particles provides limited information because the ability of the particles to infect cells remains unmeasured. The measurement of the infectivity of virus particles provides more meaningful information.

Particle Counts

Highly purified preparations of the larger viruses can be counted with an electron microscope. In one method, a known concentration of latex particles of approximately the same size as the viruses to be counted is mixed with the virus preparation. The ratio of latex to virus particles, multiplied by the concentration of latex particles, equals the concentration of virus particles (Fig. 10–17).

An alternate method for estimating virus particles employs the property of some viruses to cause agglutination of red blood cells. If twofold dilutions of virus preparation are incubated with red blood cell suspensions, the highest dilution of virus causing hemagglutination can be determined.

Infectivity Assays

A measure of the infectivity of viruses can be obtained by inoculating embryonated eggs, cell cultures, or animals with dilutions of virus sus-

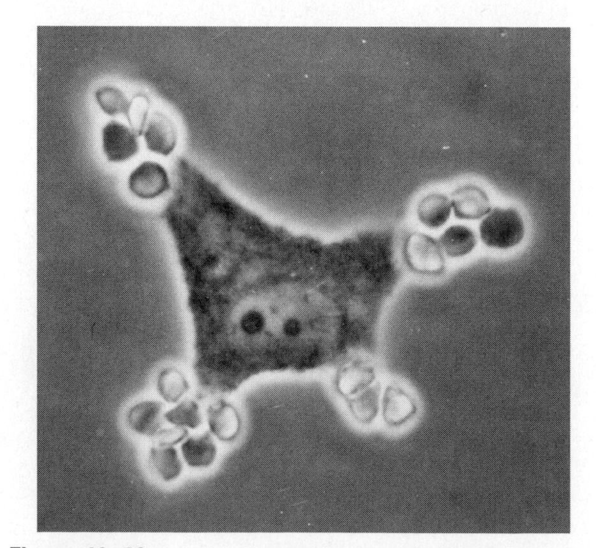

Figure 10–16 ◆ Adsorption of bovine red blood cells to a virus-infected cell.

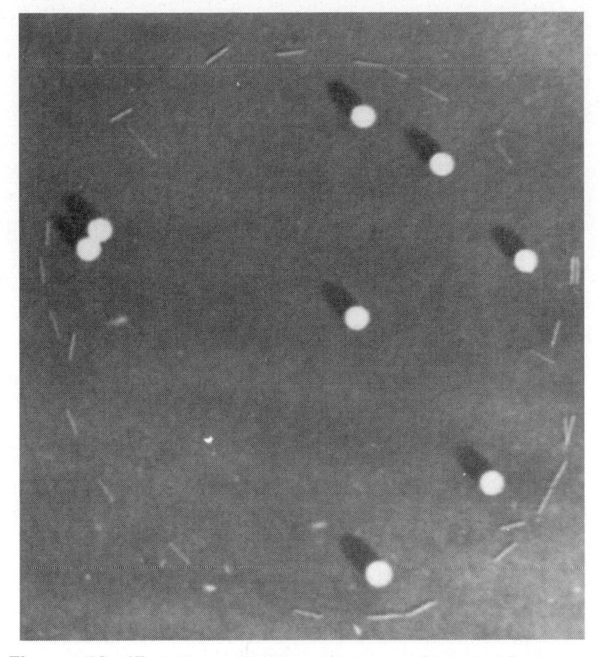

Figure 10–17 ◆ Enumeration of viruses by particle count. The ratio of latex particles (spheres) to tobacco mosaic viruses (rods) multiplied by the concentration of latex particles equals the concentration of viruses.

pensions. Effects, attributable to virus infection, are analyzed after appropriate incubation. The highest dilution of virus causing a noticeable effect contains at least one infective particle. The titer is expressed as the 50 percent infectious dose (ID_{50}). The titer is the reciprocal of the highest dilution that causes an effect due to a virus in one half of the embryonated eggs, cell cultures, or animals. For example, if 0.1 ml of a dilution of a virus suspension infected 50 percent of the test animals, the titer would be expressed as

$$\frac{1}{0.1 \times 10^{-6}} = 10^7\ ID_{50}/ml$$

Large numbers of tests are frequently necessary to obtain valid results.

A more precise and less costly estimation of viral infectivity is obtained by the plaque method. Dilutions of viral suspensions are added to monolayers of susceptible cells or, in the case of phage counting, to nutrient agar seeded with susceptible bacteria. Nutrient agar is sometimes added to monolayers of animal host cells. The growing host cells produce a "lawn" of growth interrupted by clear areas called **plaques** (Fig. 10–18). Each plaque is produced by the progeny of a single infectious particle called a **plaque-forming unit** (PFU). When compared with physical counts, the number of PFU is greater for phage particles than for animal viruses. The **efficiency of plating** (EOP) is obtained by comparing the ID_{50} with the electron microscope count.

THE MAJOR DNA VIRUSES OF VERTEBRATES

All the DNA viruses of vertebrates contain double-stranded DNA in the virion with the exception of the parvoviruses and the hepadnaviruses. The parvoviruses have a single strand of DNA and the hepadnaviruses are only partially

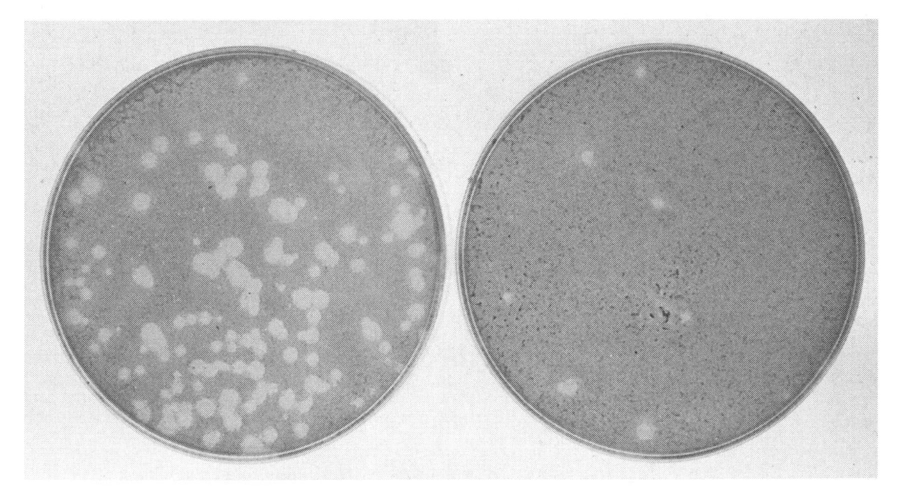

Figure 10–18 ◆ Typical plaque formation in a monolayer of human kidney cells infected with adenovirus 12. Each plaque represents a plaque-forming unit (PFU), where cells have been destroyed by progeny of an infective particle.

double-stranded. All except the poxviruses have icosahedral nucleocapsid symmetry.

Parvoviruses

The members of the parvoviruses are the smallest of the DNA viruses. They have cubic symmetry and have a naked nucleocapsid. DNA of the progeny is transcribed from the intermediate DNA, which has one strand of parental DNA (Fig. 10–19). Although a phase of replication occurs in the cytoplasm, capsid assembly takes place in the nucleus of the host cell. Some parvoviruses are so small that they depend on a helper virus to initiate infection. Parvoviruses are best known as causes of animal diseases, such as Aleutian disease of mink, canine parvovirus disease, and feline panleukemia. Vaccines are available for both the canine and feline infections.

Parvovirus B19 is the etiologic agent of contagious erythema infectiosum, sometimes called "fifth disease," in children. The same virus has been shown to be responsible for a type of aplastic anemia. The suppression of bone marrow function causes a depletion in circulating red blood cells.

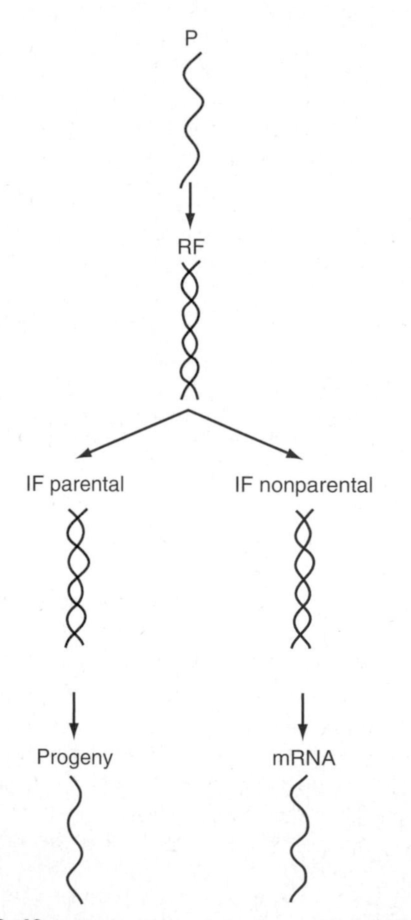

Figure 10–19 ◆ Replication of single-stranded DNA viruses. Parental DNA (P) serves as a template for the complementary strand of a replicative form of DNA (RF). Intermediate forms of DNA (IF) serve as templates for mRNA and progeny.

Hepadnaviruses

The enveloped virions of the hepadnaviruses are only partially double-stranded, but once inside a host cell, the single-stranded portion is restored to being double-stranded by a DNA polymer present in the core. The lipoprotein spikes of the envelope constitute the surface antigen (Hb_sAg). The replicative cycle uses a reverse transcriptive step in duplicating the viral genome in a procedure somewhat like that of the RNA-containing retroviruses. DNA replication occurs in the cytoplasm, but DNA transcription occurs in the nucleus of the host cell. The most studied hepadnavirus is hepatitis virus B (HVB).

The major polypeptide of the virion of HVB is the surface antigen known as HB_sAg. Core proteins HB_cAg and HB_eAg are immunologically distinct from the surface antigen. The HB_sAg is the first to appear and can be detected in active or chronic hepatitis B. HB_sAg by itself is noninfectious and is used in a currently licensed vaccine for HVB. About 2 to 10 percent of adults having hepatitis B infections develop chronic liver disease. An infant infected with HBV has an 80 to 85 percent chance of developing a chronic infection. Chronic carriers can transmit HBV through contact with body fluids and in utero to infants. The incidence of liver cancer is high in chronic carriers of HBV.

Papovaviruses

The papovaviruses, like other DNA viruses except the parvoviruses and hepadnaviruses, contain double-stranded DNA. However, unlike other DNA viruses, the nucleic acid is circular rather than linear in structure. The double-stranded DNA serves as a template for mRNA and progeny (Fig. 10–20). The naked icosahedral viruses replicate in the nucleus.

The papovaviruses produce tumors or tumor-like lesions in a number of animals, including

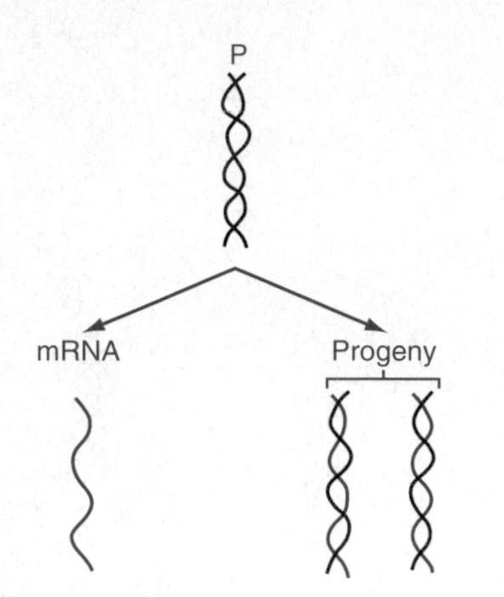

Figure 10–20 ◆ Replication of double-stranded DNA viruses. Parental DNA (P) serves as a template for mRNA and progeny.

humans. One group of papovaviruses, known as papillomaviruses, cause benign (harmless) and malignant (cancerous) warts in humans. Certain of the papillomaviruses are major suspects as causes of cervical cancer. DNA from papillomaviruses are found in dysplasia (abnormality of tissue development) in cervical epithelial cells and in invasive cancer of the cervix.

Adenoviruses

Members of the adenoviruses are icosahedral naked viruses containing double-stranded DNA in linear form. Replication occurs in the nucleus. There are at least 42 human adenoviruses. However, only half of those viruses have been demonstrated to cause disease. Adenoviruses are responsible for respiratory, gastrointestinal, and genitourinary infections, particularly in children, and for a severe eye infection, sometimes known as "shipyard eye." Adenoviruses can remain in tissue for long periods of time.

Herpesviruses

The herpesviruses are large, enveloped icosahedral DNA viruses. The envelopes are acquired by budding from the nuclear and plasma membranes of host cells. They replicate in the nucleus of infected cells. Some herpesviruses appear to have empty cores, but the significance of the barren cores is not clear (Fig. 10–21).

All herpesviruses possess the characteristic of latency, which permits them to lie dormant for a lifetime in host tissue. Upon activation they cause recurrent disease in their hosts. The viruses of fever blisters, genital herpes, chickenpox, cytomegalovirus infection, and infectious mononucleosis belong to the herpesvirus group. One herpesvirus, the Epstein-Barr virus (EBV), is the major cause of infectious mononucleosis, but it is also associated with Burkitt's lymphoma, a type of cancer found in limited areas of Africa and New Guinea. EBV has also been implicated in one type of nasopharyngeal cancer in southern China. The reasons for the geographic specificity of EBV-associated cancers are unclear.

The herpesviruses become reactivated in response to changes outside their immediate environment. Ultraviolet light, x-rays, heat, cold, hormonal imbalance, immune deficiencies, and physical or emotional stress can trigger recurrent infections. The presence of latent herpesviruses poses a special threat to bone marrow recipients and immunosuppressed patients.

Poxviruses

Not only are the poxviruses the largest of all DNA viruses, but they exhibit the most complex nucleocapsid symmetry. All poxviruses contain double-stranded DNA, protein, and lipids. They are the only DNA viruses that replicate only in the cytoplasm. Both a DNA-dependent RNA polymerase and a DNA-dependent DNA polymerase are associated with the virion.

Poxviruses include the viruses causing smallpox (now eliminated), vaccinia, and a benign tumor in humans known as molluscum contagiosum.

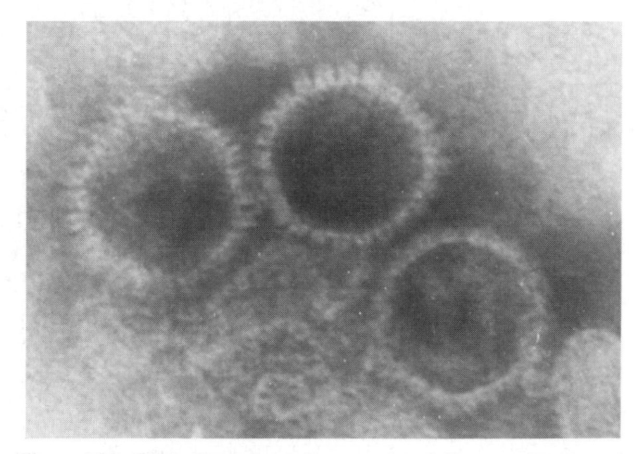

Figure 10–21 ◆ Electron micrograph of herpes simplex viruses showing barren cores.

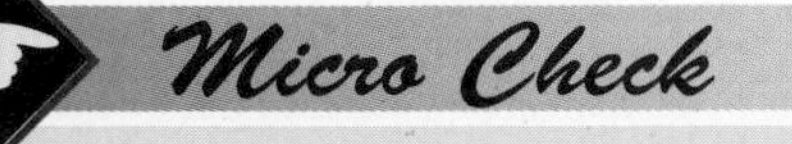

- Which of the DNA viruses causes an infection in children known as "fifth disease"?
- What are the major antigens detectable in HBV infections?
- What two characteristics of herpesviruses make them unique among the DNA viruses?

THE MAJOR RNA VIRUSES OF VERTEBRATES

The RNA viruses of vertebrates, with the exception of the reoviruses, contain single-stranded RNA. Some are without envelopes, and others have distinct envelopes. The group contains examples of both helical and icosahedral nucleocapsid symmetry. The mechanisms of replication are more complex than those for DNA viruses, often involving replication intermediates (RIs) and RNA-DNA hybrids. RNA-DNA hybrids contain one strand each of RNA and DNA. Most hybrids replicate in the cytoplasm, but a few are able to multiply in the cytoplasm or nucleus. The retroviruses continue to attract widespread attention because the AIDS virus belongs to that group. RNA tumor viruses have been isolated from chickens, rodents, cats, and humans.

Reoviruses

The reoviruses were once considered "respiratory enteric orphans" because they were not associated with particular diseases. Like many orphans, they now have found adoptive human hosts. Human reoviruses have icosahedral nucleocapsids and replicate only in the cytoplasm of host cells. They are the only double-stranded RNA viruses. The genome serves as a template for progeny and mRNA (Fig. 10–22). The discovery of reoviruses, also known as rotaviruses, in 1973 brought attention to reoviruses as causes of serious disease. At least a half-dozen rotaviruses are responsible for countless infant deaths in developing countries. The often severe vomiting and diarrhea cause rapid dehydration. Rotaviruses are also one cause of "traveler's diarrhea."

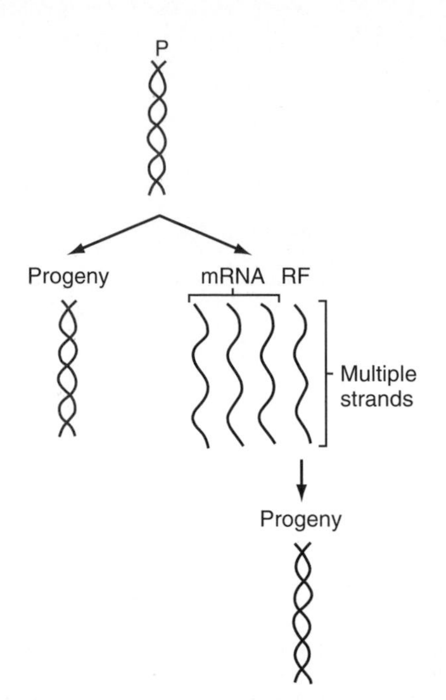

Figure 10–22 ◆ Replication of double-stranded RNA viruses. Parental RNA (P) serves as a template for multiple strands of mRNA, replicative forms (RF), or progeny. Newly synthesized RF can also serve as a template for progeny.

Picornaviruses

The picornaviruses are the smallest of the RNA viruses. They are naked viruses with icosahedral nucleocapsids. They replicate only in the cytoplasm of host cells. The single strand of RNA acts directly as mRNA or as a template for a replicative form (RF) (Fig. 10–23). Single-stranded RNA progeny, identical to parental RNA, are also formed from the RI. Progeny RNA can function, in turn, as mRNA or as a template for more RFs or proteins. Synthesis of an RNA-dependent RNA polymerase is cell-coded.

The viruses causing poliomyelitis, coxsackie disease, hepatitis A, and many enteric infections belong to the picornaviruses. The group also contains over 100 rhinoviruses, which are the cause of most common colds.

Togaviruses

Togaviruses are enveloped particles with icosahedral nucleocapsid symmetry. Many are not only transmitted by arthropod vectors, but can replicate in the cytoplasm of both vectors and animal hosts. The differences in size of togaviruses may be a reflection of variability in the deposition of

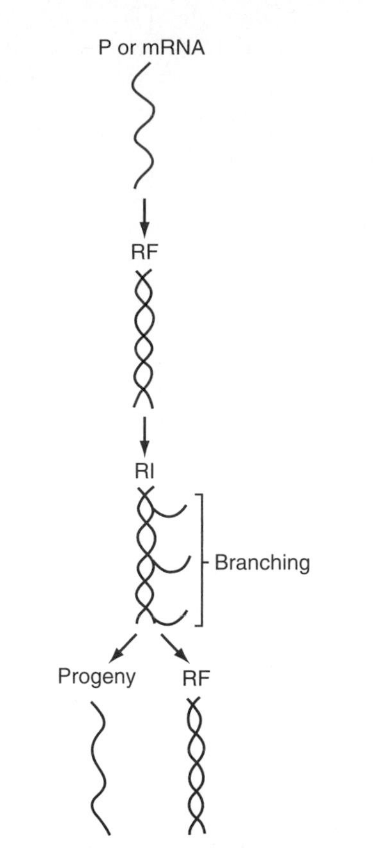

Figure 10–23 ◆ Replication of single-stranded RNA viruses. Parental RNA (P) acts directly as mRNA or as a template for a replicative form (RF), which in turn is transcribed into a replicative intermediate (RI). Progeny RNA can function as mRNA or as a template for more RF.

lipoprotein in the envelope during budding from plasma membranes of host cells. The mode of replication varies among togaviruses. With some, the single-stranded RNA can serve as mRNA, but in others, the method of replication has not been clearly demonstrated. The viruses causing rubella, eastern equine encephalitis (EEE), and western equine encephalitis (WEE) belong to the togaviruses.

Flaviviruses

Flaviviruses resemble togaviruses in structure, having envelopes and icosahedral symmetry. They also replicate alternately in the cytoplasm of their arthropod vectors and vertebrate hosts. The flaviviruses differ from the togaviruses in their method of replication. The genes coding for proteins are located at the 5′ end of the genome. Maturation of particles appears to occur within vesicles of the endoplasmic reticulum. Togaviruses and flaviviruses share one or more common antigens. Yellow fever, St. Louis encephalitis, Japanese B encephalitis, and hepatitis C are caused by flaviviruses. Hepatitis C virus (HCV) has been linked to chronic liver disease in many parts of the world.

Orthomyxoviruses

The orthomyxoviruses are roughly spherical, have envelopes, and demonstrate helical nucleocapsid symmetry. The envelopes contain two glycoproteins: a hemagglutinin antigen (HA) and a neuraminidase antigen (NA). Spikes are often seen radiating from the surface of the virions. Replication occurs in both the nucleus and cytoplasm of host cells. RNA, complementary to virion RNA, serves as mRNA, a template for progeny, and a RI (Fig. 10–24).

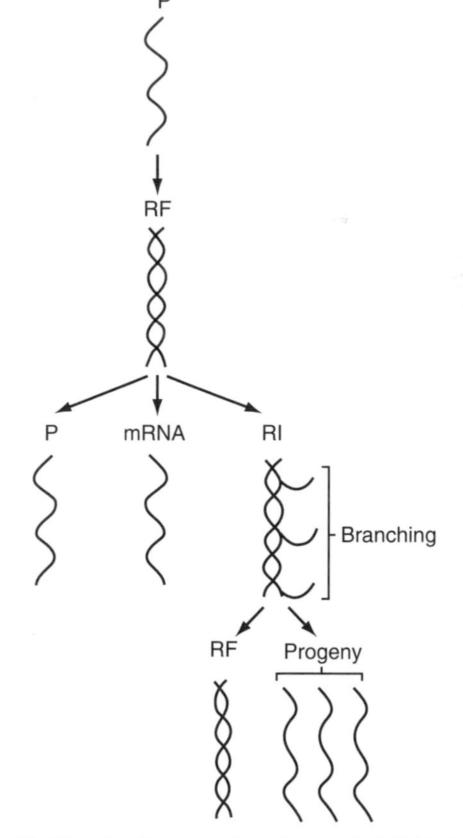

Figure 10–24 ◆ Replication of single-stranded RNA viruses in which mRNA is complementary to virion RNA. The replicative form (RF) can act as a template for the mRNA, progeny, or a replicative intermediate (RI). The RI can serve as a template for RF or progeny.

Influenza virus types A, B, and C are orthomyxoviruses. The antigenic alterations in the glycoproteins of the envelopes of types A and B permit the emergence of different virulent strains every year or two. The occurrence of recombinant variants in mixed infections is known as **antigenic shift.** A more subtle variation in influenza A virus appears to be caused by mutation. Mutant strains have a growth advantage in their hosts. An alteration occurring as consequences of mutation is called an **antigenic drift.** The H and N designation following an influenza virus letter name indicates a change in the hemagglutinin or neuraminidase antigens. Each year's influenza vaccine contains the two types of A and one type of B viruses most likely to circulate in the upcoming winter.

Paramyxoviruses

Paramyxoviruses are highly pleomorphic, enveloped viruses with helical nucleocapsid symmetry. Replication usually occurs in the cytoplasm in a manner similar to that for the orthomyxoviruses. Viral antigens are frequently found on plasma membranes of infected cells. Virus particles are released by budding. The viruses of measles, mumps, and respiratory syncytial viruses are members of the paramyxoviruses. The availability of an attenuated measles virus was thought to have practically eliminated measles in the United States as a public health threat. However, measles outbreaks have occurred in previously vaccinated school-aged children and college students. A four-dose schedule of measles vaccine is now recommended for all children.

Rhabdoviruses

All rhabdoviruses have a distinctive bullet shape. They are enveloped and have helical nucleocapsid symmetry. The viruses multiply in the cytoplasm. The replication cycle is similar to that found in the orthomyxovirus and paramyxovirus groups.

One rhabdovirus has the distinction of causing an agonizing, and almost invariably fatal disease called rabies. In the twentieth century, there was only one known case of human rabies in which the victim survived. The best way to prevent rabies in humans is to immunize domestic pets. It is virtually impossible to eliminate the infection among wild animals. The rabies vaccine has undergone much change since Pasteur saved the life of the boy Joseph Meister, who had been bitten so savagely by a rabid dog. Prompt administration of vaccine in persons exposed to the rabies virus can prevent the dreaded disease.

FOCAL POINT

Role of Swine in Virulence of Human Influenza Viruses

At first glance pigs might not seem to have much in common with humans except both belong to the same class (Mammalia) and are vertebrates. Yet pigs constitute mixing vessels for the reassortment of human and swine genes of influenza A virus in dual infections. There are at least 126 possible combinations of the genes for hemagglutinin (H) antigens and neuraminidase (N) antigens. The devastating pandemic of 1917–1918 was without doubt caused by an H1N1 strain of influenza virus A. The ability of pigs and humans to support both human and nonhuman strains of influenza virus A allows exchanges of surface antigens. Type B and C viruses are not known to undergo antigenic shifts. However, they can undergo antigenic drifts due to point mutations.

Influenza A virus, not unlike some other viruses, undergoes continuous mutations, causing antigenic drift in infected individuals with persistent infections. Variations in H antigens are also known to occur during attachment. Every new pandemic is caused by a change in the H antigen on the surface of the influenza A particle. New strains shall continue to emerge as long as animal reservoirs exist and mutations occur in human hosts.

Most attention has been focused on prevention of type A influenza infections, but epidemics of type B influenza also occur. Administration of vaccines containing inactivated viruses of influenza H or N antigen-specific A and/or B viruses is the best means to prevent epidemics or pandemics of influenza.

Clin Microbiol Rev 5(1):74–92, 1992.

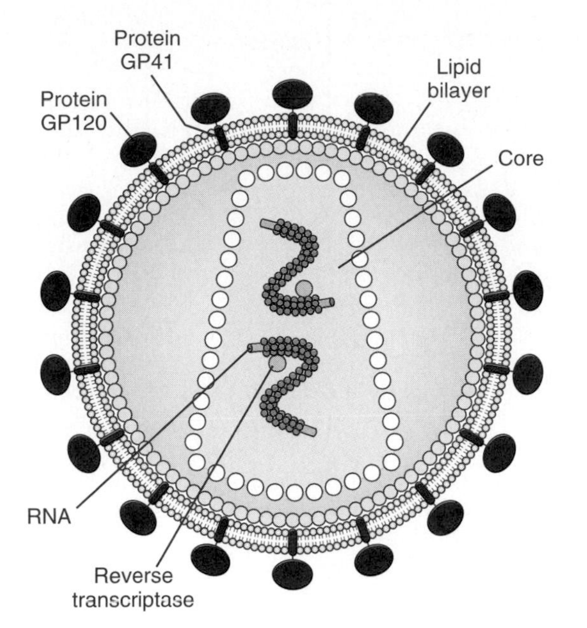

Figure 10–25 ◆ Structure of the human immunodeficiency virus (HIV).

Bunyaviruses

The bunyaviruses, long known as causes of hemorrhagic fever and kidney dysfunction in animals, are the largest group of mammalian viruses. They resemble influenza viruses both morphologically and in their ability to evolve by antigenic drift or shift. Bunyaviruses replicate in the cytoplasm and produce buds in Golgi complexes. Most members of the group are transmitted by mosquitoes, sandflies, or ticks. Diseases caused by them include human encephalitis, sandfly fever, Rift Valley fever, and hantavirus pulmonary syndrome. The hantaviruses are usually borne by symptom-free rodents and excreted in saliva, feces, and urine. Transmission appears to be by aerosolized excreta.

Rift Valley fever (RVF) is a particularly devastating hemorrhagic disease that has occurred in East and South Africa. Mosquitoes are the likely vectors because outbreaks of RVF have followed periods of heavy rains. During the Korean war, thousands of soldiers developed hemorrhagic fever with kidney involvement. The etiologic agent was subsequently found to be a bunyavirus named Hantaan. A hantavirus surfaced as a cause of an acute respiratory disease in 1993 in the United States. Because rodent control is difficult, if not impossible, a vaccine is clearly needed.

Retroviruses

Retroviruses get their name from the quite different series of events that occur during their replication. It has been known for more than 80 years that some members of the group cause cancer in animals. Retroviruses have spherical virions and helical ribonucleoprotein with icosahedral nucleocapsids. The capsids are surrounded by host-derived envelopes containing spikes of virus-coded glycoproteins (Fig. 10–25). Retroviruses replicate in the nucleus, forming both RNA-DNA hybrids and DNA intermediates. The DNA intermediates are incorporated into the host cell genome (Fig. 10–26).

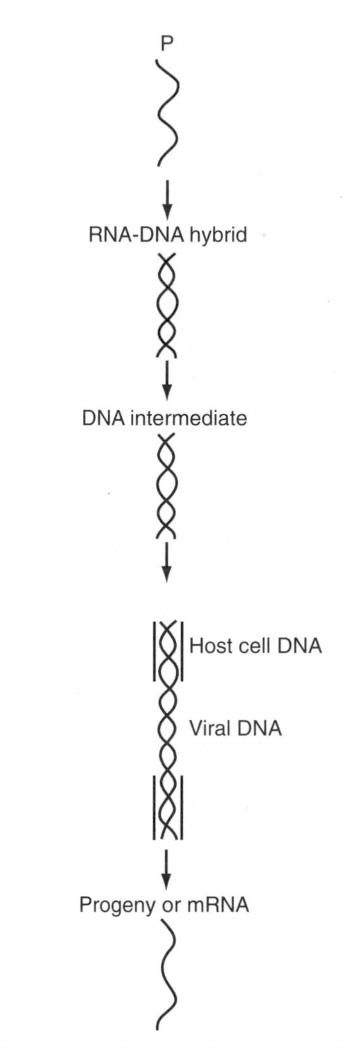

Figure 10–26 ◆ Replication of single-stranded RNA viruses having RNA-DNA hybrids and double-stranded DNA intermediates. The DNA intermediate is integrated into the host cell genome. Progeny or mRNA can be transcribed from integrated viral DNA.

A remarkable characteristic of retroviruses is their ability to code for reverse transcriptase, an enzyme that is responsible for transcription of DNA from RNA. The DNA copy of retrovirus RNA may exist as a **provirus** within host cells. A provirus can be activated by irradiation, certain chemicals, or immunological stimulation. The oncogenic (cancer-causing) retroviruses act rapidly, sometimes causing death in animals within weeks. That property is attributed to **oncogenes** (cancer-causing genes) of the retroviruses. Much attention has focused on the retrovirus that causes AIDS. That virus, known as the immunodeficiency virus (HIV), destroys a population of human cells with $CD4^+$ receptors, including the very immune cells necessary to initiate and sustain an immune response.

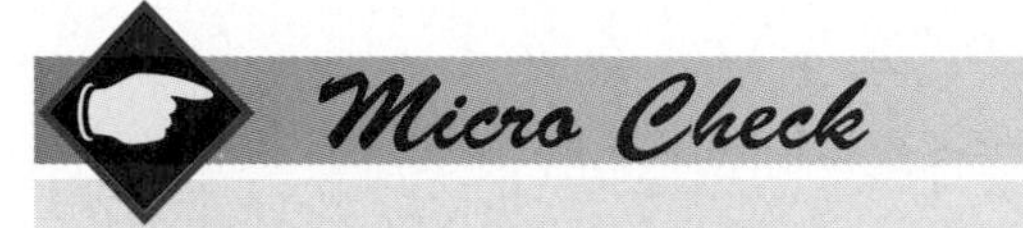

- To what major group of viruses do the more than 100 rhinoviruses belong?
- What is meant by "antigenic shift" and "antigenic drift" when referring to influenza viruses?
- What makes retroviruses unique among the RNA viruses?

Lesser Known Viruses

Some lesser known viruses are the members of the filovirus, arenavirus, and calcivirus groups. They are double-stranded RNA virions. All appear to cause zoonoses, but the animal reservoir of the filoviruses Marburg and Ebola remains a mystery. Twenty-five German laboratory workers, who handled monkey kidney cell cultures, contracted hemorrhagic fever in 1967. The monkey kidney cells were from monkeys imported from East Africa. Subsequent cases of a hemorrhagic fever occurred in the Sudan and Zaire almost a decade later. The etiologic agents, named for a city in Germany (Marburg) and a river in Zaire (Ebola), consist of identical long pleomorphic linear RNA filaments, but they are antigenically distinct from one another.

In 1969, a hemorrhagic fever, subsequently named Lassa fever, was reported in three missionary nurses living in the town of Lassa in eastern Nigeria. The cause of the disease was found to be an arenavirus.

Calciviruses are somewhat larger than picornaviruses and cause a variety of animal and human diseases. The Norwalk agent produces gastroenteritis in humans. Common source outbreaks have been traced to contaminated water supplies, food handlers, and seafood. Person-to-person transmission occurs by the fecal-oral route.

FOCAL POINT

The Challenges of Treating Viral Infections

Progress in antiviral therapy has been slow because of the difficulty in finding drugs capable of inhibiting viruses while leaving host-cell functions intact. By 1980, the drug acyclovir was found to be nontoxic enough to treat herpesvirus infections. Successful antiviral agents must reach target organs without disturbing cell function. The search for antiviral agents has been fueled by the unrelenting AIDS epidemic.

All the steps of the replicative cycle of viruses are potential targets for interference. Inhibition of synthesis of viral or host-coded enzymes necessary for replication have been popular targets for research. Among targeted enzymes have been reverse transcriptase, DNA or RNA polymerases, and nucleoside kinases.

A number of antiviral agents resemble natural nucleosides used in DNA synthesis. The drugs compete with nucleosides for substrates of enzymes. Unfortunately, some drugs inhibit DNA synthesis in uninfected cells. Acyclovir affects only virus-infected cells and zidovudine (ZDV) specifically interferes with reverse transcriptase, an enzyme not present in uninfected cells. Other enzymes, found only in virus-infected cells, represent potential targets for drugs as yet undeveloped.

Sometimes it is not possible to achieve concentrations of drugs in vivo that interfere with replication of viruses, but if symptoms can be minimized, antiviral agents can be deemed useful. Hyperimmune globulins (antibodies) and immune modulators (substances regulating immune responses) show promise in treatment of viral infections. Immune responses are critical to recovery from viral infections. When those responses fail to resolve viral infections, combination therapy with available drugs is a plausible alternative. Often drugs in combination delay the emergence of resistance to either drug and are associated with less toxicity.

Clin Microbiol Rev 5(2):146–182, 1992.

VIRUSES AND HUMAN CANCER

Cancer is a multicausal and complex disease. The exact role of viruses in human cancer has been difficult to explain. It is likely that Burkitt's lymphoma, one type of nasopharyngeal cancer, T-cell leukemia, cancer of the liver, and perhaps, cervical cancer are caused by viruses. It is impossible to fulfill Koch's postulates to establish definitive proof. The presence of a particular virus in human cancer may only be a risk factor. Environmental and host cofactors have important roles in establishing the disease.

VIROIDS, VIRUSOIDS, AND PRIONS

A number of infectious particles smaller than viruses have been discovered. They include viroids, virusoids, and prions. At one time the subviral entities were described as "slow viruses," but it is now known that at least some of the particles can grow quite rapidly under appropriate conditions.

Viroids

The viroids range in size from 15 to 100 nm. Some consist of single-stranded RNA only; others have an envelope surrounding the nucleic acid. Viroids replicate in plant cell nuclei and cause serious disease in palm trees, potatoes, tomatoes, and cucumbers.

Virusoids

The virusoids are satellite RNAs of helper viruses close in size to viroids. They are always found associated with a larger RNA plant virus that provides the genetic information for their replication.

Prions

Other smaller infectious particles, known as prions, contain protein only. Some scientists have questioned the existence of prions because proteins are not known to replicate, as do nucleic acids. The particles have been associated with mad cow disease, scrapie, a disease of sheep, and two human neurological diseases, known as kuru and Creutzfeldt-Jakob disease.

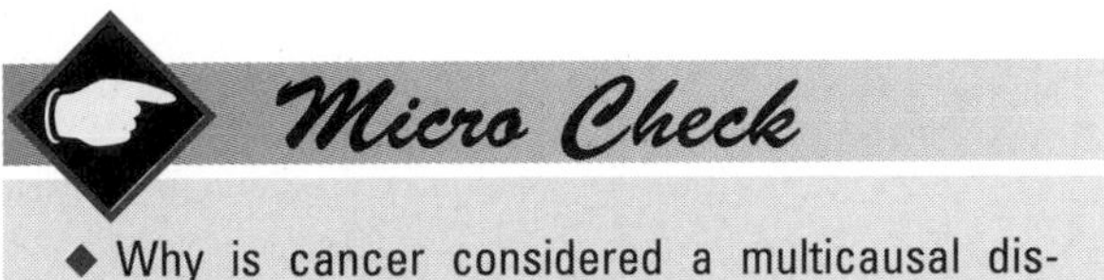

- Why is cancer considered a multicausal disease?
- Why are viroids, virusoids, and prions called subviral entities?
- Why are prions unique infectious agents?

Understanding Microbiology

1. How does a virion differ from a replicating form of a virus?
2. Explain what is meant by lysogenic conversion.
3. Describe the difference between a positive and negative sense strand of RNA.
4. What is the hallmark of herpesviruses?
5. Describe the major components of viroids, viruses, and prions.

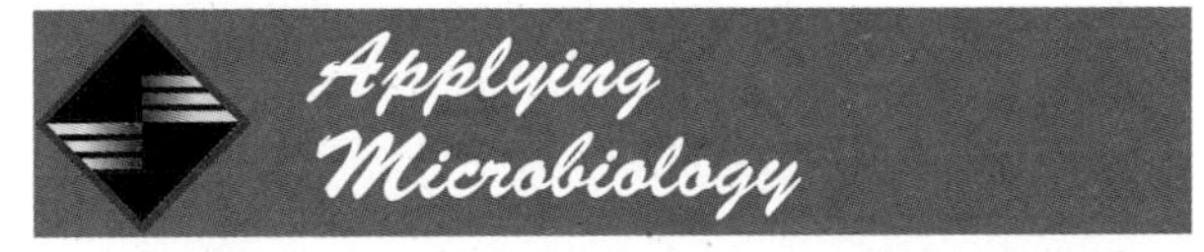

6. Prepare a statement of not more than five sentences designed to convince a senior citizen of the need for obtaining a flu vaccine every year.

Unit 4

Host-Parasite Relationships

Chapter 11

Epidemiology of Infectious Diseases

Chapter Outline

- **CLASSIFYING COMMUNITY DISEASES**
- **METHODS OF EPIDEMIOLOGY**
  - Descriptive Epidemiology
  - Analytical Epidemiology
  - Experimental Epidemiology
- **ASSESSMENTS OF DISEASE FREQUENCY**
  - Prevalence and Incidence
  - Morbidity and Mortality Rates
- **TYPES OF INFECTIOUS DISEASES**
  - Primary and Secondary Diseases
  - Opportunistic Diseases
  - Latent Diseases
  - Acute, Subacute, and Chronic Diseases
  - Local and Disseminated Diseases
  - Community- and Hospital-Acquired Diseases
- **RESERVOIRS OF INFECTIOUS AGENTS**
  - Biotic Reservoirs
  - Abiotic Reservoirs
- **MODES OF TRANSMISSION**
  - Direct Contact
  - Indirect Contact
  - Role of Air Currents
- **PORTALS OF ENTRY AND EXIT**
- **REPORTING COMMUNICABLE DISEASES**
- **RECOMMENDATIONS AND REGULATIONS FOR BLOODBORNE PATHOGENS**

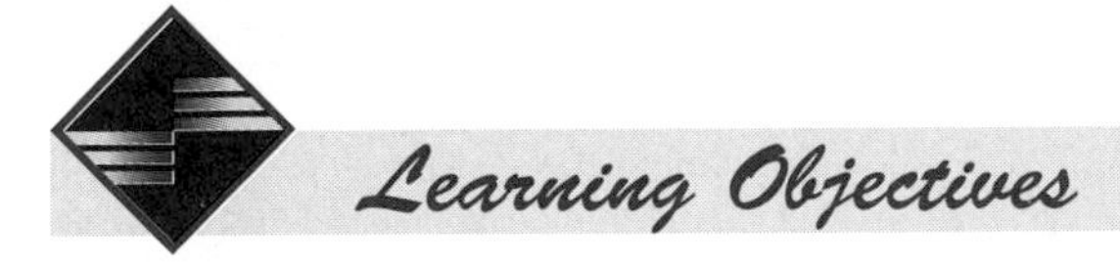

Learning Objectives

After you have read this chapter, you should be able to:

1. Differentiate between an infectious disease and a communicable disease.
2. Define epidemic, pandemic, and endemic.
3. Explain the role of carriers in communicable diseases.
4. Describe three types of epidemiological investigations.
5. Explain how infectious diseases are classified.
6. Differentiate between a reservoir and a mode of transmission.
7. Contrast the role of the Centers for Disease Control and Prevention (CDC) with that of the Occupational Safety and Health Administration (OSHA) in public health.

Epidemiology is the study of diseases occurring within populations. Our interest here is limited to the epidemiology of infectious diseases. Epidemiologists specializing in infectious diseases are concerned with causes, times, and locations of certain of these microbial and helminthic diseases.

The early pioneers of microbiology were interested in causes of infectious diseases, but did not have ready access to the numbers of cases occurring within a particular community or time period. It is unlikely that the status of communication in the nineteenth century would have permitted accurate numbers to be obtained. John Snow (1813–1858), a British physician, was the first to identify a **common source** for bacteria causing cholera in 1856.

In 1849, over 500 people died in London of cholera within a 10-day period. Snow carefully followed the epidemic and noted that most of the victims were limited to a geographic area in Golden Square served by the Broad Street pump (Fig. 11–1). Water from that pump came from an upper area of the Thames river where untreated sewage was diverted. Snow suspected that the sewage contained the microorganisms causing cholera. He therefore proposed that the handle be removed from the Broad Street pump so that it could not be used. The epidemic subsided once the pump was no longer in service.

Snow's methodical approach to the epidemic of cholera showed the importance of geographic distribution and pointed to a common source. Looking for a common source is an important part of epidemiological studies. Most epidemics are **propagated epidemics,** however, in which infected individuals transmit a disease to susceptible hosts. The number of cases from a common source peaks sharply early, whereas there is a more gradual increase in numbers of cases in a propagated epidemic (Fig. 11–2). The municipal water supply of Milwaukee proved to be the common source when over 400,000 persons in that city developed a protozoan disease, known as cryptosporidiosis, in 1993.

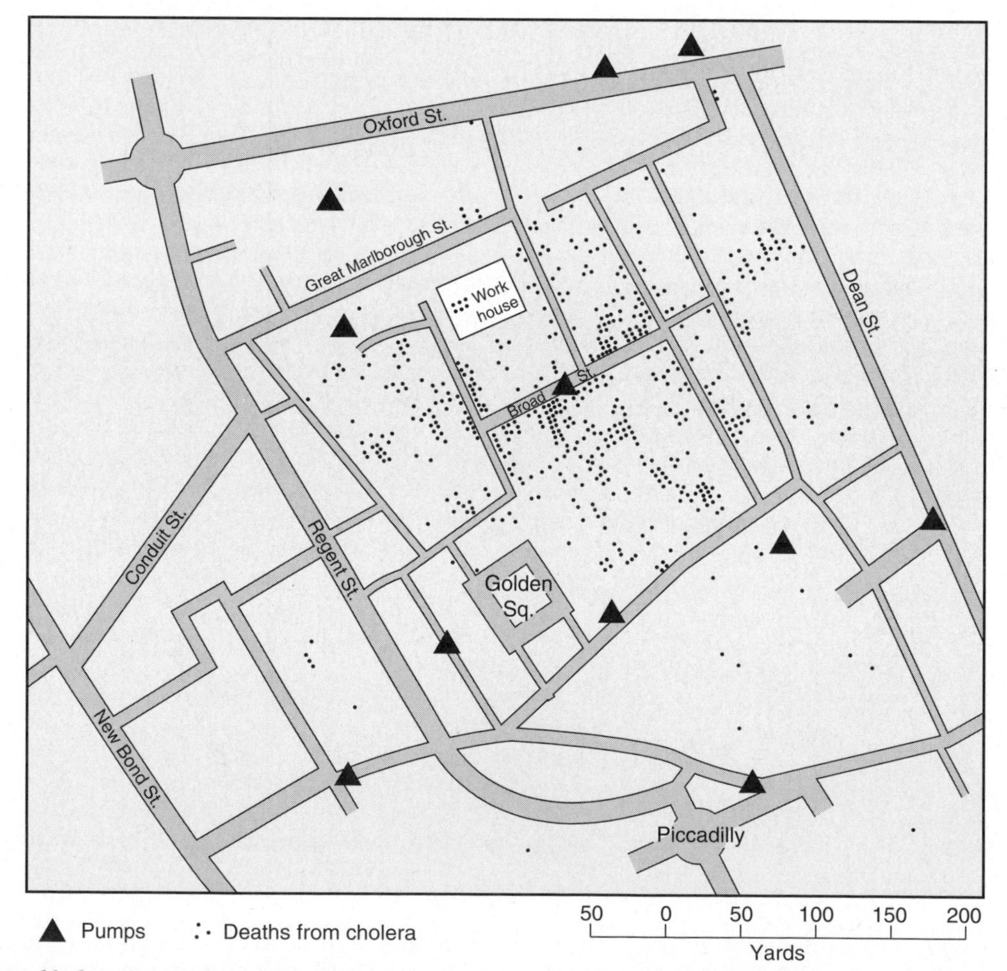

Figure 11–1 ◆ The deaths in London from cholera during 1854 were clustered around the Broad Street pump. Removal of the handle from the pump ended the epidemic by eliminating accessibility to sewage-contaminated water.

FOCAL POINT

Russia's Newest Enemies are Microbes

Since the end of the Cold War and the reduced threat of a nuclear war with Western countries, the Russian people are rediscovering old microbial adversaries. The countries of the former Soviet Union once had almost eliminated preventable infectious diseases through vaccination programs, but many diseases are returning with a vengeance. The economic base to support governmental intervention programs no longer exists. Diphtheria, anthrax, and cholera are appearing in epidemic proportions in Russia and in Georgia. The number of cases of tuberculosis increased 26 percent in the first half of 1993 over the previous six months. Life expectancy has declined and the infant mortality rate is rising. Some Russians fear taking any injectable substances since a 1989 episode in which 41 infants were given the human immunodeficiency virus (HIV) by reuse of syringes contaminated with the bloodborne virus. It is difficult for Americans to understand such carelessness in the practice of medicine. With financial assistance from the United States, it is hoped that syringes designed for a single use can be supplied.

Modern communications systems allow an epidemiologist to collect large amounts of data quickly. That data may include age, sex, occupation, socioeconomic status, history of immunization, eating habits, and high-risk behaviors of individuals having reportable infectious diseases. Epidemiologists often use these data to identify common sources for infectious agents and recommend preventive measures. Patterns of infectious disease emerge when data are accumulated over prolonged periods. Such information is valuable in formulating long-term plans for prevention or treatment of the diseases.

All communicable diseases are infectious, but not all infectious diseases are communicable. Diseases caused by preformed toxins of infectious agents or by normal flora are not communicable, whereas diseases caused by respiratory pathogens are readily transmitted from one individual to another. If a disease is highly communicable, it is described as a contagious disease. Influenza and the pneumonic form of plague are examples of contagious diseases.

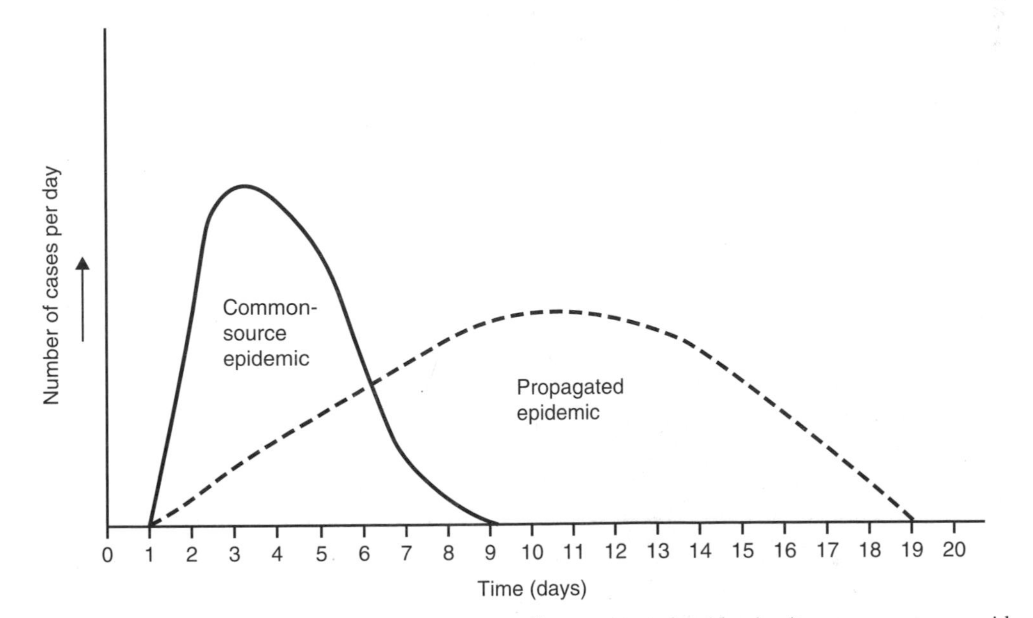

Figure 11–2 ◆ Difference between a common source and a propagated epidemic. A common source epidemic peaks early in the course of an epidemic, but a disease spreads gradually in a propagated epidemic.

CLASSIFYING COMMUNITY DISEASES

An unusually large number of cases of a particular disease occurring in a community within a short time constitutes an **epidemic.** Childhood diseases, such as poliomyelitis, measles, and mumps, used to occur in epidemic proportions in the United States before vaccination programs were instituted. The number of persons in whom disease develops during an epidemic is determined by the immunity of a population. That type of immunity in a population is called **herd immunity.** The immunity may have been obtained by having the disease or by receiving an immunizing agent. Herd immunity limits the spread of an infectious disease because there are fewer susceptible people.

Chlamydial infections, gonorrhea, and AIDS still occur in epidemic proportions in major cities of the United States. Infectious diseases that still occur in epidemic proportions produce either little or no natural immunity or are diseases for which there are no available immunizing agents.

When an epidemic spreads throughout many parts of the world, it is called a **pandemic.** Pandemics of plague are believed to have affected the course of history. During the fourteenth century almost one third of the world's population died of the disease then known as Black Death. Untold deaths have occurred in the seven pandemics of cholera occurring over the last two centuries. The seventh pandemic emerged in Indonesia in 1961 and reached Latin America in 1991. Epidemic cholera has not occurred in the United States since the nineteenth century. The AIDS pandemic continues to evolve. Infections caused by HIV are increasing worldwide at a rate approximating 9 percent a year. Nearly 90 percent of the new cases are occurring in developing sub-Saharan and Asian countries. It is estimated that a new HIV infection occurs every 13 seconds in the world. The medical, social, and economic consequences of the AIDS pandemic will prevail for years.

If a limited number of cases of an infectious disease is present at all times within a geographic area, the disease is said to be **endemic.** A fungal disease, known as coccidioidomycosis, is endemic in the southwestern part of the United States. If a particular disease occurs without regularity in a community, it is described as **sporadic.** Sporadic cases of meningococcal meningitis occur in most areas of the United States.

An individual who harbors an infectious agent in the absence of disease is a **carrier.** Some persons are resistant to the organisms themselves, but transmit the infectious agents to susceptible individuals. Other individuals are reservoirs for infectious agents before illness occurs and long after recovery is complete. The microorganisms are shed in body secretions or excreta for varying periods of time. A **transient carrier** sheds pathogens for several days or months; a **chronic carrier** can transmit an infectious agent for months or years.

METHODS OF EPIDEMIOLOGY

Epidemiologists use three methods in compiling information: (1) descriptive, (2) analytical, and (3) experimental. The information contained in their reports is valuable in following patterns of communicable diseases. Some hospitals employ persons, known as infectious disease practitioners, to gather information on community- and hospital-acquired diseases.

Descriptive Epidemiology

Descriptive epidemiology is a retrospective study on the frequency, places, times, and special circumstances of disease. Special circumstances might be related to particular occupations, eating habits, socioeconomic status, sexual behaviors, or seasonal variations in climate. A retrospective study is based on past events. Heavy, late, spring rains in Florida have led to large populations of the mosquito species that transmits eastern equine encephalitis (EEE) in the summer months. The number of cases of the disease in horses and humans reflects the wet weather, which allows surface water to collect and act as a breeding ground for mosquitos. Data are collected over a given period of time for long-term studies.

Analytical Epidemiology

Analytical epidemiology attempts to establish a cause-and-effect relationship from the information collected. Epidemiologists frequently compare age, sex, socioeconomic status, occupation, behavior, nutritional state, and ethnicity of ill people with a matched group of healthy individuals called **cohorts.** Such studies may show, for example, that a disease is more common in men than in women or in particular age groups, occupations, or geographic areas. Analytical studies may be **retrospective** if information is studied after an epidemic has subsided or **prospective** if information is collected on an ongoing epidemic. It is often possible to establish a hypothesis by carefully analyzing the factors surrounding an epidemic.

Rapid identification of isolates from outbreaks or epidemics of a particular disease is possible with the use of molecular techniques. Nucleic acid sequencing may relate outbreaks in widely separated geographic areas as having a common origin.

Experimental Epidemiology

The epidemiologist is often able to zero in on possible common sources and expand investigative studics to test a hypothesis. Such a study might involve comparing information from a similar outbreak of the same disease to test a hypothesis. Such unplanned experiments often answer pertinent questions. Most experimental epidemiology is, therefore, an observational science. An exception would be in conducting large-scale studies of various sources of food or water for the presence of a particular infectious agent. In the 1993 outbreak of cryptosporidiosis in Milwaukee, surface water was implicated as the source of the etiologic agent.

All three types of epidemiological studies are critical to an appropriate response to the welfare of a nation's citizens. Computers have made it easier to accumulate data and make predictions for the future. Much has been learned from epidemiological studies on the distribution of infectious diseases and predicted health care needs of particular geographic areas.

ASSESSMENTS OF DISEASE FREQUENCY

Prevalence and Incidence

The two most common assessments of disease frequency are prevalence and incidence. They may be expressed as numbers or percentages. The **prevalence** of a disease is the total number of cases or percentage of individuals with the disease at a point in time. For example, if 26 people out of 218 persons who attended a banquet come down with a foodborne illness on a given day, the prevalence would be 26, or 12 percent.

$$\text{Prevalence} = \frac{\text{Total cases}}{\text{Total population}} \times 100$$

Incidence is the rate of new cases of a disease that occur during a specified time interval compared with a healthy population. Incidence is reported nationally in terms of numbers of cases per 10,000 or 100,000 of a total population. For example, if a state of 250,000 reported 945 cases of a foodborne illness in one year, the incidence of that foodborne illness for that year would be 945 or 3.7 percent per 100,000.

$$\text{Incidence} = \frac{\text{New cases over given period}}{\text{Total population}} \times 100$$

When studies of incidence at various sites are compared, over periods of time, trends in overall incidence emerge. When incidence rates of group B streptococcal (GBS) disease in newborns at four geographic sites were studied recently, it revealed a 24 percent decline in cases per 1000 over a three-year period (Fig. 11–3). The decreasing incidence was attributed to implementation of preventive strategies. Much more data would need to be collected to assess national trends of GBS disease in newborns.

Look for graphs of incidence and prevalence for other diseases in the chapters ahead or in your local newspapers. Expressing data in graph form provides a way for readers to quickly assess problems in particular geographic areas and to observe trends. It is advisable to keep in mind,

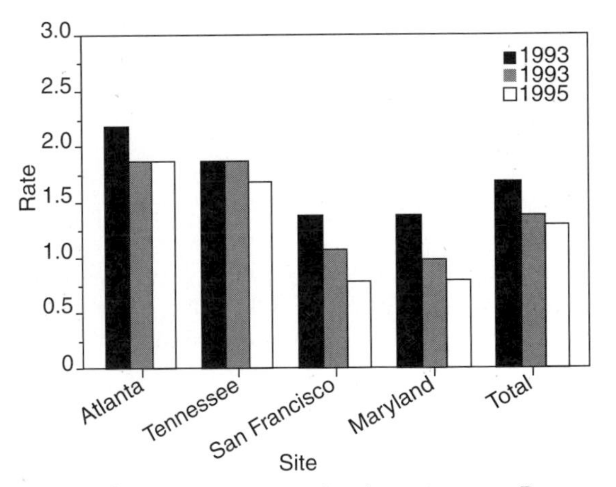

Figure 11–3 ◆ Incidence rate of early onset group B streptococcal (GBS) disease by year and selected sites, 1993–1995.

however, that true incidence and prevalence are not known because of probable underreporting. Available information does make it possible for local, state, and federal public health departments and medical advisory councils or regulatory agencies to make recommendations to protect public health.

Morbidity and Mortality Rates

Assessments on rates of **morbidity** (illness) and **mortality** (death) from infectious diseases is an important part of surveillance programs. Morbidity rate is the incidence of a disease as calculated previously. Mortality rate is the percentage of deaths from a disease when compared with the total number of persons who contracted the disease.

$$\text{Mortality rate} = \frac{\text{Deaths from a disease}}{\text{Total number with the disease}} \times 100$$

The morbidity and mortality rates reflect ecological opportunities, evolutionary pressures, economic conditions, surveillance efforts, and intervention strategies. Major declines in both morbidity and mortality rates of infectious diseases occurred with the availability of immunizations and antibiotics. As control measures have promoted the abatement of diseases like smallpox, diphtheria, and polio, other diseases are emerging or reemerging to threaten millions, particularly in developing countries. As emergency situations arise, it is important to have ready access to a common and comprehensive database.

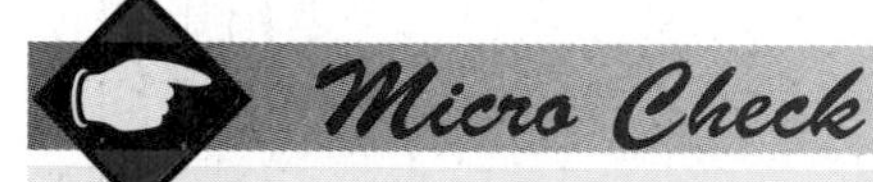

- How does an epidemic differ from a pandemic?
- In what two ways are frequency of a disease assessed?
- What are three major methods used by epidemiologists?

TYPES OF INFECTIOUS DISEASES

The primary classification of infectious diseases is based on an etiologic agent once a definitive diagnosis has been made. Other classifications of infectious diseases provide less specific, but important, information that reflects the immune status of the host, virulence of a microorganism, or time sequence in multiple infective states. Unfortunately, in some instances, it is impossible to implicate a particular etiologic agent despite the presence of disease.

Primary and Secondary Diseases

A **primary disease** is the initial disease caused by a microbial invader. It can occur on or within any part of the body. If, as a consequence of weakened host defenses or drug therapy, another infectious disease occurs, it is called a **secondary disease.** Bacteria sometimes follow viruses as secondary invaders. For example, viral respiratory infections often precede bacterial pneumonia, such as that caused by *Streptococcus pneumoniae.* The microorganisms causing the secondary disease may be part of the normal flora or may have an environmental origin.

Opportunistic Diseases

Infectious diseases caused by microorganisms that usually live in harmony with hosts, nonpathogenic environmental organisms, or pathogens that take advantage of weakened hosts are called **opportunistic diseases.** Opportunistic pathogens can cause primary or secondary disease. Opportunistic infectious diseases are often superimposed upon an already serious disease. Diseases caused by usually harmless microorganisms are increasing as survival rates are improving in immunocompromised populations. Opportunistic pathogens in more specific disease states are described in Chapter 12.

Latent Diseases

If host-defense mechanisms fail to eliminate a microbial invader completely, the disease may persist as a **latent disease.** Malaria, Brill's disease, and diseases caused by herpesviruses are examples of latent infectious diseases. Malarial parasites often persist in the liver for many years and cause subsequent attacks of malaria when an individual is subjected to physiological stress. Brill's disease is a mild disease occurring some time after what appears to be a complete recovery from typhus fever. The rickettsial organisms can become lodged in lymph nodes or other parts of the body and are activated by unknown forces. Most individuals harbor herpes simplex and varicella-zoster viruses. Both environmental and host factors are known to reactivate the viruses.

Tuberculosis can be a latent infectious disease if viable bacilli, causing that disease, remain within calcified lesions known as tubercles. When the resistance of the host is compromised by age, malnutrition, irradiation injury, underlying disease, or treatment with cortisone, the tubercle bacilli may be reactivated.

Acute, Subacute, and Chronic Diseases

An **acute disease** is serious, but of relatively short or limited duration. Acute infections are often life-threatening if appropriate treatment is not instituted promptly. Diphtheria and meningococcal meningitis are examples of acute diseases. Meningococcal meningitis has a sudden onset of headache, stiff neck, and vomiting. If not diagnosed and treated promptly, it may culminate in rapid death. Diphtheria is characterized by pharyngitis and systemic intoxication. It can last as long as six to ten weeks or may cause an individual to succumb quickly owing to blockage of air passages or effects of toxemia (toxin in the blood).

A **subacute disease** is one that is present before definitive signs or symptoms are exhibited. It does not come on rapidly or progress as fast as acute disease. Subacute bacterial endocarditis (inflammation of the membrane lining the heart) is an example of a disease that develops slowly. A mild fever may be the only sign of disease in early stages. A majority of cases of subacute bacterial endocarditis are caused by one group of streptococci.

A **chronic disease** is often milder in nature and of less immediate threat, but persists for months or even years. Kuru, a prion disease, and athlete's foot, a persistent fungal disease, are examples of chronic infectious diseases. Kuru is characterized by progressive brain degeneration and culminates inevitably in death, usually within a year. Sometimes the fungi of athlete's foot are so tenacious as to defy elimination.

Local and Disseminated Diseases

A **local disease** remains contained at a specific site. The nature of the invading agent, the site of the infection, and the immune status of the host contribute to the inability of the organism to spread. Most boils are examples of local disease. If, for any reason, infectious agents spread to other parts of the body, the disease is described as a **disseminated disease.** Entrance of microorganisms into blood or lymphatic vessels permits widespread dissemination. Coccidioidomycosis is a local infectious disease if lesions are confined to the lung. If dissemination occurs, bone, blood, and other organs may be affected.

Community- and Hospital-Acquired Diseases

Diseases in hospitalized patients are classified as community- or hospital-acquired diseases. The terms **hospital-acquired, hospital-associated,** and **nosocomial** are used interchangeably to describe an infectious disease contracted by a person during a hospital stay. The word "nosocomial" is the more commonly used term. If a patient enters the hospital with apparent signs and symptoms of an infection, the disease is classified as **community-acquired.**

The source of an infectious disease contracted by a hospitalized patient is not always easy to ascertain. Different infectious diseases have varying incubation periods. Persons admitted to health care facilities often become colonized by resident microorganisms of the institution. Trauma from surgery, intubation, or catheterization provides portals of entry for environmental microorganisms.

One nationwide epidemic of hospital-acquired sepsis focused attention on intravenous fluids as a source of infection. Although the supply of blood and blood products is the safest in the world, in the United States there are periodic episodes of illness and death in patients receiving contaminated products. Any type of injectable material or equipment used for that purpose can be involved in the accidental transfer of microorganisms. The sources of contamination may be **intrinsic** (present prior to use) or **extrinsic** (introduced in use) (Fig. 11–4).

Nosocomial infections occur in about 2 million hospitalized patients annually in the United States. Nosocomial diseases prolong hospital stays and are costly. The microorganisms that cause nosocomial diseases may be known pathogens, normal flora of patients, or hospital-associated microbial residents (Table 11–1). The infective sites may vary in a hospital setting. For example,

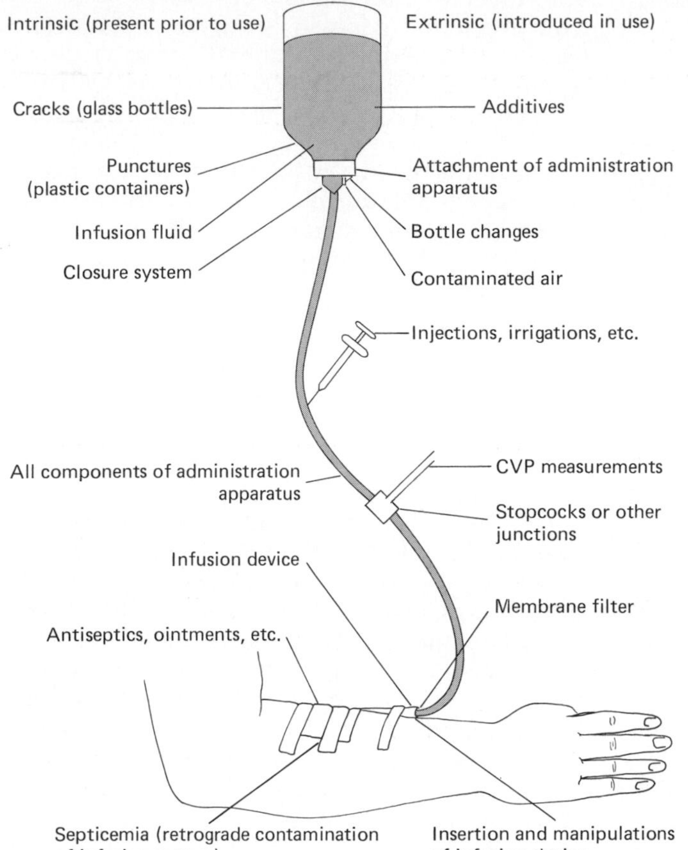

Figure 11–4 ◆ Potential intrinsic and extrinsic sources of contamination of intravenous infusion systems.

community-acquired *Streptococcus pyogenes* usually causes a pharyngitis; nosocomial disease caused by the same organism usually affects skin or gains entry to a wound.

Table 11–1
COMMON BACTERIAL ISOLATES FROM NOSOCOMIAL INFECTIONS

Acinetobacter calcoaceticus
Moraxella catarrhalis
Clostridium difficile
Enterobacter aerogenes
Escherichia coli
Klebsiella pneumoniae
Legionella pneumophila
Proteus vulgaris
Pseudomonas aeruginosa
Burkholderia cepacia
Serratia marcescens
Staphylococcus aureus

Micro Check

- ◆ What is an opportunistic disease?
- ◆ How does acute disease differ from chronic disease?
- ◆ Could an opportunistic disease also be a nosocomial disease?

RESERVOIRS OF INFECTIOUS AGENTS

A *reservoir* is a local environment or host that supports growth and multiplication of an infectious agent. A reservoir may be **biotic** (living) or **abiotic** (nonliving). The biotic reservoirs for human disease are humans and animals. The major abiotic reservoirs are water and soil. Food may become a secondary reservoir if it becomes contaminated.

Table 11–2
ANIMAL RESERVOIRS OF INFECTIOUS DISEASES

DISEASE	IMPORTANT RESERVOIRS	MANIFESTATION IN ANIMALS
Campylobacteriosis	Dogs, cats, hamsters	Asymptomatic
Cat scratch fever	Cats	Asymptomatic
Chlamydiosis	Birds	Diarrhea, pneumonia, conjunctivitis
Histoplasmosis	Dogs	Asymptomatic
Leptospirosis	Dogs	Fever, vomiting, lack of appetite
Plague	Dogs, cats, rodents	Variable
Salmonellosis	Turtles, lizards, snakes, poultry	Diarrhea or asymptomatic
Toxoplasmosis	Cats	Diarrhea, pneumonia, encephalitis
Tuberculosis	Cats	Fever, weight loss
Tularemia	Rabbits	Decreased activity
Yersiniosis	Dogs, cats, pigs, cows, rabbits	Diarrhea, respiratory distress, seizures

Biotic Reservoirs

The reservoirs for most human pathogens are other humans. Humans are reservoirs for the agents of AIDS, measles, syphilis, gonorrhea, typhoid fever, and numerous other diseases. Many human reservoirs of microbial diseases may display no signs or symptoms of disease. Both wild and domestic animals are reservoirs of animal and human diseases, such as rabies, plague, tularemia, Lyme disease, and anthrax. Household pets are often unsuspected reservoirs of infectious diseases (Table 11–2). Unfortunately, pets also may be asymptomatic. Certain insects and arachnids are reservoirs for protozoa, microfilarial worms, or rickettsial agents.

Abiotic Reservoirs

Soil and natural waters supply nutrients that support microbial growth and multiplication. Moist soil promotes the growth of large numbers of heterotrophic microorganisms. In the absence of favorable growth conditions, some soil pathogens produce spores that survive for hundreds of years. Air does not provide necessary requirements for microbial growth, but may contain large numbers of microorganisms. Atmospheric microorganisms are transient residents dependent on air currents for dispersal to environments with favorable growth conditions. The positive pressure supplied by heating and air-conditioning units can distribute microorganisms throughout large office or apartment buildings. On windy days soil pathogens, especially spores of fungi, can be distributed far from the original source.

Soil pathogens include the agents of anthrax, tetanus, botulism, and a variety of diseases caused by fungi. Water is the major reservoir for agents of cholera, cryptosporidiosis, typhoid fever, amebic dysentery, and other enteric pathogens. Wa-

FOCAL POINT

Air Quality in Airplane Cabins

The safety of air quality in cabins of airplanes has been questioned by the Department of Transportation (DOT) and the Centers for Disease Control and Prevention (CDC). At the center of the CDC investigation is a Continental Airlines attendant who was diagnosed as having active pulmonary tuberculosis. Two other members of her flight crew tested positive for tuberculosis. Three other investigations are under way on passengers with tuberculosis who traveled on Northwest, Delta, and Alaska airlines.

Concern about tuberculosis stems from an increasing incidence of the disease and the appearance of multiresistant strains of tubercle bacilli in recent years. The investigation by the CDC revealed that less fresh air is being circulated in cabins of planes built after the mid-1980s. In earlier aircraft, airlines provided cabins with 100 percent fresh air every three minutes. Newer models provide a mixture of 50 percent fresh air and 50 percent recirculated air every seven minutes. The DOT has pledged to work with the CDC to assess the potential dangers of recycled air.

ter does not remain a reservoir if nutrients are depleted or if repeated contamination does not occur. In most instances, the source of waterborne pathogens is improper sewage disposal or animal wastes. Most microorganisms store reserve material that allows them to survive for at least several days in the absence of required nutrients.

MODES OF TRANSMISSION

Infectious diseases may be transmitted by **direct** or **indirect contact** with an infected individual, an infected animal, or a carrier. Persons who come in direct contact with infected individuals or animals are at risk for contracting the same disease unless they have had the disease or been immunized against it. A number of microorganisms can be transmitted indirectly by contact with contaminated food, water, or inanimate objects. Survival for many pathogens is dependent on transfer to a susceptible human or animal host.

Direct Contact

Common forms of direct contact are touching, shaking hands, kissing, and sexual intercourse. Body contact is necessary for transmission of the virus causing the skin disease known as molluscum contagiosum. There is a high incidence of this skin disease in body contact sports, such as wrestling. The mites of scabies are also transmitted by skin-to-skin contact.

Enteric diseases, such as hepatitis A, shigellosis, and typhoid fever, are often transmitted by contaminated hands of infected food workers or carriers who practice poor personal hygiene. Adoption of procedures for safe handling of food in restaurants and regular inspections are important for the protection of consumers. Outbreaks of foodborne diseases do occur sporadically, even in some of the most elegant establishments.

Many pathogens gain access to human hosts through kissing. Infectious mononucleosis was once called the "kissing disease" because the Epstein-Barr virus (EBV) is transferred by saliva exchanged during kissing.

Sexually transmitted diseases (STDs) are usually spread by intimate contact during sexual intercourse. AIDS, genital herpes, gonorrhea, and syphilis are a few of the microbial diseases transmitted in this manner. Crab lice can also be transmitted to a sexual partner.

Direct contact can involve direct inoculation through the bite or an injectable substance. The bite of a rabid animal is fatal without prompt immunological intervention. Although most dogs and cats have been vaccinated for rabies, dog or cat bites can become infected with normal oral flora of those animals. The major potential pathogens in the oral flora of cats and dogs are *Staphylococcus aureus, Pasteurella multocida,* and streptococci belonging to groups D, G, L, and N. Arthropods are responsible for transmission of a large number of life-threatening diseases. Tropical diseases, such as malaria, African sleeping sickness, and yellow fever are only a few diseases spread by arthropod vectors in tropical climates. Arthropods are also associated with transmission of diseases such as typhus fever, viral encephalitis, and Lyme disease in temperate climates.

Some viruses, bacteria, and protozoa can be transmitted vertically to a fetus during pregnancy. Toxoplasmosis, rubella, syphilis, and AIDS are examples of diseases transmitted by placental transfer. Nine out of 10 children infected with HIV in the United States acquire the virus from their mothers at birth. HIV can also be transmitted by breast milk from infected mothers.

Indirect Contact

Transmission by indirect contact involves an intermediate material or inanimate (nonliving) object that has had contact with an infected host or their body fluids. Water and food can be both reservoirs and modes of transmission. The organisms causing enteric diseases are transmitted most often by contaminated water or food. A few enteric diseases, some skin diseases, eye infections, and one type of meningitis are caused by contact with contaminated natural water or that contained in swimming pools and hot tubs.

Foods often involved in transmission of pathogens include raw milk, shellfish, and improperly cooked poultry, eggs, or meat. There has been an increase in numbers of cases of salmonellosis related to consumption of raw or improperly cooked shell eggs in recent years. It is no longer recommended that eggs be served "sunny side up." Food also may be contaminated when mechanical vectors, such as flies, carry pathogens accidentally from animal wastes to food intended for human consumption.

Inanimate objects responsible for transmission of infectious agents are called **fomites.** Fomites can be contaminated cutting boards, utensils, instruments, syringes, needles, toys, bedding, towels, clothing, and even doorknobs. Toys are often implicated in outbreaks of infectious diseases in day care centers. Young children do not wash their hands thoroughly, most of the time, and are apt to put shared toys in their mouths.

Air can be a vehicle for transmitting pathogens released in coughing, sneezing, or talking. Small particles of mucus or saliva remain suspended as **aerosols** for varying lengths of time. The dried remnants of aerosols, called **droplet nuclei,** travel short or long distances, depending on vehicles available for transportation. Droplet nuclei can travel long distances on shoes for example (Fig. 11–5).

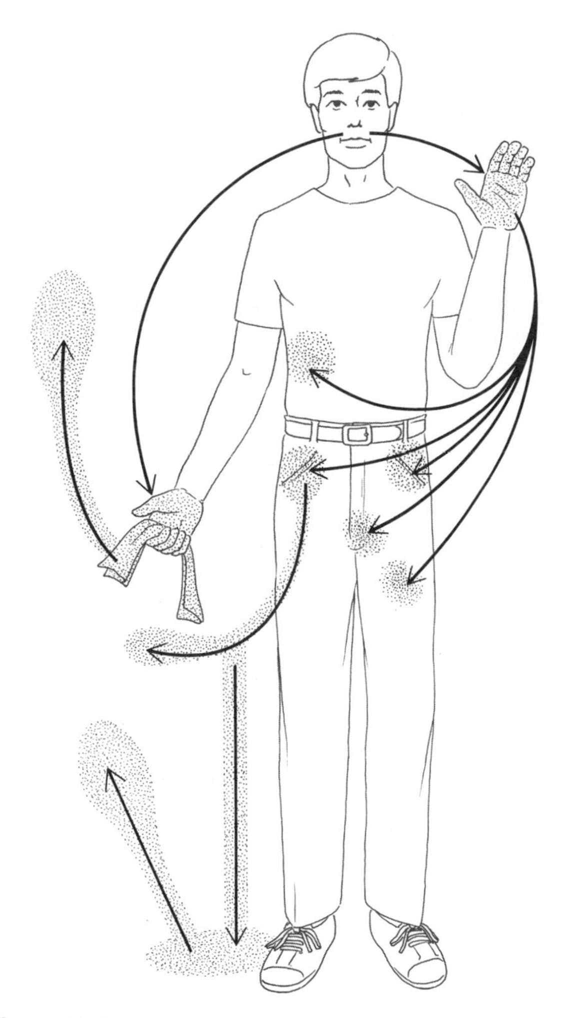

Figure 11–5 ◆ Dissemination of microorganisms by aerosols of nasal secretions. The larger aerosols can settle to the floor or shoes and be transported far away from the point of origin.

Role of Air Currents

The direction of outside and inside air currents is an important factor in the spread of respiratory diseases, such as tuberculosis, legionellosis, and influenza. Air-conditioning units disperse aerosols or droplet nuclei in indoor environments and may disperse spores of fungi as well.

Special needs exist for clean air in operating rooms, isolation units, and nurseries of hospitals. The rate of air circulation currently required in operating rooms is eight changes per hour, but many have ventilation rates of 15 or more changes per hour. Frequent changes of air can be supplied by a directed-flow ventilation system with minimal turbulence. Such systems, called laminar flow systems, operate with low, but uniform, velocities of filtered air (Fig. 11–6). Installation of unidirectional flow ventilation is costly but may prevent some nosocomial diseases.

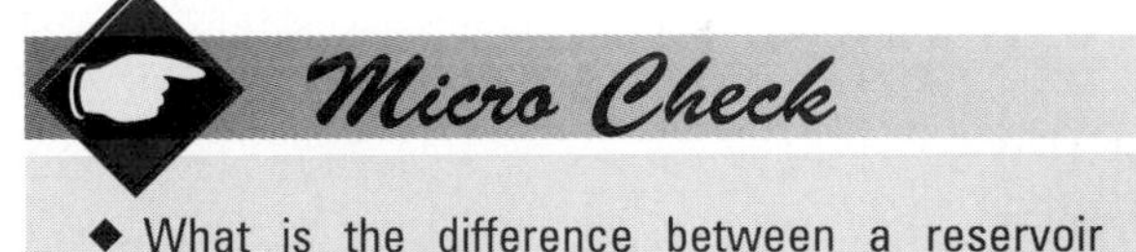

- ◆ What is the difference between a reservoir and a mode of transmission?
- ◆ What is the source of waterborne pathogens?
- ◆ What is the difference between a direct and an indirect method of contact?

PORTALS OF ENTRY AND EXIT

Most microorganisms enter the body through the digestive, respiratory, or genitourinary tract; others gain access to human tissue through a break in the skin. Less often, microorganisms are introduced by the bite of an insect or arachnid or directly into the blood through contaminated needles, syringes, or infusion sets. The most effective route for a microorganism is by direct inoculation into blood. A few pathogens can gain entrance by more than one route.

Infectious agents leave the body by way of the same systems used as portals of entry. Waste products, such as stool, urine, sputum, saliva, pus, or secretions, provide excellent vehicles of transportation for microorganisms. Bloodborne pathogens can remain viable in spilled blood or on contaminated instruments for varying lengths of time. Sharp instruments containing blood are

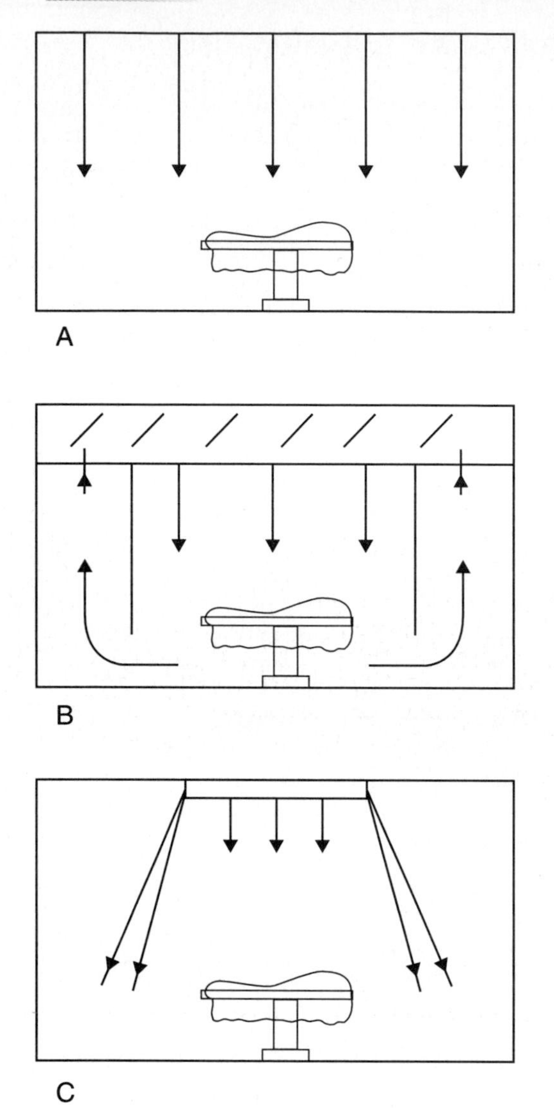

Figure 11–6 ◆ Vertical air flow in an operating room. *A,* Whole room with small lamps to minimize turbulence. *B,* Recirculating system with plastic curtains defining work area. *C,* Downflow confined within a set of higher velocity air jets.

of particular concern as potential hazards. Shedding of pathogens may persist long after signs and symptoms of disease have disappeared. Shedding has even been reported to occur following vaccination with living rubella viruses.

REPORTING COMMUNICABLE DISEASES

The list of reportable communicable diseases varies in different countries, but public health agencies in the United States are guided by the U.S. Department of Health and Human Services with headquarters in the Centers for Disease Control and Prevention (CDC) in Atlanta, Georgia. Most frequently, the system of reporting functions at several levels, with communicable diseases first being reported to a local public health agency. The local agency may be a city, county, or district department of public health. Data are next collected by the state health departments and, ultimately, forwarded to the CDC in weekly communications or on an emergency basis.

Diseases reportable to the CDC include some bacterial, viral, protozoal, and diseases caused by worms (Table 11–3). Numbers of cases of illness and death are published in the *Morbidity and Mortality Weekly Report* (MMWR) (Fig. 11–7). In addition, weekly reports also contain accounts of outbreaks of particular diseases, environmental hazards, or unusual cases of infectious disease.

Summaries of data collected from state health departments are published annually. The annual publication shows trends of communicable diseases, including emerging patterns of disease, which may be associated with travel or specific geographic areas. National health authorities cooperate with the World Health Organization by reporting certain communicable diseases so that worldwide patterns may be available for further study and action. Reports of the World Health Organization may be found in the *Weekly Epidemiological Record.*

RECOMMENDATIONS AND REGULATIONS FOR BLOODBORNE PATHOGENS

The CDC adopted a series of recommendations to prevent transmission of HIV in medical care facilities in 1987. The recommendations were based on the need to consider blood and certain other body fluids as hazardous materials (Table 11–4). Because it is unknown, in a majority of instances, whether a patient is a carrier of HIV or of another bloodborne infectious agent, the precautions apply to all patients. The "do's" and "don'ts" of recommended procedures, known as **universal precautions,** are presented in Table 11–5.

Transmission of HIV, hepatitis B, and hepatitis C has occurred in health care workers despite compliance with universal precautions. Most

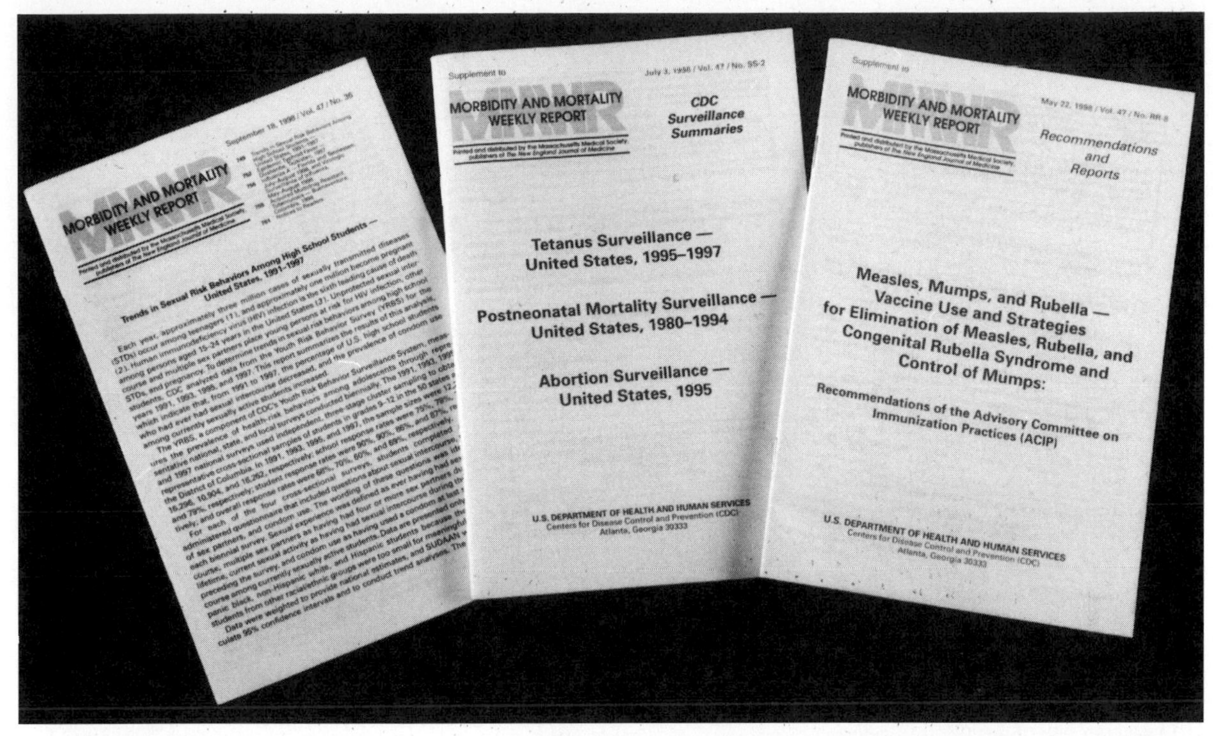

Figure 11–7 ◆ Three publications of the U.S. Department of Health and Human Services, Centers for Disease Control and Prevention (CDC). The publications include a weekly report, periodic surveillance summaries, and recommendations and reports.

Table 11–3
REPORTABLE COMMUNICABLE DISEASES—UNITED STATES

Acquired immunodeficiency syndrome (AIDS)
Amebiasis†
Anisakiasis†
Anthrax*
Babesiosis†
Botulism (infant, foodborne, wound)*
Brucellosis
Campylobacteriosis†
Chancroid
Chlamydial infections
Cholera*
Ciguatera fish poisoning*
Coccidioidomycosis
Colorado tick fever†
Conjunctivitis, acute infectious of the newborn, specify etiology†
Cryptosporidiosis†
Cysticercosis
Dengue*
Diarrhea of the newborn, outbreaks*
Diphtheria*
Domoic acid poisoning (amnesic shellfish poisoning)*
Echinococcosis (hydatid disease)
Ehrlichiosis
Encephalitis, specify etiology: viral, bacterial, fungal, parasitic†
Escherichia coli O157:H7 infection*
Foodborne disease†‡
Giardiasis
Gonococcal infections
Haemophilus influenzae, invasive disease†
Hantavirus infections*
Hemolytic uremic syndrome*
Hepatitis, viral
  Hepatitis A†
  Hepatitis B (specify acute case or chronic)
  Hepatitis C (specify acute case or chronic)
  Hepatitis D (delta)
Hepatitis, other, acute
Kawasaki syndrome (mucocutaneous lymph node syndrome)
Legionellosis
Leprosy (Hansen's disease)
Leptospirosis
Listeriosis†

Table continued on following page

Table 11–3
REPORTABLE COMMUNICABLE DISEASES—UNITED STATES *Continued*

Lyme disease
Lymphocytic choriomeningitis†
Malaria†
Measles (rubeola)†
Meningitis, specify etiology: viral, bacterial, fungal, parasitic†
Meningococcal infections*
Mumps
Nongonococcal urethritis (report laboratory-confirmed chlamydial infections as chlamydia)
Paralytic shellfish poisoning*
Pelvic inflammatory disease (PID)
Pertussis (whooping cough)†
Plague, human or animal*
Poliomyelitis, paralytic†
Psittacosis†
Q fever†
Rabies, human or animal*
Relapsing fever†
Reye syndrome
Rheumatic fever, acute
Rocky Mountain spotted fever
Rubella (German measles)
Rubella syndrome, congenital
Salmonellosis (other than typhoid fever)†
Scabies (atypical or crusted)*§
Scombroid fish poisoning*
Shigellosis†
Streptococcal infections (outbreaks of any type and individual cases in food handlers and dairy workers only)†; invasive group A streptococcal infections including streptococcal toxic shock syndrome and necrotizing fasciitis†§ (do not report individual cases of pharyngitis or scarlet fever)
Swimmer's itch (schistosomal dermatitis)†
Syphilis†
Tetanus
Toxic shock syndrome
Toxoplasmosis
Trichinosis†
Tuberculosis†
Tularemia
Typhoid fever, cases and carriers†
Typhus fever
Vibrio infections†
Viral hemorrhagic fevers (e.g., Crimean-Congo, Ebola, Lassa, and Marburg viruses)*
Water-associated disease†
Yellow fever*
Yersiniosis†
OCCURRENCE OF ANY UNUSUAL DISEASE*
OUTBREAKS OF ANY DISEASE*

Notification Required of Laboratories (CCR §2505)
Chlamydial infections
Cryptosporidiosis†
Diphtheria*
Encephalitis, arboviral†
Escherichia coli infection, O157:H7 or sorbitol negative*¶
Gonorrhea
Hepatitis A, acute infection, by IgM antibody test or positive viral antigen test†
Hepatitis B, acute infection, by IgM anti-HBc antibody test
Hepatitis B surface antigen positivity (specify gender)
Listeriosis†
Malaria†
Measles (rubeola), acute infection, by IgM antibody test or positive viral antigen test†
Plague, animal or human*
Rabies, animal or human*
Syphilis†
Tuberculosis†¶
Typhoid†¶
Vibrio species infections

No symbols: Report within seven (7) calendar days from the time of identification by mail, telephone, or electronic report.
*Report immediately by telephone.
†Report by mailing, telephoning, or electronically transmitting a report within one (1) working day of identification of the case or suspected case.
‡When two (2) or more cases or suspected cases of foodborne disease from separate households are suspected to have the same source of illness, they should be reported immediately by telephone.
§Reportable to local public health departments.
¶Bacterial isolates and malarial slides must be forwarded to the DHS Public Health Laboratory for confirmation. Health care providers must still report all such cases separately.
Source: Public Health Letter 21(1), 1999. Los Angeles County, Department of Health Services, Los Angeles, CA.

Table 11–4
HAZARDOUS BODY FLUIDS

Amniotic fluid
Blood
Pericardial fluid
Peritoneal fluid
Pleural fluid
Semen
Spinal fluid
Synovial fluid
Vaginal secretions

cases of hospital-acquired infections in health care workers have occurred in persons exposed to blood of infected patients by needlestick injuries. Extreme care must be exercised in handling any sharp instrument or object contaminated with blood or other body fluids.

Protection of laboratory workers who handle infectious materials and agents is of major concern. Guidelines established by the CDC include the development of biosafety levels and practices for handling infectious agents. Life-threatening agents, such as the Ebola, Marburg, and Lassa viruses, require maximum containment facilities and special handling procedures. Laboratories designated as maximum containment facilities must be housed in separate buildings having appropriate ventilation and waste management systems. Inoculations are done in biosafety cabinets and protective clothing is worn (see Color Plates 23 and 24).

In 1991, the Occupational Safety and Health Administration (OSHA) adopted requirements designed to prevent transmission of bloodborne pathogens in the work environment (Table 11–6). The regulations apply to employees who have occupational risks of exposure. OSHA is a governmental regulatory agency and its approach is quite different than that of the CDC, a public health agency. OSHA can fine health care facilities for noncompliance with regulations.

Table 11–5
DO'S AND DON'TS BASED ON CDC GUIDELINES

Do use appropriate barrier precautions routinely to prevent skin and mucous membrane exposure when contact with blood or other body fluids of any patient is anticipated.
Do wear gloves for touching blood and body fluids, mucous membranes, or nonintact skin of all patients, for handling items of surfaces soiled with blood or body fluids, and for performing venipuncture and other vascular access procedures. Gloves should be changed after contact with each patient.
Do wear masks and protective eyewear during procedures that are likely to generate droplets of blood or other body fluids to prevent exposure of mucous membranes of the mouth, nose, and eyes. Gowns should be worn during procedures that are likely to generate splashes of blood or other body fluids.
Do wash hands and other skin surfaces immediately and thoroughly if contaminated with blood or other body fluids. Hands should be washed immediately after gloves are removed.
Do take precautions to prevent injuries caused by needles, scalpels and other sharp instruments. To prevent needlestick injuries, needles should not be recapped, purposely bent or broken by hand, removed from disposable syringes, or otherwise manipulated by hand. After they are used, all sharp instruments should be placed in a puncture-resistant container for disposal, located as close as possible to the use area.
Although saliva has not been implicated in HIV transmission, to minimize the need for emergency mouth-to-mouth resuscitation, mouthpieces, resuscitation bags, or other ventilation devices should be available for use in areas where the need of resuscitation is predictable.
Although pregnant nurses are not known to be at greater risk of contracting HIV infection during pregnancy, the infant is at risk of infection resulting from perinatal transmission. Because of this risk, pregnant nurses should be especially familiar with and adhere strictly to precautions to minimize risks.
Do check your hands for any cuts, abrasions, or breaks in skin and cover with waterproof dressing. Health care workers who have exudative lesions or weeping dermatitis should refrain from all direct patient care and from handling patient care equipment until the condition resolves.

Source: Captain J: Universal precautions: AIDS and other infectious diseases. Calif Nurs Rev *10*(3):28–33, 1988.

Table 11–6
REGULATIONS ON OCCUPATIONAL EXPOSURE TO BLOODBORNE PATHOGENS FROM OCCUPATIONAL SAFETY AND HEALTH ADMINISTRATION

Develop an exposure-control plan that identifies employees who have occupational exposure.

Train all employees in how to recognize occupational risks and methods to reduce risk.

Maintain records of employee training and medical evaluations.

Use warning labels and signs to identify hazards, indicate when universal precautions are needed, and explain safe handling of sharps, specimens, contaminated laundry, and regulated waste.

Provide voluntary hepatitis B vaccination at no cost to employees who can "reasonably anticipate" contact with blood or other potentially infectious materials.

Provide medical evaluation after exposure incidents.

Provide personal protective clothing and equipment.

Source: Adapted from American Hospital Association, Division of Quality Resources: OSHA's Final Bloodborne Pathogens Standard: A Special Briefing. Chicago, American Hospital Association, 1992.

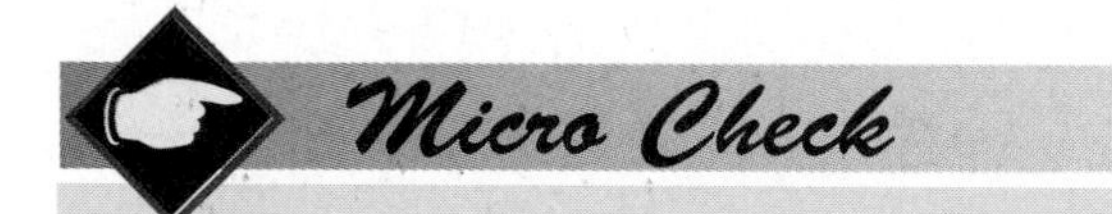

- How do pathogens exit human or animal hosts?
- Why are numbers of reportable diseases not necessarily total numbers for diseases?
- How would you characterize CDC's and OSHA's approach to preventing transmission of bloodborne pathogens?

Understanding Microbiology

1. What is the difference between an infectious disease and a communicable disease?
2. What are the two most common measures of disease frequency?
3. Why is it important to identify infectious disease in hospital patients as community- or hospital-acquired?
4. How do the roles of the CDC and OSHA differ in protecting public health?
5. What is meant by universal precautions?

Applying Microbiology

6. Review how microorganisms are transmitted and list five things that you can do to reduce the risk of infection for yourself and family members.

Chapter 12

The Nature of Pathogenicity

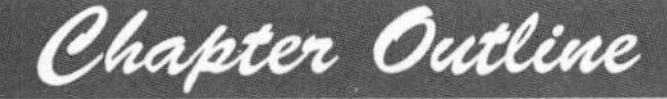

- **DETERMINANTS OF INFECTIOUS DISEASE**
  - Virulence
  - Quantity of Microbial Invaders or Toxins
  - Resistance of the Host
- **DETERMINANTS OF VIRULENCE**
  - Genetic Determinants
  - Microbial Factors
  - Host Factors
- **OPPORTUNISTIC PATHOGENS**
- **CLINICAL MANIFESTATIONS OF DISEASE**

Learning Objectives

After you have read this chapter, you should be able to:

1. Differentiate between pathogenicity and virulence.
2. Describe three major factors for development of infectious disease.
3. Identify genetic factors for virulence.
4. List microbial factors responsible for virulence.
5. List host factors responsible for virulence.
6. Differentiate between exotoxins and endotoxins.
7. Define an opportunistic pathogen.

Microorganisms have been blamed for the ravages of infectious diseases since the time of Pasteur. Certain genetic properties of the microorganism allow it to survive and flourish on or within another species. The pathogenic microorganism bypasses or destroys the host's cellular and molecular defenses that normally inhibit other microorganisms that live in or on the host. Host factors contribute to the infectious process as well. A complex set of interactions between a pathogen and a host affects the ability of the pathogen to gain entry, establish residency, colonize, and spread on or in a host.

DETERMINANTS OF INFECTIOUS DISEASE

The ability of a microorganism to cause disease is called **pathogenicity.** Various strains of pathogens differ in their disease-producing ability; this degree of pathogenicity is called **virulence.** Two characteristics that allow microorganisms to cause disease or injury to a host are invasiveness and toxigenicity. **Invasiveness** is the ability of microorganisms to gain entry and spread in host tissue. **Toxigenicity** is the capacity of microbial products, known as toxins, to cause injury to a host. More virulent organisms have one or more invasive or toxigenic properties.

Blood, lymph, cerebrospinal fluid, and most internal organs are free of microorganisms. The presence of a microorganism in these sterile fluids and tissues usually indicates an infection by that microorganism.

Various other parts of the body become contaminated with microorganisms shortly after birth. The mucous membranes of the upper respiratory tract, the gastrointestinal tract, and some parts of the genitourinary tract are colonized by bacteria and other microorganisms. Those microorganisms residing on or in the healthy human host without causing infection are **indigenous** microorganisms, or simply, **normal flora.** Sometimes normal flora challenge, or interfere with, the foreign invader or pathogen. The invader must find a surface for attachment, compete for nutrition and sometimes oxygen, and resist harmful products present in the environment. If the pathogen is not successful in finding a niche and colonizing the host, it cannot flourish and thus no infection occurs. Normal flora play a role in preventing certain pathogens from establishing an infection.

The potential for an infection begins when foreign microorganisms gain entrance to a host, or when species of the normal flora enter a new area or gain dominance at their normal site, causing an **opportunistic infection.** Some pathogens escape host defenses, colonize on particular tissues, begin an infection, but do not cause disease. It is only when the microbial invaders do harm that an infection becomes a disease.

Progression of an infection into a disease is dependent on factors such as the virulence factors of microorganisms, quantity of microbial invaders or their toxins, and the resistance factors of the host.

Virulence

Virulence is not a stable characteristic for all pathogens. The reasons for the emergence of more virulent strains of particular organisms are not always known, but many organisms undergo mutations that allow them to evade host defenses more effectively.

Frequent mutations in the genes for surface molecules on the influenza virus offer a good example. Slight changes in the structure of hemagglutinin (H) or neuraminidase (N) molecules on the virus surface result in many different influenza strains. The changes in H and N molecules provide an escape path from destruction by host defensive antibody molecules. The antibody molecules attach to specific H and N structures and destroy the virus. Production of antibody molecules depends on a previous infection or an influenza vaccination. If the infection or vaccination was produced by a different influenza virus strain, the antibody molecules may not protect the human host against the new strain. Each spring season, epidemiologists study the frequency and types of influenza virus infections occurring worldwide in order to recommend the particular combination of influenza virus strains for use in the winter vaccination program.

Quantity of Microbial Invaders or Toxins

The numbers of pathogens or amounts of microbial toxins gaining entrance to a host are significant factors as determinants of disease. A measure of the virulence of an organism or the ability of a toxin to cause harm is the LD_{50} (lethal dose for 50 percent of the hosts). Obtaining the LD_{50} value for a microorganism or its toxin is made by injecting susceptible test animals with different amounts and observing the animals for signs of disease. Results in test animals must not be considered as an absolute measure for human hosts. A few human pathogens such as the bacteria causing cholera, shigellosis, and gonorrhea are not known to cause disease in other species, and LD_{50} values are not available.

Quantities of pathogens or their toxins to which an individual is exposed also influence incubation times of a disease. An **incubation time** is the time period between exposure to a pathogen and the early appearance of signs and symptoms of disease (Table 12–1).

Resistance of the Host

The resistance of the host is another important factor in the progression of an infection to disease. Some of us have lifetime immunity to a particular disease from having had the disease or from receiving certain vaccines. Equally important in the immune status of an individual are general health factors such as age, diet, nutritional status, stress, and environmental factors. One idea in wellness theory is that a person in

Table 12–1
INCUBATION TIMES FOR SOME MAJOR PATHOGENS

MICROORGANISM	DISEASE	INCUBATION TIME
Salmonella typhi	Typhoid fever	1–2 Weeks
Vibrio cholerae	Cholera	2–3 Days
Neisseria gonorrhoeae	Gonorrhea	2–10 Days
Herpes simplex II (HSV-II)	Genital herpes infection	3–5 Days
Coccidioides immitis	Coccidioidomycosis	10–21 Days
Treponema pallidum	Syphilis	10–21 Days
Mycobacterium tuberculosis	Tuberculosis	4–6 Weeks
Yersinia pestis	Pneumonic plague	3–4 Days
Hepatitis B virus (HBV)	Hepatitis B	45–60 Days
Neisseria meningitidis	Meningococcal meningitis	2–10 Days

generally good health who eats a balanced diet with adequate exercise probably has a functioning immune system of defenses and may be less susceptible to infectious disease.

Immune responses are often diminished by existing disease or by drug therapy. Although microorganisms are known to invade and damage human tissues, many human host factors contribute to the infectious process. Nonspecific and specific immune defenses are discussed in Chapter 13. Altered functioning of the immune system is discussed in Chapter 14.

Micro Check

- Explain the difference between invasiveness and toxigenicity.
- When does an infection become a disease?
- How does the quantity of microorganisms or their toxins influence the course of an infectious disease?

DETERMINANTS OF VIRULENCE

Microorganisms are continuously developing new offense and defense strategies that enable them to cope with the hostile environment of their hosts. This adaptive process involves exploiting weaknesses in host defenses. Certain lifestyles, high densities of human populations in urban areas, and some practices of modern medicine alter the ability of humans to defend against microbial invaders. An understanding of the dual nature of virulence can be gained by examining microbial and host factors.

Genetic Determinants of Virulence

Plasmids and bacteriophages often have major roles as carriers of virulence factors (Table 12–2). Although they may not have the sole determining role in disease, the contribution of transferred DNA segments carrying virulence genes is important. Gene transfer mechanisms such as transformation, transduction, and conjugation, and gene rearrangements and interruptions by transposons are common occurrences among bacteria. The introduction of new DNA segments may result in the sharing of virulence genes among large groups of bacteria ranging from plant to animal and human pathogens.

Table 12–2
GENETIC DETERMINANTS OF VIRULENCE

Determinants carried by bacteriophages
Corynebacterium diphtheriae (diphtheria) toxin
Clostridium botulinum (botulism) neurotoxin
Streptococcus pyogenes (scarlet fever) erythrogenic toxin
Enterohemorrhagic *Escherichia coli* (hemolytic uremic syndrome) Shiga-like toxin
Determinants carried by plasmids
Shigella (dysentery) invasiveness
Clostridium tetani (tetanus) neurotoxin
Enterotoxigenic *Escherichia coli* toxin and adhesins
Bacillus anthracis (anthrax) toxins

Chromosomal genetic determinants of virulence in bacterial pathogens often reside in large regions of the DNA called **pathogenicity islands.** These islands are not found in the nonpathogenic members of the same genus. Similar clusters, or islands, of genes for virulence factors occurring on plasmids in enteric pathogens such as *Shigella flexneri* (bacterial dysentery) are found on the chromosomal DNA of *Escherichia coli* and *Salmonella typhimurium* (typhoid-like disease). Expression of such genes depends on favorable environmental conditions. Expression of these pathogenicity islands leads to hemolysin production, invasion of nonphagocytic cells, cell death, ability to adhere to cells, and other properties allowing the disease process to occur.

Microbial Factors

The ability of any one microorganism to cause disease cannot be attributed to a single factor. Most virulent pathogens have developed multiple strategies for survival and colonization in the host. Surface molecular components of particular organelles of the microorganism assist in its adherence and colonization. Other surface components have antiphagocytic activity. Many pathogens produce enzymes to degrade specific substrates of host tissue; others produce **toxins** that damage host tissue or interfere with specific organ functions. Pathogens producing **siderophore** compounds compete with their hosts for iron.

SURFACE COMPONENTS

Components of capsules, pili, cell walls, and plasma membranes are important for adherence, colonization, and antiphagocytic activity. The filaments of **M protein** on the surface of *Streptococcus pyogenes* are involved in antiphagocytic activity (Fig. 12–1). Some bacteria and yeast produce polysaccharide layers, or capsules, around the cell to protect them from phagocytosis by host defensive cells.

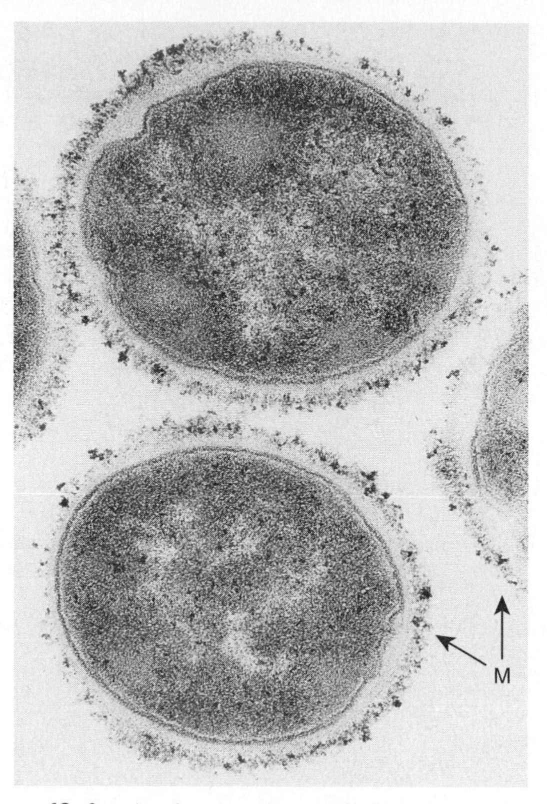

Figure 12–1 ◆ An electron micrograph through a streptococcal cell showing the M protein on the outer edge of the wall.

Some bacteria adhere to mucous membranes by means of pili. Adhesin molecules on the bacterial surface or on pili may account for the selective adherence of some bacteria to specific surfaces. *Staphylococcus saprophyticus* attaches to cells of urogenital origin, and toxigenic strains of *E. coli* adhere to human ileal cells.

Adhesins are not solely responsible for attachment. An interaction must occur between the microorganisms and host cells. In studies with enteropathogenic *E. coli* (EPEC), the leading cause of bacterial diarrhea in the world, the bacteria and host cooperate. EPEC uses one type of adhesin to attach to intestinal cells. The host cell responds to the attachment by moving actin filaments to produce a pedestal under the bacterium. A second adhesin from EPEC attaches to the host cell pedestal to make a firm attachment to the intestine. The bacterial cell begins to multiply in its stabilized location.

Lectins are proteins that bind to specific carbohydrates in human intestinal mucus and epithelial cells. The plasma membrane of invasive strains of *Entamoeba histolytica,* the cause of amebic dysentery, contains a galactose-specific **lectin.** Pathogenic strains of *Giardia lamblia,* another protozoan pathogen of the intestine, contain two mannose-binding lectins.

In natural environments, populated by several kinds of organisms, bacteria produce tangled fibers of polysaccharides that form a **glycocalyx** layer around individual cells or colonies of cells

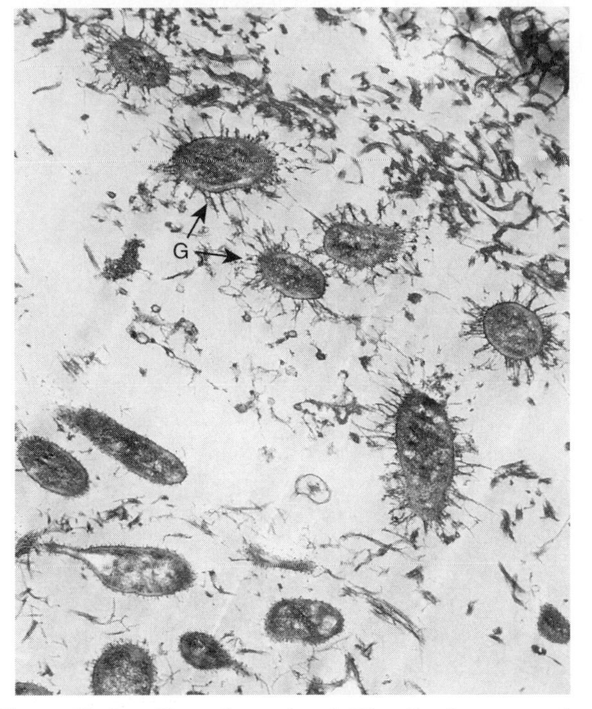

Figure 12–2 ◆ Glycocalyx-enclosed (G) cells of gram-negative pathogens from urine.

(Fig. 12–2). Glycocalyx is formed only in a competitive environment and not under the artificial conditions of growth in the laboratory. Environments of the healthy human body such as the upper respiratory tract and the gastrointestinal tract contain large numbers of competing microorganisms. Bacteria producing the glycocalyx layer adhere to the tooth surface, the lung, mucous membranes of the urethra, or "brush border" of the intestinal mucosa. The glycocalyx may offer protection from both antibodies and antimicrobial agents.

Specific proteins on the envelopes or capsids of viruses attach to receptor molecules on specific host cells. This is a highly specific mechanism by which the virus attaches to the host(s) in which it can enter and replicate.

When a microorganism shares surface molecules with those of host cells, the phenomenon is called **molecular mimicry.** The consequences can be important in the progression of disease or cause immune responses that harm the host. Molecular mimicry may allow a pathogen to go unrecognized as an invader so the disease continues without host interference. If shared components elicit an immune response, the antibodies could react with host tissue, producing irreparable damage. Molecular mimicry is a factor in certain autoimmune diseases and may have a role in the progression of HIV infection to AIDS.

ENZYMES

A number of enzymes secreted by bacteria contribute significantly to virulence. Many gram-positive bacteria secrete **hyaluronidase,** an enzyme that acts on the hyaluronic acid of the host connective tissue matrix increasing invasiveness into deeper tissues (Fig. 12–3). Members of the genus *Clostridium* secrete copious amounts of **collagenase,** an enzyme that acts on the protein col-

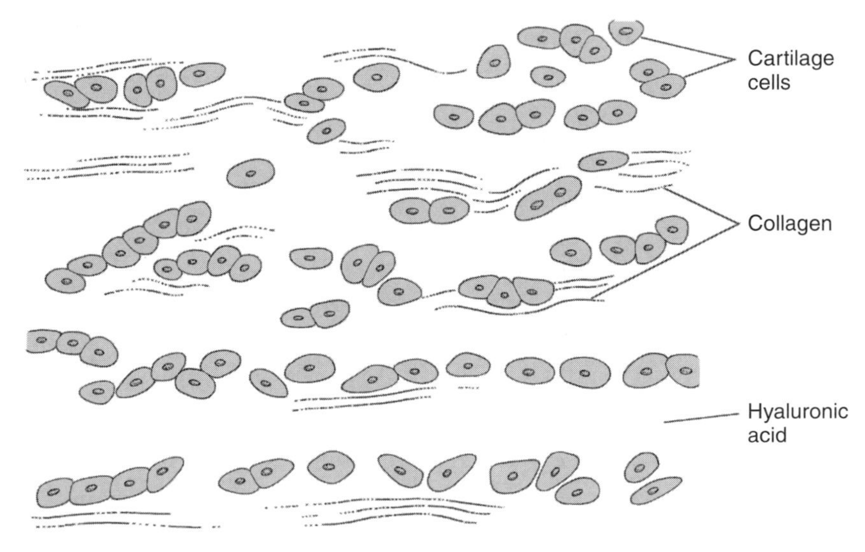

Figure 12–3 ◆ Cells of cartilage distributed throughout a matrix containing hyaluronic acid and collagen.

lagen, found in skin, bone, and cartilage. The destruction of hyaluronic acid and collagen is not necessary for invasion but greatly improves the chances of spread through the body.

The enzyme **lecithinase,** also known as **alpha toxin,** is associated with virulence of *Clostridium perfringens,* the causative agent of gas gangrene. It can destroy several types of tissues, but red blood cells are most often affected. The enzyme, **elastase,** produced by *Pseudomonas aeruginosa,* can degrade many human proteins, including elastin in tissues. Activity of the enzyme is enhanced as it leaves the outer membrane of the bacterial cell.

Other enzymes interfere with the clotting of blood. **Kinases** dissolve human fibrin, the protein network established in a blood clot to stop blood flow. Kinases catalyze the conversion of plasminogen to plasmin. Kinases are produced by a number of gram-positive bacteria, but the streptokinases have received the most attention. Medical research has developed a procedure to reduce the chance of blood clots developing in a patient's circulation by using streptokinase therapy.

Virulent strains of *Staphylococcus aureus* are known for **coagulase** enzyme, which promotes clotting of plasma in the presence of a plasma coagulase-reacting factor (CRF). The virulence of the staphylococci, however, cannot be explained by coagulase production only.

EXOTOXINS

A number of bacterial exotoxins, usually proteins, are secreted into the environment by cells of gram-positive and gram-negative pathogens. Most exotoxins have a specific action. **Hemolysins** lyse red blood cells; **leukocidins** degranulate certain white blood cells; **enterotoxins** act on the brain to induce vomiting. The exotoxins of *S. aureus* and many gram-negative bacilli are typical enterotoxins. Ingestion of preformed exotoxins can cause disease without establishing an infection. **Exofolins** promote the shedding of epidermal cells of the skin. The toxins causing the diseases botulism and tetanus affect the host's nerve cells, inducing paralysis and other effects.

FOCAL POINT

A New Drug for Muscle Hyperactivity

One of the most potent neurotoxins, botulinum toxin A, was approved by the U.S. Food and Drug Administration in 1989 for treatment of muscle hyperactivity. Toxin A, ironically, causes severe illness and death in foodborne botulism. The toxin blocks the action of acetylcholine at myoneural junctions. Death is caused by paralysis of respiratory muscles. The neurotoxin is administered to relieve involuntary muscle movements, including facial twitching, crossed eyes, writer's cramp, hand tremors, and stuttering. Administration of 20 units of the toxin intramuscularly relieves involuntary muscle movements for at least a few months. Larger doses of the toxin can affect neighboring muscles. Low doses can be repeated when muscle spasms return. Only 12 of over 7000 patients have developed antibodies to toxin A. Other microbial neurotoxins are being investigated for possible use in medicine. If approved, such toxins could be valuable for patients developing toxin A antibodies.

ENDOTOXINS

Endotoxins are present in the cell walls of some gram-negative bacteria. They are released only when cells are damaged or die. Although a few endotoxins are composed solely of protein, most are made up of both protein and lipopolysaccharide (LPS). The LPS of gram-negative bacilli, such as *Escherichia, Salmonella,* and *Shigella,* consist of a core polysaccharide (common antigen), specific polysaccharide (O antigen), and lipid A (Fig. 12–4). The lipid A component causes fever, immunosuppression, and sometimes shock.

Very small amounts of endotoxin are detectable in a patient's peripheral blood by the *Limulus* amoebocyte assay. In this assay, the lipid component of LPS precipitates the aqueous extract from the blood cells (amoebocytes) of the horseshoe crab, *Limulus polyphemus.* The assay is very sensitive and detects fewer than 1000 bacteria in a milliliter.

The properties of bacterial exotoxins and endotoxins are summarized in Table 12–3.

FOCAL POINT

Lipopolysaccharide: Toxin Behind Mimic's Mask.

Lipopolysaccharide (LPS) is unlike bacterial protein exotoxins in that it "doesn't do anything." Instead, it waits for the host to do something—namely, to mistake LPS ingredients for those of the host and, thus fooled, to succumb to their toxic effects. Mammalian hosts mount a series of responses to LPS, including fever and other fairly mild responses, as well as more severe responses, such as tissue necrosis, bleeding, toxic shock, and death. The more toxic effects depend on the LPS structure being intact, especially the lipid A portion. For example, if "piggyback" lipids are removed enzymatically from lipid A, it can cause fevers in mammals, but no longer produces shock or death. Robert Mumford of the University of Texas Southwestern Medical School, Dallas, and Robert Mandrell of the Veterans Administration Medical Center, San Francisco, found an enzyme in human cells that removes fatty acids from lipid A. The enzyme "detoxifies" but leaves its other activities intact. *Neisseria gonorrhoeae* (gonorrhea) carries an elaborate lipooligosaccharide (LOS) on its surface. LOS mimics materials found in the human hosts. This mimicry may lead the host defenses to mistakenly recognize the gonococcus as "self," thus inviting access to host tissues.

ASM News, 56:8, 1990.

Table 12–3
COMPARATIVE CHARACTERISTICS OF EXOTOXINS AND ENDOTOXINS

CHARACTERISTIC	EXOTOXIN	ENDOTOXIN
Major chemical component	Protein	Lipopolysaccharide
Source	Gram-positive and gram-negative organisms	Primarily gram-negative organisms
Antigenicity	High	Low
Means of release	Secretion by cell	Lysis of cells
Degree of specificity	High	Low

SIDEROPHORES

The growth and survival of bacteria in a host require the acquisition of iron. The majority of iron in a host would not be available immediately to bacteria were it not for chemicals, known as **siderophores,** secreted by pathogens in response to iron stress. The siderophores compete with iron-binding compounds of the host to obtain needed iron. Production of some hemolysins by pathogens is regulated by obtainable iron. If iron is limited in quantity, synthesis of certain hemolysins is increased. Production of some toxins and membrane proteins of pathogens is also depen-

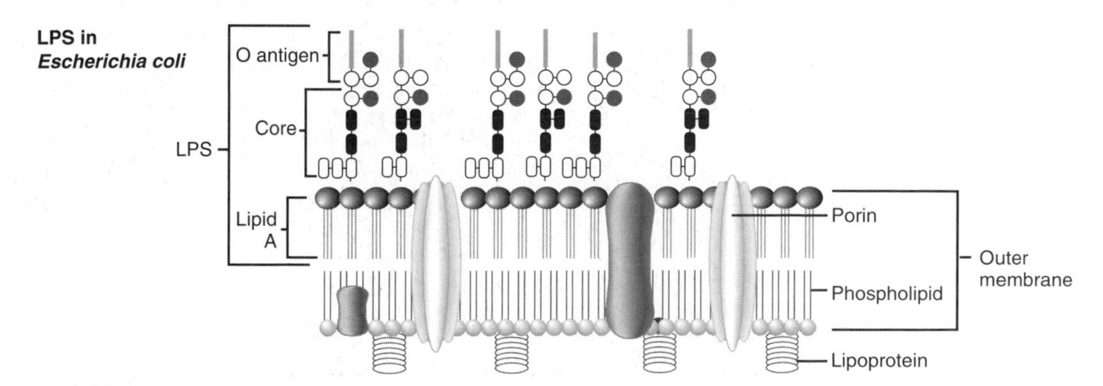

Figure 12–4 ◆ Major components of endotoxin in *E. coli* are the specific polysaccharide (O antigen), the core polysaccharide (common antigen), and the lipid *A*.

dent on available iron. The mechanisms of iron regulation to meet microbial requirements are prime examples of adaptive responses to nutritional deficits.

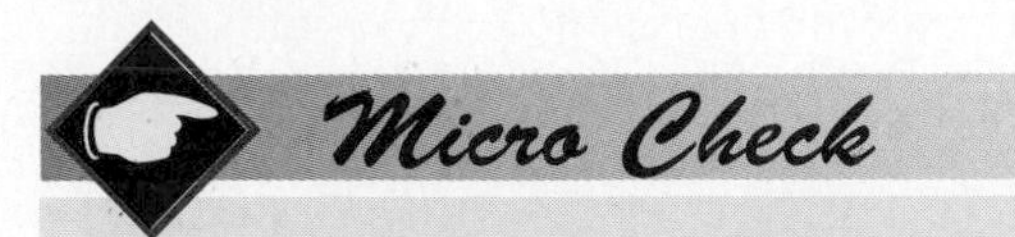

- What structural factors of microorganisms affect virulence?
- How do microbial enzymes affect virulence?
- How do siderophores contribute to virulence?

Host Factors

The anatomy and physiology of the human host provide advantageous sites for colonization and rapid transit for microorganisms in the circulatory system. The anatomic sites, favoring microbial growth, often have overlapping boundaries and are subject to some variations. Pathogenicity reflects a combination of host-microbial factors at a particular time. Even small changes in the microenvironment, supplied by the host, can affect vulnerability to infectious agents.

SKIN AND MUCOUS SECRETIONS

The spread of microbial invaders in epithelial cells of the epidermis and dermis layers of skin is relatively slow normally. However, if skin is moist, infection can spread to parts quite distant from the original site of invasion. Sometimes scratching provides the means for hands to act as transport vehicles for the dissemination of surface organisms.

Secretions help to spread microorganisms on the mucous membranes of the respiratory and genitourinary tracts. Too much moisture interferes with the ciliary action of respiratory epithelium causing microorganisms to enter the lower respiratory tract. Coughing and sneezing redistribute organisms on the mucous membranes.

ADHERENCE FACTORS OR HOST RECEPTORS

The attachment and adherence of microorganisms to mucosal surfaces are significant factors in pathogenesis. In natural habitats, attachment of organisms to a surface results in a higher rate of multiplication than when organisms are free-floating in water. The attachment of particular microorganisms depends on specific receptor sites on the host tissue. A microorganism alone cannot determine effective sites for attachment and successful colonization.

Contributions of host and microbial factors in the phenomenon of adherence are important. Host factors are responsible for adherence of certain gram-positive bacteria to human epithelial cells. For example, cells of *S. aureus* adhere to nasal mucosal cells with greater tenacity in individuals identified as carriers than in those who are noncarriers (Fig. 12–5). Other studies indicate that individuals who develop rheumatic fever after streptococcal pharyngitis have pharyngeal cells with a particular avidity (strength of binding) for rheumatic fever–associated strains of streptococci.

LYMPH VESSELS AND NODES

Microorganisms or their products enter capillaries of the lymphatic system and reach lymph nodes within minutes (Fig. 12–6). The mouth, lung, and nasopharynx are supplied by a particularly large number of lymph vessels. Phagocytes of the lymph nodes wage their attack on incoming organisms (Fig. 12–7). Most microorganisms are trapped and destroyed by phagocytes in the lymph nodes, but some viruses and rickettsias multiply in the lymph nodes and disseminate

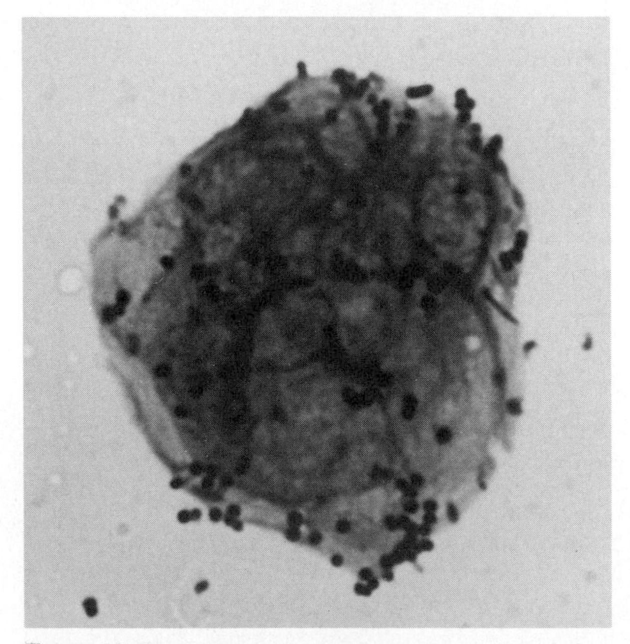

Figure 12–5 ◆ Cells of *Staphylococcus aureus* adhering to a nasal mucosal cell in a carrier.

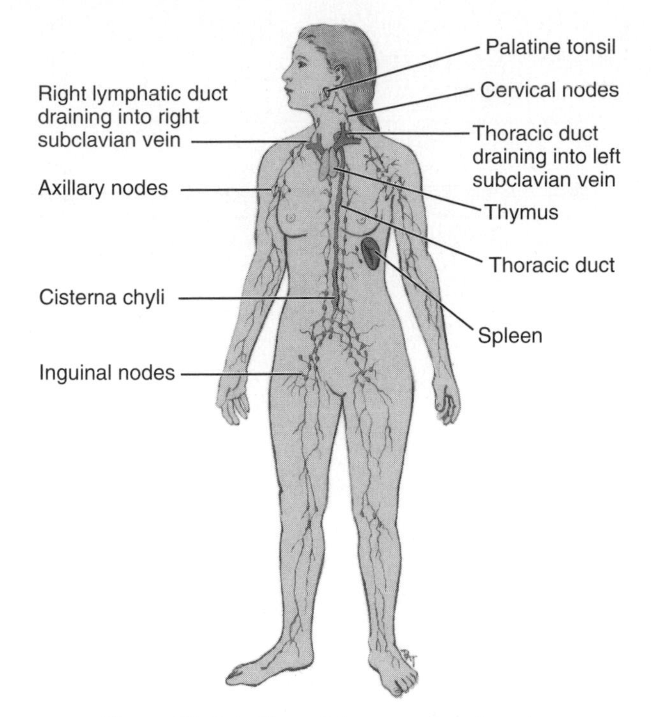

Figure 12–6 ◆ Sites of the major lymph nodes.

freely. Swollen and tender lymph nodes are often the result of host-microbial interactions.

BLOOD

In addition to providing transportation of microorganisms or their products to distant points, blood is an excellent culture medium. Microorganisms are transported in the plasma or within blood cells (Table 12–4). Some protozoa circulate in the plasma; protozoa, a few bacteria, and many viruses grow and multiply in lymphocytes and monocytes; malarial parasites find refuge in red blood cells.

CEREBROSPINAL FLUID

The cerebrospinal fluid (CSF) flows slowly compared to blood. Microorganisms, leaking into the CSF compartment, can cross into the subarachnoid space, lining of the ventricles, or spinal canal with ease. CSF, like blood, is an excellent culture medium. Invasions of the brain and spinal cord are sure to follow if aggressive treatment is not initiated rapidly.

NERVE TISSUE

A few microorganisms, such as the rabies virus, and some microbial toxins affect nerve tissue. Peripheral nerves frequently serve as reservoirs for some viruses or as pathways for particular toxins. Viruses may travel far from invasion sites along peripheral perineural lymphatics, through interspaces of a nerve, by sequential infection of the Schwann cells, or by means of axons (Fig. 12–8).

Toxin-producing bacteria often remain localized at the point of entry, but microbial toxins travel to distant anatomic sites. The tissue spaces may provide the major corridor for transporting toxins. Tetanus toxin spreads to the anterior horns of the spinal cord.

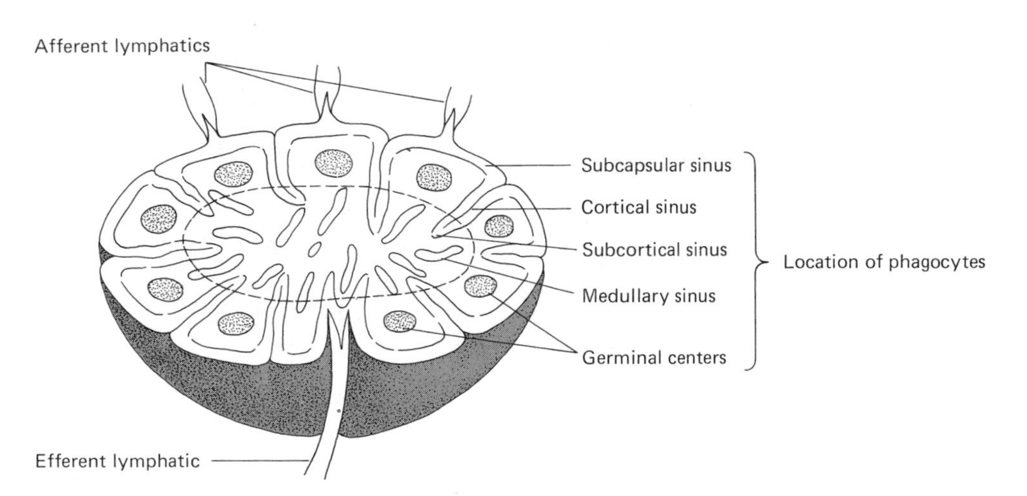

Figure 12–7 ◆ Cross section of a lymph node showing location of phagocytes within sinuses.

Table 12–4
COMPARTMENTS OF BLOOD TRANSPORTING PARTICULAR MICROORGANISMS

		WHITE BLOOD CELLS	
PLASMA	**RED BLOOD CELLS**	**Mononuclear Cells**	**Polymorphonuclear Cells**
Streptococcus pneumoniae	*Plasmodium* species	*Mycobacterium leprae*	*Staphylococcus aureus*
Bacillus anthracis	Colorado tick fever virus	*Listeria monocytogenes*	
Borrelia recurrentis		*Brucella abortus*	
Leptospira interrogans		*Leishmania donovani*	
Trypanosoma species		*Toxoplasma gondii*	
Polio virus		Measles virus	
Yellow fever virus		Smallpox virus	
		Herpes simplex virus	
		Cytomegalovirus	

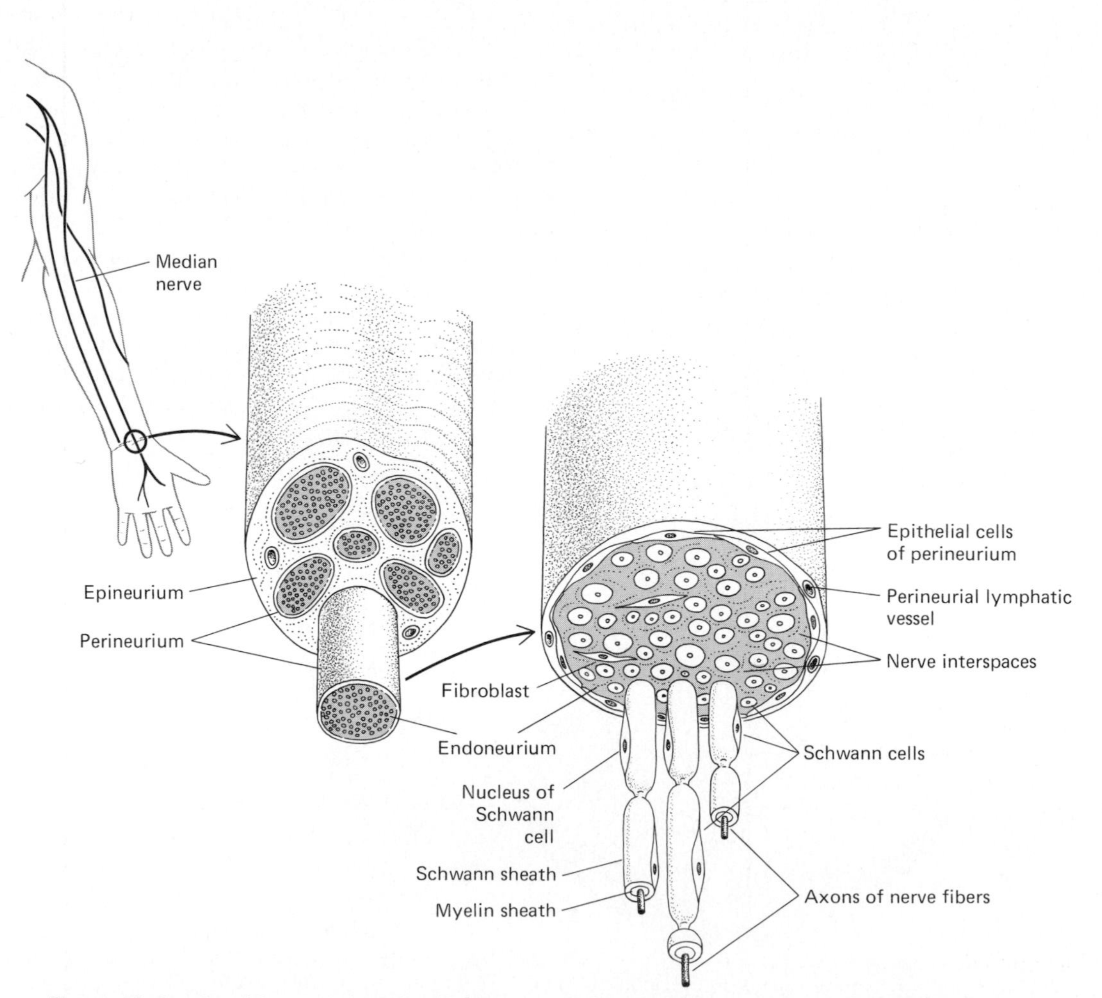

Figure 12–8 ◆ Possible routes for microbial invasion of the central nervous system via peripheral nerves.

An alternate method for microorganisms to gain entrance to tissues of the central nervous system (CNS) is by way of blood. Bloodborne microorganisms sometimes exit capillaries in the dorsal root ganglia. A few viruses actually travel across the blood-brain barrier. The major factor blocking the passage of most microorganisms from cerebral capillaries to brain tissue itself is anatomical (Fig. 12–9). Endothelial cells of cerebral capillaries are so close to one another that extremely tight junctions are formed between adjacent cells. The presence of a substantial basement membrane, separating capillaries from supporting tissue of the CNS, contributes to the barrier. Furthermore, the basement membrane is almost completely surrounded by extensive cytoplasmic processes or footplates of nerve cells known as **astrocytes.** Presumably, viruses travel across the blood-brain barrier with greater ease in children because the basement membrane is less well developed while capillaries grow.

MUSCLE TISSUE

Muscle tissue supplies conditions which attract certain protozoa and viruses. The protozoan causing Chagas' disease migrates to cardiac, skeletal, and smooth muscle tissue. Some arthropod-borne viruses find refuge in striated muscle tissue.

PERITONEUM AND PLEURA

The peritoneum is the membrane lining the abdominal cavity and covering the abdominal organs. It extends from the diaphragm to the pelvic floor. If microorganisms enter the peritoneal cavity, they can spread rapidly to any organ in the cavity on the moist surfaces of the lining.

The pleura is the membrane lining the chest cavity and enclosing the lungs. Microorganisms gaining entrance to the chest cavity can spread on the moist surfaces of the pleura.

Phagocytic cells, known as macrophages, line

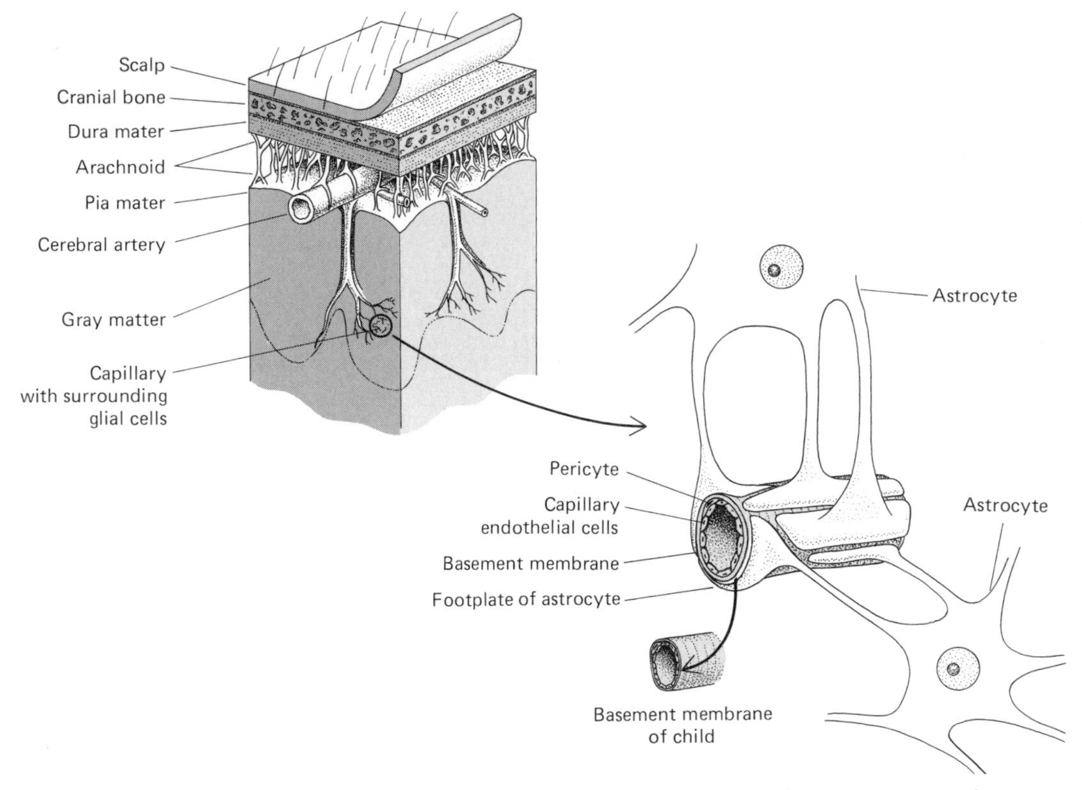

Figure 12–9 ◆ Anatomic factors contributing to the blood-brain barrier. Footplates of astrocytes almost completely surround a well-defined basement membrane and densely packed endothelial cells of cerebral capillaries in the adult. In a child, the basement membrane of cerebral capillaries is not fully developed.

both the peritoneal and pleural cavities, but a large number of microorganisms introduced by a wound in the abdominal or chest cavity may overwhelm the macrophages.

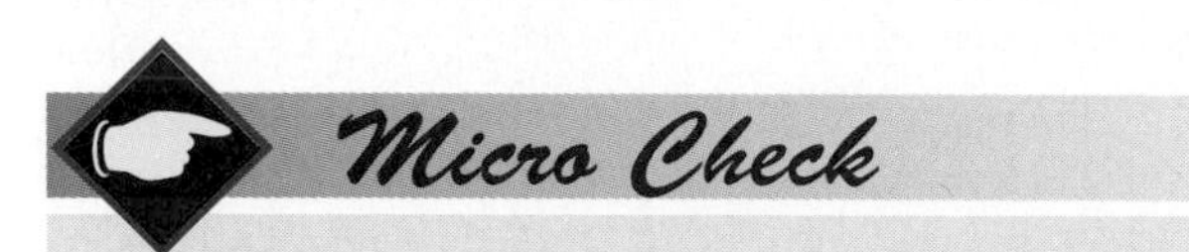

- How are microorganisms transported in the human host?
- How do microorganisms gain access to the CNS?
- How does moisture contribute to the spread of microorganisms?

OPPORTUNISTIC PATHOGENS

Immunodeficiency states, arising from genetic disorders, medical intervention, or underlying disease, provide unusual opportunities for all microorganisms to cause serious disease. Organisms usually not associated with pathogenicity in healthy hosts or pathogens that take advantage of weakened hosts are designated as **opportunistic pathogens.** Infectious complications by opportunistic pathogens are a major cause of death in individuals whose immune defense mechanisms are impaired. Diseases caused by opportunistic pathogens serve to accentuate the role of host defense factors in infectious disease.

A number of inherited immunodeficiency states predispose persons to opportunistic pathogens. Fortunately, diseases directly affecting the immune response are rare. The most commonly recognized inherited disease is severe combined immunodeficiency disease (SCID). Lymphocytes, which contribute to host defense, are affected. Parents first become aware of the deficiency when a child has frequent or severe infections.

Other inherited diseases also affect the frequency and seriousness of infectious disease. Cystic fibrosis is a disease of genetic origin occurring primarily in Caucasians. The disease is characterized by thick mucus, which accumulates in the digestive tract and lungs. The mucus sometimes interferes with the flow of pancreatic juices and bile and obstructs respiratory passages. The unusually thick mucus allows opportunistic pathogens, such as *Pseudomonas aeruginosa,* to colonize in large numbers and contribute to respiratory distress.

Immunodeficiency states occurring as a result of the use of cytotoxic or immunosuppressive drugs are more common than inherited immunodeficiency. Some drugs interfere with bone marrow activity and cause a reduction of circulating white blood cells; others destroy competing microorganisms normally present in or on particular body sites.

Antibiotic-associated pseudomembranous colitis is a serious intestinal disease usually precipitated by the oral administration of particular antimicrobial drugs. The interference with normal microbial flora allows another common intestinal resident, *Clostridium difficile,* to multiply without competition. The severe inflammatory response to *C. difficile* causes formation of a pseudomembrane covering the entire mucosa of the colon. There are many more examples of drug-induced infectious disease caused by opportunistic pathogens, but those capable of elaborating potent toxins, such as the toxin A of *C. difficile,* are of particular concern.

The emergence of AIDS is a significant factor in increasing the incidence of opportunistic infections. The human immunodeficiency virus (HIV), causing AIDS, progressively cripples the body's defenses against invading microorganisms. For reasons unknown, the opportunistic pathogens that cause disease in AIDS patients differ from those in other immunodeficiency states. An opportunistic fungus, *Pneumocystis carinii,* is responsible for death in some AIDS patients. *P. carinii* lives in harmony in the lungs of healthy adults. There has not been a single case of *P. carinii* pneumonia (PCP) reported in an otherwise healthy individual. In the United States, the two most common opportunistic infections in AIDS patients are cryptococcal meningitis and toxoplasmosis. Other opportunists occur in worldwide AIDS (Table 12–5). Unfortunately, the opportunistic pathogens return again and again to cause life-threatening diseases.

CLINICAL MANIFESTATIONS OF DISEASE

The presence of microbial invaders is often not recognized until signs or symptoms of an infectious process occur. **Signs** are findings that are apparent on physical examination of a patient. Signs include blood pressure anomalies, swollen lymph nodes, fever, and a rash. **Symptoms** are subjective complaints described by a patient and not easily detected by the health care professional. Headache, nausea, and weakness are symptoms. A **syndrome** is a collection of signs and symptoms characteristic of a disease.

Table 12–5
OPPORTUNISTIC PATHOGENS IN AIDS

Fungi
Candida albicans
Cryptococcus neoformans
Coccidioides immitis
Histoplasma capsulatum
Pneumocystis carinii
Bacteria
Mycobacterium avium-intracellulare
Mycobacterium tuberculosis
Protozoa
Cryptosporidium parvum
Entamoeba histolytica
Giardia lamblia
Isospora belli
Toxoplasma gondii
Viruses
Cytomegalovirus (CMV)
Epstein-Barr virus (EB)
Herpes simplex I and II
Varicella-zoster virus (VZV)

Perhaps the most frequent and familiar response to microbial invasion is fever. It is not always clear if fever is beneficial or harmful to an infected host. Although some bacteria are inhibited by fever temperatures, other bacteria actually multiply more rapidly at temperatures reached in fever.

Infectious agents may produce enlargement of the liver and spleen. The presence of other pathogens may induce hemorrhage or intravascular coagulation.

A local reaction caused by the presence of an irritant of microbial or nonmicrobial origin is known as **inflammation.** An inflammatory response can occur in any part of the body where an irritant is lodged. To identify a local inflammation the suffix **-itis** (inflammation of) is added to the name of the organ or body part; thus, the word "dermatitis" is a nonspecific term for an inflammatory response of the skin (derma).

The inflammatory response is a continuum of processes that begins with injury and terminates with healing, if the invading particles do not overwhelm the defense mechanisms of the host. The four "cardinal" signs of inflammation are calor (heat), rubor (redness), tumor (swelling), and dolor (pain).

During inflammation, the polymorphonuclear white blood cells (PMNs) mobilize at the scene of insult in large numbers. PMNs and the microorganisms they attack are known as **exudate,** commonly called **pus.** A **purulent exudate** (pus) always contains larger numbers of PMNs and bacteria; it has both a high protein content and a high specific gravity. Purulent exudates are usually associated with serious infections. In milder infections a watery fluid, known as a **serous exudate,** containing fewer PMNs and less protein and having a lower specific gravity, is produced. Exudates must be distinguished from **transudates,** which are noncellular fluids of blood or lymph that leak into surrounding tissues. The immune response following microbial invasion is a cooperative effort of many different cell types discussed in Chapter 13.

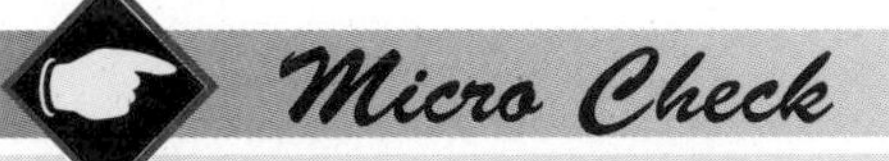

- Why are some microorganisms known as opportunistic pathogens?
- What factors predispose individuals to opportunistic pathogens?
- What is the difference between a sign and a symptom?

Understanding Microbiology

1. When does an infection become a disease?
2. What role does a host have in adherence?
3. Differentiate between the ways that exotoxins and endotoxins affect a host.
4. How do plasmids, bacteriophages, and pathogenicity islands contribute to virulence?
5. What are the four cardinal signs of inflammation?

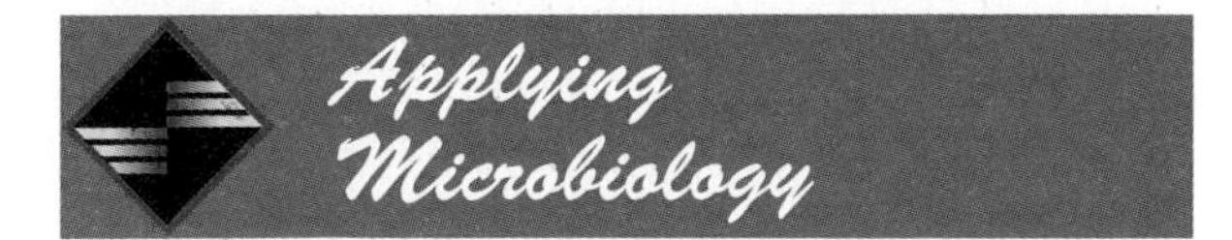

6. Write an essay of not more than 250 words explaining how concepts of pathogenicity and virulence have changed since the time of Pasteur. What new information is available to us that was not available a century ago? You may want to go to the library to obtain additional resource material.

Chapter 13

The Immune Response

Chapter Outline

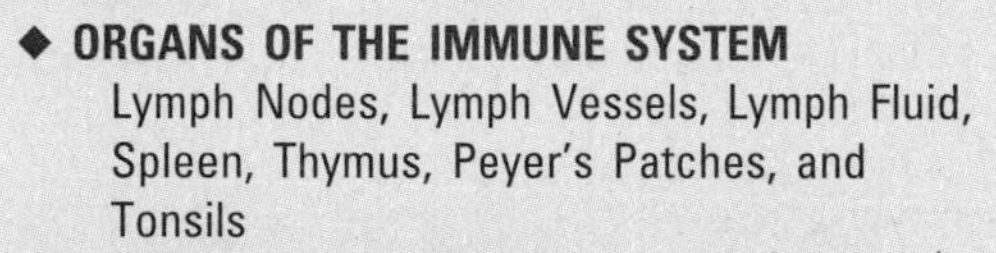

Learning Objectives

After you have read this chapter, you should be able to:

1. Compare and contrast specific and nonspecific immune responses.
2. Describe the actions of the types of leukocytes participating in immune responses.
3. Distinguish between humoral and cellular immunity.
4. Distinguish between the five classes of immunoglobulins.
5. Compare and contrast the primary and secondary immune responses.
6. Identify the roles of antigen, antibody or immunoglobulin, superantigen, cytokines, interferons, complement, B cells, T cells, macrophages, and NK cells in immunity.

The immune system has evolved over millions of years into a number of diverse interactive reactions to control microbial invasion. Antimicrobial immunity can be thought of as a series of defenses with increasing levels of sophistication (Fig. 13–1). Physical barriers such as the skin and mucous membranes lining the oral area and respiratory, gastrointestinal, and urinary tracts do not require specific identification of the invading microorganism to prevent entry. If these barriers

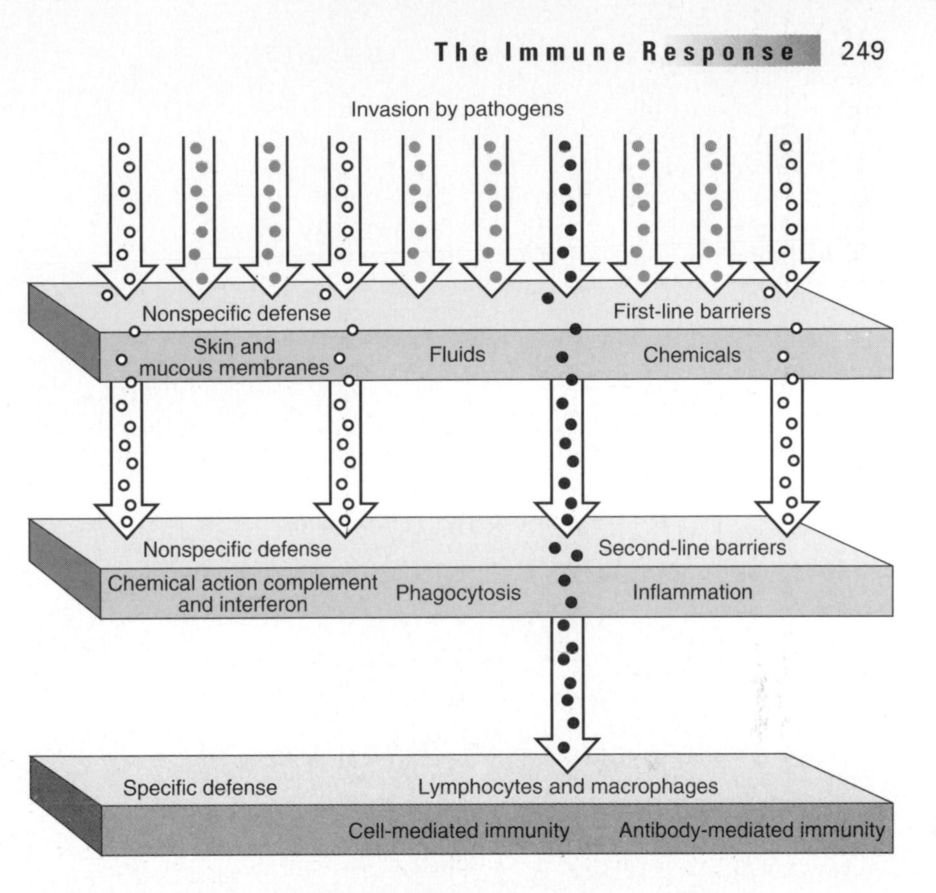

Figure 13–1 ◆ The three levels of immune defense. First- and second-line barriers form the innate or nonspecific immune system. Specific immune system defenses form the third line of defense.

are breached, however, the microorganism encounters a more specialized defense mechanism, the phagocytic leukocytes (white blood cells). Physical barriers and phagocytic leukocytes form part of the **innate** or **nonspecific immune system.**

As invading microorganisms encounter the nonspecific immune system, the **specific immune system** is activated. Specific immunity, also called **acquired** or **adaptive immunity,** activates particular immune defense cells, the lymphocytes, and molecules to act against the invader. Organs of the lymphatic system and the bone marrow are involved in the development of defensive cells.

The specific immune system also has a memory function that increases its power in defense of the body. The immune defense cells remember a previous encounter with an organism such as the bacterium *Staphylococcus aureus* and are ready for rapid action for the next invasion by the same microorganism. The specific immune system attacks *S. aureus* much more aggressively in subsequent invasions.

ORGANS OF THE LYMPHATIC SYSTEM

The lymphatic system is a group of organs and vessels distributed within the body. The primary organs of the system, the lymph nodes, are connected by lymphatic vessels that circulate the lymph fluid and various immune defense cells (see Fig. 12–6). The mammalian lymphoid system has a secondary system, the mucosal immune system located in the mucous membranes of the intestines, respiratory system, and other organs. The cells of the mucosal membranes take up foreign molecules and invader cells, digest them, and present the digested foreign material to immune defense cells.

Lymph Nodes, Lymph Vessels, Lymph Fluid

Lymph nodes are small, shaped like a bean, and usually less than 2.5 cm long (see Fig. 12–7). They are located along lymphatic vessels but are not found in the central nervous system. In the groin, axilla, and neck, lymph nodes are closer to the body surface and, when infected, can be felt easily under the skin. The lymphatic fluid travels through the thin-walled lymphatic vessels; the fluid filters through lymph nodes where large populations of lymphocytes are located. Invading microorganisms are carried in the lymph fluid to the nodes where they make contact with the lymphocytes.

Spleen, Thymus, Peyer's Patches, and Tonsils

The spleen is the largest lymphatic organ; it is located in the upper left abdominal cavity, just below the diaphragm. The spleen filters blood, receiving 200 to 300 ml per minute. About 25 percent of lymphocytes are found in the spleen, where they react to pathogenic organisms in the circulation and destroy them. Phagocytic cells, such as macrophages, remove cell debris, damaged cells, and other large particles.

The thymus has two symmetrical lobes shaped somewhat like a pyramid; it is located behind the sternum with its base resting on the pericardial surface of the heart and extending upward (Fig. 13–2). The thymus is at its largest size in infants and young children; after puberty, it begins to decrease in size, becoming quite small in the adult. The main function of the thymus is to process and develop mature lymphocytes, specifically, the thymus-derived **T lymphocytes.** When mature, T lymphocytes leave the thymus to enter the bloodstream for immune defense.

About 1000 individual lymphatic nodules called Peyer's patches are concentrated in the terminal portion of the ileum, forming part of the gut-associated lymphoid tissue (GALT). GALT encounters foreign molecules and cells transported from the lumen of the intestine across the mucosal epithelium by means of specialized M cells. The M stands for microfold for the appearance of the cell surface. The macrophages in the Peyer's patch protect against pathogens.

Inhaled foreign material and cells encounter the mucosal lymphoid tissue of the tonsils and adenoids. These mucosal tissues form the nasopharyngeal-associated lymphoid tissue (NALT). Foreign substances entering by the oral or nasal route are transported into these tissues by M cells to induce an immune response by lymphocytes and other cells.

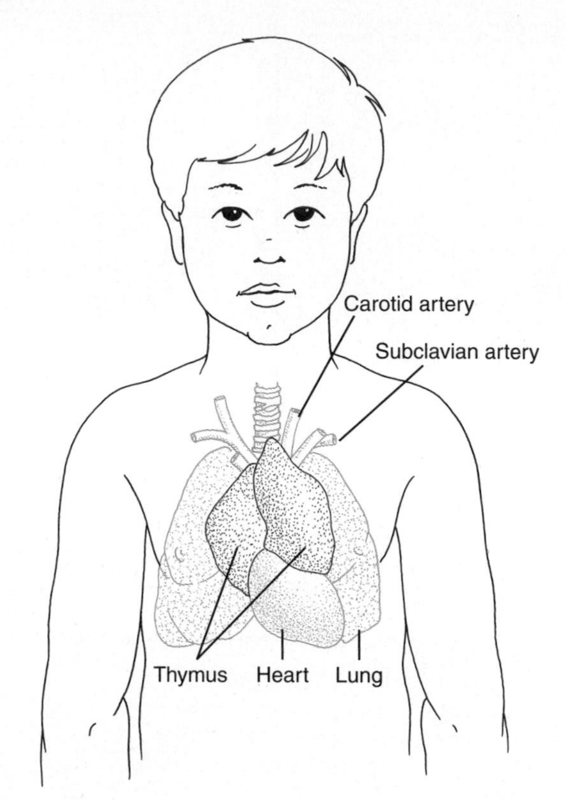

Figure 13–2 ◆ The thymus has two lobes. It is located partly behind the lungs and sternum and in front of the aorta.

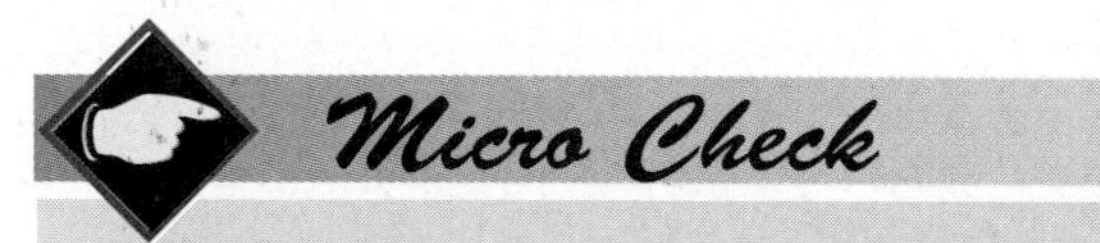

- Describe the location and role of the thymus in immune defense.
- Describe the location and role of the lymph nodes in immune defense.
- Describe the role of M cells.

LEUKOCYTES INVOLVED IN THE IMMUNE SYSTEM

The blood contains leukocytes (white blood cells), erythrocytes (red blood cells), platelets (thrombocytes), and the fluid of the blood called **plasma.** When blood is clotted, the cells are trapped in the clot by a fibrin protein network, and the liquid that surrounds the clot is the blood **serum.** Blood plasma contains the fibrinogen and other compounds required to produce a

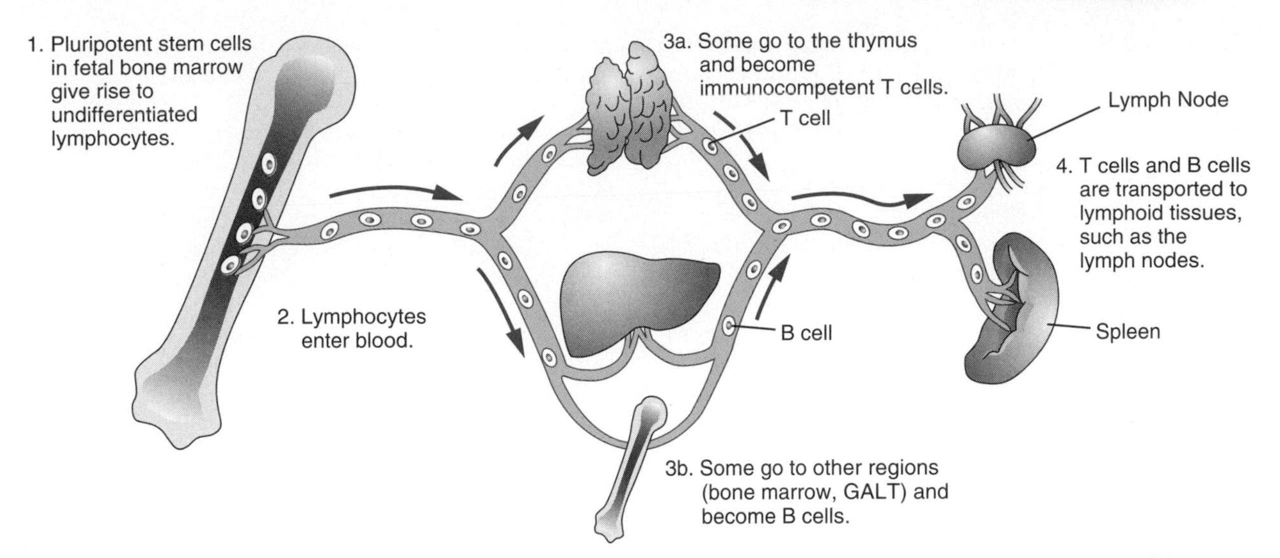

Figure 13–3 ◆ Development of lymphocyte types. After development from stem cells in the bone marrow (1), lymphocytes enter the circulation (2) for more development in either the thymus (T cells) (3a) or in other lymphoid organs such as the bone marrow and intestinal lymphoid systems, the gut-associated lymphoid tissue (GALT; B cells) (3b). Then, mature T and B cells reside in lymph nodes (4).

fibrin clot. When these compounds are removed by forming the clot, blood fluid is called serum.

Origin of Blood Cells

Before birth, blood cells are formed primarily in the liver and spleen, with some cells developing in the thymus, lymph nodes, and red bone marrow. After birth, the cells of the blood are generated in the red bone marrow by the action of **stem cells** (Fig. 13–3). Some leukocytes are produced in lymphoid tissue. Stem cells have the potential to produce any type of blood cell so they are called pluripotential. They divide actively to produce immature blood cells that will develop into the different cell lines released from the bone marrow into the circulating blood (Table 13–1).

The erythrocytes carry oxygen gas to the tissues and carbon dioxide gas from the tissues. Platelets are important in the formation of blood clots to stop blood flow and repair wounds. Leukocytes have various roles in immune defense. To

Table 13–1
BLOOD CELLS

CELL TYPE	NUMBER IN BLOOD	FUNCTION
Erythrocyte	4.5 to 6.0 million/mm^3	Transport oxygen and some carbon dioxide
Leukocytes	5000 to 9000/mm^3	Immune response
Neutrophil (PMN)	60 to 70% of total	Phagocytosis
Eosinophil	2 to 4% of total	Counteract histamine in allergy; destroy parasitic worms
Basophil	<1% of total	Release histamine and heparin; tissue form is the mast cell
Lymphocyte	20 to 25% of total	B cells produce antibodies; T cells function in cellular immunity
Monocyte-macrophage system	3 to 8% of total	Phagocytosis; tissue form is the macrophage
Thrombocyte	250,000 to 500,000/mm^3	Blood clotting; also called platelets

identify different leukocytes in stained blood smears, the size, shape, and color of the nucleus and the presence and color of granules in the cytoplasm are examined (Fig. 13–4).

Granulocytic Leukocytes: Neutrophils, Basophils, Eosinophils

Leukocytes or white blood cells (WBCs) have no colored pigments. The nucleus is distinctive in size, shape, and appearance for each leukocyte type. Leukocytes such as **neutrophils, eosinophils,** and **basophils** with granules in their cytoplasm are known as **granulocytic** cells. The granules contain potent hydrolytic enzymes. Neutrophils are the most common WBCs. Because they have a nucleus with multiple sections or lobes, neutrophils are called **polymorphonuclear leukocytes (PMNs)** (see Color Plate 25). PMNs are actively phagocytic; their numbers increase significantly in acute infections. The eosinophils are important in the destruction of parasitic worms and in allergies (see Chapter 14). Their granules release chemicals that neutralize histamine. Basophils that leave the blood and enter the tissues of the body are called mast cells. Mast cells secrete histamine to dilate blood vessels during infections,

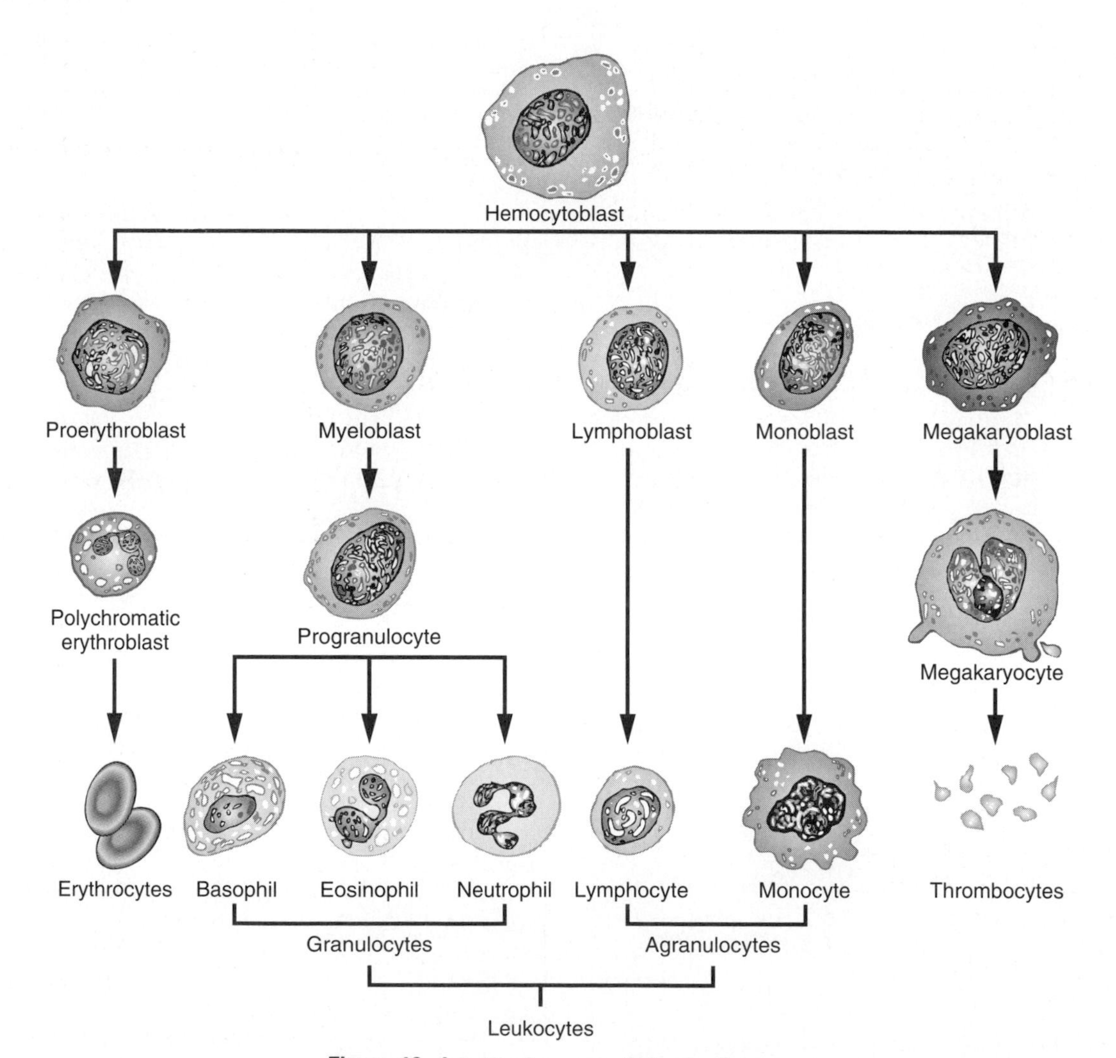

Figure 13–4 ◆ Development of blood cell types.

in damaged tissues, and in allergies. Heparin is secreted by mast cells to inhibit blood clot formation.

Agranulocytic Leukocytes: Lymphocytes, Monocyte-Macrophage System

Lymphocytes and the monocyte-macrophage system of cells have no cytoplasmic granules (**agranulocytic**) (see Color Plates 26 and 27). Lymphocytes are divided into two major subpopulations of cells depending on the organ or tissue in which they mature: **B lymphocytes (B cells)** and **T lymphocytes (T cells)**.

The majority of circulating lymphocytes are influenced by a maturation period in the thymus. These are the thymus-derived T lymphocytes. The B lymphocytes are derived from the bone marrow and migrate to the spleen and lymph nodes to attain maturity. The lymphocytes are the major defensive cells participating cooperatively with **macrophages** with unparalleled sensitivity, precision, and efficiency.

The **monocyte-macrophage system** refers to two forms of the same line of cells. Monocytes develop into macrophages ("big eaters") when they migrate from the circulating blood into other body tissues. Macrophages are excellent at phagocytizing microorganisms, viruses, and worn-out cells. Activated macrophages can phagocytize about one half of their own weight in a 30-minute period.

Platelets (Thrombocytes)

Platelets are not complete cells; they are fragments of very large cells called megakaryocytes. Their function is to form platelet plugs to close breaks and tears in blood vessels. Blood clotting is initiated by platelets.

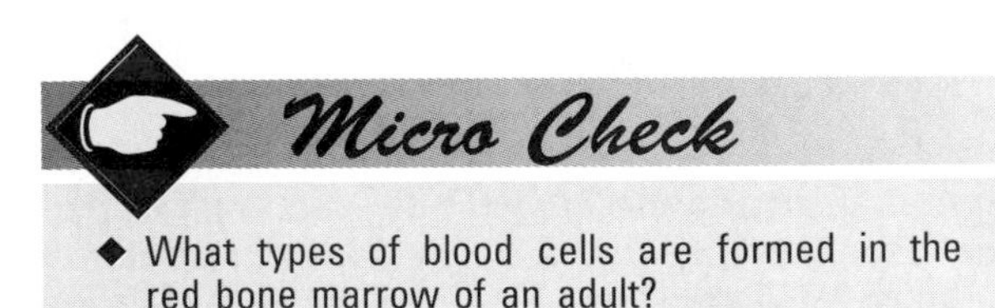

- What types of blood cells are formed in the red bone marrow of an adult?
- What is the function of the neutrophil?
- What are the two types of lymphocytes?

INNATE OR NONSPECIFIC IMMUNITY

The innate immune system almost certainly evolved before the more complex specific immune system. Physical barriers and macrophages are just two of several immune defense mechanisms present from birth and are referred to as innate immunity (Fig. 13–5). Innate immunity is also called nonspecific immunity because it does not respond with specificity; it recognizes invading microorganisms in a general manner and treats them all the same. For example, the innate immune system responds to all microorganisms in the same way over and over again. Innate immunity takes care of the bulk of microbial invaders. The various elements of the innate immune system are always there or can be made in the body in hours.

Primary Barriers to Infection of the Body

Preventing the entry of microbial pathogens into the host is the best way to avoid disease. The largest barriers to entry are the skin and mucous membranes. Skin is composed of multiple layers of flattened epithelial cells with tight junctions between cells to enhance barrier function. The rapid cell turnover and constant sloughing of skin cells prevents local infections from gaining hold. In addition, glands in the skin produce sweat to cleanse the epithelium.

Apocrine cells common to the face, the axillae, and hair follicles produce fatty secretions that preserve the epithelial barrier and inhibit the growth of some bacteria. Washing removes these protective secretions, a possible concern for health care professionals who must wash their hands frequently. Hand lotions help to preserve the skin barrier by limiting skin cracking.

Another major physical barrier to microbial entry is the mucosal epithelium covering the eyes, airways, and gastrointestinal and genitourinary tracts. Secretion of the sticky substance mucus helps to trap microorganisms, preventing their adherence to the epithelium. The mucosal epithelium of the bronchial airways is covered with rapidly beating cilia that sweep microorganisms up and out of the airways.

The bladder is protected in part by urination, which flushes out microorganisms that are mov-

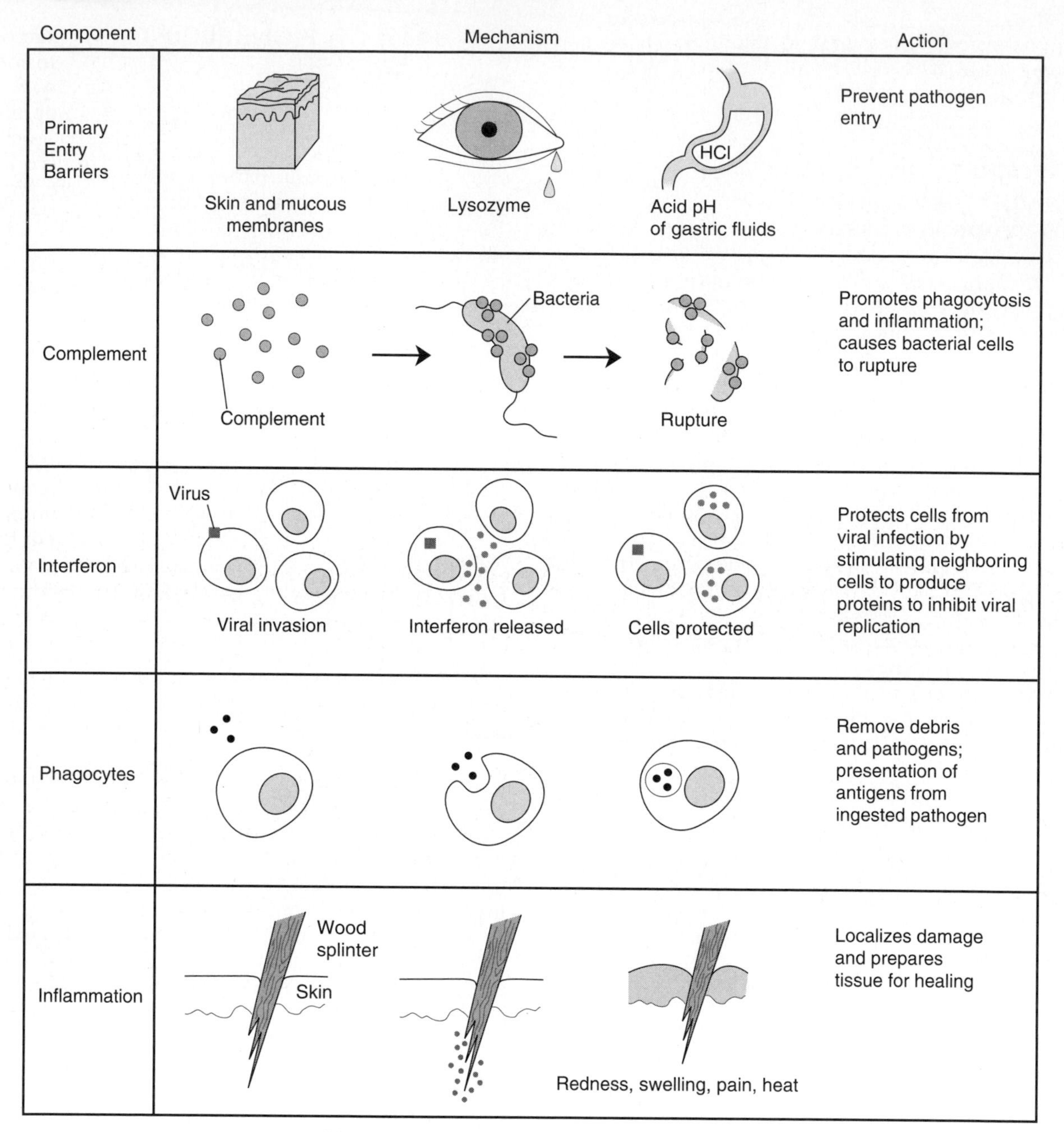

Figure 13–5 ◆ Nonspecific defense mechanisms.

ing up the urethra. Tears from the eyes have the proteolytic enzyme lysozyme to digest cell walls of gram-positive bacteria. Eyelids keep out debris, which could otherwise easily rip holes in the fragile mucosal barrier covering the eyes.

Most communicable infections are transmitted by individuals touching their eyes, nose, or mouth with contaminated hands. Because of their constant use, hands carry all kinds of microorganisms, including viruses. Thus, health care professionals in particular who daily encounter patients with infectious diseases should not touch their eyes, nose, or mouth before washing their hands.

Secondary Barriers to Invasion into the Body

Phagocytosis and inflammation provide a second barrier against microorganisms that have entered the body by crossing the skin and mucosal barriers. Wounds or abrasions are common entry mechanisms bringing dirt and a variety of microorganisms into the deeper tissues of the body.

PHAGOCYTOSIS

Macrophages are mobile WBCs that constantly patrol tissues to destroy the microorganisms in the body by phagocytosis. The phagocytic cell membrane surrounds a bacterial cell or other particles to produce a pocket that eventually closes tightly around the bacteria (Fig. 13–6). This internalized pocket is a vacuole called the phagosome. Lysosomes merge with the membrane of the phagosome to produce a combined vacuole called the phagolysosome. The lysosomal enzymes in the vacuole digest the bacterial cell into its component molecules. These components are deposited onto the surface of the macrophage in an antigen presentation phase to be described in the section on specific immunity.

Most of the time macrophages and neutrophils function as low-level garbage collectors, phagocytizing both dead host cells and the few microorganisms present (Fig. 13–7; see Color Plate 65). However, when macrophages encounter excessive numbers of bacteria or pathogenic bacteria, they become activated to produce more intracellular compounds for killing phagocytized microorganisms.

INFLAMMATION: ROLE OF MACROPHAGES, NEUTROPHILS, AND CYTOKINES

To recruit more phagocytic cells to the scene, activated macrophages also initiate an inflammatory response. Inflammation is characterized by redness, swelling, pain at the infected site, and fever in many cases (Fig. 13–8). All of these symptoms are the effects of chemicals called **proinflammatory cytokines** produced by activated

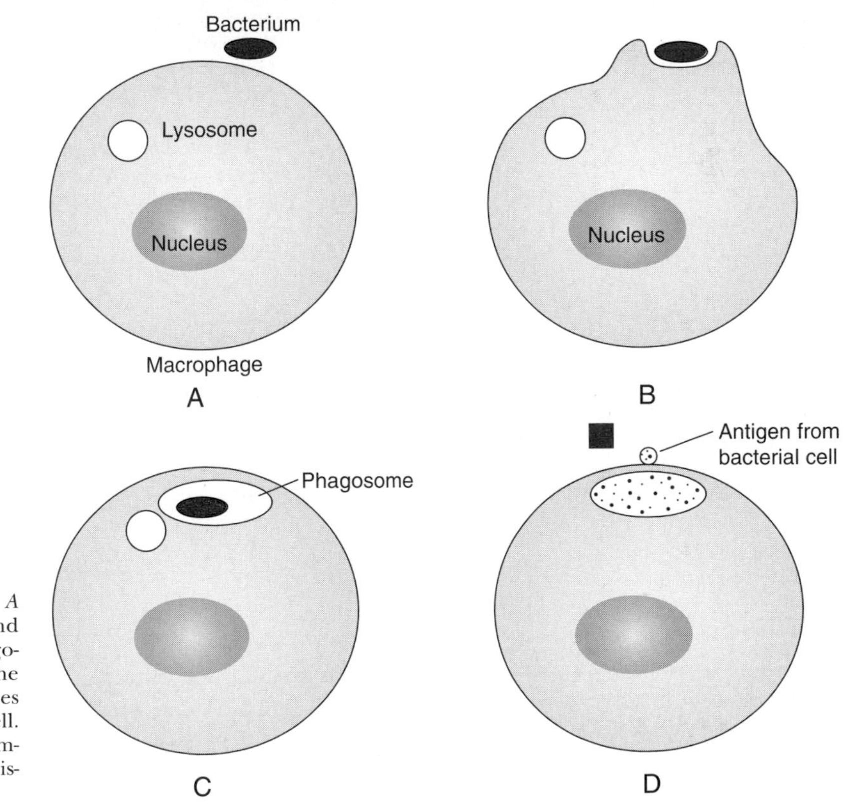

Figure 13–6 ◆ Process of phagocytosis. *A* and *B*, The macrophage surrounds and encloses the bacterial invader in a phagosome. *C*, A lysosome merges with the phagosome, releasing digestive enzymes into the space around the bacterial cell. *D*, The bacterial cell is digested into component molecules, and antigens are displayed on the macrophage surface.

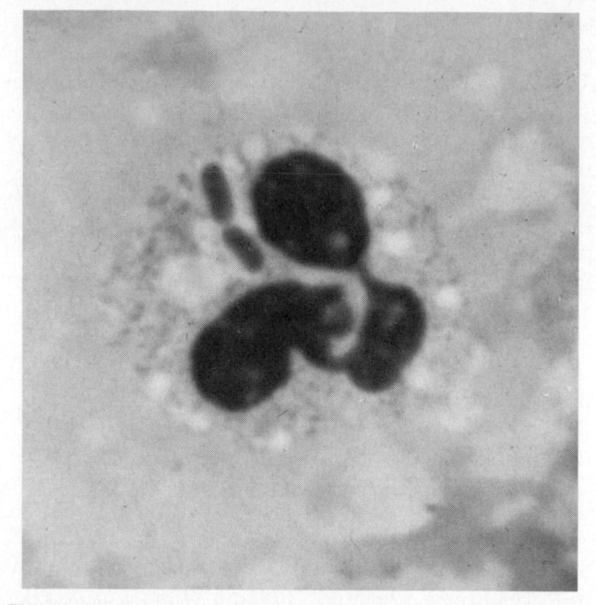

Figure 13–7 ◆ A typical neutrophil, which has engulfed two cells of *Clostridium perfringens.*

macrophages. These cytokines and those produced by other cells are listed in Table 13–2. Because they are rather small proteins (weighing about 20,000 mw) and highly soluble, proinflammatory cytokines quickly travel from the inflamed area through the blood to other organs of the body. These cytokines activate other immune defense cells to travel to the inflamed sites, activate a response by the liver, and induce fever to fight the microbial infection.

Activated macrophages produce the cytokine tumor necrosis factor (TNF) and **interleukin (IL-1),** IL-6, and IL-8. TNF increases the blood supply, resulting in local redness and swelling. IL-1 and IL-6 are produced somewhat later. IL-8 is rapidly produced, attracting another phagocytic cell type, the PMNs, to the area.

PMNs are more specialized than macrophages for phagocytosis. PMNs are normally found in the blood; but when stimulated by IL-8, they migrate through blood vessel walls at the site of inflammation. TNF and other proteins released

Table 13–2
ACTIVITIES OF SELECTED CYTOKINES

CYTOKINE	SOURCE	FUNCTION
Interleukin-1 (IL-1)	Monocytes Macrophages	Promotes proliferation of T cells
Interleukin-2 (IL-2)	$CD4^+$ T cells	Stimulates growth of T cells Activates B cells
Interleukin-3 (IL-3)	$CD4^+$ T cells	Stimulates growth of stem cells and mast cells
Interleukin-4 (IL-4)	$CD4^+$ T cells	Stimulates growth of B cells and some T cells Enhances expression of major histocompatibility complex antigens
Interleukin-5 (IL-5)	$CD4^+$ T cells	Stimulates growth of B cells Promotes secretion of immunoglobulin Stimulates growth and differentiation of eosinophils
Interleukin-6 (IL-6)	$CD4^+$ T cells and others	Promotes T-cell activation and IL-2 production Stimulates B cells and stem cells
Interleukin-7 (IL-7)	Fibroblasts, endothelial cells, some T cells	Stimulates growth of pre-T and pre-B cells
Interleukin-8 (IL-8)	Many cell types	Attracts granulocytes
Interferon-gamma (IFN-gamma)	$CD4^+$ T cells	Activates cytolytic T lymphocytes and natural killer (NK) cells
Colony-stimulating factors	$CD4^+$ T cells Monocytes	Stimulates growth of granulocytes and macrophages
Transforming growth factor (TGF)	$CD4^+$ T cells Monocytes	Inhibits activation of T cells and monocytes Stimulates production of IgA
Tumor necrosis factors (TNF)	$CD4^+$ T cells Monocytes Macrophages	Activates many immune and nonimmune cells

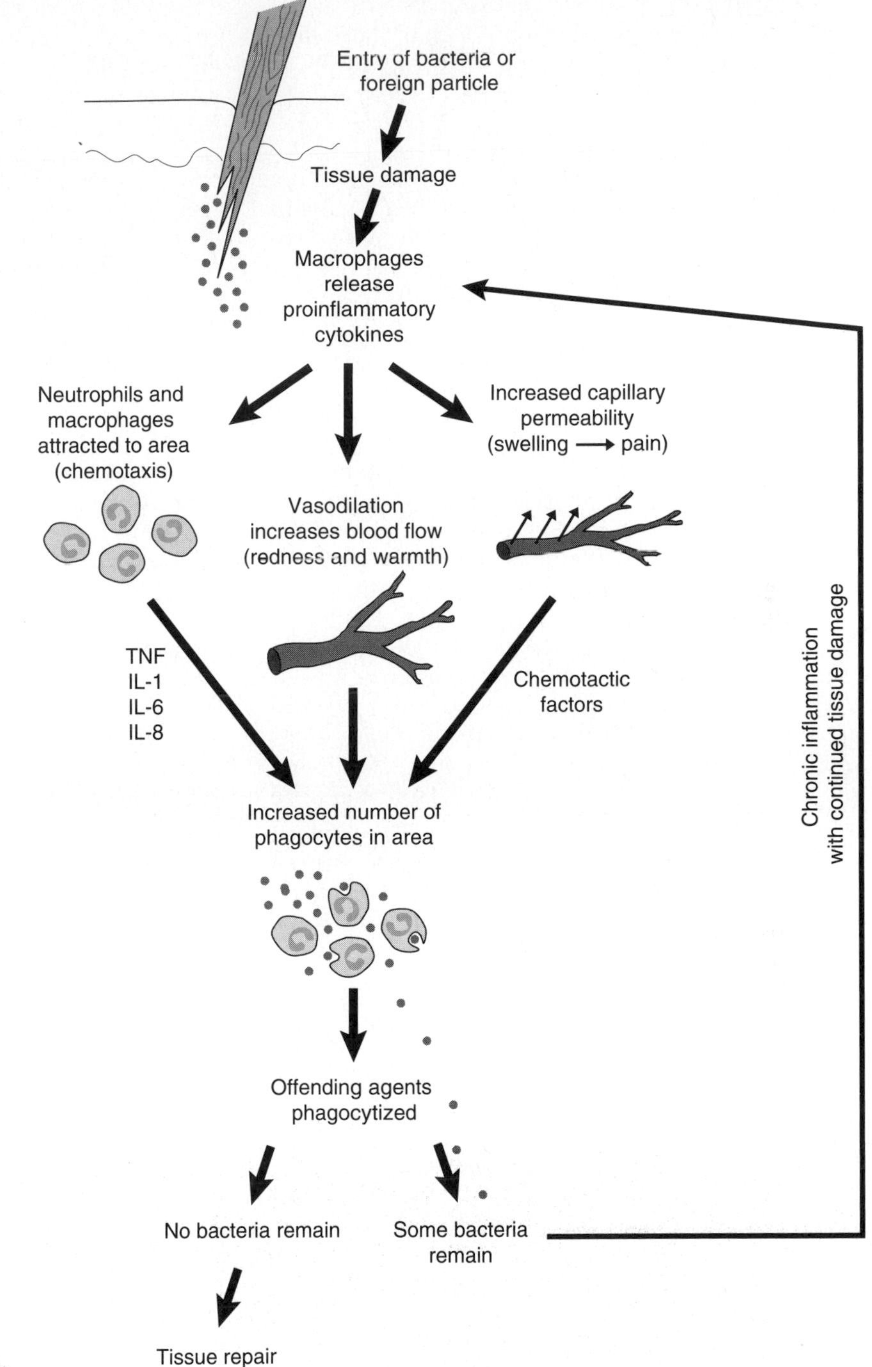

Figure 13–8 ◆ Steps in inflammation.

at the site of an infection cause endothelial cells lining blood capillaries to become very sticky. PMNs passing by in the blood adhere at the sticky sites, squeeze through the capillary wall, and enter the inflamed tissues.

In the wounded tissue, the proinflammatory cytokines activate the PMNs, increasing their phagocytic and digestive enzyme activity. Even normal tissue may be destroyed by the microbial toxins and enzymes released from activated neutrophils. Pus that forms at an infected site is largely composed of neutrophils that have died during action against invading microorganisms.

THE COMPLEMENT SYSTEM

Recruitment of phagocytic cells to the inflamed site is aided by a collection of protein molecules called **complement (C)** that always circulate in the blood. Complement plays a major role in both innate and specific immunity. Activation of complement results in opsonization (preparation for phagocytosis) of bacteria and other particles, inflammatory action, and lysis of cells by proteins called the **membrane attack complex (MAC).**

Complement consists of over 30 proteins, including enzymes, regulatory and inflammatory proteins, peptides, and the MAC proteins. The major complement proteins are named C1, C2, C3, C4, C5, C6, C7, C8, and C9. The numbering reflects the order of discovery, not the order in which they become active. Intact complement proteins are inactive. On activation, many of these proteins become proteases that split the next complement protein in the activation sequence. Fragments derived from the intact complement protein after protease splitting are named by adding lower case letters. For example, complement protein 3 (C3) fragments are named C3a, C3b, . . . C3i. These rules for naming the proteins make it easier to understand which one is being discussed.

Complement proteins can be grouped into three main sets that are each activated in an orderly sequence called the complement cascade (Fig. 13–9). Two sets of complement proteins, the **classical pathway** and the alternative pathway, generate the C3b fragment, leading to opsonization. When plasma proteins such as complement or immunoglobulin act as opsonins, they bind to an antigen, then phagocytic cells bind to the complement-antigen complex more readily, leading to phagocytosis and initiating host defenses.

The classical pathway can also be initiated by the MBLectin pathway, which binds to sugars in the capsules of microorganisms. Ultimately, the C3b fragment is generated. When C3b is generated, the final set of proteins, MAC, is activated, causing cell lysis. The discussion here is focused on only the classical pathway, involving proteins C1, C4, C2, and C3, in order.

When C1 attaches to a large complex association of antibody molecules bound to antigen molecules, the pathway is activated. Antibody molecules are produced by B cells in response to

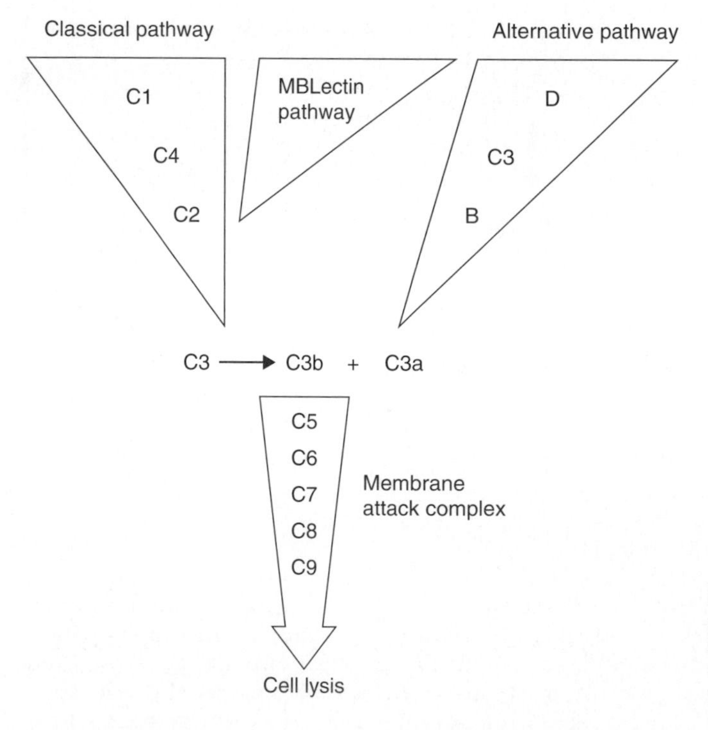

Figure 13–9 ◆ Complement activation pathways. Production of complement fragment C3b by either the classical pathway or the alternative pathway activates the membrane attack complex (MAC). The MBLectin pathway activates C4 and C2 of the classical pathway.

invasion by foreign microorganisms. Antigen molecules are derived from the chemicals of the invader's cell structures and the molecules it produces. Antigens, antibody molecules, and their specific binding action are discussed in a later section of this chapter. For our purposes at this point, these molecules form large complex binding arrangements that attract the complement proteins.

After C1 binds to the antibody molecule in the large complex, a series of reactions (a cascade) produce C3b fragments. Microorganisms bound to C3b are more easily phagocytized. The C3a fragment released into solution attracts more phagocytic cells to the scene. The microbe-bound C3b also continues the activation of the remaining components of the complement cascade. Cleaving of C5 generates C5a, which powerfully attracts phagocytic cells. Continuing through the cascade of reactions, the MAC produces pores through the cell's outer wall, resulting in osmotic lysis of the microorganism.

ACUTE PHASE RESPONSE OF LIVER IN INFLAMMATION

The proinflammatory cytokine IL-6 triggers an acute phase response by the liver. During the acute phase of an infection, the liver produces clotting factors, complement components, and other chemicals to replace those consumed by inflammatory action. Clots in inflamed areas trap and wall off bacteria.

ROLE OF FEVER

Fever is a sign of inflammation induced by the proinflammatory cytokines. The role of fever in protection from microbial disease is not certain but may inhibit bacterial growth. Induced fever was used to treat neurosyphilis before the antibiotic era. Fever also signals host cells to produce heat-shock proteins that enhance host cell survival in the presence of adversity and stress.

Body temperature measurement is used by the clinician to help discriminate between bacterial and viral infections. Viral infections do not activate macrophages nearly as effectively as bacteria, resulting in less proinflammatory cytokines and, consequently, little or no fever. The acute phase response of the liver and fever are excellent examples of the power of proinflammatory cytokines in innate immunity.

INTERFERONS AND NATURAL KILLER CELLS IN VIRAL INFECTIONS

Although phagocytic cells and proinflammatory cytokines are the major players in innate immunity to microorganisms, in viral infections the cytokine interferon alpha and natural killer (NK) cells are important. In contrast to cellular organisms, viruses cannot reproduce on their own. They use host cellular metabolism and ribosomes to produce multiple viral particles. During takeover of host cell metabolism, viruses trigger their hosts to produce interferon alpha. The interferon shuts down the host cell metabolism that allows virus replication (Fig. 13–10). However, if the host cell has already been infected with virus, NK cells kill the host cell to stop viral production.

Although NK cells look much like lymphocytes, they may have a distinct lineage. The NK cell is the first line of defense against intracellular microorganisms, tumor cells, and virus-infected cells. Interferon alpha and beta produced by virus-infected cells attract NK cells to areas of inflammation. NK cells kill virus-infected cells such as epithelial cells. Uninfected epithelial cells are protected from attack by carrying cell surface chemicals that do not attract NK

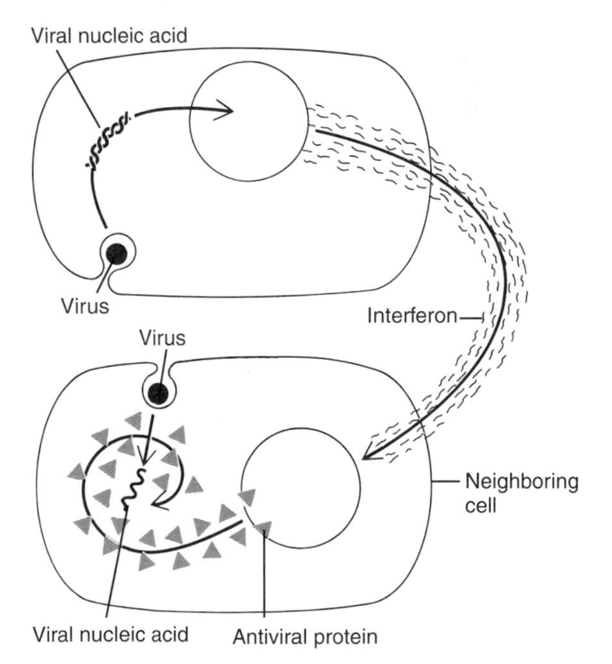

Figure 13–10 ◆ Viral infection induces interferon (INF) production by infected cell. Interferon stimulates neighboring cells to produce antiviral proteins that block viral replication.

cells. The surface chemicals are called the **major histocompatibility complex (MHC) class I** antigens. These are protein antigens produced by the cells of the body that serve as specific antigens for each human. The MHC proteins are extremely important in specific immunity and are discussed in a later section of this chapter.

The MHC-peptide complexes enable the NK cells to recognize and destroy virus-infected cells. NK cells may also carry specific antibody molecules, allowing them to bind to virus components left on the surface of an infected cell and kill the cell. Neutrophils kill cells in this same manner; the process is called **antibody-dependent cell-mediated cytotoxicity (ADCC).**

NK cells kill their targets using at least three mechanisms: (1) by secretion of proteins called perforins, which make holes in cell membranes, similar to MAC; (2) by delivering cytotoxic granules into host cells to activate the host cell to commit a type of suicide, called programmed cell death or apoptosis; and (3) by an interaction between a specific protein on the host cell surface and a protein made by the NK cell that induces apoptosis of the cell.

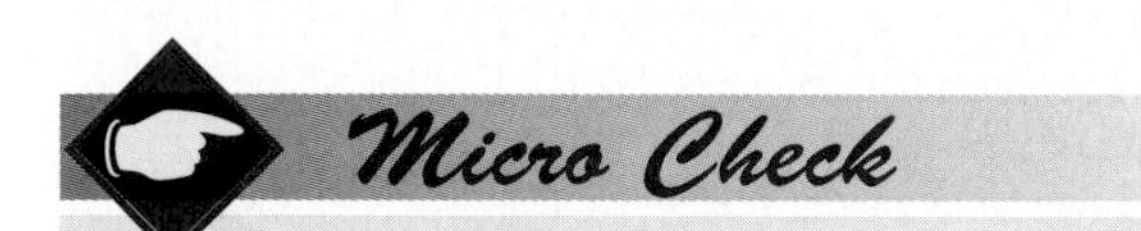

- What cells carry out phagocytosis?
- What is the role of complement in immune defense?
- Identify the role of five cells or molecules in the inflammation response.

SPECIFIC IMMUNITY

The strength of the specific immune response lies in two main phenomena. The first is the truly remarkable ability to produce defensive cells and molecules that will attack the invading microorganism, and no others, a phenomenon known as **specificity.** The second is the capability to remember past infections and react rapidly to defend against a subsequent invasion, a phenomenon called **immunological memory.**

The specific action is directed against the molecules found on the invading microorganism's surface, appendages, and secretions, such as enzymes and toxins. These molecules are foreign to the host and are called **antigens** or **immunogens** because they are capable of stimulating an immune response. As an example, a bacterial invader has dozens of antigens on its cell surface, flagella, pili, and secretions for the human host to respond to immunologically (Fig. 13–11). Each species of microbial invader has its unique set of antigens that activate particular B and T cells to grow and divide rapidly, increasing the numbers of B and T cells of a particular type (Fig. 13–12). Most B cells of the large clone mature into fully active **plasma cells.** The molecules produced by the host's plasma cells to attack the foreign antigens are called **antibody** molecules or **immunoglobulins.** Some activated B and T cells develop partial activation into **memory B** and **memory T** cells; they carry the capacity for memory by remaining in the circulation ready to respond quickly to a second and subsequent invasions by the same invader.

The specific immune system has two main types of responses carried out by the two types of lymphocytes: **humoral immunity** and **cellular immunity.** The antibodies produced by the plasma cells are responsible for humoral or, a more descriptive phrase, antibody-mediated immunity. Antibody molecules circulate freely in the blood and lymph. These fluids were once called **humors,** and immune defense was associated with these fluids until antibodies were discovered.

Macrophages, T cells, NK cells, and other cells and the cytokines they release are responsible for **cellular immunity.** As they release numerous cytokines, other cells are drawn into the battle against the invader. Cellular immunity is particularly important in the destruction of virus-infected cells, cancer cells, cells of organ transplants, and eucaryotic pathogens. Our discussion begins by introducing antigens and antibodies

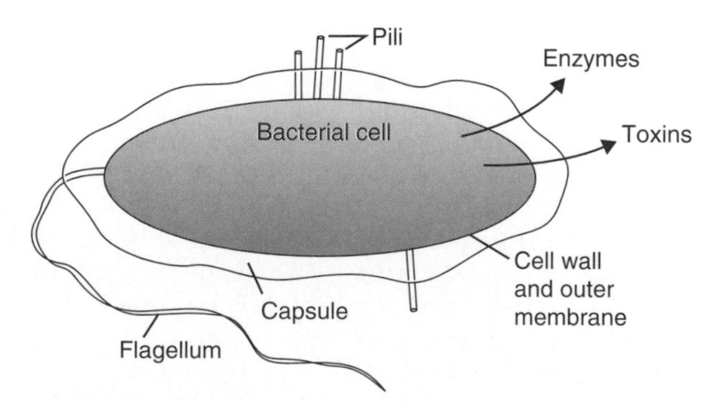

Figure 13–11 ◆ Cell structures that are the source of some bacterial antigens. Fungi, plants, animals, and other humans are sources of an infinite number of antigens.

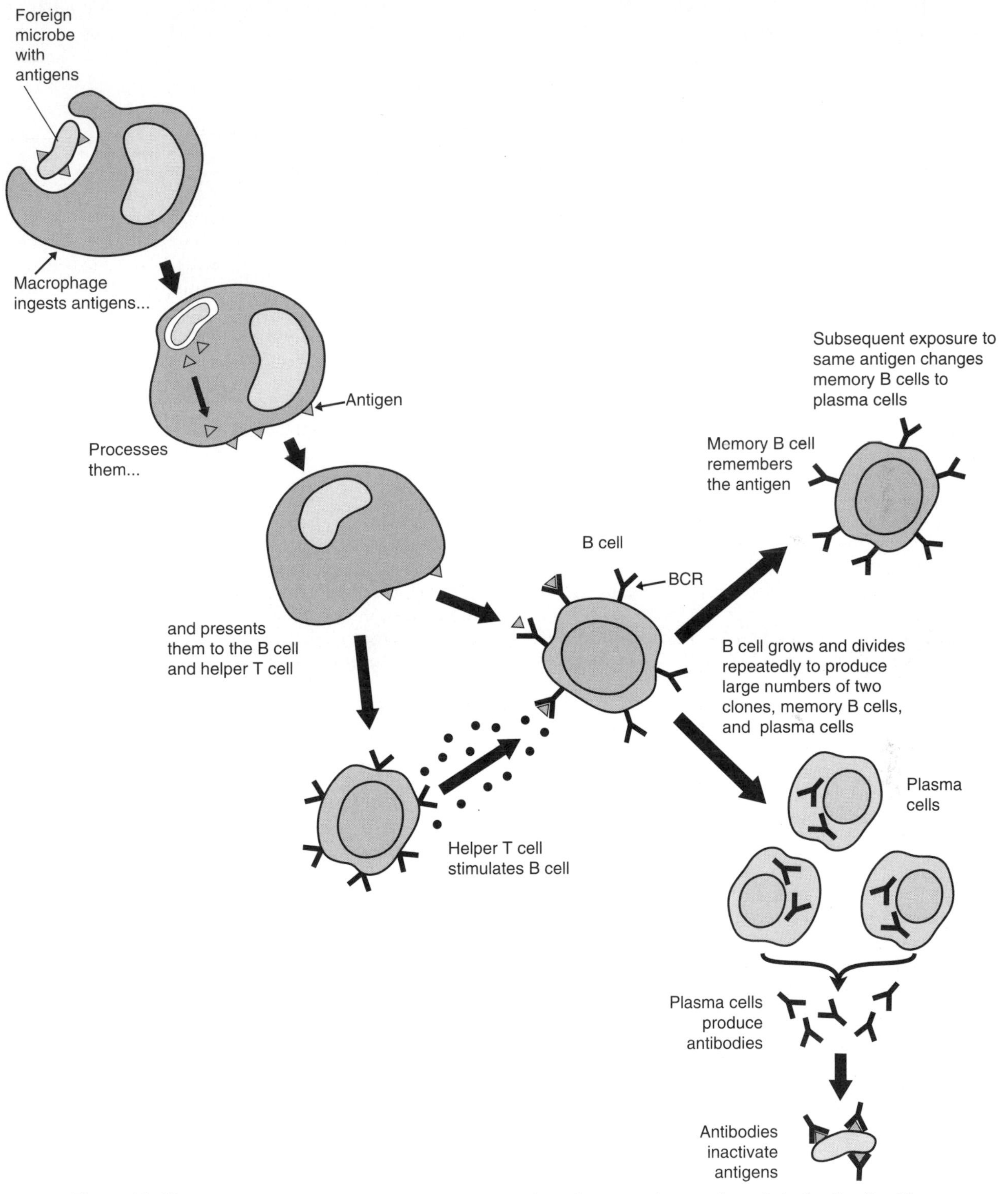

Figure 13–12 ◆ Lymphocyte activation by antigen presented on the macrophage surface. Only the B cells with a B cell receptor (BCR) for the antigens presented bind to the antigen and become activated. Activated B cells grow and divide, rapidly expanding the numbers of the specific B cell clone. Most B cells develop into plasma cells that produce large quantities of antibody molecules specific for attacking the invader. Some B cells are partially activated to become memory B cells. A similar mechanism occurs to activate specific T cell clones and to produce memory T cells.

followed by the role of macrophages and lymphocytes in the specific attack against a microbial invader.

Antigens

Most antigen molecules are large with molecular weights of 10,000 or more. Antigens may be proteins, polysaccharides, lipoproteins, and glycoproteins. Proteins are very effective antigenic molecules. Substances of low molecular weight stimulate immune responses only if they are bound to a carrier protein. Such substances are called incomplete antigens or **haptens.** Antigens have distinctive chemical groups or structural arrangements of atoms called **determinants,** or **epitopes,** that bind to receptor molecules on immune defense cells and to antibody molecules.

Most of what we know about the specific immune response is related to protein antigens that are large enough to be recognized and processed by antigen-presenting cells (APCs). Microorganisms also contain unique carbohydrates and lipids. The immune response to carbohydrate antigens is not well understood. Carbohydrates that are very large, composed of many repeating units, link multiple chemical receptor molecules on B cells, the **B cell receptors (BCRs).** Such binding or cross-linking of BCRs triggers the B cell to produce carbohydrate-specific IgM antibodies in two to three days without activating T cells.

Because many microorganisms have carbohydrate antigens in their cell walls, antibody production without T cell involvement may help the innate immune response. The combination of carbohydrates complexed with protein is highly immunogenic so it stimulates a strong immune response. Knowledge of this effect influences the design of vaccines that stimulate an immune response to provide protection without ever experiencing the disease. *Haemophilus influenzae* vaccine is designed with both protein and carbohydrate; it is more immunogenic than the carbohydrate given alone, especially in infants.

Fats, including lipids and glycolipids, are generally considered to be poor antigens. However, investigators have recently identified the capacity of phagocytic cells for reacting with lipids and glycolipid antigens to destroy the microorganism. Recognition of fat-containing substances on microorganisms may be important in cell-mediated immunity active against microbial pathogens having significant lipid components, such as *Mycobacterium tuberculosis* and *M. leprae.*

SELF AND NONSELF

It is necessary to introduce the concept of **self** and **nonself** and to explain how these terms relate to antigen and immune responsiveness. An individual's own cells and tissues contain cell surface molecules that are antigenic, capable of stimulating an immune response, but not in the individual. These antigens are called self antigens, and they are not recognized by the individual's own immune system. They do not stimulate an immune response except in certain autoimmune disease states where the immune system attacks an individual's own tissues (see Chapter 14). If the tissues and organs of an individual donor are transplanted to another person, they will stimulate the immune system of the recipient.

Sources of antigens that enter the body through contact, eating, drinking, or through cuts, wounds, and abrasions are recognized by the immune system as nonself. They stimulate first a nonspecific immune response followed by a specific immune defense.

SELF ANTIGENS OF THE MAJOR HISTOCOMPATIBILITY COMPLEX

Erythrocytes, leukocytes, and all cells and tissues of the body have unique chemicals on their surfaces that are self antigens. Erythrocytes carry blood group antigens on their surfaces corresponding to the individual's blood type. Other tissue cells have antigens coded for by the MHC of genes on human chromosomes 6 and 15. The proteins of the MHC genes are cell surface antigens that are important in specific immunity. They bind foreign antigen fragments and display them on the cell surface for contact with immune defense cells.

Two classes of MHC proteins are produced: **MHC class I** and **MHC class II** (Fig. 13–13). The proteins making up the MHC class I antigen include a polymorphic heavy chain with alpha-1, alpha-2, and alpha-3 proteins and the light chain, a beta-2 microglobulin molecule, which together form the assembled unit, the self-peptide antigen. The MHC-I heavy chain is attached to the cell membrane and extends into the cytoplasm. The

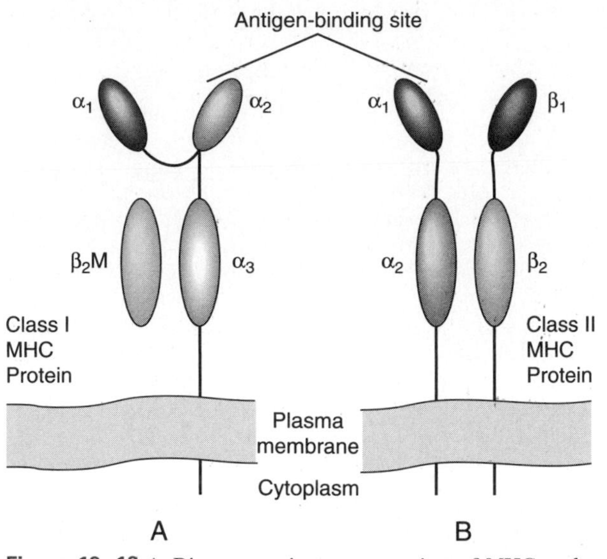

Figure 13–13 ◆ Diagrammatic representation of MHC molecules. *A,* MHC class I proteins with the antigen-binding site between the alpha-1 and alpha-2 proteins. The heavy chain (alpha-1, alpha-2, alpha-3) extends through the plasma membrane. The beta-2M forms the light chain of MHC I structure. *B,* MHC class II proteins with the antigen-binding site between the alpha-1 and beta-1 proteins. The alpha and beta chains extend through the plasma membrane.

MHC class II antigen consists of two protein chains, alpha (alpha-1 and alpha-2) and beta (beta-1 and beta-2) chains, inserted into the cell membrane. Computer-drawn images of MHC class I and class II proteins allow us to see the similarities of the portions that bind peptide antigens. The class II alpha and beta protein chains are superimposed on the class I alpha proteins (see Color Plate 28).

Each individual inherits two sets of MHC genes, one from each parent. The MHC genes that express protein antigens on human leukocytes are called human leukocyte antigens (HLA). For instance, MHC class I genes in humans are designated HLA-A, HLA-B, and HLA-C; their antigens are expressed on most nucleated cells of the body. MHC class II genes are designated HLA-DR, HLA-DQ, and HLA-DP; they are expressed on macrophages, B cells, and dendritic cells. These cells recognize and bind nonself antigens and process and display (present) them within the MHC molecules on their surfaces. For these functions, they are called **antigen-presenting cells** (Fig. 13–14).

Although each person inherits two genes for the HLA region, there are many possible variants of the genes, called alleles. Genes with multiple alleles are polymorphic, making the MHC genes the most polymorphic genes known to humans, with some genes having 150 alleles. Polymorphism of MHC genes provides a large number of variations in the MHC complex, which guards against the possibility of infection by a pathogen that no human immune system can destroy. Because of the polymorphic MHC genes, at least some individuals in the population will have an MHC antigen pattern that will initiate an immune defense against an invading pathogen.

IMMUNOLOGIC TOLERANCE

The question of how self can be distinguished from nonself is important in understanding the action of immune defense cells such as T and B cells. When lymphocytes do not become activated by foreign substances, the phenomenon is called **immunologic tolerance. Self tolerance** is the inability of an individual's own antigens to generate an immune response.

The tolerance to self antigens occurs during embryological development. Self antigens either do not activate the lymphocytes designed to recognize them or the self antigen–specific lymphocytes are destroyed early in life. In the thymus, developing T cell clones acquire a specific **T cell receptor (TCR).** The TCR recognizes antigen and binds to it. To acquire self tolerance, the T cells undergo two selection processes: positive and negative selection. The T cells that do not

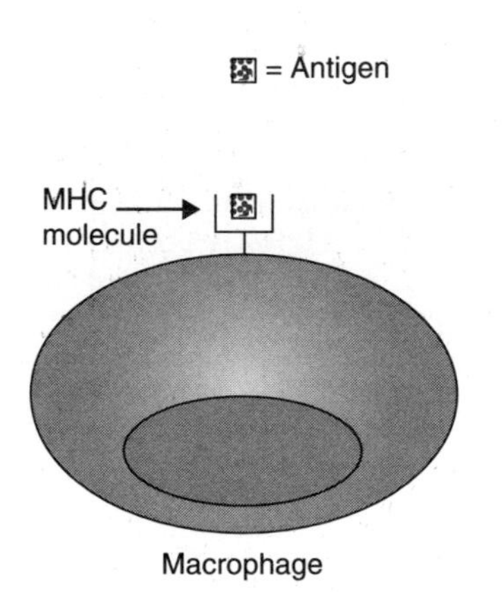

Figure 13–14 ◆ Antigen presentation. Antigen is held in MHC molecule on the surface of a macrophage.

FOCAL POINT

Diversity in Our MHC Genes Provides a Better Defense

The major histocompatibility complex (MHC) is the collection of genes coding for MHC class I and class II antigens found on the cells of vertebrate organisms. Human MHC gene products expressed on the human white blood cells are known as human leukocyte antigens (HLA). The HLA antigens serve the very important function of displaying peptide antigens from foreign organisms on the surface of antigen-presenting cells. This presentation of antigen alerts T cells to interact and begin an immune defense. Research suggests that persons with a large diversity in their HLA genes have a selective advantage for surviving malaria, hepatitis B, human immunodeficiency virus (HIV) and other infections. They may succeed in avoiding the acquired immunodeficiency syndrome (AIDS) if exposed to HIV.

About a dozen HLA genes, located on chromosomes 6 and 15, code for antigens. The genes have many different forms, or alleles, with some genes having more than 150 alleles. Each person has a unique set of HLA genes derived from both parents. Having different alleles in a gene pair is known as a heterozygous condition. When someone carries an identical pair of HLA alleles, the person is homozygous for a gene. In persons carrying homozygous genes, fewer HLA antigen types are produced.

Recent research conducted by Mary Carrington and her coworkers selected alleles of the HLA-A, HLA-B, and HLA-C genes to study in relation to HIV infection and AIDS. In their study, persons who were homozygous for one to three of these HLA genes had an increased progression to symptoms and active disease compared with persons who were heterozygous for these genes.

The same study showed that people carrying the HLA genes identified as B*35 and Cw*04 progressed more rapidly to AIDS than persons with other patterns of alleles studied. However, if a person carried just one of the B*35 or Cw*04 alleles, the progression to AIDS was slower than when both alleles were present.

Is there an explanation? Because the HLA antigens present peptides such as those from the HIV-1 virus to the T cells, more variety in our HLA antigens leads to a more effective immune system. However, some combinations of alleles may reduce the effectiveness of the immune response. Persons carrying the HLA alleles identified as B*35 and Cw*04 had reduced activity in their cytotoxic T lymphocytes, and symptoms of AIDS occurred earlier. Because almost half of the population is homozygous for these alleles, understanding the significance of these genes in HIV infections may help to develop appropriate drugs and vaccines.

*Modified with permission from Carrington M, Nelson G, Martin MP, et al: HLA and HIV-1: Heterozygote advantage and B*35-Cw*04 disadvantage. Science 1999; 483:1748–1752.*

pass these tests are destroyed. In positive selection, only T cells with TCRs that bind to MHC molecules will survive.

In negative selection, T cells must not recognize MHC molecules on certain APCs. The T cells that bind to MHC proteins on these APCs very weakly are allowed to survive; those that bind strongly are killed. T cells that bind to an MHC molecule associated with self peptides are also killed. Negative selection is a major mechanism for inducing tolerance to self antigens. Remaining T cell clones continue in the body; they recognize nonself peptide antigens of almost any type.

After differentiation into full-fledged T and B cells, these cells locate in the lymph organs where they can recognize antigens. This process is complete in the human fetus by six months of intrauterine life. At birth, the newborn has T and B cell clones to respond to any antigen it will ever encounter in a lifetime even though the antigens have not yet entered the body.

Tolerance can be induced later in life by certain drugs and by radiation therapy. A nonresponsive immune system leads to a state of anergy, a failure to respond, that can cause serious health problems.

NONSELF ANTIGENS

Antigenic molecules of microorganisms and viruses are nonself antigens. Other nonself antigens are present on the cells and tissues of humans and animals that serve as blood and tissue donors. A normally functioning immune system will not tolerate the introduction of foreign cells as in a blood transfusion of the incorrect blood type, or a transplant of heart, lung, skin or other tissues that do not match the tissue type of the patient (see Chapter 14). Drugs to suppress the immune system are administered to a transplant patient to maintain a transplanted organ.

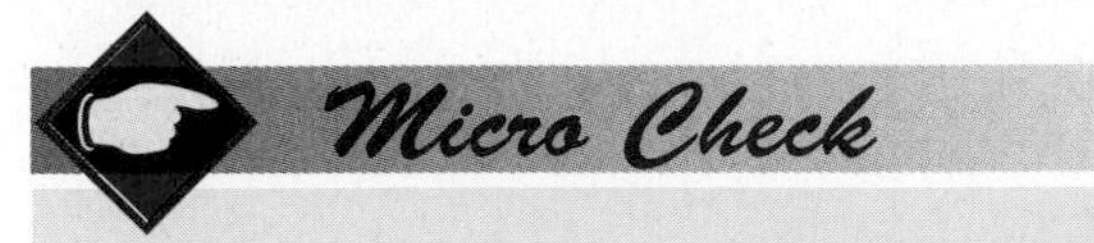

- Write a list of three physical and chemical properties of an antigen.
- Which cells carry the MHC class II antigens?
- What advantage is provided by the polymorphic MHC genes?

Five Classes of Antibody or Immunoglobulin Molecules

Antibody molecules are proteins of the gamma-globulin class found in blood plasma and serum; they are also called **immunoglobulins** because they protect against infection. Immunoglobulins are made by activated B cells that mature into antibody-secreting **plasma cells.** Five classes of immunoglobulin (Ig) molecules are known: IgA, IgD, IgE, IgG, and IgM (Fig. 13–15). Their properties are listed in Table 13–3.

The IgG molecule is the most common in the blood. Each IgG has two identical heavy (H) polypeptide chains and two identical light (L) polypeptide chains held together by disulfide bonds (Fig. 13–16). The association of the light chains with the heavy chains forms two identical antigen-binding regions that look like the two

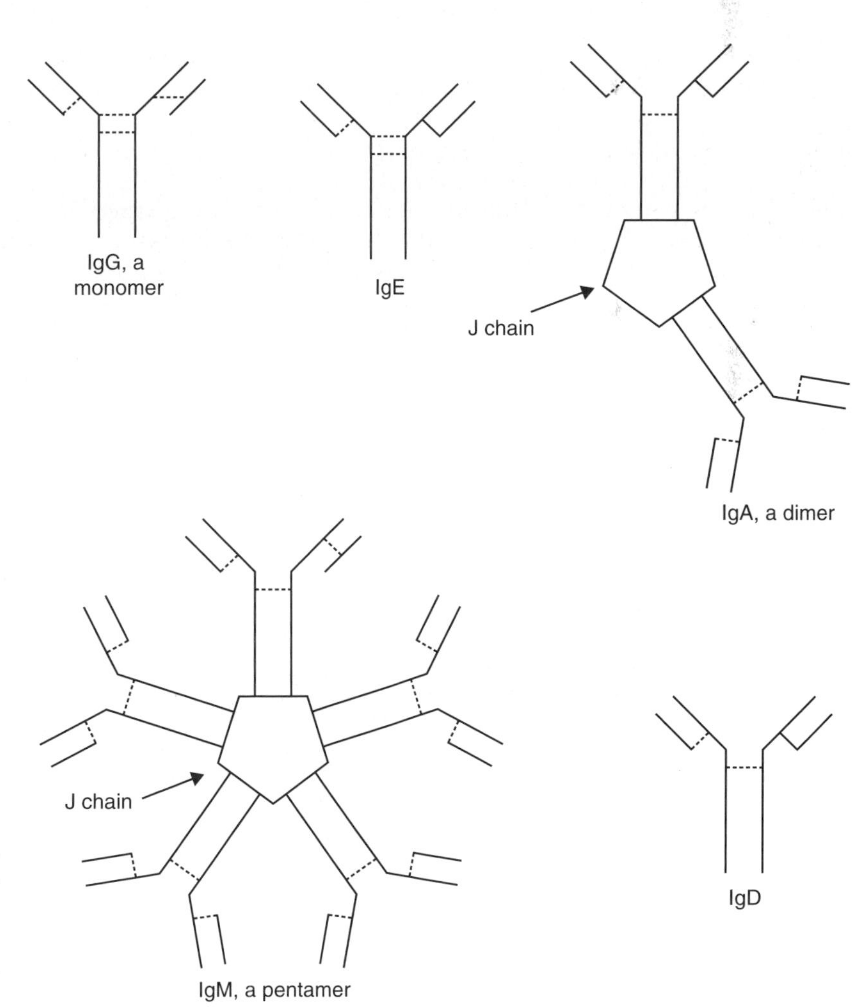

Figure 13–15 ◆ Generalized diagrams of the five classes of immunoglobulin molecules. IgG, IgE, and IgD are monomers. IgA is a dimer with the two units joined by a J chain. IgM is a pentamer with a J chain linking the five units.

Table 13-3
SOME PROPERTIES OF HUMAN IMMUNOGLOBULINS

	IgG	IgM	IgA	IgD	IgE
Molecular weight	150,000	900,000	170,000	150,000	200,000
Serum concentration (g/dl)	1.2	0.4	0.12	0.003	0.0005
Placental transfer	+	−	−	−	−
Distribution	Blood, body fluids	Blood	Blood, body fluids, secretions, breast milk	Blood	Skin, respiratory and gastrointestinal tracts, blood
Complement binding (fixing)	+	+	−	?	−
Opsonization	+	+	+	?	−

branches of a Y-shaped structure. The trunk of the Y is known as the fragment, crystalline, or **Fc** region of the molecule because the protein chains in this region can crystallize with each other. The two ends of the Y shape bind to antigen, so they are called fragment, antigen-binding, or **Fab.** IgG has two Fab regions that each bind identical antigens. A hinge region is located at the junction of the Y shape where the branches begin. The proteins of the hinge region allow flexibility in the immunoglobulin molecule for binding to antigen at both Fab sites.

The amino acid sequence of the Fab sites on one type of immunoglobulin molecule is very different from the amino acid sequence of the Fab of another immunoglobulin type. This region of the protein chains, both H and L chains, is termed the variable region. The variable region of an immunoglobulin molecule binds to a specific type of antigen. This variable region is responsible for the specificity of the interaction between an immunoglobulin and one type of antigen molecule. Below the Fab region of each protein chain the amino acid sequence is relatively identical regardless of the antigens they bind. This portion of the H and L chains is called the constant region.

The Fc end of different immunoglobulin classes have different properties. For example, complement binds to the Fc region of IgM and IgG,

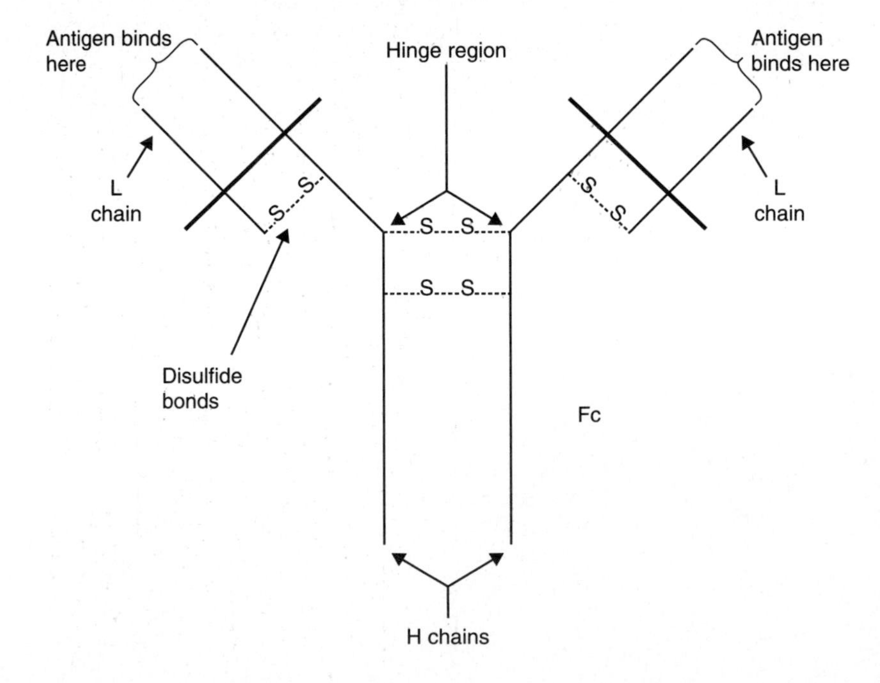

Figure 13-16 ◆ The IgG molecule has two identical heavy (H) chains and two identical light (L) chains linked by disulfide bonds, S-S (*dotted lines*). The antigen-binding sites, Fab, are at the ends of the Y-shaped structure. The crystallizable fragment, Fc, is at the base of the Y-shaped molecule. The heavy lines across the arms of the Y shape separate the variable region of the Fab from the constant regions of the chain. The variable region of each chain has a unique amino acid sequence for each IgG type. The constant region of each chain shares the same amino acid sequence among similar Ig types. The hinge region allows flexibility in the binding of IgG to antigen.

but not to IgA or IgE. Macrophages and B cells have receptors that bind to the Fc region of an IgG molecule; they are called Fc receptors. Mast cells and basophils are involved in allergy; they have Fc receptors for IgE.

The IgG structure is called a monomer, a single unit; two or more of these units form other immunoglobulins. IgG is found in high levels in serum, protecting against extracellular bacteria that cross the skin and enter the blood. The IgG class persists in the blood for long-term protection against the specific invader to which it binds.

IgM is the largest immunoglobulin molecule, composed of five identical IgG-like units, making it a pentamer. Because each of the five units has two antigen-binding sites (two Fab ends), an IgM molecule has 10 identical antigen-binding sites. IgM has a unique peptide molecule called the J chain because it joins the monomeric units together. IgM is the first antibody class produced during the primary antibody response to antigen, followed by B cells that produce IgG, IgA, or IgE.

IgA is a dimer with its monomers joined by a J chain. IgA is found in high amounts in mucosal secretions, protecting the eyes, nose, throat, and gastrointestinal system from microbial entry. Specific IgA antibodies play a very important role in protection against infection by microorganisms because mucosal surfaces are a prime entry point into the body. Breast milk supplies newborns with protective IgA antibodies.

IgE is a monomer; it is produced in very low amounts and has a role in the allergic response (see Chapter 14). IgE molecules also protect against infection with parasites by their location on mast cells and other cells that have the capability to kill parasites.

IgD molecules are monomers expressed on B-lymphocyte surfaces. The function of IgD is less well known; it may possibly induce TCRs, enhancing T helper cell action or perhaps induce the function of APCs.

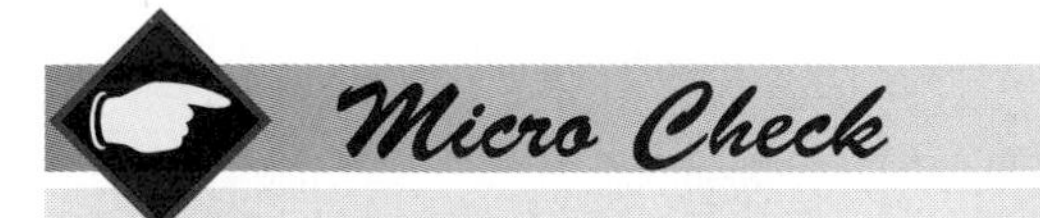

- Which cells produce antibody (immunoglobulin) molecules?
- Which class of immunoglobulin molecule is produced early in an infection?
- Identify one property for each class of immunoglobulin molecule.

PHASES OF THE SPECIFIC IMMUNE RESPONSE

The specific immune response is studied in well-recognized phases of activity. The first phase involves the recognition of antigen by APCs followed by the antigen presentation. The next phase is the activation of lymphocytes and other immune defense cells. The rapid destruction of the invading microorganism is associated with the effector phase when specific lymphocytes and immunoglobulin molecules along with complement destroy the invading organisms. The memory phase allows for development of partially activated memory T and B cells to provide protection should a subsequent invasion by the same pathogen occur months or years in the future.

Antigen Recognition Phase

To recognize antigen, T and B cells have specific receptor molecules that bind to antigen distributed across their surfaces. TCRs are composed of two polypeptide chains called alpha and beta. BCRs, on the other hand, are a membrane form of the antibody molecules that the activated cells will ultimately produce. Each type of BCR binds to a specific microorganism or microbial antigen directly on contact. TCRs bind to antigen when it is bound to MHC molecules on the surface of an APC.

At the individual cell level, however, each T and B cell can recognize only a small part of the antigen, its determinant. There are so many potential antigens in the world that it would take a vast number of antigen-specific T and B cells to fight off every possible invader.

An elegant mechanism for T and B cells to respond specifically to a microbial invader is **clonal selection** (see Fig. 13–12). Only the individual T and B cell clones that recognize the antigens on the invader by their receptor molecules are selected. They then undergo rapid proliferation to increase their numbers, followed by their rapid elimination of the microbial invader. Other clones of T and B cells remain in a resting state, because antigens of the type to stimulate them are absent.

Three main populations, or subsets, of T cells circulate in the bloodstream; they are identified by chemicals, called **markers**, on their plasma membranes. The markers are genetically determined surface proteins involved in interactions between cells and in the activation of lympho-

Table 13–4
LYMPHOCYTES AND NATURAL KILLER CELLS

CLASS	SELECTED CD MARKERS	ALTERNATE DESIGNATIONS FOR THE CELLS
B cells	CD19, CD21, Class II MHC	
T cells		
T helper (TH)	$CD3^+$, $CD4^+$, $CD8^-$	$CD4^+$ T helper, helper T cell
TH1		
TH2		
Cytolytic T	$CD3^+$, $CD4^-$, $CD8^+$	CTL, $CD8^+$ cell, cytotoxic T
Natural killer cells	CD16, receptor for IgG	NK, killer T

CD = cluster of differentiation

Note: Suppressor T (T_s) cells inhibit immune responsiveness; they are $CD8^+$ but may not be a separate subset.

cytes. Each type of marker is identified by a **cluster of differentiation (CD)** number representing a different surface antigen of leukocytes (Table 13–4).

The **T helper cell (TH)** is a **$CD4^+$** (or CD4) cell because it has the cluster of differentiation marker 4 on its membrane. The other T cells are **$CD8^+$** cells, including the **suppressor T cells (T_s)**, the **cytolytic T lymphocytes (CTLs),** and **memory T cells**. The $CD4^+$ helper cells interact with the antigen-presenting macrophages to initiate the immune response (Fig. 13–17). $CD4^+$ helper cells release interleukins to regulate the immune response of other leukocytes (see Table 13–1).

The $CD4^+$ helper cells and $CD8^+$ suppressor cells have a precisely controlled relationship in a healthy individual. The $CD4^+$ cells activate B cells, other T cells, macrophages, and NK cells. When microbial intruders have been conquered, the $CD8^+$ suppressor lymphocytes slow the immune response. In a healthy individual, the ratio of $CD4^+$ helper cells to suppressor T lymphocytes

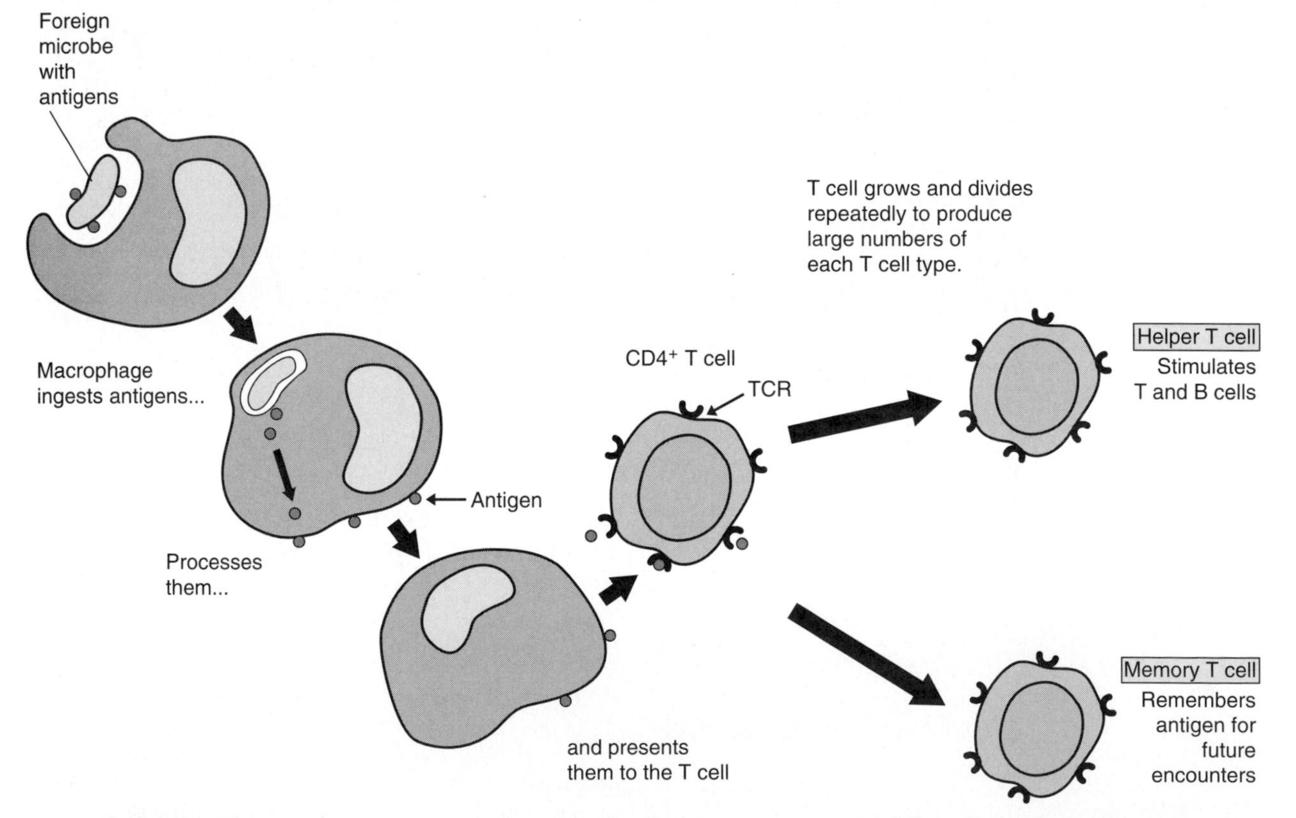

Figure 13–17 ◆ Interaction between $CD4^+$ T helper cell and macrophage. The TCR of a $CD4^+$ T helper cell interacts with the peptide antigen and the MHC molecule on the macrophage, an antigen-presenting cell, to activate cellular and humoral immunity. The CD4 molecule on the T cell interacts with the MHC molecule to complete the binding.

is about 2:1. CTLs are $CD8^+$; they trigger the lysis of virus-infected cells and tumor cells.

Antigen Presentation Phase

Once foreign microorganisms have been recognized and phagocytized by macrophages, their molecules are digested into smaller units, such as short peptides from larger protein antigens. These peptides are positioned into MHC molecules, forming an MHC-peptide complex that is then deposited onto the surface of the macrophage in the process called **antigen presentation.**

The presented antigen is recognized by specific T cells having a TCR capable of binding to the MHC-antigen complex (Fig. 13–18). By binding to the APC, the T cell begins the specific immune response.

When viruses infect epithelial or other body cells, the infected cell either fills the spaces within its MHC class I molecules with viral antigen peptides or reduces the amount of MHC I proteins on its surface. These changes lead to recognition and activation of immune defense. Computer images representing the binding of viral peptides, such as the antigens of the influenza virus, with the MHC molecules help us to visualize the precise manner in which viral antigen is held on the surface of the APC (see Color Plate 29).

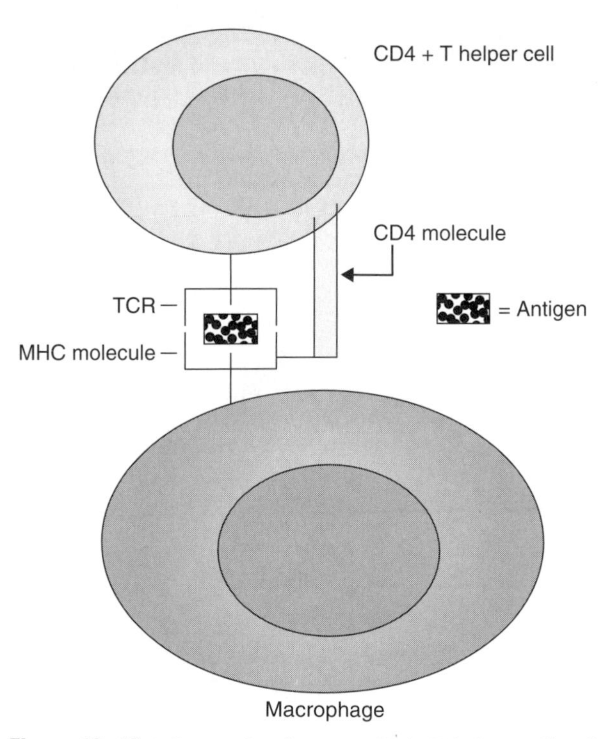

Figure 13–18 ◆ Interaction between $CD4^+$ T helper cell and macrophage. The TCR binds to the antigen when it is associated with the macrophage MHC molecule. The CD4 molecule on the T cell forms a necessary link to the MHC molecule for activation of the T cell.

Activation Phase

Binding of the T cell to the presented antigen or the B cell to antigen directly activates rapid cell division to produce large numbers of identical cells, or **clones,** of each activated B and T cell type. The clones of $CD4^+$ T helper cells enhance the rapid division of the specific B cells that are capable of reacting with the antigens. The B cell clones rapidly increase and then mature into plasma cells that produce large quantities of specific immunoglobulins. A small proportion of activated B cells become memory B cells (to be described in a later section of this chapter).

Binding of the antigen to the BCR is the first signal for the activation phase. A second signal is direct contact between the TCR of the specific $CD4^+$ T helper cells and the antigen-BCR complex. After the B cell is activated in this manner, the T cell secretes cytokines for B cell proliferation (IL-2) and differentiation (IL-4, IL-5, IL-6) into antibody-producing plasma cells. The processes of recognition, presentation, activation, proliferation, and differentiation take a few days, and then the cells are fully active as effector cells.

Effector Phase

The effector B cells are plasma cells; they rapidly secrete large amounts of immunoglobulin molecules. Immunoglobulin molecules circulate in the body fluids and bind to corresponding antigen wherever it is located. The immunoglobulin-antigen complexes attract phagocytic cells, complement components, and NK cells for destruction of the invader. The cytokines of effector $CD4^+$ T cells increase the functions of macrophages, B cells, NK cells, and $CD8^+$ T cells. Effector $CD8^+$ T cells kill virus-infected cells. Production of large numbers of specific effector T and B cells takes five to seven days after first exposure.

Two types of effector $CD4^+$ T cells produce

cytokines: **TH1** and **TH2.** TH1 cells increase cellular immunity by producing interferon gamma to activate macrophages and facilitate the elimination of intracellular microoganisms such as *Mycobacterium tuberculosis.* TH1 cytokines also enhance the killing action of CTL cells on virus-infected cells. TH2 cells increase humoral immunity by producing IL-4, Il-5, and IL-6 to enhance antibody production. TH2 cells also produce IL-10, which suppresses generation of TH1 cells.

FOCAL POINT

Eating Mud Pies May be Good for Children's Immune System

Wouldn't you know it? Just when you think you understand the importance of rearing healthy children in a clean environment, scientists propose another view about children playing in the dirt. Some scientists find that bacteria and other microbes, including worms, that do no harm actually stimulate the immune system and keep it functioning in a balanced fashion. In fact, they suggest that these nonpathogenic organisms encountered from the mud pies children make and eat, or by gardening, playing in the dirt, running in the field, and getting dusty and dirty, provide practice sessions for the immune system to develop its potential.

The balance between the types of $CD4^+$ T helper cells, called TH1 and TH2, is the subject under study by scientists who propose the hygiene hypothesis. This provocative hypothesis suggests that young children require frequent early exposures to dirt and certain microorganisms to obtain a balanced development of TH1 and TH2 and a healthy immune system. They suggest the balanced TH1 and TH2 systems result in fewer children having allergies, asthma, and some autoimmune diseases.

What's the background on these ideas? Scientists have noted a rise in the prevalence of allergies, asthma, and autoimmune diseases among young children in the past 20 years, which also correlates with much cleaner households and cleaner play areas. Some of these children have a stronger TH2 system primed to overreact to allergens.

Statistical studies have shown that children who live on farms are less likely to have hay fever than urban or rural children who do not live on a farm. Even exposure to other children in day care centers and to siblings in a large family seems to reduce the risk of allergies. It is likely that frequent exposure to other children brings more dirt and microorganisms into the environment.

According to scientists, newborns have a functioning TH2 system that provides antibody protection and drives allergic responses to foreign organisms. As a young child grows, the TH1 system develops strength either through fighting infections or through exposure to certain harmless microbes in dirt. If young children do not receive these exposures, their TH1 system may not develop fully and they may be more susceptible to the allergies and other immune system disorders produced by the stronger TH2 system in response to foreign invaders.

Not all scientists agree with the hygiene hypothesis; the more widely held view opposes the hypothesis, saying that infections help to initiate some autoimmune diseases and a cleaner household reduces the incidence of these diseases. Both sides of this issue seem to agree that environmental toxins also prompt autoimmune diseases. Most agree that children should still be reared in a clean environment because serious diseases are still a problem of a dirty environment. Science may be able to develop a solution that will make the best of both of these opposing views on how to develop a healthy immune system without risking serious illness.

These findings on the cytokines of effector T cells have directed research on vaccines against pathogens such as the human immunodeficiency virus (HIV). The basic principle is to find those factors that increase cellular immunity (TH1) instead of TH2 activity because it is known that HIV antibodies are not protective against the disease.

After the invader has been eliminated, T and B cells directed against the invader diminish in number. Clonal selection of a different set of T and B cells will occur when a new invader with a different group of antigens invades the body.

Primary and Secondary Immune Responses

The first time cells of the specific immune system respond to antigen is called the **primary immune response.** The primary immune response requires a few days to begin to generate protective antibodies by first producing IgM molecules and later IgG molecules (Fig. 13–19). IgM disappears from the bloodstream within days to weeks, and IgG molecules persist for a much longer period of protection.

The innate immune system continues to provide protection until enough specific T and B clones are generated for protection and to allow time for **memory B** cell and **memory T** cell development. Memory B cell development can take weeks, but these cells survive for a long time. Memory cells are very specific; they respond only to the antigen to which they were previously exposed in the primary response.

The specific immune system responds rapidly and vigorously to subsequent exposures to infections by the same microorganism; this is called the **secondary immune response** or, more aptly, the **memory response** carried out by the memory B and T cells. The **memory response** results in a fast and steep rise in immunoglobulin concentration in the blood serum, with IgM and IgG concentrations increasing quickly. Then IgM diminishes early but IgG persists in concentrations that are often higher than that achieved for the primary response. The IgG molecules protect for a long period of many years, in some cases.

Newborns are more susceptible to infection because they lack memory T and B cells. Antigen exposure is required for memory cell development, and most exposure occurs after birth. Vaccination to induce memory cells significantly reduces infant mortality. Vaccines generate immunological memory without having to suffer through the actual disease. Booster doses of the vaccine are given to increase further the numbers of memory T and B cells. Boosters also function to increase serum and mucosal levels of antibodies that are maintained in low, but protective, levels for years.

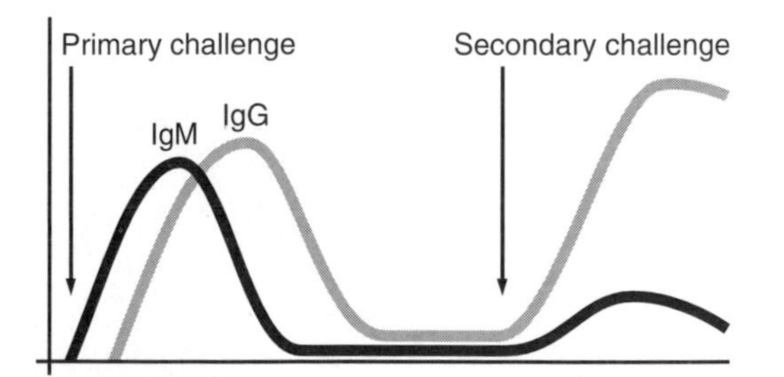

Figure 13–19 ◆ Primary and secondary immune response. In the initial contact, or challenge, with an antigen, IgM concentration increases first, then drops. IgM is followed by IgG molecules that reach a higher concentration for a longer period. In the secondary response, to subsequent contacts, secondary challenge, with the same antigen, the memory cells produce IgG and IgM quickly. IgG reaches a higher concentration than in the primary response and persists longer.

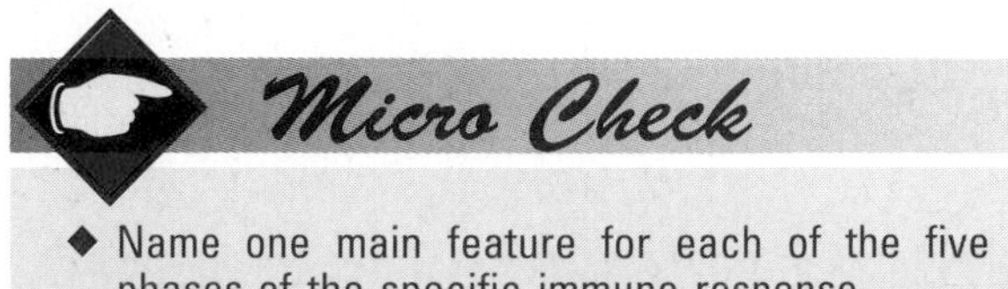

- Name one main feature for each of the five phases of the specific immune response.
- What is meant by antigen presentation?
- What is the importance of the memory response?

INTERACTIONS OF TCRs WITH SUPERANTIGENS

The specific immune response is a protective system to quell infections and restore the body to good health quickly. However, certain antigens induce a wildly exaggerated immune response that sends the body into shock. These antigens are called **superantigens.**

Normally, an antigen is packaged within a groove formed between the MHC molecule on an APC and the TCR. In the normal position, an average viral antigen would activate between one in 100,000 to 1 million T cells. The peptides of certain bacterial toxins and retroviruses are classified as superantigens. The superantigen binds to the outside of the MHC molecule rather than into a groove within the MHC (see Color Plate 30). In this more exposed position, the superantigen is a larger target to the TCR.

The presence of the superantigen alongside a segment of the TCR activates 5 percent of all T cells, which amounts to activating tens of millions of different T cells. The massive T cell response releases large quantities of cytokines such as IL-2 and TNF, causing drastic reactions. Staphylococcal infections leading to food poisoning and toxic shock syndrome result in a severe immunological reaction to a staphylococcal enterotoxin that is a superantigen. An explosive, severely damaging cellular immunity response develops instead of a protective one.

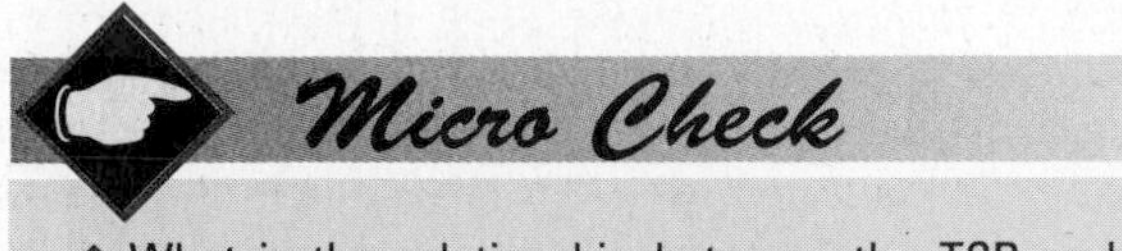

- What is the relationship between the TCR and MHC-antigen complex?
- Why does a superantigen produce such a violently harmful reaction rather than a protective one?
- What is the relationship between the TCR and an MHC-superantigen complex?

FOUR CATEGORIES OF ACQUIRED IMMUNITY

Acquired immunity may develop naturally or artificially, resulting, in both cases, in the production of circulating immunoglobulins. Immunity may be produced by either an active or passive mode, resulting in four categories of acquired immunity (Fig. 13–20).

Naturally Acquired Active Immunity

When a person becomes ill and recovers, it is due to the natural immune response and active production of specific immunoglobulin molecules. Active mode implies that the individual has produced his or her own immunoglobulins during the natural course of the disease. In addition, the IgG molecules and memory cells provide long-term protection should the same pathogen be encountered again. Recovery from some diseases results in many years of immunity.

Naturally Acquired Passive Immunity

The natural process by which maternal IgG molecules cross the placenta to enter the fetal circulation is a prime example of immunity ac-

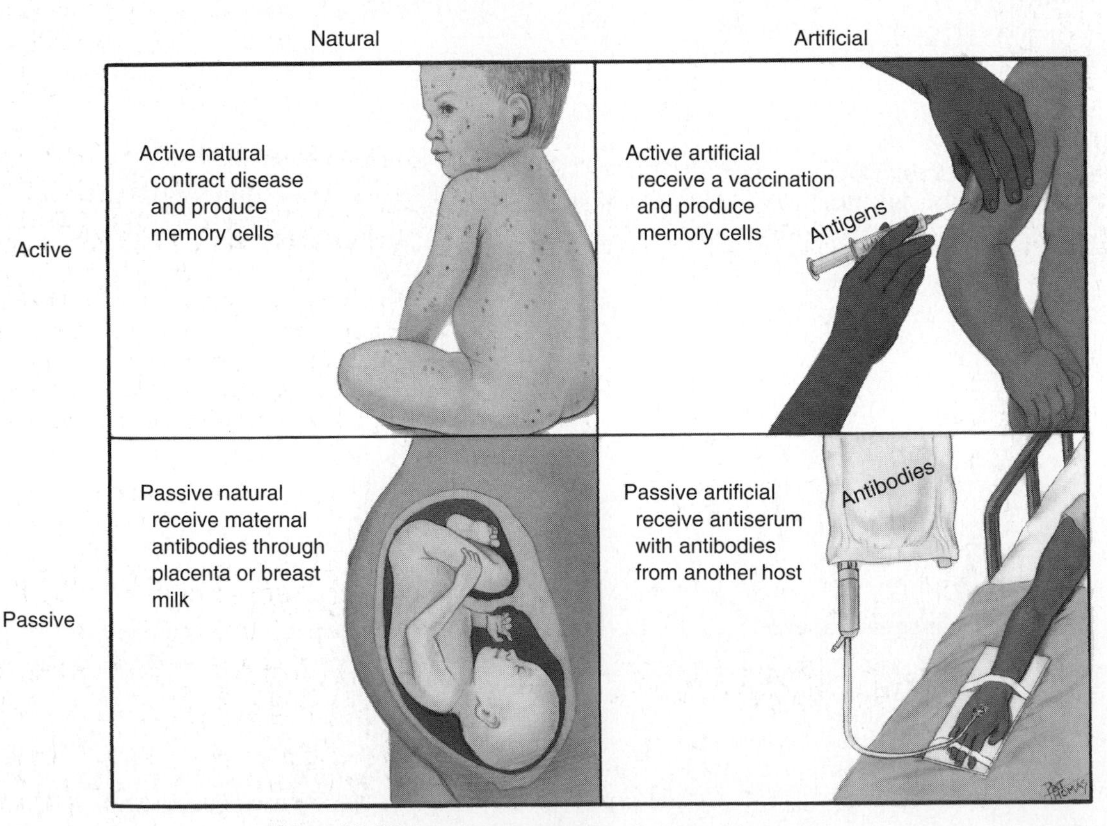

Figure 13–20 ◆ The four categories of acquired immunity.

quired passively and naturally. Infants are immune to the same infectious diseases as their mothers for 6 to 12 months after birth. If newborns are breast-fed, they receive additional protection by the maternal IgA antibodies in passive transfer from the breast milk.

Artificially Acquired Active Immunity

The administration of vaccines or injections of attenuated (weakened) products of microorganisms cause an active immune response under the artificial conditions of an injection. This immunization process allows the individual immune system to develop immunoglobulins actively without becoming ill. The actual protection afforded by immunizations required by state and national immunization programs has raised the general level of public health in developed nations.

Artificially Acquired Passive Immunity

When protective antibodies are injected into an individual who is very ill and needs immediate protection, the immunity is provided immediately, not by the patient, but by donor immunoglobulin molecules. This is the primary means for artificially acquired passive immunity. Human immune serum globulin, antitoxin, and hyperimmune serum are examples of products used for passive immunizations. The immunity obtained in this manner is not of long duration, but it is effective when time is short.

An example of the therapeutic use of globulins to prevent disease is the human rabies immune globulin. This globulin is obtained from persons immunized against rabies; it is given to all individuals exposed to the bite of a wild animal and to certain individuals who have received bites on the face or neck or to those bitten by domestic animals that have not received a rabies vaccination. The immediate protection of the anti-rabies immunoglobulin molecules prevents the development of rabies.

Micro Check

- What immune protection is available to the fetus?
- Describe the process by which one acquires a naturally acquired active immunity.
- Give an example for active and passive artificially acquired immunity.

Understanding Microbiology

1. Name the major phagocytes in the human host.
2. Where are antigens processed for presentation to T cells?
3. What is the role of MHC antigens in the immune response?
4. Explain the roles of each T cell type in the immune response.
5. Why is a secondary response to an antigen more rapid and of greater magnitude than a primary response?

Applying Microbiology

1. A child was bitten by a skunk while camping in the forests of San Luis Obispo County in California. The skunk escaped. Because skunks usually do not show aggressive behavior, but rather run and hide from people, the medical professionals considered that the child might have been exposed to rabies. What treatment might be used to give immediate protection against rabies?

Chapter 14

Alterations and Applications of the Immune Response

Chapter Outline

- **STATES OF IMMUNODEFICIENCY**
  - Primary Deficiencies
  - Secondary Deficiencies
- **AUTOIMMUNE DISEASES**
- **EXAGGERATED IMMUNE RESPONSES**
- **TYPES OF HYPERSENSITIVITIES**
  - Type I Antibody-Mediated Anaphylactic Hypersensitivity
  - Type II Antibody-Mediated Cytotoxic Hypersensitivity
  - Type III Antibody-Mediated Immune Complex Hypersensitivity
  - Type IV Cell-Mediated Delayed Hypersensitivity
- **APPLICATIONS OF THE IMMUNE RESPONSE**
  - Monoclonal Antibodies
  - Diagnostic Tests
    - Unlabeled Immunoassays
    - Labeled Immunoassays
    - Fluorescence-Activated Cell Sorting
    - Western Blot Assays
  - Vaccine-Preventable Diseases

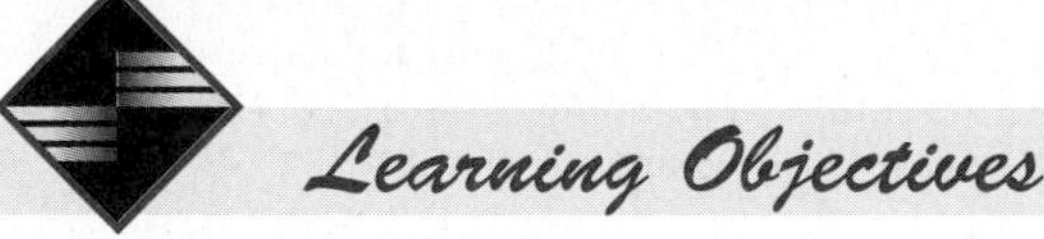

Learning Objectives

After you have read this chapter, you should be able to:

1. Differentiate between primary and secondary immunodeficiencies.
2. Contrast antibody- and cell-mediated hypersensitivities.
3. Explain a basic mechanism for each of the three types of antibody-mediated hypersensitivities.
4. Differentiate between immune reactions of transplant rejection and graft-versus-host reactions.
5. Describe advantages of immunological tests over cultural methods in the diagnosis of infectious diseases.
6. Explain the continuing need to provide early childhood vaccinations.

The immune response is a remarkable example of a cooperative effort of immune cells to defend us against microbial invasion. You may wonder what would happen if any of the participants were absent or functionally impaired. The answer depends on the identity of the impaired team member and the seriousness of the impairment. The altered immune responses are a consequence of too little or too much immunity. They are caused by deficiencies of participating cells or heightened activities of certain immune cells when exposed more than one time to particular antigens.

STATES OF IMMUNODEFICIENCY

The altered immune responses involving deficiencies are divided into primary and secondary diseases depending on their origin. If the disorder is present at birth, it is classified as a primary disease; if it is acquired during the lifetime of an individual, it is classified as a secondary disease. The cause of secondary disease may be a consequence of infections, malignancies, or forms of treatment such as irradiation or chemotherapy. The impairments may affect innate or acquired immunity and occasionally affect both types of immunity.

Primary Deficiencies

Deficiencies in phagocytes, complement, and B or T lymphocytes or both types of lymphocytes are examples of primary deficiencies. Sometimes the names of the disorders reflect the cause of the defect; at other times the names of the disorders have proper names that reflect the name of the discoverer or the name of the first patient identified with the deficiency.

PHAGOCYTIC DISORDERS

Phagocytic disorders may be caused by deficiencies of extrinsic activators, such as cytokines, or by errors of the metabolism of phagocytes. Such errors diminish the ability of phagocytes to destroy pathogens, permitting them to exist intracellularly.

In **chronic granulomatous disease,** a deficiency of reduced nicotinamide-adenine dinucleotide (NADH) oxidase or nicotinamide-adenine dinucleotide phosphate (NADPH) oxidase interferes with production of hydrogen peroxide and superoxide necessary to kill ingested microorganisms. Patients with chronic granulomatous disease have an increased susceptibility to bacteria and fungi of relatively low virulence.

COMPLEMENT-DEFICIENCY DISEASES

A deficiency of the C3 component of complement affects innate and acquired immunity. Persons lacking that component suffer from recurrent bacterial infections. Patients with deficiencies in C5 to C8 components are particularly susceptible to infections caused by *Neisseria* species. Deficiencies in C1, C2, and C4 are characteristic of diseases in which patients make antibodies to their own antigens. Protection from diseases in which complement is required for complexing of antigen with antibody is severely impaired in deficiencies of any complement component.

AGAMMAGLOBULINEMIA AND HYPOGAMMAGLOBULINEMIA

Agammaglobulinemia and **hypogammaglobulinemia** are caused by a deficiency in numbers or activity of B cells. Agammaglobulinemia, or Bruton's disease, is linked to the X chromosome and occurs in males only. After maternal-derived antibodies are gone, there is an absence of all classes of immunoglobulins. Individuals with this disease may live to the age of 30 with periodic injections of IgG, but they often die earlier from some form of lung disease.

Hypogammaglobulinemia may be transient or permanent. The transient form of the disease often occurs in premature infants and is caused by an immaturity of $CD4^+$ cells. The infants have a normal number of B cells, but they cannot function without the aid of the helper T cells. Sometimes intervention with injections of IgG is necessary until the T cells reach a functional level of maturity. By the age of two most infants recover without serious consequences.

A permanent form of hypogammaglobulinemia has an onset in persons aged 15 to 35. The nature of the defect in B cells or their activity is variable. The cause is not known, but individuals with the dysfunctional response are highly susceptible to some infections and have a high incidence of other immune disorders.

DIGEORGE SYNDROME

In **DiGeorge syndrome** there is a deficiency in T cells caused by an error in embryonic development affecting both the thymus and the parathyroid glands. Persons with the syndrome usually have normal numbers of B cells, but they lack the ability to respond to antigenic stimulation. Transplantation of fetal thymus glands can restore numbers of functioning B cells by activating helper T cells.

WISCOTT-ALDRICH SYNDROME

Wiscott-Aldrich syndrome is a congenital form of combined immunodeficiency disease in which there are reductions in the numbers of B cells, T cells, and platelets. The defective gene is linked to the X chromosome. The affected boys are not able to make antibodies to polysaccharides. Patients with the disease often have eczema, are particularly susceptible to infections caused by encapsulated bacteria, and have repeated episodes of bleeding. Without bone marrow transplants to correct deficiencies, the children seldom live beyond the age of three.

SEVERE COMBINED IMMUNODEFICIENCY DISEASE

Persons with **severe combined immunodeficiency disease** (SCID) are unable to mount B- and T-cell defenses against infectious diseases. SCID is caused by an X-linked chromosome or **autosomal** recessive gene. In the autosomal recessive form of the disease there is a deficiency of the enzyme adenosine deaminase. In those patients, correction can be made by supplying the missing enzyme, but in the majority of instances bone marrow transplantation is necessary to restore normal function. A novel approach to treatment is gene-insertion therapy to restore the missing enzyme.

One of the most publicized cases of SCID was a child from Texas often referred to as David, the Bubble Boy (Fig. 14–1). David Vetter was placed as an infant in an environment free of microorganisms within a plastic bubble. Although his activities were severely restricted, David was described as a well-adjusted child. When it was decided to correct the deficiencies with bone marrow from his sister, David was 12 years old. Unfortunately, unknown to his doctors, the sister's bone marrow contained the Epstein-Barr virus. David died a few months later from a type of cancer caused by that virus.

Secondary Deficiencies

Devastating immune consequences occur after infection with the human immunodeficiency virus (HIV). This virus destroys $CD4^+$ cells required for immunological competence. Persons having the acquired immunodeficiency syndrome (AIDS) are susceptible to a large number of opportunistic infections and malignancies. More information on AIDS is found in Chapter 20.

B-CELL MALIGNANCIES

Multiple myeloma, macroglobulinemia, and **heavy-chain disease** are examples of diseases caused by an abnormal proliferation of B lymphocytes and plasma cells. The disorders are associated with production of large amounts of a

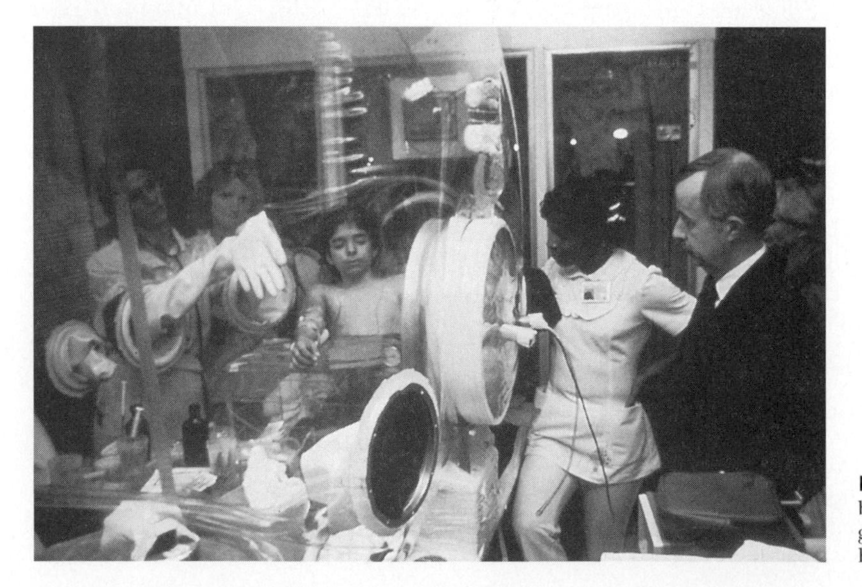

Figure 14–1 ◆ David Vetter, a Texan boy with SCID, in a specially designed germ-free "bubble" and members of his health care team.

particular whole or partial immunoglobulin, often at the expense of other immunoglobulins.

Multiple myeloma is the most common disease associated with high numbers of plasma cells that may infiltrate more than one organ system. The malignant cells originate from a single clone. The immunoglobulin synthesized is a reflection of the specificity of that clone. The disease is characterized by the excretion of large amounts of partial immunoglobulins known as **Bence Jones proteins.** The proteins precipitate at 45° to 60° C but resolubilize on cooling.

In macroglobulinemia there is an overabundance of IgM, causing an increase in viscosity of the blood. The subsequent slowing of blood flow predisposes individuals to obstruction in blood flow from intravascular clotting. There is an associated hypogammaglobulinemia that causes an increase in susceptibility to infections.

Heavy-chain disease is characterized by excess production of heavy chains of IgG, IgA, or IgM. The runaway production of partial immunoglobulins is at the expense of producing whole functional immunoglobulins. Infiltration of malignant cells into the bone marrow is reflected by deficiencies of functional red and white blood cells.

AUTOIMMUNE DISEASES

Antigens occurring on the surfaces of our own cells do not normally stimulate an immune response. The inability to respond to "self" antigens known as **immunological tolerance** is discussed in Chapter 13. Tolerance is characteristic of a healthy immune system. If the body fails to distinguish self from nonself antigens and does battle with self antigens in an attempt to eliminate them, the consequence is an **autoimmune disease.** Target tissues containing the embattled antigens sustain varying degrees of damage. If defects occur in the $CD8^+$ cell population, B-cell activity is enhanced. We shall discuss a limited number of autoimmune hypersensitivity reactions that produce serious disease. Some lesser-known autoimmune diseases and their target tissues are listed in Table 14–1.

EXAGGERATED IMMUNE RESPONSES

Exaggerated immune responses are heightened immune responses that occur on more than one exposure to the same antigen. The first-time exposure sensitizes an individual to the allergen, but no discernible signs or symptoms appear. Subsequent exposure causes mild to severe symptoms of allergy that differ with the degree and location of the altered immune response. Certain self or nonself antigens promote excesses in activity of immune cells that are damaging to tissue. The altered states of immunity are called **hypersensitivities** or **allergies.** The antigens promoting the altered responses are called **allergens.** You may have a friend who has an allergy or maybe you have one. If so, you are familiar with the discomfort and possible life-threatening consequences associated with allergies. Susceptibility to some allergens appears to have a genetic basis. Such allergies are called **atopic allergies,** but the mode of inheritance is not clear. The location of the altered immune response is responsible for the symptoms exhibited by the allergic patient.

TYPES OF HYPERSENSITIVITIES

Although states of hypersensitivity are frequently categorized as **immediate** or **delayed,** depending on the time required after exposure to

Table 14–1
EXAMPLES OF HUMAN AUTOIMMUNE DISEASES

DISEASE	TARGET TISSUE	CHARACTERISTIC
Addison's disease	Adrenal gland	Adrenocortical hormone deficiency
Allergic encephalitis	Brain	Cerebral inflammation
Autoimmune spermatogenesis	Spermatozoa	Low sperm count
Hashimoto's disease	Thyroid	Hypothyroidism
Pernicious anemia	Intrinsic factor	Impaired development of red blood cells
Primary biliary cirrhosis	Liver	Duct obstruction
Sjögren's syndrome	Salivary gland	Dryness of mouth and eyes

an allergen for symptoms to occur, the altered states of responsiveness clearly fall into antibody- or cell-mediated hypersensitivities. Four types of tissue-damaging reactions are recognized. The antibody-mediated hypersensitivities (types I, II, and III) depend on the interaction of antigens with IgE, IgG, or IgM immunoglobulins. The reactions tend to occur relatively soon after contact with the antigen. A single classification (type IV) is used to categorize cell-mediated hypersensitivities. The TH2 cells stimulate IgE synthesis; the TH1 cells promote synthesis of IgG and IgM. Both subsets are involved, therefore, in immediate types of hypersensitivity. TH1 and CD8+ cells have roles in delayed types of hypersensivity. Reactions of delayed-type hypersensitivity usually occur several hours to several days after exposure to antigens. The four types of hypersensitivity reactions are not mutually exclusive. Individuals exposed to the same allergen can exhibit symptoms associated with more than one type of hypersensitivity.

Type I Antibody-Mediated Anaphylactic Hypersensitivity

Anaphylactic-type (nonprotective) reactions occur when allergens combine with membrane-associated antibodies of the IgE class on the surface of mast cells or circulating basophils. Mast cells are especially abundant in connective tissue of the skin, lymphoid organs, eyes, nose, mouth, intestines, and respiratory tract. An estimated 100,000 to 500,000 receptors for IgE are present on the surface of mast cells. For reasons that remain unknown, some individuals make immunoglobulins of the class IgE in response to an initial contact with certain antigens. The initial contact with the allergen promotes the processing by antigen-presenting cells (APCs) and combination with Class II major histocompatibility complex (MHC) molecules. The T_h1 cells secrete cytokines that activate phagocytes and a clone of IgE-secreting B cells. The encounter sensitizes an individual to the allergen, but there are no identifiable adverse reactions. Subsequent exposure to the same allergen causes an exaggerated response and often life-threatening symptoms (Fig. 14–2). An anaphylactic response requires presynthesized IgE immunoglobulins from a **sensitizing dose** of the allergen and exposure to the same antigen as a **provocative dose** that triggers the release of preformed mediators from mast cells or basophils. An explosive degranulation and release of biologically active agents occurs when allergens and IgE molecules combine on the surface of target mast cells and basophils. Additional mediators, formerly called **slow-reacting substances of anaphylaxis (SRSs-A),** are synthesized by activated mast cells and basophils. The newly formed mediators, such as leukotrienes and prostaglandins, are able to sustain responses initiated by the preformed chemicals stored in the granules.

SYSTEMIC ANAPHYLAXIS

A sudden, sometimes fatal, vasomotor collapse occurring on exposure to a previously sensitizing allergen is called **systemic anaphylaxis.** The chemicals initiating the anaphylactic response are called **mediators.** The most important mediator released from mast cells and basophils into surrounding tissue is **histamine.** Histamine causes contraction of smooth muscle, principally in the lungs, dilation of capillaries, increased vascular permeability, and, ultimately, collapse due to shock.

Histamine secretion occurs in two stages, the first of which involves cyclic adenosine monophosphate (AMP) as a second messenger. It is believed that the antigen-antibody reaction interferes with the activity of membrane-bound adenyl cyclase of the target cells. As a result, cellular levels of cyclic AMP are decreased. The diminution of cyclic AMP triggers the second stage in which histamine is actually secreted. The second stage is calcium dependent and related to microtubule activity; it is an energy-requiring reaction. Histamine, released by basophils and mast cells, inhibits additional release of the potent vasoactive agent by a feedback mechanism.

Histamine is rapidly degraded after release, but other mediators serve to prolong the muscle contraction and capillary dilation. Leukotrienes are present in minute quantities, but their punch is responsible for many of the distressing symptoms of anaphylaxis. Systemic anaphylaxis sometimes occurs in sensitized humans after the administration of penicillin or after an insect bite. The ensuing circulatory collapse can be reversed by prompt treatment with epinephrine and antihistamines.

LOCALIZED ANAPHYLAXIS

Asthma, hay fever, and urticaria (hives) are examples of localized IgE-mediated reactions occurring after more than one exposure to an exogenous allergen. The symptoms are the result of the release of histamine, leukotrienes, and pros-

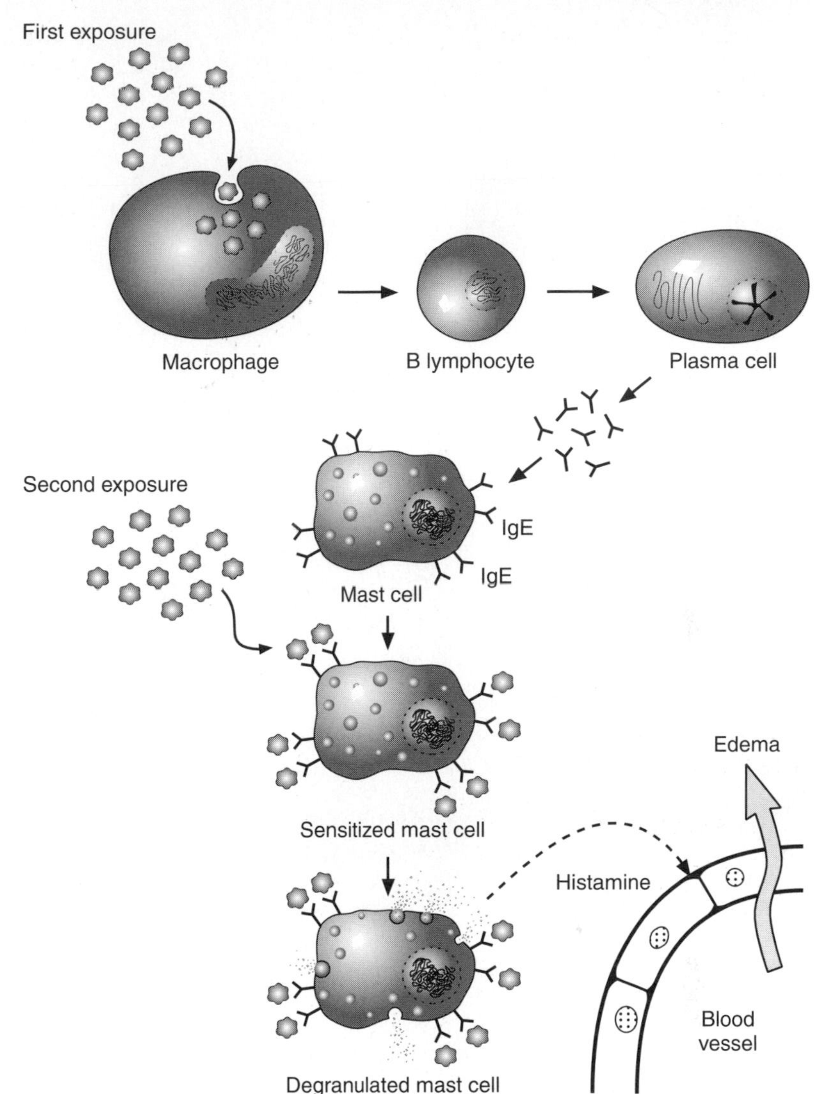

Figure 14–2 ◆ Type I hypersensitivity reaction showing role of IgE. When allergen binds to IgE on mast cells, histamine is released, increasing permeability of blood vessels.

taglandins from mast cells of the involved tissues. The reactions occur in the respiratory, conjunctival, or intestinal mucosa. Asthma and hay fever, particularly, appear to run in families. Leukotrienes are the primary mediators of antihistamine-resistant asthma. Common allergens are pollen, spores of molds, animal dander, and the house dust mite. Allergies to food are less well defined and may manifest themselves as urticaria or intestinal allergies. The raised, red, wheel-like lesions of urticaria are believed to be caused by histamine and leukotrienes. Prostaglandins are more important mediators of intestinal allergies. The proteins in cow's milk are often incriminated in food allergies. Intrinsic asthma, in which no nonself antigen can be identified, appears to be more complex.

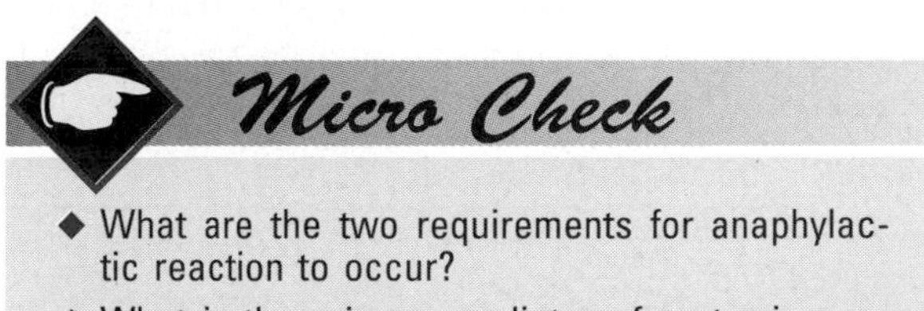

Micro Check

- What are the two requirements for anaphylactic reaction to occur?
- What is the primary mediator of systemic anaphylaxis?
- Give three examples of localized anaphylaxis.

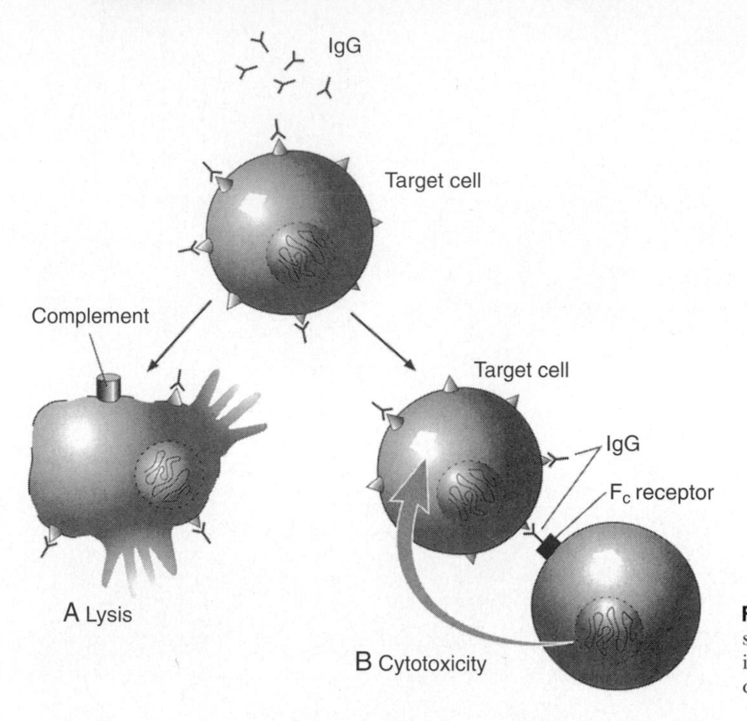

Figure 14–3 ◆ Type II hypersensitivity reaction showing binding of IgG to surface cell antigen. Binding activates complement, causing (*A*) lysis or (*B*) cytotoxicity.

Type II Antibody-Mediated Cytotoxic Hypersensitivity

Cytotoxic-type reactions occur when self antigens react with antibodies of the classes IgG or IgM and complement, causing cell destruction. The antigens are frequently bound to red blood cells, white blood cells, and platelets, but they may be present on the surface of other somatic cells.

The antibodies promote contact with phagocytes and activate complement. The complexing of antigen and antibody with complement at a single site causes lysis or cytotoxicity of red blood cells (Fig. 14–3). Other somatic cells are more resistant to destruction in this manner but may be altered by the immunological encounter. It is the destruction or alteration of cells containing the allergen that distinguishes type II hypersensitivities.

TRANSFUSION REACTIONS

The major antigens present on human red blood cells are the basis for blood typing (Table 14–2). The blood groups are A, B, AB, and O. It is somewhat paradoxical that persons lacking A

Table 14–2
ABO BLOOD GROUP ANTIGENS AND ANTIBODIES

			PERCENT FREQUENCY IN UNITED STATES			
BLOOD GROUP	RED BLOOD CELL ANTIGEN	SERUM ANTIBODY	Native Americans	Asians	Blacks	Whites
A	A	anti-B	16	28	27	40
B	B	anti-A	4	27	20	11
AB	A, B		<1	5	4	4
O		anti-A, anti-B	79	40	49	45

or B antigens on the surfaces of their red blood cells have natural circulating antibodies against both of those antigens. The presence of anti-A and anti-B antibodies can be demonstrated as early as six months of age. It has been postulated that early encounters with small amounts of antigenic determinants of blood types in food or in microorganisms may stimulate antibody production. Exposure to noncompatible antigens of the ABO groups can occur by receiving a transfusion with the wrong type of blood. Complement is activated, and transfused red blood cells are hemolyzed (Fig. 14–4). Patients under those circumstances often experience pain, nausea, vomiting, low blood pressure, fever, and even kidney damage. The antibodies may be produced in response to accidental transfusion with the wrong type of blood or from exposure to fetal antigens. In either case cytotoxic reactions can occur on more than one exposure to the incompatible blood group antigens.

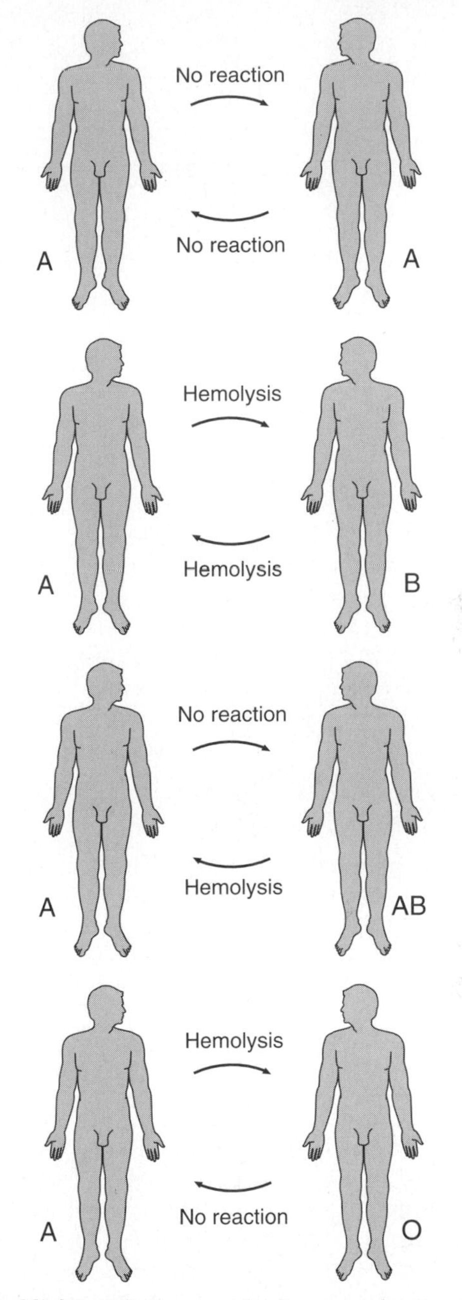

Figure 14–4 ◆ ABO human blood groups showing transfusion reactions between groups. Transfusion between incompatible groups causes hemolysis of red blood cells if recipient has antibodies to the antigen on the surface of donor cells.

ABO AND Rh INCOMPATIBILITIES OF PREGNANCY

An ABO incompatibility of maternal and fetal red cell antigens can promote an immune response in the mother. Fetal red blood cells enter maternal circulation in greater numbers just before and after delivery. The antibodies produced are primarily of the IgG class, readily cross the placenta, and bind to fetal red blood cells, causing hemolysis.

ABO incompatibilities that stimulate antibody synthesis sufficiently to cause damage are not as common as Rh antigen incompatibilities. Although no natural antibodies are associated with the Rh system, anti-Rh antibodies are made by Rh-negative individuals in response to D antigen, one of the Rh factors present on red blood cells. Rh incompatibilities of pregnancy occur most frequently when the mother is Rh negative (Rh^-) and the fetus is Rh positive (Rh^+) for the D antigen. Rh^- mothers become sensitized to the Rh antigen when exposed to fetal red blood cells at the time of birth. The high titers of Rh antibodies, produced in response to massive exposure, can cause hemolysis of fetal red blood cells in a subsequent pregnancy (Fig. 14–5). The anemia occurring as a result of hemolysis of an infant's red blood cells is called **hemolytic disease of the newborn.** If a large number of red blood cells are destroyed, stillbirth may occur. If the infant survives, complications such as mental retardation, deafness, or spasticity may be secondary to accumulation of bilirubin, a product of degradation of hemoglobin. However, Rh^+ cells can be eliminated from the maternal circulation by the administration of a small amount of immune serum specific for the D factor (RhoGAM)

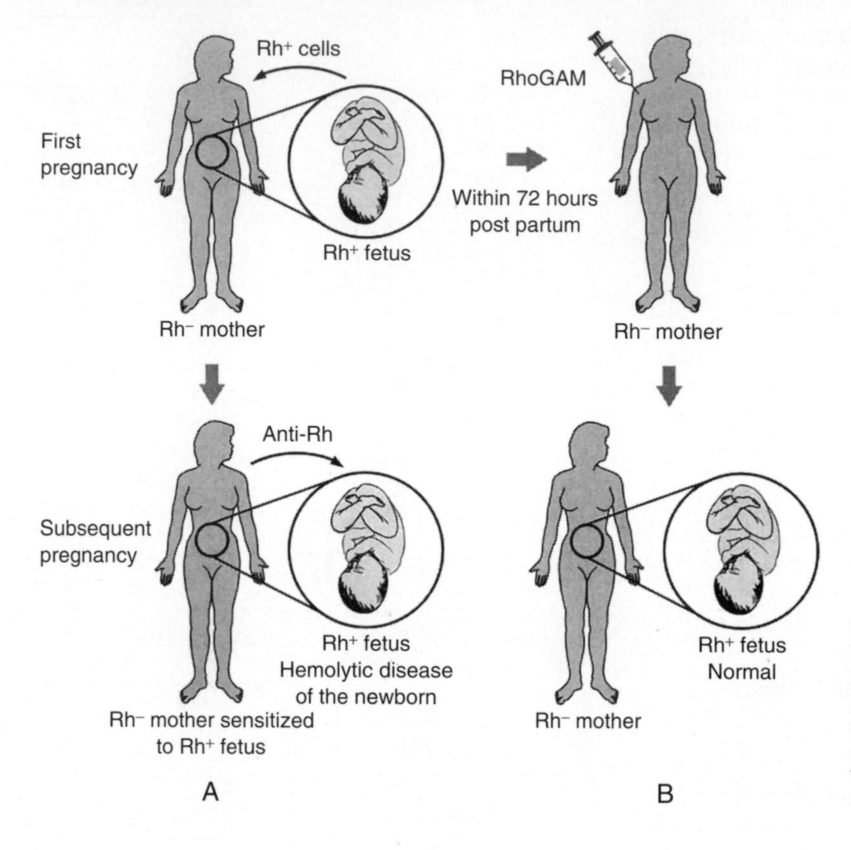

Figure 14–5 ◆ Effects of Rh incompatibility in first and subsequent pregnancy: *A,* without administration of anti-D immunoglobulin (RhoGAM) and *B,* with administration of the prophylactic immune serum. Without intervention, the infant will be born with hemolytic disease of the newborn.

within 72 hours after delivery. The Rh antibodies prevent maternal antibody synthesis by eliminating Rh^+ cells from the circulation. A subsequent pregnancy with a maternal-fetal Rh incompatibility is not complicated by the presence of antibodies.

AUTOIMMUNE HEMOLYTIC ANEMIA

Autoimmune hemolytic anemia, in which an individual develops antibodies to antigens on his or her own cell membranes, may be acquired as a consequence of exposure to certain drugs, infectious agents, or cancer. It is believed that antigens on red blood cells are altered, making them nonrecognizable as self. The antibodies produced sometimes are limited in their ability to fix complement. The inability of bone marrow to replenish the red blood cell population in persons with hemolytic anemia makes it necessary to give multiple blood transfusions or bone marrow stimulants.

THROMBOCYTOPENIA

Some individuals, for reasons not completely understood, produce antibodies to certain drugs or infectious agents that react with antigens on **thrombocytes** (platelets). When complement is activated, the thrombocytes are lysed. The decrease in circulating thrombocytes causes bleeding from the capillaries to body cavities or organs. Hemorrhaging into the skin is associated with the appearance of small, purple spots called **petechiae.** Other individuals make antibodies to their own platelets. The consequences are indistinguishable from those initiated by exogenous agents.

MYASTHENIA GRAVIS

Myasthenia gravis is an autoimmune disease characterized by the presence of antibodies to acetylcholine receptors of neuromuscular junctures. Nerve impulses are blocked by antigen-antibody complexes at receptor sites. Individuals with the disease experience progressive muscle weakness. Chewing, swallowing, and breathing become increasingly difficult. The identity of the initiating antigen that stimulates antibody production is unknown, but molecules that cross-react with acetycholine receptors have been found on cells of enlarged thymus glands.

FOCAL POINT

What's in a Tea Bag? A Case of Thrombocytopenia Induced by Chinese Herbs

Many health benefits are attributed to the traditional herbal medicine called *Jui*. *Jui* contains five Chinese herbs and is often packed for distribution in tea bags. A 51-year-old Japanese woman with a history of high blood glucose levels took *Jui* for several days before her annual health examination in the hopes of attaining a normal blood glucose. *Jui* did not lower her blood glucose, but after taking it for a third year, she developed a severe bleeding problem. Her first diagnosis was thrombocytopenia of unknown etiology. Subsequent tests revealed a high platelet-associated immunoglobulin G (PAIgG) detected by an enzyme-linked immunosorbent assay. Criteria for confirming drug- or herb-induced thrombocytopenia have not been established. With the patient's permission, however, her doctors rechallenged her with oral *Jui*. Her platelet count dropped precipitously in one day, and petechiae appeared on both legs and forearms. Treatment included oral prednisolone, intravenous IgG, and 30 units of replacement platelets. The patient recovered in two weeks. Such rechallenges are not without hazards and must not be done without a patient's consent. The discoveries made by rechallenging in this case suggest that the thrombocytopenia was induced by the herb-containing Chinese medicine in a tea bag.

The Lancet 354:304, 1999.

GRAVES' HYPERTHYROIDISM

Graves' hyperthyroidism is an autoimmune disease caused by antibodies that bind to antigens on the surface of thyroid cells. The long-acting thyroid stimulator (LATS) is actually an IgG immunoglobulin. The effect of the antigen-antibody reactions is to stimulate thyroid activity in much the same manner as thyroid-stimulating hormone (TSH) from the pituitary. Over a period of years the continued stimulation of LATS causes an enlargement of the thyroid gland called a goiter. Several studies have suggested that a deficiency of CD8+ cells may exist in patients with Graves' hyperthyroidism.

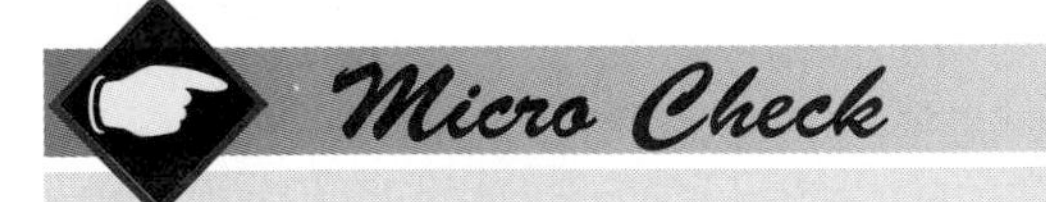

- How can the presence of natural antibodies to red blood cell antigens be explained?
- What is the cause of hemolytic disease of the newborn?
- What causes Graves' hyperthyroidism?

Type III Antibody-Mediated Immune Complex Hypersensitivity

The differences between some kinds of type II and type III hypersensitivity reactions may be subtle. Activation of complement precedes the release of chemical mediators by neutrophils. Immune complexes of type III reactions are formed in blood vessels. They may be deposited in blood vessel walls or in tissues of other parts of the body (Fig. 14–6). Small and intermediate-sized circulating immune complexes are more prone to tissue deposition than are very large complexes. The larger ones usually are cleared from the circulation by phagocytosis. The consequences of tissue deposition are necrosis (death of tissue) and neutrophil infiltration. Sometimes platelets are attracted to reaction sites, causing an obstruction in blood flow. The Arthus reac-

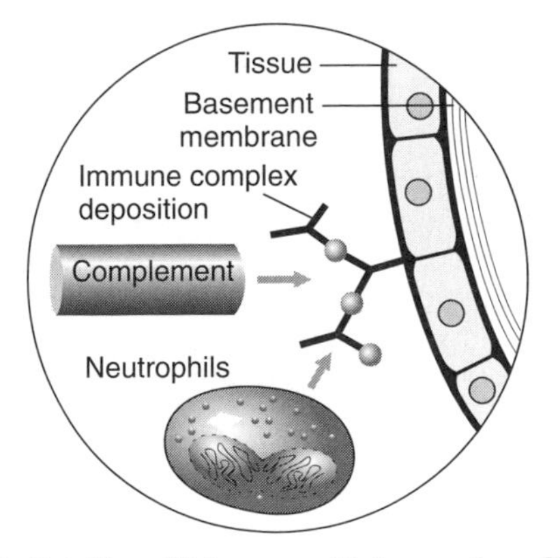

Figure 14–6 ◆ Type III hypersensitivity reaction. Circulating immune complexes bind with complement and are deposited in various tissues where they attract neutrophils.

tion and serum sickness are classic examples of type III immune complex reactions. If antibodies are made against self antigens, immune-complex deposits cause autoimmune disease.

ARTHUS REACTION

A localized response in animals to repeated injections of a soluble antigen in the presence of circulating antibody is called an **Arthus reaction.** As the aggregates increase in size, complement is activated, and neutrophils and platelets accumulate at the site of the injections. Immune complexes are deposited in walls of small arteries, causing local inflammation and necrosis. Similar localized reactions are observed in animal and human alveoli as a result of inhaled antigens. The ensuing pulmonary disease in animals or humans is called **hypersensitivity pneumonitis** (inflammation of lungs). A classic disease in which respiratory difficulties are encountered six to eight hours after exposure to moldy hay is known as **farmer's lung.** A common allergen promoting the respiratory hypersensitivity is the thermophilic actinomycete *Micropolyspora faeni.* The name of the disease may not be accurately descriptive because the disease has been observed in residents of cities from exposure to bacteria or fungi growing in air-conditioning units (Table 14–3).

SERUM SICKNESS

A disorder called **serum sickness** occurs when proteins from animal serum are used during the course of treatment. Serum sickness is rare in today's practice of medicine, but it occurred with some frequency when animal antitoxins were used for immunization. Deposits of the immune complexes caused painful joints, a rash, and swollen lymph nodes that lasted 8 to 10 days.

Table 14–3
CAUSES OF HYPERSENSITIVITY PNEUMONITIS

SOURCE	CONDITION	ALLERGEN
Animals	Furrier's lung	Animal fur
	Bird breeder's lung	Avian protein
	Rat handler's lung	Rat protein
Bacteria	Farmer's lung	*Micropolyspora faeni*
	Washing powder lung	Enzymes of *Bacillus subtilis*
Chemicals	Vineyard sprayer's lung	Bordeaux mixture
	Hard metal disease	Cobalt
Fungi	Maltworker's lung	*Aspergillus clavatus*
	Sequiosis	*Aureobasidium pullulans*

RHEUMATIC FEVER

Rheumatic fever is an active inflammatory process occurring one to five weeks after pharyngitis caused by some group A, beta-hemolytic streptococci. Antibodies to some types of the streptococci react with cardiac, muscle, cartilage, and kidney antigens similar to components of streptococcal cell walls. The serotypes responsible for rheumatic fever in the past decade have been M-1, -3, -5, -6, and -18. The streptococcal antibodies in rheumatic fever can cause arthritis, carditis, a rash, and Sydenham's chorea, a nervous disorder characterized by spasms of muscles. Sydenham's chorea, once called St. Vitus' dance because of the involuntary muscle movements and lack of coordination, was believed to be the work of Satan in the Middle Ages. If cardiac tissue is affected, the heart valves may be permanently damaged. Prompt diagnosis and treatment of group A streptococcal infections are important deterrents to the development of the misdirected attacks in rheumatic fever.

ACUTE POSTSTREPTOCOCCAL GLOMERULONEPHRITIS

Acute poststreptococcal glomerulonephritis (inflammation of glomeruli of the kidney) can follow an upper respiratory tract infection with certain group A beta-hemolytic streptococci. It may occur as soon as five days after pharyngitis or a skin infection. It is believed that antigen-antibody-complement complexes deposited on the glomerular basement membrane (GBM) attract polymorphonuclear neutrophils that promote the severe inflammatory response (Fig. 14–7). The immunologic injury increases glomerular permeability and causes degenerative changes in glomeruli. The increase in glomerular permeability permits protein and, sometimes, whole red blood cells to escape into the urine. In some cases, edema, hypertension, and renal failure are complications. Only prompt diagnosis and treatment of streptococcal pharyngeal or skin infections reduce the incidence of the immunological assault.

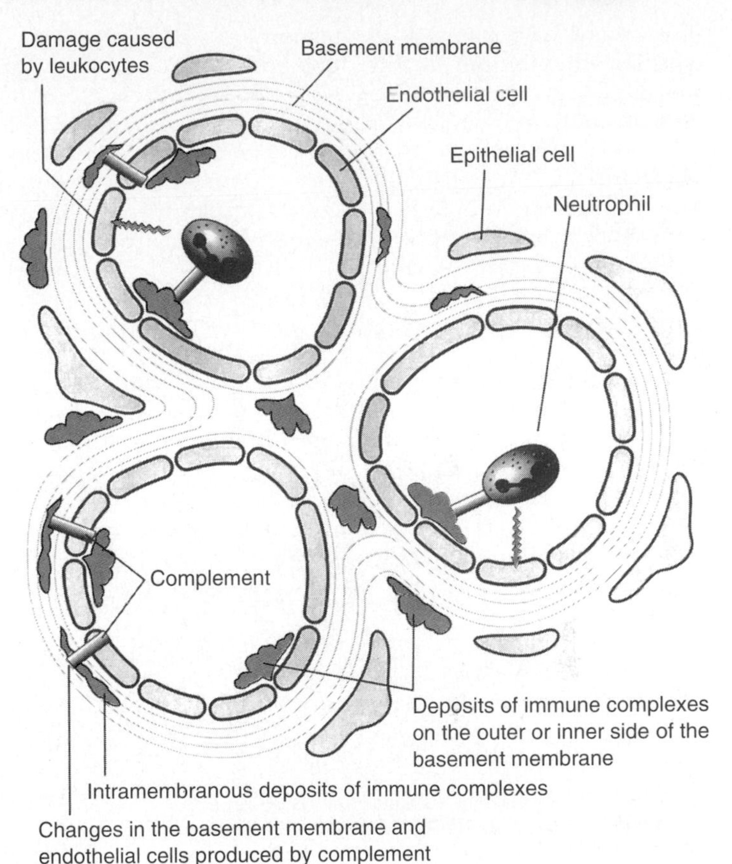

Figure 14–7 ◆ Damage produced by deposits of immune complexes containing complement and infiltration of neutrophils in acute poststreptococcal glomerulonephritis.

SYSTEMIC LUPUS ERYTHEMATOSUS

Antinuclear antibodies are produced in a disease known as **systemic lupus erythematosus** (red wolf). The antibodies do not react with intact nuclei of cells, but they may complex with antigenic components of damaged cells in the presence of complement. The immune complexes may be deposited in small blood vessels of the heart, kidneys, lymph nodes, and synovial membranes. The disease occurs primarily in women of child-bearing age and may have, as a concomitant feature, skin lesions consisting of reddish brown circumscribed soft patches. The distribution of the patches on the nose and cheeks often resembles the wings of a butterfly (Fig. 14–8).

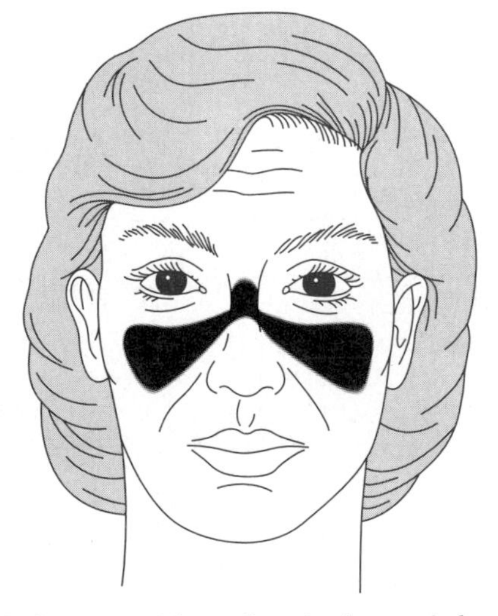

Figure 14–8 ◆ Typical butterfly rash of systemic lupus erythematosus.

RHEUMATOID ARTHRITIS

Rheumatoid arthritis is a chronic inflammatory disease of the joints. The blood of approximately

90 percent of patients with rheumatoid arthritis contains rheumatoid factors, IgM or IgG autoantibodies, that react with the Fc portion of their own antibody molecules. The initial inflammatory process in rheumatoid arthritis occurs in the synovial membranes of joints. Painful joints, limitation of movement, and atrophy of muscles are almost inevitable complications. Joints of the fingers are commonly affected.

POLYARTERITIS NODOSA

Polyarteritis nodosa is an inflammatory disease of small or middle-sized arteries containing deposits of immune complexes. The initial allergen may be a drug or part of an infectious agent but often is undeterminable. The surface antigen of hepatitis B virus (HBV) is known to initiate this type of immune complex disease.

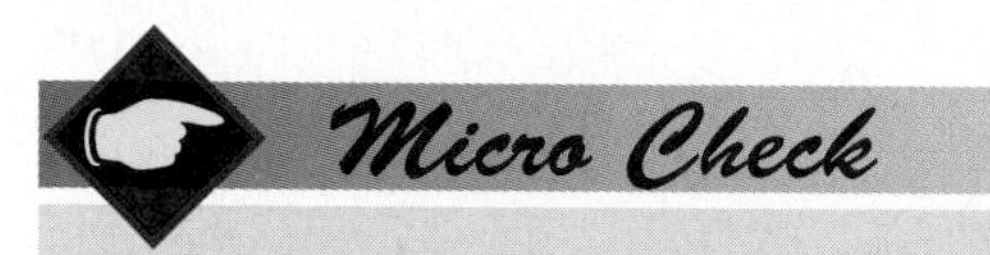

- What causes city residents to exhibit symptoms of farmer's lung?
- How can damage to human tissues or organs be explained in rheumatic fever and acute glomerulonephritis?
- How does the cause of systemic lupus erythematosus differ from that of rheumatoid arthritis?

Type IV Cell-Mediated Delayed Hypersensitivity

It is probable that Jenner observed the first cell-mediated hypersensitivity reaction in 1798 when he noted a local inflammatory response to the smallpox virus in an individual who had been previously vaccinated. The inflammatory response appeared to be maximal 24 to 72 hours after inoculation. The anticipated reaction was a decrease in inflammation in a previously immunized person. Since that first observation of what is now called cell-mediated hypersensitivity, many infections caused by viruses as well as bacteria, fungi, and protozoa have been shown to elicit the delayed hypersensitivity reaction. The reaction occurs in the absence of antibodies. The hypersensitivity response follows stimulation of TH1 cells and $CD8^+$ cells by processed antigen. Released cytokines promote a local inflammation. Like other types of hypersensitivity, cell-mediated hypersensitivity is an altered response in which immunity does not follow exposure to antigen.

The ability of specific microorganisms or their products to promote **erythema** (redness) and **induration** (hardening of tissue) in a previously sensitized individual is the basis for a variety of skin tests used for diagnostic purposes (Table 14–4).

One of the most widely used intradermal skin tests based on cell-mediated hypersensitivity is the Mantoux test for tuberculosis. The tissues of a person who has been exposed to mycobacteria are sensitized to a purified protein derivative tuberculin (PPD), a product of the etiologic agent. Erythema and induration after intradermal inoculation of PPD do not necessarily indicate active tuberculosis but merely that at one time the individual had been exposed to mycobacteria (Fig. 14–9).

Tuberculin tests are quite reliable in unvaccinated children but can be unreliable in adults who have received tuberculosis vaccinations or who have atypical mycobacterial infections. For maximum protection, all individuals with positive tuberculin skin tests should be evaluated carefully by radiological and cultural studies.

CONTACT DERMATITIS

Some chemicals may act as allergens or haptens evoking cell-mediated hypersensitivity reactions (Table 14–5). The response to such materials, after sensitization, may vary from a mild rash or erythema of the skin to weeping lesions. One

Table 14–4
DELAYED HYPERSENSITIVITY DIAGNOSTIC SKIN TESTS*

DISEASE	TEST MATERIAL
Brucellosis	Filtrate of *Brucella melitensis* or *Brucella abortus*
Candidiasis	*Candida albicans*
Coccidioidomycosis	Coccidioidin
Histoplasmosis	Histoplasmin
Leprosy	Lepromin
Mumps	Killed virus
Tuberculosis	Tuberculin
Tularemia	Protein extract of *Francisella tularensis*

*Skin tests based on delayed hypersensitivity to microorganisms or their products may indicate a current or past infection.

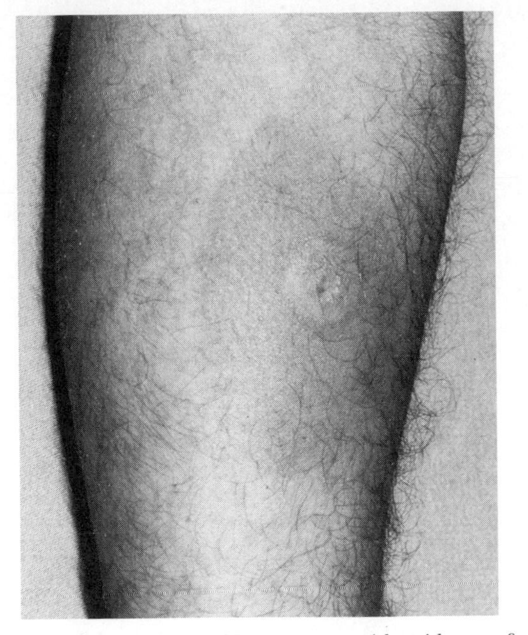

Figure 14–9 ◆ A positive Mantoux test with evidence of erythema and induration 48 hours after intradermal inoculation of tuberculin.

Table 14–5
COMMON TOPICAL ALLERGENS AND THEIR SOURCES

ALLERGEN	SOURCE
Benzocaine	Topical anesthetics
Diphenhydramine	Lotions
Formaldehyde	Nail polishes
Fragrances	Perfumes
Neomycin	Ointments
Paraphenylene diamine	Hair dyes

of the most common contact allergens is associated with poison ivy and poison oak (see Color Plate 31). The active agent, urushiol, is absorbed through the skin. Other allergens that can cause dermatitis are metals, lotions, hair dyes, soaps, perfumes, and lacquers. How do you suppose chemicals with relatively small molecules can act as allergens? Most antigens consist of molecules that are much larger. It has been proposed that small molecules are partial antigens or **haptens** that conjugate with proteins of the skin to form complete antigens. Widespread contact dermatitis of the elbows and buttocks occurred among American soldiers in Japan after World War II. The localization of the rash was curious. It was discovered to be caused by a lacquer applied to bars and toilet seats. The lacquer contained an allergen similar to urushiol that caused the reaction in individuals who had been previously sensitized to poison ivy.

FOCAL POINT

Latex Allergies: Who's at Risk?

Common to allergic reactions to natural substances is the body's need to recognize the substance. The more often the body comes in contact with the substance, the greater the opportunity to recognize and react. For the general public, the risk of an allergic reaction to latex is less than 1 percent. But because of constant exposure to latex, two groups are at greater risk—health care workers and children with spina bifida and other conditions involving multiple surgical procedures. Because latex-containing medical devices abound in surgical suites, dental offices, and other health care settings, contact with latex is an occupational hazard for health care workers. It is also part of some daily health maintenance routines and may be a problem for patients requiring special procedures such as catheterization and in the many surgeries some patients require. Dr. Jay E. Slater of Children's National Medical Center in Washington, D.C., found 25 of 64 children with spina bifida had antibodies to latex. About half of those children with the latex antibodies had a history of latex-associated allergic reactions. It is expected that allergic reactions to latex will increase over time. "Among those who had the antibody, approximately half had a history of latex-associated reactions," he says. He adds that more and more of these children will have reactions as time goes on. In rare cases, an allergic individual goes into shock; blood pressure plummets, the throat swells, and airways in the lungs constrict. Without immediate treatment, the person will die. An injection of epinephrine—the same drug used to treat severe allergic reactions to bee stings—will counteract the shock if given immediately.

FDA Consumer 26(7):16, 1992.

GRANULOMATOUS HYPERSENSITIVITY

Granulomatous hypersensitivity is a consequence of a chronic infection in which etiologic agents live within macrophages. The persistence of the antigenic stimulation of antigen causes the macrophages to enlarge and cluster around the antigen, forming palpable nodules of inflammatory tissue (Fig. 14–10). Continued antigenic stimulation leads to replacement of differentiated tissue with dense fibrous connective tissue sometimes called scar tissue. The granulomatous inflammatory response of the lungs to the bacterium *Mycobacterium tuberculosis* takes several weeks to develop.

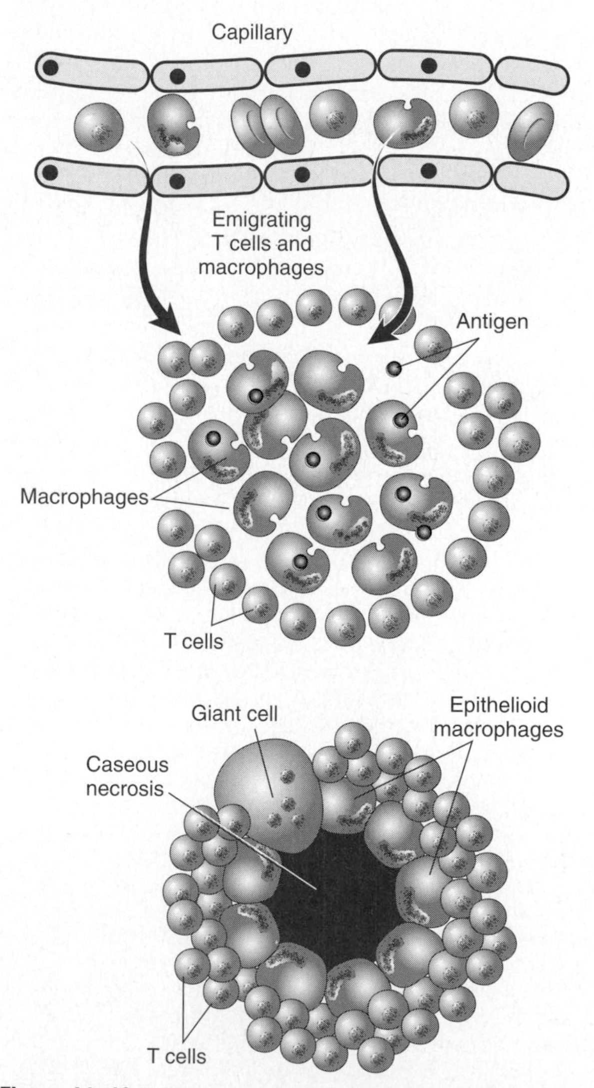

Figure 14–10 ◆ Events leading to formation of a granuloma.

TYPE 1 INSULIN-DEPENDENT DIABETES MELLITUS

A hallmark of type I **insulin-dependent diabetes mellitus** (IDDM) is a deficiency of insulin secretion by pancreatic cells. It has an early onset and also is called juvenile diabetes. Destruction of insulin-secreting cells is believed to be mediated at least in part by activated CD4+ cells. The initiating event that precedes the destruction of insulin-secreting cells is not known. Complications of long-standing IDDM include increased risks for coronary artery disease, peripheral vascular disease, renal failure, and infection.

MULTIPLE SCLEROSIS

Multiple sclerosis (MS) appears to be a chronic autoimmune disease of the central nervous system characterized by motor and sensory abnormalities and intermittent relapses. The disease is characterized by demyelination of axons of white matter in the brain, optic nerves, or spinal cord. Early lesions are infiltrated with lymphocytes and macrophages.

REJECTION OF TRANSPLANTS

Organ transplants have become an increasingly popular method of restoring a functional deficiency created by a diseased organ. The success of transplants is dependent on genetic similarities between donors and recipients. The rejection of a transplanted organ is mainly a consequence of cellular immune mechanisms. It involves a response to the MHC of transplants. The magnitude of immune responses is dependent on the degree of disparity of those antigens between donors and recipients.

A skin graft from one site to another site of the same individual is an **autograft** (Fig. 14–11). A transplant from a genetically identical individual, that is, an identical twin, is called an **isograft.** A transplant from a genetically dissimilar individual of the same species as the recipient is known as an **allograft.** A tissue graft between different species is designated as a **xenograft.** Some transplants do not generate an immune response if the site is isolated from B- or T-cell products. The anterior chamber of the eye is such a **privileged site.** For that reason, corneal replacements have been increasingly popular in restoring eye function.

Most individuals requiring transplants do not have an identical twin, so replacements of organs or tissues are almost always followed by rejection phenomena. Natural killer (NK), $CD8^+$, and cytotoxic T cells have major roles in promoting rejection. The reactive $CD8^+$ cytotoxic T cells lyse cells of transplants (Fig. 14–12). The cytokines of the TH1 cells promote the synthesis of antigraft antibodies and activate macrophages and complement. The antibodies form immune complexes that attract platelets, interfering with blood flow. The principal reaction is inflammatory, with large numbers of sensitized lymphocytes appearing in the vicinity of the graft within 6 to 10 days. Ultimately, the graft is destroyed by vascular changes that promote thrombosis. The rejection can be accentuated if individuals have been sensitized through blood transfusions or previous transplants. In the latter instance, clinical evidence of rejection may be present in minutes or hours rather than days.

Fortunately, the most drastic immunological responses to transplants can be avoided by matching antigens of potential donors and recipients and by the judicious administration of immunosuppressive agents. Most transplant patients experience some degree of rejection. Preexisting antibodies are responsible for rejection occurring within minutes after a transplant. Rejection occurring after the first week and up to several months can usually be explained by the ability of sensitized CD4+ cells to destroy donor cells. Late and progressive graft rejection can probably be explained by failure of immunosuppressive agents to modify host immune responses.

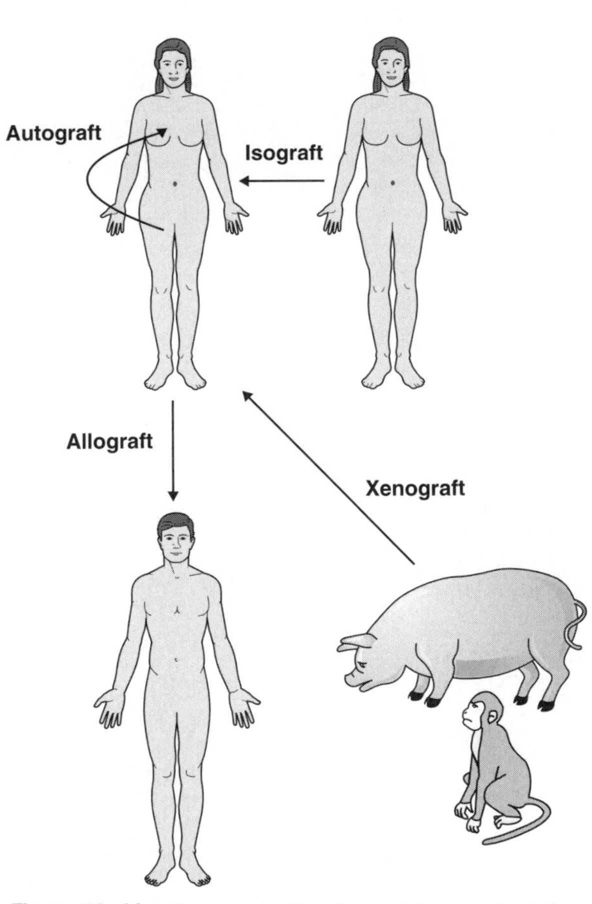

Figure 14–11 ◆ Four types of grafts used in transplantation.

GRAFT-VERSUS-HOST REACTIONS

If immunocompetent cells of a graft react against the host in a type of reverse assault, the response is called a **graft-versus-host (GVH) reaction.** NK cells predominate in GVH reactions. Those granulated cells secrete perforins, which lyse cells of the recipient. A classic syndrome, occurring in the laboratory when allogenic spleen cells are injected into neonatal animals, is called **runt disease.** Immunosuppressed adult animals develop GVH disease when injected with large doses of allogenic lymphoid cells. GVH reactions have also been observed in immunosuppressed humans. Patients receiving immunocompetent T cells in bone marrow transplants are at risk for developing GVH reactions. The consequences of such incompatibilities in humans may be enlargement of the spleen, liver, and lymph nodes, and anemia, diarrhea, and weight loss. The risk of GVH reactions may be reduced by removal of T cells from donor bone marrows.

Quite clearly, the transplantation of tissues or organs, however desirable to prolong life, is not without some hazard to the recipients. The interest in organ transplants in recent years has stimulated research in immunology.

The major characteristics of immediate and delayed hypersensitivities are summarized in Table 14–6.

Micro Check

- ◆ Explain the basis of skin tests for diagnostic purposes.
- ◆ What is the allergen in poison ivy and poison oak?
- ◆ Why are most organ or tissue transplants followed by rejection phenomena?

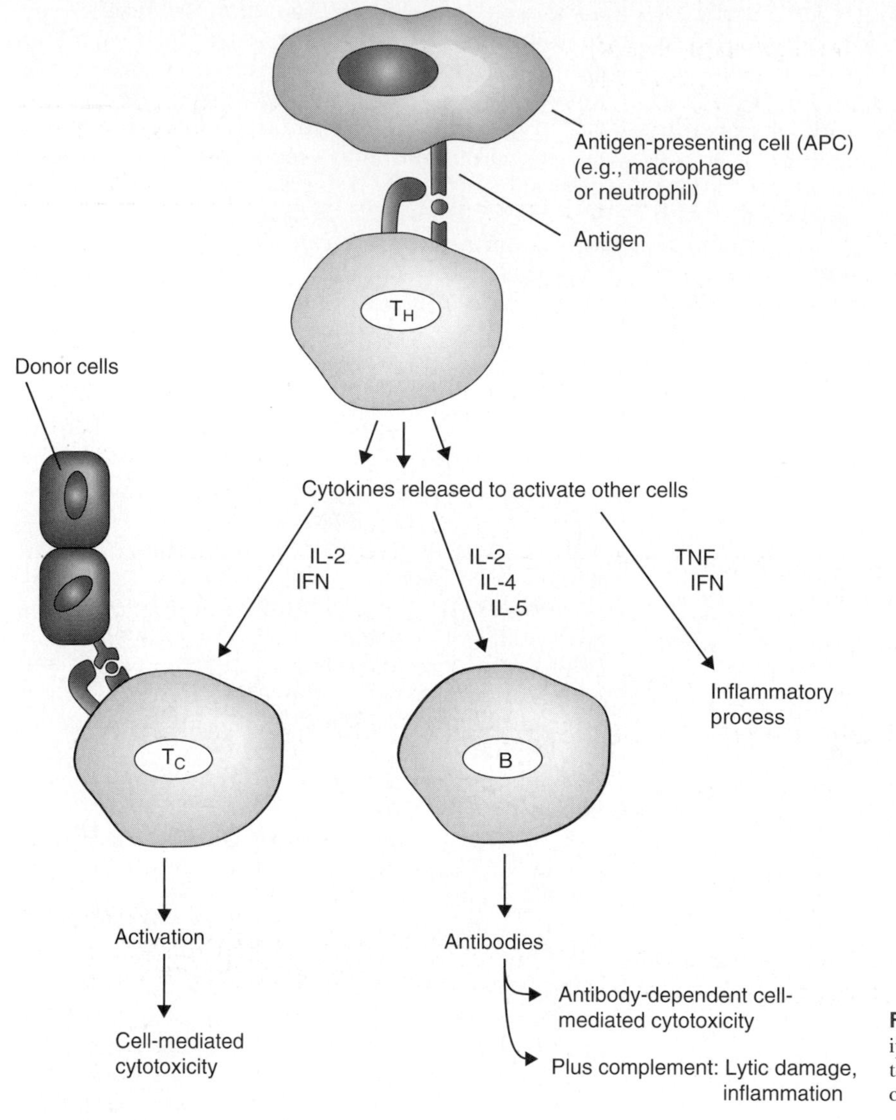

Figure 14–12 ◆ T- and B-cell participants in rejection of transplants. Cytokines secreted by T cells are indicated alongside the arrows.

APPLICATIONS OF THE IMMUNE RESPONSE

Two applications based on an understanding of the immune response have led to advancements in the diagnosis and prevention of infectious diseases. The diagnostic methods are called serological or immunological tests. The test procedures are rapid, sensitive, easy to perform, and particularly applicable to those diseases in which etiologic agents do not grow or grow with difficulty under laboratory conditions. Some infectious diseases and their consequences have been prevented by the massive administration of immunizing agents throughout the world. Other infectious diseases have been targeted for erradication within the next decade.

Monoclonal Antibodies

Many tests employed for the diagnosis of infectious diseases are based on the detection of specific antigens or antibodies. Until 1975 inoculation of laboratory animals was the only way to produce large quantities of antibodies for use in in vitro tests. At that time, George Milstein and George Kohler introduced a laboratory technique for producing antibodies of single types. They fused antibody-specific B cells and certain malignant cells of mice, called myeloma cells, to pro-

Table 14–6
A COMPARISON OF IMMEDIATE AND DELAYED HYPERSENSITIVITIES

	IMMEDIATE TYPES			DELAYED TYPE
	I	II	III	IV
Antibody Type	IgE	IgG, IgM	IgG, IgM	None
Allergen Source	Nonself	Self	Nonself, self	Nonself
Complement Participation	−	+	+	−
Response Time	2–30 min	4–10 hr	3–8 hr	24–48 hr
Examples	Anaphylaxis Asthma Hay fever Hives Food allergies	Transfusion reactions Hemolytic disease of the newborn Thrombocytopenia Graves' disease	Serum sickness Rheumatoid fever Glomerulonephritis Systemic lupus erythematosus Rheumatoid arthritis Polyarteritis nodosa	Diagnostic skin tests Contact dermatitis Transplant rejection

duce antibody-producing cells known as **hybridomas.** Because the myeloma cells are capable of dividing indefinitely, the hybrid cells continue to produce specific antibodies under laboratory conditions. The antibodies produced from a clone of single-antibody producing cells are called **monoclonal antibodies** (Fig. 14–13). The availability of monoclonal antibodies has increased the use of tests frequently called immunoassays. The assays also may be used to monitor the progress of a disease by measuring the amount of antibody present in a quantitative expression known as a **titer.** The titer is the reciprocal of the highest dilution of serum reacting with an antigen.

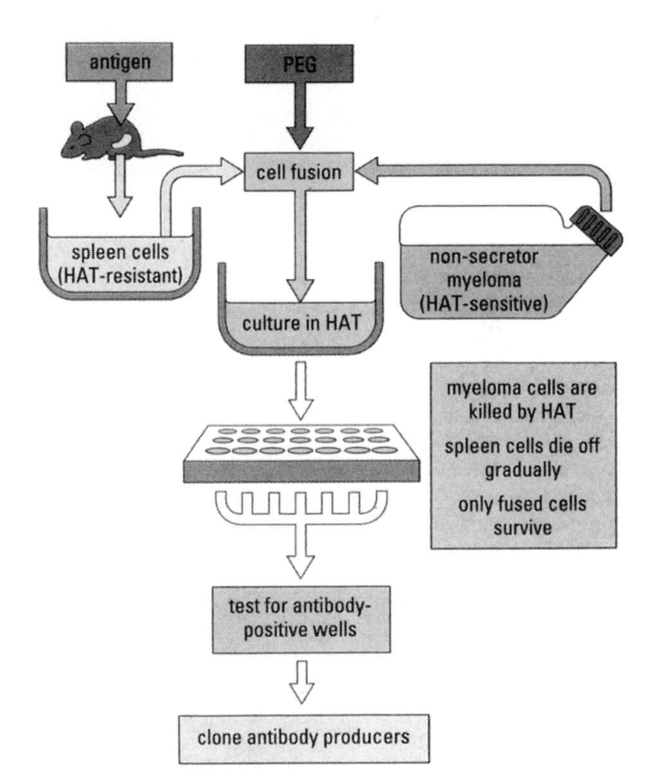

Figure 14–13 ◆ Steps in the production of monoclonal antibodies. Antibody-producing B cells are immortalized by fusion with mutant mouse myeloma cells. Fused cells are separated from the mixture by growing them in a medium containing hypoxanthine, aminopterin, and thymidine (HAT). HAT is selective for fused cells. Hybridomas are selected and cloned to obtain large quantities of specific antibody.

Diagnostic Tests

Various types of immunoassays are now used to diagnose or monitor the course of infectious diseases. The ability to tag or label antibodies or anti-antibodies with radioactive isotopes, fluorescent dyes, or enzymes has increased the sensitivity of immunoassays. The added labels make antigen-antibody complexes more visible in much the same manner that a car with headlights is easier to see in the dark than one without headlights. Immunodiagnostic tests may be classified as unlabeled or labeled immunoassays.

UNLABELED IMMUNOASSAYS

The procedures based on reactions between unlabeled antigens and antibodies require the presence of large amounts of those indicator

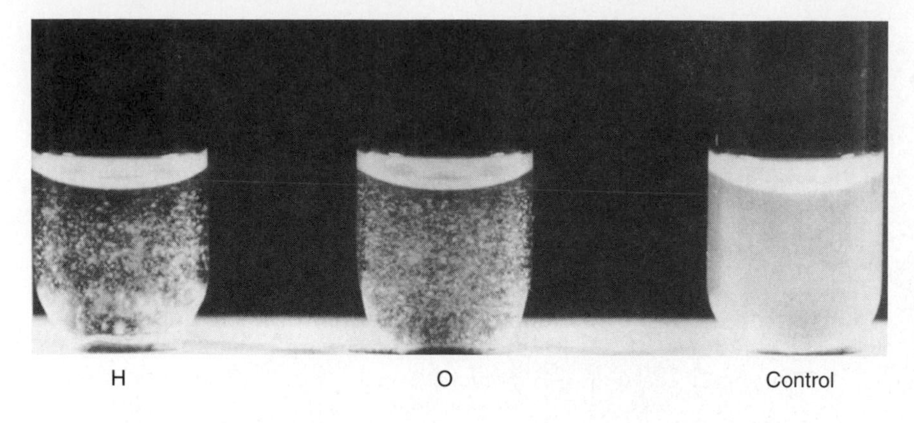

Figure 14–14 ◆ Agglutination of flagellar (H) antigens and somatic (O) antigens of bacteria compared with a nonagglutinated control on the right.

molecules for the reaction to be detected. Since one is usually looking for antibodies in a patient's serum, the tests often are referred to as serological tests.

AGGLUTINATION

Insoluble particulate antigens, such as those on microorganisms, combine with specific antibodies producing a reaction known as agglutination. The reaction is believed to take place in two stages. Antigens and antibodies first form invisible complexes. The antibody-coated antigens then undergo an alteration in surface charge and are attracted to one another in the presence of electrolytes. The antigen-antibody complexes are visible as they settle out of solution (Fig. 14–14). If the antigens are on red blood cells, the reaction is called hemagglutination. The role of components of hemagglutination is reversed in certain viral infections so that hemagglutination is inhibited in the presence of specific antibody. Some viruses possess reactive sites that combine with receptors on the surface of red blood cells to cause clumping. If specific antibodies to the receptors are present, they prevent attachment of viruses. The reaction is called hemagglutination inhibition.

PRECIPITATION

Soluble antigens and specific antibodies combine to produce insoluble complexes in a reaction known as precipitation. The precipitates

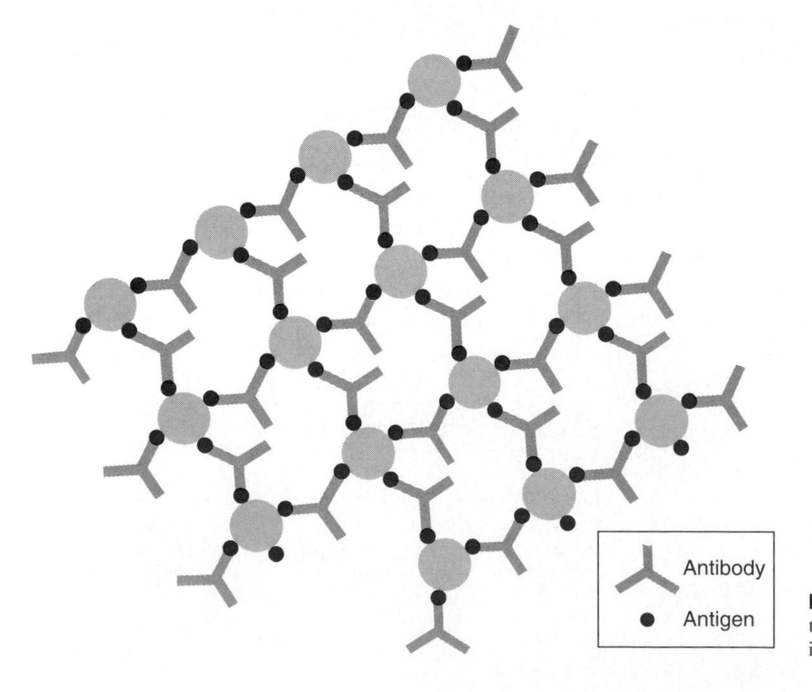

Figure 14–15 ◆ Lattice produced by formation of insoluble antigen-antibody complexes in the presence of electrolytes.

form in a solution or semisolid media called agar gels. It has been postulated that a "lattice" is produced when antigens are linked to antibodies (Fig. 14–15). When the complexes exceed a certain level, they settle out of solution. Although less sensitive than most agglutinating antibody reactions, precipitation tests are particularly valuable in forensic medicine to identify blood group antigens in stains.

COMPLEMENT FIXATION

Complement participates in many antigen-antibody reactions. Complement is said to be fixed when it binds with antigen-antibody complexes (Fig. 14–16). Fixed complement is not free to react in additional antigen-antibody reactions. If antigens are contained on the surface of cells, lysis of cells occurs, but if antigens are not associated with cells, absence of free complement can only be detected by the addition of an indicator system containing components for another antigen-antibody reaction requiring complement. Sheep red blood cells and hemolysin are often used to demonstrate the absence of free complement. Hemolysis does not occur if the complement has been fixed by another antigen-antibody reaction.

NEUTRALIZATION

Some antibodies alter the ability of microorganisms or their products to cause disease. Viruses and toxins are inactivated by a process called neutralization when antigen-antibody complexes are formed. Neutralization of viruses can be demonstrated if a virus does not grow in a cell culture or embryonated egg. Inactivation of toxins by specific antibodies requires the use of small animals bred for that purpose. If toxin is allowed to bind with specific antitoxin before inoculation, the toxin is neutralized and animals show no sign of disease.

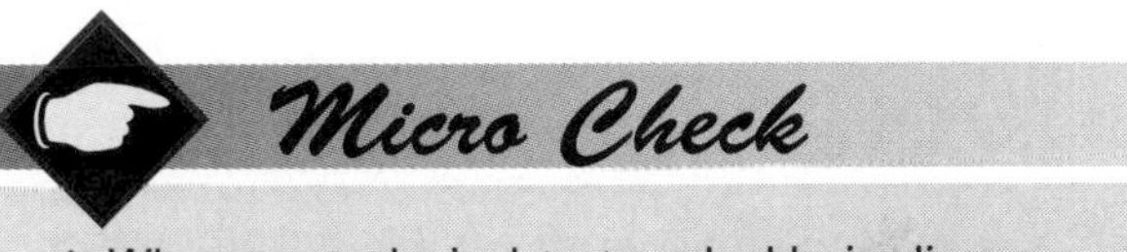

- Why are serological tests valuable in diagnostic microbiology?
- What are the components of the indicator system in complement-fixation tests?
- How can you demonstrate that a toxin has been neutralized?

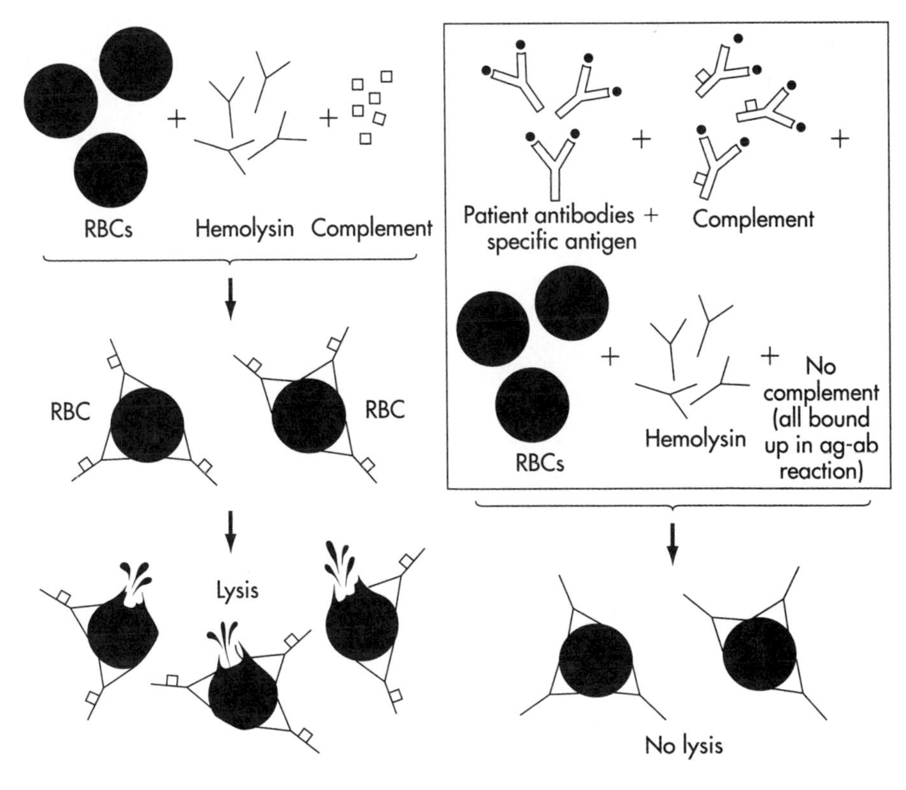

Figure 14–16 ◆ Complement fixation showing components of the primary and indicator-system reactants. If lysis occurs in the indicator system, antibodies against the primary antigen are not present. If no lysis occurs, the complement is fixed by antibodies in the primary reaction.

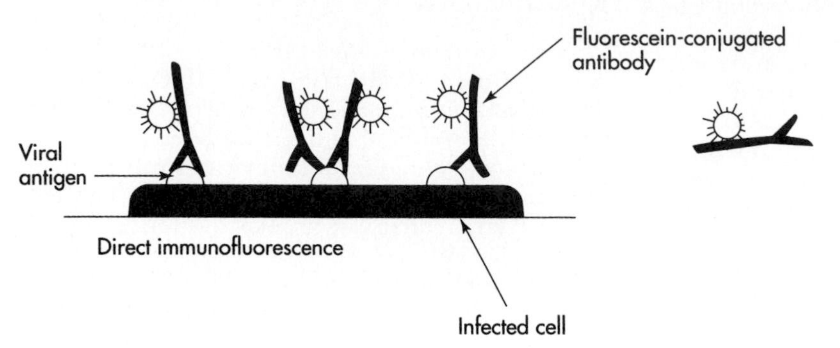

Figure 14–17 ◆ The direct method of immunofluorescence identifies antigen by allowing viral or microbial antigens to react with fluorescent antibodies.

Labeled Immunoassays

The unlabeled immunoassays are still used to diagnose or monitor the course of some infectious diseases, but they have been largely replaced by the more sensitive labeled immunoassays. Modern methods use a fluorescent dye, a radioactive isotope, or an enzyme to label antigens or antibodies. The labeled antigens or antibodies are called indicator molecules. The labels do not alter the complexing of antigens and antibodies. The tests using labels are both highly sensitive and specific. Procedures that detect the presence of antigens are called **direct** tests; tests that detect the presence of antibodies are known as **indirect** tests.

IMMUNOFLUORESCENT ASSAYS

Immunofluorescent assays are techniques by which antigens or antibodies can be detected. In the technique, antibodies or anti-antibodies are labeled by conjugation with fluorescent dyes such as fluorescein isothiocyanate or tetramethyl rhodamine. Under ultraviolet radiation both dyes appear fluorescent. Many microscopes can be adapted for fluorescence microscopy by substituting a mercury lamp for the ordinary light illuminator and using appropriate filter systems.

In the direct method fluorescent-labeled antibody is allowed to react directly with antigen on a smear prepared from a clinical specimen or imprint of tissue (Fig. 14–17). In the indirect method labeled anti-antibody is allowed to react with antigen-antibody complexes (Fig. 14–18). This method makes it unnecessary to make specific antibody conjugates for large numbers of antigens.

RADIOIMMUNOASSAYS

Radioimmunoassays (RIAs) are exquisitely sensitive serological procedures used to detect the presence of small antigens. Procedures are based on competition between radioactively labeled antigen and unlabeled antigen for antibodies. Free antigen is separated from bound antigen by the addition of an adsorbent under carefully controlled conditions. After a washing procedure, radioactivity of the adsorbent is determined. The amount of antigen present in a sample is determined by comparing the bound radioactivity with

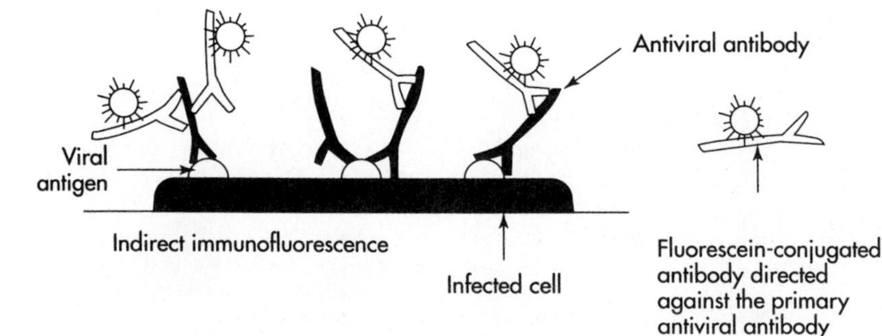

Figure 14–18 ◆ The indirect method of immunofluorescence identifies viral or microbial antibodies by allowing the antibodies to react with fluorescent anti-antibody bound to antigen.

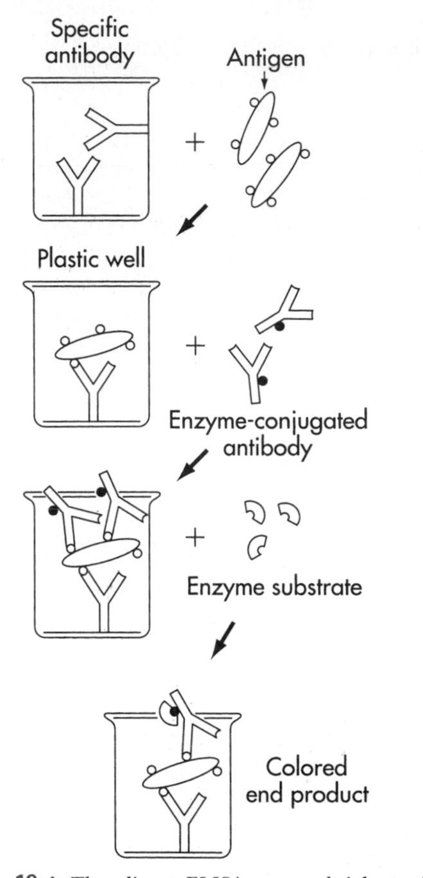

Figure 14–19 ◆ The direct ELISA or sandwich method allows fixed antibodies to complex with antigens. In a second step, enzyme-conjugated antibodies bind to the antigens, forming a "sandwich." The further addition of the enzyme's substrate produces color if antigens are present.

the radioactivity in solutions containing known amounts of antigen. RIAs require special equipment and disposal methods. It does not pay most routine testing laboratories to invest in such costly methods.

ENZYME IMMUNOASSAYS

Enzyme immunoassays (EIAs) are based on the ability of antibodies to be linked to an enzyme. The technique also depends on a solid surface to which reactants can be adsorbed. Enzyme-linked immunosorbent assay (ELISA) uses enzyme-linked antibodies or anti-antibodies. Enzymes such as peroxidase and phosphatase are often the enzymes of choice for ELISA. In the direct ELISA method or sandwich technique, antibodies are adsorbed to the bottom of wells of a plastic microtiter plate (Fig. 14–19). The test antigen is added, and unbound components are washed off. Enzyme-linked antibodies specific for the antigen are added. Bound antigen complexes with enzyme-linked antibodies. The unlabeled antibodies and labeled antibodies are like the pieces of bread in a sandwich. The filling is the antigen. When the enzyme's substrate is added to the mixture, the reaction between substrate and enzyme on the labeled antibodies produces a color reaction. The presence of color indicates a positive reaction; no color is characteristic of a negative test.

An indirect ELISA is used to test for the presence of specific antibodies. An antigen is adsorbed to the test wells. The test serum is added. If the specific antibodies are present, antigen-antibody complexes are formed. After rinsing, enzyme-linked anti-antibodies are added that bind to any antibody present. Addition of the substrate after removal of excess enzyme-linked antibodies causes a visible color change (Fig. 14–20). A color change indicates that specific antibodies are present. If no color develops, the test is negative. The indirect ELISA test is used to test for the presence of antibodies to HIV, but a confirmatory test is necessary because false-positive results occur in those infections.

Fluorescence-Activated Cell Sorting

A unique application of immunofluorescence and laser-beam technology is used to separate

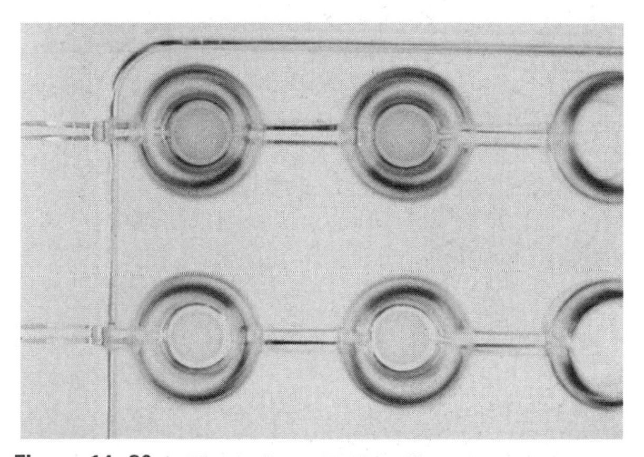

Figure 14–20 ◆ The indirect ELISA allows fixed antigens to complex with specific antibodies in a patient's serum. In a second step, enzyme-conjugated anti-antibodies are added followed by addition of the enzyme's substrate. Color development in the reaction mixtures indicates specific antibodies.

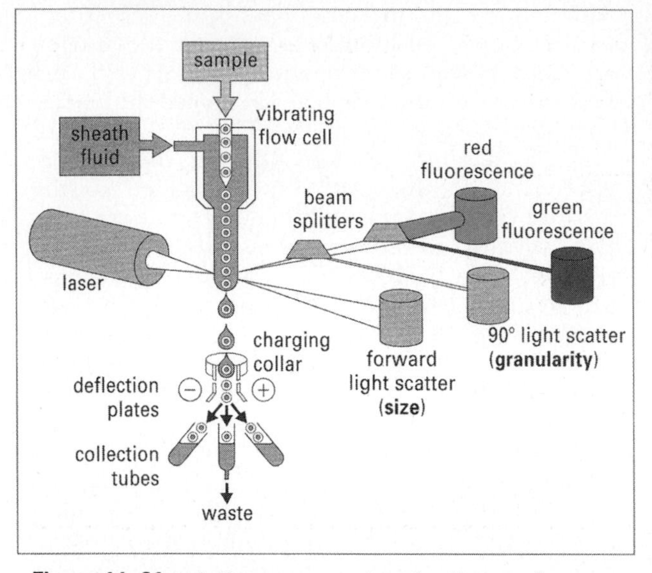

Figure 14–21 ◆ A fluorescence-activated cell sorter for separating different classes of T cells.

cells in mixed populations (Fig. 14–21). After allowing cells to react with specific-labeled antibody, fluorescing and nonfluorescing cells are subjected to a laser beam. The intensity of fluorescence causes the strength and direction of the electromagnetic field to be deflected so that fluorescent cells are separated from nonfluorescent cells. Fluorescence-activated cell sorting is extremely useful in separating populations of CD4+ and CD8+ cells in assessing AIDS patients and in monitoring their treatment.

Western Blot Assays

Western blot assays are used to identify mixtures of antigens or antibodies. The proteins are separated by a process called **electrophoresis** in gel and are blotted onto nitrocellulose paper. Radioactive or enzyme-labeled antibodies are allowed to react with the separated proteins. Radioactive or colored bands are produced when the substrate specific for the labeled antibodies is added. Western blot assays are useful as confirmatory tests in HIV screening. The bands obtained are compared with positive and negative controls (Fig. 14–22). If antibodies from at least one of three major types of HIV-1 antigens are not present, the test is reported as indeterminate.

Micro Check

- What is the primary advantage of labeled immunoassays over unlabeled immunoassays?
- What is the difference between direct and indirect labeled immunoassays?
- Why is a confirmatory test necessary if an indirect ELISA test is positive for HIV?

Vaccine-Preventable Diseases

Administration of killed or attenuated microorganisms, their parts, or inactivated products as vaccines has eliminated or controlled a number of infectious diseases and their complications throughout the world. The eradication of smallpox was accomplished largely through the efforts of the World Health Organization. Significant progress is being made in eliminating polio within the next decade. Many other diseases, such as measles, mumps, rubella, pertussis, and invasive disease caused by *Haemophilus influenzae* type b, can be substantially reduced if vaccines

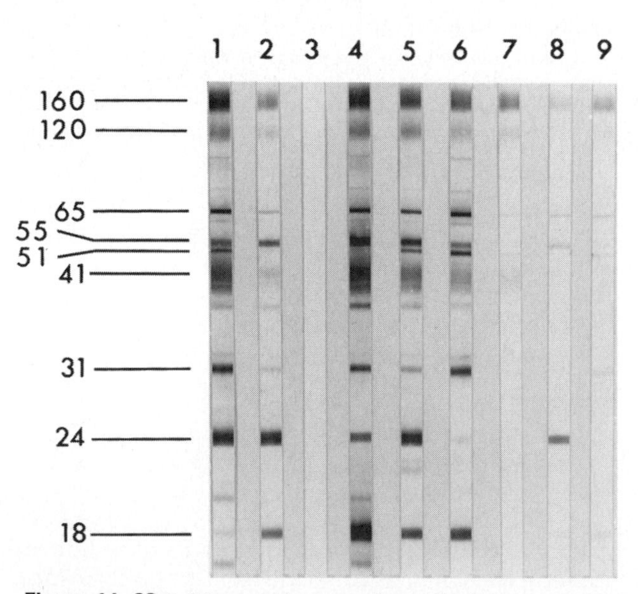

Figure 14–22 ◆ Western blot assay for antibodies to proteins and glycoproteins of HIV-1. Lane 1 is a high positive control. Lane 2 is a low positive control. Lane 3 is a negative control. Lanes 4 to 8 are positive. Lane 9 is indeterminate. Numbers on the left are the approximate molecular weights of HIV-1 antigens.

Table 14–7
RECOMMENDED EARLY CHILDHOOD IMMUNIZATIONS—UNITED STATES

DISEASE	TYPE OF IMMUNIZATION	RECOMMENDED TIME SCHEDULE
Hepatitis B	HVB surface antigen (Hep B)	1 week 2, 6, and 18 months
Diphtheria, tetanus, pertussis	Diphtheria and tetanus toxoids Whole-killed cells of pertussis or acellular pertussis preparation (DTP) or (DTaP)	2, 4, and 6 months
Meningitis	Capsular polysaccharide of *Haemophilus influenzae,* type B (Hib)	2, 4, and 6 months
Measles, mumps, rubella	Attenuated measles, mumps, and rubella viruses (MMR)	2, 4, and 6 months
Polio	Inactivated polio virus (IPV)*	2, 4, and 15 months 4–6 years
Varicella	Attenuated herpes zoster virus (VAR)	12–18 months

*The Advisory Committee on Immunization Practices (ACIP) recommends that the oral polio vaccine (OPV) no longer be used for most children in the United States starting in the year 2000.

can be brought to all of the people. Immunization programs must be maintained consistently if such goals are to be realized. Unfortunately, costs of intervention programs are high. The countries needing them most do not have money for basic necessities.

In the United States, governmental as well as private agencies are involved in recommending certain early childhood vaccinations. The Centers for Disease Control and Prevention recommends an immunization schedule for 10 vaccine-preventable diseases (Table 14–7). Some states require a

Table 14–8
RECOMMENDED ADULT IMMUNIZATIONS—UNITED STATES

DISEASE	IMMUNIZATION	INDICATION	RECOMMENDED TIME SCHEDULE
Influenza	Inactivated type A (two strains) and type B (strain) viruses	Age $\geq$ 65 years Health care workers	Annually
Hepatitis A	Inactivated HAV	Travelers	First dose—any time Second dose—one to six months later
Hepatitis B	HBV surface antigen	Health care workers Hemodialysis patients Travelers	First dose—any time Second dose—one month later Third dose—six months later
Measles, mumps, rubella	Attenuated measles, mumps, and rubella viruses	Persons born in 1957 or later Health care workers Travelers	Two doses one month or more apart
Pneumococcal disease	23 purified capsular polysaccharide antigens	Age $\geq$ 65 years Chronic disease	One time except for high-risk persons
Tetanus-diphtheria	Tetanus and diphtheria toxoids	All adults	Every 10 years
Varicella	Attenuated varicella virus	All susceptible adults	Two doses one to two months apart

minimum number of immunizations for entry into public schools and day care centers. Do you know what immunizations, if any, are required by your local school district?

Still 300 to 500 children die annually in the United States of vaccine-preventable diseases. The number of adult deaths from influenza, hepatitis B, and pneumococcal pneumonia ranges between 50,000 and 90,000 each year. Yet the diseases, like the childhood diseases, are also vaccine preventable. Adults are at risk for those particular diseases because of age, life-style, or underlying disease. There are 10 vaccine-preventable diseases for adults (Table 14–8). Immunizations in especially high-risk adults could substantially reduce the number of deaths and health care costs.

It is either difficult or impossible to develop vaccines for all infectious diseases. Many microorganisms undergo frequent mutations, continually changing their surface antigens. Global problems, such as unsafe water supplies, lack of food, and overpopulation, contribute substantially to susceptibility to infectious diseases and are difficult to solve.

A relatively large number of vaccines for infectious diseases affecting susceptible children and adults have been developed over the years. Development of new vaccines goes on even as you are studying microbiology. Most of them are for special at-risk populations. For example, individuals who share a geographic habitat with ticks of the genus *Ixodes* and who have frequent or prolonged exposure to natural vegetation could benefit from the newly developed vaccine for Lyme disease. It is prudent to be aware of your own immunization history and to discuss possible additional vaccinations with your physician if a risk factor places you in a category of persons susceptible to particular infections.

FOCAL POINT

Are There Edible Vaccines in Your Future?

Would you like to eat a spoonful of pureed bananas instead of being injected with a vaccine for your next immunization? Charles Arntzen, president of the Boyce Thompson Institute for Plant Research in Ithaca, New York, believes that could happen within the next decade. Why bananas? It is quite simple. Vaccines made from plants need to be eaten raw because heat would inactivate some antigens. Arntzen's group has induced potato plants to make proteins of a virulent strain of *Escherichia coli.* This was done by transferring a gene of that bacterium into *Agrobacterium tumifaciens,* a common soil bacterium. Cells of the potato plant were infected with the soil bacterium containing the gene responsible for the toxin of the virulent *E. coli.* When mice ate the potatoes, the toxin was recognized as "nonself" and antibodies were produced. The plants carrying the foreign gene are called transgenic plants. Studies on human volunteers as well as mice look promising. In addition to investigating the use of potatoes, cantaloupes and tomatoes from transgenic plants have been used successfully as vaccines. Indeed, probably edible vaccines are in your future, or at least in the future of your children, if molecular biologists' predictions come true.

Howard Hughes Medical Institute Report, Arousing the Fury of the Immune System. 1998, p 77.

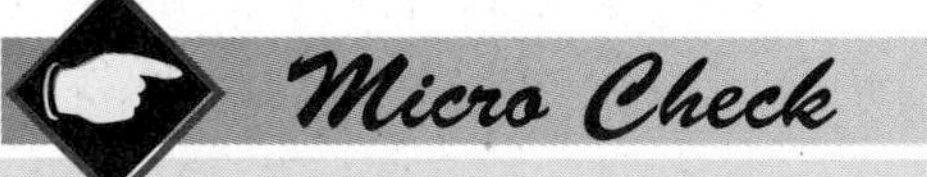

- What is the greatest obstacle to overcome in getting children immunized in developing countries?
- Why is it not possible to develop vaccines for all infectious diseases?
- What factors influence the risk of adults to vaccine-preventable diseases such as influenza, hepatitis B, and pneumococcal pneumonia?

Understanding Microbiology

1. Name three types of antibody-mediated hypersensitivity and give an example of each.
2. List three common types of localized anaphylaxis.
3. What are the primary mediators of a) systemic anaphylaxis, b) asthma, c) hay fever, d) urticaria, and e) intestinal allergies?

4. Describe the immune response in a positive test for tuberculosis.
5. Name five vaccine-preventable diseases.

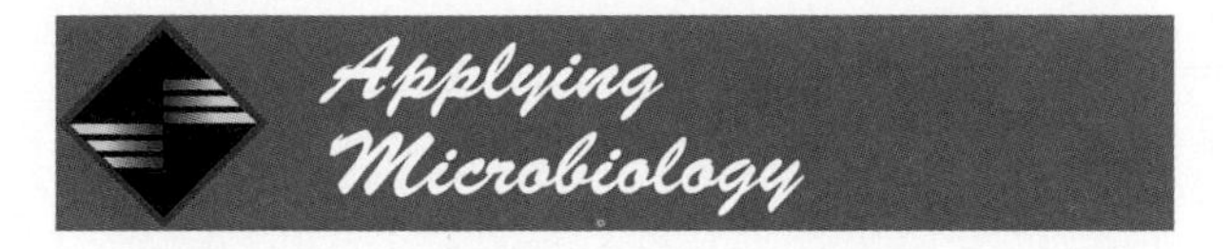

1. An otherwise healthy Rh^+ boy born to an Rh^- mother was diagnosed as having hemolytic disease of the newborn after birth. He was treated successfully, but a first-born child two years previously had no record of the blood disease despite the fact that she also was Rh^+. How can the disparity be explained?

Unit 5

Infectious Diseases of Humans

Chapter 15 Diseases of the Skin, Hair, and Nails

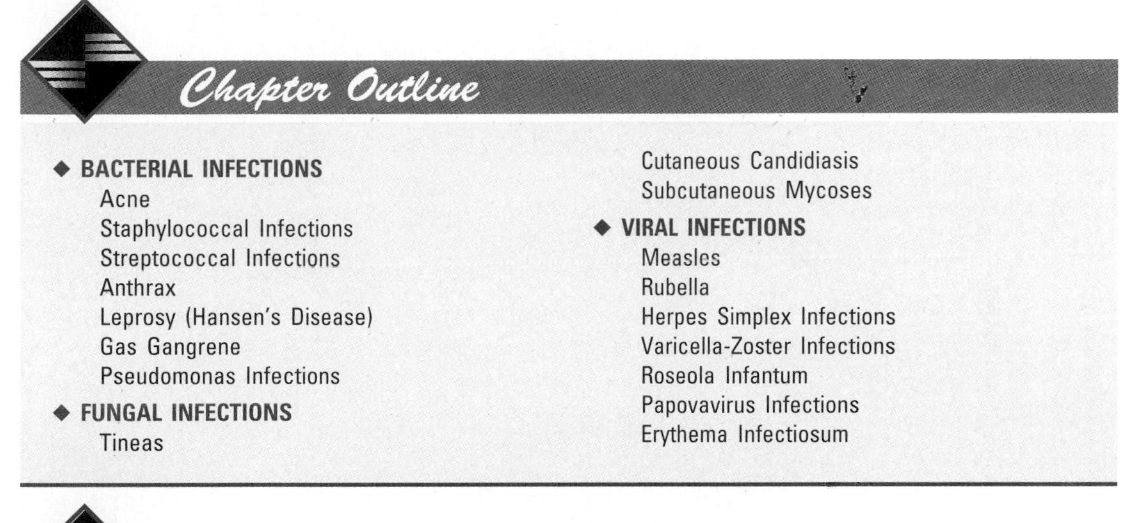

Chapter Outline

- **BACTERIAL INFECTIONS**
  - Acne
  - Staphylococcal Infections
  - Streptococcal Infections
  - Anthrax
  - Leprosy (Hansen's Disease)
  - Gas Gangrene
  - Pseudomonas Infections
- **FUNGAL INFECTIONS**
  - Tineas
  - Cutaneous Candidiasis
  - Subcutaneous Mycoses
- **VIRAL INFECTIONS**
  - Measles
  - Rubella
  - Herpes Simplex Infections
  - Varicella-Zoster Infections
  - Roseola Infantum
  - Papovavirus Infections
  - Erythema Infectiosum

Learning Objectives

After you have read this chapter, you should be able to:

1. Describe how microorganisms gain entrance through the skin.
2. Describe the lesions of the skin produced by infectious agents.
3. List the major bacterial, fungal, and viral diseases of the skin.
4. Contrast the treatment of bacterial, fungal, and viral infections of the skin.
5. Explain the recurrence of herpesvirus infections.
6. List the defects of congenital rubella syndrome.
7. Explain the persistence of pseudomonads in the hospital environment.

The skin is the largest and most important protective organ of the body. An intact skin regulates body temperature, controls loss of fluid, and prevents the entrance of foreign substances and most microorganisms. The skin consists of a layer of closely packed epithelial cells, the **epidermis,** and a layer of dense connective tissue, the **dermis** (Fig. 15–1). The dermis contains the sweat glands, sebaceous glands, nerves, and blood vessels. The skin is in contact with the mucous membranes lining several body cavities. The cells of the exposed epidermis are made up of the insoluble protein **keratin.** The epidermal cells die in the process of producing the keratin. The hair and nails are superficial structures of the skin containing even larger concentrations of keratin.

The human skin is populated with billions of microorganisms. The microbial inhabitants of the cutaneous community live in a virtual paradise with all their needs supplied. **Sebum,** a product of the sebaceous glands, and the contents of sweat provide moisture and nutrients for gram-

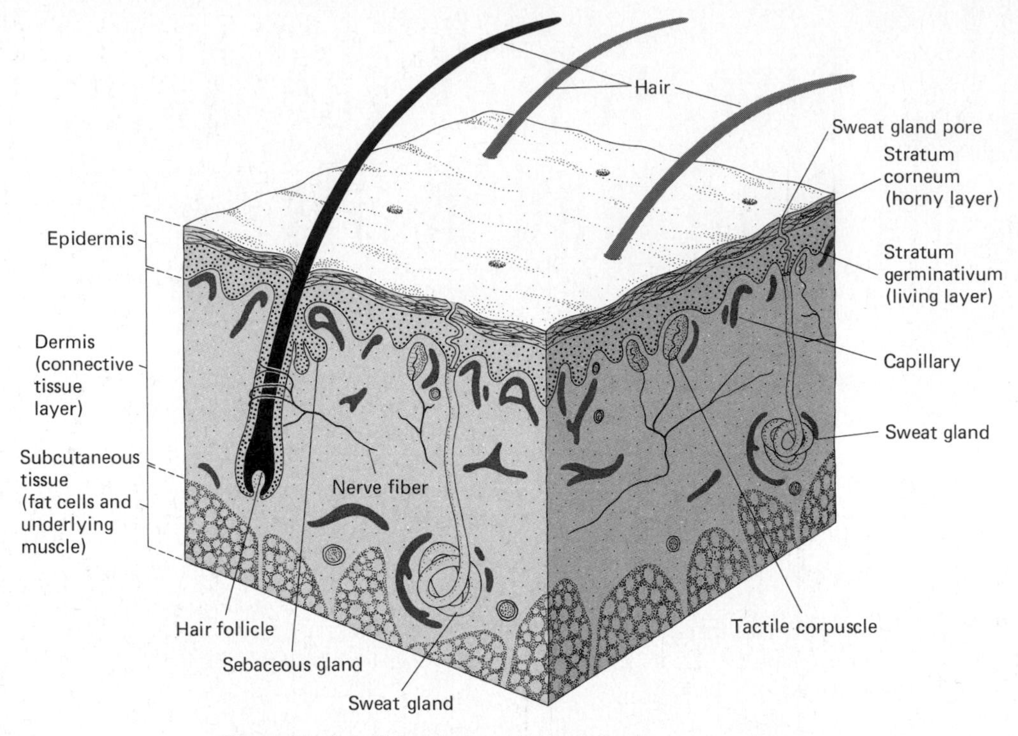

Figure 15–1 ◆ Cross section of skin and subcutaneous tissue.

positive bacteria. Most gram-negative bacteria are inhibited by the fatty acids made when gram-positive bacteria degrade the lipids of sebum. Fungi and viruses are found in limited numbers on the skin. The shedding of dead epidermal cells and their microbial inhabitants permits the dispersal of microorganisms on tiny "rafts" of skin. The journey for the microorganisms is hazardous, but some do find a favorable environment for growth.

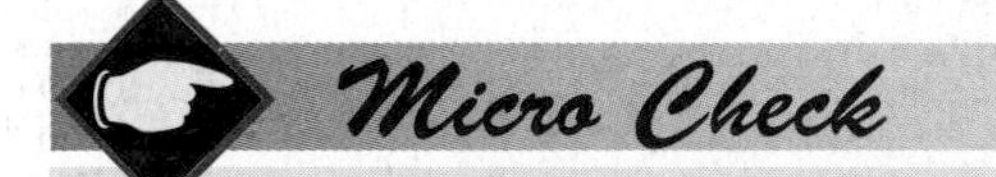

- ◆ How does physical exercise influence microbial populations of the skin?
- ◆ Why do the majority of microorganisms traveling on a raft of skin not survive?
- ◆ What parts of the body would you expect to contain the largest number of microorganisms?

The skin is exposed to an extraordinary number of additional microorganisms every day. A few of them may become transient residents, but not many can penetrate the skin unless an opening is provided. If microorganisms do gain entrance to the skin, the infections they cause are often accompanied by lesions. The descriptions of some common lesions are given in Table 15–1.

Table 15–1
LESIONS ASSOCIATED WITH INFECTIONS OF THE SKIN

TYPE OF LESION	DESCRIPTION
Abscess	Small cavity containing pus
Carbuncle	Multicentric abscess with a hard core
Erythema	Area of redness due to increase in blood supply
Furuncle	Unicentric abscess with a soft core
Macule	Small flat red or brown spot
Papule	Small raised lesion containing pus
Ulcer	Open craterlike lesion of variable size
Vesicle	Open blister containing fluid
Wart	Small localized growth of epidermal cells
Wheal	Hard, raised, red lesion

BACTERIAL INFECTIONS

Infections of the skin may be caused by permanent bacterial residents under special conditions, but most infections are caused by environmental organisms entering through an abrasion, a puncture wound, or a cut. If the infections are not treated promptly, the organisms can spread to deeper tissues and may get into the bloodstream. The infection can cause serious damage to affected body parts and may be life-threatening.

Acne

Acne is a particularly troublesome infection, which occurs primarily in teenagers. It is caused by *Propionibacterium acnes,* an organism present in subsurface epithelium and sebaceous glands. The increase in hormonal activity during adolescence stimulates the production of sebum from the sebaceous glands. The excessive amounts of sebum result in whiteheads and blackheads. The breakdown of sebum by *P. acnes* causes local inflammation and the eruption of **pimples.** Sometimes skin lesions occur with such frequency and in such large numbers that permanent scar tissue is formed.

Acne can be modified by frequent cleansing of the skin or by topical application of benzoyl peroxide and tetracyclines. Severe forms of acne may require intervention with isotretinoin, a drug that inhibits sebum formation temporarily. The drug, marketed under the trade name of Accutane, must not be used during pregnancy or in those anticipating pregnancy. Severe fetal abnormalities have been related to drug intake either during or immediately preceding pregnancy.

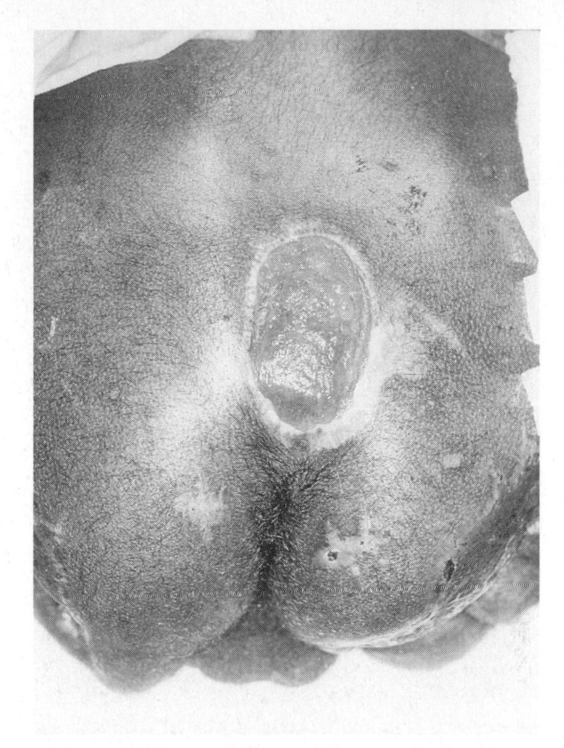

Figure 15–3 ◆ A decubitus occurring over the sacral region. This type of lesion is commonly observed in prolonged immobility.

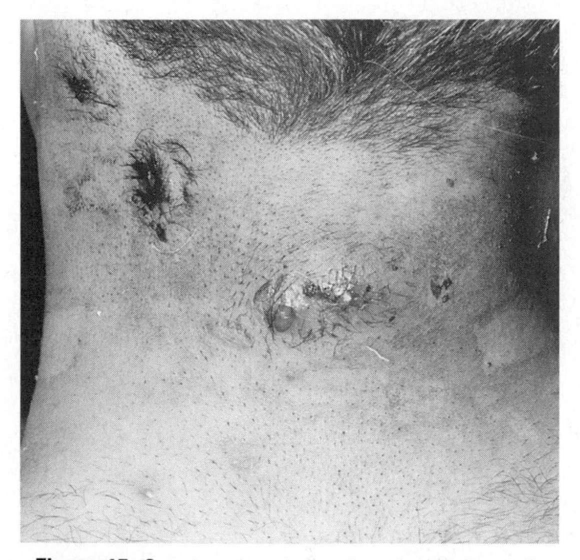

Figure 15–2 ◆ A carbuncle on the nape of the neck.

Staphylococcal Infections

Staphylococcal infections are among the most common bacterial infections of the skin. Most of us have experienced a pimple caused by the invasion of a hair follicle or a sebaceous gland with *Staphylococcus aureus.* Most pimples are no more than a nuisance, but other staphylococcal infections are more serious. If the infection extends into the subcutaneous tissue, a pus-containing lesion known as a boil appears on the surface of the skin. A boil or a **furuncle,** as it is also known, is often quite painful. Furthermore, it may spread and give rise to an even deeper seated abscess, or **carbuncle** (Fig. 15–2). If the flow of blood in capillaries is obstructed, an open lesion known as an **ulcer** is produced. Bedridden patients are at risk for developing lesions called bedsores, or **decubiti** (Fig. 15–3; Color Plate 32). Pressure points from long periods of immobility can be relieved by frequent turning and gentle massaging of irritated skin.

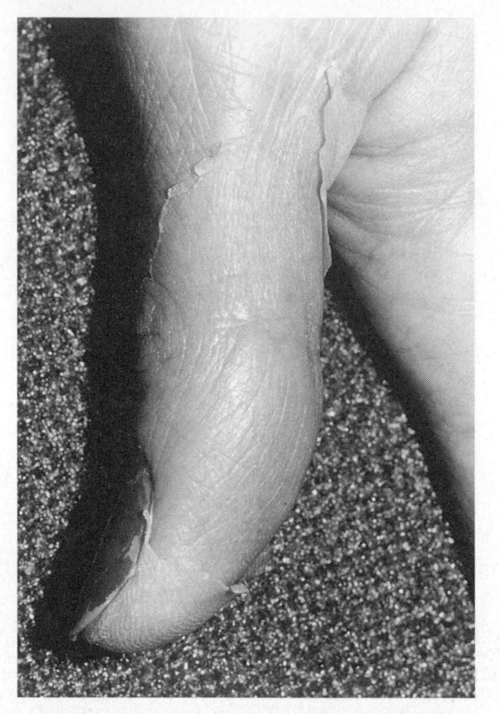

Figure 15–4 ◆ Desquamation on a thumb, occurring 12 days after onset of toxic shock syndrome.

Impetigo is a highly communicable staphylococcal infection occurring in infants and young children. Streptococcal organisms may also be present in impetigo. Rupture of the blisters or **vesicles,** induced by scratching, contributes to the rapid spread of the infection.

Another staphylococcal infection seen primarily in young infants is **scalded-skin syndrome.** The bright red color caused by the infection makes the skin appear as if it had been scalded with boiling water. The staphylococci spread rapidly and cause a scaling and loss of the outermost epidermal cells. The loss of skin is attributed to an exfoliative-toxin-producing strain of *S. aureus.* The toxin promotes the intraepidermal separation which precedes shedding of the epidermal cells.

Toxic shock syndrome (TSS) is a multisystem disease, but one of the features is a rash. Other symptoms of TSS include a fever, hypotension, vomiting, and diarrhea. A loss of epidermal cells occurs one or two weeks after onset of symptoms (Fig. 15–4). The disease was first described in children, but later appeared in women using superabsorbent tampons. Upon investigation, it was found that magnesium bound by those tampons promotes certain endogenous strains of *S. aureus* to produce the exotoxin responsible for multiple-organ dysfunction. The incubation periods for staphylococcal infections are usually four to 10 days.

Much of the success of *S. aureus* as a pathogen can be attributed to the variety of enzymes and toxins it produces. The ability of a staphylococcal organism to make coagulase separates *S. aureus* from other species belonging to the same genus. A component of the wall of *S. aureus* aids the organism in resisting phagocytosis. No doubt its survival capacity in the human host is related to both individual virulence factors and interactions among the various factors.

Gram stains of smears prepared from pus or blood agar reveal the presence of gram-positive cocci which usually occur in clusters (Fig. 15–5). Pigmentation of colonies is variable ranging from white to golden yellow. Some strains of *S. aureus* produce beta hemolysis; others are nonhemolytic. The major characteristic used to differentiate the pathogen from the normal skin resident, *S. epidermidis,* is the ability of *S. aureus* to clot rabbit plasma within four hours.

The primary purpose for using serological techniques is to confirm the diagnosis of a serious staphylococcal illness such as TSS. Strains of *S. aureus* producing toxic shock syndrome produce toxin-1 (TSST-1). A radioimmunoassay (RIA) procedure and an enzyme-linked immunoassay (ELISA) technique are sensitive methods for detecting the toxin. Illness caused by a TSST-1–producing strain can be confirmed by testing for toxin production by the organism isolated from the patient and showing the absence of antibodies to TSST-1.

Staphylococci other than *S. aureus* have been isolated from human infections, but their ability to cause serious disease is limited. *S. epidermidis*

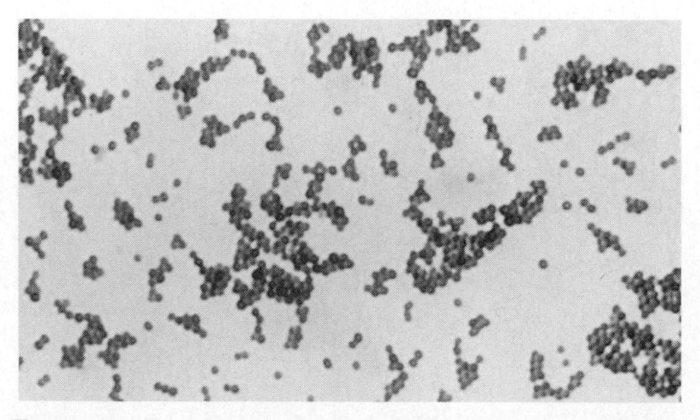

Figure 15–5 ◆ Gram-stained smear of *Staphylococcus aureus.* The cocci frequently occur in clusters.

may colonize on indwelling medical devices such as catheters and artificial valves. *S. saprophyticus* causes acute urinary tract infections in young women. It is second only to *Escherichia coli* as a cause of urinary tract infections. Both *S. epidermidis* and *S. saprophyticus* fail to cause rabbit plasma to clot.

Antimicrobial susceptibility testing is important for the selection of an appropriate drug in treatment of staphylococcal infections. Penicillin and methicillin were the drugs of choice for many years. The emergence of both penicillin- and methicillin-resistant strains of *S. aureus* has made it necessary to use other drugs for effective treatment. No longer can a universal regimen be recommended. Initial treatment must be guided by experiences of a particular care facility. Later choices of drugs can be individualized as a result of laboratory testing. The resistant strains of staphylococci may be susceptible to teicoplanin, cephalosporins, or vancomycin.

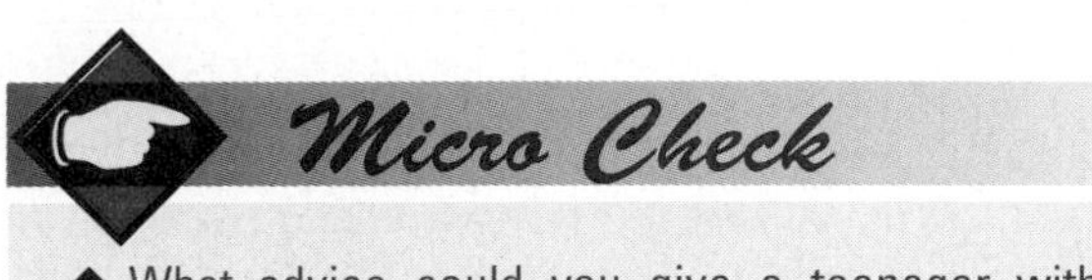

- What advice could you give a teenager with acne?
- Would you expect diet to modify the course of severe acne?
- What environmental conditions favor growth of *S. aureus* during menstruation?

FOCAL POINT

Can You Catch a Disease From a Toilet Seat?

Or a pay telephone, the handrails you touch on a bus, or any of the objects people share daily? The toilet seat question tends to drive people crazier than the others. The answer is that few diseases are transmitted through intact skin by objects, least of all toilet seats. The reason is that the human epidermis has an extremely able line of defense against harmful bacteria, fungi, viruses, and other would-be intruders.

Traditionally, skin has been thought of as just a passive envelope—a container for the most important parts of us, our birthday suit. But in the late 1970s, skin was discovered to play an active role in immunity.

For many years scientists have known that the skin is laced with Langerhans cells (LCs), named for the medical student who discovered them in 1868. But not until 1978 did studies show that these cells play a major protective role. They actually "catch" microorganisms and other antigens and present them to the T cells (a type of white blood cell), which mount an appropriate response. Besides microorganisms, allergens of many kinds are also handled by the Langerhans cells. In fact, LCs may play a larger role. There is some traffic apparently between the lymphatic system and the skin. This interaction may prove to be a kind of staging ground for many immune responses—the field where the immune cells mount their strategies for dealing with all kinds of infections. Chronic exposure to the sun reduces the efficiency of the Langerhans cells, causing them to tolerate antigens they would otherwise dispose of. Researchers are investigating the relationship between this phenomenon and skin cancer. In any case, a potential troublemaker is likely to find unbroken skin a tough terrain to penetrate.

As long as the skin of your thighs and buttocks is intact, you have almost no chance of catching a disease from a toilet seat. Sexually transmitted diseases—including AIDS—cannot be transmitted in this way, but only by direct sexual contact. One disease you might catch from an object (not a toilet seat) is the common cold, which you can pick up by touching something that has been handled by the person with the cold. Even then you would have to infect yourself by touching your nose, eyes, or the inside of your mouth.

Wellness Letter, University of California, Berkeley, March 1986.

Streptococcal Infections

Most infections of the skin caused by streptococci are secondary to a primary lesion caused by another organism. A variety of streptococci can be involved, but the organisms are usually classified on the basis of their hemolytic and serological characteristics only.

Streptococci can be classified as members of one of three groups on the basis of their ability to disrupt the red blood cells added to a basic medium, an activity known as **hemolysis. Alpha hemolysis** is characterized by the appearance of green zones surrounding streptococcal colonies. The green zones are caused by the partial lysis of red blood cells. **Beta hemolysis** is recognized by the clear zones surrounding colonies (Color Plate 33). The clear zones indicate that complete lysis of red blood cells has occurred. **Gamma streptococci** produce no detectable change around colonies because they lack the hemolysin also known as streptolysin S.

The streptococci can be divided further into serological groups based on the types of carbohydrates associated with their cell walls. The classification of at least 18 groups (A to R) was devised by the American microbiologist, Rebecca Lancefield. Human infections are caused by organisms belonging to most groups, but typically those pathogens belong to one of six groups (Table 15–2). Members of Lancefield group A are the most common causes of human infections.

The presence of streptococci and staphylococci in impetigo has already been described, but streptococci alone can cause an acute infection of the skin known as **erysipelas** (Fig. 15–6). The disease occurs with greater frequency in young children and in the elderly. The lesions of erysipelas may be small at first, but they spread rapidly when scratched. Entrance of streptococci into deeper tissues may cause a **cellulitis** accompanied by a fever and chills. The organisms may invade the bloodstream and even cause gangrene in diabetics or in patients with other vascular diseases.

Scarlet fever is a streptococcal infection of the respiratory tract with an accompanying rash. It has been described as a "strep throat" with a rash. The rash and accompanying "strawberry tongue" is caused by one of the erythrogenic toxins produced by the streptococci (Color Plate 34). Peeling of superficial epithelial cells of the skin may occur in convalescence. Some cases of toxic shock–like syndrome (TSLS) reportedly have been due to a toxin of a group A beta-hemolytic streptococci.

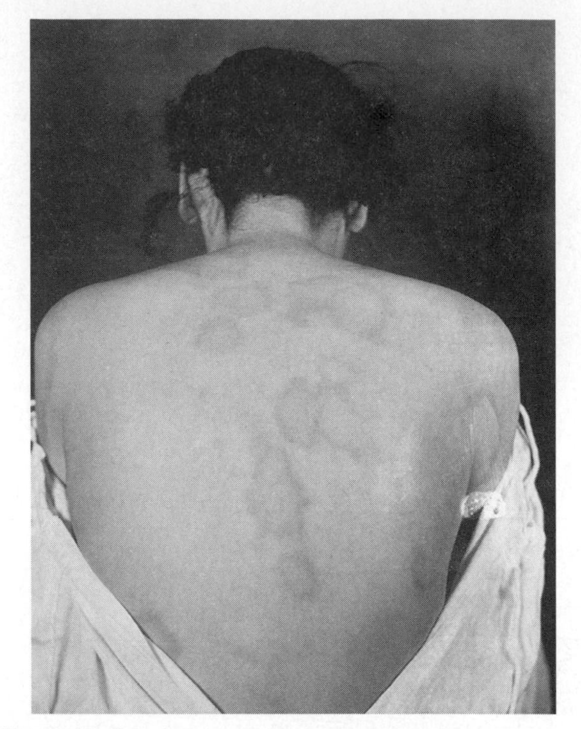

Figure 15–6 ◆ Lesions of erysipelas on the back of a patient showing dermal and subcutaneous inflammation.

Table 15–2
HEMOLYTIC REACTIONS AND PROTOTYPE SPECIES OF MAJOR LANCEFIELD GROUPS

GROUP	HEMOLYTIC REACTION	PROTOTYPE SPECIES
A	Beta	*Streptococcus pyogenes*
B	Alpha, beta, none	*S. agalactiae*
C	Alpha, beta	*S. equi*
D	Alpha, beta, none	*Enterococcus faecalis*
F	Beta	*S. anginosus*
G	Beta	Species undesignated

A highly virulent strain of *S. pyogenes* has been associated with severe, **necrotizing fasciitis.** The rapid destruction of tissue has caused journalists to call the organism a "flesh-eating" bacterium (Fig. 15–7). Destruction of tissue has been reported to occur at a rate of 2 inches per hour. The necrotizing toxin, which may be a streptococcal erythrogenic pyrogenic toxin (SPE), is responsible for 2000 to 3000 deaths every year in the United States. The incubation period for most streptococcal infections rarely exceeds three days. Reinfections are common because the immune response to streptococcal infections is minimal.

Gram stains of exudates reveal gram-positive cocci occurring singly, in pairs, and frequently in chains (Fig. 15–8). The colonies on blood agar are pinpoint, translucent, and convex. Most

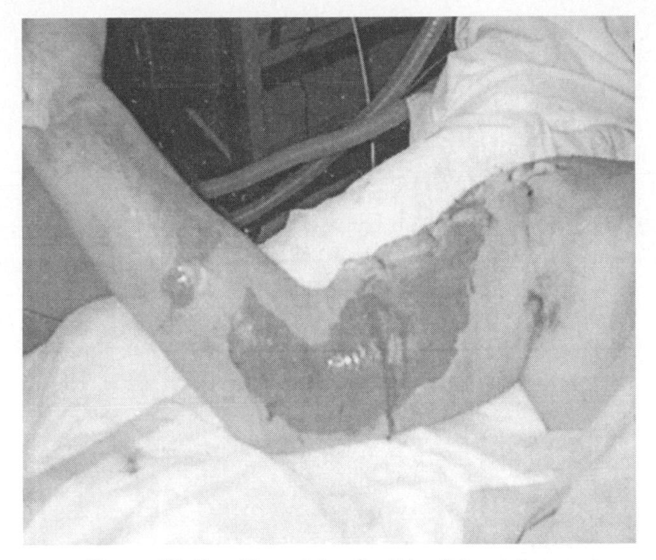

Figure 15–7 ◆ Necrotizing fasciitis of the right arm.

streptococci causing infections of the skin are beta-hemolytic.

The major Lancefield groups can be identified serologically by agglutination or coagglutination techniques. Antistreptolysin O (ASO) titers increase in acute infections caused by beta-hemolytic strains of streptococci. Tests for detection of other antibodies to streptococcal enzymes, such as hyaluronidase or deoxyribonuclease, are less frequently performed.

A group A specific antigen can be detected directly from throat swabs by an ELISA coagglutination or a DNA probe technique. Direct detection methods are useful for doctors' offices.

Penicillin is the drug of choice for most infections caused by group A streptococci. Some strains of group B streptococci are tolerant to penicillin, but susceptible to ampicillin or gentamicin. Streptococci belonging to groups C, F, or G are also generally susceptible to penicillin. Ampicillin, in combination with streptomycin, may be effective in infections caused by *Enterococcus* species, formerly classified as streptococci. High dosages and prolonged therapy may be required for deep-seated infections.

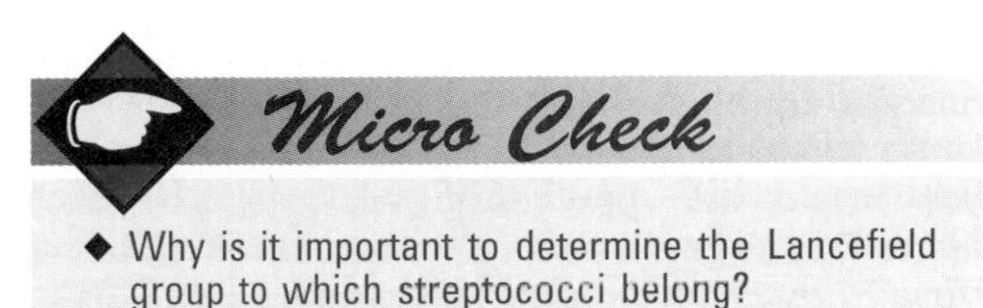

- Why is it important to determine the Lancefield group to which streptococci belong?
- What could be the cause of recurrent streptococcal infections?

Anthrax

Although anthrax is primarily a disease of cattle, goats, and sheep, it occurs in humans as cutaneous, pulmonary, or gastrointestinal disease. The most frequent form is a skin infection, which is associated with lesions ranging from small pustules to large abscesses (Fig. 15–9;

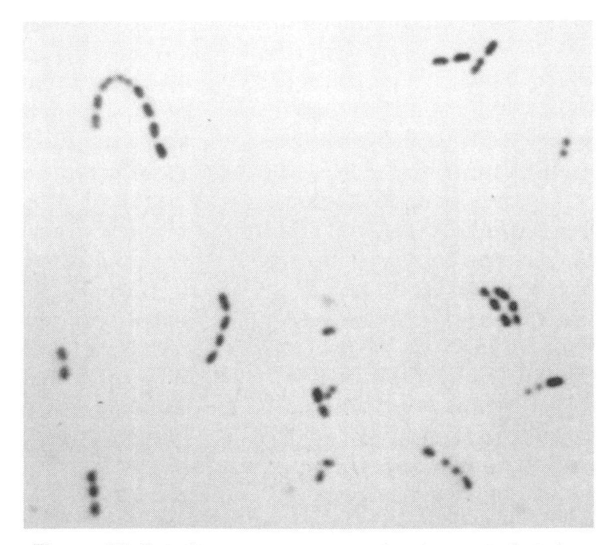

Figure 15–8 ◆ *Streptococcus pyogenes* showing typical chains.

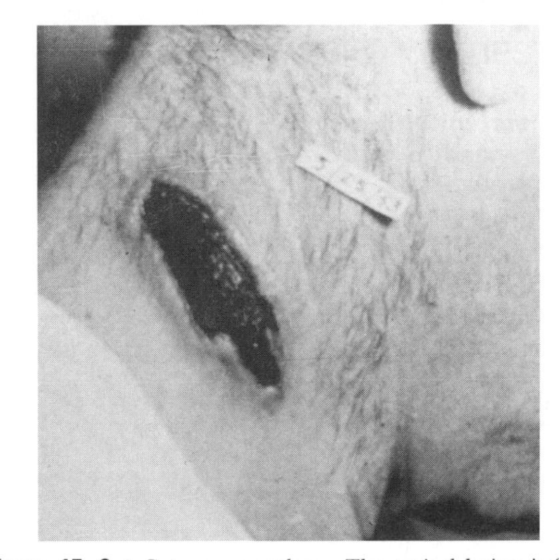

Figure 15–9 ◆ Cutaneous anthrax. The typical lesion is fully developed 7 to 10 days after contact with the causative organism.

Color Plate 35). A potent toxin promotes necrosis in surrounding areas. If prompt treatment is not initiated, systemic infection can follow. Fatality rates are as high as 20 percent.

The etiologic agent is *Bacillus anthracis*. Humans are exposed to the organism by handling animals or animal products. The spores can survive as many as 30 years in wool, yarn, hides, bristles, or soil. The disease is most prevalent in Asia, Africa, and a few countries of Europe.

Gram-stained smears of material from skin lesions reveal the presence of gram-positive bacilli appearing in long chains (Fig. 15–10). The spores can more frequently be seen on smears prepared from cultures. *B. anthracis* grows on ordinary culture media as irregular colonies with a curled internal morphology. The colonies tend to be tenacious. A battery of biochemical tests is necessary to distinguish it from the similar *B. cereus*. An indirect hemagglutination test for detection of antibodies is available at the Centers for Disease Control and Prevention in Atlanta, Georgia. Penicillin is the drug of choice to treat local lesions. It has little effect in a toxic septicemia.

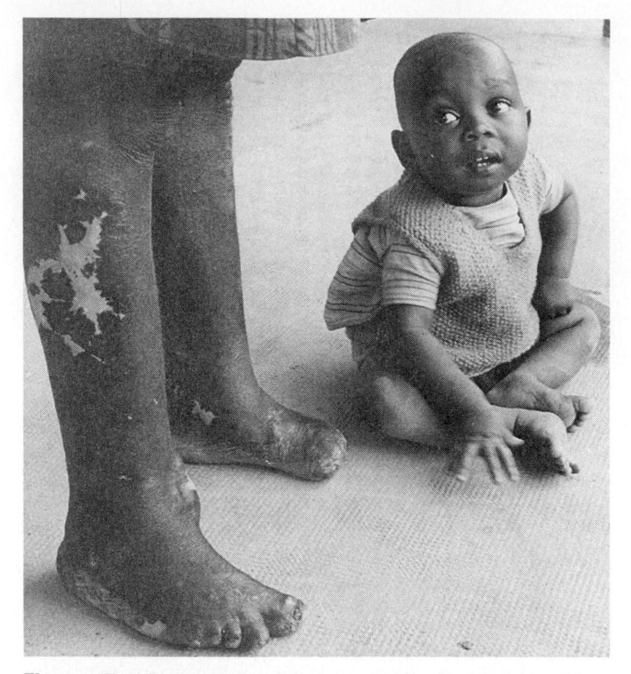

Figure 15–11 ◆ Lesions of leprosy on the feet and legs of an African mother standing beside her small boy.

Leprosy (Hansen's Disease)

Leprosy (Hansen's disease) was one of the most prevalent infectious diseases of ancient times. It still represents a major health problem in parts of Africa, Asia, the South Pacific, and some South American countries (Fig. 15–11). Leprosy, once feared as transmissible by even the slightest contact, is actually less communicable than most other infectious diseases. It is transmitted only upon close and prolonged contact with an infected individual. Cases of leprosy in the United States are largely confined to Hawaii, Louisiana, Florida, Texas, and California. Fewer than 100 new cases occur annually in the United States. The causative organism was demonstrated by Armauer Hansen to be the acid-fast bacillus *Mycobacterium leprae.*

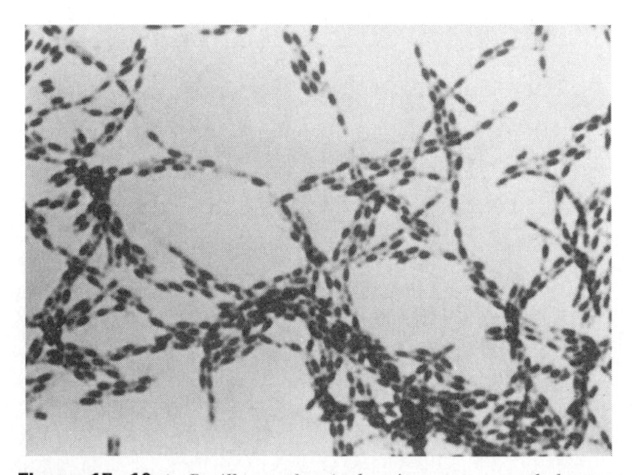

Figure 15–10 ◆ *Bacillus anthracis* showing spores and the typical arrangement of spores in chains.

The clinical entity known as leprosy or Hansen's disease has two major forms. The **lepromatous** form or progressive disease causes cutaneous lesions and frequently leads to disfigurement. Masses of granulomatous tissue, called **lepromas,** replace macules over time, and ulceration may occur. The **tuberculoid** form involves the peripheral nerves and causes impairment of sensory responses. Anesthesia is common, and severe atrophy of muscle, skin, and bones may occur in the extremities.

Hospitalization may be required in the lepromatous form of the disease. Although isolation is not essential, the services that can be provided by experts is often important for optimal health care.

Acid-fast *M. leprae* can be demonstrated on smears of skin or nasal scrapings of leprosy patients, but clinical evidence of disease is very important in establishing a diagnosis. An intradermal skin test using heat-treated lepromatous material knows as **lepromin** is sometimes useful in following the disease (Fig. 15–12). Unlike the closely related organism causing tuberculosis, Hansen's bacillus does not grow on artificial culture media.

The treatment of leprosy includes rehabilitation, education, and usually the antibacterial drug diaminodiphenolsulfone, which is continued for years. If immunity is impaired in patients, drugs must be taken over their entire lifetimes.

Gas Gangrene

Gas gangrene is an infectious disease that can be caused by a number of anaerobic bacilli belonging to the genus *Clostridium. C. perfringens,* an organism that produces large amounts of gas in devitalized tissue, has long been associated with the disease. Accumulation of gas interferes with the blood supply to affected areas, causing life-threatening disease. Soil clostridia gain entrance through a puncture wound, but infections can follow abdominal surgery. *C. perfringens* inhabits the intestines of about one-third of all healthy individuals. The incubation time is quite short, but usually ranges between one and three days.

A particularly potent exotoxin known as lecithinase is responsible for the necrosis of infected tissue (Color Plate 36). Extensive débridement of devitalized tissue may be necessary to allow a wound to be exposed to oxygen.

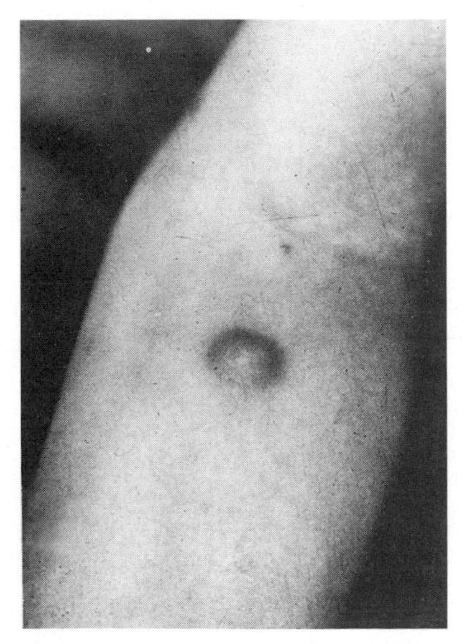

Figure 15–12 ◆ A positive lepromin reaction. A positive skin test is diagnostic for tuberculoid leprosy. A negative skin test is usually obtained with lepromatous leprosy.

Members of the genus *Clostridium* grow on anaerobic blood agar plates and in thioglycolate supplemented with hemin and vitamin K_1. Primary plating media must be incubated in anaerobic jars. GasPak jars are described in Chapter 5. *C. perfringens* produces double-zoned hemolysis on blood agar and only rarely shows spores on direct smears or those made from cultures. It produces large amounts of gas when grown in milk, a characteristic known as stormy fermentation.

Most strains of *C. perfringens* respond well to a combination of methicillin and an aminoglycoside, such as streptomycin. A procedure known as **hyperbaric oxygen therapy** has been used successfully in the treatment of gas gangrene. The patient inhales pure oxygen in a pressurized chamber. The increased oxygenation of tissues interferes with the growth of the anaerobe.

Pseudomonas Infections

The pseudomonads have become increasingly important as causes of infections following surgery and in patients with extensive burns. The most frequently implicated pathogen is *Pseudomonas aeruginosa,* but other gram-negative bacilli belonging to the same genus can invade damaged tissue. The organisms can be recovered from the gastrointestinal tracts of some healthy individuals. The pseudomonads multiply rapidly in liquid soaps, in weak disinfectants, and in containers of water in the hospital environment. The organisms grow particularly well in water of whirlpools in the absence of sufficient chemicals with germicidal activity. The time of incubation varies with the severity of burns, but infection is often evident within three to four days.

An elastase produced by *P. aeruginosa* inactivates complement and may contribute to the invasive properties of the organism. A cytotoxic exotoxin, which interferes with the action of some white blood cells, prevents a vigorous inflammatory response in the presence of the pathogen.

Certain species of pseudomonads produce blue-green, yellow-green red, or brown pigments. Nonpigmented strains do exist (Color Plate 37). The organisms are nonfermentative, and most species produce oxidase (Color Plate 38). The grapelike odor of colonies growing on primary plates is unmistakable, but is not a substitute for other tests.

Strains of *P. aeruginosa* are universally resistant to penicillin. A related drug, carbenicillin, or gentamicin is usually effective against most pseudomonads. The multiple-drug resistance demonstrated by some isolates makes it necessary to do antimicrobial susceptibility testing to select the drug of choice.

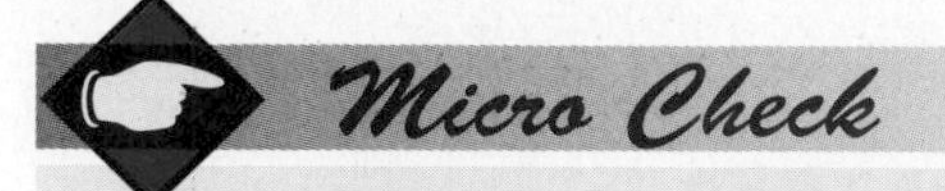

- Why are fresh flowers not an appropriate gift for a burn patient?
- Why can an infection caused by *P. aeruginosa* be life-threatening?

FOCAL POINT

Fish Fanciers' Finger

People who keep tropical fish, or clean fish tanks of those who do, can develop an infection known as "fish fanciers' finger," or tropical fish-tank granulomas. Although first described in 1962, the condition remains unknown among many tropical fish enthusiasts. Two surgeons in New South Wales, Drs. T.B. Hugh and M.J. Coleman, concerned about inappropriate antibiotic therapy or unnecessary surgical treatment of the granulomas, have coined the term "fish fanciers' finger" in the hope of bringing more attention to the malady.

In the majority of instances, the infection starts on a finger one to six weeks after a minor scratch or cut incurred while cleaning a fish tank. Small cystic swellings often occur at the site of trauma and distinct, often tender, nodules appear on the forearm along the line of the lymphatic vessels. The nodules resemble those of sporotrichosis. Disseminated disease is not known to occur in humans.

The culprit in "fish fanciers' finger" is *Mycobacterium marinum,* an acid-fast bacillus. Unlike *Mycobacterium tuberculosis,* the organism grows best at 30°C and is inhibited by higher temperatures. Daphnia, a water flea used in fish food, is a vector for the organism. No person-to-person transmission of "fish fanciers' finger" has been documented.

A diagnosis of "fish fanciers' finger" requires isolation of the organism from granulomas or demonstration of the acid-fast bacillus in biopsy specimens. Results of skin tests using antigens of *M. marinum* are not reliable because of cross-reactions occurring with other mycobacterial antigens. The disease is usually self-limiting, but can be resolved faster by treatment with trimethoprim-sulfamethoxazole. Surgical excision is not recommended. Protective gloves on the hands when cleaning fish tanks can help prevent cuts and limit exposure to the organism.

L.A. County Public Health Letter, April 1985.

FUNGAL INFECTIONS

The most important fungi that cause disease of the skin, hair, and nails are called **dermatophytes.** Some dermatophytes affect only humans, but others can also cause disease in animals. They usually do not invade the subcutaneous tissue. Soil is the natural reservoir for dermatophytes, but most are transmitted by direct contact with an infected individual or animal, or indirectly, by contact with a fomite.

The fungi that infect subcutaneous tissue gain entrance through an abrasion or puncture wound. Those fungi are inhabitants of the soil. The diseases they cause are more common in tropical countries than in temperate zones. Most cases occur in men, presumably from occupational exposure. The diseases caused by fungi are called **mycoses.**

Tineas

The superficial cutaneous infections caused by molds are called **tineas.** At one time they were thought to be caused by worms and were called ringworm. The lesions of the tineas often appear as pink circular lesions and gradually advance to form new borders. Scaling and peeling of the skin in affected areas are common. A universal feature of all tineas is the sometimes unrelenting

Table 15–3
CLASSIFICATION OF TINEAS ACCORDING TO SITE OF INFECTION

TYPE OF TINEA	SITE OF INFECTION
Barbae	Beard
Capitis	Scalp
Corporis	Any skin surface
Cruris	Groin, axillae, submammary, umbilical, perineal, or perianal areas
Manum	Hands
Pedis	Feet
Unguium	Nails

itching. Scratching may predispose individuals to secondary infections.

The many tineas are differentiated by the part of the body affected (Table 15–3). **Tinea pedis,** an infection on the feet, is better known as athlete's foot. The lesions typically occur between the toes (Fig. 15–13). **Tinea capitis** is an infection of the scalp which frequently causes hair loss. **Tinea cruris,** also known as jock itch, affects the groin. The incubation period for most tineas is seven to 10 days.

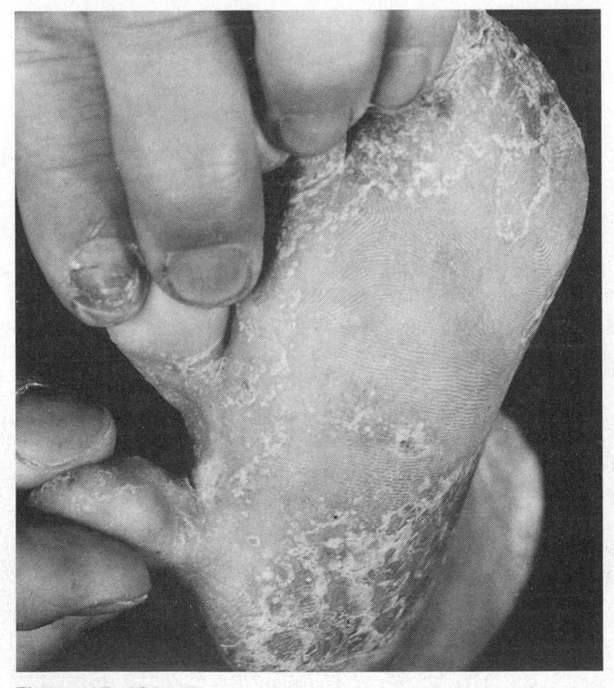

Figure 15–13 ◆ Tinea pedis showing typical lesions between the toes.

Most of the fungi causing tineas belong to three genera: *Trichophyton, Microsporum,* and *Epidermophyton*. *Trichophyton* species can cause infections of the hair, skin, or nails. Those dermatophytes belonging to the genus *Microsporum* affect the skin or hair. Isolates of *Epidermophyton* are associated with infections of the skin or nails.

None of the fungi causing superficial cutaneous infections produce toxins. Their ability to produce disease is due to their remarkable invasive potential and persistence in tissue.

Hyphae of typical fungi can be observed on smears of epidermal scales or nail scrapings placed in 10 percent potassium hydroxide (Fig. 15–14). A modified periodic acid–Schiff (PAS) stain is recommended for all negative KOH preparations. Sabouraud's agar with the antibiotics chloramphenicol and cycloheximide is an excellent medium for isolation of dermatophytes. Chloramphenicol inhibits contaminating bacteria, and cycloheximide discourages the growth of any nonpathogenic fungi that might be present. The dermatophytes grow best at 30°C and should be kept at least four weeks. Identification of a specific fungus is made on the basis of macroscopic and microscopic morphology (Fig. 15–15; Color Plates 39 and 40). The numbers and morphology of macroconidia or microconidia are helpful in assigning an organism to a particular genus (Fig. 15–16).

The only effective oral drug for treating the tineas is griseofulvin. Griseofulvin is deposited in cells of the skin, hair, and nails and prevents new fungal growth. Topical agents, such as fungicidal ointments, miconazole and clotrimazole, may be of some value.

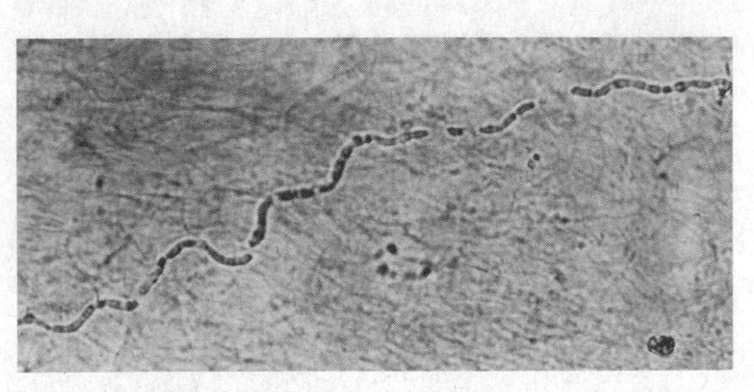

Figure 15–14 ◆ Potassium hydroxide mount of a dermatophyte showing hyphae.

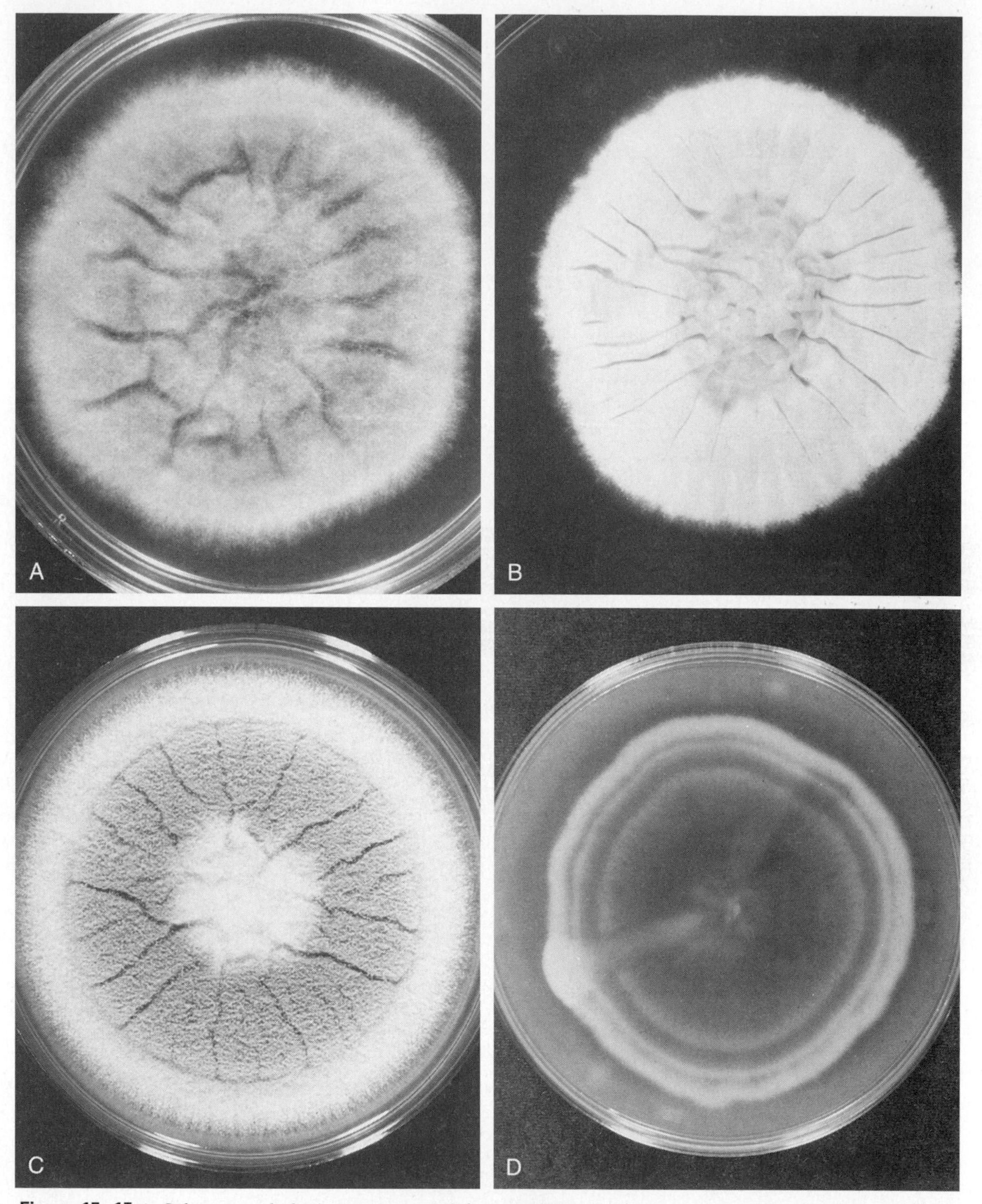

Figure 15–15 ◆ Colony morphologic appearance of dermatophytes. *A,* Cottony colony with a floccose mycelium. *B,* Velvety colony with a dense, low mycelium. *C,* Granular colony with a rough surface and an abundance of spores. *D,* Glabrous or smooth colony with a wavy appearance and no mycelium.

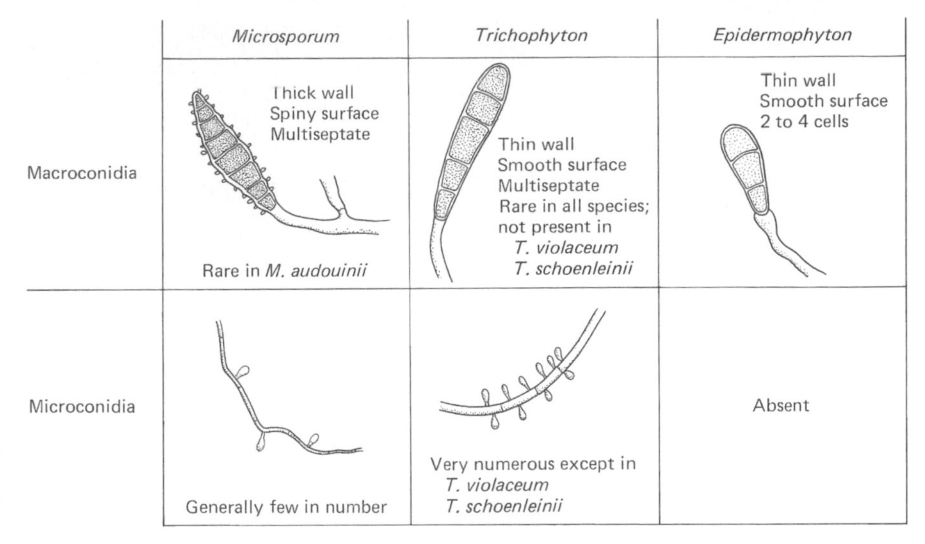

Figure 15–16 ◆ Genus differentiation of dermatophytes by numbers and morphology of macroconidia and microconidia.

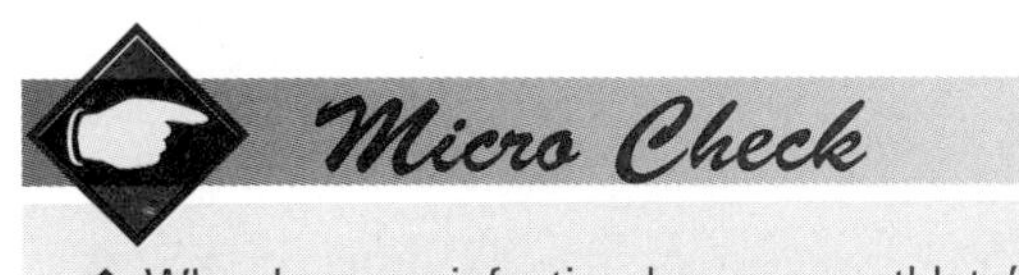

- Why does an infection known as athlete's foot tend to persist in some individuals despite treatment?
- Why should household pets be inspected frequently for evidence of fungal infections?

Cutaneous Candidiasis

The skin or nails are sometimes sites of a yeast infection known as candidiasis. It often occurs in patients compromised by underlying disease, an immune deficiency, or long-term antimicrobial therapy. Candidiasis of the oral cavity in the newborn is more commonly called **thrush.** If the tissue surrounding the nail is affected, the infection is called onychomycosis (Fig. 15–17). *Candida albicans* is the most frequent causal agent, but other species of *Candida* are being isolated with increasing frequency. Most infections are of endogenous origin because the organisms may be found in the upper respiratory tract, oral cavity, gastrointestinal tract, or vagina of healthy individuals. The time of incubation for cutaneous candidiasis is difficult to determine, but most cases of thrush occur three to five days after delivery.

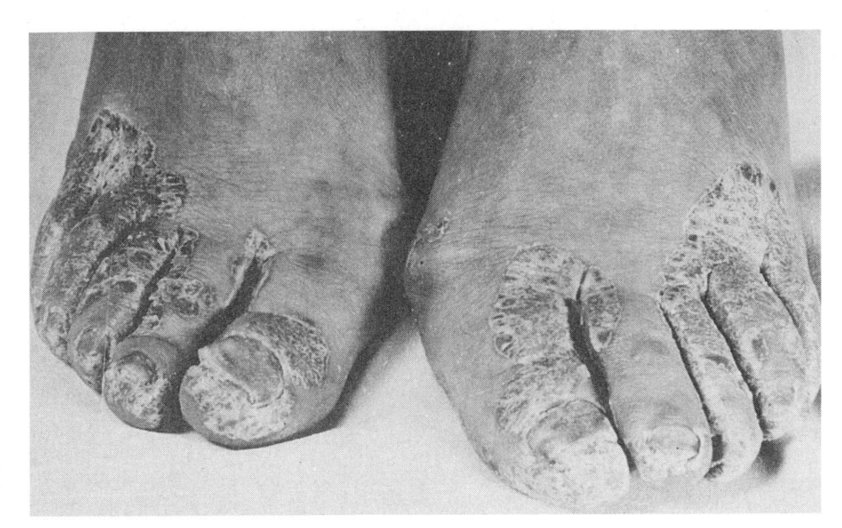

Figure 15–17 ◆ Chronic onychia caused by *Candida albicans* showing marked distortion of nails.

Candida species grow well on Sabauroud's agar, but a distinctive feature of *C. albicans* and *C. stellatoidea* is their ability to produce chlamydoconidia on corn meal agar. *C. albicans* can be differentiated from other species by its ability to form short germinating hyphae, known as germ tubes, within a few hours in sterile bovine or sheep serum (Fig. 15–18). Only a rare isolate of *C. stellatoides* will develop germ tubes. A differential primary culture medium, known as CHROMagar, provides presumptive identification of *C. albicans* and other species. Candidiasis is treated with drugs, such as nystatin and topical amphotericin B preparations.

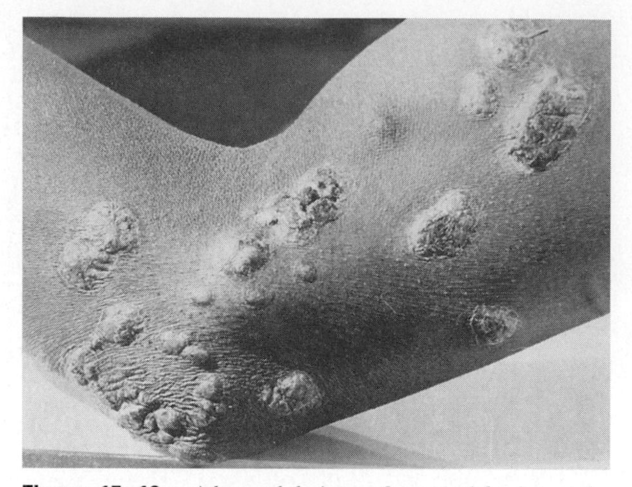

Figure 15–19 ◆ Advanced lesions of sporotrichosis on the arm and elbow.

Subcutaneous Mycoses

The subcutaneous mycoses include sporotrichosis, the chromomycoses, and certain mycetomas. Spread of the causative fungi from a subcutaneous lesion can cause severe damage to deeper tissue.

SPOROTRICHOSIS

Sporotrichosis is a chronic disease that often occurs in farmers and gardeners. A nodule or a small ulcerated lesion follows inoculation of the spores of *Sporothrix schenckii,* a dimorphic fungus found in the soil. Lymph vessels promote the spread of the organism, producing more nodules (Fig. 15–19). The disease is rarely fatal, but the infection may persist for many years.

Localized sporotrichosis responds well to a saturated solution of potassium iodide given orally in drops. The administration of amphotericin B may be required to resolve the disseminated form of the disease.

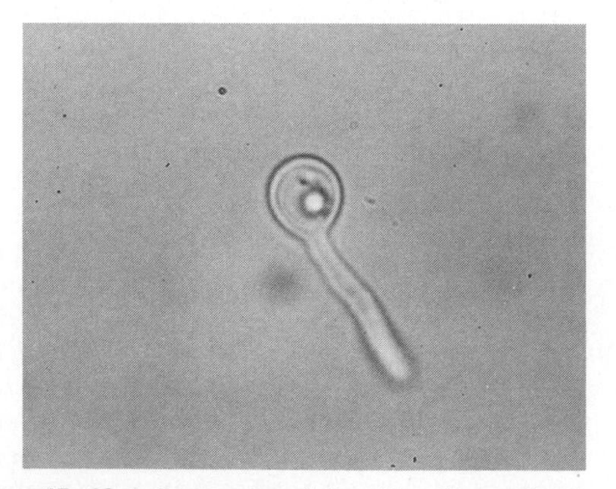

Figure 15–18 ◆ Germ tube of *Candida albicans* after incubation of the yeast cell in human serum.

CHROMOMYCOSES

The chromomycoses are localized chronic infections of the skin and subcutaneous tissue. The smallest injury, even one that is virtually invisible, is sufficient for spores of the causal fungi to enter epidermal tissue. The feet and the legs are the most frequently affected sites. The original lesion is a nodule, but subsequent crusting or ulceration is a common occurrence. Lesions may not occur for several months after injury. Scratching or lymphatic spread is responsible for additional lesions.

The chromomycoses may be caused by a variety of dimorphic dark-colored fungi, but members of the genera *Exophiala, Fonsecaea,* and *Phialophora* are common isolates. The tissue form is a sclerotic cell. The organisms grow on Sabouraud's agar producing dark-colored hyphae and distinctive conidia.

Surgical excision of nodules may be required for cosmetic reasons. Heat is of some value in early lesions, but later infiltration of lesions with amphotericin B at weekly intervals is recommended. Antibacterial drugs may be indicated to control secondary infections.

MYCETOMAS

The mycetomas begin as subcutaneous nodules after an injury, but in time they extend even deeper. As the infection progresses, the infected

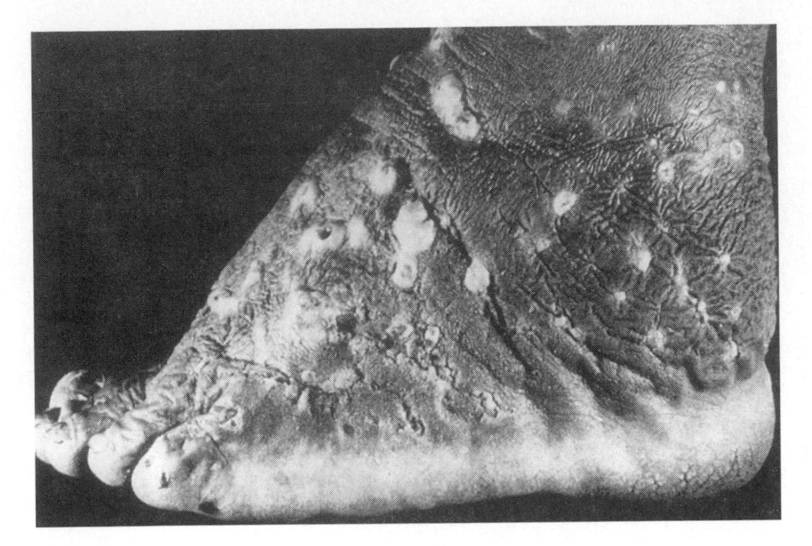

Figure 15–20 ◆ Mycetoma of a foot showing multiple nodules, draining sinuses, and swelling.

areas become swollen and develop sinus tracts. Granules containing the infectious agents are discharged when pus drains from the lesions. The hands and feet are the most frequently involved areas (Fig. 15–20). Madura foot is an old name for mycetoma of the foot. At least 20 different fungi, and some filamentous bacteria, can cause mycetomas.

The wide range of microorganisms causing mycetomas makes it impossible to predict successful treatment with any one drug. Some of the fungi isolated from mycetomas are susceptible to amphotericin B. The mycetomas caused by filamentous bacteria typically respond to treatment with streptomycin or to a combination of sulfamethoxazole and trimethoprim. Severe infections may require amputation of the affected hand or foot.

VIRAL INFECTIONS

Some viruses enter the epidermis through an abrasion or a puncture wound. More of them are introduced by the bite of an arthropod vector. In a few instances, viruses gain entrance from the bite of an animal or by a needle used for an injection, blood transfusion, or acupuncture. Still others spread by blood from another site of infection to cause skin lesions. The viruses of measles, rubella, and chickenpox enter the respiratory tract, but travel by the bloodstream to the epidermal cells of the skin to produce lesions.

Measles

Measles is an acute, highly communicable disease of the respiratory tract caused by a paramyxovirus. The respiratory symptoms are accompanied by a generalized rash, which appears about two weeks after exposure to the virus and usually lasts four to seven days (Fig. 15–21). Measles is generally a self-limiting disease, but it may predispose some individuals to secondary bacterial infections.

A diagnosis of measles can usually be made clinically, but the virus grows well in human and monkey kidney cell lines and agglutinates red blood cells. Several serological tests, including complement fixation, neutralization, hemagglutination inhibition, and ELISA, can be used to demonstrate rising titers of antibodies. There is no specific treatment for measles, but supportive care is important.

The use of measles vaccine has reduced the incidence of measles in the United States, but outbreaks have occurred in both previously vaccinated and in unvaccinated populations. Revaccination is recommended for persons vaccinated before 1980 or those individuals vaccinated at 12 to 14 months of age. Furthermore, a two-dose vaccination schedule has been adopted. The first dose is administered at the earlier age of nine months, and the second dose is given when a child enters school. It is hoped that implementation of those procedures will eliminate measles as a public health problem within the next decade.

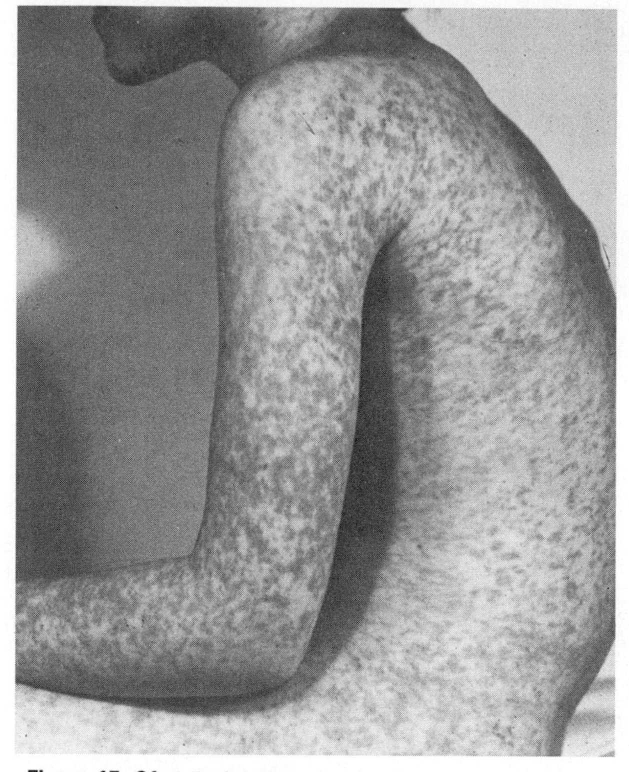

Figure 15–21 ◆ Rash of measles showing extent of lesions at peak of skin involvement.

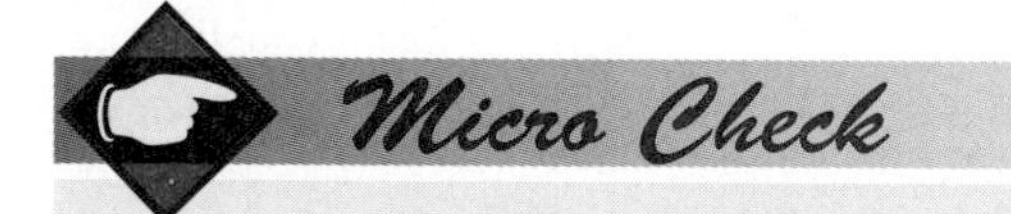

- Why has the recommended age of measles vaccinations been changed?
- What is the advantage of a two-dose vaccination schedule over a single injection of a vaccine?

Rubella

Rubella, once called German or three-day measles, is a mild, febrile, respiratory disease caused by a togavirus. A rash, resembling that of measles or scarlet fever, may or may not be associated with the disease. If rubella is acquired during pregnancy in a unprotected individual, it can produce a group of defects, known as **congenital rubella syndrome,** in the developing fetus. The defects include heart disease, mental retardation, deafness, and total or partial blindness (Fig. 15–22). The severity of the problems is related to the trimester of pregnancy in which the mother was exposed to the virus. The incubation period ranges from 14 to 23 days.

Several serological tests, such as complement-fixation, neutralization, hemagglutination inhibition, and ELISA, may be used to detect antibodies to the rubella virus. Paired serum samples must be used to indicate an active infection. Single serum samples may be used for immune status screening. The presence of antibodies indicates previous exposure to the virus and probable immunity.

Most infants receive rubella vaccine as a part of the combined measles, mumps, and rubella (MMR) immunizations. It is important that all women of child-bearing age have antibodies as a result of having had the disease or of vaccination with the attenuated virus. The availability of antibodies in fetal blood prevents congenital rubella syndrome if exposure to the virus occurs during pregnancy.

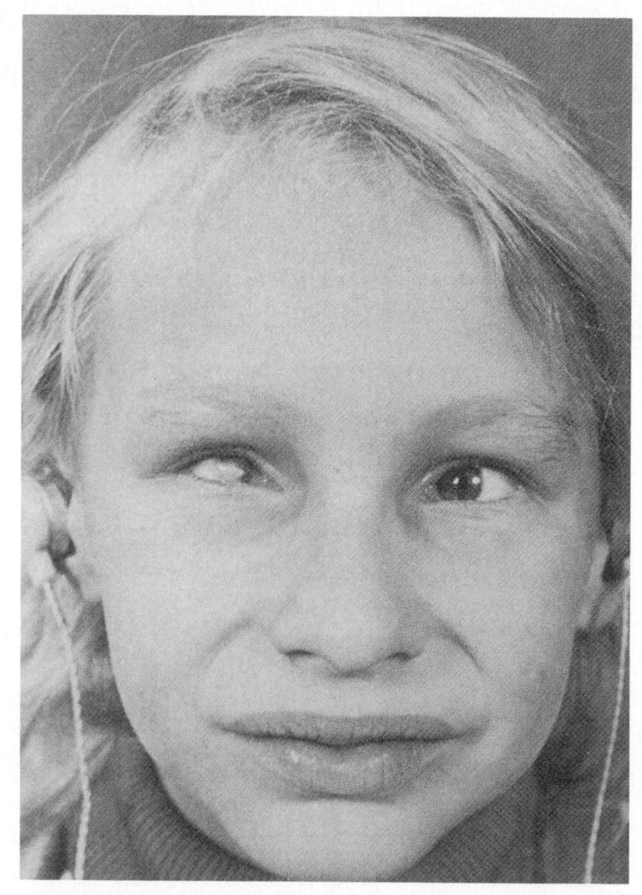

Figure 15–22 ◆ Congenital rubella syndrome showing severe bilateral deafness and severe bilateral visual defects.

Herpes Simplex Infections

Two herpes simplex viruses, HSV-1 and HSV-2, cause human skin disease. Initial infections with HSV-1 generally occur in children under two years of age. The infections may be asymptomatic or be characterized by vesicles on the lips or in the mouth. Lesions on the lips are known as **cold sores** or **fever blisters** (Fig. 15–23). HSV-2 is more commonly the cause of lesions on the genital organs. Genital herpes is discussed in greater detail in Chapter 18.

An important characteristic of all herpesviruses is their ability to remain latent in ganglia of sensory nerve fibers. Subsequent infections, therefore, may be of endogenous or exogenous origin. The mechanisms that are responsible for reactivation of HSV-1 and HSV-2 are not well understood. Ultraviolet light, x-ray, heat, cold, hormonal imbalance, and emotional disturbances may induce viral multiplication and recurrent disease. HSV inclusions are recognizable by light or fluorescent microscopy in material obtained from typical lesions. IgG antibodies to HSV-1 and HSV-2 can be detected by an ELISA technique, but cross reactivity occurs because antigens are shared by the two HSV types. Acyclovir is the drug of choice for the treatment of infections caused by either of the viruses. The drug has no effect on the ability of the virus to establish latency or on the frequency of recurrent infections.

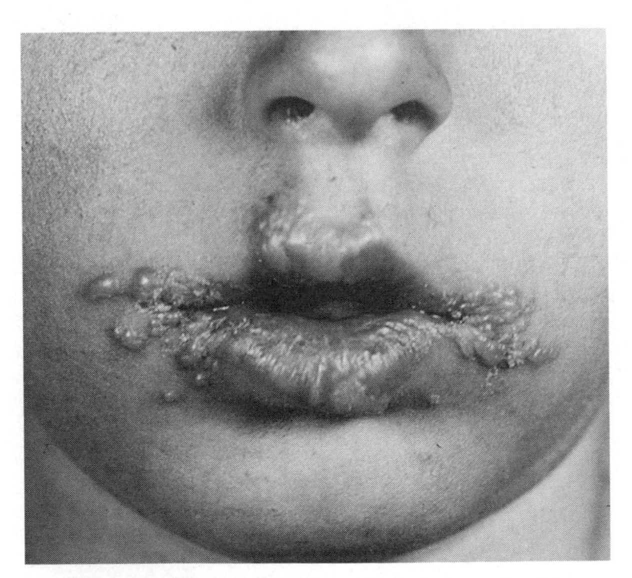

Figure 15–23 ◆ Multiple herpetic lesions on the lips.

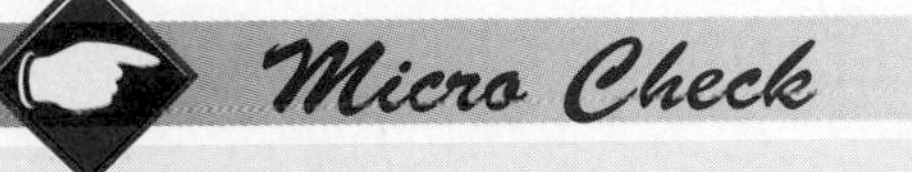

◆ Why are AIDS patients so susceptible to herpes simplex infections?
◆ Why are herpes simplex infections arrested, but never cured?

Varicella-Zoster Infections

Chickenpox (varicella) and shingles (zoster) are caused by a herpesvirus known as the varicella-zoster virus (VZV). The virus is transmitted by contact with secretions of the respiratory tract of an infected individual. Chickenpox is the primary disease and tends to be relatively mild in children. The disease is usually more severe when it affects adults. The incubation period is usually two to three weeks. Shingles is the recurrent form of the infection caused by activation of the latent virus.

The lesions of both diseases begin as a rash and proceed to vesicles. The lesions of chickenpox appear on the trunk, extremities, face, and scalp. The rash in shingles most often erupts along the distribution of a single sensory nerve (Fig. 15–24). The lesions occur most frequently on the trunk and are often quite painful.

Chickenpox and shingles are usually diagnosed clinically, but if laboratory confirmation is needed, an ELISA method for IgG antibodies may be performed.

Management of chickenpox in children includes relief from itching, as scratching may lead to secondary bacterial infections. Analgesics for pain may be necessary for patients with shingles. Acyclovir may be of some value in both diseases. The availability of a vaccine for chickenpox is expected to substantially reduce the numbers of cases of chickenpox and shingles.

Roseola Infantum

Roseola is a self-limiting disease of infants characterized by a high fever and a generalized body rash caused by herpesvirus 6. The high fevers, which last three to five days, often lead to febrile convulsions. As the fever subsides, the rash disappears. There is no form of immunization or antiviral drug available for treatment, but encouraging fluid intake may avoid the risk of

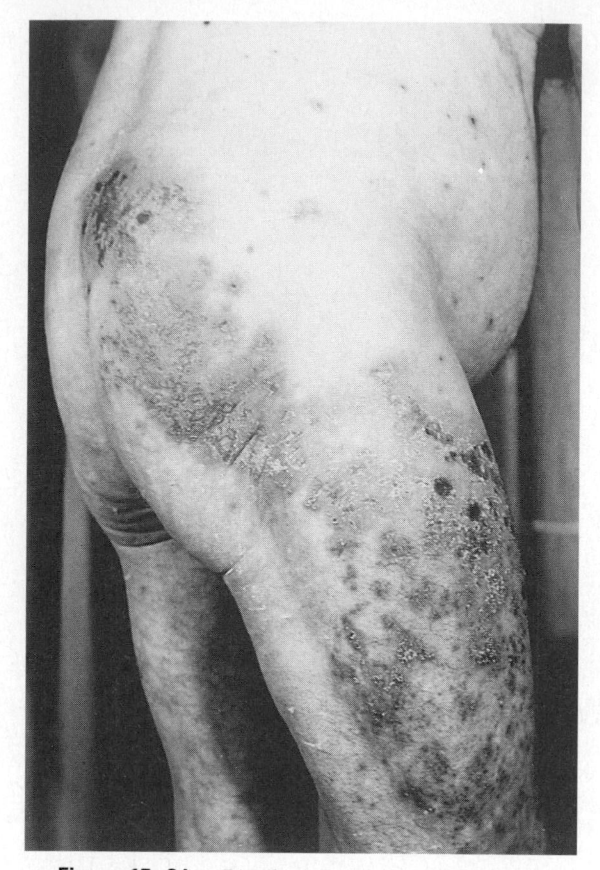

Figure 15–24 ◆ Distribution of lesions in shingles.

dehydration. Acetaminophen is recommended for reduction of fever.

Papovavirus Infections

The viruses that cause warts in humans are papillomaviruses belonging to the papovavirus group. Warts are benign tumors often found on the hands, fingers, or around the nailbeds (Fig. 15–25). The virus is transmitted by direct contact with an infected individual or a fomite. The incubation time is usually two to three months, but may extend up to 20 months. Sometimes autoinoculation is responsible for the spread of warts.

Warts tend to disappear with time, but their unsightliness has often led to remedies surrounded by mystery. Tom Sawyer's dead-cat-in-the-cemetery-at-midnight treatment for warts had no curative effect, but it stirred the imagination of the reader. Warts can be removed by excision or chemicals, such as trichloroacetic acid. Prompt treatment can prevent the spread of the largely nuisance lesions to other individuals. Genital warts (condylomata acuminata) have occurred with increasing frequency in recent years. The problems presented by the papillomaviruses causing genital disease are discussed in Chapter 18.

Erythema Infectiosum

Erythema infectiosum (EI), also known as fifth disease, is a mild, childhood illness caused by parvovirus B19. Most cases occur in children five to 14 years of age during winter or spring. The children typically develop a rash on the face, trunk, and extremities. Like the four major diseases of childhood, respiratory secretions appear to be involved in transmission of the disease. The infection can also be transmitted by fomites, by blood transfusions, and from mother to fetus. Joint disease, transient inhibition of blood cell

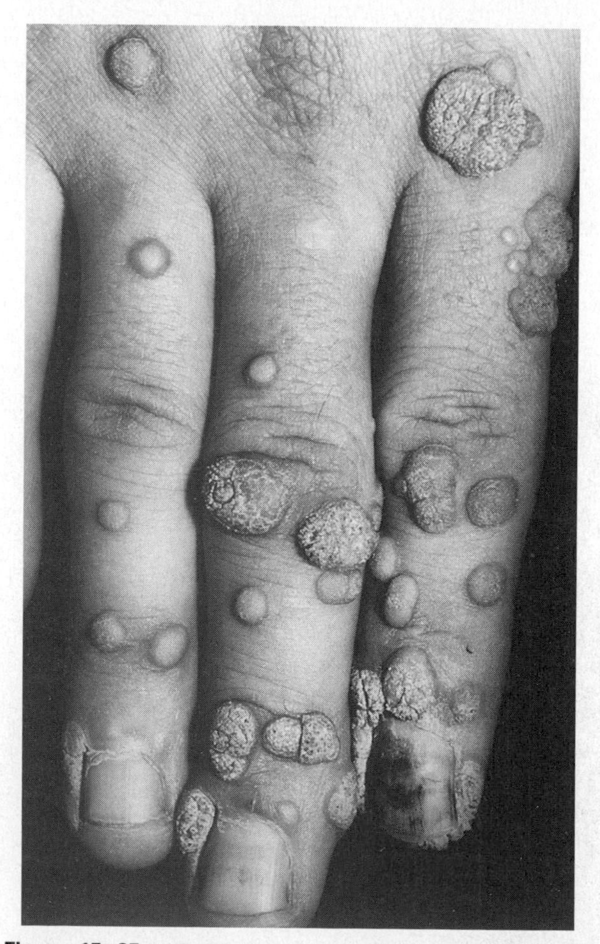

Figure 15–25 ◆ Common warts on the hand and fingers. Proliferation of epithelial cells infected with a papovavirus and progressive keratinization cause the solid growths.

production, and fetal death are complications of parvovirus B19 infection. No treatment or vaccine is currently available.

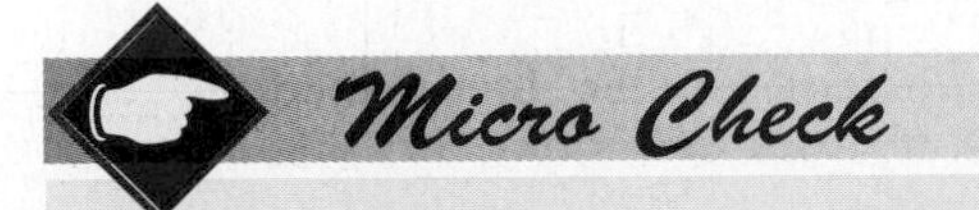

Micro Check

- How does the distribution of lesions differ in chickenpox and shingles?
- How does the rash of roseola differ from that of chickenpox?
- Why is erythema infectiosum referred to as fifth disease?

The major microorganisms causing diseases of the skin, hair, and nails are summarized in Table 15–4.

Understanding Microbiology

1. Why is it advisable to perform antimicrobial susceptibility studies to determine a drug of choice in staphylococcal infections?
2. How can you explain the occurrence of measles in some college populations in recent years?
3. What danger does rubella pose in pregnancy?
4. How does the mode of transmission for measles, rubella, and chickenpox vary from the mode of transmission of the tineas?
5. What is the importance of relieving itching in any infectious skin disease?

Table 15–4
SUMMARY OF MAJOR MICROORGANISMS CAUSING DISEASE OF SKIN, HAIR, AND NAILS

MICROORGANISM	DISEASE	TREATMENT
Bacteria		
Propionibacterium acnes	Acne	Tetracycline
Staphylococcus aureus	Furuncles, carbuncles, decubiti, impetigo, ulcers, scalded-skin syndrome, toxic shock syndrome	Methicillin Vancomycin
Group A streptococci	Erysipelas, impetigo, cellulitis, scarlet fever, toxic shock–like syndrome, necrotizing fasciitis	Penicillin
Bacillis anthracis	Anthrax	Penicillin
Mycobacterium leprae	Leprosy	Dapsone
Pseudomonas aeruginosa	Wound infections	Carbenicillin Gentamicin
Fungi		
Trichophyton sp.	Tinea of the hair, skin, and nails	Griseofulvin
Microsporum sp.	Tinea of the hair and skin	Griseofulvin
Epidermophyton sp.	Tinea of the skin and nails	Griseofulvin
Candida albicans	Cutaneous candidiasis	Nystatin
Sporothrix schenckii	Sporotrichosis	Potassium iodide
Exophiala sp.		
Fonsecaea sp.	Chromomycoses	Amphotericin B
Phialophora sp.		
Viruses		
Paramyxovirus	Measles	Supportive care
Togavirus	Rubella	Supportive care
Herpes simplex virus	Cold sores (fever blisters)	Acyclovir
Varicella-zoster virus	Chickenpox	
	Shingles	Acyclovir
Herpesvirus 6	Roseola infantum	Supportive care
Papovavirus	Warts	Trichloroacetic acid
Parvovirus	Erythema infectiosum (fifth disease)	Supportive care

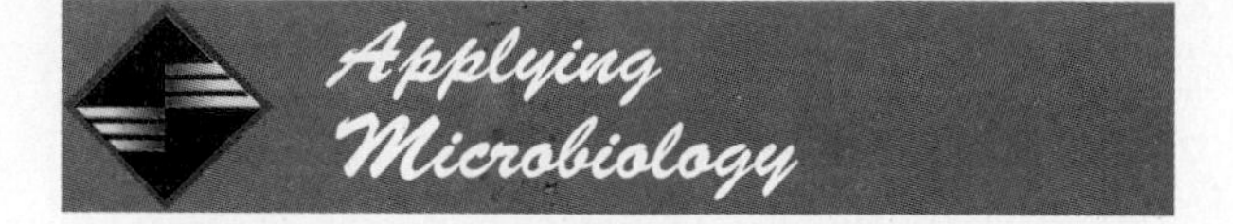

Read the following case study carefully and answer the questions: A three-year-old girl developed severe cellulitis of the left arm after an episode of chickenpox. The cellulitis and the pink-red color of the underlying lesions proceeded over the length of the arm in a single day. Some discoloration developed. The arm was extremely sensitive to touch and a foul-smelling exudate was present. A culture of the exudate revealed pinpoint translucent colonies with beta hemolysis on blood agar. A Gram stain of the colonies revealed gram-positive cocci in short chains. With intensive antibiotic treatment, the physician was able to save the arm.

6. The invasive disease and laboratory results are consistent with disease caused by which of the following:
   a. *Staphylococcus aureus*
   b. *Streptococcus pyogenes*
   c. *Pseudomonas aeruginosa*
   d. *Propionibacterium acnes*
   e. *Clostridium perfringens*
7. In the popular press the organisms causing this disease are known as the
   a. old man's friends
   b. stormy fermenters
   c. flesh-eating bacteria
   d. hot-pink cocci
   e. creeping champs
8. The toxin causing the tissue destruction is known as
   a. alpha toxin
   b. beta hemolysin
   c. coagulase
   d. SPE
   e. streptolysin
9. The most probable portal of entry was a
   a. needle prick
   b. chickenpox lesion
   c. contaminated food product
   d. rusty nail
   e. superficial burn
10. A procedure that may have prevented the risk of infection would be
    a. isolation of the child with chickenpox
    b. administration of a polyvalent vaccine
    c. gloving the child with chickenpox
    d. immunization with varicella vaccine at 12 to 18 months
    e. application of an anti-itch lotion

Chapter 16

Diseases of the Respiratory System

Chapter Outline

Learning Objectives

After you have read this chapter, you should be able to:

1. Differentiate between upper and lower respiratory tract infection.
2. Explain the conditions that permit microorganisms to cause infection of the respiratory tract.
3. List the genera of major bacteria that cause diseases of the respiratory tract.
4. Describe the role of immunization in protecting individuals from specific respiratory pathogens.
5. Compare the etiologic agents and the endemic nature of three deep mycoses.
6. Identify the major groups of viruses associated with respiratory disease.

The respiratory tract consists of the nose, pharynx, larynx, trachea, bronchi, and lungs (Fig. 16–1). With the aid of a number of accessory organs, including the diaphragm and intercostal muscles, the organs provide a passageway for the transportation and exchange of the gases of respiration. The procurement of oxygen and elimination of water and carbon dioxide are necessary to sustain life.

The exposure of the respiratory tract to microbial contaminants in the atmosphere is unavoidable. Microorganisms of varying sizes become airborne as solid or liquid particles known as aerosols. The particle size and moisture content

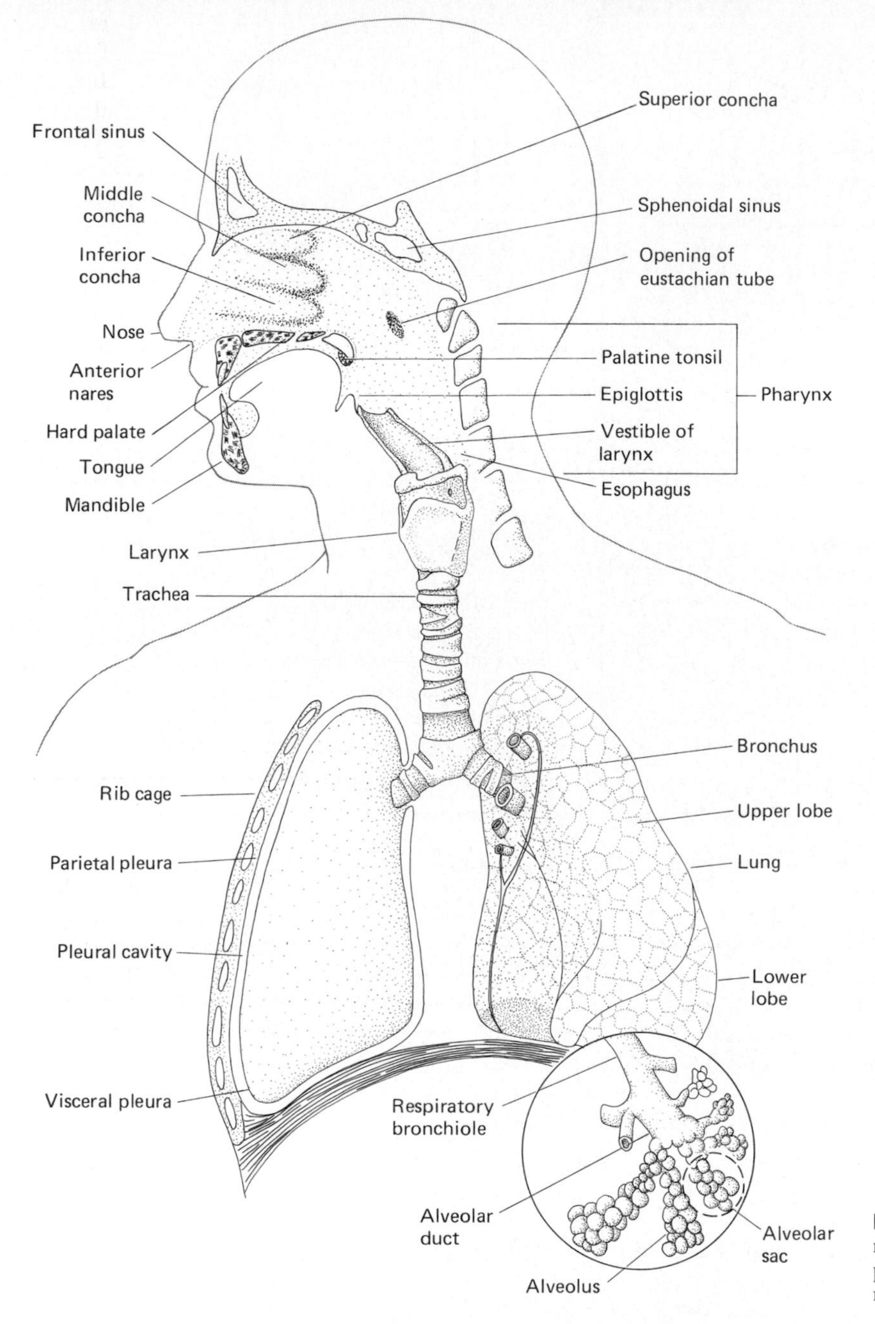

Figure 16–1 ◆ The upper and lower respiratory tract, pleura, and diaphragm. Insert shows alveoli at the terminal end of a bronchiole.

influence the deposition of aerosols following inhalation. Most particles larger than 6 μm in diameter are trapped in the nose. Of those under 6 μm, hygroscopic particles—that is, those with the capacity to absorb moisture readily—are deposited with greater frequency than nonhygroscopic particles of the same size (Table 16–1). The continuity of the mucous membrane lining of the respiratory tract provides the means for infectious aerosols to spread throughout the air passageways and even into the auditory tubes or paranasal sinuses.

Respiratory infections are known to be seasonal, but controlled experiments with human

Table 16–1
DEPOSITION OF SMALL HYGROSCOPIC PARTICLES (UNDER 6 μM DIAMETER)

ANATOMICAL SITE	PERCENTAGE OF DEPOSITION
Nose	36
Pharynx, secondary bronchi	1
Tertiary bronchi, bronchioles	25
Alveolar ducts	21
Total retained	83

Source: Adapted from Knight V: Viral and Mycoplasmal Infections of the Respiratory Tract. Philadelphia, Lea & Febiger, 1973.

subjects fail to support a common view that cold and damp weather increases susceptibility to pathogens. It is more likely that dampness and lower amounts of illumination favor preservation of aerosols. One might expect the crowded subways of big cities to be reservoirs of infectious agents, but they are surprisingly free of living airborne microorganisms. It is probable that the electric discharges of trains generate aerial disinfectants, such as ozone and oxides of nitrogen.

To some extent, the microorganisms of the nasopharynx reflect the microbial population of the skin. The variation in numbers of total flora is probably great in any one individual at different times.

Infections of the respiratory tract are classified as upper respiratory infections (URI) if the nose, paranasal sinuses, middle ear, pharynx, or tonsils are involved. The nose, pharynx, and tonsils are the most frequently affected sites. Infection of the airway can be specified as rhinitis, sinusitis, or pharyngitis, but more often the term URI is used because multiple sites frequently are involved. Lower respiratory infections involve the trachea, bronchi, alveolar spaces, or supporting interstitial tissue of the lungs. In infections of the lower respiratory tract, it is more common to differentiate the specific anatomical site of the infection.

FOCAL POINT

A Role for Anaerobes in Upper Respiratory Tract Infections

Although anaerobic organisms of the upper respiratory tract are seldom directly implicated in acute infections of the upper respiratory tract, they can be isolated regularly in cases of chronic infections of the middle ear, sinuses, and tonsils. The anaerobic gram-negative *Prevotella melaningogenicus* and *P. oralis* often establish synergistic relationships with aerobic normal flora. These organisms produce capsules and synthesize beta-lactamase, an enzyme that destroys penicillin. This often explains the failure of penicillin to resolve infections caused by more prominent aerobic pathogens, such as group A beta-hemolytic streptococci. The streptococci can even hide in the core of tonsils, where they can be protected by beta-lactamase producers and re-emerge to cause infection. The beta-lactamase-producing flora may develop rapidly following initiation of penicillin treatment. The synergy existing between aerobic and anaerobic organisms in mixed infections accentuates the need for aerobic and anaerobic cultures in materials from acute or chronic infections. If anaerobes are isolated, testing for beta-lactamase production can be recommended for isolates of both *Staphylococcus aureus* and anaerobic species. The early detection of synergism of this nature could help prevent treatment failures and recurrent infections. Clindamycin and lincomycin have been shown to be effective against mixed infections of the upper respiratory tract.

Current Hospital Topics—Upjohn, 1986.

BACTERIAL INFECTIONS

Both *Staphylococcus aureus* and *S. epidermidis* can be recovered with frequency from nasopharyngeal cultures. *S. aureus* is most often a transient resident, although it has been estimated that from 2 to 25 percent of some groups are carriers of the pathogen. Carrier rates for group A beta-hemolytic streptococci are high among children of school age. Other streptococci and gram-positive bacilli are outnumbered only by staphylococci.

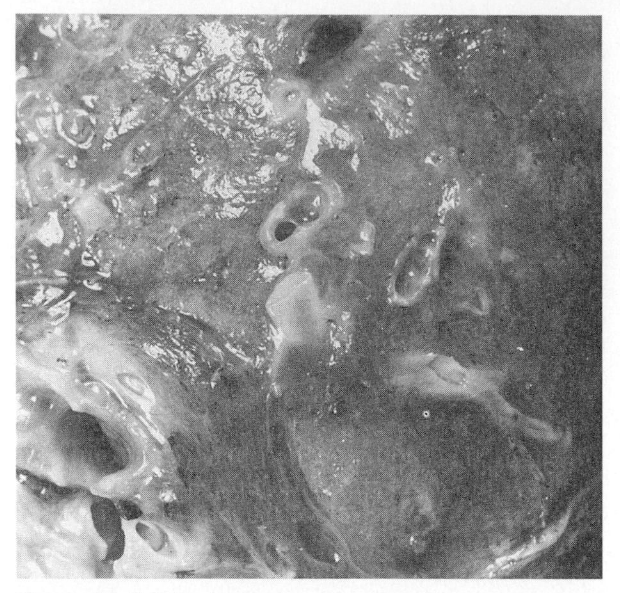

Figure 16–2 ◆ Typical lesions of a lung in staphylococcal pneumonia.

Gram-negative cocci belonging to the genera *Moraxella* and *Neisseria* are often abundant in both children and adults; the pathogens *Haemophilus influenzae* and *Streptococcus pneumoniae* frequently inhabit the nasopharynx of adults. Gram-negative bacilli are present irregularly in healthy individuals, but alteration in defense mechanisms allows the colonization of the nasopharynx by a variety of gram-negative bacilli.

The bacteria causing disease of the respiratory tract are derived from indigenous flora of the oropharynx or nasal cavities or from aerosols in coughs or sneezes of carriers or infected persons. Bacteria are small enough to gain access to alveoli, but actions of ciliated columnar epithelial cells and alveolar macrophages prevent their implantation and colonization in healthy individuals. However, inhalation of large numbers of bacteria or an immunosuppressed state provides favorable conditions for proliferation and possible invasion.

Staphylococcal Pneumonia

Staphylococci rarely cause disease of the respiratory tract in the healthy adult, but are common opportunists in the host compromised by surgical intervention, burns, or antimicrobial therapy. Staphylococcal pneumonia does not generally occur in the absence of a predisposing viral infection except in children under the age of two years. Infants become colonized with staphylococci shortly after birth. *Staphylococcus aureus* is the most frequent source, but coagulase-negative strains of staphylococci have also been implicated.

The staphylococci may be of endogenous or exogenous origin. The hospital environment is often a significant reservoir for multiresistant strains of *S. aureus*. The origin of the exogenous bacteria can be a health care worker who is a carrier or an infected patient. The time of incubation is difficult to ascertain because disease may not occur for several months after colonization. The inflammatory reaction in staphylococcal pneumonia may be absent, or edema and abscess formation may be so severe as to cause death within a few hours (Fig. 16–2).

Gram stains of sputum in staphylococcal pneumonia show numerous polymorphonuclear leukocytes (PMNs) and gram-positive cocci. Pure cultures of *S. aureus* are frequently grown on blood agar inoculated with sputum of patients with staphylococcal pneumonia (Fig. 16–3). Strains of the organism cause plasma to coagulate at 37°C within four hours. The ability to clot plasma is the accepted criterion used to separate the pathogenic *S. aureus* from other staphylococci.

Although at one time penicillin, and later methicillin, were the drugs of choice in treating staphylococcal pneumonia, an increasing number of strains are now resistant to those drugs. If a staphylococcus is resistant to both penicillin and methicillin, vancomycin is often effective.

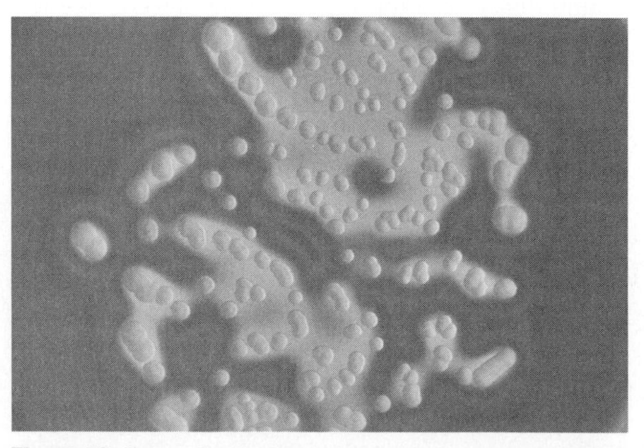

Figure 16–3 ◆ Colonies of a beta-hemolytic strain of *Staphylococcus aureus* growing on blood agar.

Streptococcal Infections

So-called "strep throat," caused by group A beta-hemolytic streptococci (GABHS), is one of the most common infectious diseases. Streptococci belonging to serological groups other than group A are rarely isolated from patients with pharyngitis or tonsillitis. The streptococci usually are spread by aerosols from a cough or a sneeze of an infected individual or a carrier. Food has been incriminated as a cause of outbreaks of streptococcal pharyngitis. It is likely that many cases go unreported, but food must be considered as a vehicle of transmission when the attack rate is high and when there is a clustering of cases. Special culinary treats served at picnics or outdoor receptions also make nutrient-rich sources of food for our unseen enemies, especially staphylococci and streptococci. A sore throat is present usually one to three days after exposure to streptococci. The disease can occur as a localized infection or as a part of disseminated streptococcal infection on membranes of the upper or lower respiratory tract. Less than 1 percent of streptococcal pneumonias are caused by *S. pyogenes.* Most usually, the posterior pharyngeal mucous membranes and tonsils are involved, but organisms can invade the middle ear, sinuses, bloodstream, joints, or heart. Increases in streptococcal bacteremia have been largely associated with the M-1 serotype.

FOCAL POINT

Jim Henson—An Avoidable Death

Jim Henson, the creator of the "muppets," was known throughout his life for the valuable ideas he taught children and young parents, but he learned one lesson in life too late. Jim Henson died in an emergency room of a New York City hospital in 1990 of a bacterial pneumonia. The microbe that ended his life was a particularly virulent strain of group A beta-hemolytic *Streptococcus.*

Henson's illness began with the flu, but developed into a secondary infection that quickly overwhelmed his whole body. The bacteria invaded his bloodstream and caused heart and kidney failure. The very talented originator of Kermit the Frog and pals experienced a fever of over 101°F, chills, and difficulty in breathing, and coughed up blood—all signs and symptoms of a serious respiratory infection.

The real reason for Henson's not seeking medical intervention sooner is not known, but it is known that he did not have a doctor and had a reputation for not wanting to inconvenience others. Only 1 percent of all pneumonias are caused by a group A beta-hemolytic *Streptococcus.* Only a fifth of those are fatal. The organism is almost always susceptible to penicillin. If he had not sought medical intervention too late, one can only speculate on the advice Kermit would have given young children and their parents in his inimitable style.

The Johns Hopkins Medical Letter, Health After 50, August 1990.

Scarlet fever is a disease of the upper respiratory system caused by an erythrogenic toxin-producing strain of group A beta-hemolytic streptococci. The distinguishing characteristic of the disease is a fine rash appearing on the chest, neck, groin, and thighs. Typically, a desquamation of skin from the fingers, toes, palms of hands, and soles of feet occurs during convalescence.

Streptococcus pneumoniae probably causes few cases of acute bacterial pharyngitis, but is a primary cause of pneumonia (Fig. 16–4). It is transmitted by aerosols or by articles freshly soiled with respiratory secretions. The time of incubation is variable. Sometimes a single lobe is involved; other times all the lobes of one lung or one lobe of both lungs are infected. There are 83 documented capsular types of *S. pneumoniae,* but only 23 cause serious disease. Pneumococcal disease is a problem in closed populations, such as military recruits, and in the elderly. It has been estimated that the fatality rate for pneumococcal pneumonia approximates 5 to 10 percent.

Gram stains of smears from throat swabs or sputum in streptococcal infections reveal gram-positive cocci in pairs or in short chains (Color Plate 41). The hemolytic reaction of streptococci is of prime importance for identification of strep-

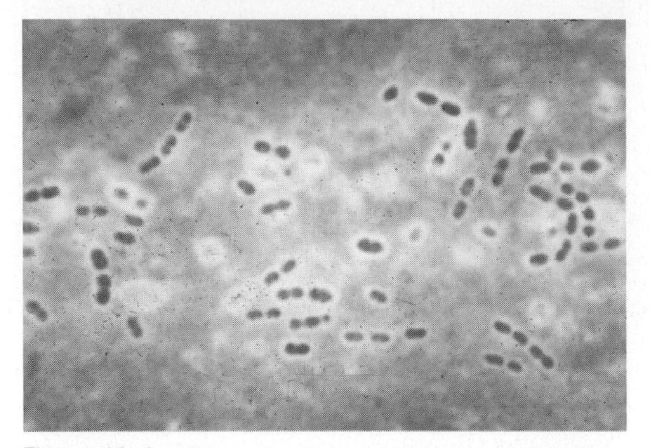

Figure 16–4 ◆ Encapsulated *Streptococcus pneumoniae* shown occurring in pairs. Capsules are produced by virulent strains of the organism.

tococci. Group A streptococci produce beta hemolysis. *S. pneumoniae* is associated with alpha hemolysis. Hemolytic characteristics of other Lancefield groups may be variable.

If an isolate is beta-hemolytic, it can be typed serologically with group A, B, C, D, F, and G antisera. *S. pneumoniae* can be differentiated from other alpha-hemolytic streptococci by its susceptibility to optochin (ethylhydrocupreine hydrochloride) (Fig. 16–5). A battery of biochemical tests can be used to confirm the presence of *S. pneumoniae* or other alpha-hemolytic streptococci. It is common practice, however, to identify other hemolytic streptococci by Lancefield group rather than attempt a species identification.

Unlike staphylococci, group A beta-hemolytic streptococci are usually susceptible to penicillin: Prompt treatment is necessary to prevent possible complications, including rheumatic fever, acute glomerulonephritis, or Sydenham's chorea, which are discussed in Chapter 14. Until recently, most pneumococcal isolates have been susceptible to penicillin, but antibiotic susceptibility tests should be performed because multiple-drug resistance does occur. A vaccine consisting of capsular material for 23 types of *S. pneumoniae* is available. It is recommended for people over 65 and for individuals with underlying disease, which makes them particularly vulnerable to the pneumococcus.

Klebsiella Pneumonia

Klebsiella pneumoniae, or Friedlander's bacillus, has long been recognized as a cause of pneumonia in males over 40 years of age and in chronic alcoholics of both sexes, but other species of *Klebsiella* may cause opportunistic infections of both the lower and upper respiratory tracts. The opportunists cause degenerative changes in the nasal and pharyngeal mucosa. *Klebsiella* species are transmitted by aerosols from an infected individual or may be endogenous in individuals receiving antibiotics or immunosuppressive agents. The time of incubation depends on the severity of impairment of host defenses. Of the klebsiellas, *K. pneumoniae* of capsular types 1 and 2 cause the most serious lung disease.

Bacilli belonging to the genus *Klebsiella* resemble the gram-negative enteric organism *Enterobacter aerogenes,* but they have large amounts of capsular material, are nonmotile, and have a mucoid appearance on the surface of the agar (Fig. 16–6; Color Plate 42). *Klebsiella* species are not fastidious in their growth requirements. They are easily isolated on MacConkey's agar and eosin methylene blue (EMB) agar. The klebsiellas can be identified by a series of biochemical tests in tubed media or by commercially available systems.

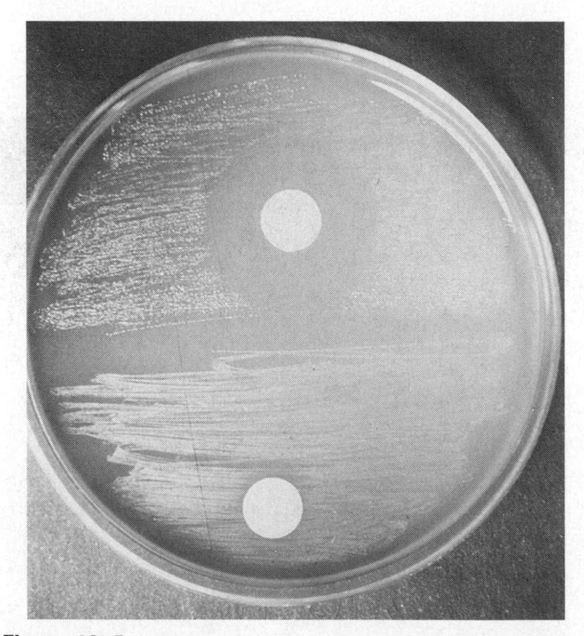

Figure 16–5 ◆ Differentiation of *Streptococcus pneumoniae* and alpha-hemolytic streptococci on a blood agar plate. The upper half of the plate demonstrates susceptibility of *S. pneumoniae* to optochin. The lower half of the plate demonstrates resistance of other alpha-hemolytic streptococci to optochin.

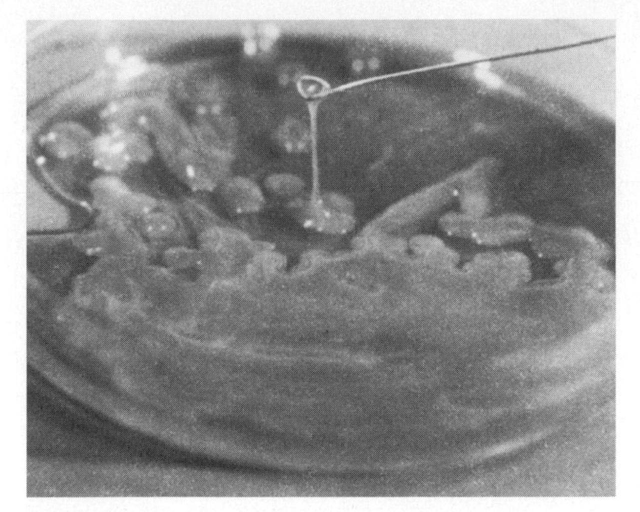

Figure 16–6 ◆ Mucoid growth of *Klebsiella pneumoniae* on Endo agar.

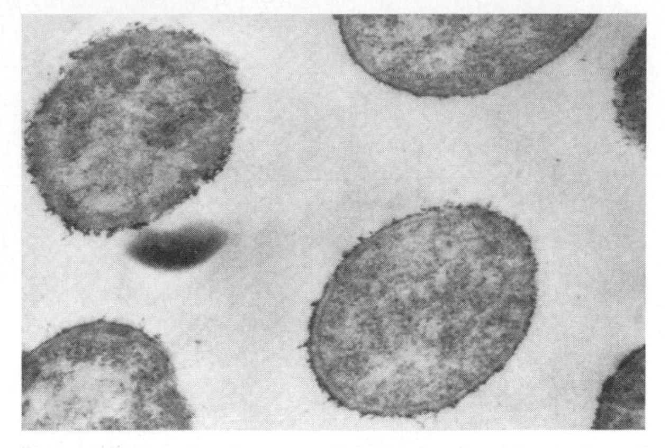

Figure 16–7 ◆ An electron micrograph of a thin section of *Haemophilus influenzae* showing encapsulated cells. The darkened area surrounding the coccobacilli consists of capsular material.

Haemophilus Infections

Haemophilus influenzae is a common cause of acute bronchiolitis in infants and young children and of chronic bronchitis in adults (Fig. 16–7). The species name *influenzae* has no etiologic significance today, but the organism was once believed to be the cause of the 1918–1919 pandemic of influenza. In 1933 the influenza virus A was unequivocally shown to be the cause of epidemic influenza. The bacterial pathogen had assumed the role of a secondary invader. Today pneumonia caused by *H. influenzae* accounts for almost all bacterial pneumonias not caused by *S. pneumoniae* or *Klebsiella* species. The primary means of transmission is by aerosols from an infected individual. *H. influenzae* and *S. pneumoniae* are sometimes isolated from the same individual. *H. influenzae* type b (Hib) is the primary serological type promoting infections in children. Meningitis is a common complication in young children with fever, lethargy, and vomiting occurring as little as two to four days after exposure.

H. influenzae is one of the smallest of the gram-negative bacilli. Some strains are highly pleomorphic and occur as coccobacilli and as long filaments. *H. influenzae* requires two growth factors: an X factor or hemoglobin component and a V factor which has been identified as the coenzyme, nicotinamide dinucleotide (NAD). Although both substances are present in blood agar, the V factor tends to be sequestered in the red blood cells. Best results are obtained when the red blood cells are lysed by heating blood agar to make chocolate agar, and inoculated plates are incubated in 5 to 10 percent CO_2. Requirement for X and V factors can be demonstrated by subculturing onto blood-free nutrient agar and applying strips containing V factor alone and strips containing both X and V factors (Color Plate 43).

H. influenzae produces a phenomenon called **satellitism** on blood agar inoculated with *S. aureus* (Color Plate 44). The colonies of *H. influenzae* are observable only in areas surrounding colonies of *S. aureus,* which supplies V factor to the fastidious *Haemophilus* organisms (Fig. 16–8). Most strains of *H. influenzae* are oxidase-positive

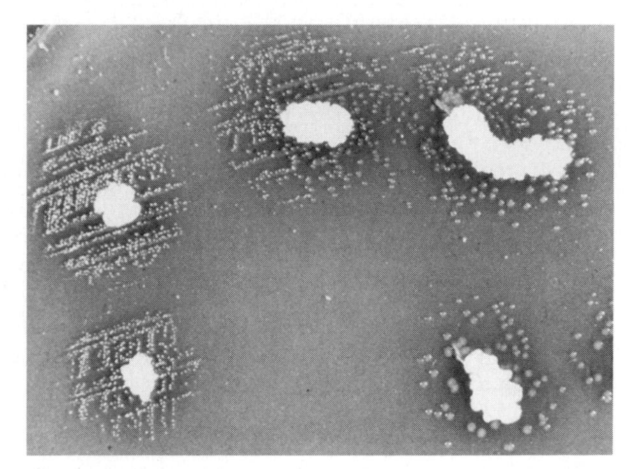

Figure 16–8 ◆ Satellism demonstrated by *Haemophilus influenzae* surrounding colonies of staphylococci on blood agar.

and catalase-positive, and will ferment glucose. Serological tests are applicable only for encapsulated strains.

Performance of antibiotic susceptibility testing is necessary to determine the drug of choice because many strains of *H. influenzae* demonstrate multiple resistance. Rifampin is used for prophylaxis now in children exposed to Hib in households or day care centers. Four doses of a polysaccharide protein conjugate vaccine are recommended for children at two, four, six, and 15 months of age.

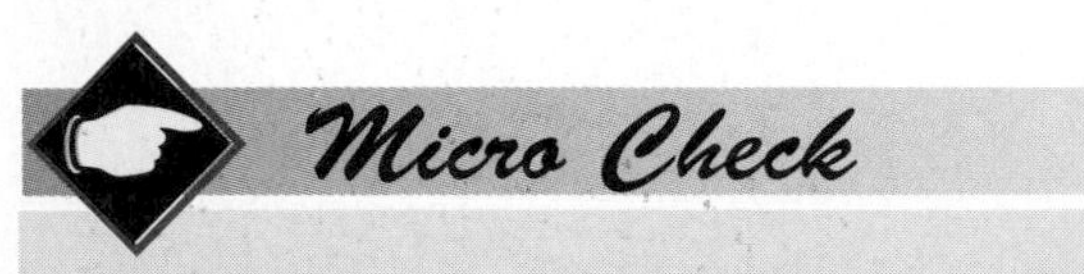

- What parts of the respiratory tract are involved in a lower respiratory infection?
- What is the source for organisms causing staphylococcal pneumonia in hospitalized patients?
- How can infections with *Haemophilus influenzae* type b (Hib) be prevented?

Whooping Cough (Pertussis)

Several *Bordetella* species have been incriminated in cases of acute bronchiolitis in both young children and adults, but the primary pathogen of the genus is *B. pertussis,* which causes whooping cough, or pertussis. The incidence of pertussis has increased in the United States since 1977, but reasons for the resurgence are unclear. There has been no decrease in vaccination coverage or significant reductions in protection afforded by vaccination. The bacteria causing whooping cough are spread by direct contact with laryngeal or bronchial discharges. The incubation period is seven to 21 days.

Whooping cough is characterized by three distinct phases. During the **catarrhal** phase, which lasts approximately two weeks, the cough is usually nonproductive and nocturnal, a rhinorrhea and low-grade fever persist, and a leukemoid reaction (an increase in leukocytes, predominantly lymphocytes) is often present. The **paroxysmal** phase, which lasts two to four weeks, is associated with paroxysms of coughing. Unlike the cough of the catarrhal phase, the paroxysmal spasms enable the patient to bring up thick mucus. Episodes of continuous coughing are often followed by a rapid inhalation of air before the glottis is fully open. The inrushing air causes a characteristic sound known as a *whoop.* The vigorous coughing is severely debilitating and may cause vomiting, and even brain hemorrhage. During the **convalescent** phase, which lasts another two weeks or longer, the cough subsides.

The specimen of choice for the isolation of *B. pertussis* is the nasopharyngeal swab. Rayon and cotton swabs should be avoided, however, because the fatty acids they contain are toxic to *B. pertussis.* Specimens collected on calcium alginate or Dacron swabs are the most satisfactory. If the swab is taken during the catarrhal stage, it is estimated that there is a 95 percent chance for recovery of the organism. The organism is very sensitive and swabs should be streaked immediately on Regan-Lowe agar, Jones-Kendrick charcoal agar, or freshly made Bordet-Gengou agar (Color Plate 45). Cultures must be incubated in a humidified atmosphere for at least 10 days. Gram stains of colonies from Bordet-Gengou agar reveal small gram-negative bacilli. Some pleomorphism may be observed, particularly in old cultures, where filamentous forms may actually predominate. The organism is hemolytic, but somewhat inert biochemically. Slide agglutination tests, using specific antiserum, can be helpful in confirming a diagnosis. A direct fluorescent antibody assay (DFA) can be used to demonstrate *B. pertussis* on smears of exudate as an alternative to culturing the organism (Color Plate 46). Complement-fixation and agglutination tests on paired sera may show rising titers of antibodies if sampling for the second specimen is done late in convalescence.

The use of antibiotics to affect the course of the disease is controversial, but erythromycin may limit spread of the infection. The cellular pertussis vaccine is combined with diphtheria and tetanus toxoids (DTP) for simultaneous immunization during infancy at two, four, and six months of age. Acellular pertussis vaccines combined with tetanus and diphtheria toxoids (DTaP) are used for the fourth and fifth vaccinations in children 15 months through six years. DtaP contains both the formaldehyde-treated pertussis toxin (PT) and filamentous hemagglutinin (FH). The side effects, including local reactions, fever, and persistent crying, occur less frequently after administration of DtaP than with the inactivated whole-cell DTP preparation, which was used for many years. Tetanus-diphtheria vaccines (Td) are recommended for adult use.

Diphtheria

The most important pathogen belonging to the genus *Corynebacterium* is an exotoxin-producing strain of *C. diphtheriae.* Only strains of *C. diphtheriae* lysogenized by a specific bacteriophage elaborate the potent toxin. It can cause disease of any part of the upper respiratory tract, but is most often the etiologic agent of a type of severe pharyngitis known as diphtheria. *C. diphtheriae* can be a part of the resident population of the upper respiratory tract in some individuals and causes no harm. It is transmitted to susceptible individuals by aerosols from carriers or infected persons. Colonization of the organisms in the pharynx and subsequent release of the exotoxin produce a localized inflammatory response usually within two to five days. The disseminated toxin causes a fever, difficulty in swallowing, and swelling of the lymph nodes. A tenacious pseudomembrane, consisting of white blood cells, red blood cells, fibrin, mucus, and dead tissue cells, may cause respiratory obstruction. A tracheotomy is sometimes necessary to restore breathing. If the toxin gets into the bloodstream, the pharyngitis is often complicated by heart, kidney, or nerve dysfunction.

Direct smears made from nasopharyngeal swabs are of little value in diphtheria. Loeffler's medium, which contains coagulated beef serum and nutrient broth, is frequently used for primary isolation of *C. diphtheriae.* Smears made from colonies growing on Loeffler's medium and stained with methylene blue reveal the presence of pleomorphic bacilli. Club-shaped and branching forms are common; irregular staining caused by an abundance of granules is characteristic (Fig. 16–9). Biochemical tests will confirm the identification. In addition, a virulence test must be performed to demonstrate toxigenicity of the isolate. An in vivo test using guinea pigs or a modified Elek in vitro procedure based on immunodiffusion may be used to show production of toxin. The clinical diagnosis and treatment of diphtheria should not await laboratory confirmation.

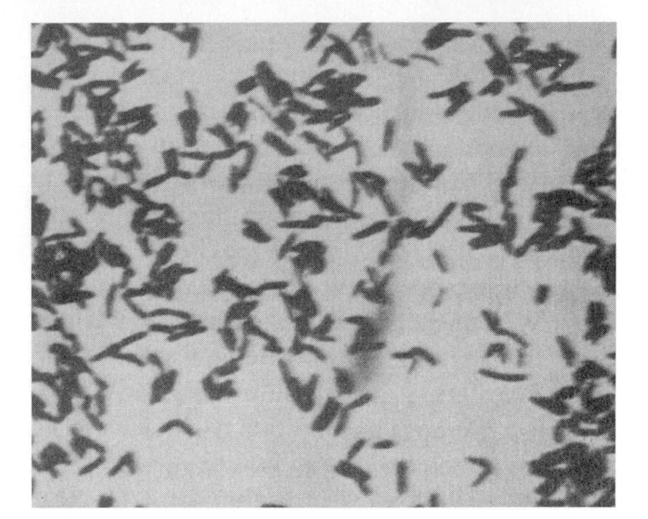

Figure 16–9 ◆ Gram stain of *C. diphtheriae* showing pleomorphism.

Early administration of diphtheria antitoxin (DAT) is required to neutralize the toxin of *C. diphtheriae.* Penicillin or erythromycin is effective against the diphtheria bacilli and, therefore, is usually included in a treatment regimen. The carrier rate varies from 1 to 15 percent in individuals who do not receive antibiotics.

The use of diphtheria toxoid in DTP preparations has eliminated diphtheria as a major threat in the United States. Diphtheria remains a problem in some Third World countries, where it is difficult to reach certain geographic areas with preventive immunization. The Schick skin test can be used to detect susceptibility for the toxin of *C. diphtheriae.* In the test, a small amount of diluted purified toxin is injected intradermally on the forearm. If a localized inflammatory response occurs within four to seven days, it is a positive Schick test and indicates absence of immunity.

Tuberculosis

Tuberculosis is caused by the acid-fast bacillus, *Mycobacterium tuberculosis,* but several other species, particularly *M. avium* and *M. intracellulare* (MAI), cause pulmonary disease that is indistinguishable from tuberculosis. Disseminated MAI infections are common in AIDS patients. The number and percentage of tuberculosis cases among foreign-born persons in the United States have been increasing in the last decade (Fig. 16–10). The increases are related to immigration from high-prevalence countries, incidence of HIV infections, and development of multiple-drug-resistant strains of *M. tuberculosis.* Mycobacteria are spread by aerosols from a person with active pulmonary disease. They are probably only rarely transmitted by contaminated materials from a patient.

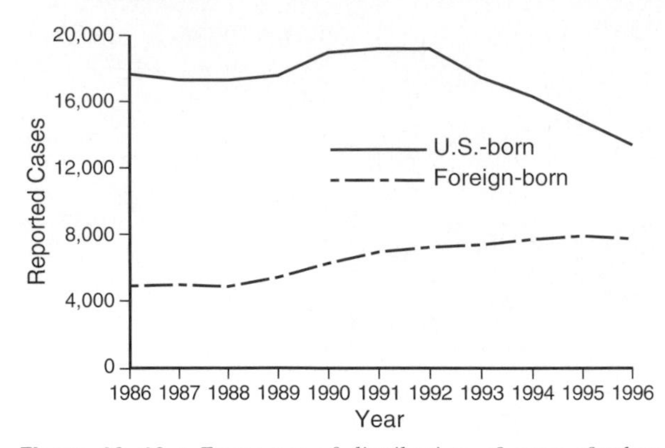

Figure 16–10 ◆ Frequency of distribution of cases of tuberculosis in United States–born and foreign-born persons, United States, 1986–1996.

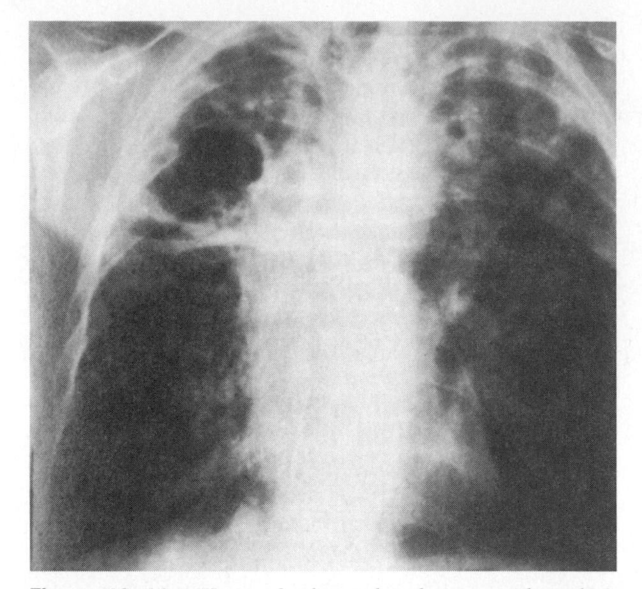

Figure 16–11 ◆ X-ray of advanced pulmonary tuberculosis with cavitation of both upper lobes and scattered patches of infiltrates.

Travel on commercial airlines with symptomatic tuberculosis patients has been determined to be a risk factor in exposure to *M. tuberculosis.* The risk, however, does not seem to be greater than in other confined spaces. Long international flights, particularly those originating in developing countries, would favor transmission of the pathogen from any infected passengers.

In the early stages of tuberculosis, individuals may be asymptomatic or may have only a low-grade fever. Later symptoms include a higher temperature, a cough, fatigue, lack of appetite, weight loss, and pulmonary hemorrhage. Distinct lesions of the lung cannot be demonstrated for four to 12 weeks after exposure to the acid-fast bacilli. If untreated, the tubercle bacilli disseminate within the lung and may spread to other organs.

Skin tests and chest x-rays are of importance in screening large numbers of persons in high-incidence populations for pulmonary tuberculosis (Fig. 16–11). Individuals with tuberculosis demonstrate a cell-mediated type of hypersensitivity to a purified protein derivative (PPD) of tuberculin. The Mantoux skin test is described in Chapter 14. Positive findings on x-rays, seen as shadows on chest films, constitute only presumptive evidence for the presence of the disease. The confirmatory diagnosis requires isolation and identification of the etiologic agent from sputum or gastric washings. The presence of acid-fast bacilli on smears supports a presumptive diagnosis (Fig. 16–12). Mycobacteria can also be demonstrated by fluorescent microscopy using auramine. With appropriate filters, the organisms appear yellow against a dark background. A polymerase chain reaction (PCR) assay can detect the bacilli in sputum, gastric washings, cerebrospinal fluids, and tissue biopsy specimens. None of the available PCR tests can identify drug-resistant strains of *M. tuberculosis,* so tests for antibiotic susceptibility must be performed.

Successful isolation of *M. tuberculosis* or other *Mycobacterium* species is time-consuming. Sputum

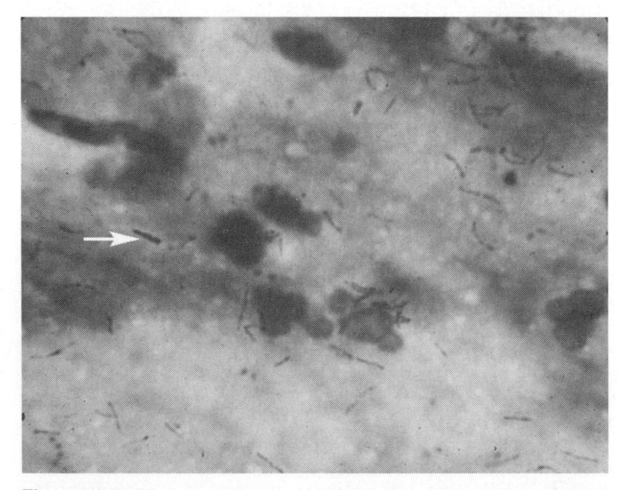

Figure 16–12 ◆ A microscopic field showing numerous acid-fast bacilli stained by the Ziehl-Neelsen method. With this technique the bacilli can be observed as brilliant red rods (arrow) against a blue background.

and gastric washings require processing with a digestant and a decontaminant to reduce viscosity and destroy other microorganisms. Sediments, obtained by centrifugation, are transferred to an egg medium, such as Lowenstein-Jensen medium. Growth frequently takes six to eight weeks (Color Plates 47 and 48). Species identification requires biochemical testing.

Drugs such as isoniazid, rifampin, pyrazinamide, and ethambutol are used to treat tuberculosis. Initial therapy may involve use of all four drugs for prolonged periods of time to eradicate the acid-fast bacilli from sputum. No treatment for illness caused by MAI in AIDS patients prolongs survival.

The vaccine BCG (Bacille Calmette and Guérin), developed by the French scientists Calmette and Guérin early in the twentieth century, has been employed successfully in many parts of the world to prevent tuberculosis. The vaccine, which contains an attenuated bovine strain of the tubercle bacillus, has not been used on a large scale in the United States. The tuberculin sensitivity resulting from use of the vaccine negates the usefulness of diagnostic skin tests.

An alternate preventive measure, in the event of high risk because of age, underlying disease, or prolonged immunosuppressive therapy, is the administration of isoniazid. Isoniazid is particularly effective in preventing relapse in arrested cases of tuberculosis. This form of chemoprophylaxis is, however, too expensive for entire communities.

Mycoplasmal Pneumonia

Mycoplasmas have been known for many years to be important pathogens of animals, but the major human pathogen is *Mycoplasma pneumoniae*, the cause of primary atypical pneumonia. The infection is sporadic and primarily affects older children and young adults. *M. pneumoniae* is transmitted by aerosols from an infected person, but it is not highly communicable. It sometimes takes weeks for it to spread even among members of the same family. The risk of infection is greater in congested areas. Outbreaks in military recruits and college populations suggest that repeated contact with respiratory secretions may be necessary for transmission to occur.

M. pneumoniae can be isolated from sputum on media enriched with yeast extract and horse serum, but it grows slowly. Colonies of *M. pneumoniae* can be observed in one to three weeks on solid media after incubation at 37°C. They typically have a "fried-egg" appearance and are visible only with magnification (Fig. 16–13). Cold agglutinins are present in the blood of approximately 50 percent of individuals with mycoplasmal pneumonia. Specific antibodies to *M. pneumoniae* can be detected by complement fixation (CF), enzyme immunoassay (EIA), and immunofluorescence (IF). Both a DNA probe method and a PCR technique have been developed for rapid detection of the mycoplasmas in clinical specimens, but use of them is limited.

Because mycoplasmas have no cell walls, penicillin is not effective in the treatment of infections caused by *M. pneumoniae.* Both erythromycin and tetracycline have been used to resolve the infection. Despite antibiotic therapy, a paroxysmal cough may last for several weeks.

Legionellosis

Legionellosis is a multisystem illness characterized by an atypical form of pneumonia. It was thought to have made its first appearance as an outbreak of a mysterious pneumonia in Philadelphia in the summer of 1976 and was given its

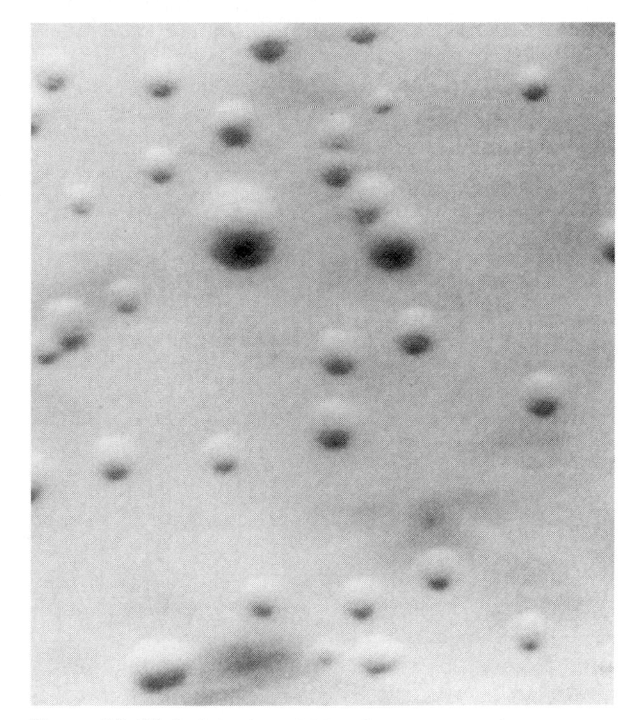

Figure 16–13 ◆ Colonies of *Mycoplasma pneumoniae* grown on PPLO agar.

name because individuals affected were attending a state American Legion convention. It now appears that the pulmonary infection is widespread and occurred as early as 1947.

The bacterium causing the outbreak of respiratory illness in Philadelphia was subsequently named *Legionella pneumophila* (Fig. 16–14). Since 1976 a number of other *Legionella* species have been implicated in pneumonic and nonpneumonic infections. The bacteria are widely distributed in nature and have been isolated from water supplies, humidifiers, and air-conditioning equipment. Ventilation systems appear to disperse aerosols containing *Legionella* species. No person-to-person transmission has been documented. The incubation period varies from two to 10 days.

The atypical pneumonia caused by *L. pneumophila* is characterized by fever, cough, difficulty in breathing, and chest pain. The mortality rate approximates 20 percent. Legionellosis also occurs as a nonpneumonic, self-limited febrile disease. Nosocomial infections have been reported in immunocompromised patients especially in recipients of organ transplants.

L. pneumophila is a gram-negative pleomorphic bacillus, but it does not stain well by the usual Gram stain procedure. If basic fuchsin is used as the counterstain instead of safranin, satisfactory results can be obtained. Coccobacillary and filamentous forms are not infrequent (Fig. 16–15). A direct fluorescent antibody (DFA) technique for staining smears is more specific for demonstrating the organisms (Color Plate 49). Buffered charcoal yeast extract agar is the preferred medium for isolating *L. pneumophila*. Biochemical tests are required to differentiate the organism from other *Legionella* species, but the slow growth

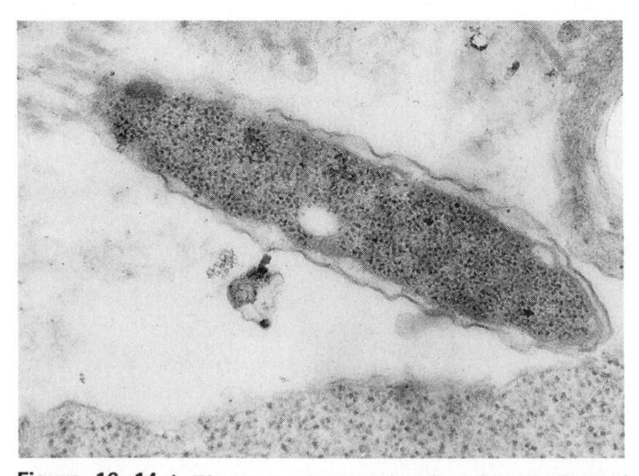

Figure 16–14 ◆ Electron micrograph of a thin section of *Legionella pneumophila* in the yolk sac of an embryonated egg.

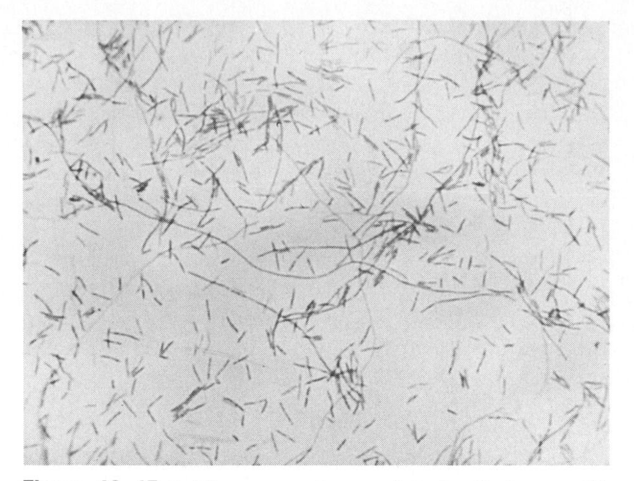

Figure 16–15 ◆ Filamentous forms of *Legionella pneumophila* stained by a modified gram-stain procedure.

and relative inertness of the organism limits the application of such tests. An indirect fluorescent antibody (IFA) or an enzyme immunoassay (EIA) can be used for detection of antibodies in serum. A DNA probe for *L. pneumophila* is available.

L. pneumophila appears to be susceptible to a number of antibiotics, but most success in treatment has been with erythromycin and rifampin. There is no accurate method for detecting antibiotic susceptibility in the laboratory.

Psittacosis (Ornithosis)

Psittacosis or ornithosis was a disease at one time thought to be limited to the parrot family, but many kinds of birds can harbor the etiologic agent, *Chlamydia psittaci*. Many of the infections in birds remain latent, surfacing only under conditions of stress. *C. psittaci* is spread from bird to bird and bird to human by aerosols, by contact with discharges from an infected bird, or by the bite of an infected bird. The incubation period is four to 15 days. In some birds *C. psittaci* is transmitted vertically from parents to offspring in sex cells. Human-to-human transmission is rare. Psittacosis may be a relatively mild disease, a severe pulmonary infection, or a septicemia in humans. The early symptoms of pulmonary disease vary, but a headache and a fever are fairly constant. Later a nonproductive cough is present. It is not easily differentiated from other types of lung infections.

A diagnosis of psittacosis can be made by CF, IF, or neutralization in cell cultures. The chlamydias will grow in cell cultures, but recovery of the organisms from clinical specimens is difficult if antimicrobial therapy has been instituted prior to specimen collection. A PCR method is available for identifying *C. psittaci* in cell culture.

Administration of tetracycline results in marked improvement in 24 to 72 hours. Radiological evidence of disease may persist up to two weeks after symptoms disappear. Shedding of *C. psittaci* may go on for months.

Chlamydial Pneumonia

Chlamydial pneumonia emerged in the 1980s as an acute respiratory disease, but the organism had probably caused pneumonia for many years. The etiologic agent, once known as the TWAR (Taiwan acute respiratory) agent causes a febrile illness characterized by a sometimes productive cough, sore throat, and painful swallowing.

The organism, now named *Chlamydia pneumoniae,* grows in cell cultures and is distinct from other chlamydial species. Both IgM and IgG antibodies can be detected by an indirect fluorescent (IF) technique. Tetracycline and erythromycin are drugs of choice.

A pneumonitis occurring in newborn infants is caused by *C. trachomatis.* The infants acquire the pathogen during delivery from a mother with a cervical chlamydial infection. Babies develop some congestion and a cough, but usually no fever. Chlamydias may be grown from respiratory secretions or identified by immunofluorescent procedures. The pneumonitis responds to treatment with tetracycline or erythromycin.

Q Fever

Q fever (query fever) is an acute febrile influenza-like disease caused by *Coxiella burnetii.* It is endemic in California, Arizona, Oregon, and Washington, but has also been reported in other states and in countries on five continents. The disease is transmitted by aerosols containing excreta of infected animals. Cattle, sheep, goats, ticks, and some wild animals are natural reservoirs of *C. burnetii.* The organism can tolerate dry conditions and remain viable for many years in contaminated soils. Raw milk is frequently incriminated as a mode of transmission for the rickettsial agent. Infected ticks pass the organism to offspring transovarially and to humans by a bite, but transmission from person to person is rare. The incubation period is dependent on the infective dose, but generally symptoms appear within two to three weeks after exposure to the chlamydias. Symptoms are variable, but a high fever is generally present. A cough, chest pain, nausea, vomiting, a headache and diarrhea are common. Most cases of Q fever are self-limiting with a resolution in one to two weeks after onset. However, chronic infections, particularly in persons with underlying diseases, are known to occur.

Because *C. burnetii* has been transmitted in laboratory settings, the recommended diagnostic procedures are serological. The most widely used test is for complement-fixing antibodies, but IFA tests and ELISA techniques are also valuable. Rising titers can be demonstrated by the second or third week after onset.

Prompt treatment with tetracycline is effective in shortening the course of the acute phase of Q fever. An inactivated vaccine is available for laboratory workers or other high-risk groups.

Pulmonary Actinomycosis

Pulmonary actinomycosis is a suppurative or granulomatous disease caused by the aspiration of the endogenous organism *Actinomyces israelii* from the pharynx. Production of a purulent or blood-streaked sputum and the formation of abscesses and multiple draining sinus tracts are characteristic of the infection. The filamentous organisms are often organized into sulfur granules in affected tissues (Fig. 16–16).

Thioglycolate broth is used for the initial isolation of *A. israelii.* The gram-positive bacilli vary in

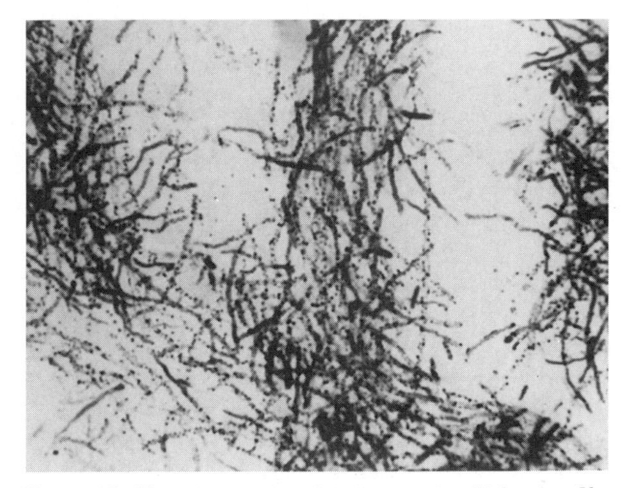

Figure 16–16 ◆ Gram stain of *Actinomyces israelii* showing filaments.

size from short rods to long, thin filamentous forms. The organism will grow on phenylethyl alcohol (PEA) blood agar under anaerobic conditions. Biochemical tests must be performed to differentiate *A. israelii* from other anaerobic bacilli.

Infections caused by *A. israelii* usually respond well to penicillin or tetracycline. Particularly purulent **loci** may require surgical intervention.

Nocardiosis

Nocardiosis is a chronic disease most often originating in the lungs. It begins rather insidiously several months after exposure with a cough and fever. The primary etiologic agent is *Nocardia asteroides*. The partially acid-fast actinomycete is not known to be endogenous in humans. Pulmonary nocardiosis is spread by inhalation of the organisms in dust-laden air. The soil is the natural reservoir of the organism. There is no known animal-to-animal or person-to-person transmission of *N. asteroides*. The organisms commonly spread via the bloodstream to the brain or kidney, but can disseminate to virtually any part of the body. Invasion of the brain by *N. asteroides* is almost always fatal.

N. asteroides is a gram-positive pleomorphic bacillus that may be coccoidal or filamentous. Most strains are acid-fast when grown in the presence of sufficient protein. The organism grows on Sabouraud dextrose agar, blood agar, and Lowenstein-Jensen medium (Color Plate 50). *N. asteroides* does not hydrolyze casein, xanthine, or tyrosine.

Prompt treatment of pulmonary nocardiosis with trimethoprim-sulfamethoxazole can prevent dissemination of the infection. Antibiotic susceptibility studies are not practical because of technical problems associated with the procedure for actinomycetes.

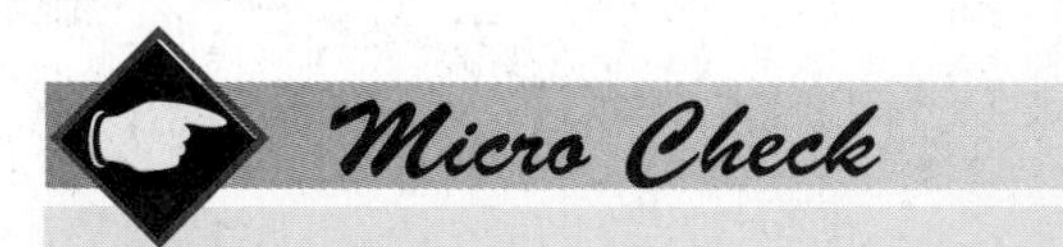

- How can the increased incidence of tuberculosis be explained?
- How do air-conditioning units contribute to the transmission of legionellosis?
- Why is penicillin not effective in the treatment of mycoplasmal pneumonia?

FUNGAL INFECTIONS

The conidia of a large number of fungi are inhaled by most individuals, but except for some yeasts, most do not colonize extensively on the mucous membranes of the respiratory tract. If colonization does occur, the infections may go unrecognized. Respiratory disease caused by fungi occurs under special conditions, only some of which are understood.

Other than the skin, hair, and nails, the most common primary sites of fungal infections are the lungs. The fungi that infect deep tissues and internal organs are distinct from those which cause superficial infections. The diseases they cause are called **deep mycoses.** The major deep mycoses—histoplasmosis, coccidioidomycosis, and blastomycosis—are caused by dimorphic fungi.

Histoplasmosis

Acute pulmonary infections caused by *Histoplasma capsulatum* occur in all age groups of both sexes, but are more frequent in adult males, probably because of greater occupational exposure. It is often seen as a systemic, debilitating disease in AIDS patients. *H. capsulatum* is transmitted by inhalation of airborne conidia of the fungus. Soil around old chicken houses, starling roosts, and caves harboring the common brown bat serve as reservoirs for the organism. The disease is contracted mostly by persons in rural areas of the Mississippi and Ohio river valleys, but it also occurs in immunosuppressed individuals in other geographic areas. Symptoms of disease occur most frequently about 10 days after exposure.

The symptoms and clinical course of histoplasmosis resemble those of tuberculosis. Primary histoplasmosis may be asymptomatic. A heavy exposure to the fungi cause fever, headache, and a nonproductive cough. The progressive systemic form of the disease is most often observed in the very young, the aged, or those with immunological deficiencies. It differs from tuberculosis in that favorable resolution of the infection is more frequent.

The mycelial phase of *H. capsulatum* may be obtained on Sabouraud dextrose agar, whereas the yeast phase grows well on blood agar (Color Plates 51 and 52). A white aerial mycelium that turns brown with age is characteristic of the mycelial phase (Fig. 16–17). Large spherical tuberculate macroconidia are important in the identi-

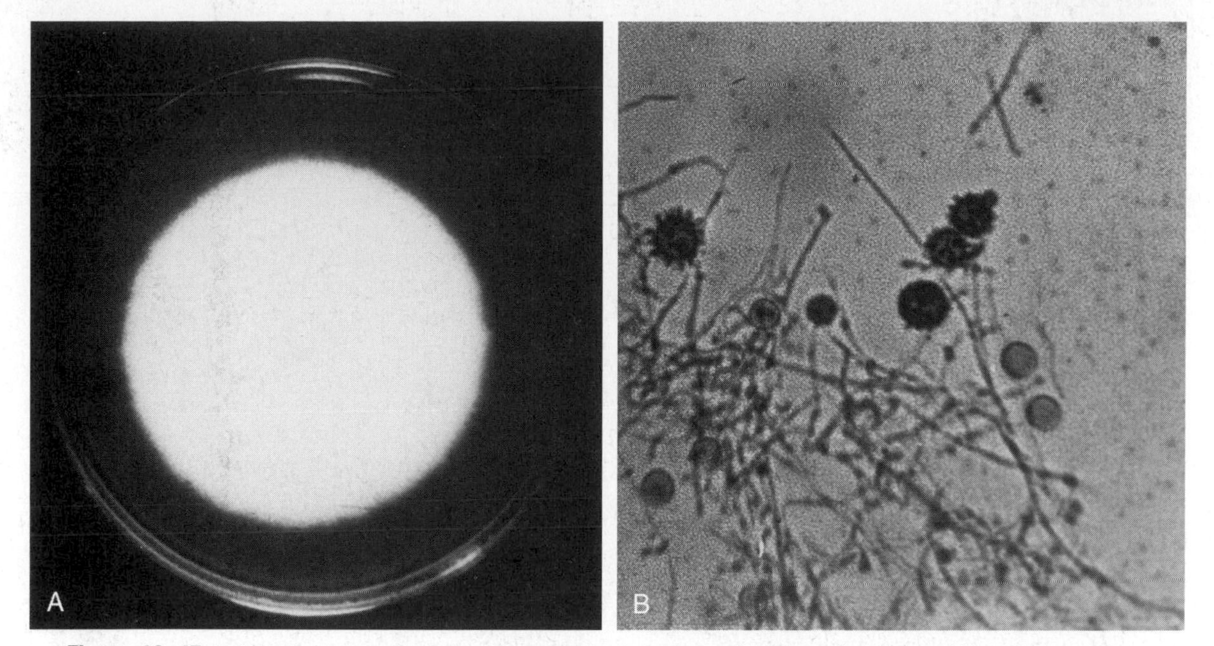

Figure 16–17 ◆ *Histoplasma capsulatum. A,* Macroscopic view of mycelial phase showing a white aerial mycelium. *B,* Microscopic view showing tuberculate macroconidia.

fication of the organism. A number of serological tests are available for detection of antibodies to *H. capsulatum.* A skin test with histoplasmin, a protein analogous to tuberculin, may also be employed in the diagnosis of histoplasmosis.

Amphotericin B and fluconazole are the drugs of choice. Ketoconazole is generally not effective in AIDS patients with histoplasmosis.

Coccidioidomycosis

Coccidioidomycosis is endemic in the Southwestern United States and some parts of Central and South America. It is the cause of a severe pneumonia in AIDS patients, but may also involve the meninges, joints, liver, lymph nodes, or skin. It is not known if the disease in AIDS patients is from reactivation or new exposure.

The etiologic agent, *Coccidioides immitis,* grows in soil as a mold. The organism infects cattle, dogs, sheep, burros, pigs, rodents, and humans. *C. immitis* is transmitted by inhalation of arthroconidia from soil, dust, or plants from arid areas. An increased incidence of coccidioidomycosis occurred after the Northridge earthquake in California early in 1994. The dust stirred up from falling concrete and bricks released spores into the atmosphere. It is also readily transmitted from cultures in the laboratory. The white, cottony mycelium on laboratory cultures bears abundant infectious conidia and should be handled only by experienced personnel. There is no evidence that the organism is transmitted by an infected individual to a susceptible person.

Only a relatively few people who have contact with the arthroconidia develop symptoms of respiratory disease. Symptoms occur in one to four weeks in primary infections. Fever is almost always present, and there may be a nonproductive cough. The disease is self-limited in most individuals, and no treatment is required. The disseminated form of coccidioidomycosis, which occurs more frequently in dark-skinned individuals, can be fatal.

Direct examination of sputum may reveal thick-walled spherules that contain numerous endospores (Fig. 16–18; Color Plate 53). Definitive diagnosis requires culturing the organism on Sabouraud dextrose agar and demonstrating arthroconidia on wet mounts (Fig.16–19; Color Plate 54). Precipitating antibodies are produced early in the disease, but complement-fixing antibodies are not present until four to eight weeks following onset. Intracutaneous administration of coccidioidin produces induration in pulmonary infections and only a weak reaction or no reaction in disseminated infections.

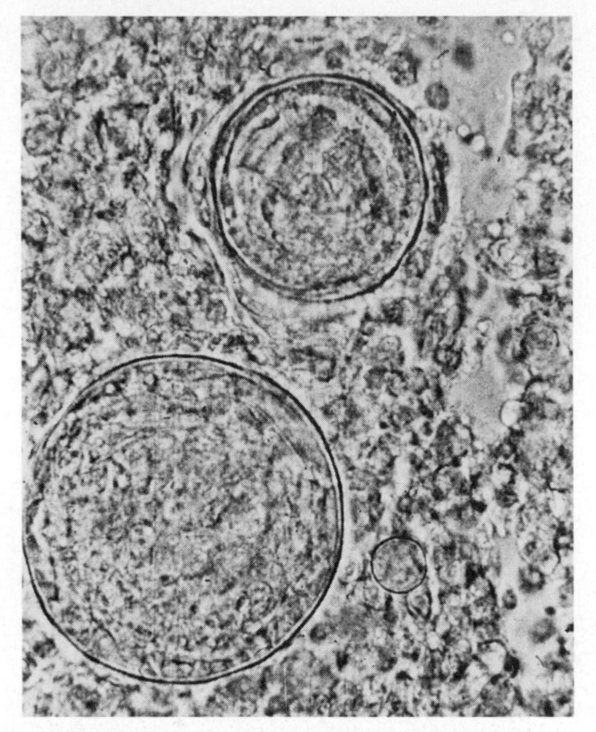

Figure 16–18 ◆ Thick-walled spherules of *Coccidioides immitis* in unstained wet mount of sputum.

Amphotericin B has remained the drug of choice in coccidioidomycosis for years, but fluconazole and itraconazole are less toxic than amphotericin B and may prove to be equally effective.

Blastomycosis

Blastomycosis is an acute or chronic respiratory disease of the lungs or skin caused by *Blastomyces dermatitidis* in North America. Blastomycosis occurs most frequently in the Southeastern United States and in the Mississippi River valley.

The conidia of the mycelial phase of *B. dermatitidis* from soil reservoirs are probably inhaled in dust, but the organism has not been isolated from soil with any regularity. There is no evidence that blastomycosis is transmitted directly from person to person. The time of incubation varies in individuals. It may be as short as one month or as long as several years.

The pulmonary form of the disease varies from a mild and often unrecognized infection to a severe disease resembling tuberculosis and histoplasmosis. A low-grade fever, weight loss, and a cough may be present. The cutaneous form of the disease usually follows systemic involvement.

Smears of sputum, pleural fluid, exudates, or biopsy material often reveal large, spherical thick-walled yeast cells in blastomycosis. The mycelial phase of *B. dermatitidis* grows on Sabouraud dextrose agar producing terminal or lateral conidia. The yeast phase can be obtained on blood agar. Cells of *B. dermatitidis* produce single buds with broad bases (Fig. 16–20). Multiple buds on narrow bases are formed by cells of *Paracoccidioides brasiliensis,* which causes a similar disease in Central and South America (Fig. 16–21). The appearance of the large, spherical cells of the organism has been likened to the wheel of a ship. Both precipitating and complement-fixing antibodies are produced in North American blastomycosis. Blastomycin skin tests are of little help in the diagnosis of blastomycosis.

Amphotericin B is effective against systemic blastomycosis, but milder cases may respond to ketoconazole.

Pulmonary Aspergillosis

Pulmonary aspergillosis is caused by one or more species of *Aspergillus,* a mold found on de-

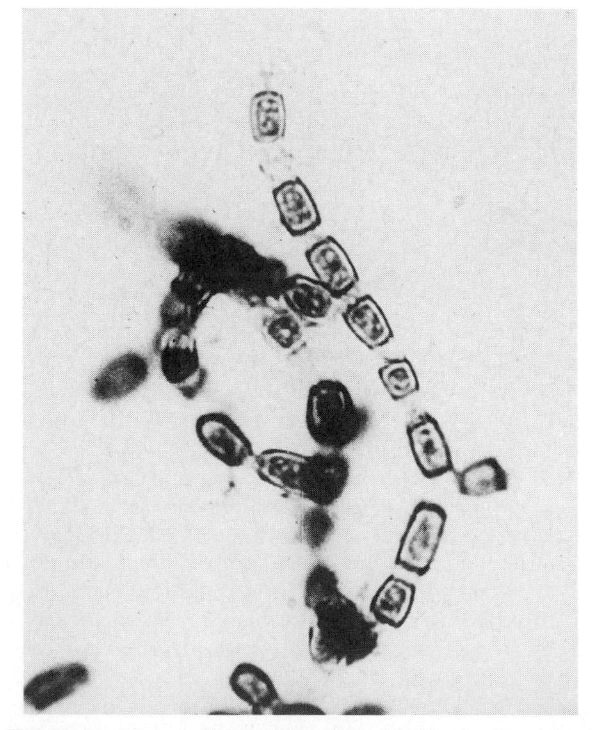

Figure 16–19 ◆ Arthroconidia of *Coccidioides immitis* stained with lactophenol cotton blue in a wet mount.

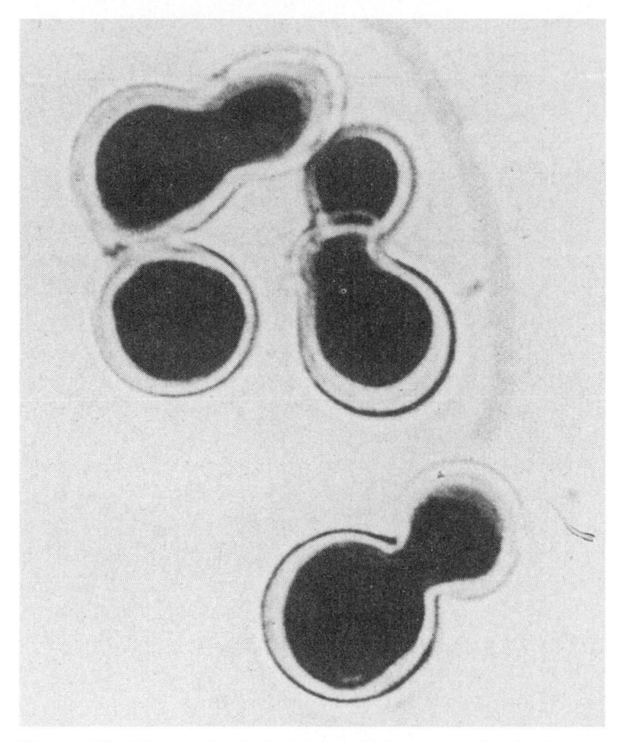

Figure 16–20 ◆ Spherical, thick-walled yeast cells of *Blastomyces dermatitidis* stained with lactophenol cotton blue in a wet mount.

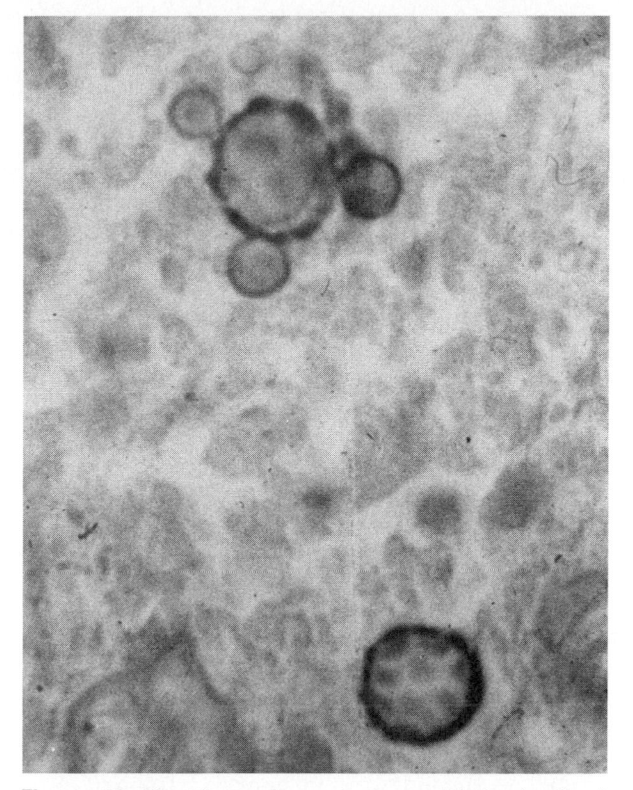

Figure 16–21 ◆ Yeast phase of *Paracoccidioides brasiliensis* stained with methenamine silver, showing multiple budding.

caying plants, in stored hay, and in cereal grains. The most important human pathogen is *A. fumigatus,* but other species occasionally are isolated from the lung. *Aspergillus* species are transmitted in inhalation of the conidia in dust. There is no evidence of person-to-person transmission. Symptoms may occur a few days after exposure or may be evident only after several months.

Four major forms of pulmonary disease have been designated as aspergillosis: (1) primary acute pneumonia, (2) formation of a "fungus ball" within a previously existing cavity, (3) allergic bronchopulmonary aspergillosis, and (4) secondary pulmonary aspergillosis occurring as an opportunistic infection. Certain toxic metabolites, known as **aflatoxins,** produced by some species of *Aspergillus,* cause serious liver disease in animals.

A. fumigatus can be observed often in wet mounts of sputum, but only short fragments of hyphae are usually visible in biopsy material (Fig. 16–22). The organism grows rapidly on Sabouraud dextrose agar as a dark blue or green mold. Its flask-shaped vesicles and a single row of conidia differentiate it from other species. Unlike other *Aspergillus* species, *A. fumigatus* grows at 50°C.

Amphotericin B alone or with 5-fluorocytosine is the drug of choice for all forms of aspergillosis. Surgical excision may be necessary when a "fungus ball" is present.

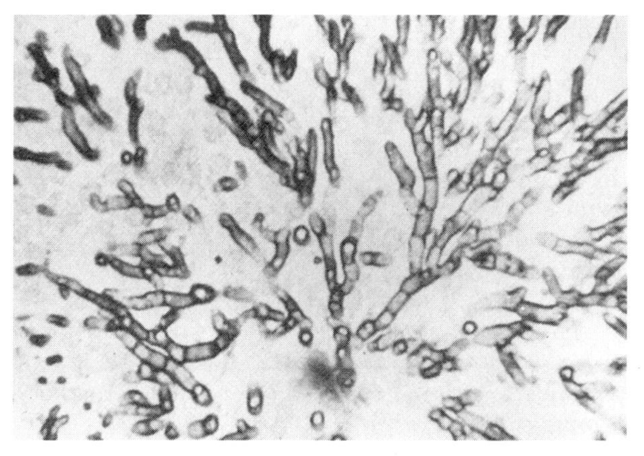

Figure 16–22 ◆ Human lung tissue showing short fragments of hyphae of *Aspergillus fumigatus.*

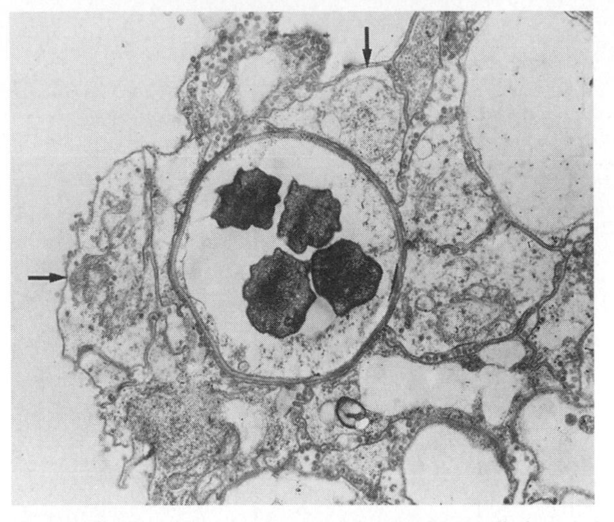

Figure 16–23 ◆ Electron micrograph of a thick-walled cyst of *Pneumocystis carinii* containing sporelike bodies. The surrounding thin-walled cysts (indicated by arrows) display marked variation in configuration suggestive of a pliable outer limiting membrane.

Pneumocystis carinii Pneumonia

An extracellular fungus, once classified as a protozoan, occurs as a primary invader in premature infants and as an opportunistic respiratory pathogen in AIDS patients. The disease is known as *Pneumocystis carinii* pneumonia (PCP). PCP is a common opportunistic infection in AIDS patients and frequently proves to be fatal.

The mode of transmission for *P. carinii* has not been definitely established, but the fungus appears to be widespread in nature. It is likely that the organism is airborne and that it can reside in the nasopharynx of asymptomatic individuals. In institutional outbreaks, incubation periods of one to two months have been recorded.

The fungus causes interstitial plasma cell pneumonia, which is characterized by infiltration of alveoli with plasma cells, exudate, and the fungi. There is often progressive difficulty in breathing, but fever may not be present. Like other opportunistic microorganisms, the ubiquity of *P. carinii* makes control measures difficult.

Definitive diagnosis of PCP requires that materials from the lung be obtained. Cysts can be seen on smears stained with a silver-nitrate stain. Four forms of cysts have been described: (1) a precyst, (2) a mature cyst, (3) a cyst liberating trophozoites, and (4) an empty collapsed cyst. When electron microscopy is applied to biopsy material, intracystic bodies can be observed within the cysts (Fig. 16–23).

The drugs of choice are pentamidine and trimethoprim-sulfamethoxazole. Pentamidine is used in an aerosolized form to prevent PCP. Prednisone, a corticosteroid, is an accepted form of treatment in moderate to severe PCP, but must be limited to short-term use. Long-term administration of corticosteroids causes immunosuppression. Drugs greatly improve the chances for survival in PCP except in severely compromised patients.

FOCAL POINT

Prevention of *Pneumocystis carinii* Pneumonia

The old adage of a "stitch in time saves nine" applies to the prevention of *Pneumocystis carinii* pneumonia (PCP) in HIV-infected individuals. Repeated episodes of PCP in persons with AIDS has caused repeated hospital admissions, untold suffering, and enormous costs. PCP is the most life-threatening opportunistic infection associated with AIDS. For that reason, preventive measures are recommended for all persons with less than 200 CD4$^+$ T cells per μl for anyone with unexplained fever or thrush, and individuals who have recovered from a documented episode of PCP.

Either a dose of double-strength sulfamethoxazole-trimethoprim (800 mg of sulfamethoxazole and 160 mg of trimethoprim) daily or aerosolized pentamidine (300 mg once a month or an initial regimen of five 60-mg doses over a two-week period with a 60 mg dose bimonthly) is recommended.

Before aerosolized pentamidine is administered, patients must be evaluated for the presence of tuberculosis. Sulfamethoxazole-trimethoprim is the preferred choice for prophylaxis if it can be tolerated by a patient. A rash, with or without itching, depression of circulating blood cells, or elevations of liver enzymes are contraindications for continuing use of this drug. Patients must continue preventive intervention for life.

Morbidity and Mortality Weekly Report, 41:RR-4, 1992.

Table 16–2
MAJOR GROUPS AND SEROTYPES OF RESPIRATORY VIRUSES

VIRUS	SEROTYPES	MAJOR DISEASE
Adenovirus	1, 2, 3, 4, 5, 6, 7, 14, and 21	Acute respiratory disease
Hantavirus		Hantavirus infection
Orthomyxovirus		
Influenza	A, B	Influenza
Paramyxovirus		
Parainfluenza	1, 2, 3, 4	Croup
Respiratory syncytial (RS)	1	Bronchiolitis
Picornavirus		
Coxsackievirus	A2, A4, A5, A6, A7, A12, and A21; B2, B3, and B5	Pharyngitis
Rhinovirus	1–100	Common cold

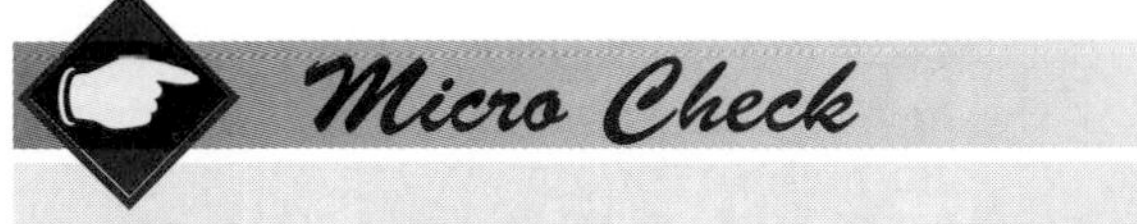

- What is the most common site of infection in the deep mycoses?
- Why must cultures of dimorphic fungi be handled with care in the laboratory?
- What measure is recommended for AIDS patients to prevent *Pneumocystis carinii* infections?

VIRAL INFECTIONS

A large number of viruses are probably transient residents of nasopharyngeal cells. Infection of cells is not always synonymous with disease. Many infections are inapparent because no symptoms occur. The majority of virions reaching the lungs are destroyed by alveolar macrophages. When a viral disease is established, infectious particles may be shed in oropharyngeal secretions for varying periods even after symptoms disappear.

It has been estimated that at least 90 percent of acute upper respiratory infections and nearly 50 percent of lower respiratory infections are caused by viruses. A number of viruses have been isolated from human respiratory tract disease (Table 16–2).

The multiplicity of viral agents involved in acute respiratory illnesses, along with the varying symptoms produced in humans, complicates the identification of specific etiologic agents. However, at least 13 viruses are now known to cause serious lower respiratory tract disease: influenza A and B, respiratory syncytial virus, parainfluenza virus types 1, 2, 3, and 4, and more than 20 adenovirus types (Fig. 16–24). The over 100 serotypes of rhinoviruses and several strains of coronaviruses colonize in cells of the upper airways. Most viral infections do not respond well to chemotherapy and do, therefore, have life-threatening potential.

Influenza

Influenza viruses rank as primary causes of epidemics and pandemics of respiratory tract infection. The viruses are transmitted by aerosols

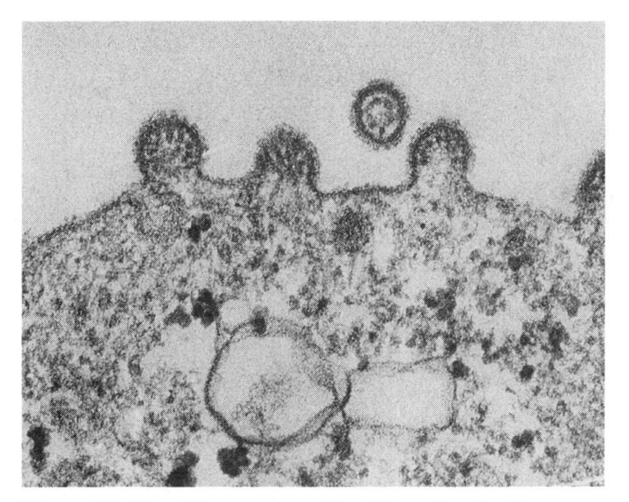

Figure 16–24 ◆ The process of budding whereby viruses are released in a green monkey kidney cell infected with a respiratory syncytial (RS) virus.

from an infected individual. An encephalopathy, known as Reye syndrome, has occurred as a complication in children with influenza or chickenpox who are treated with aspirin. The role of aspirin in promoting Reye syndrome remains controversial. The consequences of the brain disease are so severe, however, that the Surgeon General of the United States has recommended that salicylate and salicylate-containing medications should not be given to children with influenza or chickenpox.

The influenza viruses are divided into three major groups based on antigens associated with the capsid. Type A and type B cause outbreaks that have occurred in regular cycles throughout the world. Outbreaks of influenza in which type A has been implicated have recurred every two to four years, whereas epidemics associated with type B have cycled every four to six years. Type C influenza virus almost never causes severe disease.

Influenza A virus can be divided into additional groups according to the type of glycoproteins associated with spikes of the envelope (Fig. 16–25). The hemagglutinin antigens (HA) promote clumping of red blood cells and binding to other eucaryotic cell membranes. The neuraminidase antigens (NA) facilitate the release of viruses from infected cells. These antigens are unstable and undergo changes with time. If the change is minor, the phenomenon is called **antigenic drift.** If the alteration in antigenic identity is sufficient to interfere with a type-specific antibody reaction, the phenomenon is called **antigenic shift.** Influenza viruses are identified by the major group to which they belong and arabic numbers for their H and N antigens.

As new strains of the influenza virus emerge, preceding strains disappear or become sequestered for long periods of time. It was feared that a swine virus resembling the strain involved in the pandemic of 1918–1919 would spread in epidemic proportions when it surfaced briefly in the United States in the 1976–1977 season, but such an epidemic did not materialize. Influenza has an incubation time of only one to three days and is most often characterized by an abrupt onset of fever, chills, headache, and muscle aches.

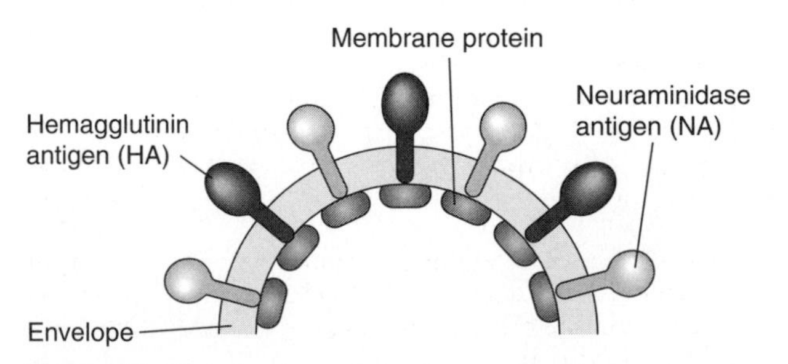

Figure 16–25 ◆ Portion of envelope of influenza virus A. Hemagglutinin antigens (HA) and neuraminidase antigens (NA) are contained on the spikes of the envelope.

Specific diagnosis of influenza depends on the location of viruses from nasal washings in tissue cultures or at least a fourfold increase in antibody titer in convalescent sera when compared with sera obtained during the acute phase of the disease. Antibodies to the influenza viruses can be identified using a hemagglutination inhibition (HI) test, a neutralization technique (NT), a complement fixation (CF), test, or an enzyme immunoassay (EIA).

Amantadine and rimantadine, antiviral drugs, limit the duration of influenza caused by type A strains of influenza virus if administered during the incubation period. The drug interferes with uncoating of the viruses in cells. Universal immunization with vaccine consisting of type-specific inactivated virus has never been deemed practical. The procedure is recommended for the elderly, the very young, or other high-risk groups, which include medical personnel and institutionalized individuals, in places where influenza can spread rapidly. New vaccines are continually in development because vaccines rapidly become obsolete because of antigenic shift and drift.

The Common Cold

The common cold is a frequent infection of the upper respiratory tract that can occur at any time of the year, but the incidence of the annoying disability increases in the fall and late spring. The most frequent cause is one of the 100 or more rhinoviruses. The sometimes slight fever, headache, sore throat, coughing, sneezing, and nasal discharge that occur within two days after exposure to the etiologic agent are usually self-limiting. Although aerosol transmission can occur, the disease may be spread with greater frequency by contaminated hands or fomites. Because of the mild nature and short duration of the common cold, specific etiologic agents are rarely identified. There is no specific treatment, but secondary bacterial infections require prompt intervention with appropriate antibiotic therapy.

Viral Pneumonia

Viral pneumonia can follow a viral infection of the upper respiratory tract or may occur as a complication in postsurgical patients. A number of viruses can be involved as etiologic agents. Serotypes 3 and 7 of the adenoviruses and respiratory syncytial virus (RSV) have been responsible for the high incidence of pneumonia in infants and in the elderly with underlying pulmonary disease. The time of incubation is related to the infective dose and the severity of impairment of host defenses, but usually ranges from one to six days. Deep breathing, early ambulation following surgery, and use of **nebulizers** can prevent pooling of lower respiratory secretions and limit the opportunity for infection.

Viral pneumonia begins insidiously with headache, malaise, hoarseness, fever, and cough. Later infiltration may be observed on chest x-rays. Bacterial pneumonia often follows lung disease caused by viruses.

Adenoviruses and RSV can be grown in tissue cultures, but the methods are time-consuming. Complement-fixing and neutralizing antibodies can be detected in adults. It is impossible to prevent exposure of susceptible individuals to aerosols containing potentially infective particles, but respiratory therapy can encourage deep breathing and clearing the lungs of fluid containing microorganisms.

Hantavirus Pulmonary Syndrome

An outbreak of acute respiratory disease caused by a hantavirus, named Sin Nombre (no name) virus, occurred in the spring of 1993 among residents of the "four corners" region of the United States, along the borders of Utah, New Mexico, Arizona, and Colorado. The pulmonary syndrome, accompanied by fever, muscle aches, headache, and cough, progressed rapidly to respiratory failure. A 50 percent mortality rate occurred in diagnosed cases. The hantavirus, a bunyavirus reported previously to cause disease in Korea, is transmitted by inhalation of salivary or fecal aerosols of infected rodents. There is no evidence of person-to-person transmission in the United States, but during an outbreak in Argentina in 1996, the virus passed through individuals having no exposure to rodents. Although intravenous ribavirin has been effective in treating hantavirus infections in other parts of the world, it is not licensed for intravenous use in the United States. The virus does not cause apparent infection in rodent hosts. Deer mice are suspected as primary reservoirs, but pinon mice, brush mice, and western chipmunks also carry the hantavirus.

There is insufficient evidence to restrict travel to endemic areas, but persons who camp or hike should take precaution to reduce their possible exposure to potentially infectious materials (Table 16–3).

The major microorganisms causing respiratory disease are summarized in Table 16–4.

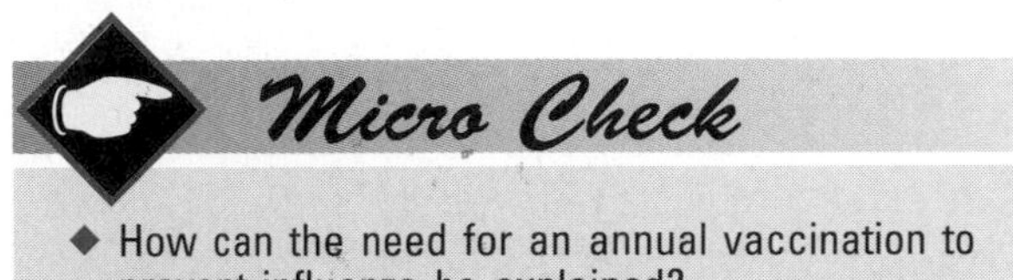

- How can the need for an annual vaccination to prevent influenza be explained?
- What viruses are the most frequent cause of the common cold?
- How does respiratory therapy aid in prevention of viral pneumonia?

Table 16–3
REDUCING THE RISK OF HANTAVIRUS INFECTION FOR HIKERS AND CAMPERS

Avoid coming into contact with rodents and rodent burrows or disturbing dens (such as pack rat nests).

Do not use cabins or other enclosed shelters that are rodent infested until they have been appropriately cleaned and disinfected.

Do not pitch tents or place sleeping bags in areas in proximity to rodent feces or burrows or near possible rodent shelters (e.g., garbage dumps or woodpiles).

If possible, do not sleep on the bare ground. Use a cot with the sleeping surface at least 12 inches above the ground. Use tents with floors.

Keep food in rodent-proof containers.

Promptly bury (or preferably burn followed by burying, when in accordance with local requirements) all garbage and trash, or discard in covered trash containers.

Use only bottled water or water that has been disinfected by filtration, boiling, chlorination, or iodination for drinking, cooking, washing dishes, and brushing teeth.

Source: MMWR *42*(RR-11):11, 1993.

Table 16–4
SUMMARY OF MAJOR MICROORGANISMS CAUSING DISEASES OF THE RESPIRATORY TRACT

MICROORGANISM	DISEASE	TREATMENT
Bacteria		
Staphylococcus aureus	Pneumonia	Methicillin, vancomycin
Group A beta-hemolytic streptococci	"Strep throat," scarlet fever	Penicillin
Streptococcus pneumonia	Pneumonia	Penicillin
Klebsiella pneumoniae	Pneumonia	Cephalothin, kanamycin
Haemophilus influenzae	Bronchiolitis, bronchitis, pneumonia	Based on susceptibility tests
Bordetella pertussis	Whooping cough	Erythromycin
Corynebacterium diphtheriae	Diphtheria	Diphtheria antitoxin, penicillin, erythromycin
Mycobacterium tuberculosis	Tuberculosis	Isoniazid, pyrazinamide, rifampin, ethambutol
Mycoplasma pneumoniae	Pneumonia	Erythromycin, tetracycline
Legionella pneumophila	Legionellosis	Erythromycin, rifampin
Chlamydia psittacii	Psittacosis	Tetracycline
Chlamydia pneumoniae	Chlamydial pneumonitis	Tetracycline
Coxiella burnetii	Q fever	Tetracycline
Filamentous bacteria		
Actinomyces israelii	Pulmonary actinomycosis	Penicillin, tetracycline
Nocardia asteroides	Nocardiosis	Sulfonamides
Fungi		
Histoplasma capsulatum	Histoplasmosis	Amphotericin B, fluconazole
Coccidioides immitis	Coccidioidomycosis	Amphotericin B, fluconazole, itraconazole
Blastomyces dermatitidis	Blastomycosis	Amphotericin B, ketonazole
Aspergillus fumigatus	Pulmonary aspergillosis	Amphotericin B, 5-fluorocytosine
Pneumocystis carinii	Interstitial plasma cell pneumonia	Pentamidine, trimethoprim-sulfamethoxazole, prednisone
Viruses		
Influenza viruses A and B	Influenza	Amantadine, rimantadine
Rhinoviruses	Common cold	None
Adenoviruses, respiratory syncytial virus and others	Viral pneumonia	Respiratory therapy
Hantavirus	Acute respiratory disease	None

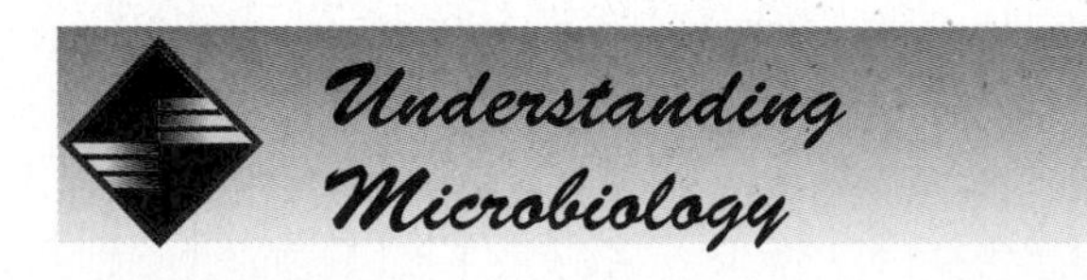

1. How does particle size and moisture content influence the deposition of microorganism-laden aerosols?
2. How do the etiologic agents of mycoplasmal and chlamydial pneumonia differ from typical bacteria causing pneumonia?
3. What are the three primary deep mycoses affecting the respiratory system?
4. What individuals are at risk for *Pneumocystis carinii* pneumonia (PCP)?
5. Why is immunization not a practical approach for the prevention of the common cold?

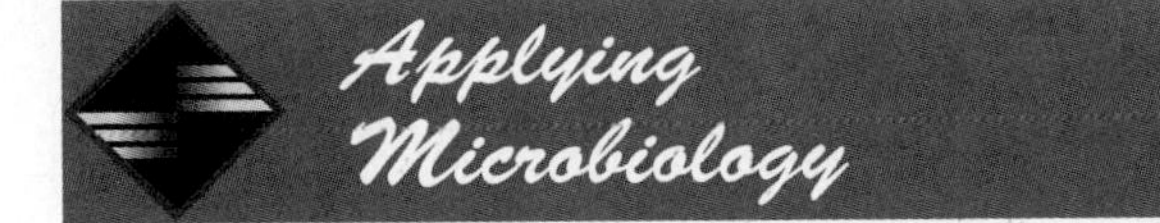

Read the following case study carefully and answer the questions: A 68-year-old man with a sore throat was seen at a Los Angeles County Health Department Clinic. He complained of a sore throat and some difficulty in breathing. Questioning revealed that the man had no history of immunizations. When a pharyngeal pseudomembrane was discovered, a culture from membrane fragments was taken, and the patient was referred to the Los Angeles County–USC Medical Center. A slender, non–spore-forming, pleomorphic gram-positive bacillus was cultured. The Elek test for toxigenicity was positive.

6. The clinical symptoms and laboratory findings are consistent with a diagnosis of
   a. strep throat
   b. rubella
   c. legionellosis
   d. diphtheria
   e. pneumonia
7. The etiologic agent was
   a. *Streptococcus pyogenes*
   b. *Legionella pneumophila*
   c. *Haemophilus influenzae*
   d. *Corynebacterium diphtheriae*
   e. *Listeria monocytogenes*
8. The disease could have been prevented by administration of a preparation known as
   a. Td
   b. BCG
   c. DEV
   d. HIG
   e. OPV
9. The ability of particular strains of this organism to cause disease is associated with a process known as
   a. conjugation
   b. zygotic induction
   c. lysogenic conversion
   d. transformation
   e. serological conversion
10. A frequent complication of this type of pharyngitis is
    a. rheumatic fever
    b. heart dysfunction
    c. acute glomerulonephritis
    d. persistent skin lesions
    e. Graves' disease

Chapter 17

Diseases of the Gastrointestinal Tract

Chapter Outline

- **BACTERIAL DISEASES**
  - Dental Caries
  - Gingivitis and Periodontal Disease
  - Salmonelloses
  - Shigellosis (Bacillary Dysentery)
  - Travelers' Diarrhea
  - Bloody Diarrhea
  - Cholera
  - Campylobacteriosis
  - Peptic Ulcers
  - Gastrointestinal Yersiniosis
  - Pseudomembranous Colitis
  - Staphylococcal Food Poisoning
  - Botulism
  - Perfringens Food Poisoning
  - Halophilic Vibrio Poisoning and Infection
- **VIRAL INFECTIONS**
  - Mumps
  - Cytomegalovirus Infection
  - Hepatitis
- **ALGAL AND FUNGAL TOXIN-ASSOCIATED DISEASE**
- **PROTOZOAL INFECTIONS**
  - Amebiasis (Amebic Dysentery)
  - Giardiasis
  - Balantidiasis
  - Cryptosporidiosis
  - Cyclosporiasis

Learning Objectives

After you have read this chapter, you should be able to:

1. List the genera of major microorganisms that colonize the gastrointestinal tract.
2. Discuss the causes and prevention of dental caries and periodontal disease.
3. Differentiate between a food infection and a food poisoning.
4. List the major viruses causing infections of the gastrointestinal tract and their target organs.
5. Describe the primary features of protozoal infections of the gastrointestestinal tract.
6. List methods that can be used to prevent gastrointestinal disease while traveling in Third World countries.

The gastrointestinal tract, or alimentary canal, is a continuous tube that begins with the mouth, includes part of the pharynx, esophagus, stomach, small intestine, large intestine, and ends with the anus. The accessory organs are the teeth, tongue, salivary glands, liver, gallbladder, and pancreas (Fig. 17–1).

The gastrointestinal tract and its accessory organs are responsible for the processes of digestion of food, absorption of nutrients, and elimi-

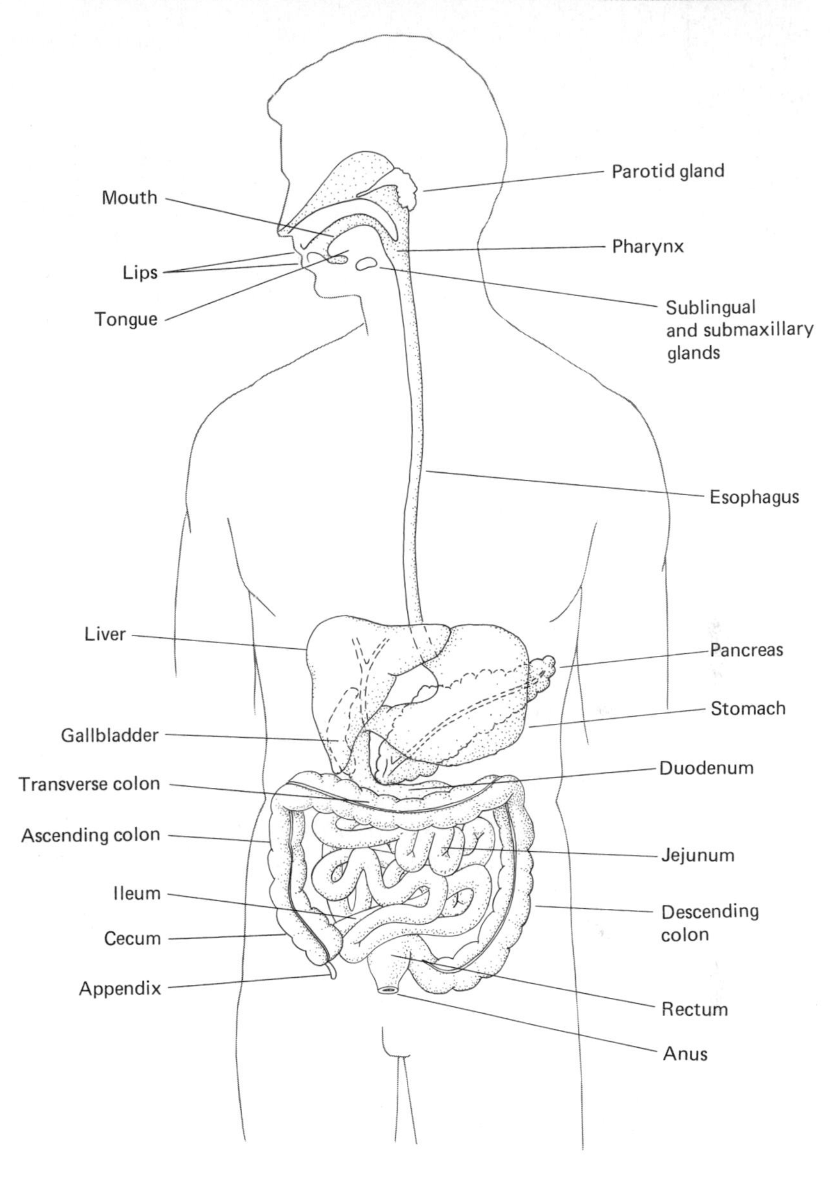

Figure 17–1 ◆ Organs of the gastrointestinal tract and accessory organs of digestion.

nation of undigested food. Some organs that lie outside the alimentary canal contribute to the processes by secretion or storage of digestive juices. The salivary glands, liver, gallbladder, pancreas, and their secretions are normally sterile; the mouth, esophagus, stomach, small intestine, and large intestine are contaminated soon after birth.

We are usually not aware of the large numbers of microorganisms that enter the mouth with food. Saliva contains solubilized buffers that keep the oral cavity close to neutral despite highly acid or alkaline contents of foods. It has been estimated that saliva contains approximately 1 billion bacteria per milliliter. That count does not take into consideration bacteria that attach to epithelial surfaces of the mouth or gingiva or those that prefer the surfaces of the teeth for colonization. Crevices and pits of the teeth provide environments where oxidation-reduction potentials are low enough to support the growth of obligate anaerobes. Both aerobic and anaerobic gram-positive cocci are abundant in the mouth. Gram-negative cocci belonging to the genus *Moraxella* frequently colonize the mucous membranes of the oropharynx. Of the anaerobic organisms, species of the genus *Bacteroides, Prevotella,* and *Veillonella* are common isolates of oropharyngeal secretions.

Gram-positive bacilli of the genus *Lactobacillus* colonize the oral cavity soon after birth; they may be homofermentative or heterofermentative. The homofermentative strains produce lactic acid, while heterofermentative strains produce alcohol, acetic acid, and carbon dioxide in addition to lactic acid.

Filamentous branched forms of anaerobes belonging to the genus *Actinomyces* are also common in the oral cavity, growing on or near dental plaque. Their numbers are usually few enough to present no difficulty (Fig. 17–2).

The oral spirochetes are common inhabitants in adults with normal **dentition,** but their prevalence increases to nearly 100 percent as gingival recession occurs. A competitive environment keeps the oral spirochetes from attacking mucosa of the oropharynx. Fusobacteria, spirilla, vibrios, and mycoplasmas are also common oral residents.

Candida albicans is the most prominent permanent fungal resident of the oral cavity. It occurs in approximately one-half of the general population. It is more common among women than men. Colonization of the protozoan *Entamoeba gingivalis* is equally prevalent in mouths of men and women; the trophozoites are found in approximately one-tenth of clean, healthy mouths. *E. gingivalis* forms no cysts (Fig. 17–3).

The stomach does not harbor many viable microorganisms. Most bacteria cannot survive in the acid environment of the stomach. A few organisms can escape the bactericidal action of the

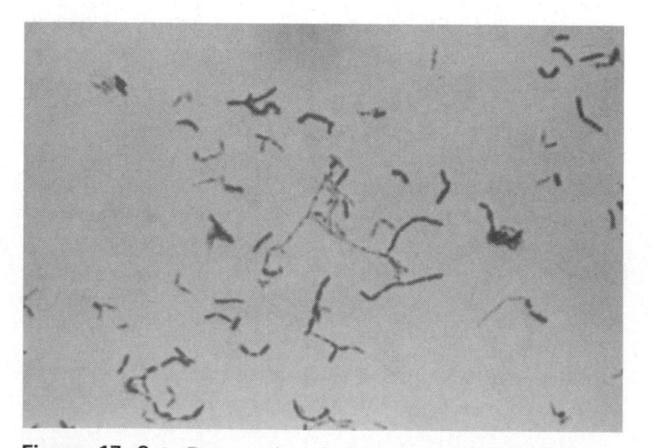

Figure 17–2 ◆ Gram stain of *Actinomyces odontolyticus* from the oral cavity. Members of the genus are gram-positive, filamentous bacilli.

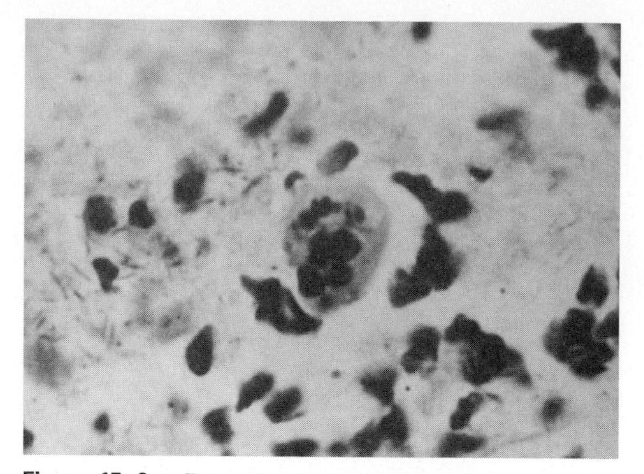

Figure 17–3 ◆ *Entamoeba gingivalis.* Although the ameba is found in approximately one-tenth of clean, healthy mouths, the organism can promote periodontal disease.

gastric juices by being enmeshed in food particles. They also may survive if a reflux of intestinal contents into the stomach occurs because of intestinal obstruction. Only then is alkalinity provided to promote the growth of bacteria of oropharyngeal origin.

Few bacteria colonize the upper part of the intestine, but the numbers increase progressively with distance from the duodenum to the colon. The jejunum may contain streptococci, lactobacilli, and diphtheroids. Small numbers of *Candida* also commonly reside in the small intestine. The yeasts flourish only when antibiotics that inhibit the growth of other enteric organisms are given orally. The formation of intestinal pouches, known as **diverticula,** permits proliferation of microorganisms in a protected environment (Fig. 17–4). Most individuals with diverticula are asymptomatic. However, diverticulosis can be hazardous should an inflammatory process develop which affects adjacent areas.

The colon constitutes a large fermentation vessel in which numbers of bacteria approximate 100 billion per gram of feces. Anaerobic gram-negative and gram-positive bacteria are the most abundant organisms. *Bacteroides, Prevotella,* and *Fusobacterium* species rank high in frequency of gram-negative bacilli found among microorganisms of the gastrointestinal tract. A gram-positive, anaerobic, spore-forming bacillus, *Clostridium perfringens,* colonizes the large intestine of approximately one-third of healthy individuals with no apparent harm, although this organism commonly causes infection in traumatized tissue.

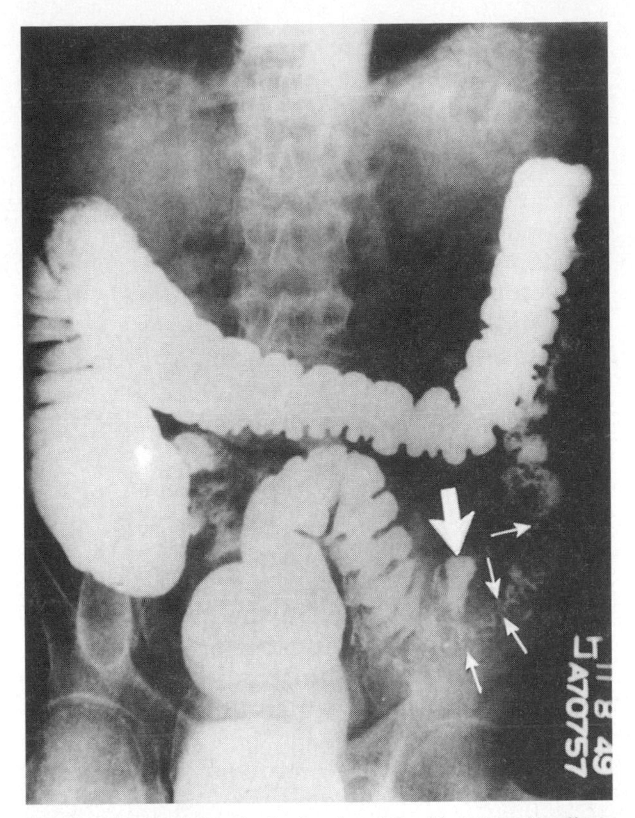

Figure 17–4 ◆ Diverticula in the sigmoid colon (small arrows). Extravasation of barium through a perforated diverticulum (large arrow).

Other *Clostridium* species are easily recoverable from stool specimens and have similar potentials for causing disease.

Species of *Peptostreptococcus* (anaerobic streptococci) and *Peptococcus* (anaerobic staphylococci) abound in the large intestine. Group D streptococci, including enterococci, are recoverable from stool specimens of all healthy individuals, but *S. aureus* in feces is usually associated with nasopharyngeal carriers. *Candida* species frequently colonize the large intestine. Both *S. aureus* and *Candida* species tend to flourish when antibiotic therapy destroys competing microorganisms.

Although the ratio of facultative, anaerobic gram-negative bacilli to obligate anaerobes is 1:300 in the large intestine, attention has been focused on the facultative gram-negative bacilli for many years. *Escherichia coli,* for example, is universally recoverable from stool specimens of healthy individuals. *Klebsiella, Enterobacter, Proteus,* and *Pseudomonas* species, all gram-negative bacilli, also can be found in the intestinal **microbiota.** The ubiquity of microorganisms and the basic human need for food and water make it impossible to avoid disease-producing organisms.

Bacteria cause disease by the effects of preformed toxin ingested with food or by actual colonization of organisms within the intestinal tract. Once established, some bacteria secrete enterotoxins that interfere with intestinal tract functions. Preformed toxins are the cause of diseases classified as food poisonings, such as botulism and staphylococcal food poisoning. Cholera, bacillary dysentery, and the salmonelloses are more appropriately called infections.

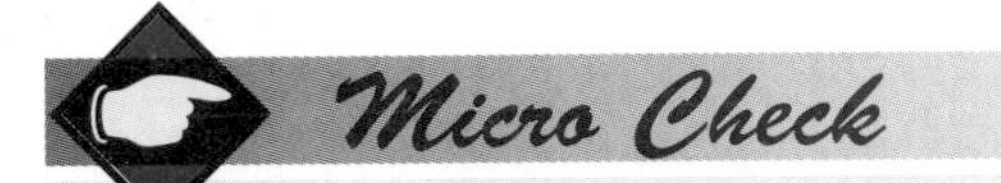

- ◆ What accounts for the high microbial counts in saliva?
- ◆ Why is gastric juice not a suitable culture medium for microorganisms?
- ◆ Why is it impossible to prevent pathogens from entering the gastrointestinal tracts?

BACTERIAL DISEASES

The diseases caused by bacteria range from dental caries and periodontal disease to diarrheal disease. Dental caries and periodontal disease are largely preventable by attention to diet and by the practice of good oral hygiene. The prevention of diarrheal disease is more complex. Several geographic and socioeconomic factors play roles as determinants of gastroenteric disease in particular populations. Diarrheal disease caused by bacteria is still a major cause of illness and death, particularly in developing countries without access to safe drinking water. The prevalence of certain parasitic diseases in Third World countries causes persons in those areas to be more susceptible to bacteria as secondary invaders. The incidence of enteric disease caused by bacterial pathogens tends to be higher in tropical than in temperate climates, but just as people travel with greater ease than a few decades ago, so do the bacteria that cause human infections. Whatever the geographic factors, the availability of clean water, adequate sewage disposal, and a balanced diet influence the incidence of enteric disease more than the climate.

Dental Caries

Dental caries, or tooth decay, has a complex etiology. Unlike many infectious diseases, it cannot be attributed to the presence of a single bacterium in the mouth. Genetics, diet, and oral hygiene also contribute to the production of dental caries. The role of diet in the development of dental caries was attributed by Aristotle to tooth damage from small particles of figs lodged between the teeth. Figs are not, of course, uniquely responsible for tooth decay. The incidence of dental caries is related to the amount and frequency of sugar intake. Sucrose is considered to be more **cariogenic** (caries-producing) than other sugars, but other fermentable carbohydrates are also cariogenic.

A number of bacteria indigenous to the mouth can ferment carbohydrates, but most attention has been focused on *Streptococcus mutans.* It is likely that other streptococci and lactobacilli contribute to tooth decay. Frequent brushing, flossing, and professional cleaning to remove the bacteria which adhere to the surface of the teeth as **dental plaque** are important in reducing the potential for dental caries (Fig. 17–5).

Dental caries are characterized by gradual and localized demineralizations of tooth enamel and destruction of **dentin** and **cementum.** *S. mutans* is believed to have a major role in destroying enamel surfaces of teeth. Not only do the streptococci adhere to one another and other bacteria, but also produce acids which dissolve calcium. No drugs are available to treat tooth decay, but consumption of a balanced diet, and the limitation of sugar-containing food to mealtimes, combined with good oral hygiene can afford some protection against dental caries. Fluoridation of community water and addition of fluorides to toothpastes and powders has reduced tooth decay by as much as 50 to 60 percent in the last decade. A vaccine directed against *S. mutans,* currently under investigation, holds some promise for reducing the incidence of dental caries further.

Gingivitis and Periodontal Disease

Gingivitis is an inflammation of the gums associated with the accumulation of dental plaque on tooth surfaces. If the periodontal membrane and bone are involved, it leads to **periodontal disease.** Streptococci, spirochetes, corynebacteria, and filamentous bacteria belonging to the genus *Actinomyces* may have roles in establishing the inflammatory process.

The degenerative process often begins with an inflammation of the gums with gradual tissue destruction, bone resorption, and loss of teeth. Unlike dental caries, nutrition appears to have a modifying rather than an initiating role in the development of disease.

Some inflammatory processes of tissues supporting the teeth may require use of antibiotics, such as penicillin or tetracycline. Attention to oral hygiene and consumption of a nutritionally balanced diet helps to maintain the integrity of the supporting tissues of teeth. Toothpastes that contain fluoride are responsible for hardening of the enamel, thereby providing protection from acids. It hardens enamel thereby providing pro-

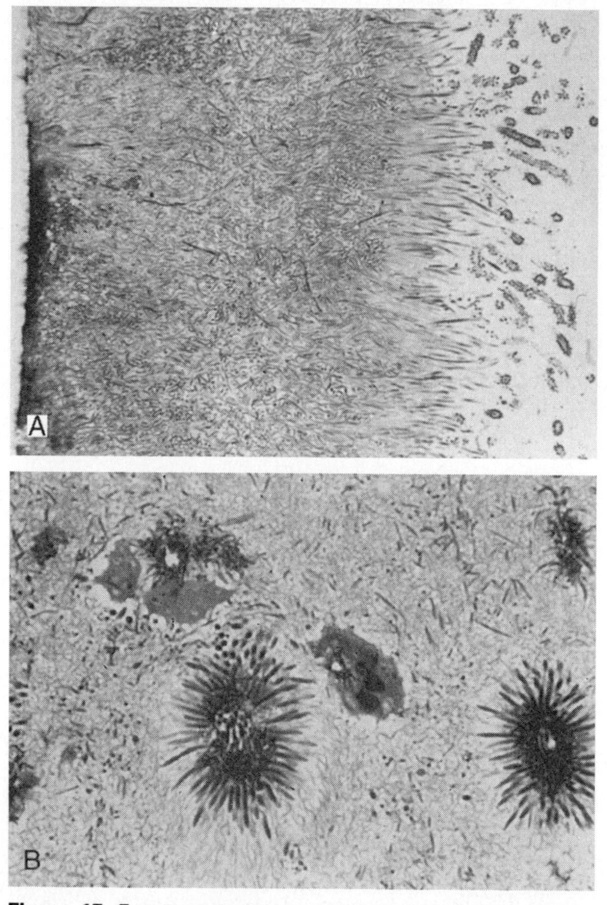

Figure 17–5 ◆ Dental plaque. *A,* Supragingival plaque showing dense, predominately filamentous bacterial mass in "corncob" formations adherent to the enamel surface. *B,* Cross section through "test-tube" formations of subgingival plaque. The adherent flora are less filamentous than the supragingival plaque.

tection from acids. Vaccines against strains of *S. mutans* may one day eliminate this most common bacterial infection.

Salmonelloses

The widespread dissemination of salmonellas makes them among the most prominent of the enteric pathogens. Domestic fowl constitute the largest single reservoir of salmonellas, but other domestic and wild animals also harbor the organisms. Human *Salmonella* infections, or salmonelloses, produce three forms of disease: enteric fever, gastroenteritis, and a septicemia. It has recently become acceptable to consider three species of *Salmonella* as the etiologic agents: *S. typhi* is the cause of the enteric fever known as typhoid; *S. choleraesuis* and *S. enteritidis* both cause gastroenteritis. Septicemia is observed with infections caused by both *S. typhi* and *S. choleraesuis*. The multiple serotypes of salmonellas are considered to be antigenic variations of *S. enteritidis*. Although approximately 1800 serotypes of *S. enteritidis* have been identified, most human disease in the United States is caused by eight subspecies (Table 17–1).

Table 17–1

COMMON ETIOLOGIC AGENTS OF SALMONELLOSIS IN HUMANS

ORGANISM	REPRESENTATIVE SUBSPECIES	MAJOR HUMAN DISEASE
Salmonella choleraesuis	*arizonae* *choleraesuis*	Septicemia
Salmonella typhi		Typhoid fever
Salmonella enteritidis	*paratyphi A.* *schottmuelleri* *dublin* *typhimurium* *enteritidis* *newport*	Gastroenteritis

The salmonellas are transmitted indirectly by contaminated poultry, eggs, meat, and water or directly by the fecal-oral route. In recent years eggs have been incriminated more frequently as sources of salmonellas. In a recent study most people contracted the pathogens in a restaurant, at a banquet, or in a hospital setting. Domestic pets, including cats, birds, dogs, and even turtles and iguanas, host a wide variety of salmonellas. Although fruits and vegetables are not usually vehicles for *Salmonella* transmission, cantaloupes and tomatoes have been implicated. Any fruit or vegetable grown on the ground may be contaminated with soil or animal wastes. If produce is not thoroughly washed, the numbers of organisms present may increase upon incubation on a salad bar even at room temperature. Undetected carriers of typhoid may unknowingly spread the disease.

FOCAL POINT

The Notorious Typhoid Mary

Have you ever wondered about the true identity of the notorious Typhoid Mary? Typhoid Mary was an Irish woman named Mary Mallon, who worked as a cook in homes in New York state in the early 1900s. She contracted typhoid in 1901, recovered, and became a carrier for the etiological agent. Everywhere that Mary went, outbreaks of typhoid were sure to follow. It is likely that the true numbers for morbidity and mortality from typhoid for which Mary was responsible were never recorded. Mary changed jobs frequently to avoid the investigations by public health authorities of households where typhoid occurred. When the New York City Health Department finally caught up with her, she refused to provide a stool sample for testing as a possible carrier of typhoid. That refusal caused her to be forcibly confined to a hospital for testing. Typhoid bacilli were found in the stool samples, and the source was a bacilli colonization in her gallbladder. Surgical removal was the only option in 1907. Mary refused to have surgery and was sent to prison. She was released and promised never to work as a cook again. Mary broke that promise and took a job as a cook in a hospital. An outbreak of typhoid soon occurred, but Mary walked off her job before a member of the health department arrived to investigate the outbreak. When she was located, she was quarantined for life in a hospital on an island in the East River. She died there at the age of 70 in 1938, but the story of Typhoid Mary lives on.

Nausea, abdominal cramps, fever, and diarrhea typically occur within 12 to 36 hours after ingestion of contaminated food or water in salmonelloses other than typhoid fever. The incubation time in typhoid fever may be up to two weeks. Diarrhea may be absent, but the fever is often high and of long duration.

Salmonellas can be recovered from stool or blood during the acute phase of disease. *S. typhi* can sometimes be isolated from urine during peak periods of bacteremia. Direct microscopic examination for the gram-negative bacilli is of no value since they are indistinguishable from nonpathogens.

The salmonellas grow on bismuth sulfite agar, MacConkey's agar, and in enteric enrichment broths. A fluorescent reagent can be used to flood plates of H_2S-positive colonies. Fluorescence occurs in the presence of the enzyme C8 esterase. Biochemical properties are used for identification, but serological confirmation is required. The more common salmonellas belong to one of six serological types (groups A, B, C, C_1, D, or E). A probe for a nucleotide, associated with the most virulent strains of *S. enteritidis,* can detect salmonellas in water and food.

The drug of choice for typhoid fever is chloramphenicol, but it must be used with some caution because of toxic side effects. Drug susceptibility tests often reveal multiple-drug resistance, but are valuable in finding alternative drugs for treatment. Other salmonelloses do not usually require antibiotic therapy. Replacement of fluids and electrolytes may be necessary if diarrhea has been profuse or persists.

The salmonellas are killed by exposure to a temperature of 68°C (145°F). Immunization with killed typhoid bacilli is recommended for travelers to endemic areas, for household contacts of carriers, and for laboratory personnel. Vaccines for other salmonellas have not proved to be effective in prevention of gastroenteritis or septicemia.

Shigellosis (Bacillary Dysentery)

The shigellas, unlike the salmonellas, are found only in humans. The species of *Shigella* are represented by four major serological types. Although all shigellas produce a common endotoxin, a potent neurotoxin is elaborated by *Shigella dysenteriae,* type 1, as an exotoxin. *S. sonnei* is the most prevalent cause of bacillary dysentery in the United States. Most bacillary dysentery is transmitted by contaminated water, milk, and food. Both flies and food handlers have been incriminated in the spread of the disease. However, documented cases of sexual transmission are increasing in incidence among homosexual men. More aggressive searches for means of enteric disease-transmission may reveal that other enteric infections can spread sexually.

Shigellosis, or bacillary dysentery, is characterized by an onset of abdominal cramps, fever, and diarrhea one to four days after ingestion of the organisms. Blood and mucus are almost always present in stool specimens. The large numbers of white blood cells in the feces distinguish bacillary dysentery from amebic dysentery, which is discussed later in this chapter.

Unlike the salmonellas, shigellas can be iso-

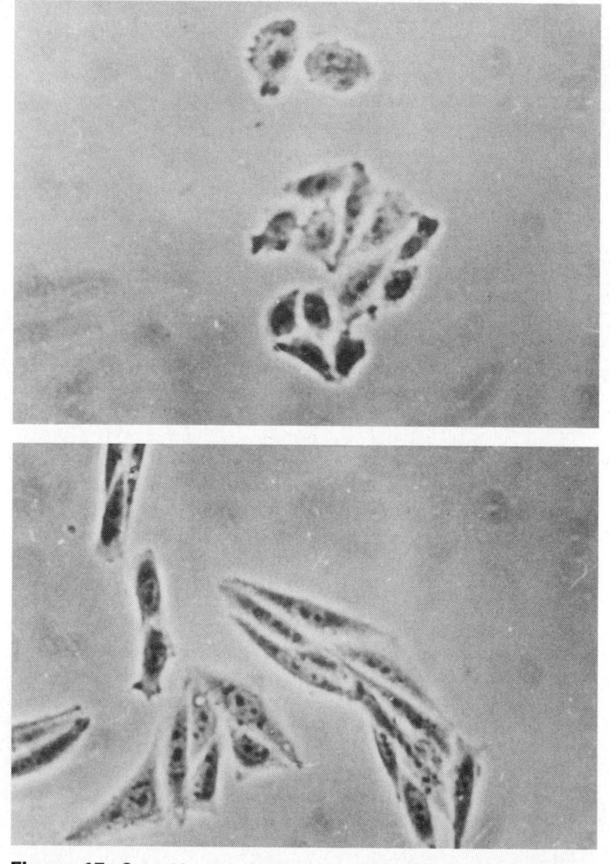

Figure 17–6 ◆ Chinese hamster ovary (CHO) cells 24 hours after exposure to the culture filtrate of nontoxigenic *Escherichia coli* (top) and enterotoxigenic *Escherichia coli* (bottom). The cells exposed to heat-labile toxin (LT) appear elongated and no longer possess knoblike projections.

lated only from stool specimens during the acute phase of disease. Direct microscopic examination is of no value, but the organisms will grow on MacConkey's agar. Identification depends on biochemical tests and serological typing. Shigellas belong to one of four serological types (groups A, B, C, or D).

Shigellosis is usually a self-limiting infection, but ampicillin and trimethoprim-sulfamethoxazole are drugs of choice in severe infections. It is important to perform antibiotic susceptibility tests since multiresistant strains are isolated with increasing frequency. Replacement of fluids and electrolytes may be required if dehydration is present.

Travelers' Diarrhea

One of the least appealing aspects of international travel, particularly in developing countries, is the probability of experiencing diarrheal disease. It is estimated that approximately half of all persons traveling in Third World countries get travelers' diarrhea.

One of the most frequent causes of travelers' diarrhea is enterotoxin-producing strains of *Escherichia coli.* Two enterotoxins, a heat-labile toxin (LT) and a heat-stable toxin (ST) have been identified. Some toxigenic strains produce both enterotoxins. A cytotoxin-producing strain has also been isolated. The enterotoxin-producing strain of *E. coli* is transmitted by contaminated food and water. It is likely that flies may spread the organisms. Careful attention in selection of beverages and food can reduce the risk of developing travelers' diarrhea.

The diarrheal disease is characterized by an abrupt onset of watery diarrhea, nausea, vomiting, fever, chills, and cramps, within 48 hours of ingestion of an infective dose of an enterotoxin-producing strain of *E. coli.* The disease is usually self-limiting in two to three days, but fluid and electrolyte therapy may be required in severe cases.

The toxin-producing strains of *E. coli* are indistinguishable from indigenous strains of the organism by the usual laboratory methods (Color Plate 55). An enzyme-linked immunosorbent assay (ELISA) or tissue cultures may be used to demonstrate LT (Fig. 17–6). An ELISA or an immunodiffusion test has largely replaced the suckling mouse assay once required to confirm the presence of ST. The ST promotes the loss of intestinal fluid in the animals. Serotyping of *E. coli* is reserved for epidemic forms of travelers' diarrhea.

Bismuth subsalicylate, the active ingredient of Pepto-Bismol, is effective in mild cases. If symptoms persist, treatment with trimethoprim-sulfamethoxazole may be indicated. Treatment of water to be used for drinking or cooking with a dilute solution of chlorine or tincture of iodine can prevent travelers' diarrhea (Table 17–2).

FOCAL POINT

Good News for Travelers: Hold the Pepto-Bismol

The most common cause of diarrhea in travelers to developing countries are strains of enterotoxigenic *Escherichia coli* (ETEC). Both a heat labile (HL) toxin and a heat-stable (HS) toxin have been incriminated in the travelers' disease. The HL toxin is closely related to the toxin produced by the cholera organism in antigenicity and mode of action. A recent trial of a cholera vaccine in Bangladesh was found to also protect persons from ETEC diarrhea for at least three months. Although the vaccine was deficient in producing long-term immunity, it may have use in protecting travelers visiting developing countries for less than three months. A research team from Finland reported protection of 23 percent from ETEC diarrhea among 615 travelers to Morocco and a 71 percent protection for infections with ETEC and other enteric pathogens.

Lancet 338:1285, 1991.

Bloody Diarrhea

Shiga-like toxin-producing *E. coli* (SLTEC) are well recognized causes of bloody and nonbloody diarrhea. *E. coli* 0157:H7 is the most common isolate, but a strain designated as 0104:H21 has also been implicated. Eating improperly cooked hamburgers and drinking raw milk have been implicated as primary means of transmission in several outbreaks. Healthy cattle may serve as a

Table 17–2
TREATMENT OF WATER WITH CHLORINE OR TINCTURE OF IODINE

TREATMENT	DROPS PER QUART OR LITER	
	CLEAR WATER	CLOUDY WATER
Chlorine solution*		
1%	10	20
4–6%	2	4
7–10%	1	2
Unknown	10	20
Tincture of iodine, 2%	5	10

*Most chlorine bleach solutions have 4 to 6 percent available chlorine. Water treated with chlorine or iodine should be allowed to stand for 30 minutes before using. Water treated with chlorine is less reliable than that treated with iodine.

reservoir for SLTEC. The disease usually begins with watery diarrhea and severe abdominal cramps within hours of ingesting the toxin produced by the bacterium. The toxin resembles one produced by a *Shigella* species. Blood may appear in the stool one to eight days later. A serious complication of *E. coli* 0157:H7 infections is kidney failure. The kidney disease is known to cause death in very young or elderly patients. Asymptomatic infections are known to occur.

Screening for the *E. coli* 0157:H7 can be done by inoculating MacConkey-sorbitol agar with stool specimens. *E. coli* 0157:H7 does not ferment sorbitol. Sorbitol-negative colonies can be selected for further study. An antiserum is available that will agglutinate *E. coli* 0157:H7. More sophisticated studies, including DNA probes or animal studies, can be used to identify the toxin. Although the organism appears to be susceptible to most antibiotics, drug therapy is not usually beneficial. Replacement of fluid and electrolytes as well as blood transfusions may be necessary.

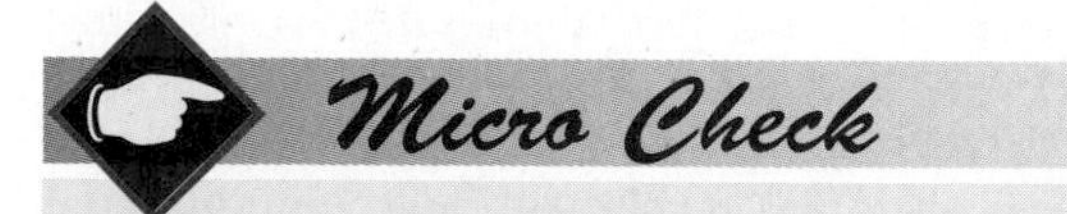

- What specimens may be required for the diagnosis of a salmonellosis?
- Why is it particularly inadvisable to give a young infant or an elderly person food containing raw eggs?
- How can you explain a failure to isolate shigellas from a suspected case of shigellosis?

Cholera

Cholera, like shigellosis, has been described in humans only. It is endemic in Asia and India, but also occurs sporadically in other parts of the world. An epidemic of major proportion was reported in Peru and neighboring countries in 1991. The etiologic agent, *Vibrio cholerae,* multiplies rapidly in the intestinal tract and ruptures, releasing a potent enterotoxin and an enzyme, neuraminidase.

The vibrios of cholera are spread by the fecal-oral route, most often by contaminated water, raw or partially cooked fish or shellfish, or uncooked vegetables. Illness typically occurs within two to three days, but can be experienced after only a few hours. An English physician, John Snow, first recognized the role of "spoiled water" in 1854 as the mode of transmission for cholera. He succeeded in controlling the spread of the disease by removing the handle of London's Broad Street pump (see Fig. 11–1).

Cholera is characterized by a sudden onset of vomiting and profuse watery stools with rapid dehydration, acidosis, and possible circulatory collapse resulting in death. In severe cases, as much as 15 percent of the body weight can be lost in just a few hours. Replacement of lost fluid and electrolytes is important in cholera.

Darkfield microscopy of stool can be used to detect the vibrios of cholera (Fig. 17–7). Thiosulfate citrate bile salts (TCBS) agar is the plating medium of choice. An enrichment broth of alkaline peptone water adjusted to a pH of 9.0 inhibits the growth of other enteric pathogens and

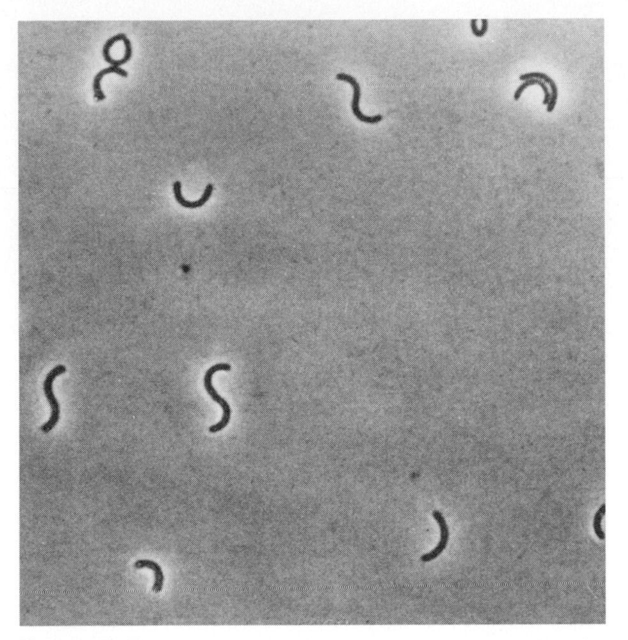

Figure 17–7 ◆ Appearance of *Vibrio cholerae* observed under the dark-field microscope.

coliforms. A slide agglutination test using cholera antiserum is available for confirming the identification of *V. cholerae.*

Tetracycline is the drug of choice except in Tanzania and Bangladesh, where tetracycline-resistant strains have been recovered. With prompt treatment, the fatality rate is less than 1 percent. A vaccine, consisting of heat-killed vibrios, administered in two doses provides only temporary immunity. Cholera vaccination is not recommended routinely, as it has been shown to provide immunity in only about half of those who receive it. The discovery of *V. cholerae* in the marshes along the Gulf of Mexico in the United States has revived interest in cholera, which was once considered a foreign or an imported disease.

Campylobacteriosis

Enteric campylobacteriosis is rivaling the salmonelloses as a cause of sporadic bacterial diarrhea. The most frequent cause of the enteric form of campylobacteriosis is the gram-negative vibrio *Campylobacter jejuni* (Fig. 17–8). The pathogen is cosmopolitan in that it is found in both tropical and temperate areas. The organism has been isolated from the intestines of a variety of domestic and wild animals. About 40 percent of dairy cattle harbor the organism in their intestinal tracts. The 43°C body temperature of many birds is close to the optimal growth temperature of the organism. *C. jejuni* persists in poultry processed for market. Improperly cooked poultry, hot dogs, raw milk, and contaminated water have been implicated as sources of the vibrio. Person-to-person transmission can also occur.

Classic symptoms of enteric campylobacteriosis include fever, abdominal pain, and bloody diarrhea. The two- to five-day incubation period is longer than that for the salmonelloses. The disease is usually self-limiting, but arthritis may occur as a complication in children.

Optimal environmental conditions for the recovery of *C. jejuni* include a temperature of 42°C and an atmosphere containing 5 to 10 percent CO_2 and oxygen in a concentration no greater than 6 percent. A special hydrogen and CO_2–generating envelope for providing that atmosphere in a GasPak jar is available commercially. Several selective plating agars containing reducing salts and antibiotics, such as Campy-BAP, are available. A battery of biochemical tests can be used for species identification. An RNA probe can identify *C. jejuni.* The drug of choice is erythromycin if symptoms are severe or persist.

Peptic Ulcers

One of the surprising discoveries of the last decade has been the infectious nature of peptic ulcers. Once thought to be associated with a stressful life-style, often accompanied by smoking

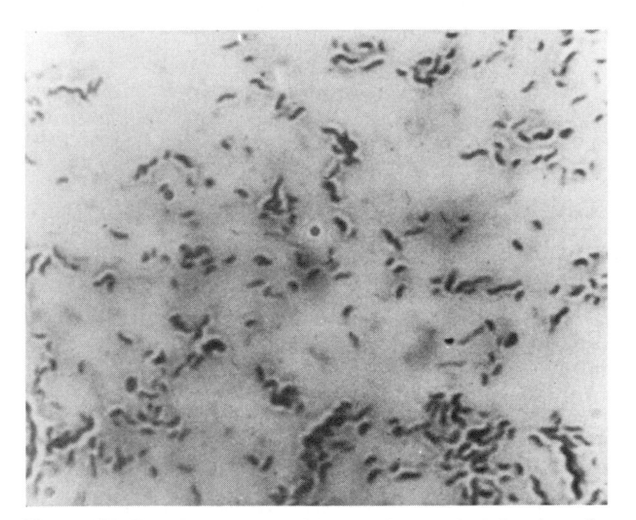

Figure 17–8 ◆ Gram stain of *Campylobacter jejuni* showing pleomorphic forms.

and alcohol consumption, it is actually caused by a gram-negative vibrio, *Helicobacter pylori,* in 70 to 90 percent of the cases. The disease, once considered chronic, consists of ulceration of the gastric mucosa or any part of the gastrointestinal tract coming into contact with gastric juices. The presence of the vibrios in the gastric mucosa causes an increase in mucus secretion and makes the mucosa more vulnerable to damage. The bacteria may be protected from effects of acidity because they produce the enzyme urease, which catalyzes the liberation of ammonia from urea. The urease may also destroy cells lining the gastrointestinal tract. It is not uncommon for perforation of the intestinal wall and subsequent peritonitis to occur. Symptoms usually include pain one to three hours after eating and often nausea, vomiting, and halitosis. Weight loss is often a long-term consequence of prolonged infection.

A noninvasive **urea breath test** (UBT) has gained popularity in screening persons for gastric urease. One hour after ingestion of ^{14}C-labeled urea, the breath is analyzed for the presence of $^{14}CO_2$. The amount of labeled CO_2 is proportional to the magnitude of the *H. pylori* infection. IgG antibodies to *H. pylori* may be elevated in infections, but test results are difficult to evaluate. For reasons not completely understood, antibody levels are sometimes higher in the absence of symptoms.

Peptic ulcers can be successfully treated by inhibiting gastric acid secretion, and by eliminating the presence of *H. pylori* with appropriate antibiotics.

Gastrointestinal Yersiniosis

Gastrointestinal yersiniosis appears to have been a disease of the twentieth century, but its presence may have been obscured by preoccupation of microbiologists with shigellosis and the salmonelloses. The most common etiologic agent is *Yersinia enterocolitica,* which is widely distributed in the environment and in a variety of domestic and wild animals. It produces a heat-stable (ST) enterotoxin which is unaffected by a temperature of 100°C for 20 minutes. If the organisms are present in sufficient numbers, some can survive heat-processing. Ingestion of improperly cooked pork and raw milk have been implicated in outbreaks of the enteric disease. Children and young adults appear to be more susceptible than mature healthy adults.

Gastrointestinal yersiniosis manifests itself as two distinct entities. A self-limiting diarrheal disease, indistinguishable from that produced by other pathogens, occurs within several days after ingestion of contaminated food. Stools are usually watery but do not contain blood or mucus. Symptoms typically disappear in five to 10 days.

A more serious illness of shorter duration closely resembles staphylococcal food poisoning. It begins with an abrupt onset of nausea, cramps, vomiting, and diarrhea. A fever is frequently present. The symptoms may subside within 24 hours or may precede extraintestinal infections. The mesenteric adenitis that occurs in some young adults may be confused with appendicitis.

Y. enterocolitica can usually be recovered by use of blood agar and most media selective for gram-negative bacilli. Confirmatory biochemical tests can differentiate strains of *Y. enterocolitica* from other species of *Yersinia.* Antibodies for specific serotypes are produced in acute gastrointestinal yersiniosis. In the United States, serotype 08 is the antigen of choice in testing for specific agglutinins.

Antibiotic susceptibility tests should be performed to determine the drug of choice because if septicemia develops prompt treatment is required. The enteric disease appears to run its course without the intervention of antibiotics, but fluid and electrolyte replacement may be necessary if diarrhea is severe.

Pseudomembranous Colitis

Pseudomembranous colitis is a serious intestinal disease that occurs as a complication of antibiotic therapy. It is caused by enterotoxins A and B elaborated by the indigenous anaerobe, *Clostridium difficile,* when administration of antibiotics reduces the numbers of competing intestinal microorganisms. Toxin A is responsible for most enterotoxic activity of *C. difficile,* whereas toxin B causes an impairment in the cytoskeleton of cells.

The enterotoxins cause sloughing of intestinal tissue, ulceration of mucosa, hemorrhaging, and plaques containing white blood cells, which are characteristic of pseudomembranous colitis. The disease is self-limiting in most individuals, but perforation of the colon can occur.

Gram stains of smears from individuals with pseudomembranous colitis reveal large numbers of polymorphonuclear white blood cells. Sometimes gram-positive bacilli with or without terminal spores can be seen. *C. difficile* will grow on prereduced fructose–egg yolk agar containing cycloserine and cefoxitin in a GasPak jar. A rapid latex agglutination procedure can identify toxin A in stool extracts. Vancomycin is the drug of choice, but most strains are susceptible also to penicillin and ampicillin.

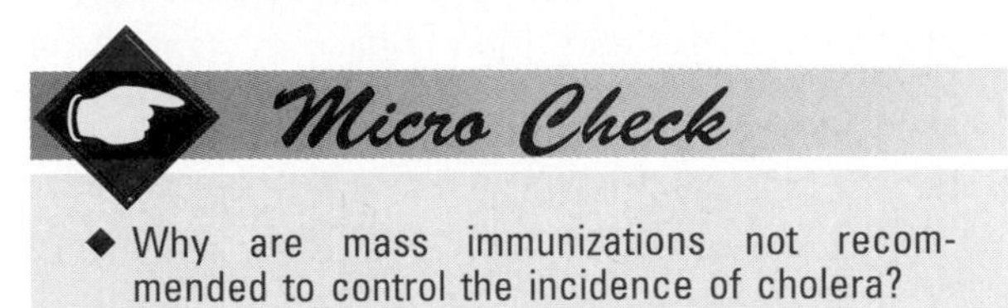

- Why are mass immunizations not recommended to control the incidence of cholera?
- What are two environmental requirements necessary for the isolation of campylobacters?
- What two forms of illness are caused by yersinias?

Staphylococcal Food Poisoning

It is important to differentiate between staphylococcal enteritis and staphylococcal food poisoning. The cocci are found in limited numbers in the gastrointestinal tract of healthy individuals. In the absence of effective competition by other indigenous flora, the staphylococci proliferate and produce sufficient enterotoxin to cause enteritis. Enterotoxin-producing staphylococci gain entrance to food from persons or animals with staphylococcal disease or from carriers of *Staphylococcus aureus.* The cocci grow especially well in dairy products, cream-filled pastries, custards, ham, sausage, and mayonnaise-containing salads or sandwich spreads. After contamination, food must stand at room temperature for several hours to permit sufficient growth of *S. aureus* for enterotoxin production.

Staphylococcal food poisoning is caused by ingestion of enough preformed enterotoxin to cause nausea, vomiting, and diarrhea. The symptoms usually occur two to six hours after eating contaminated food, but do not last longer than a day or two. Food poisoning was at one time referred to as *ptomaine poisoning.* Ptomaine is a nitrogenous product derived from putrefactive action of bacteria. The enterotoxin elaborated by certain strains of *S. aureus* is not a product of putrefaction, nor are other enterotoxins derived from bacterial metabolism. True ptomaine poisoning is probably rare, because evidence of putrefaction is usually recognizable by distinctly unpleasant odor or taste.

Samples of food or lesions on the skin of a food handler in suspected staphylococcal food poisoning may be cultured on blood agar or selective media, such as mannitol salt (MS) agar. The microscopic appearance of staphylococci is described in an Chapter 15. Strongly positive coagulase-producing staphylococci will cause normal plasma to coagulate within four hours. Not all coagulase-positive staphylococci produce enterotoxin, however. In order to incriminate staphylococci as etiologic agents, cultures should be sent to a public health laboratory so serological and phage typing can be performed. Replacement of fluid and electrolytes may be necessary. No antibiotic therapy is indicated. Storing of susceptible foods at temperatures below 4.4°C (40°F) is important in the prevention of staphylococcal food poisoning. Preformed toxin is not destroyed by the usual cooking temperatures. The enterotoxin can withstand boiling for 20 to 60 minutes. Individuals with suspected or diagnosed staphylococcal lesions should refrain from active involvement in preparing or serving food.

Botulism

Like staphylococcal food poisoning, botulism is not classified as an infection, but rather as an intoxication from a potent exotoxin of *Clostridium botulinum.* The effect of the toxin is not limited to the gastrointestinal tract, but botulism is included here because of the toxin's portal of entry. Most foodborne botulism outbreaks in the United States have been traced to home-processed foods in which heating has been inadequate to kill *C. botulinum* cells or to inactivate preformed botulinal toxin. A temperature of 100°C for 10 minutes is sufficient to destroy the toxin. Home-canned lamprey, beans, mushrooms, fermented salmon eggs, smoked fish, and commercially processed tuna fish and beef stew have been incriminated as sources for the neurotoxin in outbreaks of botulism. Honey has been implicated as a source for botulinal organisms in infant botulism.

When the exotoxin of *C. botulinum* is ingested, it is absorbed by the stomach and small intestine. The toxin disseminates within 18 to 36 hours and blocks release of acetylcholine by nerve fibers. Symptoms include facial paralysis, difficulty in speaking, muscle weakness, vertigo, double vision, nausea, vomiting, and respiratory failure. The high fatality rate for botulism, which approximates 20 to 30 percent in the United States, is related to the irreversible "fixing" of toxin to efferent nerve endings. Minute amounts of type A botulinum toxin are used for treatment of several neuromuscular disorders. The toxin effectively blocks the muscular responses to nerve impulses causing the dysfunctions.

Botulism has recently been reported as a "new disease" in infants with constipation and profound muscle weakness. The disease appears to be the result of intraintestinal production of toxin by *C. botulinum.* In most cases the source of the organisms remains a mystery. To date, all recognized cases of infant botulism have recovered without neurological complications.

A clinical entity called "wound botulism" has also been described in recent years in the United States. The spores of *C. botulinum,* abundant in soil, presumably gain entrance through a deep puncture wound. Neurological effects are evident only after sufficient time has elapsed to permit multiplication of the organisms. After four to 14 days, sufficient exotoxin may be produced to cause sensory disturbances in an affected extremity.

Botulism is usually diagnosed clinically on the basis of symptoms and recent history of consuming suspected food within the past several days. If samples of food are available they should be sent to a public health laboratory. Food extracts or serum from a patient can be injected intraperitoneally into mice. The mice exhibit neurological symptoms and die within several hours. Seven types of botulinum toxin have been identified, but most cases of botulism are caused by type A, B, or E toxin. If some mice are immunized with type A, B, or E toxin before being inoculated with suspected toxin, the serological type of the toxin can also be determined. An enzyme-linked coagulation assay (ELCA) can detect toxins A, B, and E from crude culture filtrates with the sensitivity of mice bioassays.

Treatment consists of trivalent ABE antitoxin. The antitoxin can neutralize only unbound toxin. Antibiotics are of little use, but penicillin may be of value for individuals with type E toxin–producing *C. botulinum.* Recovery is often delayed if neurological impairment is substantial. Mechanically assisted respiration may be required for an extended period of time. Wound botulism may require débridement of affected tissue.

Perfringens Food Poisoning

Perfringens food poisoning ranks second as a cause of food poisoning in the United States. Only *S. aureus* is responsible for more outbreaks of food poisoning than *Clostridium perfringens.* Contaminated meat or poultry products are responsible for most cases of perfringens food poisoning. Lack of attention to personal hygiene also contributes to the transmission of the *C. perfringens* from human sources. Five types of exotoxins have been identified, but only type A is associated with foodborne disease. The enterotoxin is synthesized during late stages of sporulation.

Abdominal pain, diarrhea, and nausea usually occur within eight to 12 hours after ingestion of contaminated food. Fever is usually absent. The illness does not usually last more than 24 hours.

A diagnosis of perfringens food poisoning can be established by culturing large numbers of *C. perfringens* from food samples or stool. Isolates must be typed serologically to confirm the presence of type A *C. perfringens.* Several commercially available assay kits are available. Quantitative analysis of food samples is sometimes performed by public health laboratories to support a diagnosis of this type of food poisoning.

No antibiotics are indicated, but fluid and electrolyte replacement may be necessary for infants or the elderly. Thorough cooking of foods containing meat or poultry and prompt refrigeration of unused portions can reduce the risk of perfringens food poisoning.

Halophilic Vibrio Poisoning and Infection

Facultative halophilic (salt-loving) vibrios have been associated with a type of food poisoning or infection in both Japan and the United States. The marine vibrio, *Vibrio parahaemolyticus,* is responsible for over 50 percent of food poisoning occurring during the summer months in Japan. Sushi, a vinegar-treated rice ball, topped with raw fish, is frequently implicated. An explosive watery diarrhea is a hallmark of the disease. At least three biotypes of *V. parahaemolyticus,* based on biochemical and antimicrobial susceptibility characteristics, have been recognized. A heat-stable (HS) toxin has been isolated from virulent strains of *V. parahaemolyticus,* but its role in producing diarrhea is not known.

In the United States halophilic vibrio infection is transmitted by ingestion of raw oysters or improperly cooked crab, shrimp, clams, or scallops. *V. vulnificus* thrives in warm sea water, particularly in the Gulf of Mexico. The halophilic bacterium causes a septicemia and is most often associated with consumption of raw oysters.

The onset of symptoms of halophilic vibrio poisoning or infection may be rapid or delayed as long as eight to 10 days after ingestion of contaminated seafood. All cases, except one in the United States, have originated in an ocean-bound state.

Direct microscopic examination of stool specimens or culturing of stool in suspected cases of halophilic vibrio poisoning or infection is not always recommended. The organism will grow on bromthymol blue "teepol" (BBT) or thiosulfate citrate bile salts sucrose (TCBS) agar or in alkaline peptone water adjusted to a pH of 9.4. Most enteric culture media do not contain sufficient salt for isolation of halophilic vibrios. Biochemical tests are required to identify pathogenic *Vibrio* species.

Specific antibiotic therapy is not usually recommended in *V. vulnificus* septicemia. Fluid and electrolyte replacement may be necessary. Control measures are aimed at keeping the numbers of marine vibrios or their products below the minimal infective dose in seafoods. However, it is impossible to rid the oceans of the pathogenic vibrios, and thus, eating raw fish should be avoided. Special care should be taken not to allow seafoods to stand at room temperature for long periods of time.

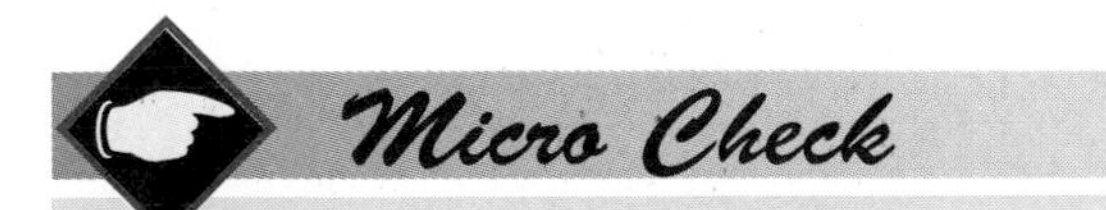

- How do the symptoms of staphylococcal food poisoning differ from those of botulism?
- What value does botulinal toxin have in treatment of neuromuscular disorders?
- Why do the usual culture media not support the growth of the halophilic vibrios?

VIRAL INFECTIONS

There is no doubt that the digestive system provides a major portal of entry for viruses. Several viruses are merely transient residents of the alimentary tract, but some become sequestered in crypts of the intestinal tract. If intestinal cells contain specific receptors, an infection can be established. Those that produce gastrointestinal disease are acid- and bile-tolerant.

Symptoms resulting from viral invasion of the gastrointestinal tract may resemble those arising from bacterial invasion or toxigenicity. In the absence of a specific bacterial etiologic agent, a virus is usually assumed to be the agent of disease. If symptoms are mild and recovery is rapid, the specific virus is almost never identified.

Rotavirus (reovirus) and the Norwalk virus (calicivirus), are the major causes of diarrheal disease. Rotaviruses account for at least one third of deaths in young children in developing countries. The Norwalk virus has been implicated as a cause of viral diarrhea in other children and adults in the United States. Vomiting may also be present. Rotavirus infections are sometimes called "stomach flu." Influenza, or "flu" as we are prone to call it, is a respiratory disease usually not characterized by diarrhea or vomiting. There is no such disease as stomach flu. Replacement of fluids and electrolytes may be needed in severe cases. Rotaviruses and Norwalk-like agents may be detected by several immunoassays and PCR techniques. An oral, live, tetravalent, rhesus-based rotavirus vaccine (RRV-TV) is licensed for infants in the United States. The recommended three doses are given at 2, 4, and 6 months of age. Many other viruses cause asymptomatic infections, but others cause more serious disease of accessory digestive organs or even other systems (Table 17–3).

Mumps

Mumps is an acute viral infection that usually affects the parotid gland. It is caused by a paramyxovirus that is able to multiply in the upper respiratory tract before it enters the bloodstream. The virus is transmitted by oral or respiratory secretions from an infected individual.

The symptoms do not usually appear for two to three weeks after exposure to the virus. The swelling is accompanied by a fever, a headache, and generalized muscle aches. Typically only one parotid gland exhibits swelling early in the disease (Fig. 17–9). Later bilateral involvement is common. The virus can spread and affect a variety of organs including the brain. **Orchitis** (inflammation of a testicle) is a common complication occurring in 20 to 25 percent of adult males. It sometimes causes atrophy of the testicle and subsequent sterility. About one-third of persons having mumps are asymptomatic or experience only mild respiratory symptoms.

Mumps is usually diagnosed clinically, but the

Table 17–3
MAJOR GROUPS AND SEROTYPES OF GASTROINTESTINAL VIRUSES

VIRUS	SEROTYPES	MAJOR DISEASE
Calicivirus		
Norwalk virus		Enteritis, Norwalk virus syndrome
Picornavirus		
Coxsackievirus	A1–123, B1–6	Undifferentiated febrile disease
Echovirus	1–31	Enteritis, epidemic diarrhea
Enterovirus	1–69	Gastroenteritis, hepatitis A
Hepadnavirus	1–4	Hepatitis B
Herpesvirus		
Cytomegalovirus	1–2	Cytomegalovirus infection, inapparent infection
Reovirus		
Rotavirus	1–5	Gastroenteritis
Flaviviruses	Unknown	Hepatitis C

virus can be isolated from saliva, urine, and sometimes cerebrospinal fluid (CSF), and grows in embryonated eggs, or in tissue cultures. Serological tests are used to identify the virus in cell cultures. A number of serological tests are available to detect antibodies to the mumps virus.

Mumps is usually a self-limiting disease, but supportive therapy may be helpful. There is no specific antiviral drug. Mumps is becoming a rare disease since the introduction of an attenuated mumps vaccine. The vaccine may be administered at any time after 12 months of age, but is ineffective after exposure has occurred.

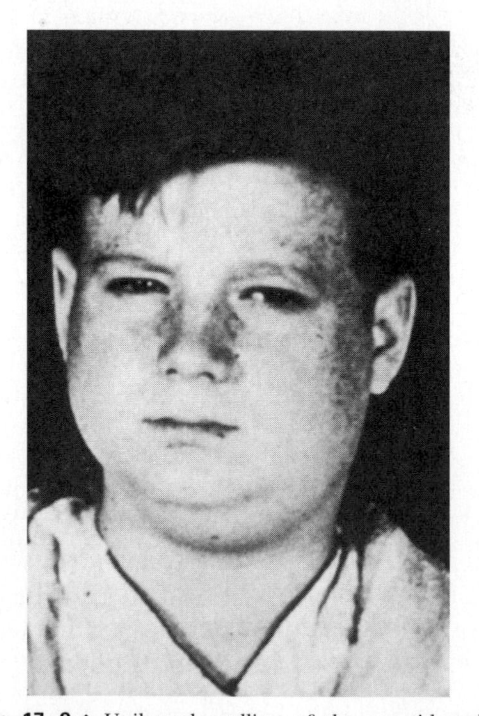

Figure 17–9 ◆ Unilateral swelling of the parotid and submaxillary glands in mumps.

Cytomegalovirus Infection

Cytomegalovirus infection can affect any organ, but commonly involves the gastrointestinal tract. It is caused by a herpesvirus known as the cytomegalovirus (CMV). The virus can be transmitted across the placenta from mothers with inapparent infections, but it also can be acquired throughout life. The virus is transmitted by kissing, sexual intercourse, blood transfusions, organ transplants, and fomites. Approximately one-half of all persons living in developed countries test positive for CMV antibodies by the age of 50. Except in newborns, the healthy individual has no symptoms in about 90 percent of the cases when the virus is first acquired. Like other herpesviruses, the virus remains latent and may return to cause serious disease.

CMV infection is a frequent complication in AIDS patients. Gastrointestinal CMV disease in AIDS patients include colitis, esophagitis, gastritis, and hepatitis. In disseminated disease, the virus is shed in aerosols and urine. The time of incubation is variable. Neonatal infections occur within three to 12 weeks after delivery. Post-transfusion infections may occur three to six weeks following receipt of CMV-positive blood.

The virus causes increases in cell size of the invaded tissue. Motor aberrations, mental retardation, and loss of sight are common **sequelae** in surviving infants.

A diagnosis of CMV infection can be established by culturing throat washings, urine, autopsy material, or biopsy material in cells. The intranuclear eosinophilic inclusion bodies in large cells are observable in infected cells (Fig. 17–10). Cell cultures can be stained with fluorescent antibodies for more rapid identification of CMV antigen (Color Plate 56). Agglutinating, complement-fixing (CF), and immunofluorescent (IF) IgG antibodies develop in one to two weeks in primary CMV infections. Paired serum samples must be used to demonstrate a rising titer. The presence of IgM antibodies to CMV indicates recent infection.

A CMV hyperimmune globulin may modify the severity of CMV infection, but cannot prevent it. Gastrointestinal CMV infection responds to the drug ganciclovir.

Hepatitis

Hepatitis is an inflammatory disease of the liver which can be caused by a variety of viruses. The most common forms of the disease are classified as hepatitis A, B, and C. The virus which causes hepatitis A is a picornavirus called enterovirus 72. The etiologic agent of hepatitis B is one of a group of DNA viruses, known as hepadnaviruses, which cause liver disease in humans and animals. The cause of hepatitis C has been identified as a flavivirus. The hepatitis A virus (HAV) is transmitted by the fecal-oral route. Hepatitis B virus (HBV) was once thought to be transmitted only by contaminated blood or needles, but the virus has been detected in urine, saliva, tears, semen, breast milk, and skin lesions of infected individuals. Hepatitis C virus (HCV) is transmitted by the **parenteral** route.

The onset of hepatitis A is abrupt with fever, anorexia, nausea, and abdominal discomfort occurring 15 to 40 days after ingestion of HAV. Jaundice is evident after a few days. The illness is usually mild, but can be very serious in the elderly. The onset of hepatitis B is more insidious and usually occurs 60 to 160 days after exposure to HBV. The symptoms include nausea, vomiting, anorexia, and sometimes extreme fatigue, a skin rash, and even arthritis. A fever may be mild or absent. Jaundice may be present as the disease progresses.

Hepatitis C usually occurs following blood transfusions. Hepatitis C can be quite severe and cause rapidly fulminating disease. Hemophiliacs, intravenous drug abusers, male homosexuals, hemodialysis patients, and laboratory workers constitute high-risk groups for HBV and HCV infections. In the parenterally transmitted infection, symptoms are less severe and more often lead to a chronic state. Most mild cases of hepatitis C resolve spontaneously. About 10 percent of cases of hepatitis C progress to cirrhosis. Other characteristics of the three types of hepatitis are outlined in Table 17–4.

A particle known as the delta agent has been isolated from the nuclei of liver cells infected with HBV. The delta agent is a defective virus in that it can only replicate with the help of HBV. Infection of a chronic HBV carrier with the delta agent can cause acute hepatitis. It is likely that some initial cases of hepatitis B are caused by a co-infection of both viruses. Hepatitis E virus (HEV) was identified in 1990 as a cause of waterborne epidemics of hepatitis in developing countries. It closely resembles caliciviruses but has characteristics differing from members of that group. It causes a mild, self-limiting form of hepatitis.

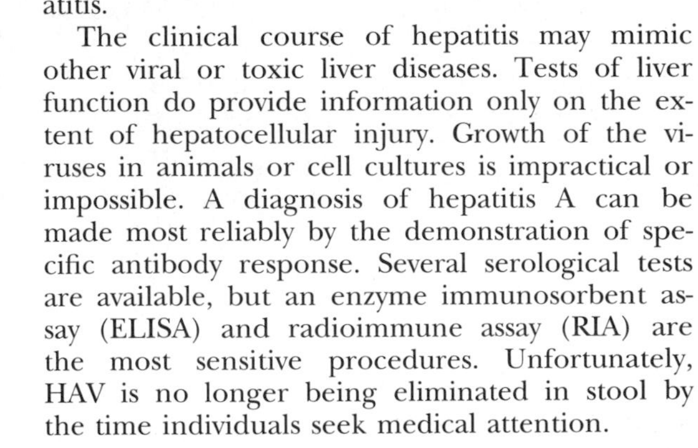

The clinical course of hepatitis may mimic other viral or toxic liver diseases. Tests of liver function do provide information only on the extent of hepatocellular injury. Growth of the viruses in animals or cell cultures is impractical or impossible. A diagnosis of hepatitis A can be made most reliably by the demonstration of specific antibody response. Several serological tests are available, but an enzyme immunosorbent assay (ELISA) and radioimmune assay (RIA) are the most sensitive procedures. Unfortunately, HAV is no longer being eliminated in stool by the time individuals seek medical attention.

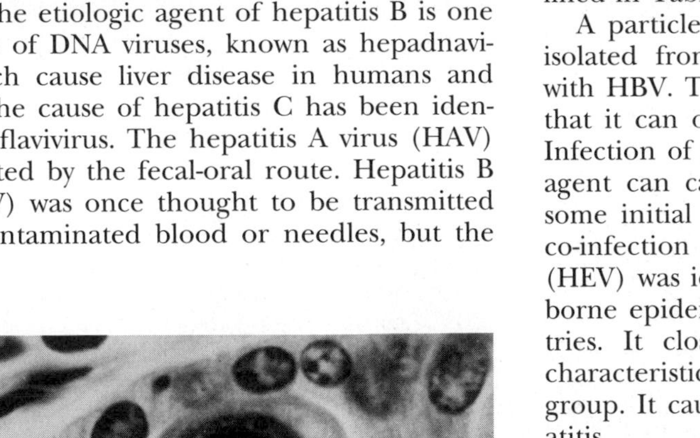

Figure 17–10 ◆ Intranuclear and intracytoplasmic inclusions in an epithelial cell of a salivary gland duct infected with cytomegalovirus.

Table 17–4
CHARACTERISTICS OF MAJOR TYPES OF HEPATITIS

CHARACTERISTIC	HEPATITIS A	HEPATITIS B	HEPATITIS C
Communicability	Highly contagious	Mildly contagious	Mildly contagious
Incidence	Autumn and winter	Year round	Year round
Incubation period	15–40 days	60–160 days	14–84 days
Onset	Abrupt	Insidious	Insidious
Type of infection	Acute	Acute to chronic	Acute to chronic
Carrier state	Absent	Present	Present
Marker	Specific IgM antibody Hepatitis A vaccine viral RNA	Surface or core antigens and antibodies	HCV antibodies viral RNA
Immunizing agent	Human immune globulin (HIG)	Hepatitis B vaccine	Human immune globulin (HIG)

A number of serological tests are available for the detection of HBV antigens and their specific antibodies. The most sensitive technique is a RIA for identifying the hepatitis B surface antigen (HB_sAg). The core antigen (HB_cAg) is present during acute stages of hepatitis B. A number of PCR procedures for HBV have been described.

IgM antibodies to HCV can be detected with an ELISA technique. An RNA probe also is available for HCV. Identification of viral RNA in serum is the principal marker since there are no reliable culture methods. No immunoassays are available for HEV. Interferons are used to treat HVB and HVC infections. Immune serum globulin (ISG) may minimize symptoms of hepatitis A in an individual if it is administered within a few days of exposure to HAV, but it has not been effective in community-wide outbreaks of hepatitis A. An inactivated hepatitis A vaccine is protective against HAV and should be used in states or countries with high incidences of the infection. A vaccine for hepatitis B is recommended for high-risk groups and children.

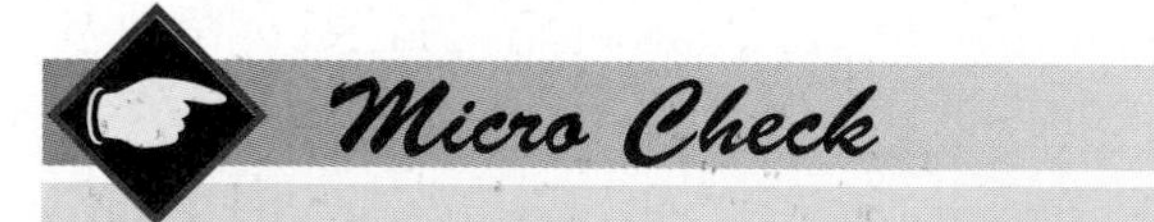

- Why does mumps constitute a serious disease in adult males?
- Why are AIDS patients so susceptible to cytomegalovirus infections?
- What groups are at risk of being exposed to hepatitis B or hepatitis C?

ALGAL AND FUNGAL TOXIN-ASSOCIATED DISEASE

Despite the ubiquity of both algae and fungi in the human environment, toxigenic algae and fungi have not been studied as much as toxigenic bacteria. Evidence has accumulated during recent years, however, which incriminates cyanobacteria, eucaryotic algae, and a variety of fungi in animal and some human toxin-associated diseases. Blooms of cyanobacteria belonging to the genus *Anabaena,* for example, have been responsible for some serious wildlife and livestock poisonings. Moldy grains have long been associated with toxicosis in domestic birds, sheep, and cattle. *Aspergillus flavus, A. parasiticus,* and *Penicillium notatum* frequently contaminate animal feed. The toxic products of the fungi, called **mycotoxins,** cause severe poisoning with liver damage. It is likely that ingestion of the toxins in moldy grain, nuts, or milk is the cause of human liver disease in many parts of the world.

PROTOZOAL INFECTIONS

Pathogenic protozoa have probably been significant causes of diarrheal disease and dysentery throughout the history of the world. Although it is not possible to incriminate any one protozoan, it is likely that protozoa were among the etiologic agents of the epidemic diarrheal diseases that decimated Napoleon's troops during the Russian campaign and severely hampered efforts of the British soldiers in India at one time.

Amebiasis (Amebic Dysentery)

The pathogenicity of *Entamoeba histolytica* for humans was established early in the twentieth century. At one time *E. histolytica* was believed to be the sole etiologic agent of amebic dysentery, but six other amebas are known to cause human disease. Most amebiasis is transmitted by ingestion of food- or water-containing cysts of *E. histolytica* (Fig. 17–11). Ingested cysts are resistant to the highly acid gastric juice, but their walls are ultimately digested by the action of intestinal enzymes. Upon excystation, vegetative forms, known as **trophozoites,** are liberated. The trophozoites migrate to the large intestine where stasis contributes to their ability to colonize. The time of incubation may vary from a few days to several weeks.

Amebiasis can mimic a variety of intestinal disorders. There may be only mild diarrhea followed by intermittent periods of constipation or an acute, fulminating dysentery with fever and chills. The dysenteric form of the disease is accompanied by ulceration of the lining of the large intestine (Fig. 17–12). The trophozoites can disseminate to the brain, liver, or lungs. The vegetative forms undergo the metamorphosis from trophozoites to cysts outside the host.

Diagnosis of amebiasis is made by demonstrating trophozoites or cysts of *E. histolytica* in wet or permanent mounts prepared from fresh stool tissue biopsy samples or hepatic aspirates. The trophozoites often contain red blood cells in otherwise refractile cytoplasm (Color Plate 57). The cysts are variable in size and contain glycogen vacuoles and dark-staining cigar-shaped chroma-

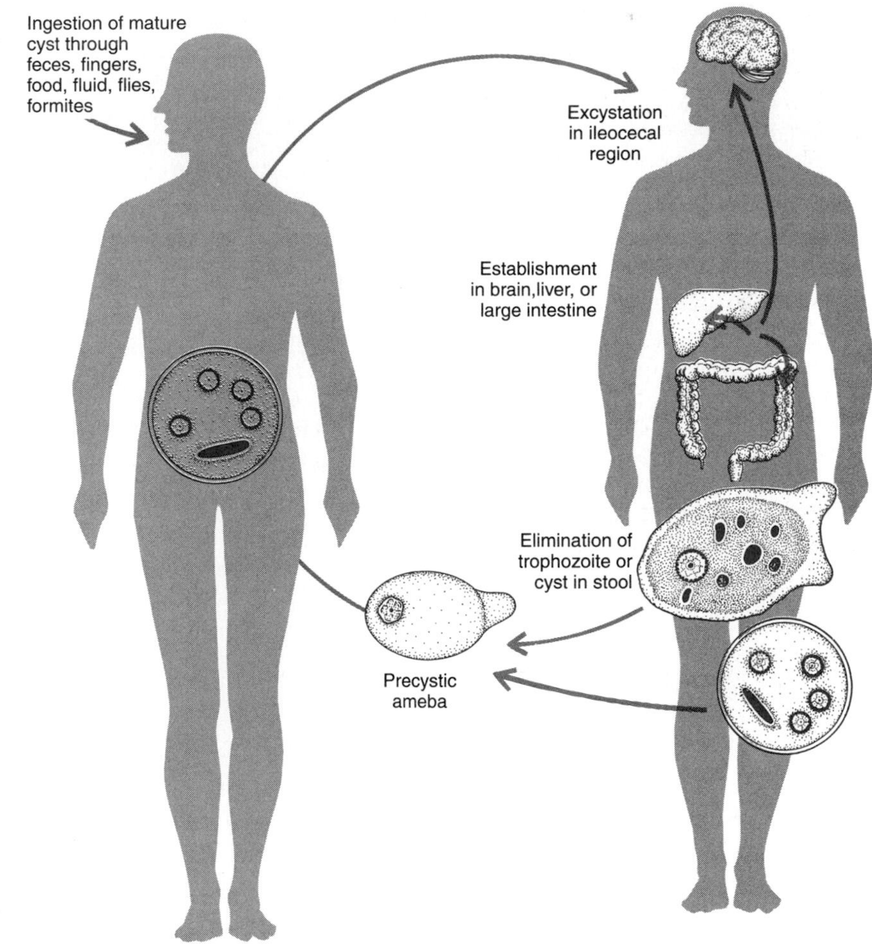

Figure 17–11 ◆ Life cycle of *Entamoeba histolytica.*

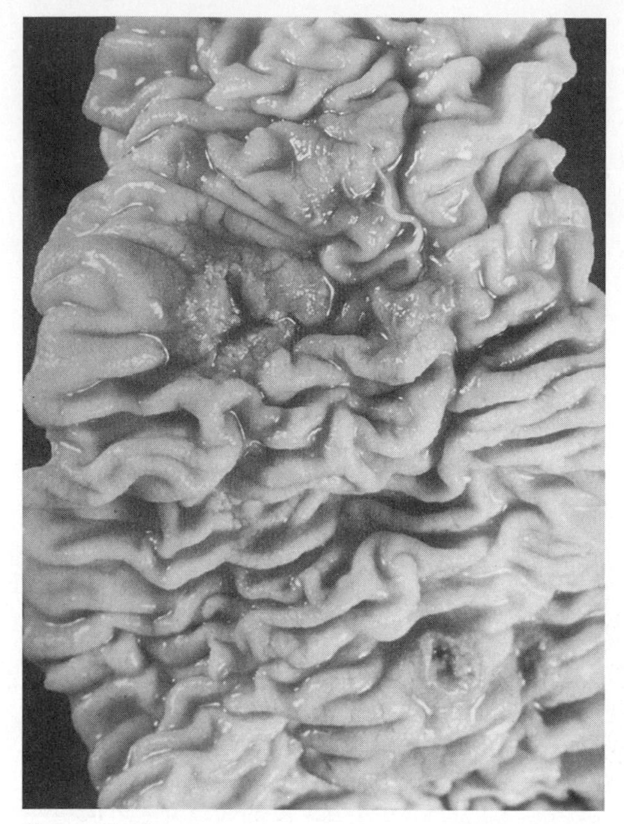

Figure 17–12 ◆ Typical buttonhole ulcers of the large intestine showing irregular margins.

toidal bodies. The cysts rarely have more than four nuclei bounded by chromatin on the inner nuclear membranes. Small central karyosomes can be seen within nuclei. Antigens may be detected in stools by an enzyme linked immunosorbent assay (ELISA) technique. Serological tests are especially useful for extraintestinal amebiasis. Iodoquinol and diloxanide furoate act on amebas in the intestinal lumen. Metronidazole, chloroquine, and dehydroxyemetine are effective in invasive amebiasis.

Giardiasis

Giardiasis is an infection of the duodenum or jejunum of humans caused by the flagellate *Giardia lamblia.* The cyst constitutes the infective stage almost without exception. Giardiasis is transmitted by food or water contaminated with cysts of *G. lamblia* or directly from person to person by the fecal-oral route. Campers often become infected when they drink contaminated ground or surface water.

It is likely that many people harbor the protozoan without any symptoms of disease. *G. lamblia* is found in 4 to 18 percent of homosexual males. If the *G. lamblia* parasites are present in sufficient numbers, abdominal cramps, **flatulence,** and a watery diarrhea occur one to four weeks after exposure. Acute giardiasis may be self-limiting, or may last for up to 32 months. In the chronic form of the disease, symptoms may be intermittent and go on for many years.

Diagnosis of giardiasis is made by demonstrating the cysts in stained, wet, or permanent mounts made from formed stool specimens. Trophozoites are found in liquid stools or duodenal contents. The trophozoites are pear-shaped and are bilaterally symmetrical (see Fig. 9–11). The anterior end is rounded and the posterior end is tapered (Color Plate 58). There are two prominent nuclei and four pairs of flagella. The cyst is ellipsoidal, has a smooth, readily visible wall, and has two to four nuclei (Color Plate 59). However, *Giardia* trophozoites and cysts are shed in stool irregularly so a negative result may not rule out the infection. A string test is a unique approach if stool sample findings are negative. A tightly wound string in a weighted capsule that contains gelatin is swallowed and one end of that string is taped to the cheek. After 5 hours the string is removed. Material adhering to the string is used to prepare wet or permanent mounts. Occasionally duodenal aspiration or a biopsy may be necessary.

Monoclonal antibodies are available for detection of *Giardia* antigens by an enzyme immunoassay (EIA) technique and for demonstration of intact organisms by indirect immunofluorescence (IF) (Color Plate 58). Metronidazole, furazolidone, or quinacrine relieves the symptoms of giardiasis and eradicates the protozoan from the small intestine.

Balantidiasis

Balantidiasis is a rare cause of dysentery in humans, but of considerable interest, because it is caused by the only pathogenic ciliate, *Balantidium coli.* The cysts of the ciliate are transmitted by contaminated food or water. Pigs are the most important reservoir of *B. coli,* but poorly cooked pork has been implicated only rarely in the transmission of the protozoan. The organism lives mainly in the ileum or cecum of the host and is able to penetrate the intestinal mucosa with apparent ease. Penetration may be minimal, with hyperemia the only effect, or it may be deep enough to cause marked ulcerations. The time of incubation is unknown.

Individuals infected with *B. coli* exhibit diarrhea, abdominal pain, nausea, vomiting, and weight loss. Balantidiasis can take a rapidly fulminating course in immunocompromised individuals.

Direct saline wet mounts of stool are preferable for observing trophozoites or cysts of *B. coli.* Trophozoites are more frequently observed and are unmistakable because of their large size and saclike shape (Color Plate 61). Both a micro- and a macronucleus are observable. The cilia are sometimes difficult to see. The cysts, if present, are spherical or oval. A distinct cell wall is visible, but the cilia are retracted. Oxytetracycline or iodoquinol are effective in eliminating the protozoan from the intestines.

Cryptosporidiosis

Cryptosporidiosis has been recognized as a diarrheal disease in animals for a long time, but it has in the last decade surfaced as a cause of human diarrheal disease. It is caused by the protozoan *Cryptosporidium parvum.* The protozoan is believed to be transmitted by water, food, or fomites contaminated with the oocysts of the organism and may be transmitted sexually, as well, in homosexual males. The incubation period is five to 10 days. Cryptosporidiosis is a frequent opportunistic infection in AIDS patients and has occurred in epidemic form in day care centers. *Cryptosporidium* may also cause respiratory tract infections in immune deficiency states.

The symptoms of cryptosporidiosis include a low-grade fever, nausea, vomiting, abdominal cramps, anorexia, five to 10 watery, frothy bowel movements a day, and periods of constipation. The diarrhea is usually self-limiting in otherwise healthy individuals and lasts from several days to two weeks. In immunosuppressed persons, the diarrhea may become chronic and weight loss may occur.

Concentrated fresh stool specimens can be observed in wet mounts for *Cryptosporidium* oocysts by phase-contrast microscopy (Fig. 17–13). The oocysts, which measure 4 to 6 μm in diameter, are highly refractile and contain one to six dark granules. A modified acid-fast technique or auramine can be used successfully to demonstrate the oocysts on heat-fixed smears of stool specimens (Color Plate 62). The organisms stain pink to deep red against a blue background with the acid-fast staining technique. An ELISA technique is less time-consuming for examining multiple stool specimens for the parasite. No effective treatment is yet available for cryptosporidiosis.

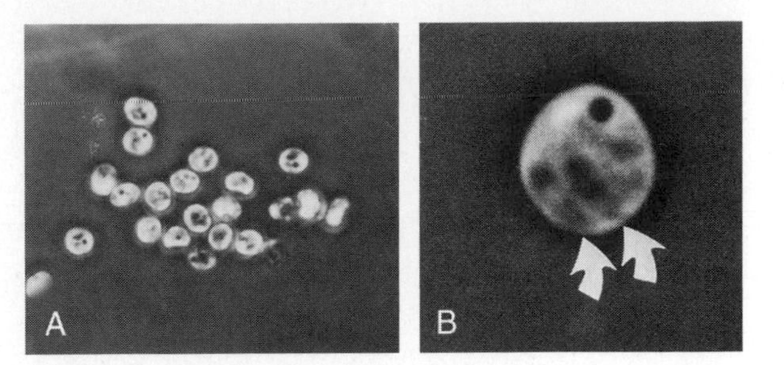

Figure 17–13 ◆ Phase-contrast micrograph of oocysts of *Cryptosporidium* from human feces concentrated by Sheather's sugar flotation *(A)*. Phase-contrast micrograph of a single oocyst after one week at room temperature *(B)*.

Cyclosporiasis

An increasing number of cases of explosive diarrheal disease in humans has been attributed to the protozoan *Cyclospora cayetanensis.* It was first reported to occur in travelers and immunosuppressed patients, but an epidemic in the United States in the summer of 1996 showed more general susceptibility. Raspberries imported from Guatemala were the prime suspects as a

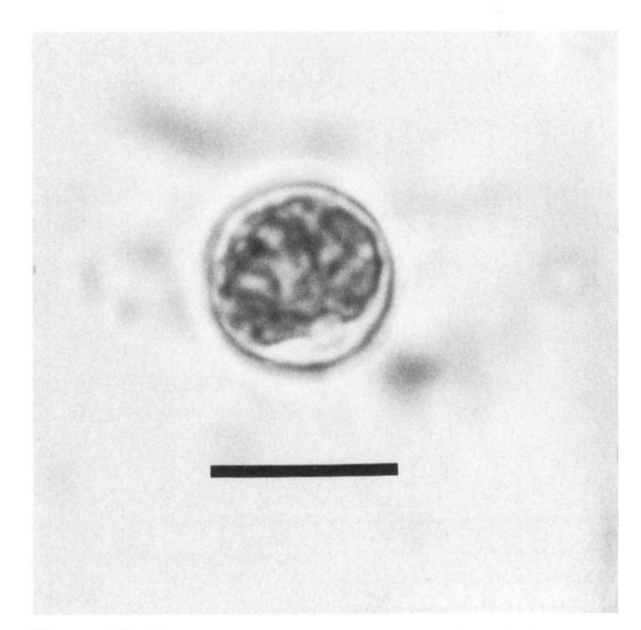

Figure 17–14 ◆ An iodine-stained oocyst of a *Cyclospora* organism. Internal granules take up iodine.

source for the intestinal parasite. It is believed that *C. cayetanensis* can also be transmitted by drinking water. The diarrheal disease differs from most others by having an extended incubation period and frequent relapses.

The oocysts of *C. cayetanensis* are approximately twice the size of those seen in cryptosporidiosis, stain with iodine, a modified acid-fast procedure, and fluorescent stains (Fig. 17–14; Color Plate 63). The illness can be treated with a seven-day course of trimethoprim-sulfamethoxazole, but is frequently self-limiting.

Table 17–5
SUMMARY OF MAJOR MICROORGANISMS CAUSING DISEASES OF THE GASTROINTESTINAL TRACT

ORGANISM	DISEASE	TREATMENT
Bacteria		
Streptococcus mutans	Dental caries	Filling
Bacteria found in dental plaque	Periodontal disease	Removal of plaque
Salmonella sp.	Salmonellosis	Replacement of fluid and electrolytes
Salmonella typhi	Typhoid fever	Choramphenicol
Shigella sp.	Shigellosis	Replacement of fluid and electrolytes Ampicillin Trimethoprim-sulfamethoxazole
Escherichia coli	Travelers' diarrhea	Replacement of fluid and electrolytes Pepto-Bismol Trimethoprim-sulfamethoxazole
Escherichia coli 0157:H7	Bloody diarrhea	Replacement of fluid and electrolytes Blood transfusion
Vibrio cholerae	Cholera	Replacement of fluid and electrolytes Tetracycline
Campylobacter jejuni	Campylobacteriosis	Erythromycin
Yersinia enterocolitica	Gastrointestinal yersiniosis	Fluid and electrolyte replacement
Clostridium difficile	Pseudomembranous colitis	Vancomycin
Staphylococcus aureus	Staphylococcal food poisoning	Fluid and electrolyte replacement
Clostridium botulinum	Botulism	Trivalent ABE antitoxin
Clostridium perfringens	Perfringens food poisoning	Fluid and electrolyte replacement
Vibrio parahaemolyticus	Halophilic vibrio poisoning	Fluid and electrolyte replacement
Vibrio vulnificus	Halophilic vibrio poisoning	Fluid and electrolyte replacement
Viruses		
Mumps virus	Mumps	Supportive care
Cytomegalovirus (CMV)	Cytomegalovirus infection	Ganciclovir
Hepatitis A virus (HAV)	Hepatitis A	Human serum globulin
Hepatitis B virus (HBV)	Hepatitis B	Interferons
Hepatitis C virus (HCV)	Hepatitis C	Interferons
Protozoa		
Entamoeba histolytica	Amebiasis	Iodoquinol Diloxanide furoate Metronidazole Chloroquine Dehydroemetine
Giardia lamblia	Giardiasis	Metronidazole Quinacrine
Balantidium coli	Balantidiasis	Tetracycline
Cryptosporidium parvum	Cryptosporidiosis	None
Cyclospora cayetanensis	Cyclosporiosis	Trimethoprim-sulfamethoxazole

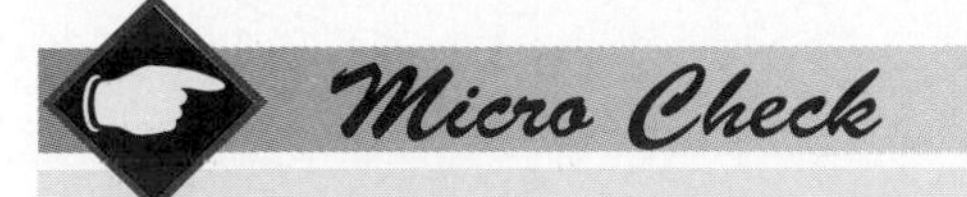

Micro Check

- How is it possible to differentiate between amebic dysentery and bacillary dysentery (shigellosis)?
- What animal is the primary reservoir for the only pathogenic ciliate?
- What staining techniques may be used to demonstrate oocysts of *Cryptosporidium* and *Cyclospora?*

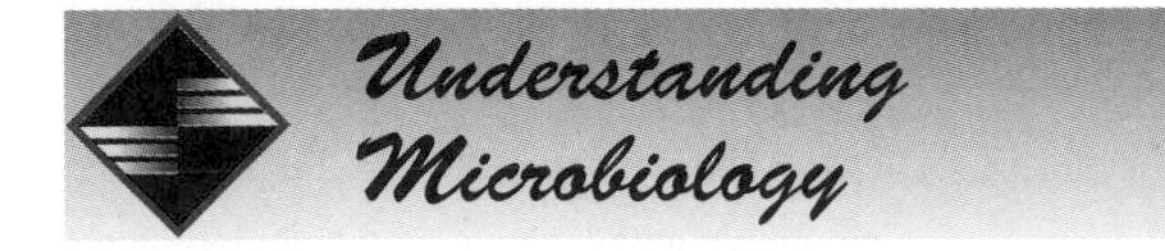

Understanding Microbiology

1. How do microorganisms escape the action of gastric juice in the stomach?
2. What is the role of diet in dental caries and periodontal disease?
3. Why does botulism qualify as a food poisoning rather than a food infection?
4. How can diarrheal disease be differentiated from dysentery?
5. How can thorough handwashing prevent infectious gastrointestinal disease?

Applying Microbiology

Read the following case study carefully and answer the questions: A 42-year-old man was treated for profuse watery diarrhea, vomiting, and dehydration at an emergency room. Two days earlier he had eaten approximately 12 raw oysters from a local processing plant. Approximately 36 hours after eating the oysters, he had a sudden onset of symptoms and passed 20 stools during the day before seeking medical attention. The oysters came from a bay off the coast of Louisiana. Eight other persons ate the oysters, but did not become ill. The patient was given fluid and electrolytes intravenously and recovered without incident.

6. The name of the disease is most probably
   a. amebic dysentery
   b. halophilic food poisoning
   c. cholera
   d. salmonellosis
   e. botulism
7. The etiologic agent can be described as a (an)
   a. gram-negative bacillus
   b. gram-positive coccus
   c. gram-positive bacillus
   d. gram-negative vibrio
   e. acid-fast bacillus
8. A condition required for growth of the etiologic agent is
   a. an alkaline environment
   b. eosin methylene blue
   c. blood
   d. a microaerophilic environment
   e. a temperature of 20°C
9. A life-threatening feature of this disease is
   a. hemorrhaging
   b. unrelenting fever
   c. paralysis of intercostal muscles
   d. loss of fluid and electrolytes
   e. opportunistic pathogens
10. The most practical method to prevent acquiring infectious diseases from shellfish is
    a. thorough washing of hands
    b. massive immunization programs
    c. reporting diarrheal diseases
    d. administration of Hib
    e. thorough cooking of shellfish

Chapter 18 Diseases of the Genitourinary Tract

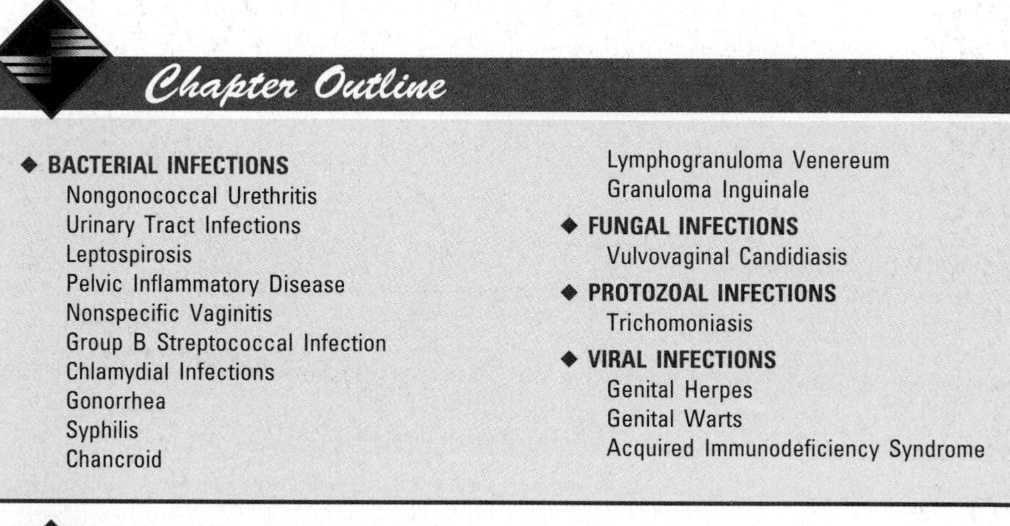

Chapter Outline

- **BACTERIAL INFECTIONS**
  - Nongonococcal Urethritis
  - Urinary Tract Infections
  - Leptospirosis
  - Pelvic Inflammatory Disease
  - Nonspecific Vaginitis
  - Group B Streptococcal Infection
  - Chlamydial Infections
  - Gonorrhea
  - Syphilis
  - Chancroid
  - Lymphogranuloma Venereum
  - Granuloma Inguinale
- **FUNGAL INFECTIONS**
  - Vulvovaginal Candidiasis
- **PROTOZOAL INFECTIONS**
  - Trichomoniasis
- **VIRAL INFECTIONS**
  - Genital Herpes
  - Genital Warts
  - Acquired Immunodeficiency Syndrome

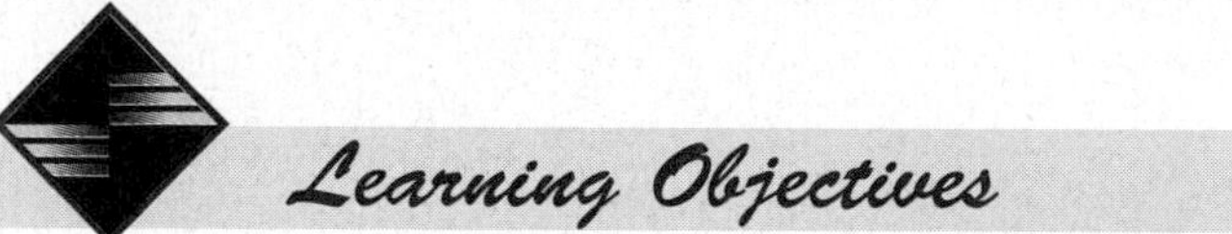

Learning Objectives

After you have read this chapter, you should be able to:

1. Explain why urinary tract infections are more common in women than in men.
2. Name the most common isolates of urinary tract infections.
3. Name several bacteria associated with pelvic inflammatory disease.
4. Explain the significance of penicillinase-producing *Neisseria gonorrhoeae* and chromosomally mediated resistant *N. gonorrhoeae.*
5. Name one fungus and one protozoan that cause vaginitis.
6. Explain why genital herpes infections may be of exogenous or endogenous origin.

Although the genital (reproductive) and urinary systems perform different functions, the anatomical proximity of the organs and their environment provides ample opportunities for microorganisms to invade one or both systems. For this reason we can conveniently combine the study of infections of both systems as diseases of the genitourinary tract.

The urinary system in both sexes consists of the kidneys, ureters, urinary bladder, and urethra (Fig. 18–1). The Skene's glands consist of two tubular glands near the orifice of the female urethra. The genital organs of the male include the scrotum, testes, seminal vesicles, prostate gland, and the paired Cowper's glands, which are located anteriorly to the prostate gland (Fig. 18–2); those of the female include the ovaries, fallopian tubes, uterus, vagina, vulva, clitoris, and Bar-

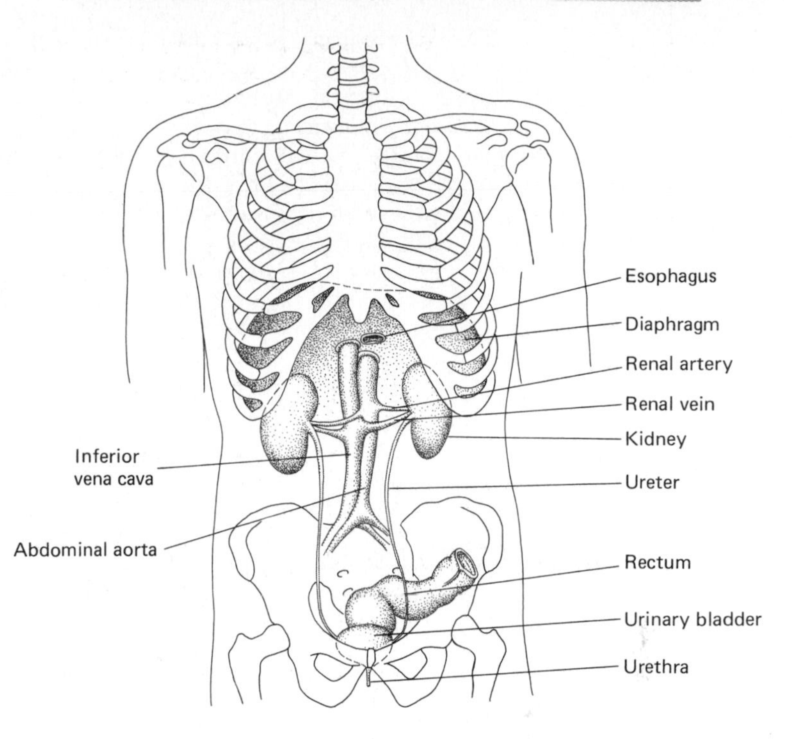

Figure 18–1 ◆ Organs of the urinary system.

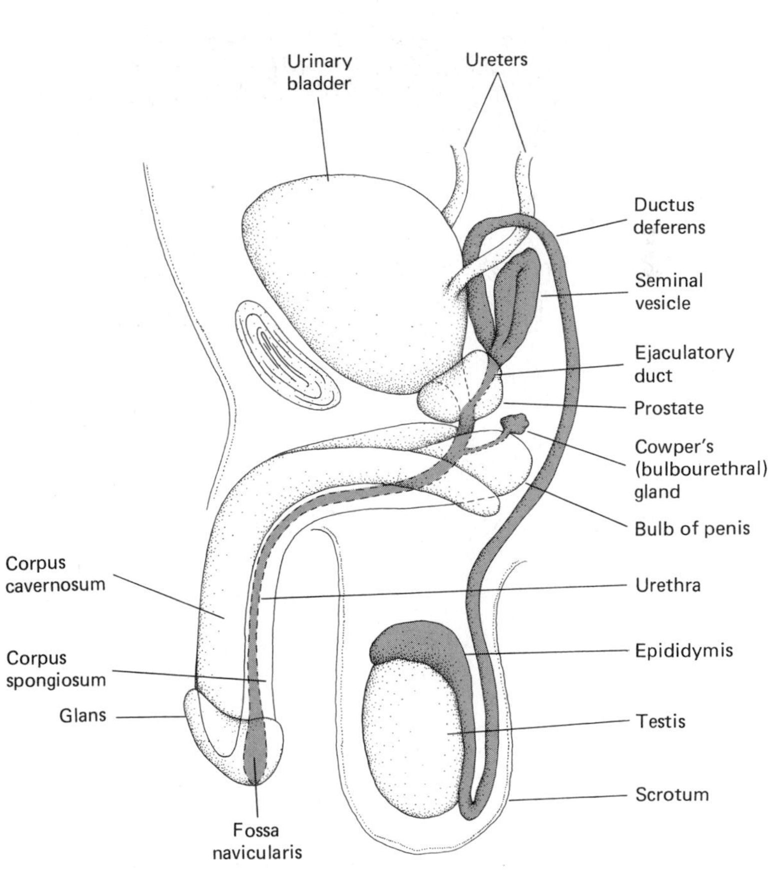

Figure 18–2 ◆ Genital organs of the male.

tholin's glands, which are the counterparts of the male Cowper's glands (Fig. 18–3).

The area bounded by the buttocks and thighs in both sexes is called the **perineum.** It can be divided into a **urogenital triangle,** which contains the external genitals, urethral orifice, and surrounding tissue, and an **anal triangle,** which contains the anus and surrounding tissue (Fig. 18–4).

There are no microorganisms normally residing in the kidneys, ureters, or urinary bladder. In both sexes the numbers of bacteria near the distal end of the urethra are relatively few. The flora are largely a reflection of the organisms of the skin, but often include organisms of intestinal origin as well. Microorganisms inhabiting these anatomic sites in both sexes and the vagina in women constitute the reservoirs for organisms causing urinary tract infection.

The microbial flora of the vagina varies with age and even during the menstrual cycle. Microaerophilic lactobacilli, sometimes called Döderlein's bacilli, colonize the vagina shortly after birth, but disappear as effects of maternal progesterone dissipate. They return to populate the vagina again with the beginning of menses. The vaginal lactobacilli tend to be heterofermentative, but maintain the pH of the vagina below 5.0 (Fig. 18–5). Coliforms are inhibited by the acid environment, but more tolerant anaerobic *Bacteroides, Clostridium,* and *Peptostreptococcus* species survive and sometimes flourish. In addition, enterococci, staphylococci, and diphtheroids may be recovered with regularity from vaginal secretions.

Mycoplasmas are ubiquitous inhabitants of male and female genital tracts. Genital mycoplasma colonization increases with the number of sexual partners. *Mycobacterium smegmatis,* an acid-fast bacillus, has been recovered from secretions of male and female genitals.

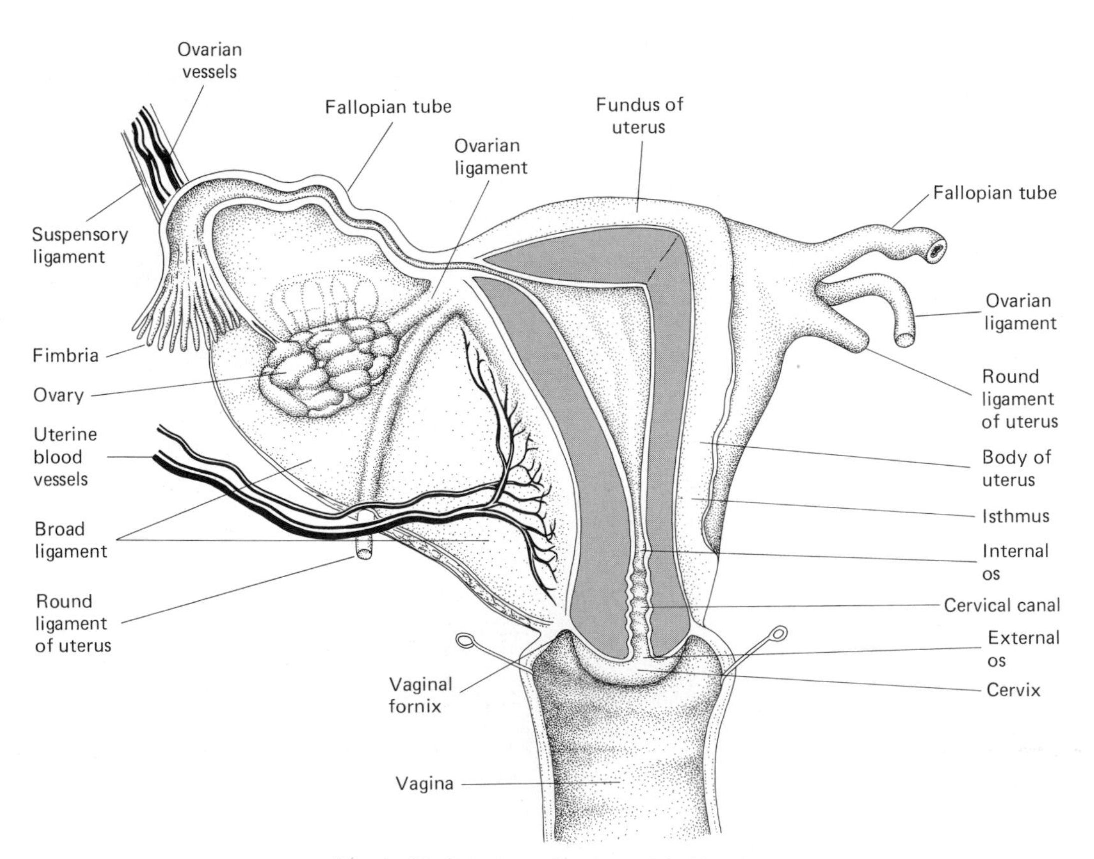

Figure 18–3 ◆ Genital organs of the female.

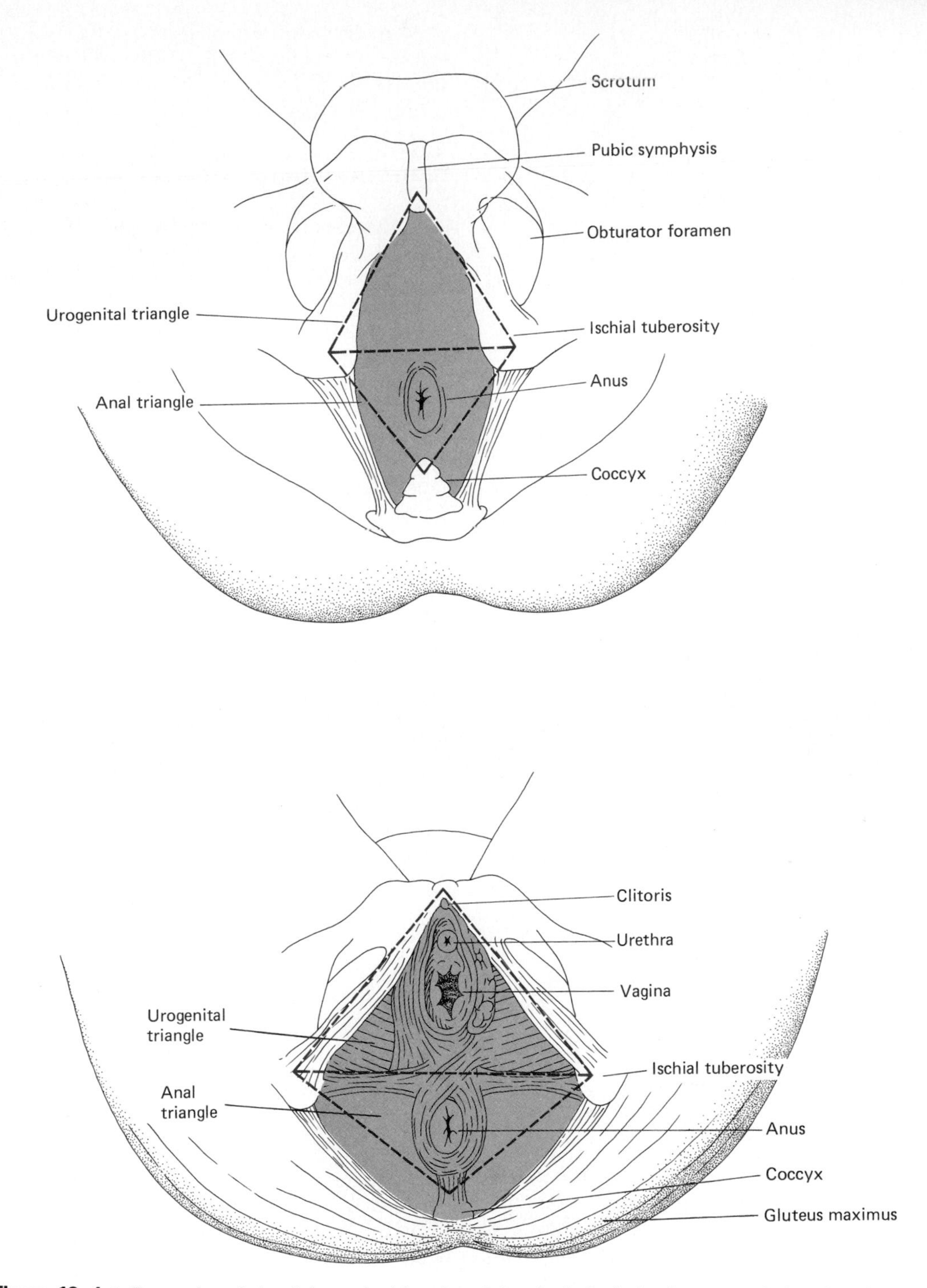

Figure 18–4 ◆ External genitals of the male (above) and female (below) showing urogenital and anal triangles of the perineum in both sexes.

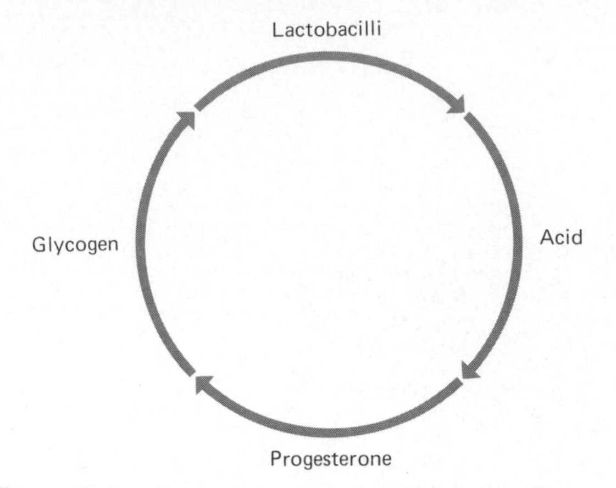

Figure 18–5 ◆ Interrelationship of vaginal factors. Progesterone increases the glycogen content of vaginal epithelium. Lactobacilli break down products of glycogen hydrolysis to maintain an acid environment.

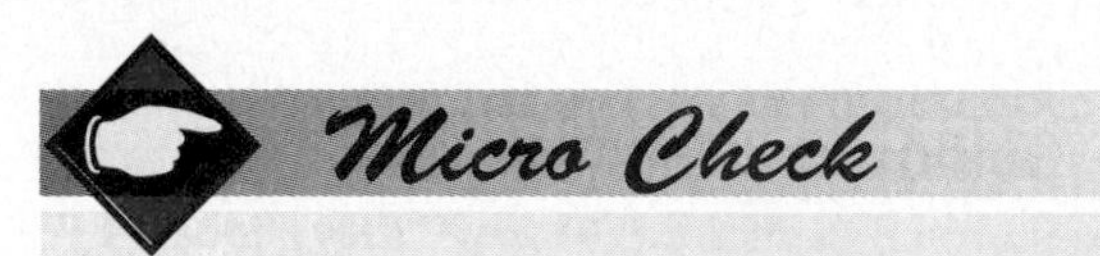

- What parts of the urinary tract are normally sterile?
- What are the primary reservoirs of microorganisms causing urinary tract infections in women?
- Why does the vagina constitute an unfavorable environment for coliforms?

BACTERIAL INFECTIONS

Urinary tract infections (UTIs) can affect men and women at any age. The number of urinary tract infections in women is about 30 times greater than the number reported in men. Incidence of bacteriuria is as high as 10 percent in the elderly. The relatively short female urethra and warm, moist conditions of the perineum favor microbial growth. Sexual intercourse may injure the short urethra and provide a means for bacteria of the perineum to gain entrance. Following invasion of the bladder mucosa, microorganisms can multiply in bladder urine. Bacteria or their endotoxins can interfere with peristaltic action and permit reflux of urine into ureters. Organisms or their products can migrate in this manner against the pressure gradient to the kidneys.

Sexually transmitted diseases (STDs) constitute the most serious infectious diseases of the genital tract. If untreated, the invading microorganisms can cause severe disease and even death.

Nongonococcal Urethritis

Nongonococcal urethritis (NGU) is an infection of the urethra caused by a microbial agent other than the gonococcus. Bacterial agents include staphylococci, streptococci, mycoplasmas, chlamydias, gram-negative cocci, and gram-negative bacilli. The most prevalent cause of NGU in the United States is *Chlamydia trachomatis. C. trachomatis* causes about 50 percent of NGU among men. Chlamydial infections are discussed in greater detail later in this chapter. The mycoplasmas causing NGU are *Mycoplasma genitalium, M. hominis,* and *Ureaplasma urealyticum* (Fig. 18–6). The time of incubation is variable, but often it is less than one week. The symptoms of NGU include discomfort, pain, and burning on urination, as well as frequency of urination. The urethra may be inflamed.

Microscopic examination of Gram-stained smears of urethral discharge reveal the morphologic appearance and staining characteristics of bacteria, other than chlamydias or mycoplasmas, if they are present in sufficient numbers. A fluorescein-conjugated monoclonal antibody reagent may be applied directly to clinical specimens for direct detection of *C. trachomatis.* A nucleic acid (NA) probe is available for detecting amplified frag-

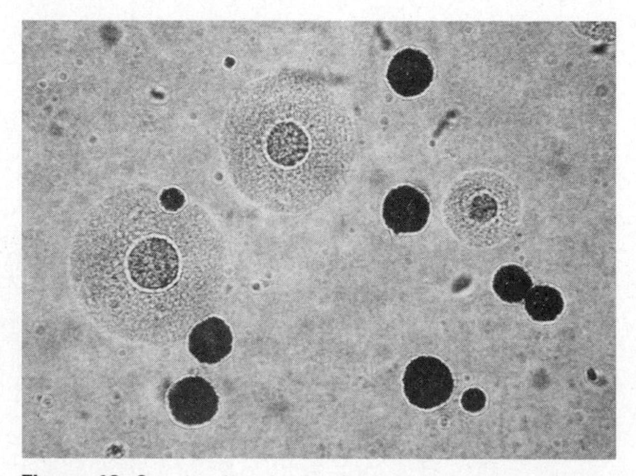

Figure 18–6 ◆ A mixture of colonies of *Mycoplasma hominis* and *Ureaplasma urealyticum* on a differential agar medium. The deep colored colonies of *U. urealyticum* can be differentiated easily from the colorless colonies of *M. hominis.*

ments of the organism's deoxyribonucleic acid (DNA).

Mycoplasmas cannot be detected by microscopic examination. All the bacteria except chlamydias and mycoplasmas can be recovered by using selective media, such as blood agar and eosin methylene blue (EMB), and can be identified by appropriate biochemical tests. Mycoplasmas can be grown on special media, but isolation of chlamydias requires special cell lines, embryonated eggs, or laboratory animals. The time and expense involved preclude most laboratories from culturing chlamydias or mycoplasmas in cases of NGU.

NGU requires prompt treatment to prevent ascending urinary tract infection or recurrence of an infection. Evaluation and treatment of sex partners is often required. Tetracycline, erythromycin, and azithromycin are the drugs of choice.

Urinary Tract Infections

The most important urinary tract infections are **cystitis** (infection of the urinary bladder) and **pyelonephritis** (infection of the kidney). They usually are caused by gram-negative bacilli of intestinal origin. *Escherichia coli* is the most frequently isolated organism, but *Proteus, Enterococcus, Enterobacter, Citrobacter, Klebsiella,* and *Pseudomonas* species are also isolated with regularity. *Enterococcus faecium,* an intestinal organism, sometimes presents problems because of its resistance to most antibiotics. Staphylococci and streptococci are isolated less frequently. *Staphylococcus epidermidis* and *S. saprophyticus* are normal skin residents. Anaerobic streptococci, *Bacteroides* species, and *Clostridium* species are rarely isolated, but when present, these anaerobes may act synergistically with other bacteria to produce necrosis.

Most UTIs are acquired by the ascending route. Incomplete emptying of the bladder predisposes individuals to UTIs because urine is a good culture medium. Retention of urine can occur when pressure of a "drooping" uterus or an enlarged prostate obstructs elimination. Even slight trauma to the urethra in women, which can occur during intercourse, is believed to be sufficient to attract bacterial migrations. Wiping from back to front with toilet tissue introduces enteric organisms into the female urethra. Inadequate cleansing of the genital area, coupled with the warmth and moisture of such a protected environment, contributes to increased colonization of the urethra in both men and women. Bacteria in the blood rarely invade healthy kidneys or the bladder. The period of incubation is usually between one and five days.

Cystitis causes varying degrees of pain and tenderness. Frequency and burning on urination are common complaints. Renal infections may be associated with loin pain. Unfortunately, both cystitis and pyelonephritis may be asymptomatic.

The bacteria causing UTIs can be isolated from catheterized, clean, voided midstream urine, or urine withdrawn from the bladder by special procedures. Counts greater than 10^5 CFU/ml (100,000 organisms per ml) are indicative of UTI. Several screening tests are available to laboratories for rapid detection of bacteriuria (bacteria in the urine). Most UTIs are caused by a single bacterial species that can be identified using standard cultural and biochemical tests.

Most urinary tract infections respond to sulfonamides, trimethoprim-sulfamethoxazole, quinalones, or ampicillin. Treatment of persistent infections should be based on the results of antibiotic susceptibility tests because some of the bacteria causing urinary tract infection are resistant to commonly employed drugs.

Leptospirosis

Leptospirosis is a multisystem disease that frequently localizes in the kidneys. Although mild cases of human leptospirosis probably go unrecognized, the disease is being detected with increasing frequency in the United States. The etiologic agents are spirochetes belonging to the genus *Leptospira.* In humans, the most serious disease is caused by *Leptospira interrogans* serotype *icterohaemorrhagiae.* Many domestic and wild animals, including cattle, dogs, rats, and pigs, with or without apparent infection, harbor leptospires. Dogs have become the major source of human leptospirosis in recent years. Leptospires are spread by water contaminated with urine of infected animals or by direct contact with animals with leptospirosis. The organisms can enter the body by ingestion or through dust and abrasions. The time of incubation is about 10 to 12 days.

The initial symptoms of leptospirosis may resemble influenza, but may progress to conjunctivitis, gastrointestinal distress, encephalitis, jaundice, or renal insufficiency.

Leptospires are difficult to demonstrate by direct microscopic examination, but may be observed by phase-contrast or dark-field or fluorescent microscopy if they are present in large numbers (Fig. 18–7). The organisms are helical at one or both ends and may be bent or hooked. The organisms can be isolated from blood early in the disease and from urine for several months. Most strains of leptospires will grow in media enriched with rabbit serum at 30°C. Young hamsters or guinea pigs may be inoculated as an alternate procedure. Agglutinins against leptospiral antigens are frequently detectable within two weeks after onset of illness. A PCR technique may be applied to serum, urine, aqueous humor, and cerebrospinal fluid. Leptospires respond to treatment with penicillin or tetracycline.

Table 18–1
COMMON ANAEROBIC ISOLATES FROM PELVIC INFLAMMATORY DISEASE

Gram-negative cocci	***Gram-positive cocci***
Veillonella	*Peptococcus*
Gram-negative bacilli	*Peptostreptococcus*
Bacteroides fragilis	***Gram-positive bacilli***
Prevotella melaninogenicus	*Clostridium perfringens*
Prevotella oralis	*Clostridium tetani*
Fusobacterium nucleatum	*Clostridium novyi*
Fusobacterium necrophorum	*Bifidobacterium bifidum*
	Propionibacterium

Pelvic Inflammatory Disease

Pelvic inflammatory disease (PID) occurs almost without exception in sexually active women of childbearing age. About one-quarter to one-half of the million cases of PID in the United States are caused by *Chlamydia trachomatis. Neisseria gonorrhoeae* is also commonly isolated. In other instances the cervix, uterus, fallopian tubes, ovaries, or perineum is infected with anaerobic cocci or bacilli (Table 18–1). *Bacteroides fragilis* is the most commonly recovered anaerobe, but mixed infections are not infrequent. PID is sometimes a complication of a primary ascending genitourinary tract infection, but may spread by means of lymphatic vessels. The attraction of anaerobes may be enhanced by trauma caused by injury or a primary infective agent. The time of incubation is variable, depending on the degree of trauma.

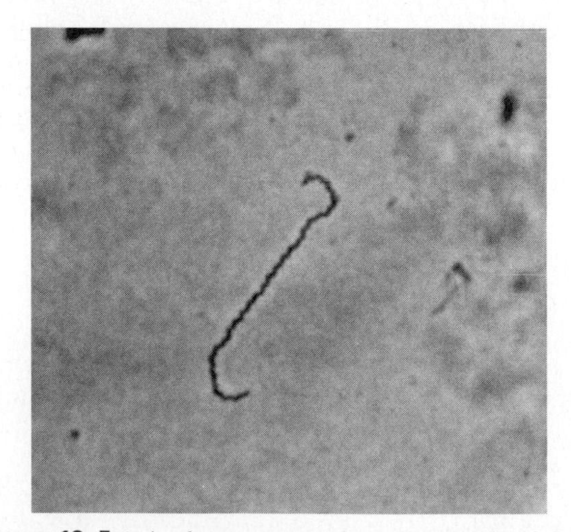

Figure 18–7 ◆ A phase-contrast photomicrograph of *Leptospira interrogans,* serotype *icterohaemorrhagiae,* the causative agent of human leptospirosis.

Symptoms of PID include fever, chills, malaise, and lower abdominal pain. A purulent (pus-containing) discharge may be present. Scar tissue may block the lumen of the fallopian tubes in severe infections. Repeated infections may lead to the chronic state as well as irreparable damage to reproductive organs.

Gram stains of smears made from purulent discharges may reveal a mixture of gram-negative bacilli and cocci and gram-positive bacilli. Most anaerobes will grow in supplemented thioglycolate broth. Specific identification procedures, however, are often time-consuming.

No single antibiotic is active against the spectrum of bacteria that can cause PID. Combination therapy with broad-spectrum antibiotics is recommended. Partners of patients with PID should be examined for sexually transmitted disease and treated promptly if disease is present.

Nonspecific Vaginitis

Nonspecific vaginitis (NSV) is an infection of the vagina characterized by a nonirritating, foul-smelling, thin, homogeneous white discharge. The cause is usually attributed to the presence of vaginal anaerobes and *Gardnerella vaginalis,* but other bacteria may also be involved. The time of incubation has not been definitely established because *G. vaginalis* is often indigenous to the vagina. The conditions that permit its proliferation are not completely understood.

Microscopic examination of vaginal fluid typically reveals the presence of small, gram-variable coccobacilli associated with epithelial cells if *G.*

vaginalis is present. The stippled or granulated epithelial cells are known as "clue cells." Although the organism can be recovered with ease, the value of cultures is debatable, as *G. vaginalis* is so commonly present in women without vaginitis.

NSV responds well to treatment with metronidazole, but the drug is contraindicated during pregnancy. Alternative drugs recommended for NSV include ampicillin and amoxicillin. Treatment is not recommended for asymptomatic carriers of *G. vaginalis*.

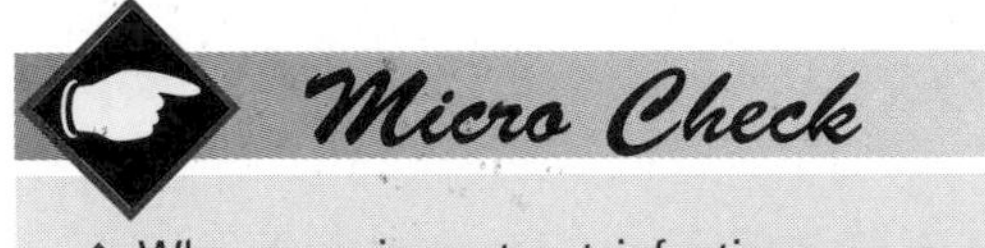

- Why are urinary tract infections more common in women?
- What is the primary cause of nongonococcal urethritis?
- Of what significance are "clue cells"?

Group B Streptococcal Infection

Group B streptococci (GBS) or *Streptococcus agalactiae* colonize the vagina of 15 to 20 percent of pregnant women. If the organisms get into amniotic fluid, consequences include sepsis, pneumonia, or meningitis in the newborn infant. Two to three newborns per 1000 live births get a GBS infection; up to 50 percent of the infants die. Unfortunately, GBS only occasionally causes vaginitis in colonized women.

GBS is usually detected late in pregnancy or during labor. Women at high risk of delivering infants with GBS infection include those having (1) premature labor, (2) premature rupture of membranes, and (3) fever during labor. Cultures should be taken from women meeting one or more of the conditions. Swabs may be taken from the cervix, vaginal walls, or anal opening.

An enriched selective medium containing 5 percent sheep blood and antibiotics to inhibit normal flora is recommended for culture. Group B streptococci secrete a so-called Camp factor that intereacts with beta hemolysin of *S. aureus* to produce an arrowhead-shaped zone of hemolysis (Color Plate 64). If subcultures on blood agar grow as typical beta-hemolytic streptococci, type-specific antisera will demonstrate agglutination. GBS are usually susceptible to ampicillin.

Chlamydial Infections

Genital infections caused by *Chlamydia trachomatis* are common among sexually active young women in the United States. States with metropolitan areas have the largest case rates (Fig. 18–8). The numbers of cases in men are assumed to be much higher than those actually reported. It is estimated that the number of chlamydial infections is 3 million to 5 million cases annually in the United States, making it the most common of STDs. Infection with the bacterium is commonly seen in NGU, but may also cause cervicitis, acute salpingitis, epididymitis, proctitis, pelvic inflammatory disease (PID), ectopic (outside the uterus) pregnancy, and infertility. The risk of infertility increases significantly with each new infection.

Genital chlamydial infections may be mild. Most women are asymptomatic, but a yellow exudate may accumulate in the entrance to the cervix. Sometimes there is a vaginal discharge. Men usually have a watery or purulent urethral discharge one to three weeks after exposure. There may be increased frequency of urination in both men and women. The bacterium is transmitted sexually in adults, but an infected mother can transmit it to a newborn during a vaginal delivery, causing **conjunctivitiis** (an inflammation of the membrane that lines the eyelid) or pneumonia.

A number of tests are available to detect the presence of chlamydial infections. Isolation of *C. trachomatis* in cell culture is a sensitive procedure when combined with a staining technique. Elementary bodies (EBs), a stage during replication of the chlamydia, within cells can be seen. Chlamydial antigen can be detected by direct fluorescent antibody (DFA) methods and enzyme-linked immunosorbent assays (ELISA) (Color Plate 63).

A tetracycline, such as deoxycline, azithromycin, or erythromycin is used to treat chlamydial infections. Treatment of sex partners is also recommended. Unfortunately, reinfections are common among sexually active individuals.

Gonorrhea

Gonorrhea remains one of the most prevalent STDs; despite steady declines since the mid-1970s. It is worldwide in distribution. More than half a million cases of gonorrhea are reported in the United States alone annually (Fig. 18–9). Because many cases go unreported, the true incidence is much higher. It is probable that there is a high frequency of coexisting chlamydial and

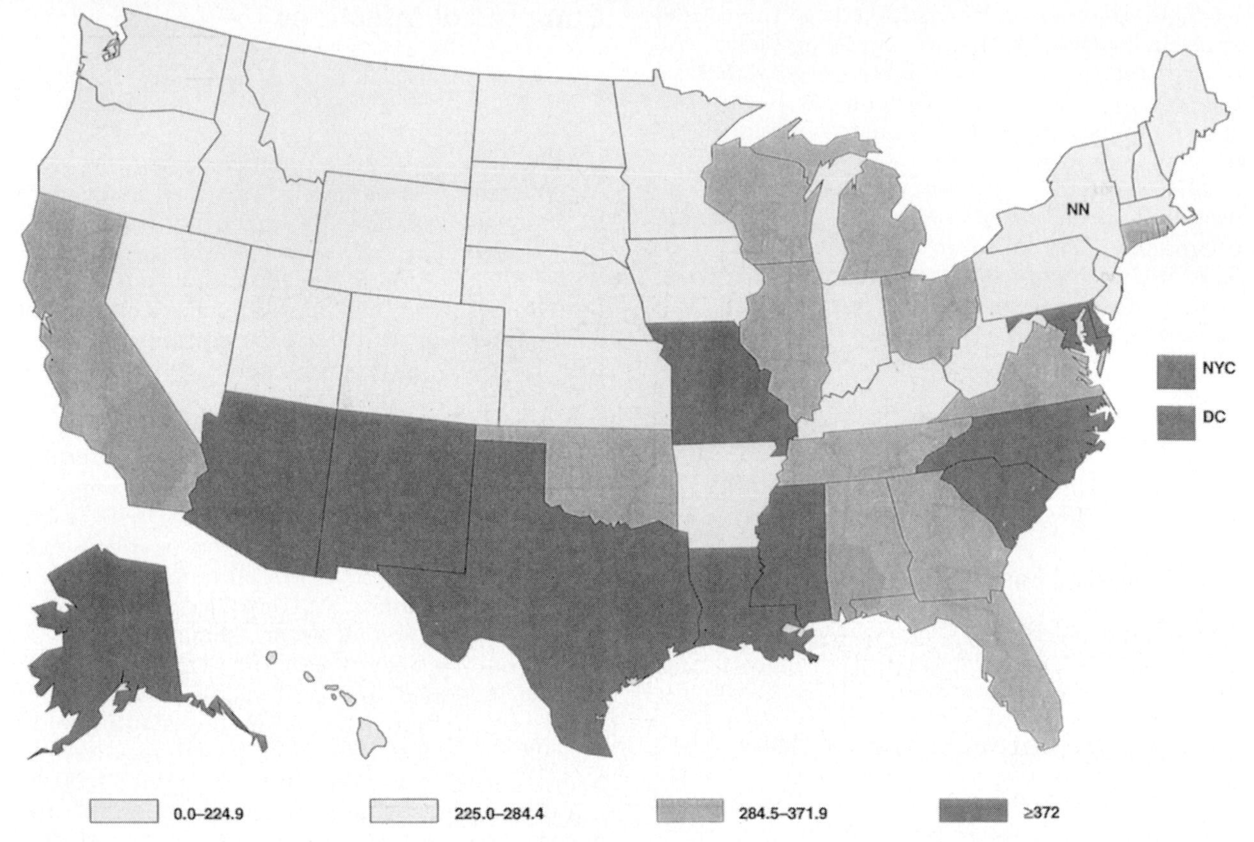

In 1997, the chlamydia rate among women was 322.1 cases per 100,000 population. The rates for men are not presented because reporting for men is more limited than it is for women.

Figure 18–8 ◆ Reported cases of *Chlamydia* infections, United States, 1997.

gonococcal infections among young sexually active individuals. The etiologic agent of gonorrhea is *Neisseria gonorrhoeae.* The organism invades the epithelial tissue of the genitourinary tract in adults and the conjunctiva of both adults and newborn infants. *N. gonorrhoeae* is almost universally transmitted by sexual intercourse in the adult or during delivery in the newborn. Involvement of the pharynx may follow oral intercourse; rectal involvement may follow anal intercourse. Transmission by toilet seats, bath towels, sheets, chairs, or drinking glasses is negligible. The organism is very susceptible to drying and survives only a short period of time in the external environment. The period of incubation is three to nine days.

Acute gonorrhea may involve the urethra, testes, prostate gland, or rectum in men. Invasion of tissue causes pain on urination, inflammation of the urethra, and a purulent discharge. Accumulations of scar tissue from untreated or repeated infections can lead to urethral stricture (narrowing) and make urination difficult. Sterility is a complication if the vas deferens is affected.

Gonococci may colonize the urethra, cervix, Skene's glands, Bartholin's glands, rectum, or pharynx in women. Vaginal infections occur in young girls. In contrast to the disease in men, approximately 75 to 90 percent of infected women have no symptoms. Women exhibiting symptoms are likely to have a purulent discharge from the urethra, cervix, or rectum and, possibly, painful urination or defecation. An ascending infection may involve the uterus, fallopian tubes, ovary, or abdominal tissues. Formation of scar tissue in the fallopian tubes may result in ectopic pregnancy or sterility; acute peritonitis may be fatal.

Gonococcal arthritis can occur in men or women as a consequence of genitourinary tract infection. The inflammatory process is particularly debilitating if large joints are affected.

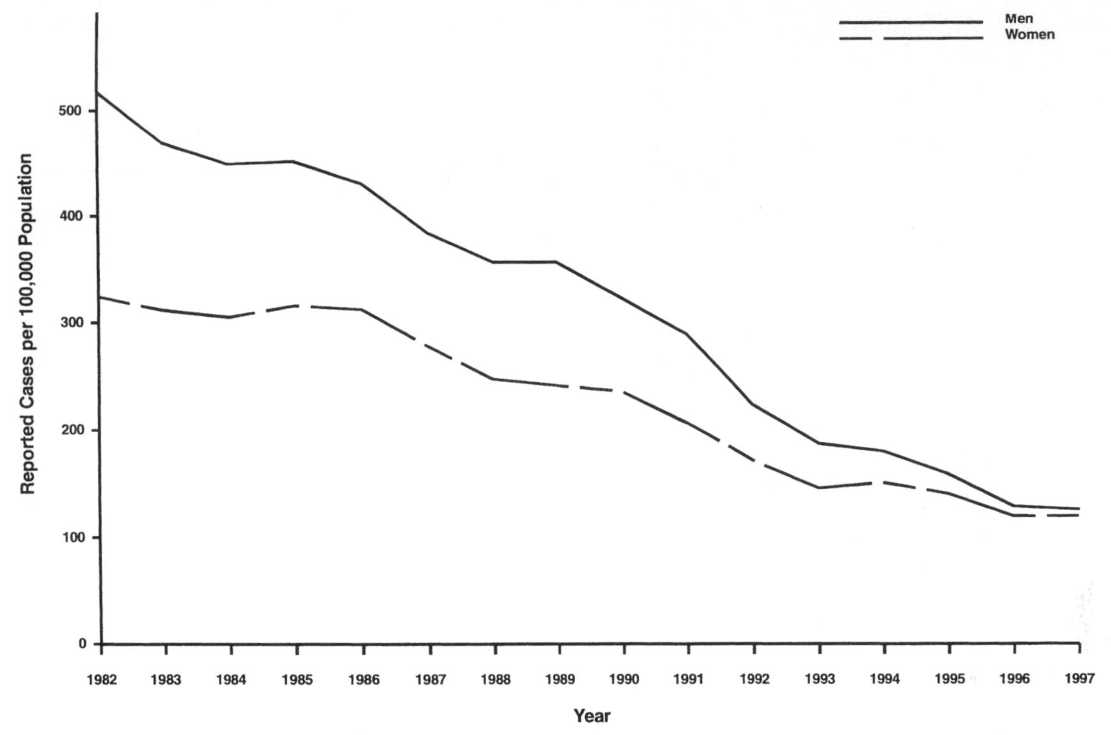

In 1997, the overall reported rate of gonorrhea in the United States was 121.4 per 100,000 population, similar to the rate of 122.8 in 1996. Among men, the rate decreased slightly from 128.5 per 100,000 population in 1996 to 125.4 in 1997. Among women, the rate increased slightly from 118.3 per 100,000 population in 1996 to 119.3 in 1997.*

*Data source: Division of Sexually Transmitted Diseases Prevention, National Center for HIV, STD, and TB Prevention.

Figure 18–9 ◆ Numbers of cases of gonorrhea in the United States from 1981 to 1997 compared by sex.

Ophthalmia neonatorum is a conjunctivitis of the newborn caused by contact with *N. gonorrhoeae* or *C. trachomatis* during delivery. If untreated, corneal ulcers or blindness may occur. Installation of a prophylactic agent into the eyes of all newborn infants is required by law in most states.

None of the recommended approaches is completely effective in preventing chlamydial or gonococcal disease. A 1 percent solution of silver nitrate prevents gonococcal ophthalmia, but not chlamydial ophthalmia. Erthyromycin (0.5 percent) is effective against both bacterial agents, but topical use does not prevent respiratory chlamydial infection. Tetracycline ointment (1 percent) has also been used successfully to prevent neonatal ophthalmia.

Gram stains of urethral or cervical exudates reveal the presence of polymorphonuclear neutrophils containing intracellular gram-negative diplococci in most cases of gonorrhea (Fig. 18–10; Color Plate 65). However, cultures are more reliable for diagnosing the infection, particularly in women. The organism grows well in an atmosphere of 3 to 10 percent CO_2 on modified Thayer-Martin (MTM) agar, an enriched medium containing vancomycin, colistin, and nystatin. *N. gonorrhoeae* produces oxidase. Species identification can be made by the pattern of carbohydrate degradation or by fluorescent antibody, co-agglutination antibody reagents, or a DNA probe method (Color Plate 66).

Public health authorities are concerned about plasmid- or chromosomal-mediated penicillin- and tetracycline-resistant strains of *N. gonorrhoeae.* Most penicillinase-producing strains of *N. gonorrhoeae* (PPNG) are plasmid-mediated, whereas most tetracycline-resistant strains (TRNG) are chromosome-mediated. An increasing number of strains are resistant to both drugs. Penicillins are no longer recommended for treatment of gonorrhea. Ceftriaxone, cefixime, and ciprofloxacin are the drugs of choice. All individuals contracting gonorrhea should have a serological test for syphilis and chlamydial infection. It is important that sexual partners be examined and treated

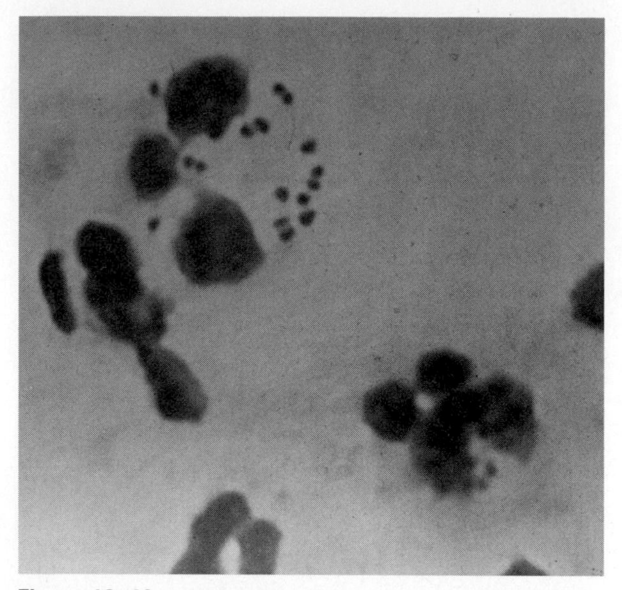

Figure 18–10 ◆ Intracellular *Neisseria gonorrhoeae* in a Gram-stained smear of urethral pus.

prophylactically to prevent the spread or recurrence of gonococcal infections.

Syphilis

Syphilis is an acute or chronic infection caused by the spirochete *Treponema pallidum* (Color Plate 67). The disease was once believed to have been introduced in Europe upon the return of Columbus and his crew in 1493. There is, however, much evidence that the disease existed in epidemic proportions during earlier times. The particularly virulent form of syphilis that spread during the century that followed the discovery of America was probably caused by a new strain, which could well have originated in the New World. The number of cases of syphilis reported annually has declined in the United States in both sexes in the last decade (Fig. 18–11). High rates of syphilis still continue to occur

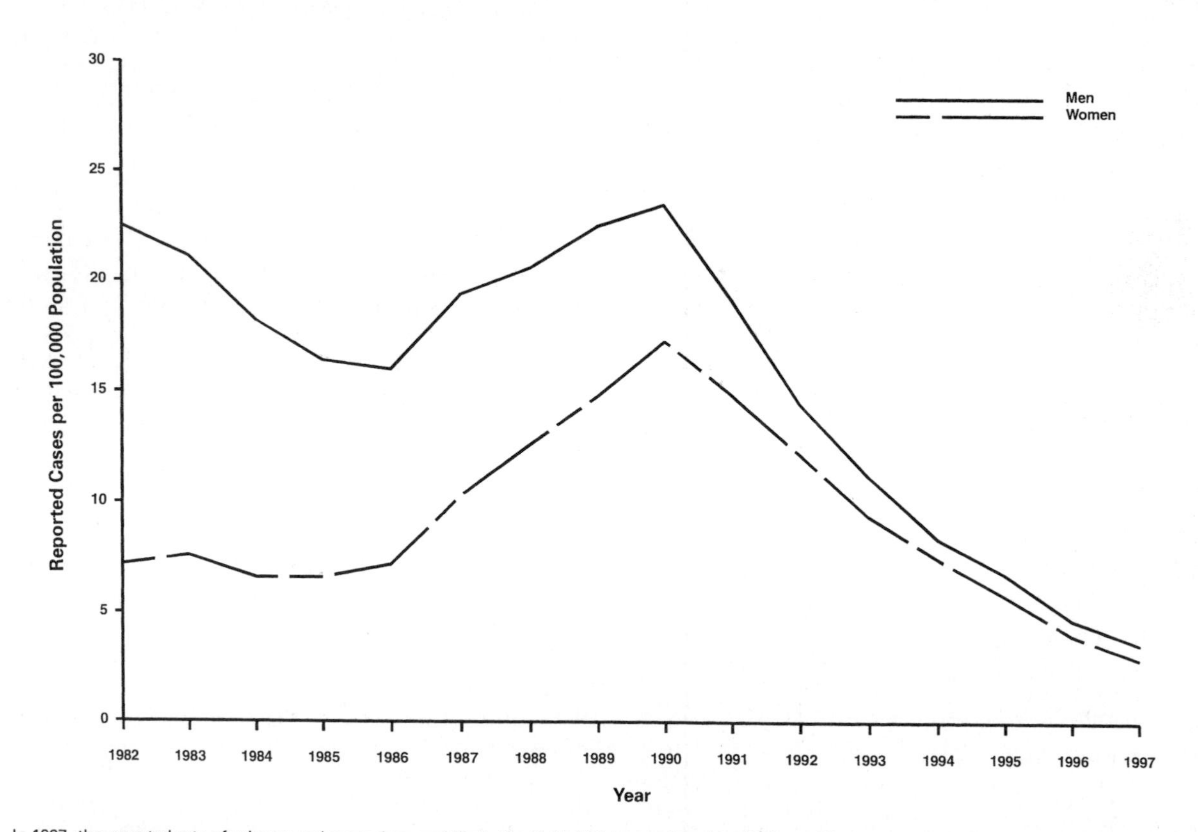

Figure 18–11 ◆ Numbers of cases per 100,000 population of primary and secondary syphilis from 1981 to 1997 showing a steady decline since 1990.

in the Southern states in places where access to health care is limited.

Approximately 95 percent of all syphilis is transmitted by direct contact with exudates or lesions of infected individuals through sexual intercourse. The rest is transmitted by kissing, placental transfer, or blood transfusions. The laboratory worker can contact *T. pallidum* through accidental exposure to blood or exudates containing the treponemes. Fortunately, such accidents are rare.

Syphilis occurs in four stages. **Primary syphilis** is characterized by a hard ulcer known as a **chancre,** occurring on the genitals 10 to 90 days after exposure to *T. pallidum.* The chancre usually develops on the tip of the penis and less frequently on the scrotum in men. A primary lesion may remain undetected in women if it develops on the inner surface of the genital organs. The chancre heals in one to five weeks with or without treatment. **Secondary syphilis** develops six to eight weeks after the appearance of the primary chancre and manifests itself as a skin rash (Fig. 18–12). The lesions of secondary syphilis are commonly present on the palms of the hands and soles of the feet, differing in that respect from other infectious skin rashes, which rarely affect the palmar or plantar surfaces. **Tertiary syphilis** may not become apparent for 10 or 20 years following the secondary stage. The disease in which there are no apparent signs of infection, even though the spirochetes may be spreading to inner organs, is called **latent syphilis.** Cases of latent syphilis may be classified as early or late latent disease. Persons acquiring syphilis within the preceding year are classified as having early latent syphilis. If more than one year has elapsed since acquisition can be documented or if time of exposure is unknown, individuals are classified as having late latent syphilis. Late latent syphilis is thought to be noninfectious except in pregnant women, who can transmit the disease to a fetus. The effects of the infection, which finally become apparent in the tertiary stage, are lesions of the cardiovascular, central nervous, or musculoskeletal systems. The soft tumorlike lesions of the tertiary stage are called **gummas.** The lesions are the result of a delayed hypersensitivity to *T. pallidum.* Persistent inflammation causes destruction of tissue as cytokines are released.

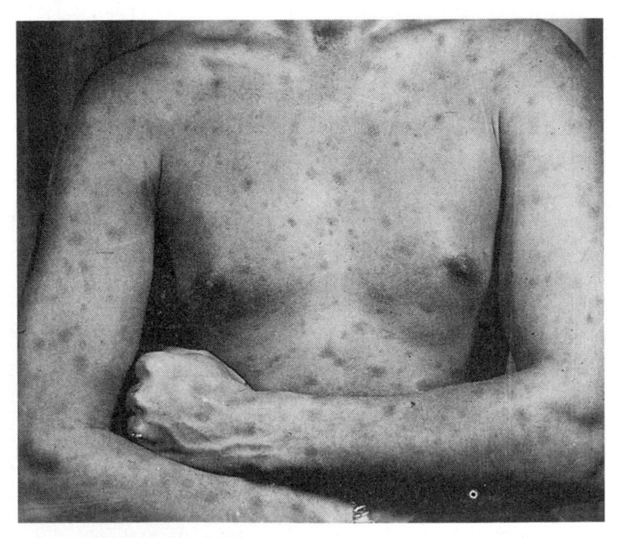

Figure 18–12 ◆ Lesions of secondary syphilis.

Tertiary syphilis is disabling, and the outcome is always fatal if undiagnosed before symptoms appear. Any organ can be invaded by the spirochetes, but the aorta, spinal cord, brain, and long bones are more commonly affected. Manifestations of aortitis include progressive aortic regurgitation, enlargement of the left ventricle, and congestive heart failure. Changes in reflexes, coordination, speech, emotions, and memory are common in neurosyphilis. In the most serious cases of tertiary syphilis, patients exhibit such severe delusions of grandeur that confinement in an institution is required.

Congenital syphilis occurs when the spirochetes penetrate the placental barrier and infect the fetus in utero. Primary or secondary maternal syphilis almost invariably causes miscarriage, stillbirth, neonatal death, or serious developmental abnormalities in the fetus (Fig. 18–13). Bullae (blisters) are present in the infant with congenital syphilis, in contrast to the maculopapular or papular lesions seen in adults with secondary syphilis.

The bacteriological diagnosis of syphilis by dark-field microscopy depends on finding helical forms of *T. pallidum* in fluid collected from a chancre (see Fig. 3–6). The organisms move slowly with winding movements in a liquid environment. *T. pallidum* does not grow in vitro, but it can be grown by scarification of hamster or rabbit skin and in rabbit testes.

Syphilis is usually diagnosed by serological methods because opportunities to do dark-field examinations on primary lesions is limited. Several serological tests for treponemal antibodies are available. The most specific test is the *Treponema pallidum* immobilization (TPI) test, but it is too cumbersome for most laboratories. A microhemagglutination test (MHA-TP) is easier to per-

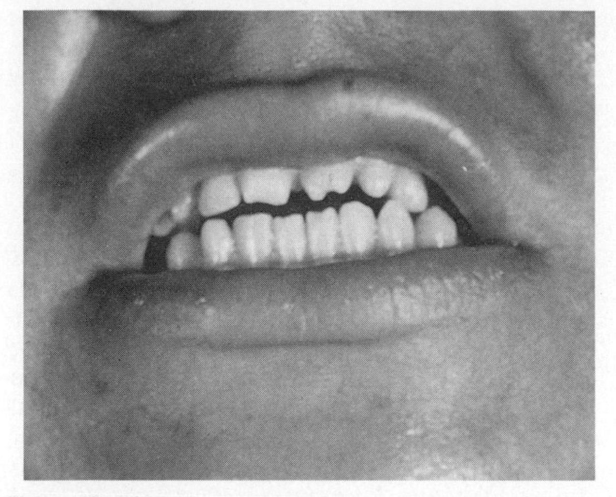

Figure 18–13 ◆ Notched teeth known as Hutchinson's teeth resulting from congenital syphilis.

form. Many laboratories do nontreponemal screening tests, such as the Venereal Disease Research Laboratory (VDRL) test or the rapid plasma reagin (RPR) card test, which are based on the presence of precipitating antibodies to a synthetic antigen. Mandatory premarital and prenatal testing for syphilis was once required by most states. It has been given up because testing programs were expensive and yielded so few positive results.

An enzyme immunoassay (EIA) procedure differentiates IgG from IgM antibody to *T. pallidum.* It is useful in diagnosing congenital syphilis and confirming a new infection in a person with a previous history of syphilis. Some patients may have low, but stable, IgG titers despite treatment. A PCR method is valuable in detecting *T. pallidum* in the amniotic fluid of pregnant women with untreated syphilis.

Primary, secondary, or latent syphilis of less than one year's duration responds to a single high dose of penicillin. Tetracycline is the drug of choice for individuals allergic to penicillin.

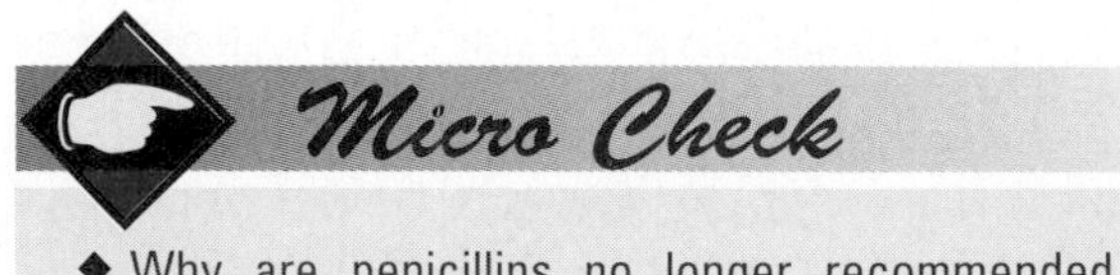

- ◆ Why are penicillins no longer recommended for treatment of gonorrhea?
- ◆ How can ophthalmia neonatorum be prevented?
- ◆ What is the drug of choice for treating syphilis?

Chancroid

Chancroid is an acute, sexually transmitted bacterial disease that is relatively uncommon in temperate climates. The primary lesion is an ulcer known as a soft chancre. It is caused by *Haemophilus ducreyi.* The infection is frequently associated with pain and suppuration of regional lymph nodes three to 14 days after exposure. Chancroid is transmitted primarily by sexual intercourse. Only rarely have dressings, instruments, or contaminated hands of attending medical personnel been implicated as a means for spreading chancroid.

Men with chancroid may have single or multiple soft chancres on the penis (Fig. 18–14). Ulcers in women are usually multiple and occur on the labia, vagina, buttocks, cervix, thigh, and perianal region. The lesions may be confused with lesions of herpes simplex virus (HSV) or those of syphilis.

Culturing material from lesions on enriched chocolate blood agar and vancomycin is the only reliable method for diagnosing chancroid, but these special culture media are not always stocked by laboratories. A clinical diagnosis of chancroid is dependent on physical findings and exclusion of genital herpes and syphilis.

The susceptibility of *H. ducreyi* to drugs differs among geographic regions, but azithromycin offers the advantage of single-dose therapy. Sex partners of infected individuals should also be treated.

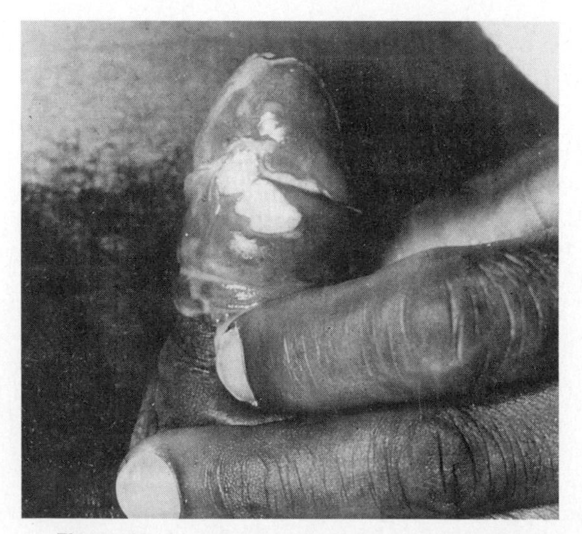

Figure 18–14 ◆ Lesions of chancroid on a penis.

Lymphogranuloma Venereum

Lymphogranuloma venereum (LGV) is a chlamydial disease that is worldwide in distribution, but more common in tropical and subtropical countries. The etiologic agents are LGV serotypes of *Chlamydia trachomatis*. The disease is transmitted by sexual intercourse or by contact with articles contaminated with material from active lesions. The incubation period varies from a week to several months.

The initial lesions of LGV commonly appear on the penis of men, but may be present on the external genitals, vaginal mucosa, or cervix in women. Spontaneous healing of the lesions is followed by enlargements of lymph nodes known as buboes. Swelling of the lymph nodes in the groin is the most frequent form of LGV observed. Complications include narrowing of the urethra or rectum and blockage of lymph vessels.

Fluorescein-conjugated monoclonal antibody reagent can be applied to smears prepared from lesion material, but a great deal of experience is required to detect *C. trachomatis* inclusions. The LGV serotypes of *C. trachomatis* can be grown in cell cultures or embryonated eggs. Several serological tests are available for detecting LVG strains of *C. trachomatis*.

Erythromycin, sulfamethoxazole, and tetracycline are active against LGV serotypes of *C. trachomatis*. Blockages may require surgical intervention. Sex partners of individuals with LGV should also receive treatment.

Granuloma Inguinale

Granuloma inguinale is an ulcerative genital infection caused by the pleomorphic, encapsulated bacterium *Calymmatobacterium granulomatis*. Granuloma inguinale is endemic in tropical and subtropical climates, but is rare in Europe and the United States. The infection is not highly communicable, but is believed to be transmitted sexually. The time of incubation varies from a week to six months.

The initial lesion of granuloma inguinale is a painless nodule, but it soon degenerates into a bleeding, tender ulcer and causes progressive ulceration of the genitals. The lesions become infiltrated with neutrophils and monocytes.

Biopsy material from the lesion found in granuloma inguinale is the specimen of choice for diagnosing the infection. Giemsa stains of that material reveal the typical coccobacilli inside vacuoles of macrophages. Cultural methods are too cumbersome to be practical because special media are required. The drug of choice is tetracycline or ampicillin.

FUNGAL INFECTIONS

Colonization of the vagina by yeast is favored by the acidity of the vagina, but except for vulvovaginal candidiasis (once called moniliasis), infections of the genitourinary tract caused by fungi are rare. However, indwelling catheters may become contaminated with *Candida albicans* and ultimately cause systemic infection. Conversely, yeast in urine may be the manifestation of disseminated fungal disease.

Vulvovaginal Candidiasis

Vulvovaginal candidiasis consists of an inflammation of the vulva and vagina; it can be caused by a variety of *Candida* species, but it is most frequently caused by *C. albicans*. Most disease originates from endogenous yeasts which proliferate in the vagina under special conditions. Sexual partners of women with vulvovaginal candidiasis can carry the yeast on the penis, but rarely become infected. Vulvovaginitis is common in diabetics. The high estrogen levels accompanying pregnancy, or administration of corticosteroids or broad-spectrum antibacterial drugs also predispose individuals to the infection. Symptoms include pruritus (itching) and a thick curdlike vaginal discharge. Candidiasis can spread readily to the perineum or perianal regions.

A wet mount of vaginal secretions in 10 percent potassium hydroxide (KOH) usually reveals the presence of budding yeasts and pseudohyphae in vulvovaginal candidiasis. *Candida* species grow on Sabouraud's agar. *C. albicans* forms short, lateral hyphal filaments called germ tubes, in beef serum (see Fig. 15–18). CHROMagar can provide presumptive evidence for the presence of more than 10 *Candida* species based on color production. An enzymatic test that detects the presence of β-galactosaminidase and proline aminopeptidase is both specific and sensitive for identifying colonies of *C. albicans*. A series of oxidative and fermentative tests on carbohydrates may be used to determine the species of yeasts, but the procedures are time-consuming.

Vulvovaginal candidiasis usually responds well to miconazole or nystatin. Symptomatic disease during pregnancy is particularly difficult to eradicate. Sometimes it is important to treat sex partners with topical anticandidal preparations.

PROTOZOAL INFECTIONS

Most pathogenic protozoa will grow in intestines or blood, where access is provided through the gastrointestinal tract or by capillary invasion following the bite of an arthropod. An exception is the flagellate *Trichomonas vaginalis,* which resides in the vagina of approximately 25 percent of American women. The parasite can invade the Bartholin's or Skene's glands, but more frequently causes urethritis, cystitis, or vaginitis.

Trichomoniasis

Trichomoniasis may occur as a single infection or may coexist with candidiasis in the inflamed vagina. The etiologic agent, *Trichomonas vaginalis,* is a flagellated protozoan with three to five anterior flagella and a single posterior flagellum. The time of incubation is four to 20 days. Sometimes there is an accompanying urethritis or cervicitis caused by gonococcal infection. It is doubtful that extrasexual transmission of *T. vaginalis* occurs with any regularity. Vaginal trichomoniasis causes itching, burning, and a frothy creamy yellow discharge.

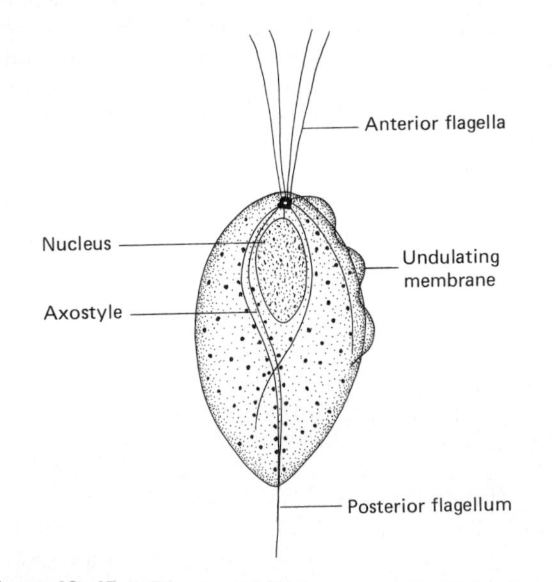

Figure 18–15 ◆ Diagram of *Trichomonas vaginalis* showing internal morphology and positions of flagella.

A saline wet mount prepared from a vaginal discharge reveals the presence of numerous polymorphonuclear white blood cells and actively motile trichomonads in the protozoan infection. The flagellates are pear-shaped and contain an undulating membrane over approximately half of the organism (Fig. 18–15). Culture is rarely necessary. Immunofluorescent (IF) and enzyme-linked immunoassay (EIA) reagents are also available, but are usually unnecessary.

Metronidazole is the drug of choice for trichomoniasis, but is contraindicated during pregnancy. Clotrimazole may produce symptomatic improvement. Male sex partners of infected individuals should be treated with metronidazole.

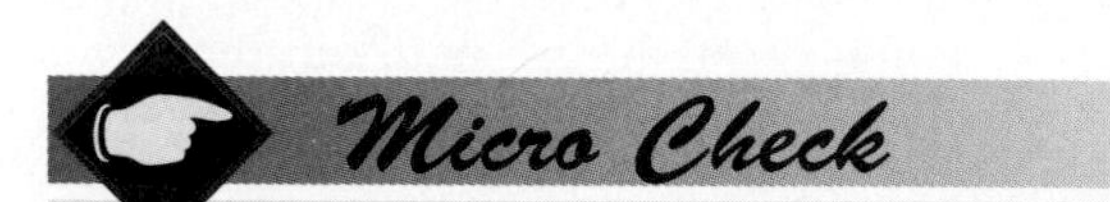

- ◆ How do the lesions of chancroid differ from the primary lesions of syphilis?
- ◆ What protozoan infection frequently coexists with candidiasis?
- ◆ What vaginal condition favors the growth of yeast?

VIRAL INFECTIONS

It is likely that the presence of many sexually transmittable viruses on the genital organs escape detection. A number of viruses, including those of mumps, rubeola, and cytomegalovirus (CMV) inclusion disease, are shed in urine. The human immunodeficiency virus (HIV) is excreted in semen and cervical secretions of infected patients.

Genital Herpes

Both the male and female genital tracts may be sites of primary and recurrent disease caused by herpes simplex viruses. Approximately 80 percent of primary genital infections are caused by herpes simplex virus 2 (HSV-2), but an increasing number of infections with HSV-1 are occurring. The actual number of genital herpes infections in the United States is not known, but it is estimated that at least 25 million individuals in the United States have or have had genital herpes infections. The primary mode of transmission is by sexual intercourse, but the possibility of autoinfection by fingers cannot be overlooked. The disease can occur as a primary exogenous infection two to 12 days after exposure or as a recurrent endogenous infection when latent HSV-1 or HSV-2 are activated. Most carriers of HSV-2 have at least six recurrences a year.

Primary lesions occur in the cervix, vulva, and vagina in women, but may be followed by lesions on the surrounding skin of the perineum, buttocks, and thighs. There may be a profuse watery discharge from the vagina. Lesions usually occur on the glans penis and less often on the perineum or scrotum in men (Fig. 18–16). The lesions in both sexes are painful and accompanied by dysuria (painful urination), fever, and swelling of lymph nodes in the groin. Ultraviolet light, heat, cold, x-ray, hormonal imbalance, immunosuppression, and even emotional imbalances can induce recurrent disease. Recurrent infections are usually less severe than primary infections.

Genital herpes infections can be diagnosed by direct examination of lesion scrapings on a Papanicolaou (Pap) smear, by immunofluorescent (IF) tests, by an enzyme-linked immunosorbent assay (ELISA), or by nucleic acid probes. The viruses can be detected in genital ulcer specimens by a PCR technique. HSV-1 and HSV-2 may be isolated in tissue cultures. Both viruses produce cytopathic effects (CPE), which consist of granulation, ballooning, and rounding within one to three days.

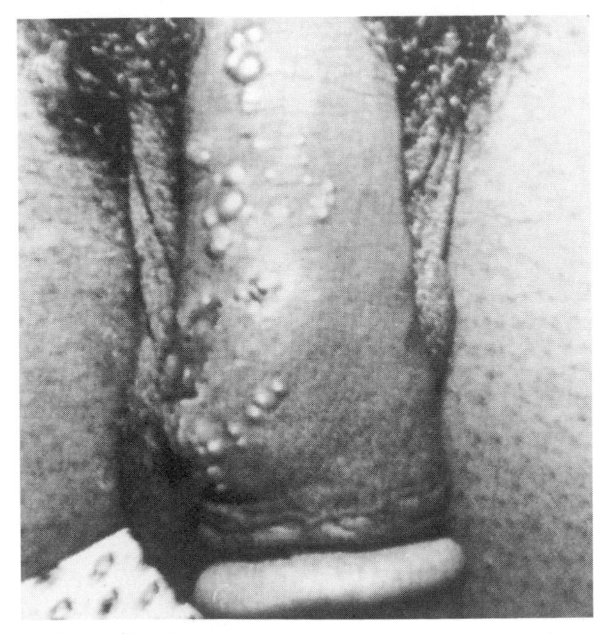

Figure 18–16 ◆ Lesions of herpes simplex on a penis.

Genital herpes infections are self-limiting but cause affected individuals a great amount of physical and mental stress. Acyclovir may alleviate some symptoms and shorten the course of primary infections, but has less effect on recurrent infections. Unfortunately, the drug does not affect the subsequent risk, rate, or severity of recurrences.

Genital Warts (Condylomata Acuminata)

The incidence of **genital warts** (condylomata acuminata) has risen dramatically in the past several years. Although there are more than 60 types of human papillomaviruses (HPVs), genital warts are caused by types 6, 11, 16, 31, 33, and 35. The viruses are transmitted sexually. The warts do not appear for two to three months after exposure to the virus. Single or multiple lesions may be present on the external genitals, and in the urethra, vagina, and cervix, or in the perianal region. Genital warts have been linked to the development of squamous cell genital cancers so Pap smears are recommended for all women with genital warts.

A diagnosis of genital warts does not require laboratory confirmation, but a special instrument may be necessary to detect intraurethral warts. Identification of the common types can be made with nucleic acid probes. Treatment may consist of cryotherapy (freezing), electrosurgery, laser vaporization, or topical application of podophyllin. Podophyllin should not be used during pregnancy. The goal of treatment is the removal of warts and relief from symptoms, not the eradication of HPVs. No form of treatment can prevent recurrences.

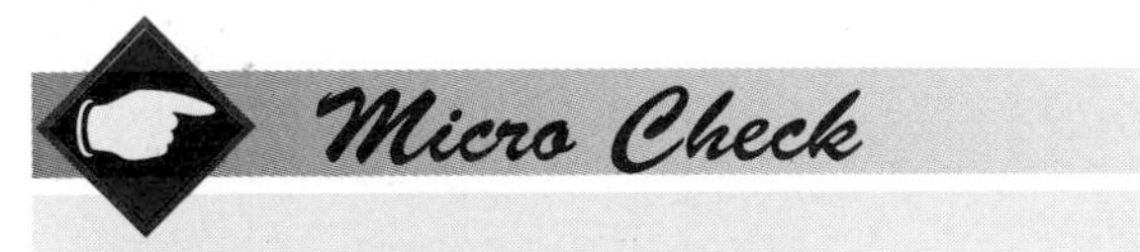

- What viruses are shed in urine?
- Why does genital herpes recur?
- Why are Papanicolaou (Pap) smears recommended for women with genital warts?

Table 18–2
SUMMARY OF MAJOR MICROORGANISMS CAUSING DISEASES OF THE GENITOURINARY TRACT

MICROORGANISM	DISEASE	TREATMENT
Bacteria		
Chlamydia trachomatis	Nongonococcal urethritis	Tetracycline
	Lymphogranuloma venereum	Erythromycin
		Azithromycin
*Escherichia coli**	Cystitis	Sulfonamides
		Trimethoprim-sulfathoxazole
Leptospira interrogans	Leptospirosis	Penicillin
		Tetracycline
Bacteroides fragilis†	Pelvic inflammatory disease	Clindamycin
Gardnerella vaginalis	Nonspecific vaginitis	Metronidazole
Group B *Streptococcus*	GBS infection	Ampicillin
Neisseria gonorrhoeae	Gonorrhea	Ceftriazone
Treponema pallidum	Syphilis	Penicillin
Haemophilus ducreyi	Chancroid	Trimethoprim-sulfathoxazole
Calymmatobacterium granulomatis	Granuloma inguinale	Tetracycline
		Ampicillin
Fungi		
Candida albicans	Vulvovaginal candidiasis	Miconazole
		Nystatin
Protozoa		
Trichomonas vaginalis	Trichomoniasis	Metronidazole
Viruses		
Herpes simplex virus 2	Genital herpes infection	Acyclovir
Papillomaviruses (types 6, 11, 16, 31, 33, and 35)	Genital warts	Cryotherapy
		Electrosurgery
		Podophyllin

* *E. coli* is the most common cause of cystitis.
† *B. fragilis* is one etiologic agent of pelvic inflammatory disease.

Acquired Immunodeficiency Syndrome

The emergence of **acquired immunodeficiency syndrome (AIDS)** in 1981 has focused attention once again on the devastating effects of epidemics. AIDS is classified as an STD, but the human immunodeficiency virus (HIV) infects helper T cells (CD4 cells). HIV infections and AIDS are discussed in Chapter 20. Other sexually transmitted diseases, such as gonorrhea, syphilis, and genital herpes, may be risk factors in heterosexual transmission of HIV. Concurrent infections of HIV and other STDs cause persistence of symptoms, despite aggressive treatment. All STDs can be substantially reduced by the consistent and correct use of condoms with water-based lubricants, such as K-Y Jelly or glycerine.

The major microorganisms causing genitourinary tract diseases are summarized in Table 18–2.

Understanding Microbiology

1. Name three factors that predispose women to urinary tract infection.
2. What risk factors are associated with GBS infections in newborns?
3. Why is penicillin no longer the drug of choice for gonorrhea?
4. How can gonococcal or chlamydial eye infections of the newborn be prevented?
5. Why is treatment of sex partners often recommended in sexually transmitted diseases?

FOCAL POINT

The AIDS of the Sixteenth Century

Modern evidence suggests that the spirochete of syphilis originated in Africa and was brought to the West Indies by dark-skinned aborigines. Although many historians feel that syphilis had been present in Europe for a long time, the numbers of cases exploded into a pandemic in the sixteenth century. The presence of syphilis in the New World was supported by a discovery of fossilized bones of a bear in Indiana a few years ago. The fossil remains of that bear who lived 11,500 years ago had holes and spikes similar to those found in syphilis. No country wanted to take responsibility for the disease. The British called it the French disease. The Germans called it the Italian disease. The year following Columbus's return, syphilis had entered France. No one can be sure if the strain of the spirochete introduced had been incubating in an unsuspecting French population for many years or, indeed, if it had traveled across the ocean to victimize Europeans. It is known that when the French king, Charles VIII, led his army of 30,000 men into Naples, the pandemic began. His soldiers were the high-risk group of their day. In Paris alone, it was estimated that a third of the population had syphilis. Schubert, Beethoven, Keats, Henry VIII, Mary Tudor, and Napoleon, all recognized for their special contributions, had the disease. It is not uncommon for microorganisms to lie dormant, or almost so, and cause resurgence of disease many years later. The origin of any disease is not nearly as important as ways to resolve the problems it presents for the millions of infected people.

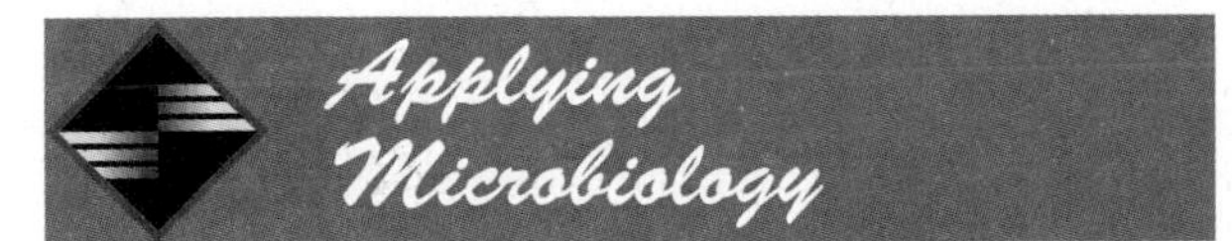

Read the following case study carefully and answer the questions: A 28-year-old woman was admitted to a hospital in Racine, Wisconsin, with a one-week history of arthritis of the left knee. Synovial and cervical cultures produced beta-lactamase. The patient had had no cervical or urethral discharge. She was treated for two days with intravenous penicillin, but when the lab results were available, her therapy was changed to ceftriaxone. She was discharged within one week after the knee had been drained.

6. Her disease should have been reported to the local health department as a case of
   a. Lyme disease
   b. gonorrhea
   c. pertussis
   d. rheumatoid arthritis
   e. syphilis
7. It is likely that treatment was changed because the organism isolated produced
   a. oxidase
   b. penicillinase
   c. decarboxylase
   d. pectinase
   e. urease
8. The organism causing the disease is classified as a (an)
   a. protozoan
   b. helminth
   c. RNA virus
   d. bacterium
   e. DNA virus
9. The mode of transmission for the disease was most likely
   a. the bite of a tick
   b. a fomite
   c. sexual intercourse
   d. kissing
   e. an aerosol
10. Another complication of the infection in women can be
    a. a persistent cough
    b. neurological damage
    c. gastrointestinal distress
    d. infertility
    e. prostatitis

Chapter 19

Diseases of the Nervous System, Eye, and Ear

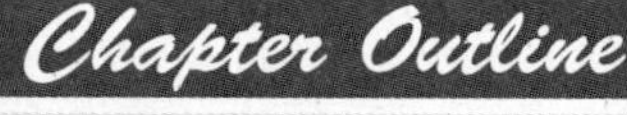

Chapter Outline

- **BACTERIAL INFECTIONS**
  - Meningococcal Meningitis
  - *Haemophilus* Meningitis
  - Streptococcal Meningitis
  - Other Bacterial Meningitides
  - Brain Abscess
  - Tetanus
  - Conjunctivitis
  - Trachoma
  - Otitis Media
- **FUNGAL INFECTIONS**
  - Cryptococcosis
  - Cerebrorhinoorbital Phycomycoses
- **PROTOZOAL INFECTIONS**
  - Amebic Meningoencephalitis
  - Toxoplasmosis
  - African Sleeping Sickness
- **VIRAL INFECTIONS**
  - Aseptic Meningitis
  - Poliomyelitis
  - Encephalitis
  - Rabies
  - Viral Conjunctivitis and Keratitis
- **PRION-ASSOCIATED DISEASES**

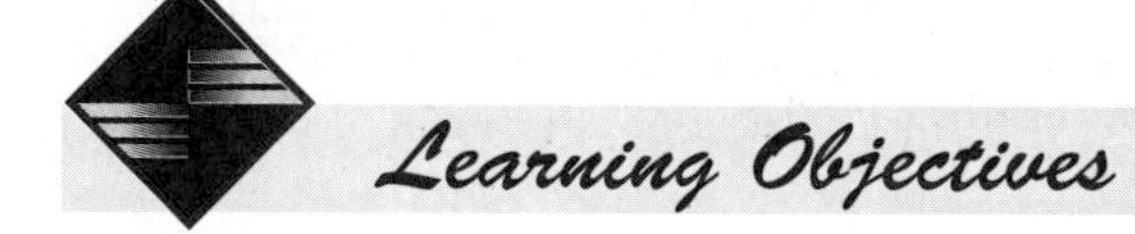

Learning Objectives

After you have read this chapter, you should be able to:

1. Describe how microorganisms gain entrance to neural tissue.
2. List the bacteria that commonly cause meningitis.
3. List the major microbial diseases and etiologic agents of eye and ear infections.
4. List the major fungi and protozoa causing diseases of the nervous system.
5. Explain how central nervous system diseases believed to be caused by prions differ from viral infections of the CNS.

The nervous system is divided into the central nervous system (CNS), consisting of the brain and spinal cord, and the peripheral nervous system making up the motor and sensory peripheral nerves (Fig. 19–1). Highly specialized receptors of peripheral nerve fibers are responsible for the special senses of smell, taste, sight, hearing, and equilibrium. The brain is contained within a vault of bone known as the **cranium;** the spinal cord is encased in a tunnel of bones known as the **vertebrae.** The spinal cord passes through the **foramen magnum,** an opening in the skull, and expands into the **medulla oblongata** or brain stem.

The brain and spinal column are covered by three membranes, called meninges. The **dura mater** is the strong outermost covering; the **pia mater** is a thin membrane adjacent to the brain

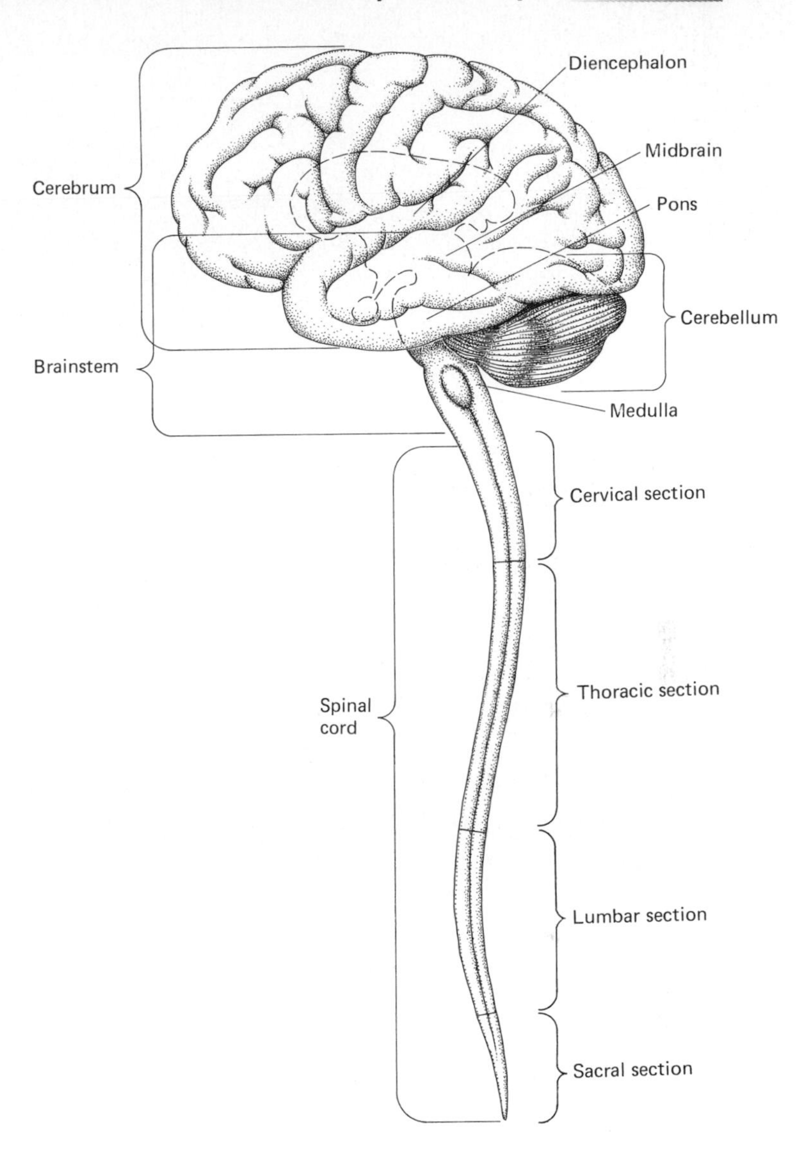

Figure 19–1 ◆ Lateral view showing major parts of the central nervous system.

and the spinal cord. The **arachnoid** is the delicate middle membrane separated from the dura mater by the subdural space and from the pia mater by the subarachnoid space (Fig. 19–2).

The hollow central canal of the spinal cord and cavities of the brain, called **ventricles,** contain the **cerebrospinal fluid** (CSF). The same fluid circulates in the subarachnoid space and also flows a short distance along sheaths of the cranial and spinal nerves.

The central and peripheral nervous systems are normally sterile. The indigenous microorganisms of the conjunctiva and external auditory canal are largely a reflection of the microorganisms indigenous to the skin (Table 19–1). Microorganisms, antibodies, and some antibiotics have difficulty in passing from the bloodstream to the brain and meninges because of selective permeability of their capillaries. The blood-brain and blood-CSF barriers serve as protective mechanisms, but are also limitations in the treatment of infections of the brain. In the event of a severe septicemia, even intact blood-brain and blood-CSF barriers cannot prevent the migration of microorganisms into neural tissue. Other ways that microorganisms or their toxins reach the CNS

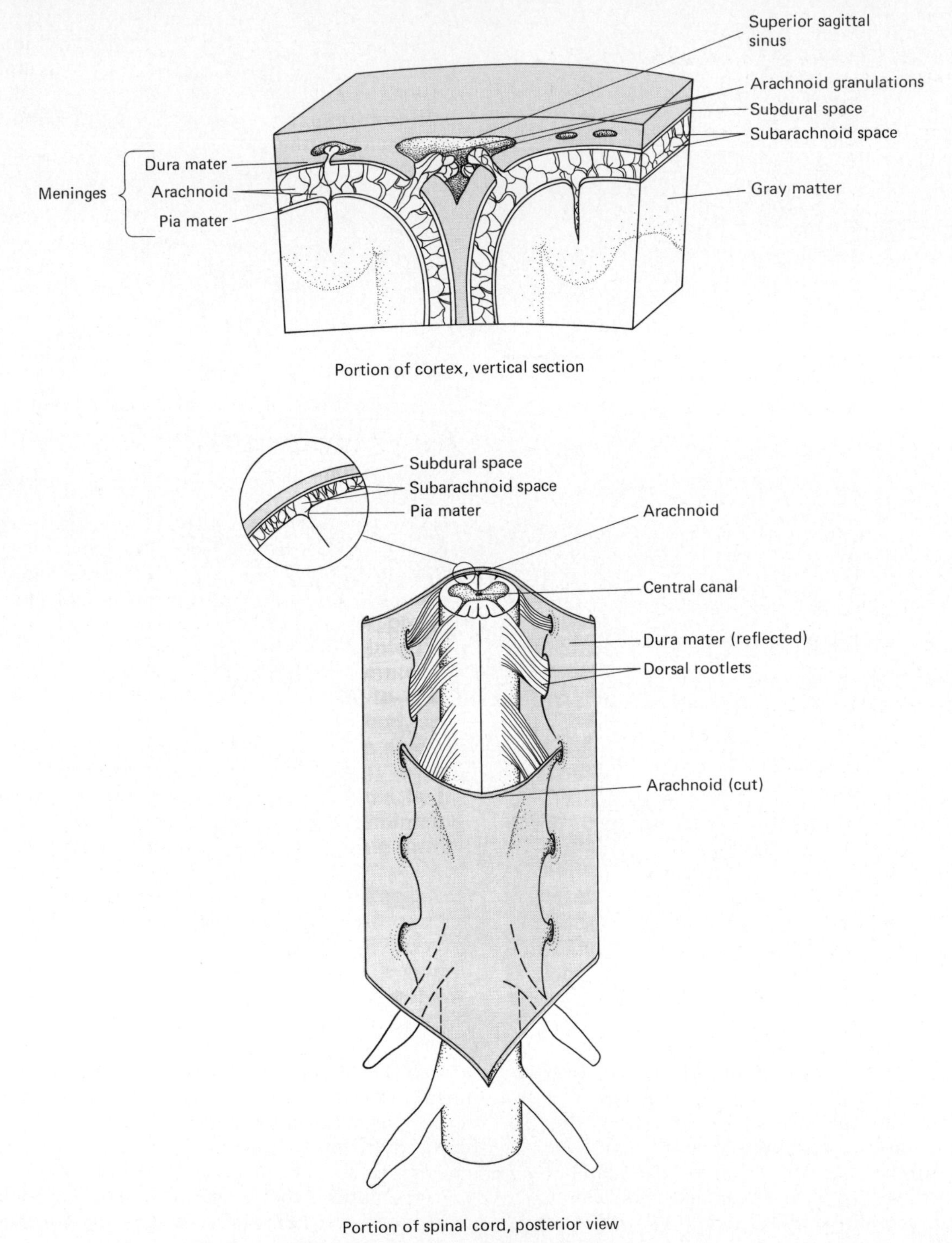

Figure 19–2 ◆ The meninges of the brain and the spinal cord.

Table 19–1

MICROORGANISMS INDIGENOUS TO THE CONJUNCTIVA AND EXTERNAL AUDITORY CANAL

GRAM-POSITIVE BACTERIA	GRAM-NEGATIVE BACTERIA
Corynebacterium species	*Moraxella catarrhalis*
Propionibacterium acnes	*Moraxella lacunata*
Staphylococcus aureus	Miscellaneous gram-negative bacilli*
Staphylococcus epidermidis	
Streptococcus species	

* Gram-negative bacilli are isolated with a frequency of 0 to 5 percent.

can be by way of the (1) eustachian tube, (2) mastoid process, (3) peripheral nerves, (4) cribriform plate, and (5) trauma.

The eye is afforded protection from invading microorganisms by the thin mucous membrane known as the conjunctiva, which covers the eyeball and lines the eyelid. The eyelid protects the eye from foreign objects and spreads lacrimal secretions over the eyeball. The secretions contain a bactericidal enzyme called **lysozyme.** Trauma to ocular tissue can provide a portal of entry for any organism. Some microorganisms reach the eye by way of the bloodstream or infected implant material. The aqueous and vitreous humors, which are the fluids of the anterior and posterior chambers of the eye, make excellent culture media. Some microorganisms demonstrate a particular affinity for a specific part of the eye or accessory structure (Fig. 19–3). No infection of the eye should be considered lightly because manifestations of the infection may be serious enough to impair vision or even cause loss of sight.

Despite the anatomical barriers provided by the tympanic membrane, microorganisms can enter the inner ear by means of a penetrating wound, the bloodstream, or through the eustachian tube (Fig. 19–4). Viral or bacterial disease of the upper respiratory system predisposes individuals, especially children, to infections of the middle ear (otitis media) and the accompanying earache. Infections of the outer ear (otitis externa) are associated with contaminated fingers, objects used in removing wax from ears, hearing aids, or swimming pool water. The protective enclosure provided by the external auditory canal provides especially favorable growth conditions.

Some diseases that ultimately affect neural tissue are discussed in the chapter concerned with portal of entry or site of primary infection. For example, the tuberculoid form of leprosy, a disease that causes impairment of peripheral nerves, is discussed in Chapter 15. Botulism is discussed in Chapter 17 with diseases of the gastrointestinal tract, and syphilis is discussed in Chapter 18 with diseases of the genitourinary tract. Diseases of the eye and ear are included in this chapter because the eyes and ears are sensory organs and represent portals of entry for more serious CNS infections.

BACTERIAL INFECTIONS

Most bacterial diseases of the nervous system involve the meninges. In most cases of meningitis there is an inflammation of the pia mater and the arachnoid. The nature of the infection can often be determined by the presence of etiologic agents in the CSF.

Meningococcal Meningitis

Meningococcal meningitis is endemic throughout the world. Although it once occurred in epidemic form in the United States, in recent years it has been observed only sporadically in small clusters or single cases. At one time epidemics of this type of meningitis were common in military recruits. Caused by *Neisseria meningitidis,* the disease is transmitted by direct contact with aerosols or nasopharyngeal discharges from an infected person or a carrier. Children are particularly susceptible to the disease. The carrier rate is much higher than the frequency of the disease. The time of incubation is two to ten days. Meningococcal meningitis is characterized by an abrupt onset of fever and nausea. Sometimes vomiting, stiff neck, and petechiae (small hemorrhagic spots on the skin) occur. In fulminating (rapidly occurring) cases of meningococcal bacteremia, adrenal hemorrhage and circulatory collapse may cause death within 24 hours. At one time fatality rates were as high as 50 percent.

Gram stains of sediment from CSF reveal the presence of intracellular and extracellular gram-negative diplococci in meningococcal meningitis. The organism grows on blood or chocolate agar

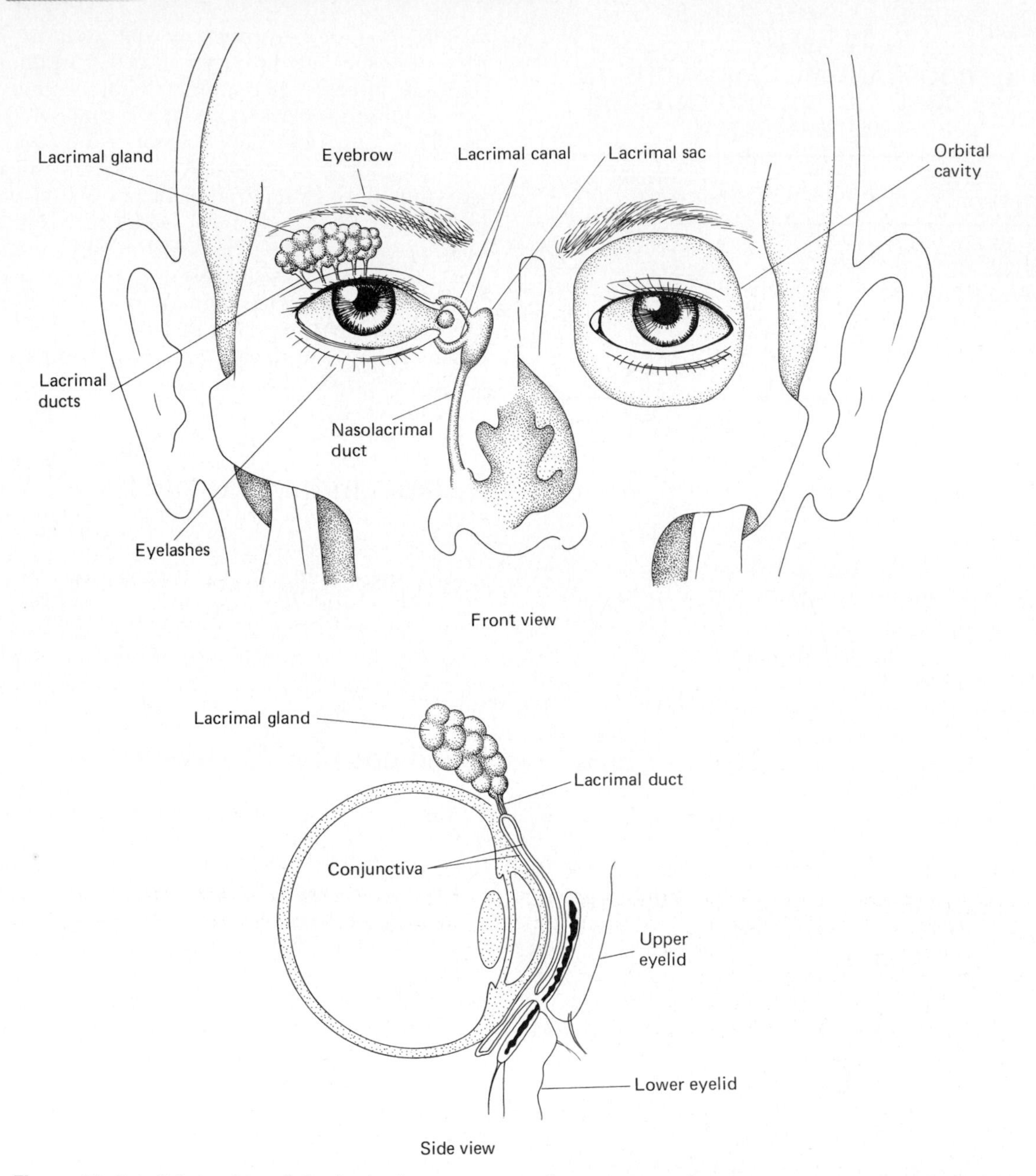

Figure 19–3 ◆ Relationship of the lacrimal apparatus to other eye parts of accessory organs as seen from the front and side. The lacrimal structures are responsible for the manufacture, secretion, and drainage of tears, which protect the eye from invasion by foreign objects.

in an atmosphere of 10 percent CO_2 (Fig. 19–5). Like *N. gonorrhoeae,* colonies of meningococci exhibit a positive oxidase reaction, but they degrade both glucose and maltose. *N. meningitidis* tests negative for β-galactosidase, and results are variable for proline aminopeptidase. Polyvalent reagents for serotypes A, B, and C may be used for direct antigen testing on CSF. Both latex and coagglutination tests are available commercially. Although direct antigen testing is of value in making a possible presumptive diagnosis, it should not be substituted for the Gram stain and culture of CSF.

Penicillin given parenterally is the drug of

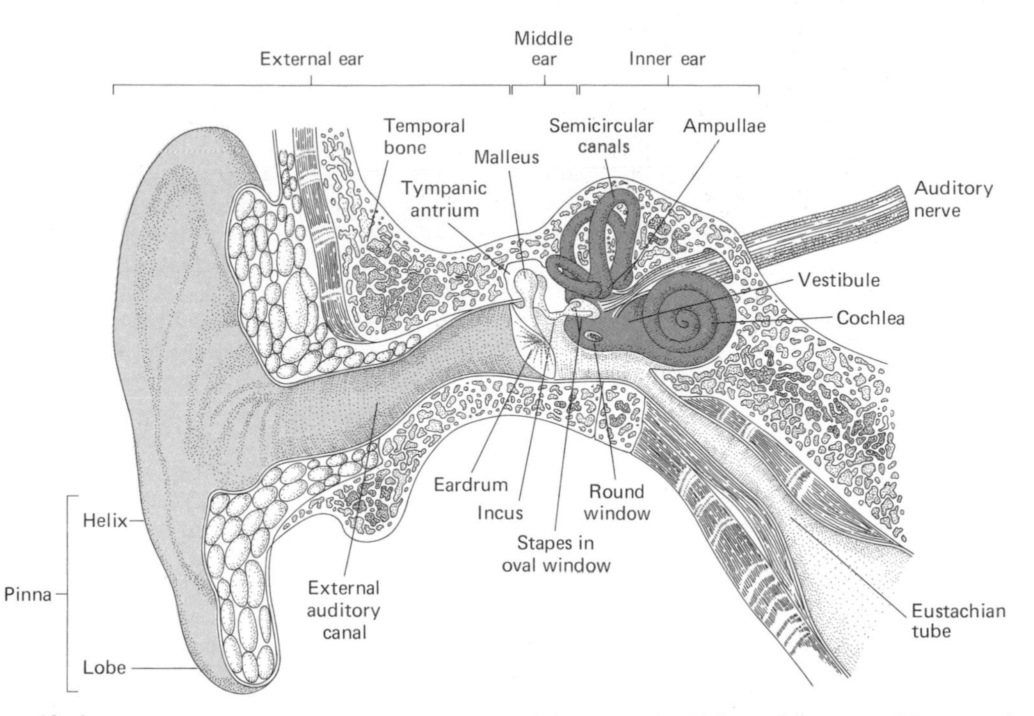

Figure 19–4 ◆ Structure of the ear showing major parts of the external, middle, and inner ear. Microorganisms enter the inner ear when the eardrum is punctured, by the eustachian tube, or by the bloodstream.

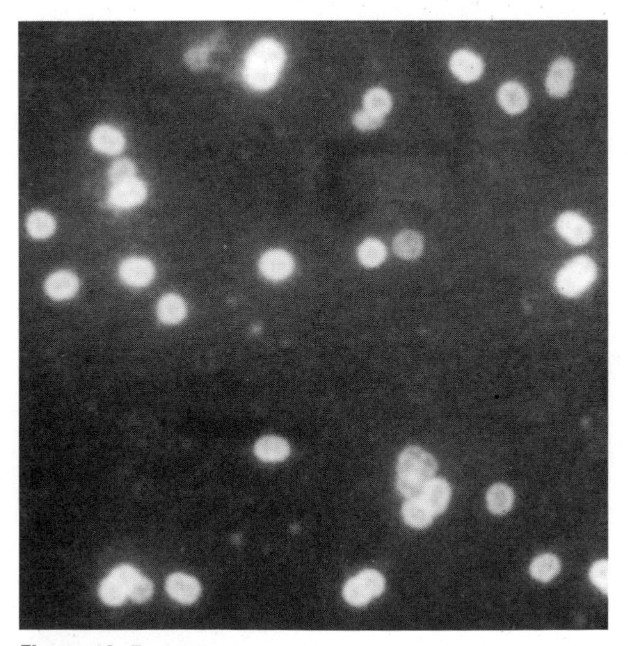

Figure 19–5 ◆ Colonies of *Neisseria meningitidis,* group C, as observed in cerebrospinal fluid using a fluorescent dye.

choice in proven meningococcal disease, but antibiotic susceptibility tests should be performed. If an isolate is sulfonamide-susceptible, intravenous sulfadiazine may be administered instead. If meningococcal meningitis is suspected, treatment should be started promptly. Monovalent vaccines of purified capsular polysaccharides against serotypes A and C and a bivalent A-C vaccine are available for selective use. Serotype C vaccine has been given to military recruits in the United States since 1971. Routine vaccination for civilians is not recommended, but it should be considered for travelers to countries experiencing epidemics of meningococcal meningitis.

Haemophilus Meningitis

Whereas a variety of microorganisms can cause meningitis, the most common cause of meningitis for years in children two months to five years of age was *Haemophilus influenzae.* type B (Hib). The availability of a vaccine in 1985 resulted in a dramatic decline in the cases of this type of meningitis. Hib is transmitted by aerosols or contact with nasopharyngeal discharges from an infected person or a carrier. The carrier rate approximates 5 percent. The period of incubation rarely exceeds two to four days. The infection usually follows otitis media or sinusitis. The onset is often sudden. The symptoms include fever, vomiting, stiff neck, and lethargy, which may proceed to stupor or coma. The fatality rate is very high if prompt treatment is not initiated.

In Gram stains of sediment from CSF, *H. influenzae* appear as gram-negative coccobacilli, but the bacteria may be few in number. The organism grows well on chocolate agar supplemented with X and V factors. The satellite phenomenon demonstrated by *H. influenzae* on blood agar is described in Chapter 16. Latex and coagglutination tests may be used to detect the presence of Hib antigen in CSF, but results must be confirmed by the isolation of the organism from CSF.

The drugs of choice for meningitis caused by Hib are ampicillin and chloramphenicol. Antibiotic susceptibility tests should be performed, because as many as 35 percent of strains of Hib are resistant to ampicillin. An Hib capsular polysaccharide vaccine prevents invasive disease. Immunization of all children aged two months to five years is recommended.

Streptococcal Meningitis

The third most common cause of bacterial meningitis is *Streptococcus pneumoniae.* It occurs more frequently in adults than in children. The signs and symptoms may be indistinguishable from other types of meningitis. It is frequently a complication of pneumococcal pneumonia, otitis media, or endocarditis.

The isolation and identification of *S. pneumoniae* is discussed in Chapter 16. Rapid antigen detection methods using latex agglutination or coagglutination tests are applied in many laboratories directly to CSF for a presumptive diagnosis of meningitis caused by the pneumococcus. Mortality rates approximate 20 percent. Penicillin is the drug of choice.

Other Bacterial Meningitides

Most other cases of bacterial meningitis are extensions of a primary infection or follow brain or spinal cord injury. A variety of gram-negative bacilli, staphylococci, *Listeria monocytogenes,* and group B streptococci are occasional isolates. Many newborns appear to acquire group B streptococci or *L. monocytogenes* congenitally. Both neonatal group B streptococcal infections and listeriosis have an early onset after birth and may be rapidly fulminating. Listeriosis has received increased attention as a result of an outbreak of foodborne listeriosis in California in 1985 in which 105 deaths occurred. Sixty-five deaths were in fetuses and newborns and the remaining cases were in older immunocompromised individuals. None of the mothers died in that outbreak.

The use of prophylactic antibiotics may be indicated in brain or spinal cord injuries. Penicillin, ampicillin, or tetracycline may be used to treat meningitis of undetermined bacterial etiology, but the actual drug of choice should be determined by antibiotic susceptibility tests.

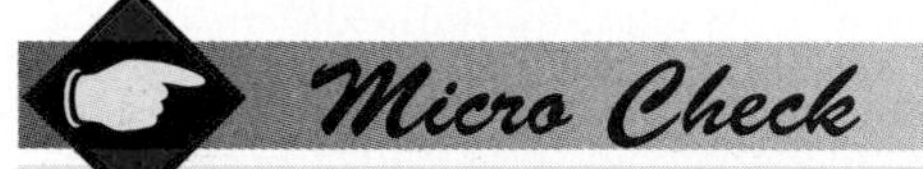

- Why do some microorganisms, antibodies, and antibiotics have difficulty in passing from the bloodstream to the brain and meninges?
- Why is meningitis caused by *Haemophilus* no longer the threat to young children that it once was?
- What bacteria are associated with congenital transmission of meningitis?

Brain Abscess

A brain abscess consists of a pyogenic local infection in the brain. It commonly occurs in the cerebrum or cerebellum as a result of trauma or as an extension of a primary infection (Fig. 19–6). Bacteria commonly isolated from CSF of patients with post-trauma brain abscesses include staphylococci, streptococci, and coliforms. Most abscesses occurring as an extension of a primary infection are caused by anaerobes. Severe headache is almost always an early symptom. Nausea, vomiting, drowsiness, confusion, and loss of consciousness may occur as the disease progresses. Surgical intervention is often necessary to drain or excise the abscess.

The techniques for isolation of anaerobes are discussed in Chapter 5. Gram-stained smears of specimens submitted to the laboratory provide valuable clues to possible etiologic agents. Both

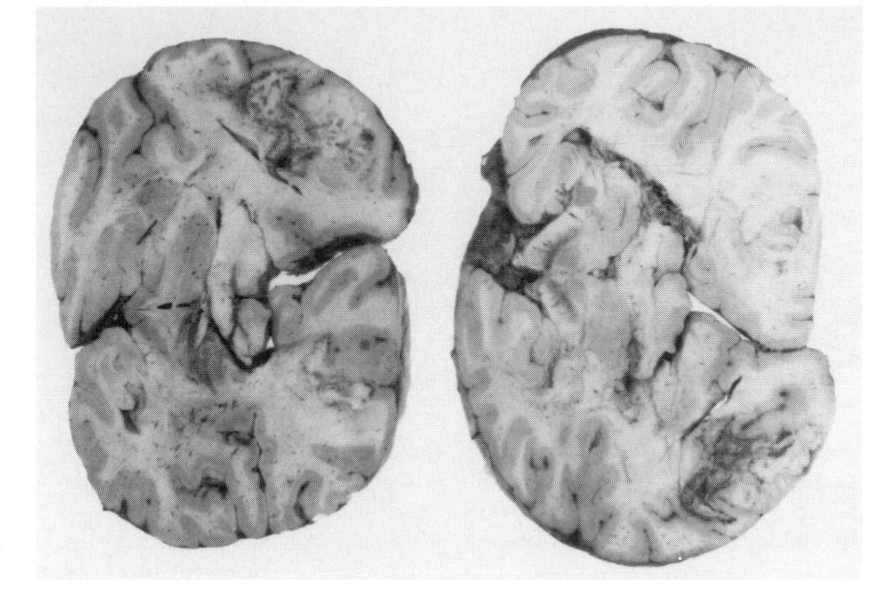

Figure 19–6 ◆ Brain abscesses in nocardiosis.

conventional and commercial systems may be used for biochemical characteristics. Many laboratories use reference laboratories specializing in anaerobic bacteriology to confirm identification of anaerobes.

Prompt treatment of ear or periodontal infections (infections of tissue supporting the teeth) can be a deterrent to dissemination of microorganisms to the brain. The administration of antibiotics following injury or surgery can sometimes prevent microbial colonization of traumatized tissue. Treatment for brain abscess depends on the specific etiology and is best determined by antibiotic susceptibility tests for aerobes. Penicillin and chloramphenicol are often used in combination. Most anaerobes have predictable patterns of susceptibility in a particular geographic area, but metronidazole is particularly effective in most instances.

Tetanus

Tetanus, a severe disease of the nervous system, is a complication of a wound infection. It is a relatively rare disease in developed countries. The etiologic agent, *Clostridium tetani,* a bacterium found in soil, produces a potent neurotoxin (Fig. 19–7). The spores of *C. tetani* are usually introduced into the body by a puncture wound. There is no person-to-person transmission. The symptoms of disease occur only after the exotoxin spreads by **retrograde axonal transport** from the initial site of infection to the CNS. The incubation period is four to 21 days. Early symptoms of tetanus may include irritability, headache, low-grade fever, and abdominal rigidity. The toxin, tetanospasmin, causes contractions of

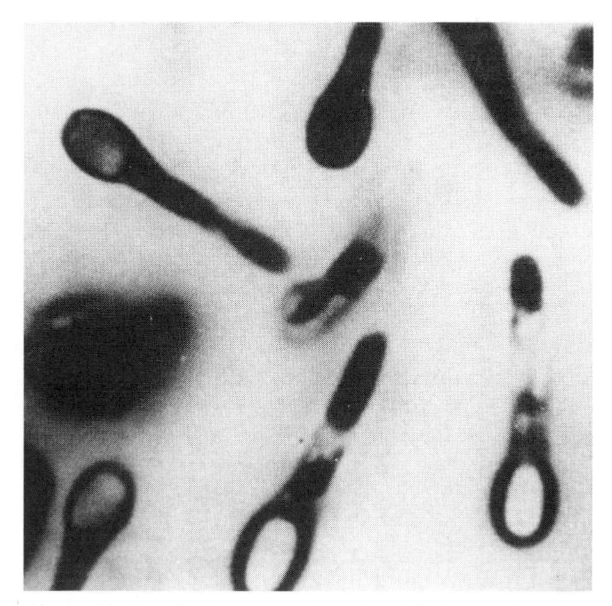

Figure 19–7 ◆ Endospores of a clostridial organism in a stained wet-mount preparation.

muscles and is often followed by respiratory paralysis and death. The jaw muscles are frequently affected. The fatality rate varies from 30 to 90 percent. A diagnosis of tetanus does not require laboratory confirmation.

Tetanus immune globulin (TIG) is the recommended treatment, but additional supportive treatment is usually necessary. Sedatives can sometimes control muscle spasms or at least minimize them. Sometimes an injection of tetanus toxoid is also given. Penicillin or tetracycline is required to eliminate *C. tetani* from wounds. Tetanus can be prevented by immunization with tetanus toxoid. The toxoid is given in three injections during the first year of life with diphtheria toxoid and pertussis vaccine. For maximum protection, initial injections are followed by boosters one year later, when the child enters school, and at 10-year intervals thereafter.

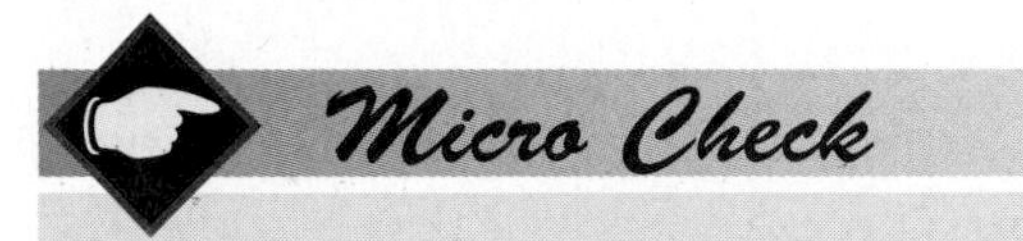

- Why is surgical intervention sometimes required in brain abscesses?
- How does the exotoxin of tetanus spread to the CNS?
- How do injuries predispose people to spores of the tetanus organisms?

Conjunctivitis

The conjunctiva is exposed to a variety of environmental bacteria. Conjunctivitis (inflammation of the conjunctiva) can be caused by a number of bacteria, but *Staphylococcus aureus,* group A streptococci, *Streptococcus pneumoniae,* some serotypes of *Chlamydia trachomatis, Haemophilus influenzae* (Hib), and *Neisseria gonorrhoeae* are all recognized as frequent causes. *H. aegyptius* (Koch-Weeks bacillus) produces the very contagious infection sometimes called "pinkeye." Neonatal conjunctivitis is caused by *N. gonorrhoeae* or *C. trachomatis.* It is discussed in Chapter 18. The etiologic agents of conjunctivitis are transmitted by fingers, linens, or other articles contaminated with conjunctival, respiratory, genital, or urethral discharges in other than neonatal infections. Cases of conjunctivitis followed by inner ear infections have occurred following lens implantation. Newborns acquire the infection from their mothers during delivery. The time of incubation is 24 to 72 hours.

The symptoms of bacterial conjunctivitis include edema and redness of the lid, photophobia, and, often, a purulent conjunctival discharge. One or both lids may be involved.

Gram stains of pus from purulent conjunctivitis usually reveal the presence of etiologic agents. Gram stains of smears from nonpurulent conjunctivitis may reveal the Gram reaction and morphology of the invading organism. However, despite the presence of oppressive symptoms, organisms often are not present in sufficient numbers to be seen on stained smears. Supplemented chocolate agar, blood agar, and an enriched thioglycolate broth may be employed for primary isolation. The cultural and biochemical characteristics of the organisms have been discussed in previous chapters. Treatment varies with the etiologic agent, but broad-spectrum antibiotics, penicillinase-resistant penicillins, and aminoglycosides are widely used.

Trachoma

Trachoma is a chronic form of conjunctivitis and is the major cause of preventable blindness in the world. The disease, which is caused by immunotypes A, B, and C of *Chlamydia trachomatis,* is widespread in India, Africa, and South America. It is common among both Native Americans and Mexican immigrants in the Southwestern United States. *C. trachomatis* is transmitted by contact with ocular or nasal discharges of infected individuals or by contaminated materials. The time of incubation is five to 12 days.

Trachoma is characterized by inflammation of the conjunctiva followed by **papillary hyperplasia,** invasion of the cornea, and progressive loss of vision. Deformities of the eyelids are seen with some frequency (Fig. 19–8).

Scrapings of epithelial cells from the conjunctiva reveal the presence of inclusion bodies in the cytoplasm using a Giemsa or immunofluorescent technique. *C. trachomatis* can be cultured in egg yolk sacs of embryonated eggs, but recovery of the organism is not feasible as a routine laboratory procedure. Serological tests are not useful in diagnosing trachoma. In developing countries, mass applications of topical erythromycin or tetracycline to the conjunctivae are employed both prophylactically and to treat active infections.

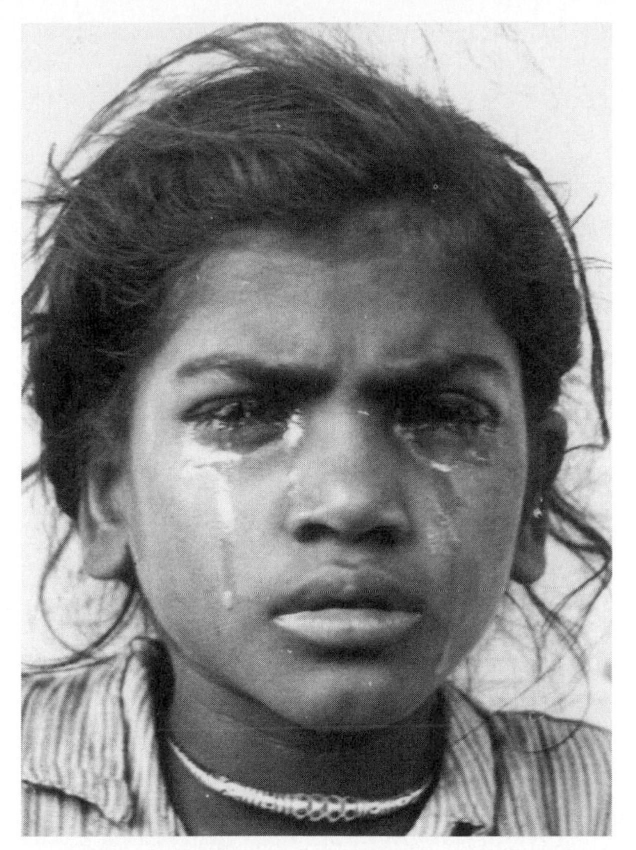

Figure 19–8 ◆ Trachoma in a young Indian girl. The suffering caused by the disease is reflected in her face.

Micro Check

- Why do infections of the eye require prompt treatment?
- What bacteria are common etiologic agents of conjunctivitis?

Otitis Media

Otitis media is an acute or chronic inflammation of the middle ear. Acute otitis media most often occurs in infants and young children. Chronic otitis media usually affects older children and adults. It is commonly caused by staphylococci, *Streptococcus pneumoniae, Haemophilus influenzae* (Hib), and *Pseudomonas aeruginosa.* In most instances, the bacteria migrate upward from the nasopharynx by way of the eustachian tube.

Fever, earache, redness, and tenderness of the eardrums may occur in both acute and chronic otitis media. Sometimes pus formation causes perforation of the eardrum, and the scarring may result in hearing impairment. Acute mastoiditis is a possible complication of acute suppurative otitis media. Other complications include meningitis and brain abscess.

Gram stains and cultures of nasopharyngeal secretions sometimes reveal the presence of pathogens, but the evidence is only circumstantial. There is no way to prove migration of a particular organism without obtaining material from the middle ear. There appears little justification for performing **tympanocentesis** (puncture of the eardrum), except if the infection does not respond to a broad-spectrum antibiotic. The drug of choice for otitis media is a broad-spectrum penicillin, such as dicloxacillin, or erythromycin.

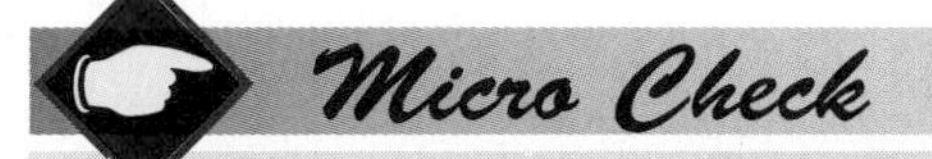

- What is the origin of bacteria that cause otitis media?
- What complications are associated with ear infections?
- Why is evidence obtained on Gram-stained smears from nasopharyngeal secretions only circumstantial?

FUNGAL INFECTIONS

Infections of the nervous system, eye, or ear caused by fungi typically occur in the immunocompromised host. The presence of underlying degenerative diseases predisposes some individuals to brain and spinal cord infections caused by fungi. The infections are almost universally fatal, and diagnosis is most often made at autopsy.

Cryptococcosis

Cryptococcosis is a worldwide mycosis caused by the yeast *Cryptococcus neoformans.* Exposure to pigeon droppings is the most important factor in transmission of cryptococcosis. The yeast cells are present in the soil in many parts of the world, but are particularly abundant in aerosols surrounding pigeon coops. There is no evidence

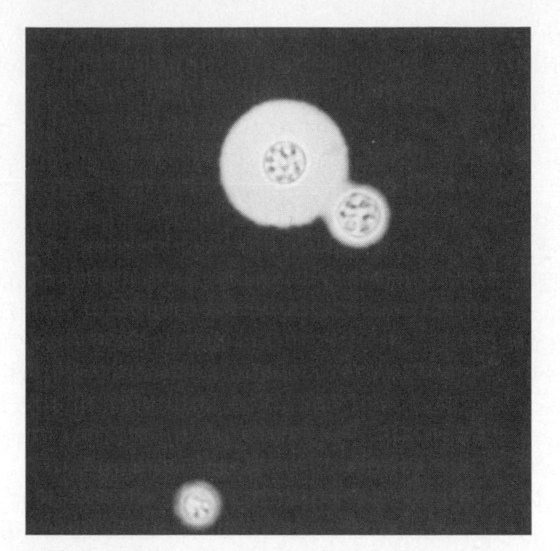

Figure 19–9 ◆ *Cryptococcus neoformans* in an India ink wet-mount preparation.

that the disease can be transmitted from person to person. The time of incubation may be months or even years.

The primary site of infection is usually the lung, and when confined to the lung, the illness is most often of a transient and uncomplicated nature. Extension of the infection to the meninges of the brain and spinal cord causes a subacute or chronic meningoencephalitis. Chronic cryptococcosis may be present over a period of 10 to 20 years but is more often a rapidly fulminating disease. The mortality rate is 100 percent in untreated cases and approximates 30 to 40 percent in individuals who receive treatment. Cryptococcosis is a life-threatening opportunistic infection in AIDS patients. Cryptococcal organisms disseminate frequently to lymph nodes, liver, kidneys, spleen, and bone marrow of patients with a serious immune deficiency.

A diagnosis of cryptococcal meningitis can be made by direct examination of sediment from CSF using India ink (Fig. 19–9). The yeast can be recognized by the large capsules that surround the organisms. *C. neoformans* grows well on Sabouraud's agar, producing mucoid colonies which turn tan to brown with age. The ability to grow in vitro at 37°C, pathogenicity for mice, and hydrolysis of urea are useful identifying characteristics (Color Plate 68). A latex particle agglutination test can detect presence of cryptococcal polysaccharide in CSF, but the cost may be prohibitive for laboratories that only rarely have the need to rule out cryptococcal meningitis. Amphotericin B and 5-flucytosine or fluconazole are used to treat cryptococcosis.

Cerebrorhinoorbital Phycomycoses

The cerebrorhinoorbital phycomycoses (CROP) are caused primarily by members of the genera *Absidia, Mucor, Rhizopus,* and *Mortierella.* The fungal infections may be the result of trauma, but most occur following a paranasal sinus infection. Diabetic acidosis and immunocompromised states appear to be important factors predisposing individuals to CROP. The etiologic agents are common in the environment. They are found on old bread, decaying fruit, and animal wastes.

The symptoms include facial pain and edema of the eyelids and conjunctivae (Fig. 19–10). Blood vessels are often invaded. Later fever, convulsions, and death may occur. An infection can reach the terminal stage within a week.

Cultures alone are not diagnostic for CROP as *Absidia, Mucor, Rhizopus,* and *Mortierella* are common contaminants. Diagnosis must be confirmed by the demonstration of nonseptate hyphae in biopsy material and culture of tissue obtained by biopsy or at autopsy.

Amphotericin B and 5-flucytosine are used to treat CROP, but unfortunately, many cases go unrecognized until the fungi are found in autopsy material.

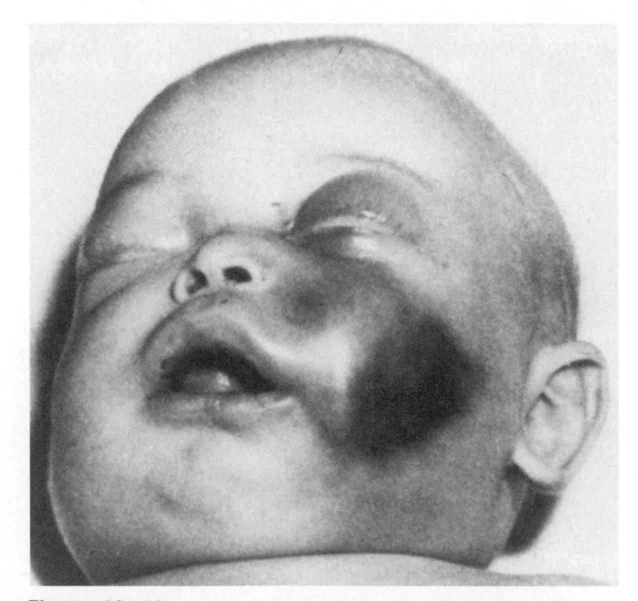

Figure 19–10 ◆ Orbital cellulitis in an infant. Occlusion of blood vessels has caused gangrene of left orbit and cheek.

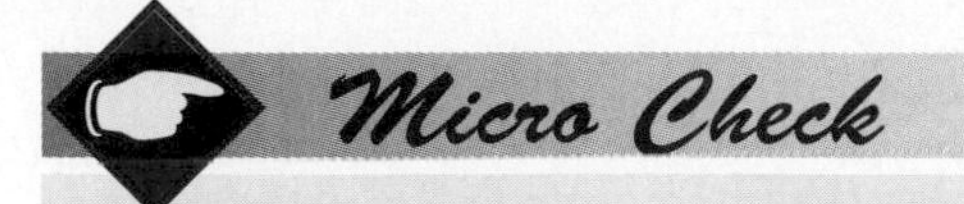

◆ What is the primary site of infection in cryptococcosis?
◆ Why does cryptococcosis frequently disseminate in AIDS patients?
◆ Why are cultures alone not diagnostic in CROP?

PROTOZOAL INFECTIONS

The migration of protozoa from intestinal or extraintestinal sites to the CNS is relatively rare. However, some trypanosomes, toxoplasmas, and amebas can gain entrance to the brain by penetrating the **cribriform plate** or can infect the meninges. The protozoa are frequently scattered throughout the brain substance. CNS involvement occurs in amebic meningoencephalitis, in disseminated toxoplasmosis, and in chronic stages of African sleeping sickness. In congenital trypanosomiasis, in toxoplasmosis, and in amebic meningoencephalitis, granulomatous lesions containing extracellular parasites can be found in the brain or on the meninges.

Other protozoal parasites, namely, *Plasmodium falciparum* and more rarely *P. vivax,* cause brain damage in quite a different manner. Red blood cells infected with the malarial organisms tend to agglutinate in cerebral capillaries, interferring with blood flow. The surrounding tissue becomes necrotic, and hemorrhaging frequently occurs around the occluded vessels. The net effect of the blood vessel damage is to produce cerebral edema and subsequent irreversible brain damage. Malaria is discussed in Chapter 20.

Amebic Meningoencephalitis

Amebic meningoencephalitis is a rare and usually fatal infection caused by free-living amebas. It has been reported in Australia, England, the United States, Africa, and Czechoslovakia, but it is likely that it occurs elsewhere as well. Trophozoites of *Naegleria fowleri* or species of *Acanthamoeba* enter nasal passages when people swim in contaminated water. The cysts of the same protozoa may enter the nasal passages during dust storms where they excyst. Trophozoites are able to penetrate the cribriform plate and migrate to the brain where they proliferate and destroy tissue. No person-to-person transmission has been documented. The time of incubation is three to seven days in infections caused by *Naegleria,* but may be much longer when species of *Acanthamoeba* are the etiologic agents.

Early symptoms of amebic meningoencephalitis include headache, fever, malaise, lethargy, and a stiff neck. Later disorientation and **ataxia** may be evident with ultimate coma followed by death within 10 days. *Acanthamoeba* may also cause infections of the eye, lungs, skin, and vagina.

Trophozoites of amebas may or may not be seen in centrifuged specimens of CSF in amebic meningoencephalitis. The amebas grow well on 1.5 percent nonnutrient agar medium prepared with Page's ameba saline and precoated with *Escherichia coli.* The lack of commercially available standardized antigens or antibodies limits the value of serological tests. No reliable treatment is available.

Toxoplasmosis

Toxoplasmosis is one of the most common infections occurring in humans throughout the world. Fortunately, it is a rare disease. Most individuals are asymptomatic despite exposure to the protozoan, *Toxoplasma gondii.* The protozoan has a complex life cycle involving cats as definitive hosts (Fig. 19–11). Other warm-blooded animals serve as intermediate hosts. Cats become infected by eating mice and birds harboring the parasite. Humans become infected by eating raw or inadequately cooked meat or poultry or by contact with cat feces. The incubation time is variable depending on the mode of transmission. Transmission by undercooked meat or poultry causes recognizable disease in 10 to 23 days. Incubation times for cat-associated transmission range from five to 20 days. *T. gondii* can also be transmitted across the placenta to the fetus. Transmission can also occur during delivery.

In adults the protozoan multiplies and encysts in the retina causing blurred vision, pain, photophobia, and exudative retinitis. Involvement of the macula may cause a severe impairment in central vision. Disseminated toxoplasmosis was rare in adults, but it is seen with increasing frequency in AIDS patients. It is believed to be a reactivated infection in those individuals. Congenital toxoplasmosis causes serious consequences when it is acquired in utero from mothers with acute infections. The amount of damage

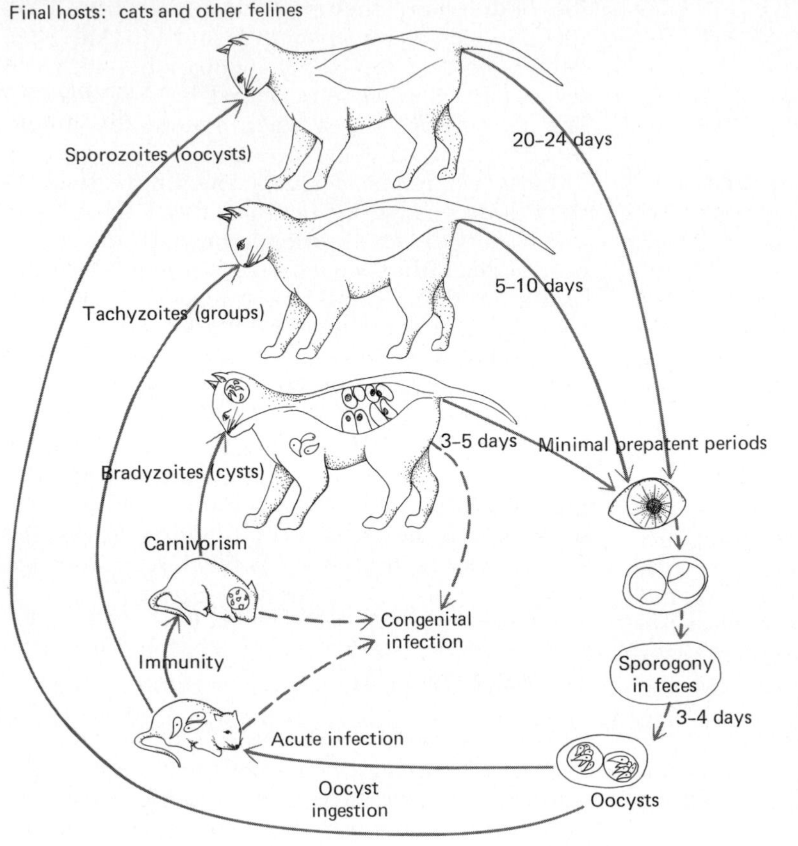

Figure 19–11 ◆ Life cycle of *Toxoplasma gondii* showing stages infective for cats and mice as well as minimal prepatent periods (days elapsing between ingestion of parasites and their appearance in feces) required for the parasites to develop in the cat.

to a fetus carried by an infected woman, with or without symptoms of disease, is related to the trimester in which the disease is acquired. Retinochoroiditis (inflammation of the retina and choroid of the eye), hepatosplenomegaly (enlargement of the liver and spleen), hydrocephalus (accumulation of cerebrospinal fluid in the ventricles of the brain), cerebral calcification, and convulsions are possible consequences of the infection in neonates.

Ocular toxoplasmosis can be recognized clinically. Serological tests are of limited value because antibody response tends to be poor in the localized infection. In disseminated adult toxoplasmosis, trophozoites or encysted forms of *T. gondii* can be observed in body tissues or fluids (Fig. 19–12). The protozoan develops extracellularly as a crescent-shaped trophozoite; intracellular forms of the parasite are smaller. Membrane-enclosed pseudocysts sometimes develop in the brain and eyes. Experience with serological tests as an adjunct in the diagnosis of disseminated disease has been limited. The diagnosis of congenital toxoplasmosis depends on the demonstration of specific IgM antibodies to *T. gondii.* Serological tests are used to screen obstetric patients for the presence of IgG antibodies. High titers of IgG antibodies indicate recent infection. The choice of a particular serological procedure de-

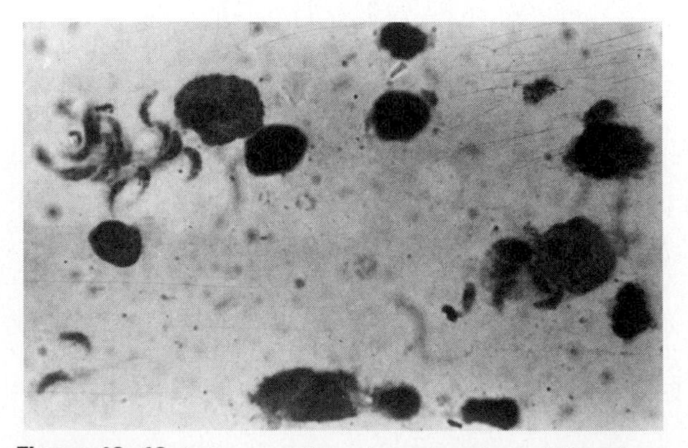

Figure 19–12 ◆ Crescent-shaped trophozoites of *Toxoplasma gondii* in pleural fluid.

pends on the purpose for which it is to be used. Pyrimethamine and sulfadiazine are used in the treatment of toxoplasmosis.

African Sleeping Sickness

African sleeping sickness is a trypanosomiasis that occurs in tropical Africa in areas where tsetse flies are found. It is caused by the hemoflagellates *Trypanosoma brucei gambiense* or *T. b. rhodesiense* (Fig. 19–13). The principal vectors are members of the genus *Glossina*. Humans are the major reservoir of the trypanosomes, but wild game may also be infected. When the tsetse flies bite infected persons or animals, blood containing the parasites is ingested. The hemoflagellates multiply in the midguts of flies and later migrate to the salivary glands. The parasites are transferred to new mammalian hosts when infected tsetse flies bite them. The time of incubation for infections caused by *T. b. rhodesiense* is about two to three weeks. Incubation times for infections associated with *T. b. gambiense* may be several months or years.

A primary chancre develops at the site of the bite. The lesion usually is self-limiting, but it is accompanied by fever, **tachycardia,** lymph node enlargement, edema, and sometimes a rash as the trypanosomes multiply and disseminate. Later when invasion of the central nervous system (CNS) occurs, there are mental disturbances, irri-

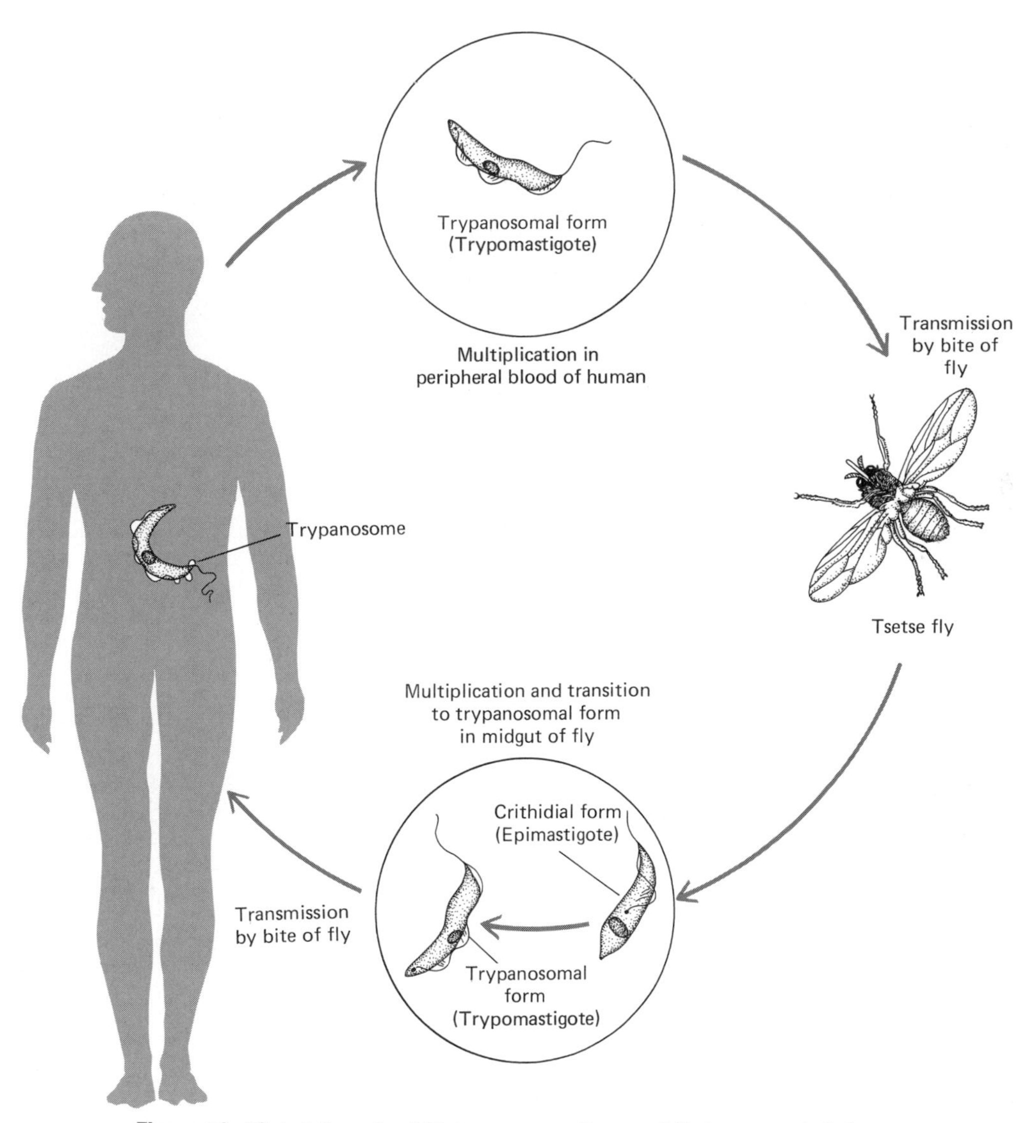

Figure 19–13 ◆ Life cycle of *Trypanosoma gambiense* and *Trypanosoma rhodesiense.*

tability, emaciation, and ultimately, coma. The comatose state may last for months or years, but is usually followed by death.

A definitive diagnosis of African sleeping sickness can be made by finding trypanosomes in blood, lymph nodes, bone marrow, or cerebrospinal fluid. The parasite is two to four times the diameter of a red blood cell in length.

The drugs of choice for parasitemia are suramin and pentamidine. When the CNS is involved, melarsoprol, an arsenic-containing compound, is administered intravenously with caution. Because complete eradication of tsetse flies has not been possible, the use of protective clothing and sleeping nets are recommended precautionary measures in endemic areas.

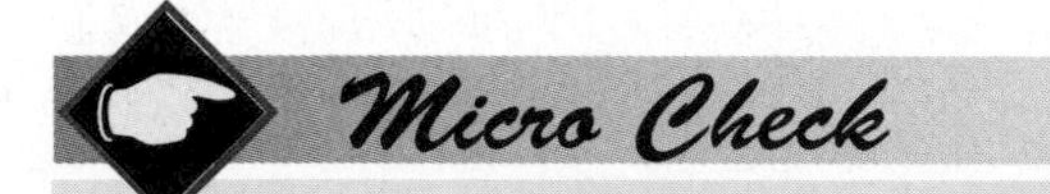

- How do some malarial parasites cause brain damage?
- How are free-living soil amebas able to migrate to the brain?
- Why can toxoplasmosis be described as both a common infection and a rare disease?

VIRAL INFECTIONS

Certain viruses have an affinity for tissue of the central nervous system (CNS); they are often called neurotropic viruses (Table 19–2). Most other viruses do not invade the CNS except under unusual circumstances. An exception would be dissemination of the measles or mumps viruses to the CNS during convalescence.

The permissive role of some peripheral nerves in housing the herpes simplex and zoster viruses during long periods of dormancy is not well understood. The nerves appear unaffected by the presence of those viruses in the inactive state.

Aseptic Meningitis

Aseptic meningitis is an inflammation of the meninges not caused by bacteria and assumed in most cases to be caused by a virus. A variety of viruses have been implicated, but enteroviruses are considered to be the most common cause of aseptic meningitis. In a majority of cases, however, etiologic agents are unknown. The viruses are most probably disseminated by the bloodstream during a period of viremia. The viruses do not appear to spread easily to other patients,

Table 19–2
MAJOR GROUPS AND SEROTYPES OF VIRUSES CAUSING DISEASES OF THE CENTRAL NERVOUS SYSTEM

VIRUS	SEROTYPES*	MAJOR DISEASE
Picornavirus		
Poliovirus	1, 2, 3	Poliomyelitis
Coxsackievirus A	1, 2, 4–11, 16–18, 22–24	Aseptic meningitis
Coxsackievirus B	1–6	Aseptic meningitis
Echovirus	1–9, 11–25, 30, 31	Aseptic meningitis
Togavirus		
Eastern equine virus (EEE)		Encephalitis
Western equine virus (WEE)		Encephalitis
Venezuelan equine virus (VEE)		Encephalitis
Paramyxovirus		
Mumps virus		Aseptic meningitis
Rubella virus		Encephalitis
Herpesvirus		
Herpes simplex virus	1	Encephalitis
Herpes simplex virus	2	Aseptic meningitis
Varicella-zoster virus		Encephalitis
Epstein-Barr virus		Aseptic meningitis
Rhabdovirus		
Rabies virus		Encephalitis

* No designation for serotype means that a single antigenic type has been identified.

family members, or hospital personnel. The time of incubation varies with the etiologic agent.

The disease has a sudden onset with an intense headache being a primary symptom. A fever, nausea, vomiting, stiff neck, sore throat, and drowsiness also occur with some regularity. Most individuals recover without incident in two weeks. In others a mild and transient paralysis may occur. Viral meningitis in newborns is more serious and may result in systemic disease or death.

CSF, stool, rectal swabs, or paired sera may be submitted to a virology laboratory. Most laboratories have a panel of serological tests available for aseptic meningitis. Usually enteroviruses that are responsible for the greater share of CNS disease are not included because of the multiple serological types. An exception is sometimes made if one or two types of enteroviruses are occurring in epidemic form in a community. There is no specific treatment other than supportive care for aseptic meningitis.

Poliomyelitis

Poliomyelitis has virtually disappeared as a public health problem in North and South America since the development of a vaccine by Jonas Salk in 1955. The last reported case occurred in Peru in the summer of 1991. This infection remains a problem in some developing countries that do not have access to the vaccine. As many as 100,000 cases of paralytic poliomyelitis occur annually worldwide.

Poliomyelitis (once called infantile paralysis) is an acute inflammation of the spinal cord and brain stem. It affects chiefly the anterior horns of the lumbar sections of the spinal cord (Fig. 19–14). The paralysis that develops in some patients distinguishes the disease from aseptic meningitis.

There are three antigenic types of polioviruses, designated as 1, 2, and 3. Type 2 is the cause of most paralytic illness. The polioviruses are transmitted by direct contact with nasopharyngeal secretions or feces of an infected individual. Water, milk, and occasionally flies have been responsible for outbreaks of poliomyelitis. A viremia is established before invasion of the central nervous system (CNS). From the blood, viruses may penetrate the blood-brain or blood-CSF barrier. The incubation period is usually seven to 14 days, but can be a month or more.

Early symptoms of poliomyelitis include a stiff neck, a sore throat, fever, headache, nausea, vomiting, and abdominal discomfort. Most infections are inapparent. Less than 1 percent of symptomatic individuals develop paralytic disease. Muscle involvement is frequently unilateral, but the sites of paralysis depend on the location of the viral invasion. Paralysis of muscles of respiration led to use of the so-called "iron-lung" to provide a mechanical means of respiration.

Poliomyelitis can be diagnosed by isolation of the virus from pharyngeal secretions early in the disease and later from stool or rectal swabs. The viruses grow readily in monkey kidney cells, producing rounding of cells, inclusion bodies, ballooning, and ultimately death of cells (Fig. 19–15). Serodiagnosis can often be made on paired sera using complement-fixation (CF) or neutralization techniques.

No drugs affect the course of paralytic poliomyelitis, but sometimes rather extraordinary methods of supportive care are required to assist in breathing or swallowing. Both an inactivated polio virus vaccine (IPV) and a live oral polio virus vaccine (OPV) are available for immunization. The IPV is given in a series of four doses during the first year of life, again before entering school, and at 5-year intervals until the age of 18. The OPV is usually given in three doses along with diphtheria-tetanus-pertussis (DTP) or DTaP immunizations. Many school districts require an additional immunization before children enter school. The once familiar deformities, braces, and "iron lungs" associated with poliomyelitis are a part of history except for the survivors of past epidemics of the once dreaded disease.

Encephalitis

Encephalitis is an inflammation of the brain characterized by altered cerebral function, including loss of consciousness. It can be caused by a number of viruses and other etiologic agents including bacteria, fungi, protozoa, and *Trichinella spiralis.* Pathogenic arthropod-borne viruses cause sporadic disease but also are associated with epidemics when mosquitoes are particularly abundant. Fatality rates vary from 5 to 60 percent, depending on the infectious agent. Eastern equine (EEE), western equine (WEE), Venezuela equine (VEE), and St. Louis (SLE) encephalitis are among the most important types of arthropod-borne encephalitis caused by togaviruses. WEE is transmitted by the mosquito *Culex tarsalis.* Birds, rodents, and other mammals may be significant reservoirs for WEE, but both horses and humans are dead-end hosts (Fig. 19–16). The

FOCAL POINT

Jonas Salk, Conqueror of Polio

From his sequestered office overlooking the Pacific Ocean, Jonas Salk sustained an abiding faith in mankind's capacity to create a better world. "I think we're generally programmed to solve problems we create," he maintains, "even though it appears we're on the verge of autodestruction." Salk's words carry unusual authority, for any survey of gifted problem solvers would almost certainly include his name. Though Salk continued to decode biological puzzles at the California research center that bears his name, he is best remembered as the scientific hero who conquered polio. Born in 1914 in a New York tenement, Salk abandoned a career as a practicing physician to conduct his own research. Asked why he pursued $1500- and $2500-a-year fellowships instead of a lucrative medical practice, he replied, "Why did Mozart compose music?" Salk's chance to compose a brilliant scientific score came in 1947 at the University of Pittsburgh where he developed a vaccine against polio. Salk became an overnight celebrity, and within seven years polio was virtually wiped out in the United States.

Page, J: Blood: The River of Life. Washington, D.C., U.S. News Books, 1981.

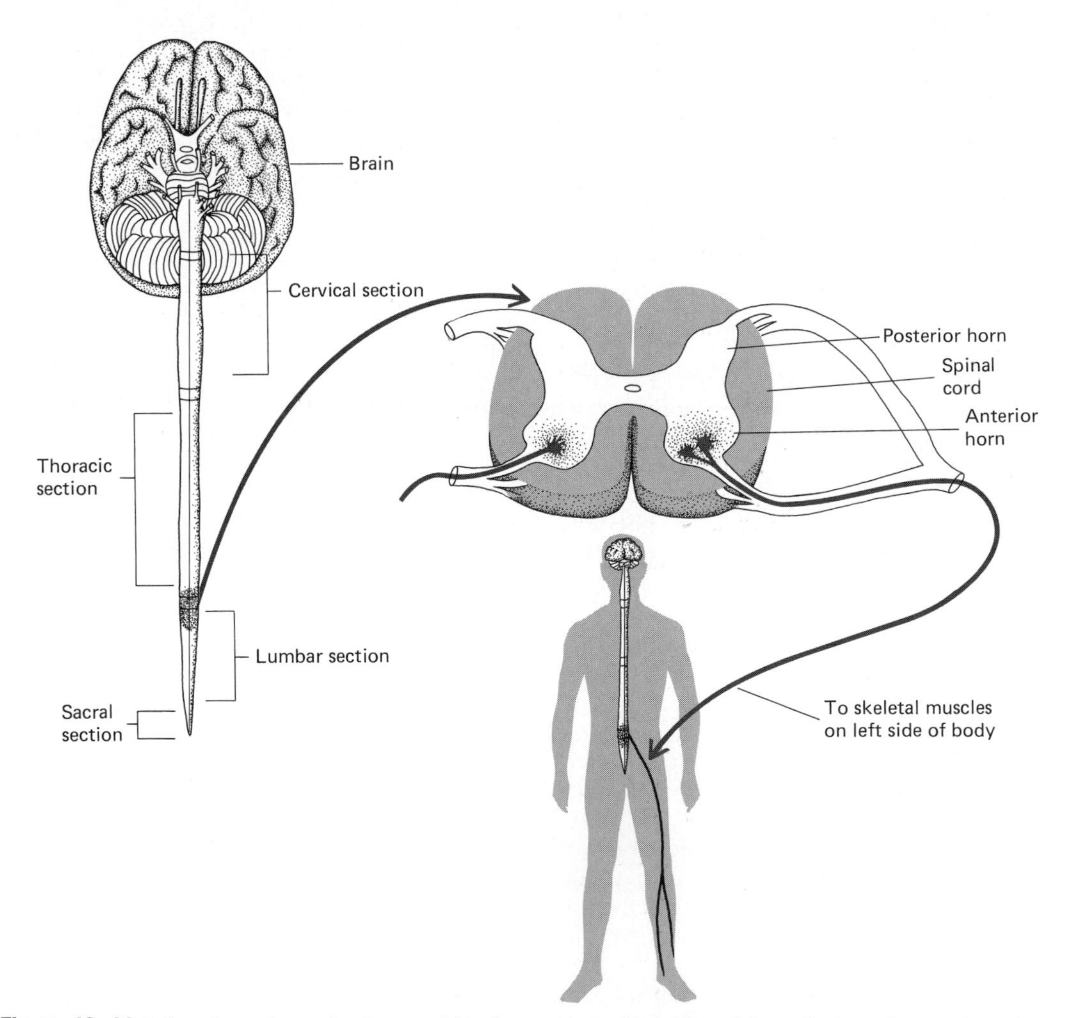

Figure 19–14 ◆ Invasion of anterior horns of lumbar section of spinal cord by poliovirus. Destruction of nerve cells frequently causes a unilateral paralysis of muscles.

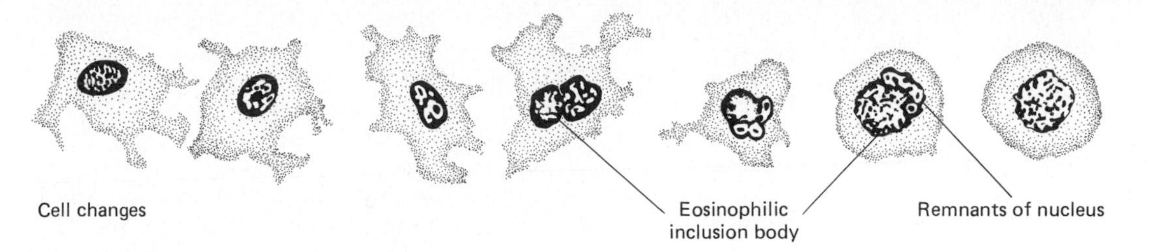

Figure 19–15 ◆ The effect of poliovirus on an infected cell. As numbers of viruses reach a maximum, an inclusion body is produced, causing ultimate cell death.

specific vectors for EEE, VEE, and SLE are not known. Encephalitis is not transmitted from person to person. The time of incubation is five to 15 days.

Symptoms of encephalitis vary in severity, but include a headache, fever, and disturbed consciousness. In severe infections, convulsions, paralysis, stupor, and even a coma may occur. Permanent neurological impairment is more frequent in children than in adults. The mortality rate is 2 to 3 percent.

Serological diagnosis can be made on paired sera from persons suspected of having encephalitis caused by EEE, WEE, or VEE agents. Complement-fixation (CF) techniques are most satisfactory for early diagnosis, but complement-fixing antibodies do not persist as long as neutralizing or hemagglutination-inhibiting antibodies. The viruses can be isolated from extracts of brain and spinal cord specimens obtained at autopsy and only rarely from blood or cerebrospinal fluid. There is no specific treatment, but supportive care is important. The use of insect repellents and elimination of breeding places for mosquitoes can minimize exposure to bites of mosquitoes carrying the virus. Surveillance programs, conducted by public health departments, are critical for providing early alerts on particular viral activity in various parts of the United States. California has reported extensive areas of WEE and SLE activity in recent years through testing of mosquitoes or serological assay in chickens.

Rabies

Rabies is a type of encephalitis caused by a rhabdovirus occurring mainly in infected dogs, cats, raccoons, skunks, bats, foxes, woodchucks, and squirrels. Since 1980, a total of 24 cases of rabies has occurred in the United States. Nine of these were believed to have been acquired out-

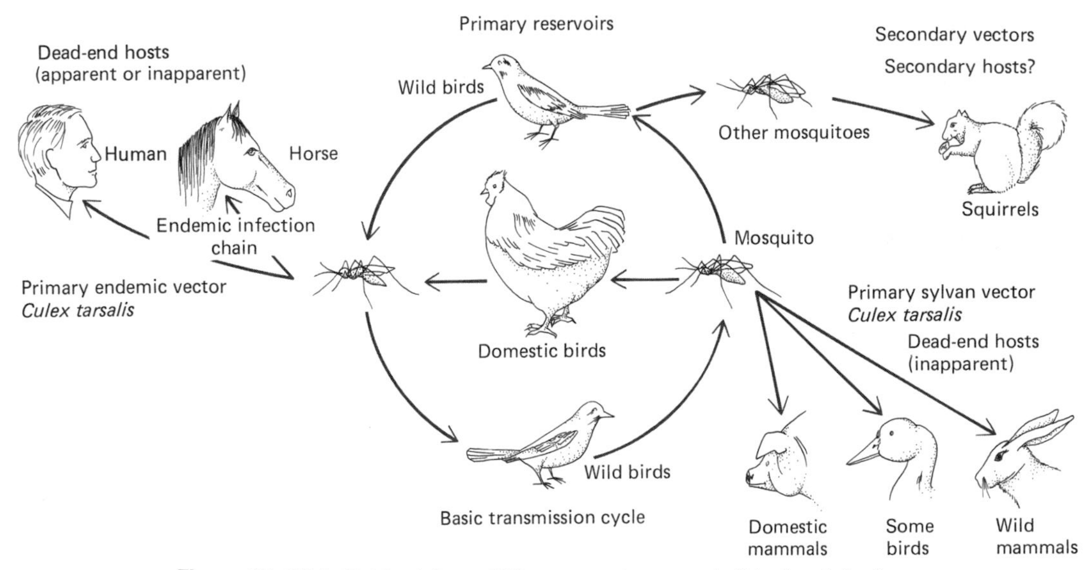

Figure 19–16 ◆ Epidemiology of Western equine encephalitis virus infections.

side the country. The disease is almost invariably fatal in humans. The virus enters through a bite, an abrasion from an infected animal, or through virus-laden aerosols. The time of incubation varies from two to eight weeks. The virus migrates to the CNS by way of peripheral nerves, so the shorter the pathway from the site of a bite, the shorter the incubation time for the disease.

Onset of rabies is heralded by apprehension, irritability, fever, malaise, and difficulty in swallowing. Often the mere sight or thought of water induces spasmodic contractions of the muscles used in swallowing. For that reason, the name **hydrophobia** (fear of water) was once used to describe the illness.

Rabies virus can be detected on brain-impression smears made from infected animals on autopsy by an immunofluorescent antibody (IFA) technique. An alternate, but less sensitive, procedure consists of demonstrating inclusions known as Negri bodies in brain-tissue smears (Fig. 19–17, Color Plate 69). The rabies virus can be recovered from saliva or nasal secretions in humans. Mice are the animals of choice for culturing the virus. The presence of rabies virus antigens on brain-impression smears using IFA confirms a diagnosis of rabies.

Two types of rabies vaccines are in use in the United States for possible exposure to the virus. Human diploid cell vaccine (HDCV) and rabies vaccine, adsorbed (RVA) are equally effective for both pre- and postexposure prevention of rabies. Rabies immune globulin (RIG) is also given in all cases of postexposure. One of the vaccines should be given as soon as possible after the suspected exposure and repeated on days 3, 7, 14, and 28 after the initial vaccination. The antibody response requires a week or more to develop and lasts for about two years. The protection afforded by RIG is of limited duration as the product has a half life of about 21 days.

The effective control of rabies requires compulsory vaccination of dogs and cats, registration of dogs, quarantine, and careful observation of animals inflicting wounds on humans. If signs of rabies develop in a quarantined animal, the animal must be sacrificed, and the head sent promptly under refrigeration to a public health laboratory for examination.

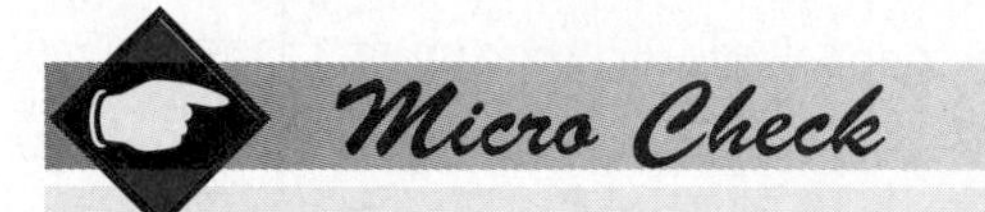

- Why is the term "aseptic meningitis" a misnomer?
- Why are "iron lungs" relics of the past?
- Which arthropod-borne togaviruses cause encephalitis?

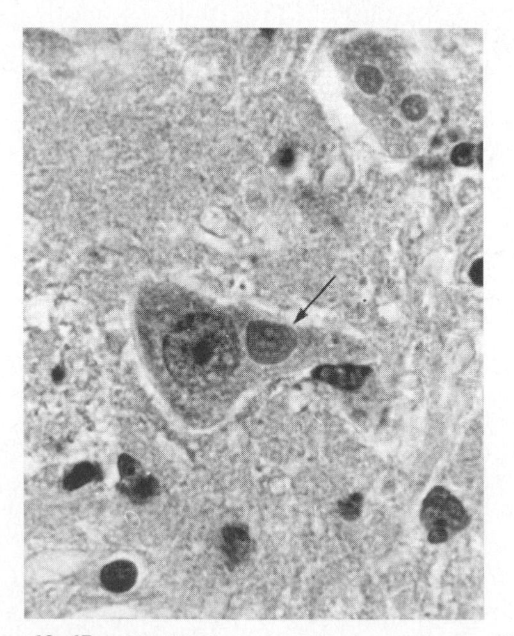

Figure 19–17 ◆ Negri inclusion body in human brain cell.

Viral Conjunctivitis and Keratitis

A number of viruses, including herpes simplex virus 1 (HSV-1), herpes simplex virus 2 (HSV-2), herpes zoster virus (HZV), adenoviruses 8, 19a, and 37, and some enteroviruses, can cause conjunctivitis with or without concurrent keratitis. Some are extensions of genital or respiratory disease transmitted by contact with body secretions. Adenovirus infections often occur in epidemic form and may be transmitted by use of common linens, contaminated hands, or ocular instruments. The time of incubation varies with the viral agent and the infecting dose. A low-grade fever, headache, inflammation, photophobia, and pain are often present in viral conjunctivitis and keratitis.

Fluorescent antibody (FA) techniques can detect the presence of herpesviruses and adenoviral antigens in conjunctival scrapings. Viral cultures can be obtained from serous discharges present in conjunctivitis. Iodo-deoxyuridine (IDU) is effective in some types of viral keratoconjunctivitis. Corticosteroids may provide some symptomatic relief.

PRION-ASSOCIATED DISEASES

Disease caused by the protein particles known as prions includes a group of infections characterized by a period of latency lasting for months or years. The first protein-particle infections described were chronic diseases of Icelandic sheep, two of which affect the central nervous system (CNS). The role of prions, which contain only protein, is puzzling since proteins are not known to replicate like the DNA or RNA of viruses.

Several prions are believed to cause disease of the CNS in humans. *Subacute sclerosing panencephalitis* (SSPE) is believed to be a delayed reaction to infection with the measles virus. Proteins of that virus have been demonstrated in brain tissues of patients with SSPE. Infections with measles before the age of two is a predisposing factor in SSPE. *Kuru,* a degenerative disease of the cerebellum, has been observed in persons practicing **cannibalism** in New Guinea. The disease produces alterations in balance, causing difficulty in walking, then tremors, and eventual death (Fig. 19–18). *Creutzfeldt-Jakob disease* (CJD) and *progressive multifocal leukoencephalopathy* (PMC) are rare human diseases associated with mental deterioration and lack of muscle coordination.

An outbreak of a variant form of CJD occurred in the United Kingdom in 1994. The disease was linked to the consumption of beef. This association helped give this outbreak the name of "mad cow disease." It is similar to bovine spongiform encephalitis (BSE), a disease of cattle. The variant form of the disease affected persons with a median age of 28 years. In the past, CJD had occurred in older individuals. No cases of the variant CJD have been reported in the United States.

Prions are the suspected etiologic agents of *multiple sclerosis* (MS), a neurological disorder in which the myelin sheath surrounding nerves is destroyed. The disease affects 500,000 individuals in the United States. Several findings suggest that the paralysis, numbness, loss of coordination, tremors, and interference with balance may be caused by an autoimmune response resulting from a previous viral infection. There is no specific treatment for these serious neurological diseases.

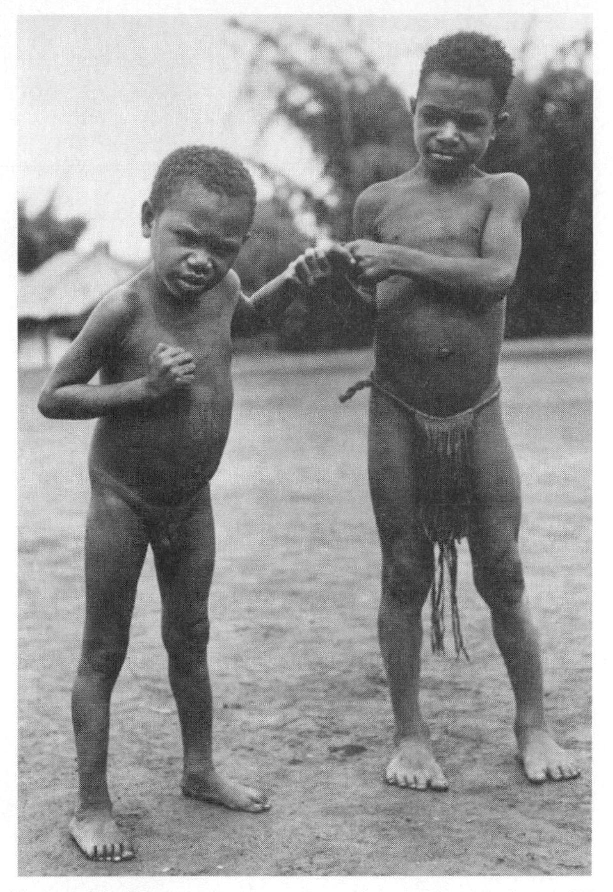

Figure 19–18 ◆ A young patient (on left) with kuru. He died at five years of age, several years before his mother developed kuru.

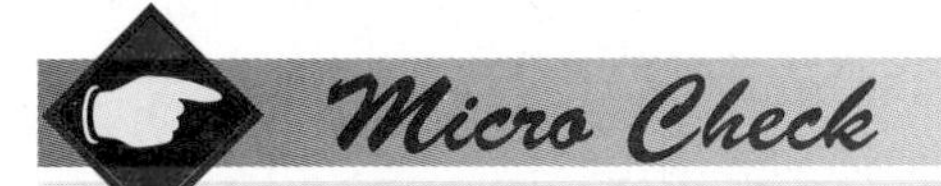

- How can a diagnosis of rabies be confirmed?
- How can you account for the rarity of rabies in the United States?
- Why is the role of prions in diseases of the CNS puzzling?

The major microorganisms causing diseases of the nervous system, eye, and ear are summarized in Table 19–3.

Table 19–3
MAJOR MICROORGANISMS CAUSING DISEASE OF THE NERVOUS SYSTEM, EYE, AND EAR

MICROORGANISM	DISEASE	TREATMENT
Bacteria		
Neisseria meningitidis	Meningitis	Penicillin
Haemophilus influenzae		Ampicillin
Streptococcus pneumoniae		Chloramphenicol
Group B streptococci		Penicillin
Listeria monocytogenes		
Staphylococci, streptococci coliforms, anaerobes	Brain abscess	As determined by antibiotic susceptibility tests
Clostridium tetani	Tetanus	Tetanus immune globulin
Staphylococcus aureus	Conjunctivitis	As determined by antibiotic susceptibility tests
Group B streptococci		
Streptococcus pneumoniae		
Haemophilus influenzae		
Neisseria gonorrhoeae		
Haemophilus aegyptius		
Chlamydia trachomatis	Trachoma	Tetracycline Erythromycin
Staphylococcus aureus	Blepharitis	Tetracycline
Staphylococcus epidermidis		Chloramphenicol Sulfacetamide
Staphylococcus aureus	Keratitis	Broad-spectrum penicillin
Streptococcus pneumoniae		Chloramphenicol
Pseudomonas aeruginosa		Gentamicin
Multiple bacteria	Endophthalmitis	As determined by antibiotic susceptibility tests
Fungi		
Cryptococcosis neoformans	Cryptococcosis	Amphotericin B 5-Flucytosine
Absidia sp.	Cerebrorhinoorbital mycosis	Amphotericin B
Mucor sp.		5-Flucytosine
Rhizopus sp.		
Mortierella sp.		
Protozoa		
Naegleria fowleri	Amebic meningoencephalitis	None
Acanthamoeba sp.		
Toxoplasma gondii	Toxoplasmosis	Pyrimethamine Sulfadiazine
Trypanosoma brucei gambiense	African sleeping sickness	Suramin
Trypanosoma brucei rhodesiense		Pentamidine Melarsoprol
Viruses		
Enteroviruses	Aseptic meningitis	Supportive care
Polioviruses 1, 2, and 3	Poliomyelitis	Supportive care
Togaviruses	Eastern equine encephalitis	Supportive care
	Western equine encephalitis	Supportive care
	Venezuelan equine encephalitis	Supportive care
Rhabdovirus	Rabies	Rabies immune globulin (RIG)
Herpes simplex 1 and 2	Conjunctivitis	Iodo-deoxyuridine
Adenoviruses 8, 19A, and 37	Keratitis	Corticosteroids
Enteroviruses	Polio	Supportive care

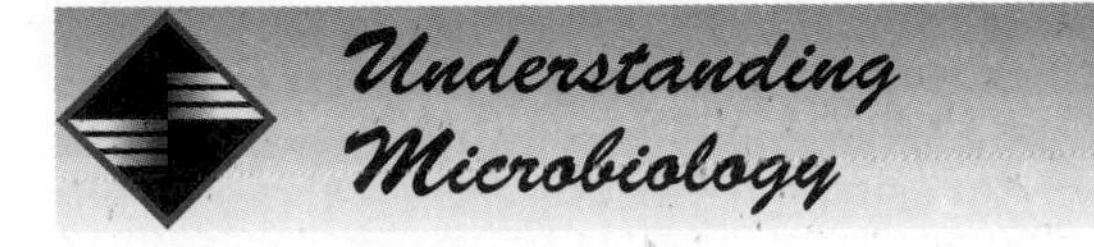

1. How does injury predispose an individual to infections of the central nervous system?
2. Of what significance are the blood-brain and blood-CSF barriers in preventing and treating infections?
3. What are the two most common causes of meningitis in newborns?
4. What factors predispose individuals to the phycomycoses?
5. What are the possible consequences of congenital toxoplasmosis?

Applying Microbiology

Read the following case study carefully and answer the questions: An HIV positive 25-year-old man complained of a severe headache, a high fever, and a stiff neck. Examination of sediment from an India ink preparation of spinal fluid revealed thick-walled spherical cells surrounded by distinct capsules. The organism produced tan mucoid colonies on Sabouraud's agar at 37°C. The patient's symptoms disappeared after treatment with fluconazole.

6. The morphology of the organism observed is typical of
   a. *Candida albicans*
   b. *Histoplasma capsulatum*
   c. *Coccidioides immitis*
   d. *Neisseria meningiditis*
   e. *Cryptococcus neoformans*
7. The reservoir of the etiologic agent demonstrated is
   a. air-conditioning systems
   b. soil
   c. backbay waters
   d. pigeon droppings
   e. air
8. It is likely that there was a primary infection of the
   a. lung
   b. gastrointestinal tract
   c. liver
   d. genitourinary tract
   e. sinuses
9. In AIDS or HIV-infected patients the infection can be described as
   a. primary
   b. opportunistic
   c. invariably fatal
   d. fulminating
   e. nosocomial
10. The etiologic agent is classified as a
    a. dimorphic fungus
    b. gram-positive bacillus
    c. yeast
    d. gram-negative coccus
    e. mold

Chapter 20

Diseases of the Blood, Lymph, and Immune System

Chapter Outline

- **BACTERIAL INFECTIONS**
  - Common Bacteremias
  - Brucellosis (Undulant Fever)
  - Plague
  - Tularemia
  - Rocky Mountain Spotted Fever
  - Other Rickettsial Diseases
  - Lyme Disease
  - Ehrlichiosis
  - Relapsing Fever
  - Cat-Scratch Disease
- **VIRAL INFECTIONS**
  - Infectious Mononucleosis
  - Acquired Immunodeficiency Syndrome (AIDS)
  - Viral Hemorrhagic Fevers
- **PROTOZOAL INFECTIONS**
  - Malaria
  - Babesiosis
  - Chagas' Disease (American Trypanosomiasis)
  - Leishmaniasis

Learning Objectives

After you have read this chapter, you should be able to:

1. Explain the role of circulating and sessile cells of the blood and lymph.
2. Compare the life cycles of malarial parasites in mosquitoes and humans.
3. Explain why malaria is still so prevalent in certain parts of the world.
4. Explain the geographic distribution of diseases of the blood, lymph, and immune system.
5. Explain why persons with HIV are so vulnerable to other infectious agents.
6. Discuss the life cycles and geographic distribution of the etiologic agents of Chagas' disease and leishmaniasis.

The blood, lymph, and immune system contain a variety of circulating and sessile cells. The circulating elements include macrophages, red blood cells, white blood cells, and platelets, which are fragments of cytoplasm derived from **megakaryocytes** found in bone marrow. Macrophages also are found in various parts of the body, including blood sinuses of bone marrow, lymph nodes, liver, spleen, adrenal cortex, alveoli, pleural membranes, peritoneum, brain, spi-

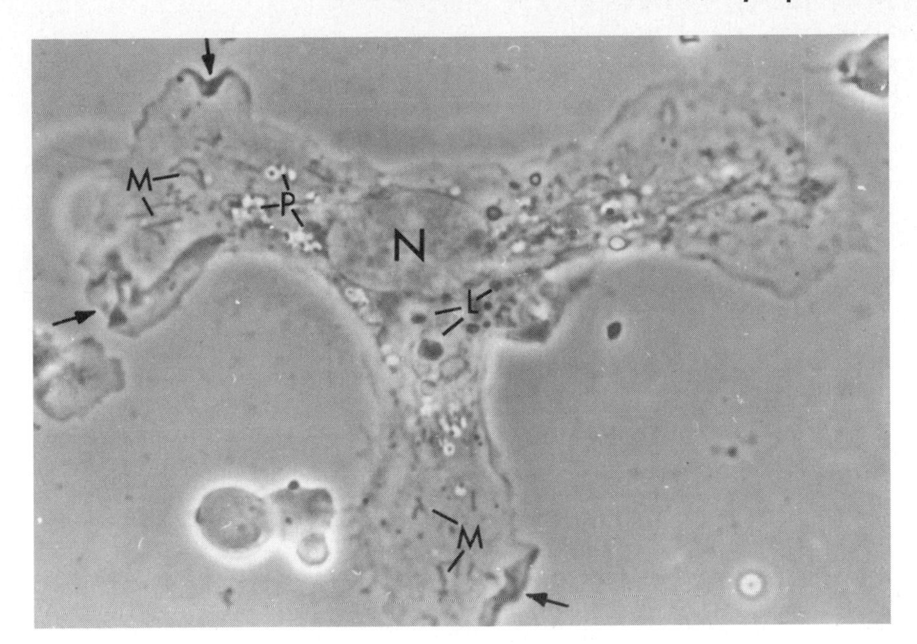

Figure 20–1 ◆ A mouse spleen macrophage two hours after removal from the animal. Structural features of the elongated cell include the oval nucleus (N), rod-shaped mitochondria (M), pinocytic vesicles (P), and lysosomes (L) of varying size.

nal cord, and subcutaneous connective tissue. Certain white blood cells and macrophages are able to phagocytize invading microorganisms (Fig. 20–1). Macrophages of the liver, bone, and nerve tissue are known as Kupffer cells, osteoclasts, and microglial cells, respectively. The organs of the body containing large numbers of macrophages are part of the immune system. Unlike other systems in which organs exist in anatomic proximity to one another, the immune system constitutes a diffuse system in which the organs share the common characteristics of containing noncirculating cells having phagocytic activity.

Like other body tissues, blood, lymph, and the organs of the immune system can become infected. Blood is an excellent culture medium supplying both nutrients and an appropriate temperature for the rapid proliferation of microorganisms. Moreover, blood transports microorganisms to points far distant from the portal of entry (Fig. 20–2). A complex network of lymphatic vessels can also transport microorganisms from the blood or subepithelial layers of the skin to lymph nodes where many infectious particles are removed by filtration (Fig. 20–3). Some microorganisms escape phagocytic action and multiply within the regional lymph nodes, producing lesions known as **buboes.** A large array of microorganisms can invade the bloodstream as a com-

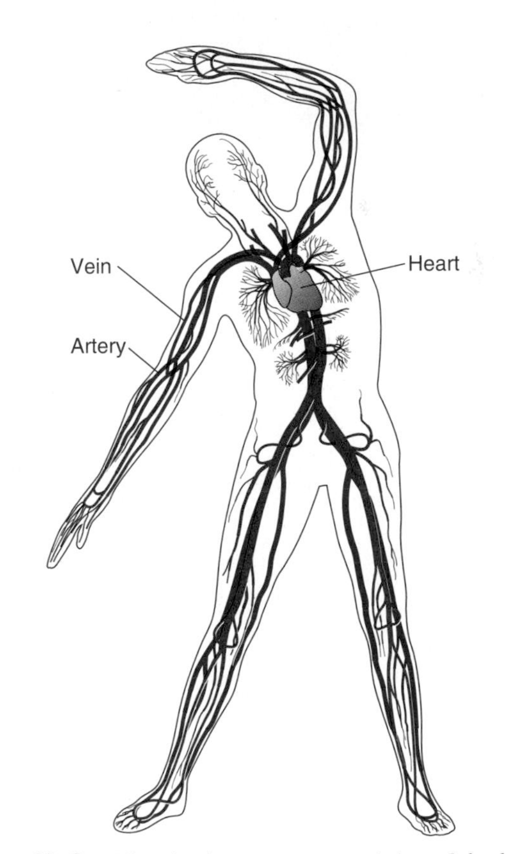

Figure 20–2 ◆ The circulatory system consisting of the heart and blood vessels provides a means for microorganisms to be transferred far from a portal of entry.

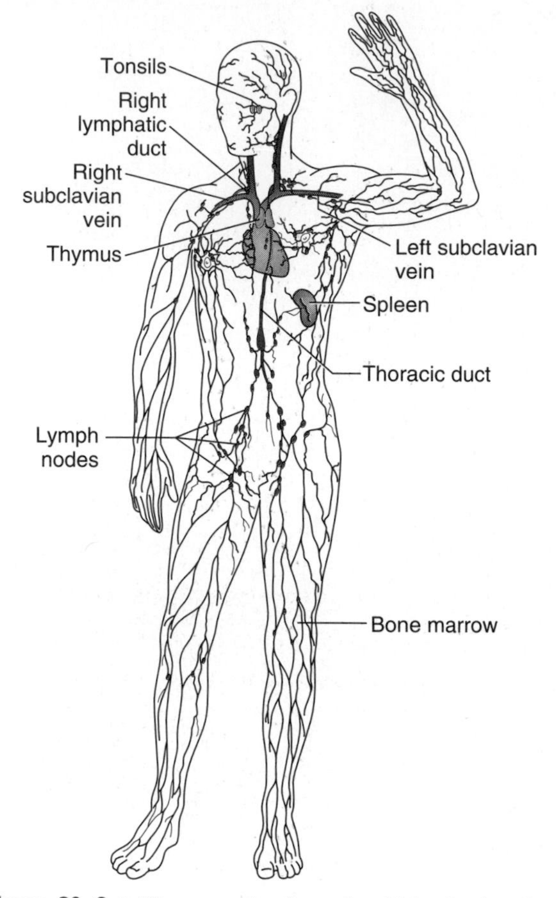

Figure 20–3 ◆ The network of vessels within the lymphatic system transports microorganisms to lymph nodes where the infectious particles are removed by filtration.

plication of a primary infection of other organs. This chapter is devoted to infectious diseases that occur as primary infections of the blood, lymph, and immune systems.

BACTERIAL INFECTIONS

In primary bacteremias (presence of viable bacteria in the blood), the etiologic agents gain access to the bloodstream through wounds, burns, and bites of infected animals or penetrate the skin directly (Color Plate 70). The types of bacteria causing primary infections vary with geographic area, type of services rendered in health care, and level of patient care. Positive blood cultures are always significant because blood is normally sterile.

Common Bacteremias

Both gram-positive and gram-negative organisms are common isolates in patients with bacteremias. Etiologic agents include *Staphylococcus aureus,* streptococci, *Clostridium* species, *Escherichia coli, Pseudomonas aeruginosa,* and *Klebsiella* species. Risk factors consist of the administration of broad-spectrum antibiotics, steroid or immunosuppressive therapy, invasive procedures, anatomical obstruction, and chronic disease states. In recent years, colonization of prosthetic devices, such as artificial heart valves, with *S. epidermidis* has been a problem. Fever is the most frequent sign of sepsis. A lipopolysaccharide (LPS) of the outer membrane of gram-negative bacteria can cause marked hypotension and circulatory shock. Enriched broth media, such as trypticase soy broth, in vented (aerobic) and unvented (anaerobic) bottles, are usually inoculated with 10 ml samples of blood. A minimum of three blood cultures with blood taken at different sites and times is recommended. Bottles must be examined for evidence of growth daily. Aerobic bottles need to be subcultured after six to 18 hours of incubation.

Growth of bacteria can be recognized by presence of turbidity or gas in enriched broth media, growth of colonies on sedimented layer of blood, or hemolysis of blood. Gram stains of positive cultures provide important information on possible etiology. Several automated systems monitor blood cultures continuously for the production or consumption of gas. Appropriate biochemical, serological, or molecular tests can be chosen for identification of the bacteria. Appropriate therapy can be determined by antibiotic susceptibility testing.

In addition to the common pathogens just listed, other bacteria that cause specific diseases can be isolated from blood or seen on stained blood smears. Although the incidence of some of the specific diseases is relatively rare in the United States, travel to endemic areas makes it necessary to rule them out in any differential diagnosis.

Brucellosis (Undulant Fever)

Brucellosis (undulant fever) is one of the oldest infections of animals. The incidence of brucellosis has been markedly reduced in the United States by pasteurization of milk. Three species of the genus *Brucella* cause most infections: *B. abor-*

tus from cattle, *B. melitensis* from goats, and *B. suis* from pigs. During recent years most cases of brucellosis in the United States have been caused by *B. suis*. A fourth species, *B. canis,* causes disease in dog colonies and, therefore, constitutes a health hazard to animal attendants. Human brucellosis is transmitted by ingestion of contaminated meat or dairy products, by contact with infected animal fetuses, placentas, or waste products, or by inhalation of aerosols. Person-to-person transmission is probably almost nonexistent. The time of incubation varies from 30 days to months.

Brucellosis may have an abrupt or insidious onset of fever, headache, sweating, chills, generalized aches, and joint pain. There may be alternating periods of freedom from symptoms. The duration of the disease may be prolonged despite treatment.

Multiple blood cultures are often required to isolate brucellae. It is important to provide an atmosphere of 5 to 10 percent CO_2. Growth is often slow requiring as long as 30 days. Gram stains of subcultures demonstrate gram-negative coccobacilli. Confirmation of isolates as brucellae and species identification require biochemical and serological tests.

Tetracycline and streptomycin are the drugs of choice. One problem in treating brucellosis is that *Brucella* organisms persist in macrophages and can produce foci of infection in many organs. A vaccine is available for cattle, sheep, and goats. Vaccination programs for all herds of those animals could effectively eliminate brucellosis.

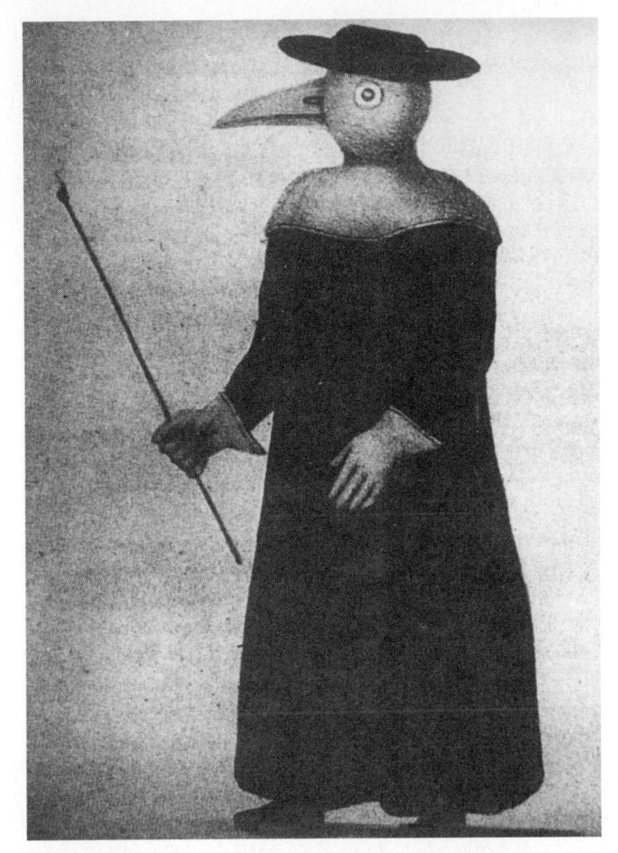

Figure 20–4 ◆ Example of a protective bird mask and clothing worn by physicians during a plague outbreak in Marseilles in 1720.

Plague

In the fourteenth century a mysterious disease, called the Black Death, destroyed as much as one quarter of the world's population. Wherever plague was found, the suddenness of death frightened people. Individuals were found dead in their beds in the morning without having apparent illness. Bodies, piled up on the streets, caused such a stench that some people walked around with flowers in their noses. Physicians in subsequent epidemics often wore birdlike costumes made of leather to protect themselves (Fig. 20–4). Centuries elapsed before it was discovered that rats were the primary reservoirs for the causative agents and that illness followed the bite of infected rat fleas (*Xenopsylla cheopis,* Color Plate 75). One rat can harbor several hundred plague bacilli in its intestines. The disease came to be known as bubonic plague.

The disease is characterized by swollen lymph nodes, particularly those of the inguinal, axillary, or cervical areas two to six days after a bite (Fig. 20–5). Hemorrhages in lymph nodes are responsible for the swelling of the lymph nodes. The swellings are called buboes. The bacteria, accumulated in the nodes, are ultimately released, causing **septicemia.** If the lungs become infected, the illness is called **pneumonic plague.** The pneumonic form of the plague is highly communicable and has been responsible for most of the devastating epidemics in the past. The bacteria can be transferred from person to person by aerosols.

Yersinia pestis can be isolated from blood and bubonic exudates. Caution should be used in handling suspected cultures of the organism. Gram stains of bubonic exudates or subcultures

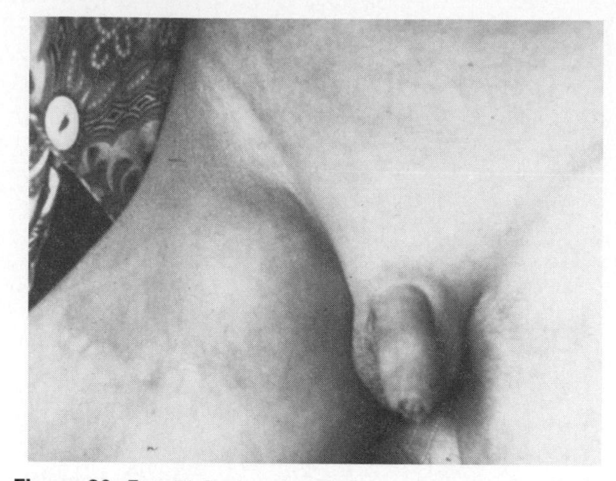

Figure 20–5 ◆ Right inguinal bubo in a seven-year-old boy with a classic case of bubonic plague.

of isolates reveal small gram-negative bacilli that tend to stain darker at the ends (Fig. 20–6). The staining phenomenon is called bipolar staining. *Y. pestis* can be differentiated from other yersiniae by biochemical tests.

Before antibiotics became available, plague was almost invariably fatal, but early treatment with streptomycin, tetracycline, or chloramphenicol is very effective. A vaccine of killed cells of *Y. pestis* is available for those traveling to or working in high-risk areas. Elimination of plague would require eradication of rodents and other wild animal reservoirs of *Y. pestis.* Massive control programs are not feasible, but periodic application of rodenticides to ships, airplanes, and buildings is advised.

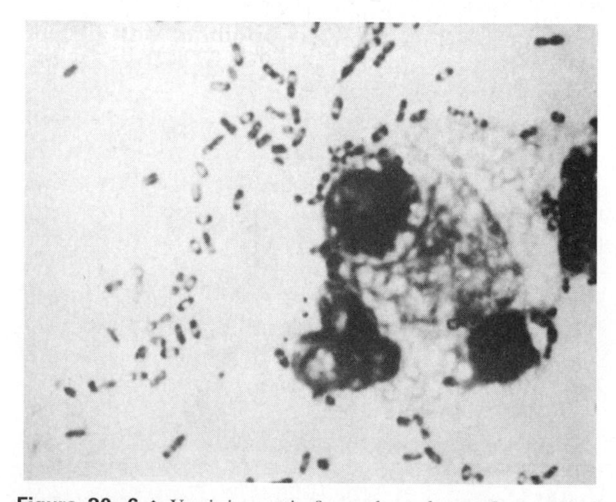

Figure 20–6 ◆ Yersinia pestis from the spleen of an experimentally infected mouse.

Tularemia

Tularemia, another zoonosis, is an infection of the blood and lymph nodes caused by *Franciscella tularensis,* which closely resembles *Y. pestis.* The febrile disease was once known as "rabbit fever" because it is most frequently transmitted to humans by handling rabbits. It is recognized that other wild animals, such as muskrats and bobcats, and some domestic animals can harbor the infectious agent. Most cases of tularemia occur as a consequence of direct inoculation of skin, conjunctival sac, or oropharyngeal mucosa, but ticks, deer flies, and mosquitoes also can transmit the organism. It is not transmitted from person to person. The time of incubation is two to 10 days. Tularemia is characterized by an abrupt rise in temperature that persists if untreated. Lymph node enlargement and septicemia are followed by lung or gastrointestinal disease.

F. tularensis grows only on media enriched with cystine and glucose. The gram-negative bacillus is highly pleomorphic and faintly bipolar. Biochemical tests are of little value, but a precipitation procedure (Ascoli test), a fluorescent-antibody reaction, or an agglutination test may be used to confirm the presence of the organism. A single titer of 1:160 is presumptive evidence of infection.

Streptomycin is the drug of choice, but tetracycline and chloramphenicol are also used to treat tularemia. Killed vaccines are of dubious value, but a live attenuated vaccine used in Russia and on a limited basis in the United States has reduced the incidence of tularemia in laboratory personnel. Preventive measures include use of rubber or plastic gloves in handling animal carcasses, covering exposed parts of the body to prevent insect bites, and thorough cooking of wild game.

Rocky Mountain Spotted Fever

Rocky Mountain spotted fever is a tickborne disease that, contrary to its name, occurs throughout the United States. It is caused by *Rickettsia rickettsii* carried by the wood tick, *Dermacentor andersoni,* and the dog tick, (Color Plate 76) *Dermacentor variabilis* (Fig. 20–7). An ulcerated lesion covered by a black scab, known as an

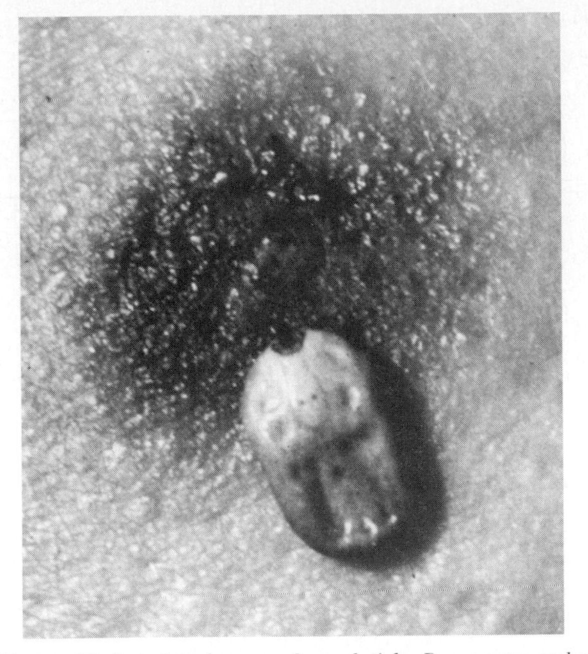

Figure 20–7 ◆ Attachment of wood tick, *Dermacentor andersoni,* to the shoulder of a victim. The tick is shown at the site of the lesion (eschar) five days after attachment. *D. andersoni* is the vector for Rocky Mountain spotted fever.

eschar, may occur at the site of a bite. The organisms enter and proliferate in the endothelial lining of arterioles and capillaries. The time of incubation is three to 14 days.

The illness is characterized by a sudden onset with a relatively high fever and a maculopapular rash on the extremities. The organism disseminates rapidly and the appearance of petechiae and hemorrhage is common. Fatality rates approximate 15 to 20 percent unless the disease is recognized and treated promptly.

R. rickettsii is a pleomorphic coccobacillus that can be seen in infected cells stained by the Giemsa method (Fig. 20–8). The organism can be isolated from blood, but the techniques required are expensive, dangerous, and available only in a limited number of laboratories. Rocky Mountain spotted fever can usually be diagnosed clinically, but agglutination tests with certain *Proteus* antigens are of some value in the Weil-Felix reaction because of some shared antigens. Specific complement-fixation (CF) and agglutination tests can confirm a diagnosis.

Tetracycline or chloramphenicol is the drug of choice. No vaccine is currently licensed for distribution in the United States. Use of insect repellents does limit exposure to tick bites.

Other Rickettsial Diseases

Rickettsial diseases of humans, other than Q fever, which was discussed in Chapter 18, and Rocky Mountain spotted fever, do not occur frequently in the United States. They are transmitted by bites of lice, rat fleas, or mites (Table 20–1). In some instances, fleas defecate rickettsias while sucking blood, thus contaminating the sites of the bite. Inhalation of rickettsias in aerosols may account for some infections. No person-to-person transmission occurs. The period of incubation varies with the disease, but is commonly 10 to 12 days. The last outbreak of louseborn typhus fever occurred in the United States in 1922, but human reservoirs of the disease persist in some parts of the world because the rickettsias may remain latent in lymph nodes.

A less severe form of the typhus, known as Brill Zinsscr disease, may recur 10 or more years after an initial infection. Fleaborne typhus fever is endemic in some parts of the United States where rats and their fleas still turn up as unwelcome guests on incoming ships. Less than 100 cases are reported annually.

A fever and a maculopapular rash are universal symptoms of rickettsial infected endothelial cells of blood vessels. In miteborne typhus fever, an eschar frequently occurs at the site of attachment of the infected mite. Patients are sometimes mentally confused and may become delirious. Fatality rates are high in untreated cases.

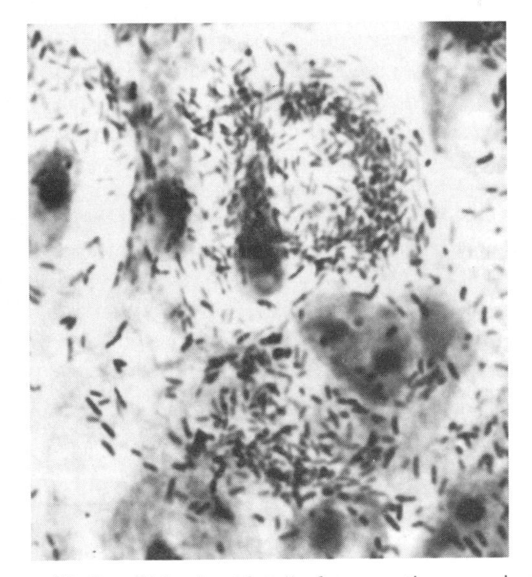

Figure 20–8 ◆ *Rickettsia rickettsii,* the causative organism of Rocky Mountain spotted fever, grown in an egg yolk sac.

Table 20–1
ARTHROPOD VECTORS AND MODES OF TRANSMISSION FOR RICKETTSIAL DISEASES

DISEASE	MODE OF TRANSMISSION	ARTHROPOD VECTOR
Epidemic typhus	Feces	*Pediculus humanus corporis* (human louse)
Endemic typhus	Feces	*Xenopsylla cheopis* (rat flea)
		Polyplax spinulosus (rat louse)
Rocky Mountain spotted fever	Bite	*Dermacentor andersoni* (wood tick)
		Dermacentor variabilis (dog tick)
Rickettsialpox	Bite	*Allodermanyssus sanguineus* (mouse mite)
Tsutsugamushi fever	Bite	*Trombicula akamushi* (larval mammalian mite)
Trench fever	Feces	*Pediculus humanus corporis* (human louse)

The technique for isolation of rickettsial organisms are cumbersome and not without danger. A variety of serological tests are available for detection of specific antibodies. Sera of individuals with some types of typhus fever agglutinate strains of *Proteus* species in the Weil-Felix reaction.

The rickettsial diseases respond to tetracycline or chloramphenicol. A necessary measure for rapid control is the application of insecticides and destruction of rodents in affected areas.

Lyme Disease

Lyme disease is a bacterial infection acquired through the bites of infected ticks that live in wooded areas. The disease got its name from the town of Old Lyme, Connecticut, where it was discovered in 1975. The primary vector for the spirochete *Borrelia burgdorferi,* which causes Lyme disease, is the tick, *Ixodes dammini,* but the organism is also carried by *I. pacificus* and *I. neotornae.*

The ticks have a two-year life cycle. Eggs are deposited in the spring and hatch into larvae in about 30 days. The larvae are dormant over the winter, maturing into second developmental stages, known as **nymphs,** the following spring. The nymphs feed on infected deer or white-footed mice and transfer the spirochetes when they bite humans. Most humans are bitten by nymphs. A minimum of a 24-hour attachment period is required for the ticks to transmit disease. Lyme disease is second only to AIDS in the United States as a public health problem of major concern. It is the most common tickborne disease in this country, but it also occurs in parts of Europe, Australia, and the Far East.

The infection in humans occurs in three stages, not all of which necessarily occur in each patient with the disease. The first stage is characterized by the appearance of an expanding "bull's eye" rash two to five weeks after the tick bite (Fig. 20–9). The circular lesions may be accompanied by influenza-like symptoms. The second stage may occur weeks to months later when symptoms of neurological, cardiac, or joint disease may be present. The third stage consists of repeated and severe attacks of arthritis over a period of years. The spirochete can cross the placenta causing fetal damage.

Although borreliae are gram-negative, a Giemsa or a fluorescent antibody stain is recommended for visualization of the spirochetes. En-

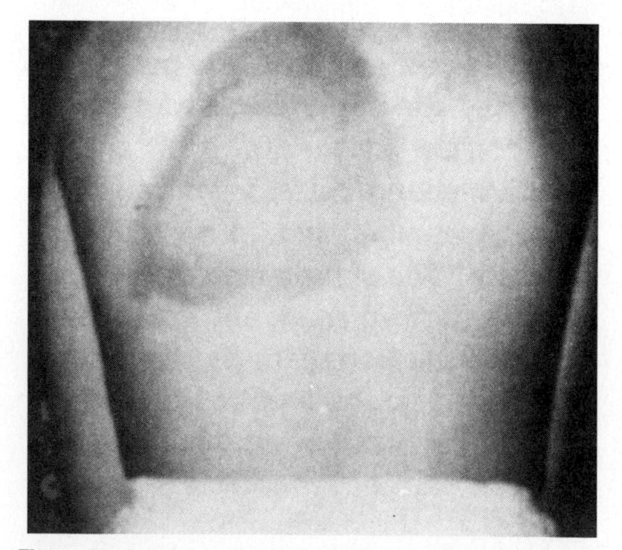

Figure 20–9 ◆ The expanding skin lesion of Lyme disease.

zyme-linked immunosorbent assays (ELISA) for IgG or IgM antibodies are most often used for diagnosis of Lyme disease, but information obtained is not always reliable. A unique outer surface protein, Osp A, found in patients with the telltale rash, can be detected in immune complexes from blood, but a commercial test is not yet available. The diagnosis of early Lyme disease in the majority of individuals remains a clinical diagnosis.

The risk of spirochetal transmission can be reduced by inspecting the skin for the presence of attached ticks and promptly removing them. The developmental stages may be no bigger than the period at the end of this sentence. A tick repellant, containing diethyltoluamide, and protective clothing can deter ticks in their quest for a blood meal.

B. burgdorferi responds to treatment with penicillin or tetracycline. If antimicrobial agents are given early in the illness, joint disease may be prevented or minimized. The neurological, cardiac, or joint complications, seen later in the disease, are not abated by the administration of those drugs.

A Lyme disease vaccine became available in the United States in 1999. It is a genetically engineered vaccine containing the outer surface lipoprotein Osp A of *B. burgdorferi*. It is effective against symptomatic and asymptomatic infections.

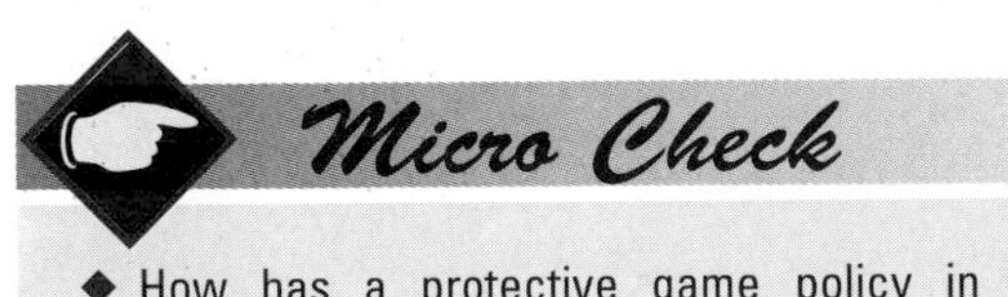

- How has a protective game policy in most parts of the United States affected deer-tick populations?
- Why would reducing the deer population not necessarily affect the incidence of Lyme disease?
- Why is a diagnosis of Lyme disease so difficult?

Ehrlichiosis

Human monocytic ehrlichiosis (HME), caused by *Ehrlichia chafeensis* and human granulocytic ehrlichiosis (HGE), caused by an organism closely related to *E. equi*, are two emerging tickborne diseases in the United States. Both dog and deer ticks have been implicated as arthropod vectors.

Both HME and HGE are acute febrile diseases characterized by **leukopenia, thrombocytopenia,** headache, and muscle pain. Only 20 percent of those affected have a rash. The causative agents are obligate parasites that grow in white blood cells and have complex developmental cycles.

Diagnosis is made by detecting antibodies in the serum of patients. Empirical treatment with tetracycline is recommended for suspected cases even before laboratory confirmation to prevent consequences of low white blood cell or platelet counts.

Relapsing Fever

Relapsing fever is a systemic febrile disease characterized by recurrent febrile episodes occurring at intervals of two to 14 days. The disease is caused by the spirochete *Borrelia recurrentis,* which can be found in blood during febrile periods. Relapsing fever is worldwide in distribution, but epidemics tend to be more prevalent in overcrowded populations with poor habits of personal hygiene. Epidemic relapsing fever is transmitted by the lice *Pediculus humanus corporis* and *P. humanus capitis* (Color Plate 77). Lice are infected by biting individuals with the disease. The lice remain infected for their lifetime, which ranges from five to six weeks. Endemic relapsing fever is tickborne. The spirochetes, which can persist in fluids and feces of ticks for years, are transmitted from one generation of tick to another. In the United States soft ticks belonging to the genus *Ornithodoros* transmit relapsing fever. The ticks feed exclusively on blood. Persons are most often bitten by the ticks at night and are often unaware of their bites. Relapsing fever is not transmitted from person to person. The time of incubation is five to 15 days. Febrile periods of relapsing fever last two to nine days with alternate afebrile periods of two to four days. The number of relapses may be as many as 10. The recurrent rises in temperature in relapsing fever are increasingly less severe and progressively shorter. Transitory petechial rashes are common in some patients.

Relapsing fever can be diagnosed by finding *B. recurrentis* in Giemsa-stained blood smears from infected individuals or rats or mice inoculated with whole blood containing the spirochetes (Fig. 20–10). Animal blood should be checked daily for appearance of the organisms. Serological tests are of limited value since antigens of *B. recurrentis* are unstable.

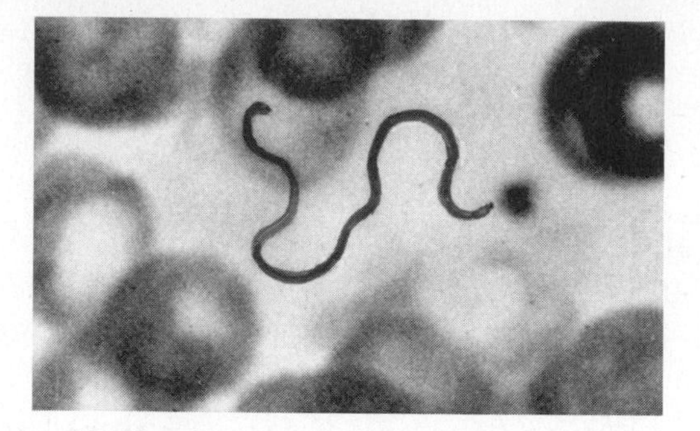

Figure 20–10 ◆ *Borrelia recurrentis* in Giemsa-stained mouse blood.

Relapsing fever responds to penicillin, tetracycline, or chloramphenicol. Control is dependent on elimination of rodent nests and use of insecticides.

Cat-Scratch Disease

Cat-scratch disease (CSD) is a subacute, self-limited disease that follows the scratch or a bite of a cat. Although the disease was recognized more than 50 years ago, the etiologic agent has only recently been recognized as a gram-negative bacillus, *Bartonella henselae.*

CSD is rarely serious, but the fever, chills, and swollen lymph nodes mimic other illnesses, including malignancies (Fig. 20–11). The appearance of excised lymph nodes has been mistaken for lymphogranuloma venereum, chronic tularemia, or tuberculosis. A primary skin lesion appears three to 14 days after a scratch or bite. Although complications are rare, they can occur. The most serious complication is suppuration, which may develop into a draining **fistula.** The organism can be grown on freshly made chocolate agar plates or other enriched media. The organism is slow-growing and requires an atmosphere of 5 to 10 percent CO_2.

Antibiotics do not alter the course of CSD. Declawing of cats could reduce the risks of infection from scratches, but the etiologic agent is suspected as being indigenous to the mouths of cats.

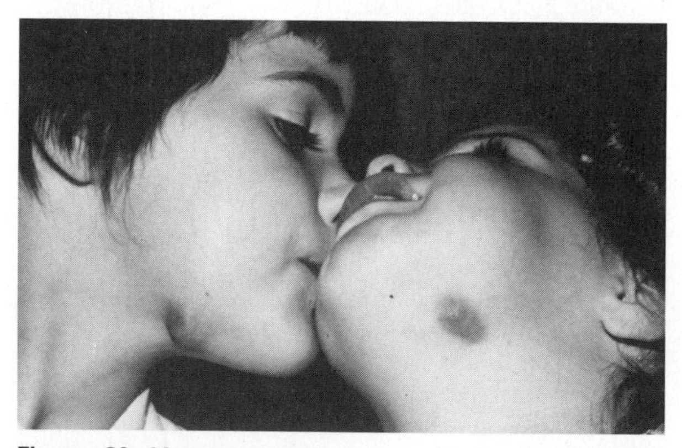

Figure 20–11 ◆ Sisters with submandibular lymphadenitis following numerous cat scratches.

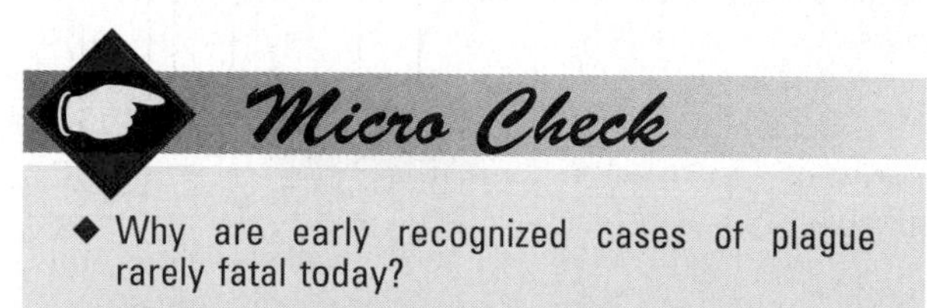

- ◆ Why are early recognized cases of plague rarely fatal today?
- ◆ What arthropods are important in the transmission of Rocky Mountain spotted fever?
- ◆ With what other diseases might cat-scratch disease be confused?

VIRAL INFECTIONS

Viral infections of the blood are particularly serious because initially the viruses may be present without any signs or symptoms of disease. Circulating viruses frequently localize in the liver, spleen, endothelial cells of capillaries, lymphocytes, or macrophages. Primary viremias are often the result of direct invasion of the bloodstream following the bite of an arthropod. A few of these viruses are highly virulent. The incidence for most life-threatening viral infections is higher in tropical and subtropical climates.

Infectious Mononucleosis

Infectious mononucleosis is usually a self-limiting disease of the lymphatic system most frequently caused by a herpesvirus known as the Epstein-Barr virus (EBV) or the cytomegalovirus (CMV). Like other herpesviruses, these viruses have a potential for latency and can cause recurrent infections. Infectious mononucleosis is chiefly a disease of young adults in developed countries. Primary infectious mononucleosis is rare in Third World countries with low standards of hygiene. The association of EBV with Burkitt's lymphoma and nasopharyngeal carcinoma in some parts of Africa is a curious phenomenon. The circumstances that permit the induction of tumors is not understood. CMV is the cause of a serious retinitis in AIDS patients and can result in blindness.

The disease is transmitted by oral contact. For that reason, the infection is commonly called "the kissing disease." EBV and CMV may also be transmitted by blood, blood products, and bone marrow transplants. The incubation period is highly variable. It may be as short as six days or as long as 60 days.

Infectious mononucleosis has an insidious onset starting with a sore throat and swollen cervical lymph nodes. Other lymph nodes also may be enlarged. A prominent feature of the disease is a proliferation of and presence of atypical lymphocytes in blood (Fig. 20–12). The most common complications are neurological disorders, such as aseptic meningitis, encephalitis, and Guillain-Barré syndrome.

It is not practical to attempt to isolate EBV or CMV. Primary infectious mononucleosis can be diagnosed by demonstration of moderate to high titers of heterophil or agglutinating antibodies. Antibodies to EBV or CMV antigens can also be measured as indicators of current or reactivated infections.

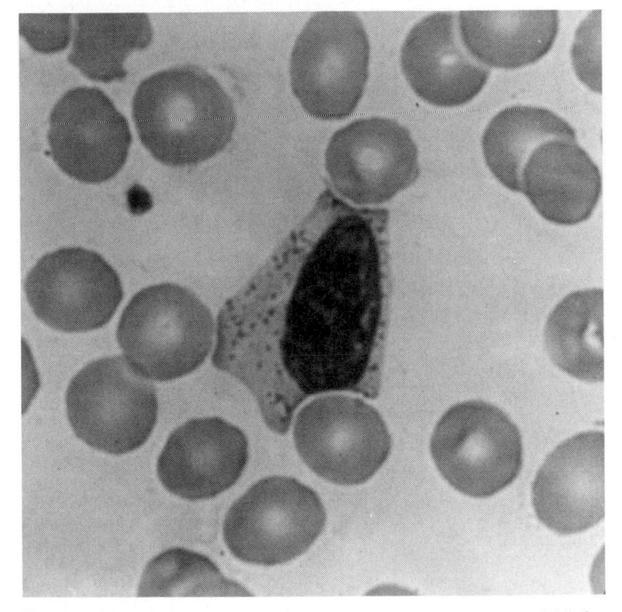

Figure 20–12 ◆ An atypical lymphocyte seen on a Wright-Giemsa stained peripheral blood smear of a patient with infectious mononucleosis. The cell frequently appears indented from contact with other blood cells. The cytoplasm is abundant with basophilic granules.

There is no treatment specific for infectious mononucleosis, but supportive care, including bed rest, is sometimes very important. Antiviral therapy is currently under investigation. Administration of steroids provides some symptomatic relief.

Acquired Immunodeficiency Syndrome (AIDS)

The first cases of a highly debilitating viral blood disease that was to destroy the lives of millions in a worldwide epidemic were recognized in 1981. At one time both CMV and EBV were suspected as etiologic agents in the disease because of their ability to cause immunosuppression.

In 1984 Luc Montagnier of France and Robert Gallo of the United States identified a retrovirus as the cause of the devastating disease. The virus was named human immunodeficiency virus (HIV) because of the severity of its ability to destroy $CD4^+$ lymphocytes (also known as helper T cells). The role of $CD4^+$ lymphocytes in the immune response is discussed in Chapter 13.

The destruction of sufficient $CD4^+$ lymphocytes makes individuals infected with HIV vulnerable to opportunistic infections. The appearance of a second similar virus in West Africa in 1985 has made it necessary to designate human immunodeficiency viruses as HIV-1 or HIV-2. Most HIV infections in the United States, Canada, and Europe are caused by HIV-1. In a few parts of Africa, both viruses have been isolated from infected individuals.

At one time AIDS was considered to be a disease of gay or bisexual men and drug abusers, but the disease is spreading among the heterosexual population in the United States. The disease occurs mainly in heterosexual populations in Third World countries. HIV is transmitted sexually, by placental or breast-milk transfer, and, more rarely, by blood transfusions. A test for antibodies to HIV has been used to screen blood for transfusion purposes in the United States since 1985. Contact with body fluids of infected patients poses a risk for health care workers. There is no evidence that the virus is spread by casual contact.

Several weeks or months after exposure to HIV, an individual may experience a slight fever, fatigue, swollen lymph nodes, muscle aches, and mild diarrhea. The infection may not progress to AIDS with $CD4^+$ counts under 200/ml and the onset of other infections for many years. The average time between initial exposure to HIV and the progression to AIDS is about 10 years. Only a few persons with HIV have remained well for longer periods. The reasons for the delay of the onset of AIDS in these individuals is not understood.

Only cases of AIDS are reportable in the United States: thus, the actual numbers of HIV infections can only be surmised. It is estimated that there are about 1 to 1.5 million Americans carrying HIV. The World Health Organization (WHO) estimates that at least 21.8 million people are infected throughout the world. The majority of those individuals live in Sub-Saharan Africa. Without knowledge of the presence of HIV in their bodies, they are unknowingly transmitting the virus to their sexual partners. About one-third of babies born to infected mothers acquire the infection by placental transfer or breast milk.

By mid-1993, more than 300,000 Americans had developed AIDS and more than 190,000 had died—nearly three times more than the number of Vietnam War casualties. AIDS is one of the leading causes of the death in women and men 25 to 44 years old. It is among the top ten causes of disease in children one to four years of age. The total number of AIDS cases in the United States continues to rise despite aggressive educational campaigns (Fig. 20–13).

The emotional and economic toll of AIDS is staggering. Most people in the united States have lost a friend or relative to the devastating disease. Of particular concern is the cost of treating persons infected with HIV or full-blown AIDS. The drugs used for treatment are expensive and the costs of hospitalization and raising children orphaned by the disease are high.

A diagnosis of HIV infection is made by finding antibodies to the virus by an enzyme-linked immunosorbent assay (ELISA) screening procedure. Antibodies can be detected in most instances within three months after exposure to the virus.

Antibodies to specific proteins associated with the virus can be demonstrated by a Western blot

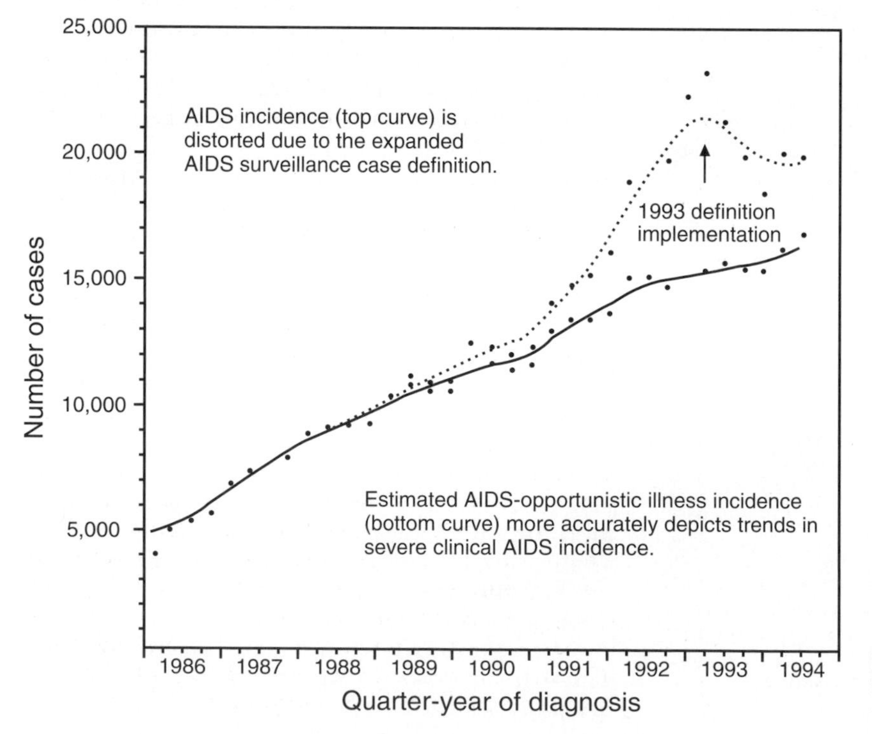

Figure 20–13 ◆ The precipitous rise in cases of AIDS seen in 1993 was due to a change in case definition.

method (Fig. 20–14). The viral proteins are separated by electrophoresis in a polyacrylamide gel and "blotted" onto strips of nitrocellulose paper. Serum is applied to the nitrocellulose strip. Any antibodies present will react with specific proteins to form a complex. Enzyme-linked antihuman globulin G is added to the bands of antigen-antibody complexes. Production of color when the substrate is added indicates positive antibodies. The presence of antibodies to the glycoprotein gp120 and gp41 confirms the presence of an HIV infection.

The ELISA and Western blot tests, when used together, are accurate more than 99.9 percent of the time. The amount of circulating HIV nucleic acid is useful as a diagnostic tool in infants because tests for antibodies fail to discriminate between those of the mother and infant. Tests that measure HIV nucleic acid are called **viral load** determinations. Diagnostic procedures for the opportunistic diseases occurring in HIV infection or AIDS are discussed in chapters on diseases of the particular systems involved.

Drugs cannot cure AIDS, but they can slow down the infection and prolong periods of wellness. Zidovudine (also known as azidothymidine, or AZT), dideoxycytidine (DDC), dideoxyinosine (DDI), stavudine (d4T), and abacavir inhibit the process of reverse transcription required for replication of HIV. AZT, given after the first trimester of pregnancy, reduces the risk of transmission of the virus from an infected mother to a fetus by 67.5 percent. A group of drugs known as protease inhibitors are often combined with AZT in treatment regimens. Those drugs are discussed in Chapter 22.

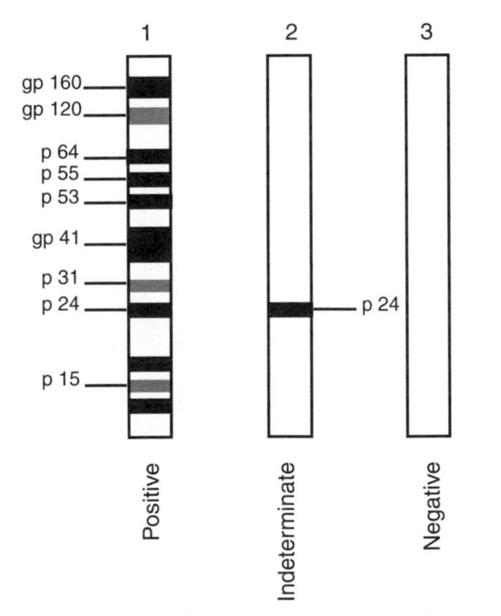

Figure 20–14 ◆ Nitrocellulose strips from a Western blot analysis. Lane 1 is positive. Lane 2 is indeterminant. Lane 3 is negative. The strips are used to confirm positive ELISA tests for HIV antibodies.

The "cocktails" of combined drugs have prolonged lives of some of the recipients by reducing the viral load in plasma. Tests for viral load are of value in adults for predicting the course of AIDS and monitoring treatment. There are several molecular amplification methods available for determining viral load. Persons with more than 100,000 copies of nucleic acid per milliliter of plasma within the first six months of diagnosis are more likely to progress to AIDS within five years. Viral load testing is usually performed every three or four months to monitor treatment.

Other drugs are available to prevent or treat opportunistic diseases (Color Plate 71). Many drugs are currently under investigation. The Food and Drug Administration (FDA) has shortened the review process for newly developed promising drugs for AIDS and organized investigational studies through which additional treatments are available.

Unfortunately, there is no vaccine for HIV, although several are being studied. Development of a safe and effective vaccine presents multiple problems. There are no appropriate animal models, and surface antigens of the virus mutate frequently. The very cells infected ($CD4^+$ cells) are the same immune cells needed to initiate an immune response.

Viral Hemorrhagic Fevers

The viral hemorrhagic fevers consist of a group of systemic diseases affecting humans, and sometimes animals; they include yellow fever (urban and sylvan), hemorrhagic dengue fever, Lassa fever, and at least seven other varieties of hemorrhagic diseases. The hemorrhagic diseases are widespread geographically, but tend to be present in larger numbers in tropical and subtropical climates. The viruses that cause hemorrhagic fevers belong to diverse groups and include arenaviruses, bunyaviruses, flaviviruses, and filoviruses. None of the etiologic agents occurs naturally in the United States, but imported cases of dengue fever are not rare. Many of the diseases are transmitted by mosquitoes and ticks.

FOCAL POINT

A Life Ended Too Soon

On September 8, 1988, in the aftermath of a brain operation, Arthur Ashe, a veteran of tennis's Davis Cup competitions, and 1975 Wimbleton winner, discovered he had toxoplasmosis. Not normally a cause for alarm, the diagnosis explained the numbness in his right hand and heralded the onset of full-blown AIDS. Only six days earlier, he had learned for the first time that he was HIV positive. Arthur Ashe had the misfortune of receiving two units of HIV-contaminated blood in 1983 during heart surgery. The blood was donated before routine testing on blood for transfusions was required. The enzyme-linked immunosorbent assay (ELISA) test for antibodies to HIV was not available until March 1985.

From the day following brain surgery for the abscess caused by *Toxoplasma gondii,* Arthur Ashe knew his days on Earth were numbered. Unfortunately, about 13,000 other people who received blood transfusions before March 1985 also were given tainted blood. Arthur Ashe soon became an expert on toxoplasmosis, *Pneumocystis carinii* pneumonia, and other manifestations of AIDS. In April 1992, he was forced to announce to the world that he had the killer disease AIDS rather than endure a media massacre when news of his illness became known. Arthur Ashe was not only a tennis champion. He was a firm advocate of justice and opportunity for black men and women and a leader in the battle against AIDS for as long as he had the strength to fight. Arthur Ashe died of pneumonia on February 6, 1993, at New York's Cornell Medical Center. Arthur Ashe's life was a life ended too soon, but the legacy of courage displayed, both on the tennis court and in his final days in facing death, will live on.

Ashe A, Rampersand A: Days of Grace, a Memoir. Alfred A. Knopf Inc., 1993.

The mosquito *Aedes aegypti* is an important vector in both dengue and yellow fever (Color Plate 78). Dengue is also transmitted by the exotic Asian tiger mosquito *A. albopictus* believed to have entered the United States in 1985 in shipments of used tires from Asia. The larvae of the mosquitoes commonly breed in standing water found in tires stored outside on their sides. It is not known if the imported Asian mosquitoes could serve as vectors for viruses causing encephalitis in the United States. The time of incubation varies with the hemorrhagic fevers, but most usually varies from three to 21 days.

The hemorrhagic fevers are extremely debilitating and some have high fatality rates. For example, average deaths of patients hospitalized with Lassa fever have been 30 to 50 percent. Hemorrhagic dengue has a fatality rate as high as 8 percent in children.

The viruses of the hemorrhagic fevers may be isolated from blood, urine, or throat swabs, but should only be attempted by experienced personnel in special laboratories. A variety of serological tests are available to detect specific antibodies.

There is no treatment specific for the viral hemorrhagic fevers. Patients need to be hospitalized and monitored carefully for signs of bleeding. Blood transfusions are often required. A vaccine consisting of an attenuated strain of the yellow fever virus is of paramount importance to residents of and travelers to endemic areas. Effective control of viral hemorrhagic fevers would require elimination of vectors. Insect repellents and protective clothing are of some value in preventing exposure to the vectors.

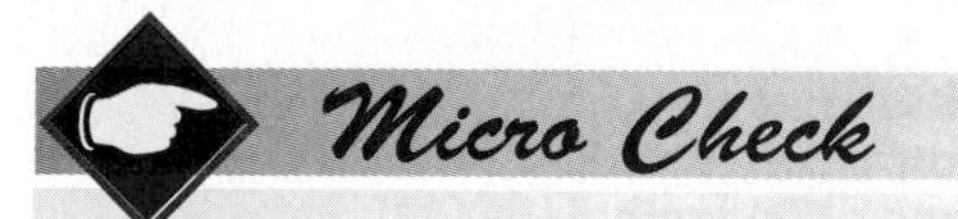

- What two viruses can cause infectious mononucleosis?
- What are the primary target cells of the human immunodeficiency virus?
- Why are public health authorities concerned about the accidental entry of the mosquito *Aedes albopictus* into the United States?

PROTOZOAL INFECTIONS

A few protozoa have a propensity for taking up residence within blood cells, plasma, lymph nodes, liver, spleen, bone marrow, or other organs. All require an arthropod to complete their life cycle. The parasites are transmitted to humans through the bite of a protozoan-infected arthropod. The intensity of the symptoms depends on the location of the parasite within the host, the migratory capacity of the protozoan, and the reaction of the host to invasion by the parasite.

Malaria

Malaria is an acute and sometimes chronic disease that at one time was a leading cause of illness and death throughout the world. It is estimated that the disease still affects some 300 million persons each year, most in tropical and subtropical climates of Africa, Asia, Central America, South America, and the islands of the Southwest Pacific. Each year over 1 million die in tropical Africa alone from malaria. Most cases appearing in the United States are related to exposure during a tour of military duty or travel to areas in which malaria is endemic.

Human malaria is caused by four species of the protozoan *Plasmodium: P. malariae, P. vivax, P. falciparum,* and *P. ovale.* All the species are carried by the female *Anopheles* mosquito (Color Plate 79). Distribution of the species is related to climate and availability of vectors (Table 20–2). The most common malarial parasite in temperate zones is *P. vivax,* which can persist in a dormant state for years in the liver. The multiplication and release of infective forms is often triggered by physical stress.

The most common means of transmission for malaria is by the bite of an infected female *Anopheles* mosquito, but the disease can also be transmitted by blood transfusion from an infected donor. Malaria has been reported to spread among drug addicts by use of a common syringe contaminated with the protozoa. In malaria originating from a transfusion or syringe, the exoerythrocytic cycle is precluded, so that symptoms appear earlier. The plasmodia do not readily penetrate the placental barrier, but a breach in the placenta can provide a portal of entry for a congenitally acquired infection. The incubation period averages 30 days for *P. malariae,* 14 days for *P. vivax,* and 12 days for *P. falciparum* and *P. ovale.*

The life cycles of the *Plasmodium* species are complex (Fig. 20–15). The human serves as the intermediate host for the phase of asexual reproduction, known as **schizogony;** the mosquito serves as the definitive host for the phase of sexual reproduction known as **sporogony.** The asexual phase of the life cycle is divided into two developmental periods: exoerythrocytic (outside red blood cells) and erythrocytic (inside red blood cells). An infected mosquito introduces infective stages of the *Plasmodium* parasite, known as **sporozoites,** into the blood when it bites a person. The exoerythrocytic period begins when the parasites are transported to the liver. Asexual progeny, known as **merozoites,** are released into the circulation in approximately eight to 12 days, depending on the species. The merozoites penetrate red blood cells, starting the erythrocytic developmental period.

Early in the erythrocytic period the parasites take the form of signet rings, but in the oxygen-rich environment of the red blood cells they soon develop into ameboid **trophozoites.** The mature trophozoites undergo mitosis and segmentation

Table 20–2
CHARACTERISTICS OF INFECTIONS CAUSED BY *PLASMODIUM* PARASITES

CHARACTERISTIC	*P. vivax*	*P. malariae*	*P. falciparum*	*P. ovale*
Geographic distribution	Temperate and tropical	Subtropical	Tropical	Tropical
Exoerythrocytic period (days)	8	12	6	9
Erythrocytic period (hours)	45±	72	48	49
Average parasitemia (per mm^3)	20,000	6,000	100,000–500,000	9,000
Severity	Mild to severe	Mild	Severe	Mild
Duration of infection (years)	1–3	10–30	0.5–1.5	—
Name of disease	Benign tertian	Quartan	Malignant tertian	Benign tertian
Prognosis	Favorable	Favorable	Guarded	Favorable

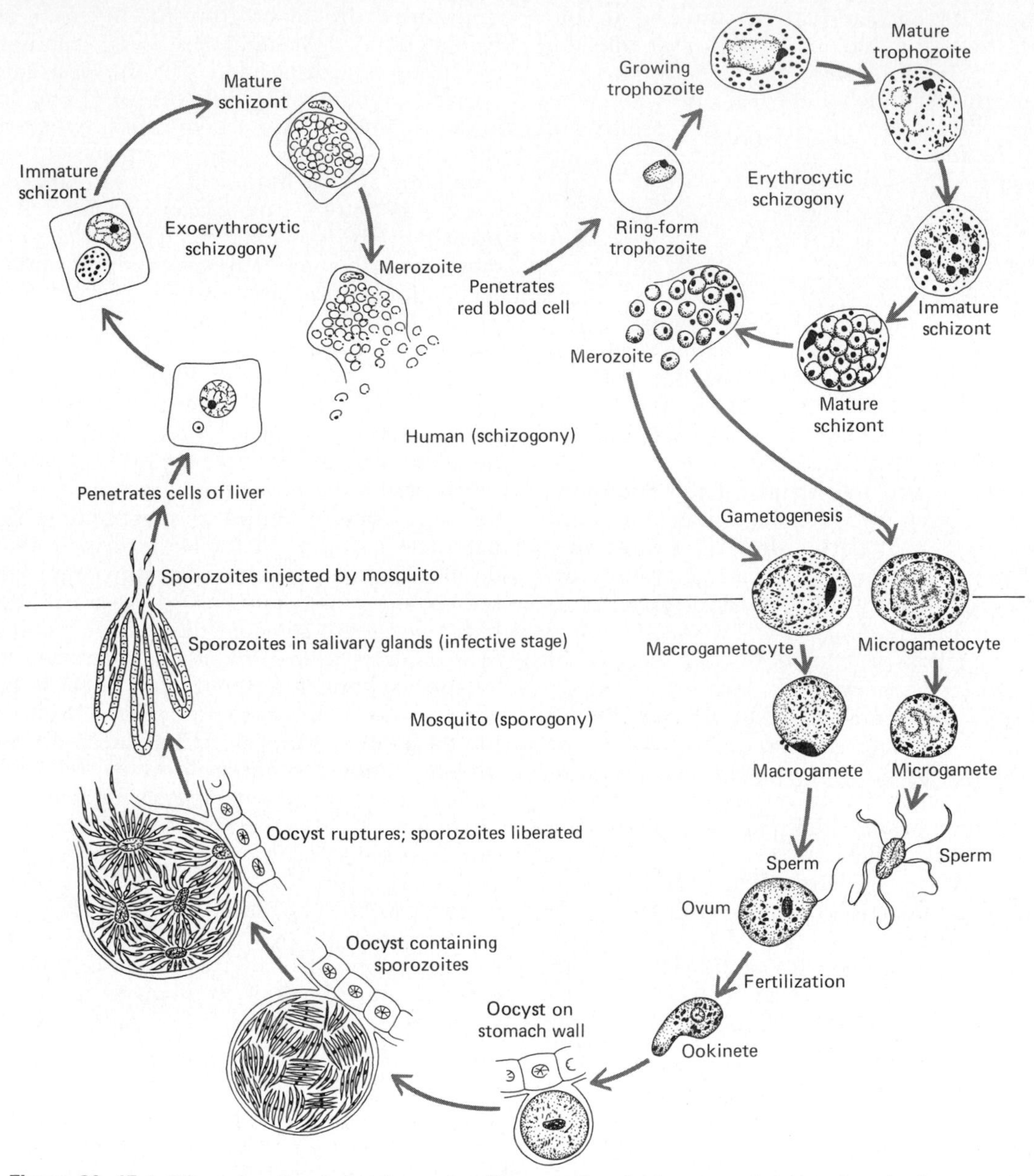

Figure 20–15 ◆ Life cycle of a malarial parasite. The sexual cycle (sporogony) takes place in the mosquito, whereas the asexual cycle (schizogony) takes place in the human.

to produce **schizonts** that contain an average of six to 20 merozoites, depending on the species (Color Plate 72). When red blood cells rupture, releasing merozoites and toxins associated with metabolic processes of the organisms, the infected host experiences a fever followed by a chill.

Although in early stages of malarial infections no periodicity in fevers and chills can be recognized, symptoms occur with greater regularity as synchrony is established in developmental cycles. The time interval required for development of *P. vivax, P. ovale,* and *P. falciparum* is 48 hours: a period of 72 hours is required for *P. malariae* (Fig. 20–16).

There is a progressive anemia as erythrocytes rupture upon completion of successive asexual

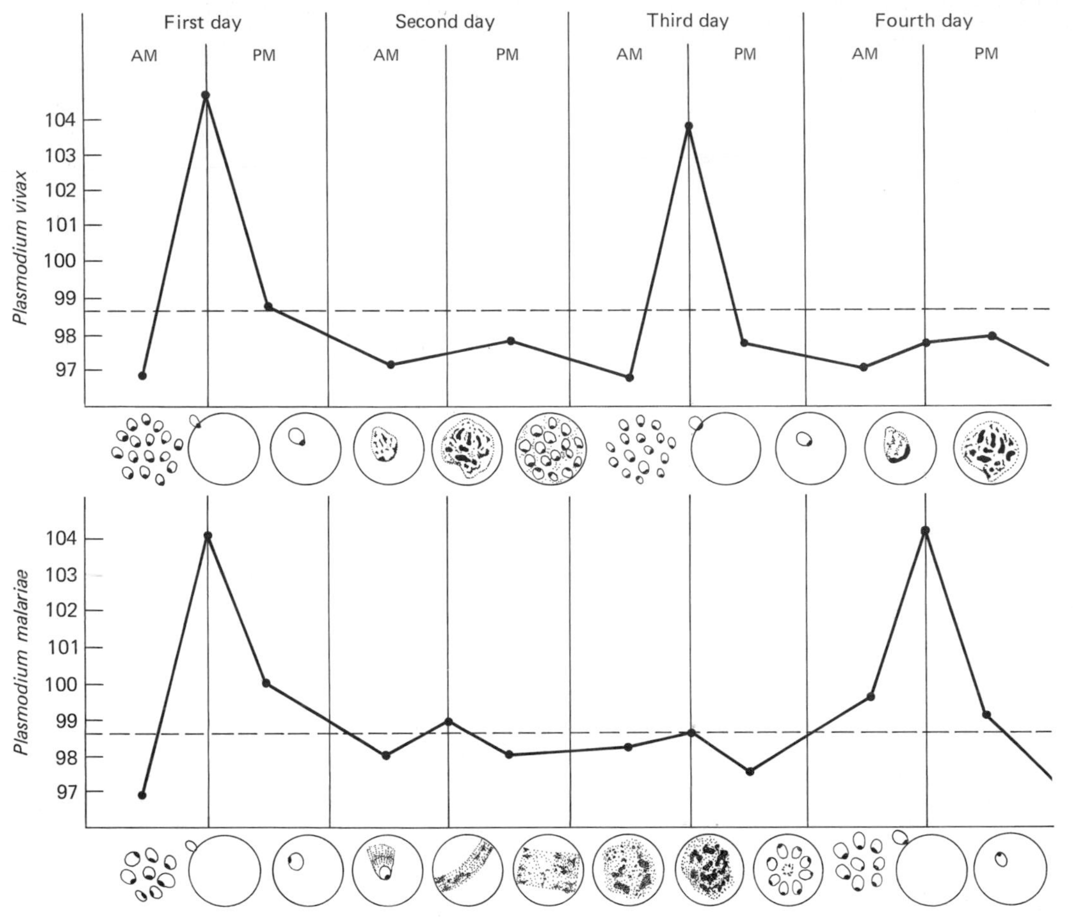

Figure 20–16 ◆ Temperature curves in benign tertian (*P. vivax*) and quartan (*P. malariae*) malaria. Temperature spikes when merozoites are released from parasitized red blood cells.

developmental periods. The most serious illness is caused by *P. falciparum.* That organism is sometimes responsible for an acute hemolytic syndrome known as **blackwater fever.** Circulatory disturbances can also complicate infections caused by *P. falciparum* when parasites block capillaries. Obstruction of cerebral capillaries causes delirium, convulsions, coma, and ultimately death.

Some merozoites differentiate within the environment of the red blood cells to form sex cells known as **gametocytes.** The gametocytes are ingested with the blood meal by a mosquito when it bites the human host.

The female gametocytes **(macrogametocytes)** and male gametocytes **(microgametocytes)** undergo a short developmental period in the stomach of the *Anopheles* mosquito during which globular *macrogametes* and motile *microgametes* are formed. Fertilization occurs when the motile microgametes enter the cytoplasm of the macrogametes to form *zygotes.* Within 12 to 24 hours the zygotes develop into **ookinetes,** elongated motile forms, which penetrate the wall of the stomach and lodge between the epithelial and muscle layers. Approximately 40 hours later **oocysts,** the encysted forms of ookinetes, are observable. A reorganization occurring within the oocysts results in the formation of thousands of sporozoites. Rupture of the sac liberates sporozoites into the body cavity of the mosquito where the actively motile forms migrate to various body parts, including the salivary glands. The life cycle is repeated when sporozoites are injected into the human host by the bite of the mosquito.

A diagnosis of malaria is made by finding the

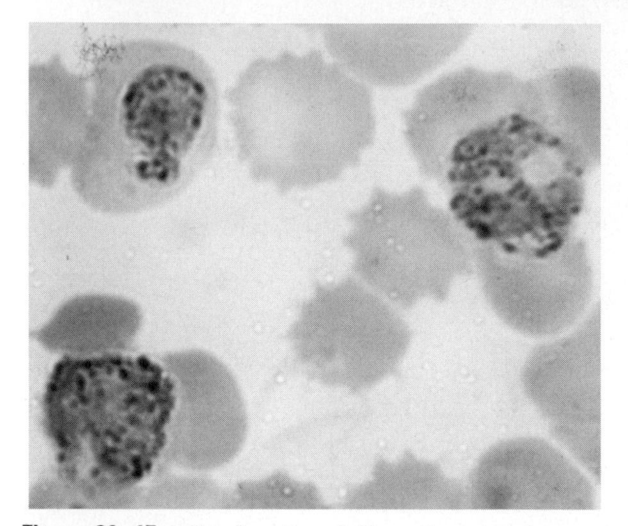

Figure 20–17 ◆ Trophozoites of *Plasmodium vivax* in a peripheral blood smear.

parasites on thin or thick blood smears after the application of Giemsa stain (Fig. 20–17). It is sometimes necessary to sample blood repeatedly in order to demonstrate the parasites. The appearance of more than one ring form in a single red blood cell is common in infections caused by *P. falciparum*. It takes a good deal of experience and careful observation to speciate malarial organisms, but a few characteristics are quite definitive (Table 20–3). DNA probes for malarial parasites appear to have value only in mass screening programs.

Chloroquine and other aminoquinoline compounds have been used both to treat malaria and as a prophylactic measure. Unfortunately, drug-resistant strains of *P. falciparum* have emerged in many endemic areas. A combination of sulfonamides and pyrimethamine has been successful against the drug-resistant parasites.

Most measures for prevention of malaria have been aimed at mosquito control, but such programs are cumbersome and difficult to administer. Attempts to develop a suitable vaccine for malaria have been hampered until recently by the inability to culture the plasmodia outside the host. Plasmodia can now be maintained in vitro almost indefinitely. However, the frequent changes in surface antigens of malarial parasites presents problems in developing a successful vaccine.

Babesiosis

Babesiosis is a rare, but serious disease occurring primarily as an infection of immunocompromised hosts. It is caused by *Babesia microti, B. bigemina,* and perhaps by other *Babesia* species. It is transmitted by *Ixodes* ticks, but is also carried by deer mice and field mice. Incubation periods of one to 12 months have been reported. The protozoa infect red blood cells in much the same manner as plasmodia. The disease is characterized by a fever, fatigue, and anemia lasting for several days or months. Most individuals with babesiosis are not as ill as those with malaria.

A diagnosis of babesiosis is made by finding the parasites on Giemsa-stained thin blood smears or inoculating susceptible animal hosts with blood from infected individuals. The ring forms of the parasite are typically smaller than those in malaria. The degree of parasitemia is usually quite low.

Chloroquine has been used to treat babesiosis, but it is not effective in eliminating parasitemia. Pentamidine reduces the degree of parasitemia and relieves some symptoms. Blood transfusions may be required in severe infections.

Table 20–3

DEFINITIVE CHARACTERISTICS OF THREE SPECIES OF *PLASMODIUM* AND INFECTED RED BLOOD CELLS

CHARACTERISTIC	*P. vivax*	*P. malariae*	*P. falciparum*
Size of infected cell	Increased	No change	No change
Shape of infected cell	Irregular	No change	No change
Parasitic forms present	All	All	Rings, gametocytes
Size of trophozoites	3+	2+	1+
Inclusions	Schüffner's granules	None	Maurer's spots

Chagas' Disease (American Trypanosomiasis)

Chagas' disease (American trypanosomiasis) is a common cause of heart disease in children of rural districts of Central and South America. Between 10 and 20 million individuals are diagnosed with Chagas' disease each year, and 50,000 deaths occur annually from the infection. The etiologic agent, *Trypanosoma cruzi,* is transmitted primarily by the blood-sucking reduviid bugs belonging to the genus *Triatoma* (Color Plate 80). The bugs defecate at the same time they bite, causing contamination of the bite wound with the infectious protozoa. Transfusion of blood containing *T. cruzi* is an alternate mode of transmission. The protozoa can also cross the placental barrier, causing congenital infection. The time of incubation is five to 14 days after the bite of the reduviid bug, but up to a month or more if infection is transmitted by a blood transfusion.

T. cruzi spends a part of its life cycle in the intestine of one or more species of the reduviid or kissing bug. **Crithidial** (epimastigote) and **trypanosomal** (trypomastigote) forms occur in the bugs. Those forms as well as **leptomonas** (promastigote) and **leishmania** (amastigote) may be present in mammals, including humans (Fig. 20–18). Leptomonads are elongated, slender, and flagellated forms. The kinetoplasts are located near the anterior end. Leishmanial forms are small, spherical, or oval nonflagellated intracellular bodies characterized by post-central nuclei and anterior kinetoplasts. Burrows of rodents and armadillos are often reservoirs of infected reduviid bugs.

Fever, rash, lymphadenitis, conjunctivitis, and **hepatosplenomegaly** (enlargement of liver and spleen) are common manifestations of Chagas' disease. Edema of the eyelids (Romañas sign) often is found in acute cases (Fig. 20–19). The meningoencephalitis or meningomyelitis occurring as a result of the infection can be life-threatening. The heart or intestines are affected in chronic cases.

Tryptomastigote forms of *T. cruzi* can be detected on Giemsa-stained, thick blood smears early in the disease (Fig. 20–20, Color Plate 73). The protozoa can be cultured on Novy, MacNeal, and Nicolle medium, but serological tests are more commonly used to establish a diagnosis. Indirect hemagglutination (IH) and complement-fixation (CF) tests are available, but cross-reactivity occurs with antibodies produced in leishmaniasis.

Nifurtimox is effective against trypomastigotes circulating in blood, but intracellular amastigotes are difficult to eliminate. Control measures include replacement of adobe housing and spraying with insecticides. Unfortunately, most poor, rural communities cannot afford to replace housing with suitable materials.

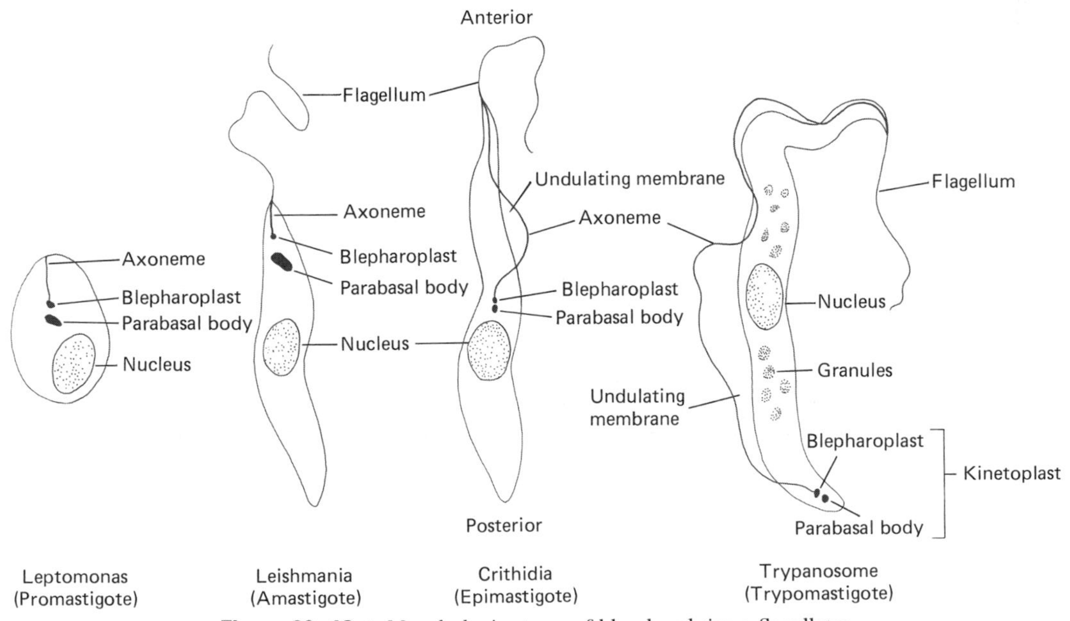

Figure 20–18 ◆ Morphologic stages of blood and tissue flagellates.

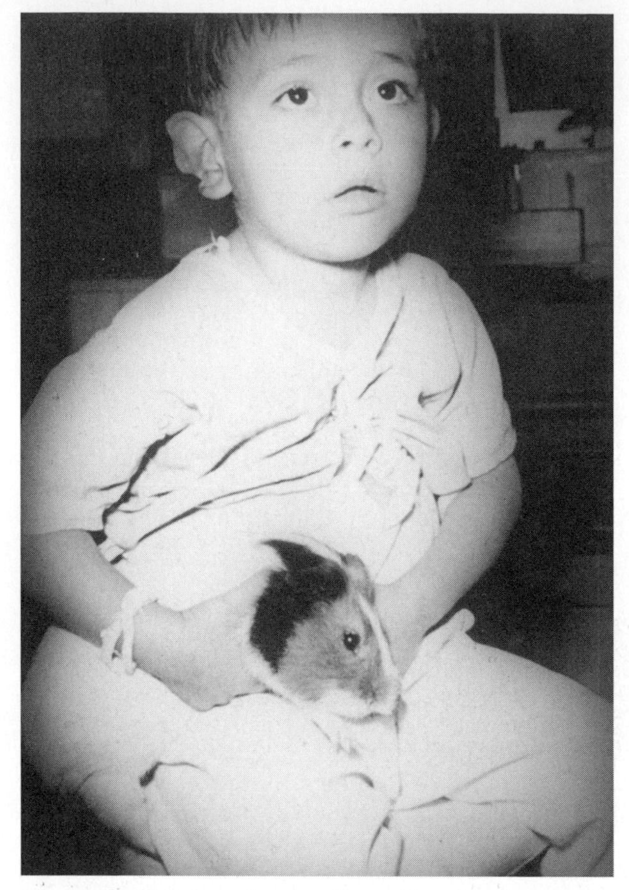

Figure 20–19 ◆ Romañas sign in a child with Chagas' disease.

the disease, and cutaneous leishmaniasis can be transmitted by direct contact with an infected person or animal. The incubation time may be as short as 10 days or as long as nine years.

Leishmania parasites exist in different morphological forms in their vertebrate and invertebrate hosts. In humans the parasites are found only in the leishmanial form (amastigote) as intracellular, nonflagellated, oval bodies; the organisms in this form are called **Leishman-Donovan** (LD) bodies. The life cycle is maintained only if amastigotes are ingested by sandflies.

Leptomonad forms (promastigotes) develop in the intestinal tract of the flies and migrate to the buccal cavity. When the sandflies bite humans, dogs, or wild animals, amastigotes develop in cells of the skin, mucous membranes, or viscera.

Visceral leishmaniasis is characterized by fever, chills, and lymph node, bone marrow, spleen, and liver dysfunction, anemia, and hemorrhage. A cutaneous nodule may be present early in the disease. The general debility associated with visceral leishmaniasis makes individuals particularly susceptible to secondary bacterial infections. If the disease is untreated, the mortality rate may be as high as 90 percent. The early lesion in cutaneous leishmaniasis, appearing two to 10 weeks after a sandfly bite, is a papule that progresses to a nodule and later to a distinct nodule (Fig. 20–21). Ulcerative metastases constitute the primary lesions in a type of leishmaniasis known

Leishmaniasis

Visceral leishmaniasis, or **kala azar,** is a chronic systemic disease in which macrophages of the spleen, liver, bone marrow, lymph nodes, intestinal mucosa, or other organs are invaded by the protozoan *Leishmania donovani.* A more limited disease, in which parasites are restricted to intracellular invasion of white blood cells and epithelial cells of cutaneous tissues or mucous membranes, is caused by *L. tropica, L. braziliensis,* or *L. mexicana* (Color Plate 74). Cutaneous leishmaniasis is endemic in some parts of Asia, North Africa, southern Europe, and both Central and South America. In Asia it is often called **Oriental sore.** Both visceral and cutaneous leishmaniasis are usually transmitted by the bite of infected sandflies belonging to the genus *Phlebotomus* (Color Plate 81). Sexual transmission has been documented in one case of the visceral form of

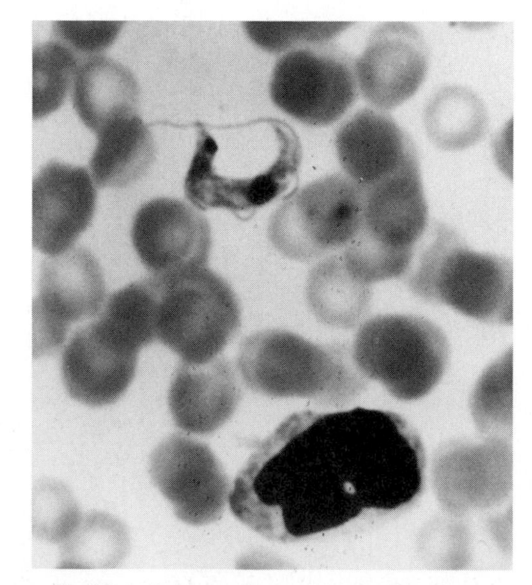

Figure 20–20 ◆ *Trypanosoma cruzi* in a thin Giemsa-stained blood smear.

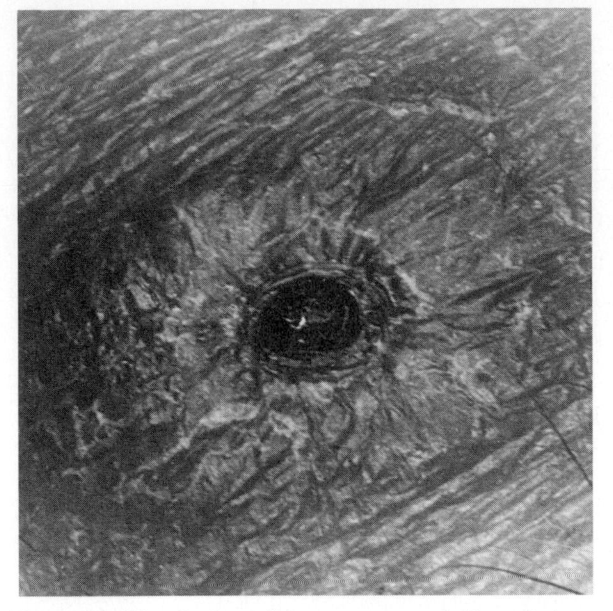

Figure 20–21 ◆ Lesion of acute cutaneous leishmaniasis, or Oriental sore.

as **espundia.** Diffuse cutaneous leishmaniasis is not common, but a lesion may last for years.

A diagnosis of visceral leishmaniasis depends on finding LD bodies in Giemsa-stained blood smears or aspirates of the spleen, liver, lymph nodes, or bone marrow. Splenic aspirates are the most reliable for diagnosing the disease. The LD bodies appear as blue, round or oval bodies; they typically contain two chromatin masses that stain red to purple (Fig. 20–22). Fluorescent-tagged antibodies also detect the presence of parasites on smears. Complement-fixation (CF) tests are of limited value.

A diagnosis of cutaneous leishmaniasis can be made by observing amastigote forms of *L. tropica, L. braziliensis,* or *L. mexicana* in scrapings from skin lesions after staining by the Giemsa technique. Tissue samples can be inoculated on a solid medium containing rabbit blood. Wet mounts must be examined for promastigotes twice a week for 30 days. Bacterial and fungal contamination due to decreasing potency of antibiotics added to the medium often negate the value of cultures. Serological diagnosis is of limited value in cutaneous leishmaniasis, but nucleic acid probes to leishmanial kinetoplasts are of value in diagnosing leishmanial disease.

Most lesions caused by *L. tropica* or *L. mexicana* heal spontaneously. Lesions due to *L. braziliensis* and visceral leishmaniasis are best treated with pentavalent antimony. Supportive care is of utmost importance in visceral leishmaniasis. It is nearly impossible in some parts of the world to eliminate vectors of leishmaniasis.

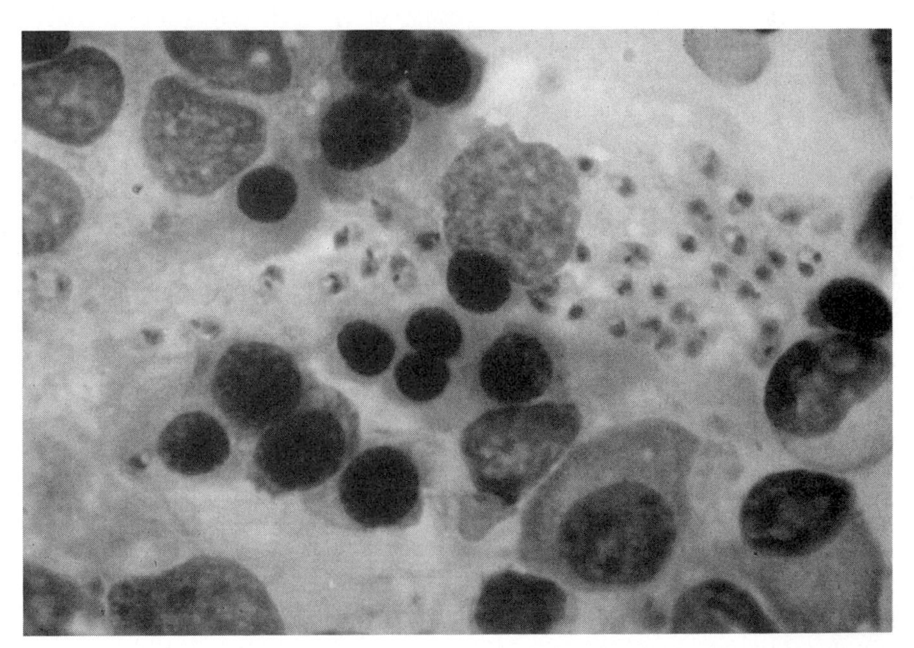

Figure 20–22 ◆ Leishman-Donovan (LD) bodies in human bone marrow smear stained with Giemsa stain.

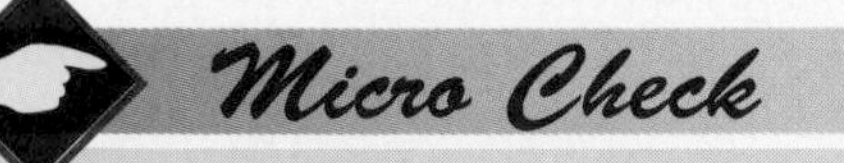

- What is the infective stage of the malarian parasite?
- Why is it difficult to eliminate reservoirs of the vectors of Chagas' disease?
- How is visceral leishmaniasis differentiated from cutaneous leishmaniasis?

A summary of the microorganisms causing diseases of the blood, lymph, and immune systems can be found in Table 20–4.

Understanding Microbiology

1. Where are the circulating and sessile cells of the immune system located?

Table 20–4
MAJOR MICROORGANISMS CAUSING DISEASES OF THE BLOOD, LYMPH, AND IMMUNE SYSTEM

MICROORGANISM	DISEASE	TREATMENT
Bacteria		
Brucella abortus	Brucellosis	Streptomycin
Brucella melitensis		Tetracycline
Brucella suis		
Yersenia pestis	Bubonic plague	Streptomycin
		Tetracycline
		Chloramphenicol
Franciscella tularensis	Tularemia	Streptomycin
		Tetracycline
		Chloramphenicol
Rickettsia rickettsii	Rocky Mountain spotted fever	Tetracycline
		Chloramphenicol
Borrelia burgdorferi	Lyme disease	Penicillin
		Tetracycline
Borrelia recurrentis	Relapsing fever	Penicillin
		Tetracycline
		Chloramphenicol
Viruses		
Cytomegalovirus (CMV)	Cytomegalovirus infection	Foscarnet
		Ganciclovir
Epstein-Barr virus (EBV)	Infectious mononucleosis	None
Human immunodeficiency virus (HIV)	AIDS	Zidovudine
		Dideoxycytidine
		Dideoxyinosine
Protozoa		
Plasmodium vivax	Malaria	Chloroquine*
Plasmodium malariae	Malaria	Primaquine
Plasmodium ovale	Malaria	Quinidine
Plasmodium falciparum	Malaria	Pyrimethamine-sulfadoxine
Babesia bigemina	Babesiosis	Chloroquine
Babesia microti	Babesiosis	Pentamidine
Trypanosoma cruzi	Chagas' disease	Nifurtimox
Leishmania donovani	Visceral leishmaniasis	Pentavalent antimony
Leishmania brasiliensis	Cutaneous leishmaniasis	Pentavalent antimony
Leishmania tropica	Cutaneous leishmaniasis	Pentavalent antimony
Leishmania mexicana	Cutaneous leishmaniasis	Pentavalent antimony

Treatment of malaria must be individualized depending on stage of the disease, severity of the symptoms, and drug resistance, particularly of *P. falciparsum*.

2. How do etiologic agents of primary bacteremias gain access to the bloodstream?
3. What is the rationale for taking multiple samples of blood from different sites in bacteremias?
4. Diagram the life cycles of the malarian parasites in the human and the mosquito.
5. How has the human immunodeficiency virus (HIV) been able to cause disease in epidemic proportions in so many countries?

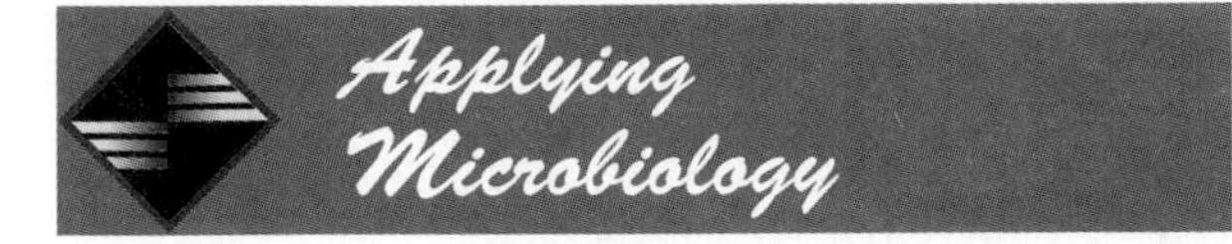

Read the following case study carefully and answer the questions: A 47-year-old female mammalogist from the United States who was traveling in Bolivia had an acute illness consisting of a severe headache, chills, fever, sweating, loss of appetite, and pain and swelling in her right axilla. She was treated with ampicillin, but the pain and swelling in the axillia increased. When she returned home three days later, she had a cough, a temperature of 101.3°F, and an enlarged lymph node in the right axilla. She was hospitalized immediately by her physician. Careful questioning revealed she had camped intermittently in rural areas of Bolivia and collected small mammals, including rice rats. The laboratory isolated a gram-negative bacillus with bipolar staining from the lymph node aspirate.

6. The symptoms and laboratory findings are consistent with a diagnosis of
   a. tuberculosis
   b. malaria
   c. PCP
   d. plague
   e. Chagas' disease
7. The probable mode of transmission was
   a. a mosquito
   b. contaminated shellfish
   c. a fomite
   d. a rat flea
   e. an aerosol
8. The usual lesion characteristic of this disease is a (an)
   a. abscess
   b. carbuncle
   c. decubitus
   d. pustule
   e. bubo
9. The reservoirs for the etiologic agent are primarily
   a. arid soils
   b. rodent populations
   c. infected humans
   d. domestic cats
   e. contaminated water supplies
10. The disease described is preventable by the administration of
    a. prophylactic penicillin
    b. a killed bacterial vaccine
    c. wearing protective clothing
    d. a polyvalent antitoxin
    e. prophylactic chloroquine

Unit 6

Control of Microorganisms

Chapter 21 Disinfection and Sterilization

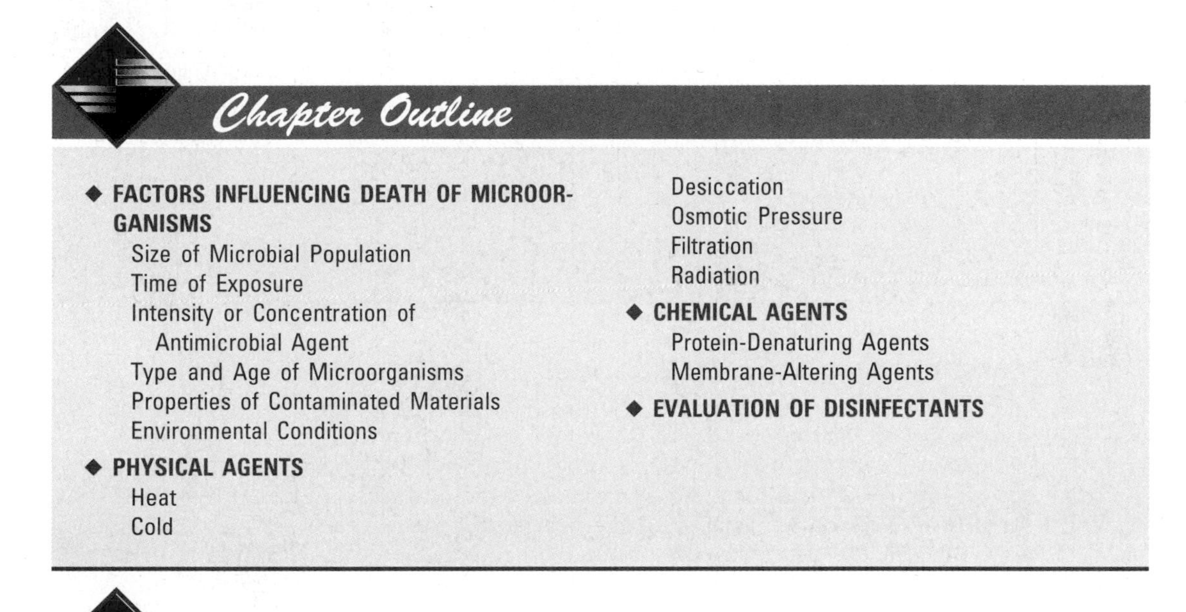

Chapter Outline

- **FACTORS INFLUENCING DEATH OF MICROORGANISMS**
  - Size of Microbial Population
  - Time of Exposure
  - Intensity or Concentration of Antimicrobial Agent
  - Type and Age of Microorganisms
  - Properties of Contaminated Materials
  - Environmental Conditions
- **PHYSICAL AGENTS**
  - Heat
  - Cold
  - Desiccation
  - Osmotic Pressure
  - Filtration
  - Radiation
- **CHEMICAL AGENTS**
  - Protein-Denaturing Agents
  - Membrane-Altering Agents
- **EVALUATION OF DISINFECTANTS**

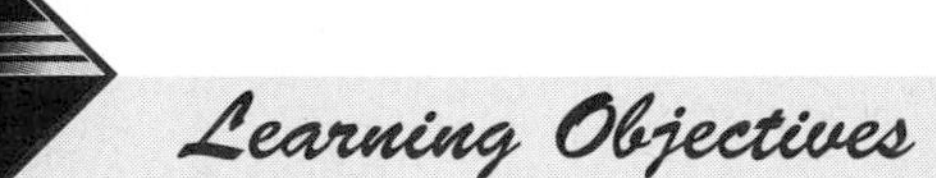

Learning Objectives

After you have read this chapter, you should be able to:

1. Differentiate between asepsis, disinfection, sanitation, and sterilization.
2. Describe the factors that influence the death of microorganisms.
3. Contrast the efficiency of the physical agents commonly employed for disinfection and sterilization.
4. Differentiate between thermal death time and thermal death point.
5. Define photoreactivation and photo-oxidation.
6. Classify the major disinfectants as protein-denaturing or membrane-altering agents.
7. Describe two standardized methods for testing the efficiency of disinfectants.

A great deal of progress has been made over the years in eliminating unwanted microorganisms from our environment. Aristotle (384–322 B.C.) instructed Alexander the Great to boil water for his armies. Campsites were moved daily to avoid both the stench and contamination from human waste. Early methods of food preservation included heating, drying, smoking, and salting. The Romans used snow to pack perishable foods around 1000 B.C.

The age of chemical control of the atmosphere began with Joseph Lister, the English surgeon, in 1867. Lister used aqueous phenol to disinfect instruments, soak dressings, and spray the air of surgical rooms. In contemporary times, a large number of physical, chemical, and me-

Table 21–1
THE TERMINOLOGY OF MICROBIAL CONTROL

TERM	DEFINITION
Antiseptic	An agent that destroys or inhibits growth or activity of microorganisms on living tissue
Asepsis	A method that prevents contamination by unwanted microorganisms
Biocide or germicide	A chemical agent that has antiseptic, disinfectant or preservative activities
Contamination	A process that allows the transfer of microorganisms to a sterile object
Disinfectant	An agent that inhibits or destroys microorganisms on nonliving objects
Disinfection	A process that destroys infectious agents exclusive of endospores and viruses
Insecticide	An agent that kills insects, such as fleas, flies, and mosquitoes, that frequently transmit infectious agents
Microbicide	An agent that kills microorganisms; the terms *bactericide, virucide,* and *fungicide* indicate action against a specific group of organisms
Microbiostat	An agent that inhibits the growth of microorganisms; the terms *bacteriostatic, virustatic,* and *fungistatic* indicate inhibition of a specific group of organisms
Molluscicide	An agent that kills mollusks, such as snails, that are important in the life cycle of certain parasites
Sanitizer	An agent that reduces the number of microorganisms present
Sterilization	A process that destroys microorganisms and viruses

chanical agents are available to eliminate or control microorganisms in our environment. There is no single agent or method that can be recommended for universal use. Some of these agents inactivate or destroy microorganisms in a microbicidal effect, such as in the term bactericidal. Other agents merely inhibit the growth of microorganisms; for example, an agent that inhibits growth of bacteria is known as a bacteriostatic agent. The terminology for categories of microbial control agents is very specific (Table 21–1). Familiarize yourself with these terms before you read further.

Aseptic techniques employed in a laboratory for the isolation of pure cultures can be successful because the conditions can be carefully controlled. The hospital environment, a communicable disease isolation unit, or an operating room presents a more challenging problem. The specific solution depends on the quantity and type of disease organism, disease type, the type of surface to be disinfected or sterilized, and the environmental factors of temperature, pH, presence of organic matter, and others.

FACTORS INFLUENCING DEATH OF MICROORGANISMS

The death of specific microbial populations is affected by microbial factors and by forces at work in the immediate environment. Microbial death occurs when an organism, or population of organisms, is no longer capable of reproduction. Microbial susceptibility to biocides are extremely variable (Table 21–2). The circumstances under which microorganisms die constitute the basis for the principles of disinfection and sterilization. Environmental factors may stimulate or inhibit growth, influence synthesis of products, cause biochemical variation, or completely destroy microorganisms. Understanding the effects of particular physical, chemical, and mechanical agents on microorganisms makes it possible to use those agents, singly or in combination, to destroy microorganisms or reduce their numbers to tolerable levels.

Size of the Microbial Population

The ability of an agent to destroy microorganisms is dependent on the size of the initial population. When large numbers of organisms are present, some may escape a direct hit by the injurious agent. Mere density of large populations may prevent penetration of harmful agents. However, a lesser density or smaller population does not necessarily increase the number affected by the agent; the probability of a direct hit lessens with the diminishing population because the action of physical and chemical agents is random. Presumably, with enough time and killing

Table 21–2
SUSCEPTIBILITY OF MICROORGANISMS TO BIOCIDES

RANK BY SUSCEPTIBILITY	GENERAL COMMENTS
Enveloped viruses	Sensitive to biocides; includes HIV
Nonsporulating gram-positive bacteria	Staphylococci and streptococci usually very susceptible, enterococci show varied responses
Large nonenveloped viruses	Enteroviruses more sensitive than smaller nonenveloped viruses
Yeasts and molds	Spores may be resistant
Nonsporulating gram-negative bacteria	Wide variation in susceptibility
Trophozoites (protozoa)	More sensitive than the cyst stage
Small nonenveloped viruses	Such as picornaviruses, parvoviruses
Cysts (protozoa)	Important parasites such as *Giardia* and *Cryptosporidium* have highly resistant cyst stages
Mycobacteria	*Mycobacterium chelonae* may be highly resistant
Spores (bacteria)	Prolonged periods of time may be necessary for large numbers of spores
Coccidia	May be highly resistant
Prions	Most resistant of all infectious agents

Source: Russell AD, Furr JR, Maillard JY: Microbial susceptibility and resistance to biocides. ASM News *63*:481–487, 1997.

power, one can destroy all microorganisms within a limited space.

Time of Exposure

Exposure of a microbial population to a lethal agent causes a progressive reduction of organisms with time. If the logarithm of the number remaining alive is plotted against time, a straight line is obtained (Fig. 21–1). The microorganisms are not all killed instantaneously nor are all cells of a population equally susceptible to antimicrobial action. There is no "rule of thumb" for estimating appropriate times of exposure for particular disinfectants without identification of the contaminating organisms. The time required for complete destruction of undesirable organisms may be as little as 15 minutes or as long as 10 or more hours.

Intensity or Concentration of Antimicrobial Agent

The intensity or concentration of an agent affects the efficiency of antimicrobial activity. The destructive power of most disinfectants increases exponentially with concentration up to a certain point only. For each chemical agent there is an optimal microbicidal concentration beyond which efficiency is decreased. A 70 percent concentration of isopropyl alcohol is generally more effective than absolute or 90 percent isopropanol. Because the microbial population of an object or environment must be assumed to contain spores, the success of any method used for sterilization is dependent on its destructive action on spores. Most chemical agents are designed to reduce the population of microorganisms and less often accomplish sterilization.

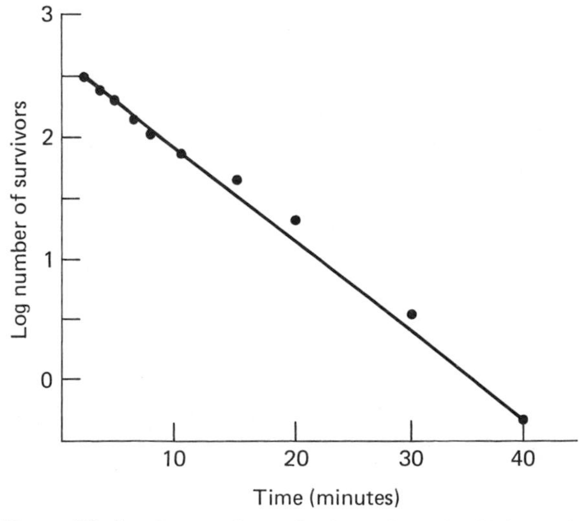

Figure 21–1 ◆ Progressive reduction of a microbial population exposed to a lethal agent.

Type and Age of Microorganisms

The various types of microorganisms vary considerably in their vulnerability to physical and chemical agents. Fungi and some viruses are more resistant to chemical agents than are vegetative cells of bacteria. The vulnerability of vegetative cells of bacteria and nonenveloped viruses to physical and chemical agents is due largely to the susceptibility of proteins to denaturation. Staphylococci and enterococci are somewhat more resistant to disinfectants than other gram-positive organisms. *Serratia, Pseudomonas, Klebsiella,* and *Enterobacter* are more resistant to disinfectants than most coliforms. Mycobacteria are less susceptible to the action of some aqueous chemical agents than other vegetative forms of bacteria. The resistance of mycobacteria is apparently related to the hydrophobic (water-avoiding) chemical nature of their cell surfaces.

Vegetative cells show varying degrees of susceptibility to chemical and physical agents during growth cycles. In general, cells in the logarithmic growth phase, when they are "physiologically young," are more susceptible to heat (Fig. 21–2). Differences in the susceptibility of *Escherichia coli* during the growth cycle have been attributed to variation in cell wall content.

Although endospores are more resistant to destruction by physical and chemical agents than vegetative cells, there are wide variations in tolerance. Not only are there differences among the various groups of spore-formers, but environmental influences active during formation of spores affect their resistance. Spores of thermophilic *Bacillus* species, often associated with food spoilage, are not destroyed as easily as those produced by mesophilic species. The age of spores can also affect their susceptibility to destructive agents. For example, spores of *Clostridium botulinum* exhibit maximum resistance after aging four to eight days.

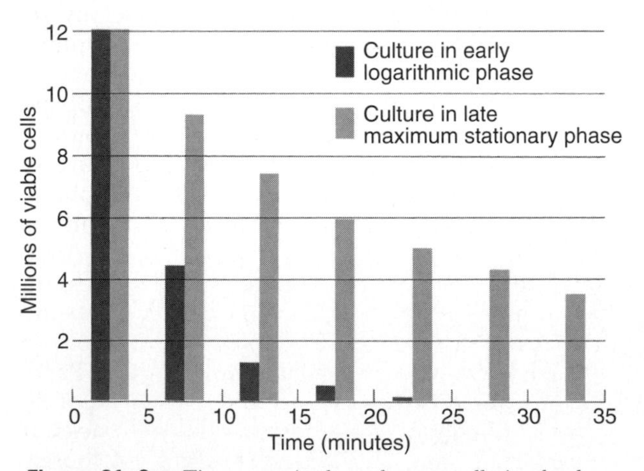

Figure 21–2 ◆ Times required to destroy cells in the logarithmic and stationary phases of growth by a lethal agent. More than one-fourth of the cells in the stationary phase remain viable after more than 30 minutes of exposure.

Properties of Contaminated Materials

The properties of materials to be disinfected or sterilized influence the choice of a particular physical or chemical agent. Plastic or rubber cannot tolerate high temperatures; cutting edges of some surgical instruments cannot withstand moist heat or corrosive chemicals. Some fabrics are too delicate for chemical disinfection. Penetration of physical and chemical agents is dependent on the consistency of molecular constituents of contaminated materials. More viscous contaminated solutions require greater exposure times than do less dense solutions. Accumulations of extraneous organic material on the surface of microbial cells increase the time required for penetration and destruction of organisms.

Environmental Conditions

Conditions of the immediate environment surrounding microorganisms can influence the efficiency of antimicrobial agents. As a rule an increase in temperature enhances the destructive ability of a disinfectant. The presence of oxygen is required for some chemicals to act upon microorganisms; an acidic environment promotes the action of other chemical agents. The synergistic effect of heat, oxygen, and acid pH often lowers the time of exposure to an antimicrobial agent required for disinfection or sterilization.

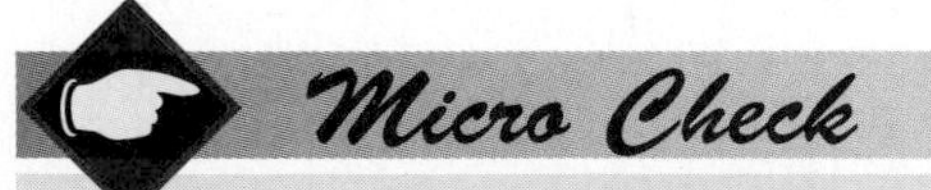

- What accounts for differences of microorganisms in susceptibility to physical or chemical agents?
- Why can there be no "rule of thumb" for exposure times in most instances?
- What is meant by synergism between an antimicrobial agent and an environmental factor?

PHYSICAL AGENTS

An understanding of the environmental factors favoring microbial growth provides a basis for the application of physical agents in the destruction of microorganisms. Many organisms grow optimally within narrow ranges of temperature, osmotic pressure, and atmospheric conditions. Some obligate anaerobic vegetative cells are extremely susceptible to oxygen. They do not tolerate even brief exposure to the concentration of oxygen found in the atmosphere. When a particular microbial contaminant is present, the method for destruction is chosen on the basis of knowledge of the physiological tolerances of that particular organism. When the nature of the contamination is unknown, as is most often the case, rather stringent methods of decontamination must be employed.

Heat

Dry heat, moist heat, and steam under pressure are among the most common methods employed for destroying microorganisms, provided that the contaminated object or material can withstand the high temperatures required. Death of microbial cells subjected to dry heat is caused by an oxidation of cell substances; moist heat, with or without pressure, causes coagulation, or clumping, of cell proteins. Bacterial toxins vary in their susceptibility to heat, but most enzymes are heat-sensitive. Some viruses, such as the encephalitis agents, are inactivated at room temperature. Other viruses, such as the agent of polio, are inactivated only when exposed to a temperature of 60°C for 30 minutes. The hepatitis viruses are inactivated by dry heat only after exposure to 180°C for an hour.

The length of time required to kill a particular microorganism at a specific temperature is called the **thermal death time.** The temperature required to kill a particular microorganism within 10 minutes is called the **thermal death point.** A knowledge of thermal death times is especially valuable in the canned food industry, in which heat processing must be adequate to destroy pathogens and spoilage bacteria.

DRY HEAT

One of the most efficient methods of dry-heat sterilization exposes objects to intense heat or direct flame. If the contaminated object, such as a wound dressing or animal carcass, is combustible and can be sacrificed, **incineration** is recommended. A platinum alloy bacteriological loop, which can withstand intense heat, can be sterilized rapidly by **flaming** (i.e., a process of placing the loop into a burner flame until thoroughly heated).

However, all materials or objects requiring sterilization either cannot withstand direct flaming or are not expendable. Exposure to temperatures of 160°C for two hours in a hot air oven sterilizes metal objects and glassware, such as Petri plates, test tubes, and pipettes. The time required for this type of dry-heat sterilization often limits its use as a method of choice.

MOIST HEAT

A moist environment permits an article to be sterilized at lower temperatures and shorter exposure times than a dry atmosphere. **Boiling** is a readily accessible method requiring no expensive equipment. Boiling for 30 minutes to 6 hours may be necessary if an object is contaminated with spores, but most vegetative cells of pathogens are killed by boiling for 20 minutes.

Flowing steam can be applied as an alternative to boiling, but prolonged exposure is necessary to destroy spores. Intermittent exposure to flowing steam, the process known as **tyndallization,** named for John Tyndall, its developer, is valuable. Tyndallization involves a 30-minute period of steaming on three successive days. The process is successful in destroying bacterial spore-formers if materials are incubated at 37°C between heating periods to allow for germination of any remaining spores into the more heat-susceptible vegetative cells.

The most efficient use of moist heat employs **steam under pressure** in an instrument known as an **autoclave** (Fig. 21–3). Raising the pressure to 15 pounds per square inch (psi) of atmospheric pressure raises the temperature of steam to 121°C, which is used for sterilization. The time required to achieve sterilization at that pressure and temperature depends on the object being sterilized. For example, 15 minutes is sufficient to sterilize most bacteriological culture media. Packs of surgical dressings require exposure times of 30 minutes or longer, depending on size of packs. It is important that each pack be wrapped loosely and that sufficient space be left around the packs in the autoclave so that the steam can penetrate all the material.

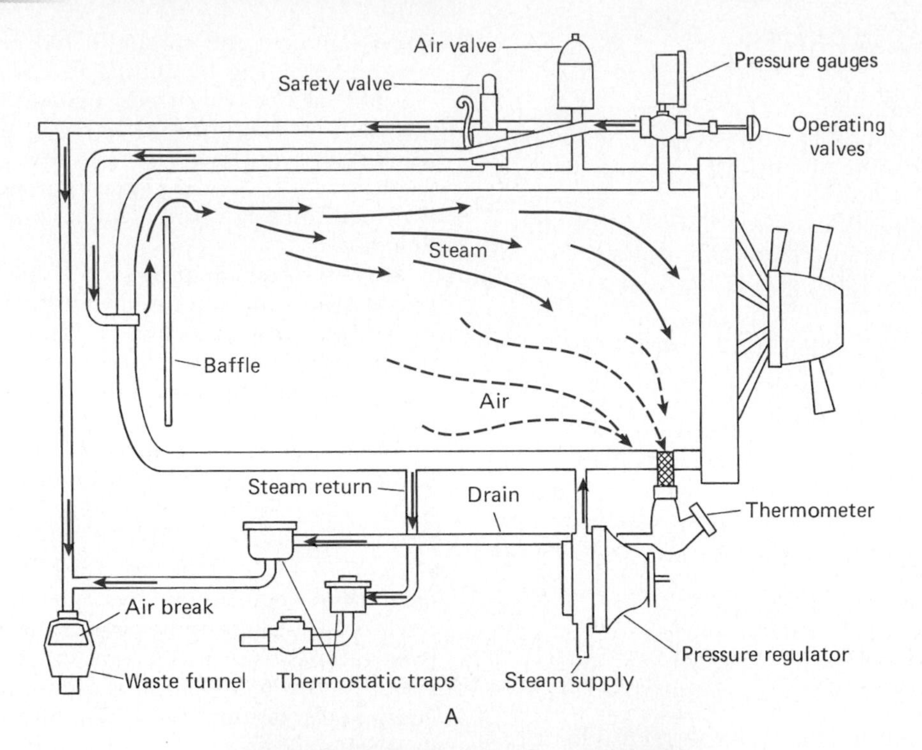

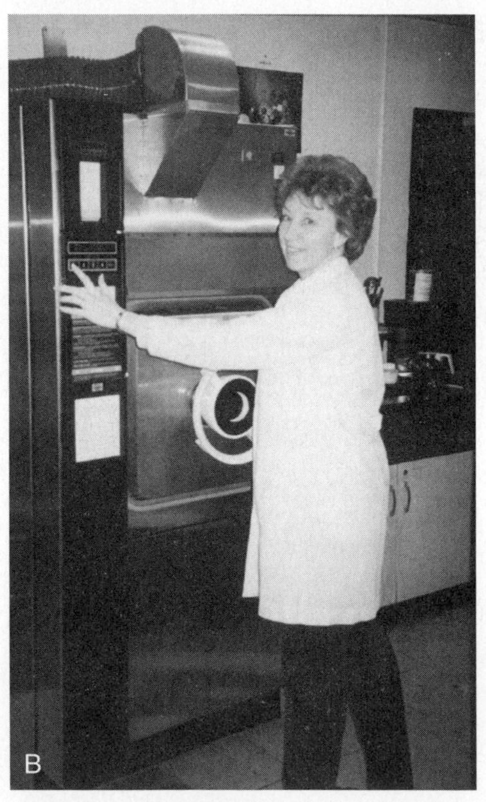

Figure 21–3 ◆ An autoclave. *A,* Diagram of a longitudinal section of an autoclave showing flow patterns for steam and air. *B,* Autoclave control panel.

Heat is used in the food industry to improve the keeping quality of foods. The temperature and times of exposure used are determined by thermal resistance of contaminants, type of food, pH, water content, and method of packaging. The processes of commercial sterilization for canned foods and pasteurization, a moist heat treatment for liquid and dried foods, are discussed in Chapter 24.

Pasteurization is sometimes used for the disinfection of respiratory therapy equipment, which cannot withstand the intense heat of the autoclave. A drawback in pasteurizing reusable equipment is that recontamination can occur during the drying period if special precautions are not taken.

Cold

Low temperatures inhibit the growth of most microorganisms, but do not necessarily kill all organisms. Low temperature methods include refrigeration (0°C to 8°C), freezing (−20°C to 0°C), and freeze-drying, or lyophilization, discussed in the following section on Desiccation. Rapid freezing is not as efficient as slow freezing because it does not allow for the formation of damaging ice crystals. A few species of bacteria and bacterial toxins demonstrate unusual tolerance for cold. Cells of *C. botulinum* type E can elaborate toxin even at temperatures as low as 3.3°C. Endospores, spores of fungi, and cells of many microorganisms in the exponential phase of growth resist freezing temperatures.

Osmotic pressure, pH, and humidity influence destruction of microorganisms at low temperatures. A high osmotic pressure is protective. A low pH contributes to the bactericidal power of cold. Too much moisture favors the survival of microorganisms. In general, microbial cells can tolerate lower storage temperatures if moisture is available.

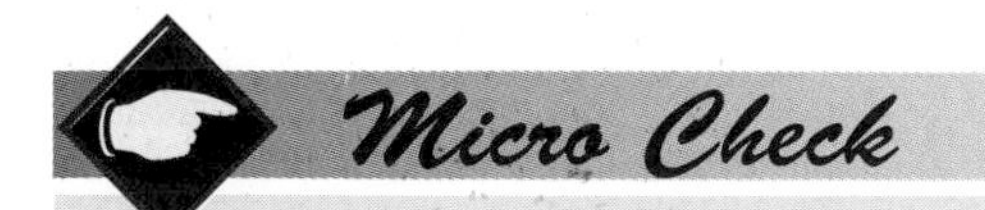

- What factors contribute to growth of fungi on food stored in the refrigerator?
- What is a definition of thermal death time?
- What is the advantage of using moist heat instead of dry heat for sterilization?

Desiccation

Many microorganisms can survive in an environment of low moisture content, but carry on metabolic processes of such a low order that spoilage of food or textiles does not occur. Anthrax spores dried on silk threads can survive as long as 20 years.

Moisture can be removed from foods or other products in a number of ways. Sun drying is still applied to certain fruits, such as apricots, figs, prunes, and raisins. Artificial drying requires the use of heated air and carefully controlled humidity.

Rapid freezing combined with desiccation, in a procedure known as **lyophilization,** is employed rather extensively in the preservation of blood serum products, enzymes, and even bacteriological cultures. Lyophilization combines rapid freezing and exposure to a vacuum for removal of water. The formation of ice crystals is avoided so that viability of cultures and activity of biological products is maintained. The minimal amount of crystallization does not impair the quality of the product.

An alternative method for maintaining stock bacteriological and tissue cultures is storage under liquid nitrogen at a temperature of −196°C (Fig. 21–4). The method is particularly suitable for storage of cell lines because they cannot survive the rigors of lyophilization. The lack of a cell wall makes animal cells more susceptible to se-

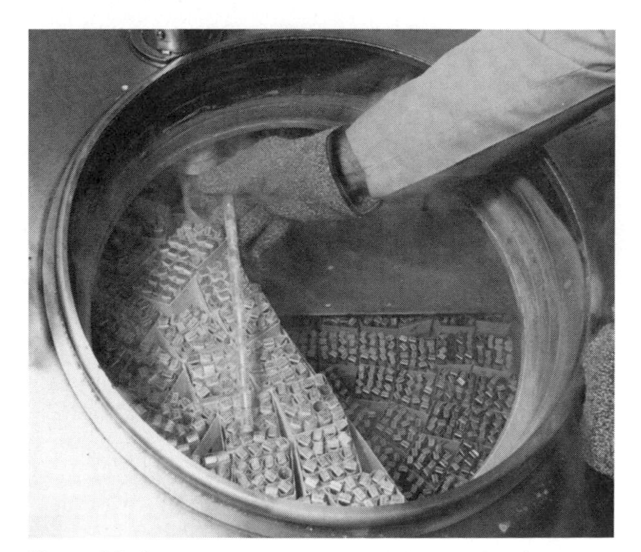

Figure 21–4 ◆ Container used for storing stock cultures under liquid nitrogen at −196°C.

vere dehydration. Some moisture is necessary to preserve the integrity of cells.

Osmotic Pressure

Most microorganisms do not tolerate an environment in which the concentration of solute (solids dissolved in a liquid) exceeds solute concentration in the cells. Humans have taken advantage of this lack of tolerance for thousands of years. Salting fish and meat preserves the food, a process in use since the days of early nomad tribes. Most microorganisms are inhibited by a 20 percent concentration of NaCl. Sucrose, in concentrations of 50 percent or higher in jams, jellies, and candy, inhibits microbial growth by a similar dehydrating effect. Organisms that can grow in media containing excess solutes are **osmotolerant;** they include the **halophilic** (salt-loving) and **saccharophilic** (sugar-loving) species.

Osmotic tolerance is usually expressed in terms of lowest water activity (a_w) permitting growth (discussed in Chapter 24). The a_w indicates the water vapor pressure in a food compared to pure water. Most fungi show greater osmotolerance than do bacteria.

Filtration

Most microorganisms can be removed from liquids by passing them through filters. Asbestos, sand, diatomaceous earth, porcelain, plaster of Paris, glass, resins or membrane filters, can be used to filter microorganisms from a liquid suspension. The membrane filters, composed of biologically inert materials, such as cellulose acetate or cellulose nitrate, and constructed so pores measure 0.01 to 10.0 μm, have largely replaced other filters. Membrane filters with pore sizes of 0.22 to 0.45 μm will remove most microorganisms (Table 21–3).

All solutions for renal dialysis, heart bypass machines, and intravenous administration must be filtered through special resins. These resins release an ion as they bind a molecule from the fluids passing across the resin surface, in a process known as ion exchange. The ion-exchange process is very effective at removing molecules that are not destroyed or removed by autoclaving or membrane filtration. Molecules such as toxins, specifically the endotoxins released from gram-negative bacteria, are a major concern. The presence of endotoxins on equipment or intravenous

Table 21–3
PORE SIZE RETENTION

PORE SIZE (μm)	RETENTION CAPACITY
5.0	Cells present in body fluids
1.2	Nonliving particles in intravenous fluids
0.8	Airborne particles
0.45	Some bacteria
0.22	All bacteria and some large viruses
0.02	Medium to small viruses

solutions introduced into a patient may induce circulatory collapse.

A microfiltration process, which combines filtration with chemical disinfection on a resin is recommended for removing protozoan cysts, such as those of *Giardia lamblia* (Chapter 19) from water of questionable quality. The device has been successful in preventing the disease giardiasis in campers and hikers who drink raw river or spring water contaminated by animal wastes. Even the clearest of mountain streams can be contaminated by this intestinal parasite.

Application of negative pressure to a flask makes filtration rapid and efficient (see Fig. 5–17). The process is applied to culture media that cannot withstand the heat required for autoclave sterilization. Highly efficient particulate air (HEPA) filters are used in laminar airflow hoods in laboratories, isolation units and some operating rooms to achieve a better quality of air (see Fig. 11–6). Frequent exchanges of air can be supplied by directed flow ventilation with minimal air turbulence to remove airborne microorganisms from particular environments (see Color Plates 23 and 24).

Radiation

The propagation of energy through space as electromagnetic waves is often called **radiation.** The electromagnetic spectrum includes radio waves, Hertzian waves, visible light, ultraviolet light, x-rays, gamma rays, and cosmic rays (Fig. 21–5). Wavelength of electromagnetic waves is usually expressed in nanometers (nm).

The radio communication waves have only slight microbicidal properties, but the ultraviolet waves of light and the emissions of x-rays, gamma rays, and cosmic rays are more highly microbicidal.

FOCAL POINT

The Child Called Manya: Discoverer of Radioactivity

Early in her life in Poland, the tiny, shy child named Manya was encouraged to study and to develop her curiosity. Who could know that she would become world famous as Madame Curie (1867–1934), the first woman to win a Nobel Prize in 1911 and one of few persons ever to receive a second Nobel Prize? The youngest of three girls in the family, Manya went to work as a governess to help her sister Bronya through medical school. It was not until she was 24 that Manya, later known as Marie, was able to study at the University of Sorbonne in Paris, France. She married the French physicist Pierre Curie (1859–1906) in 1895; she and her husband discovered the radioactive elements polonium and radium. As a busy wife and mother, she managed her household with remarkable efficiency while continuing research. The Curies refused to patent the process of purifying radium; they agreed that any financial gain would be contrary to the scientific spirit. During World War I, Madame Curie initiated a program of mobile x-ray units to assist in battlefield surgeries. Her daughters and others operated x-ray machines throughout France. She developed a serious illness, probably related to years of radiation exposure, and died in 1934. Sixty-one years later, on April 20, 1995, President François Mitterand presided over the interment of Madame Curie's remains in the Pantheon. She is the first woman ever to be interred on her own merits in the Pantheon, the national mausoleum for the "Grand Hommes" (great men) of France. Pierre Curie's remains are interred at her side.

ULTRAVIOLET RAYS

Ultraviolet radiation (UV) ranges in wavelength from 1 nm to 390 nm. The sun is a major source of UV radiation. Much of the shorter rays are filtered out by materials in the atmosphere, such as ozone, so that only those rays of higher wavelengths reach the surface of the earth. UV lamps that emit wavelengths of 260 to 270 nm are used in surgery or inoculating hoods to reduce numbers of microorganisms on surfaces.

The destruction of microorganisms by UV is caused by its action on the DNA and proteins of cells. Some bases of DNA absorb UV radiation and are altered, causing mutations in the cells. UV radiation produces dimer bonds (bonding between two neighboring bases on the same DNA strand) between two thymine bases (T-T) or a thymine and a cytosine base (T-C) (see Fig. 7–11). Formation of T-T or C-T dimer bonds is sometimes lethal because it induces errors in DNA replication or prevents replication. Protein structure and function are altered by UV exposure. The amount of injury inflicted is related to the duration of exposure and to the species. Some pigmented cells and endospores require longer periods of exposure to UV for the lethal waves to penetrate the organisms.

The amount of UV-induced injury is also related to the efficiency of two known repair mechanisms found in some organisms. One mechanism is **photoreactivation,** which operates if UV-exposed cells are placed in a sunny location or under a bright lamp. Visible light can activate a photorepair enzyme (PRE). The longer the expo-

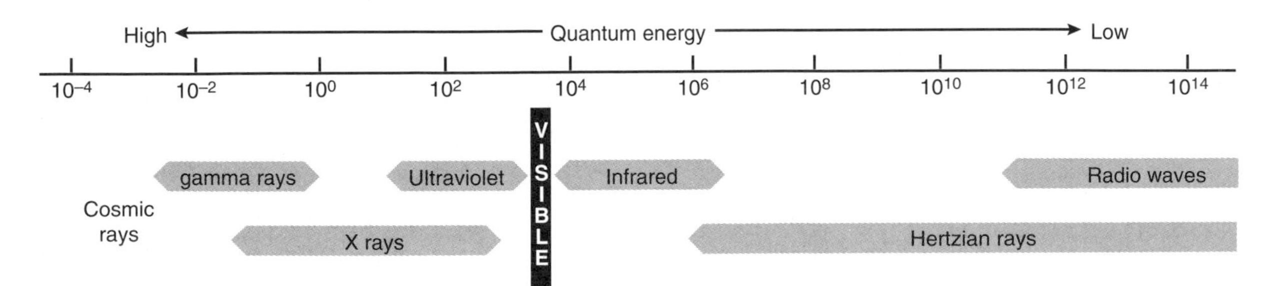

Figure 21–5 ◆ The electromagnetic spectrum showing wavelengths in nm on an exponential scale.

sure to bright light, the longer the PRE can operate to remove the damage. PRE moves along the DNA molecule, breaking the dimer bonds, allowing the bases to bond normally to their complementary base on the opposite strand. The possibility exists that all dimers may be broken by PRE with long exposure to visible light, thus reversing the effects of UV radiation. Photoreactivation is not 100 percent efficient in large populations of microorganisms damaged by UV or if a larger number of dimers are formed.

A second mechanism involves a **dark repair** set of enzymes that function when UV-exposed cells are placed in the refrigerator where it is cold and dark. After 1 to 2 days, the action of four enzymes involved in dark repair will have reduced the number of thymine dimer bonds. First, a **UV-specific endonuclease** detects the damaged region and makes a nick close to the dimer. A **DNA polymerase** synthesizes new nucleotides. The dimer is excised by **exonuclease** activity of DNA polymerase. The newly synthesized portion of DNA replaces the excised region and is bound in place by the action of **DNA ligase.** The new thymine bases bond normally with adenines on the opposite strand of DNA.

The use of UV for actual disinfection or sterilization is limited because it does not penetrate surfaces and damages human DNA as well. The repair mechanisms in human cells appear to be similar to those found in bacteria. In the human disease, xeroderma pigmentosum, there is a deficiency of the endonuclease required to identify the strand of DNA with the dimers. Affected individuals are extremely sensitive to sunlight and usually die of skin cancer before the age of 30. Fortunately, only one in 250,000 persons have this genetic disorder. Overloading repair mechanisms by too much exposure to sunlight or tanning machines used by people with the endonuclease deficiency can also cause skin cancer.

VISIBLE LIGHT

Exposure to visible light (400 to 700 nm) for prolonged periods can destroy microbial cells in the presence of oxygen. Death occurs as a result of **photo-oxidation,** the chemical changes induced by visible light exposure in an oxygen environment. The destructive effects occur when light is absorbed by cytochromes and flavins of the electron transport chain. Exposure to visible light also can result in the production of singlet oxygen (O_2^-) in the presence of pigments called photosensitizers. The singlet form of oxygen is a strong oxidant and promotes destruction of microorganisms.

Many airborne bacteria, such as *Micrococcus luteus* and *Serratia marcescens,* are highly pigmented with protective carotenoid pigments in their cell membranes. The pigments absorb light radiation, preventing the light from reaching vulnerable molecules inside the cell. Because most pathogens lack pigments, they are quite susceptible to the effects of visible light.

IONIZING RADIATION

Ionizing radiation consisting of wavelengths less than 200 nm is emitted by an x-ray machine, radioactive decay, nuclear reactors, and atomic particles from outer space. The radiation causes rapid ionization of water molecules, producing free radicals that injure essential macromolecules. X-rays, gamma rays, and high-speed electrons are the most important ionizing sources for sterilization.

Ionizing radiation affects primarily the water molecules of microbial cells. Ionization occurs when energy is transferred to the cells.

$$H_2O \longrightarrow H_2O^+ + e^-$$

Positively charged ions react with other water molecules to form additional charged molecules and hydroxyl radicals.

$$e^- + H_2O^+ + H_2O \longrightarrow H_3O^+ + OH^-$$

The electrons (e^-) react with nonionized water to form hydroxyl ions and hydrogen radicals. Hydrogen radicals are effective reducing agents; hydroxyl radicals are potent oxidizing agents. The free radicals can react with any molecules of microbial cells, but usually promote breaks in bonds of DNA molecules.

Ionizing radiation is economically feasible in only a limited number of circumstances. It is most suitable for sterilization of heat-sensitive sutures and disposable plastic items. Radiation of foods holds promise to provide longer shelf lives and to reduce the number of foodborne illnesses. Although foods do not usually become radioactive at dosages employed, many fear the occurrence of free radicals in irradiated foods and subsequent damage which could be caused in humans by the **radiolytic** products.

The **rad** is used as the primary unit of measurement for absorbed radiation. The kilorad (krad) is equal to one thousand rads. Doses of irradiation are classified as low, medium, and high, and applied to specific foods for controlling insects, pathogens, and spoilage (Table 21–4). Spores are resistant to ionizing radiation in low doses because of their dehydrated state. Some enterococci survive low doses of ionizing radiation.

MICROWAVE RADIATION

Microwaves occupy the space between the infrared and radio frequency parts of the electromagnetic spectrum (see Fig. 21–5). Such long wavelengths have little penetrating ability, but the heat generated when molecules are subjected to the electromagnetic field does not destroy some microorganisms. Microwave radiation is not a very effective means for decontamination of most materials. It has limited use in the beverage industry for pasteurization of beer and wine. A microwave oven can be used to increase the shelf life of infant formulas if bottles are exposed to 650 to 700 watts for two minutes.

Microwave radiation is the method of choice for decontamination of wood cutting boards, sponges, and dish cloths. Ten minutes of microwaving, on high, is sufficient to sterilize medium-sized wooden cutting boards. Dry cellulose sponges and dish cloths can be sterilized in 30 seconds, but periods of one to three minutes, respectively, are required for wet sponges and dish cloths. Unfortunately, no amount of microwaving can assure the safety of plastic cutting boards.

Micro Check

- What is the effect of UV radiation on cellular DNA?
- How does ionizing radiation affect the molecules of microbial cells?
- How does PRE repair UV-damaged DNA?

CHEMICAL AGENTS

Chemical agents are widely used for disinfection, but are not reliable for sterilization. Spores, some viruses, and mycobacteria are especially resistant to destruction by chemical agents. Some equipment cannot withstand autoclaving, however, and chemical agents must be employed to render equipment free from contamination. The choice of a chemical agent depends on the nature of the material to be disinfected and the type of organisms present.

Three levels of disinfection are recognized: high, intermediate, and low (Table 21–5). Only high-level biocides, or germicides, destroy endospores, the bacilli of tuberculosis, and all viruses, but they may require 24 hours to do so. The sporicidal activity of a chemical agent may vary with the origin of the endospores. Naturally occurring spores are more resistant than those which originate from cultures. In a system proposed by the Environmental Protection Agency (EPA) for classifying germicides, only disinfectants that destroy *Salmonella choleraesuis, Staphylococcus aureus,* and *Pseudomonas aeruginosa* can be recommended for hospital use.

Table 21–4
DOSE RANGES FOR FOOD IRRADIATION

DOSE RANGE	KILORADS (krads)	PURPOSES
Low	1–100	Control insects in wheat and wheat flour; inhibit sprouting in white potatoes; sterilize *Trichinella* worms in fresh pork; inhibit decay, control insects in fresh fruits and vegetables
Medium	100–1000	Destroy *Salmonella* and other bacteria in meat and poultry; control microorganisms in dried enzymes
High	1000–3000	Control insects, microorganisms in dried spices and enzymes used in food processing

Table 21–5
LEVELS OF GERMICIDAL ACTION

LEVELS	VEGETATIVE BACTERIA	TUBERCLE BACILLUS	BACTERIAL SPORES	FUNGI*	LIPID, MEDIUM-SIZED VIRUSES	NONLIPID, SMALL VIRUSES
High†	+	+	+	+	+	+
Intermediate‡	+	+	±	+	+	±
Low	+	−	−	±	+	±

Key: +, Killing effect can be expected when the normal-use concentrations of chemical disinfectants or pasteurization are properly employed; −, little or no killing effect; ±, results vary.

* Includes asexual spores but not necessarily chlamydospores or sexual spores.

† Only with extended exposure times are high-level disinfectants capable of actual sterilization of bacterial spores.

‡ Some intermediate-level disinfectants, e.g., iodophors, formaldehyde, tincture of iodine, and chlorine compounds, can be expected to exhibit some sporicidal action. Some intermediate-level disinfectants, e.g., alcohols and phenolic compounds, may have limited virucidal activity.

Protein-Denaturing Agents

Cells are vulnerable to any chemical agent that changes the configuration of their protein molecules. Proteins damaged by unfolding or incorrect looping of their chains are said to be **denatured.** The denaturation of cellular proteins by chemicals as well as physical agents is irreversible. Acids and organic solvents are protein-denaturing agents. Heavy metal derivatives, oxidizing agents, dyes, and alkylating agents alter catalytic sites on enzyme molecules by reacting with hydrogen atoms on the enzymes or on phosphoric acid residues of nucleic acids.

ORGANIC SOLVENTS

Organic solvents, such as alcohols, ethers, and acetone, denature proteins of microbial cell membranes (Color Plate 82). The alcohols, especially ethyl and isopropyl, are widely used in a concentration of 70 percent in water (Fig. 21–6). A solution of 70 percent ethyl alcohol is not effective for rapidly inactivating HIV in dried spills. Complete inactivation requires 20 minutes of contact with the alcohol. In the absence of some water, proteins are not denatured as efficiently (Table 21–6). The alcohols are safe and quite inexpensive, but have limited action against spores and viruses (Table 21–7). Both ethyl and isopropyl alcohol in concentrations of 70 percent can be applied to disinfect skin, thermometers, and anesthesia equipment. Ethers, benzene, acetone, and other ketones are highly germicidal, but are not recommended for routine use because of their irritating and carcinogenic properties.

HEAVY METAL COMPOUNDS

Soluble salts of heavy metals inactivate proteins containing sulfhydryl (SH) groups. Heavy metals include mercury, silver, copper, zinc, arsenic, and others. Derivatives of heavy metals, particularly of mercury, have been used for years. The inorganic salts, such as bichloride of mercury, are toxic, irritate tissue, and corrode metal.

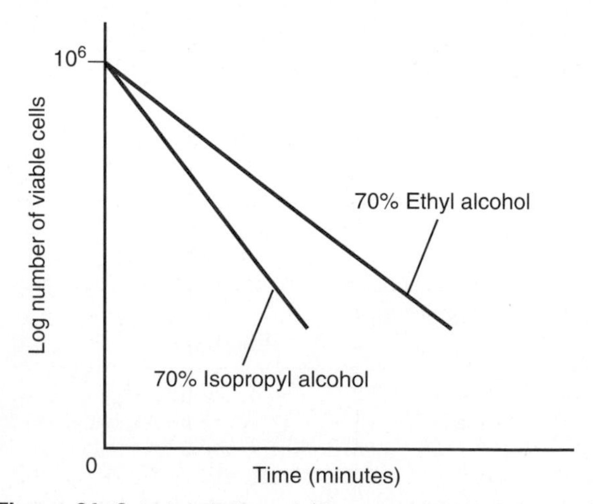

Figure 21–6 ◆ A solution of 70 percent isopropyl alcohol reduces the total number of viable bacteria on skin faster than 70 percent ethyl alcohol.

Table 21–6
THE KILLING ACTION OF VARIOUS CONCENTRATIONS OF ETHYL ALCOHOL AGAINST *STREPTOCOCCUS PYOGENES*

ALCOHOL		EXPOSURE OF TEST ORGANISMS TO GERMICIDE																
		Seconds					Minutes											
Volume (%)	Weight (%)	10	20	30	40	50	1	1.5	2	3	3.5	4	5	10	15	30	45	60
100	100	+	+	+	+	+	+	−	−	−	−	−	−	−	−	−	−	−
95	92	−	−	−	−	−	−	−	−	−	−	−	−	−	−	−	−	−
90	85	−	−	−	−	−	−	−	−	−	−	−	−	−	−	−	−	−
80	73	−	−	−	−	−	−	−	−	−	−	−	−	−	−	−	−	−
70	62	−	−	−	−	−	−	−	−	−	−	−	−	−	−	−	−	−
60	52	−	−	−	−	−	−	−	−	−	−	−	−	−	−	−	−	−
50	42	+	+	−	−	−	−	−	−	−	−	−	−	−	−	−	−	−
40	33	+	+	+	+	+	+	+	+	+	+	−	−	−	−	−	−	−
30	24	+	+	+	+	+	+	+	+	+	+	+	+	+	+	+	−	−
25	20	+	+	+	+	+	+	+	+	+	+	+	+	+	+	+	−	−
20	16	+	+	+	+	+	+	+	+	+	+	+	+	+	+	+	+	−

Key: +, growth; −, no growth.
Source: Block SS: Disinfection, Sterilization and Preservation, 4th ed. Philadelphia, Lippincott, 1991.

The organic mercurials, such as Mercurochrome and Merthiolate, are less offensive in their effects on tissue or metal, but are not any more effective than the inorganic mercurials.

Silver compounds also have limited use as disinfecting agents because of their irritating and corrosive properties. Silver nitrate in a concentration of 1 percent has a selective action on *Neisseria gonorrhoeae.* At one time it was used in eye drops to prevent gonorrheal eye infections in newborn infants delivered from an infected mother. Penicillin and erythromycin ointments have largely replaced silver nitrate as the agents of choice.

Copper salts are fungicidal and algicidal. Their use is largely limited to spraying plants and treatment of water supplies. A concentration of 2 parts per million (ppm) copper sulfate is usually employed for control of algae.

Zinc salts, especially zinc oxide, are of value in certain superficial fungal and bacterial infections. They are constituents of powders and ointments

Table 21–7
THE VIRUCIDAL ACTION OF ETHYL AND ISOPROPYL ALCOHOLS ON SEVEN VIRUSES

VIRUS	ETHYL* (%)	ISOPROPYL* (%)	LIPID ENVELOPE	LIPOPHILIC
Poliovirus, type 1	70	95 (Negative)		
Coxsackievirus B-1	60	95 (Negative)		
Echovirus 6	50	90		
Adenovirus, type 2	50	50		+
Herpes simplex	30	20	+	+
Vaccinia	40	30		
Influenza, Asian	30	30	+	+

*Lowest concentration inactivating in 10 minutes.
Source: Block SS: Disinfection, Sterilization and Preservation, 4th ed. Philadelphia, Lippincott, 1991.

used in the treatment of diaper rash and athletes' foot.

The arsenic derivative arsphenamine (salvarsan), developed by Paul Ehrlich, heralded the beginning of chemotherapy for treatment of syphilis. The discovery of penicillin and its safety and effectiveness in treating syphilis has replaced arsenic compounds. Arsenic compounds are still used in some protozoal infections.

OXIDIZING AGENTS

The oxidizing agents include the halogens, hydrogen peroxide, potassium permanganate, and peracetic acid. These agents oxidize sulfhydryl groups (SH), but may also react with amino groups (NH_2) of essential cellular proteins. Chlorine and iodine, in particular, are effective against vegetative cells, spores, fungi, and some viruses. Bromine is usually considered too toxic for general use as a disinfectant. Some organic bromides are used safely in spas or hot tubs.

Iodine preparations include tincture of iodine (2 percent iodine and 2.5 percent sodium iodide in a solution of 47 percent alcohol), aqueous iodine, and iodophors (compounds containing iodine and a detergent). A commercially available iodophor is Betadine. Iodophors release iodine more slowly than do most iodine-iodide complexes. The gradual release of iodine provides a long period of activity against microorganisms. Iodine solutions are effective disinfectants for skin, mucous membranes, suture materials, thermometers, surgical instruments, and eating utensils. Swabs, gauze pads, and surgical scrubs containing iodophors are packaged in easy-to-use disposable units. The effectiveness of iodine solutions or iodophors is not altered by the presence of organic matter.

The germicidal activity of chlorine compounds is dependent on their ability to liberate chlorine. Hypochlorite preparations are marketed as bleach for household use. Household bleach contains 5.25 percent sodium hypochlorite by weight in water. Acid-fast bacilli are not inactivated by chlorine compounds, but chlorine products are effective disinfectants for floors, bathrooms, linens, cutting boards, and dishes. Both wooden and plastic cutting boards can be sanitized by

FOCAL POINT

Survival of HIV on Environmental Surfaces

Questions often arise about the stability of HIV on environmental surfaces and its inactivation by commonly used disinfectants. Many studies have been conducted to answer these questions. The concentration of HIV used for the studies is at least five orders of magnitude greater than that encountered in clinical situations. In real-life situations, the virus is often present in small quantities, but study information can be used to assess the adequacy of routine housekeeping and infection control procedures.

The Centers for Disease control (CDC) demonstrated in their studies that drying HIV causes a 90 to 99 percent reduction in HIV concentration within several hours. In another study using a highly concentrated dried preparation of HIV, infectious virus could be recovered for up to three days. In an aqueous environment, infectious virus survived more than 15 days at room temperature. Though these results may seem alarming at first glance, it is important to understand that the objective of the study was to evaluate infection control procedures. Also, the preparation of HIV was 100,000 times more concentrated than would normally occur in the blood of an HIV-infected person.

HIV is very sensitive to chemical disinfectants. Common germicides inactivate HIV within two to ten minutes. Sodium hypochlorite (household bleach) diluted 1:10 and 70% ethyl or isopropyl alcohol inactivate HIV within 1 minute. In dried spills, complete inactivation of HIV may require 20 minutes of contact with 70 percent ethyl alcohol. For most clinical settings, the best disinfectant is a fresh 1:10 to 1:100 dilution of bleach (1/4 cup bleach in 1 gallon water). To inactivate an HIV culture or a preparation of the virus, a 1 percent available chlorine solution is recommended.

The results of these studies do not necessitate any changes in currently recommended procedures for sterilization or disinfection in health care settings or housekeeping in public, private, or health care facilities. Medical devices contaminated with blood or body fluids should be thoroughly cleaned first with soap or detergent and water to remove the organic materials. Then, appropriate disinfection or sterilization procedures should be carried out immediately.

flooding surfaces with a 1:10 solution of household bleach and allowing it to stand for several minutes before rinsing and air drying. A hypochlorite solution of 0.5 to 1 percent concentration available chlorine is recommended as a disinfectant for HIV preparations and contaminated surfaces; with a 1 percent concentration recommended for treating HIV cultures.

Dakin's solution, which is effective for cleansing of wounds, is a hypochlorite solution containing 0.5 percent chlorine. Water supplies are often chlorinated with hypochlorites or chloramines. Chlorine replaces one or more hydrogens of an amino group in chloramines. Chloramines are more stable than hypochlorites but are toxic to some fish. The presence of organic matter reduces the efficiency of all chlorine compounds.

Chlorine is widely used to purify drinking water. When chlorine gas (Cl_2) reacts with water it forms hypochlorous acid (HClO):

$$Cl_2 + H_2O \longrightarrow HClO + HCl$$

Hypochlorous acid is not stable and dissociates into a reactive form of oxygen (O), which is an oxidizing agent.

$$HClO \longrightarrow HCl + O$$

Chlorination is highly effective against bacteria. Unfortunately, the dormant stages, known as **cysts** or **oocysts,** in the life cycle of some protozoa survive chlorine treatment. The cysts of *Giardia* are especially resistant.

FOCAL POINT

Danger in Some Mixtures of Cleaning Products

In a two-year period, five episodes of chlorine gas exposure with toxicity occurred at two state hospitals in California. A total of 14 inpatients, allowed to perform cleaning duties as a part of their rehabilitation programs, were affected. Each incident involved the mixture of bleach (sodium hypochlorite) and a phosphoric acid cleaner. Exposed persons experienced a temporary illness with symptoms that included nausea, vomiting, coughing, difficulty in breathing, chest tightness, headache, and eye irritation. Some required emergency supplementary oxygen.

The label of the phosphoric acid cleaner in all five incidents did not list the active ingredient nor warn of the potential for toxic reactions when mixing phosphoric acid with other chemicals. As a result of these episodes, the Material Safety Data Sheet (MSDS) was revised in May 1991 to caution against mixing phosphoric acid cleaners with other chemicals (such as bleach or ammonia). The label does not state the possible consequences of mixing phosphoric acid cleaners with other chemicals. Some hospitals now place warning labels on their cleaning products against mixing with other cleaners. "Do not mix" signs have been posted on janitorial closet doors. In our desire to rid the environment of potentially hazardous microorganisms, new hazards may emerge for both staff and patients in hospitals. Remember that mixing of any cleaning products may constitute a health hazard.

MMWR 40:*619, 1991.*

Hydrogen peroxide, in a concentration of 3 percent, is an effective disinfectant for home or hospital use (Fig. 21–7). It has even been used to decontaminate spacecraft and is recommended for disinfecting soft contact lenses. Oxygen is released rapidly from hydrogen peroxide by catalase enzyme present in human tissues. The bubbling action effectively clears a wound of dirt particles and the oxidizing action may reduce the survival of anaerobic bacteria in deep tissues.

$$2\ H_2O_2 \xrightarrow{\text{catalase}} 2\ H_2O + O_2$$

The disinfectant is lethal to bacteria, viruses, and fungi; higher concentrations are effective against spores.

Potassium permanganate and peracetic acid are strong oxidizing agents. The potassium salt can be used as a urethral irrigant, if diluted at least 1000 times. Peracetic acid in vapor form is an efficient method for sterilizing animal cages.

DYES

Dyes are organic compounds derived from one or more substances found in coal tar; most com-

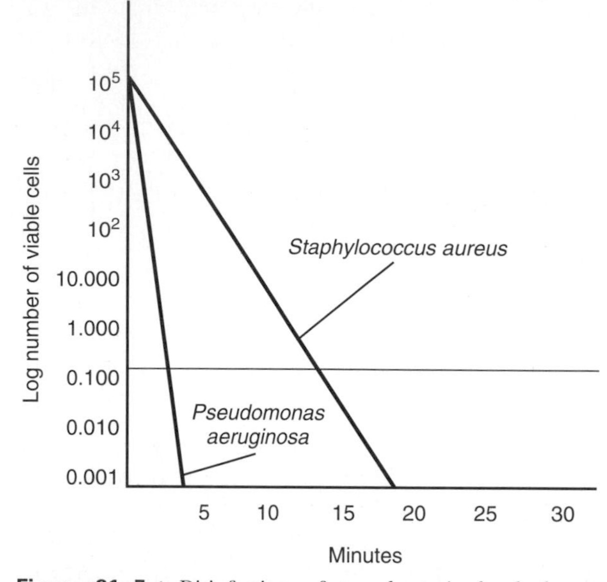

Figure 21–7 ◆ Disinfection of two bacteria by hydrogen peroxide alone. The horizontal line reflects the reduction of the original population of bacteria to a theoretical 0.5 organism/ml.

mercial dyes are distributed as dye salts. Basic dyes have a positive charge on the molecule; they are more effective microbiostatic agents than acid dyes (having a negative charge on the molecule). The basic dyes have an affinity for nucleic acids. Some aniline dyes have selective activity against gram-positive bacteria. The basic dyes, crystal violet and brilliant green, are sometimes added to culture media because they inhibit some gram-positive bacteria, allowing gram-negative bacteria to form colonies. Gentian violet is applied topically to skin infections caused by some fungi and some gram-positive bacteria to limit the spread of the infection.

ALKYLATING AGENTS

Formaldehyde, glutaraldehyde, and ethylene oxide inhibit enzyme activity by replacing hydrogen atoms on amino (NH_2), hydroxyl (OH), sulfhydryl (SH), and carboxyl (COOH) groups. They alter nucleic acids by replacing hydrogen atoms on NH_2 and OH groups. An aqueous solution of formaldehyde is called formalin.

Formalin, in concentrations of 5 to 37 percent, is active against vegetative bacterial cells, spores, fungi, and viruses. It is widely used to inactivate microorganisms in vaccines, but it is irritating to tissues, so care must be taken to eliminate traces of formalin in final products. Formalin can be used to disinfect instruments and as a vapor for gas sterilization of heat-sensitive materials.

Glutaraldehyde, in a concentration of 2 percent, is a potent antimicrobial agent. It is effective against acid-fast bacilli, other vegetative bacterial cells, spores, fungi, and viruses. It is less irritating than formaldehyde and is active even in the presence of extraneous matter. Glutaraldehyde is used extensively in the disinfection of respiratory therapy equipment. A major disadvantage of aqueous glutaraldehyde is instability at room temperature.

Ethylene oxide is used for the gas sterilization of heat- or moisture-sensitive materials. The gas is contained in a special chamber with a humidity of 25 to 50 percent and a temperature of 38° to 60°C for several hours of exposure (Fig. 21–8). Ethylene oxide is a carcinogen; it is explosive in air and must be mixed with an inactive gas, such as carbon dioxide or nitrogen. Other gases, such as beta-propiolactone or methyl bromide, can also be employed as sterilants. Installation of equipment for gas sterilization is costly, but the process is especially suitable for artificial heart valves, bedding, and spacecraft components.

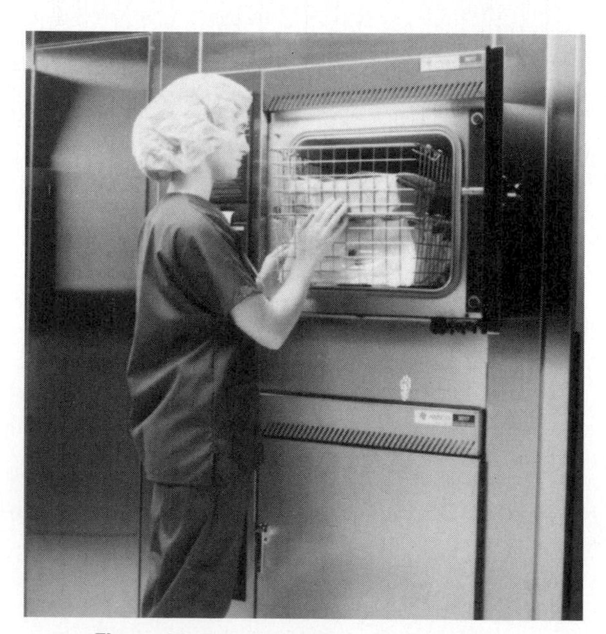

Figure 21–8 ◆ An ethylene oxide sterilizer.

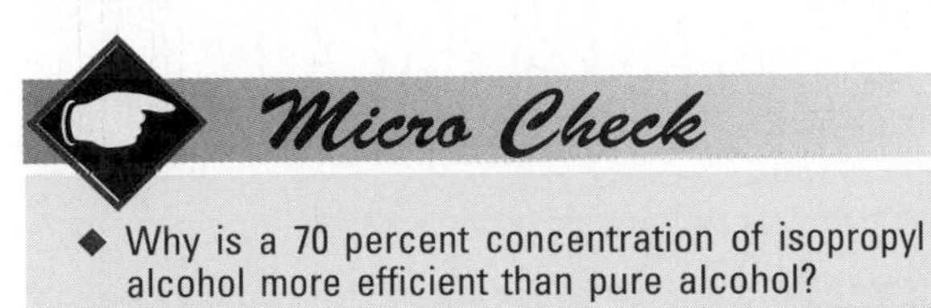

- Why is a 70 percent concentration of isopropyl alcohol more efficient than pure alcohol?
- What microorganisms can be presumed to be present in the hospital environment?
- Why are iodophors more effective than tincture of iodine?

Membrane-Altering Agents

Any structural damage to the plasma membrane of cells causes the loss of required metabolites or provides a portal of entry for harmful agents in the environment. Many useful chemicals are active on the plasma membrane surface to control microorganisms.

SURFACE-ACTIVE AGENTS

Chemical agents that reduce surface tension are called surface-active agents or detergents. Surface tension refers to the pressure or force between liquid molecules in the liquid-air surface. Surface-active agents such as soaps and detergents increase the penetration of the liquid-air surface by other molecules. Surface-active agents may dissociate to form negatively (anionic) or positively (cationic) charged molecules, or they may be nonionic. These agents are not strong disinfectants when used alone. If used with other antimicrobial agents, they have a synergistic effect. The mechanical action involved in cleansing does wash bacteria away from the surface of the skin or other objects.

Most of the effective cationic surface-active germicides are the quaternary ammonium salts ("quats"). These cationic detergents alter the charges of phospholipids on plasma membranes. Quats are effective against gram-positive bacteria, but have only limited activity against most species of gram-negative organisms. Opportunistic pathogens are remarkably resistant to the quats. Spores and mycobacteria may not be destroyed by cationic detergents. These products are highly stable, nonirritating, odorless, and relatively inexpensive.

Soaps are often used with detergents for laundry, dishwashing, preoperative scrubbing, handwashing, and cleaning of walls, furniture, and floors. Soaps without added disinfectants have only a slight inhibiting effect on microbial populations. *Pseudomonas* bacteria grow very well in liquid soaps containing detergents. Soap preparations available under a variety of trade names have been implicated as sources for hospital-acquired infections caused by gram-negative bacteria.

PHENOLIC DERIVATIVES

Although Lister introduced the use of phenol (carbolic acid) in the nineteenth century for hospital surgeries, phenol is a highly irritating and toxic substance that is not used now. Even low concentrations of phenol disrupt cell membranes. A large number of phenolic derivatives and synthetic phenolic compounds, which are less irritating and lack phenol's pungent odor, are widely used as effective antimicrobial agents, but none of the phenolic compounds are effective against spores.

Aqueous solutions of 5 percent phenol can be used to disinfect sputum, urine, feces, or contaminated glass slides because it is effective in the presence of organic materials. Other members in the family of phenol compounds have greater microbicidal activity than phenol. The popular household disinfectant sold under the trade name of Lysol, contains two phenolic compounds: cresol (ortho-phenylphenol) mixed with ortho-benzyl-para-chlorophenol.

Other phenolic compounds include alpha-phenylphenol, hexylresorcinol, hexachlorophene, and chlorhexidine. Hexachlorophene is contained in the commercial product, pHisoHex, for use in surgical scrubs. It is recommended with the caution to rinse thoroughly for infant skin care. Without thorough rinsing, there is a risk of neurological damage in the infant from the hexachlorophene. Chlorhexidine is the active ingredient in popular surgical scrubs, such as Betasept and Hibiclens. It is bactericidal against a wide variety of gram-positive and gram-negative bacteria and destroys enveloped viruses and some others. Its antimicrobial effect is long-lasting and unaffected by the presence of organic matter, such as blood. No one disinfectant is suitable as a universal biocide, but some can be recommended for particular areas (Table 21–8).

Table 21–8
RECOMMENDED CONCENTRATIONS AND APPLICATIONS OF SELECTED DISINFECTANTS

CHEMICAL AGENTS	LEVEL OF ACTIVITY*	CONCENTRATION (%)	APPLICATION
Alcohols	I	70.0–95.0	Anesthesia equipment, thermometers, skin surfaces
Chlorhexidine in alcohol	H	0.5–4.0	Surgical scrub
Chlorine compounds (sodium hypochlorite household bleach)	I	0.5–1.0	Toilets, lavatories, bathtubs, laundry, dishes, blood and body fluid spills, plastics, medical instruments, organ and tissue transplants
Ethylene oxide	H	10	Heat-sensitive objects, mattresses, pillows, shoes
Formaldehyde in alcohol	H	20.0, 70.0	Surgical instruments
Formaldehyde, aqueous	I to H	16.0	Dialysis equipment
Glutaraldehyde, aqueous	H to I	2.0–3.2	Anesthesia and respiratory therapy equipment, endoscopes
Iodophors	L to I	0.5–10	Suture materials, thermometers, surgical instruments, anesthesia equipment
Phenolic compounds	I to L	5.0	Laboratory, glassware, floors, walls, furniture
Quaternary ammonium compounds	L	0.1–0.13	Walls, floors, furniture shelves, ledges, light fixtures, dishes, laundry

* L, low; I, intermediate; H, high.

Micro Check

- Why are most soaps not good disinfectants?
- Why is there no one ideal disinfectant?
- Why are surface-active agents useful in disinfection?

EVALUATION OF DISINFECTANTS

The efficiency of a disinfectant at killing microorganisms is determined by either of two main evaluation procedures: the phenol coefficient (PC) test and the use-dilution method. In the PC method, the microbicidal power of the test disinfectant is compared with that of phenol. The phenol coefficient is determined by adding a standard inoculum of a pathogenic bacterium such as *Salmonella typhi* or *Staphylococcus aureus* to various dilutions of phenol and to dilutions of the new disinfectant under test. The dilution tubes are incubated at room temperature (20°C). Samples are removed from each tube after 5, 10, and 15 minutes of contact time and streaked onto a separate nutrient agar plate. After two days, the plates are examined for bacterial colonies. The highest dilution of disinfectant represented on the plate with no colonies is used to calculate the PC value.

The phenol coefficient (PC) is the ratio of the highest dilution of the test disinfectant killing the test organism in 10 minutes to the highest dilution of phenol with the same germicidal activity. A phenol coefficient of 10 would indicate that the test disinfectant had 10 times the efficiency of phenol; a phenol coefficient of 0.1 would mean that the test disinfectant exhibited only one-tenth as much activity as phenol against the test organisms.

The Association of Official Analytical Chemists (AOAC) recommends the use-dilution method for a more definitive result. Actual dilutions of disinfectants for practical purposes are obtained by this method. Three pathogenic bacterial cultures are commonly used as the test organisms:

Staphylococcus aureus (ATCC 6538), *Salmonella choleraesuis* (ATCC 10708), and *Pseudomonas aeruginosa* (ATCC 15442). The ATCC number represents the catalog number of the species in the American Type Culture Collection. Various chemicals are tested to determine the lowest concentration that kills the test organism; this is then identified as the "use dilution."

In the procedure sterile stainless steel cylinders, glass rods, surgical threads, or small porcelain cylinders are inoculated with the test organisms, dried, and transferred to dilutions of the test disinfectant usually for 10 minutes at 20°C. Ten replicates of each dilution are prepared in this way. When the exposure time ends, the cylinders are transferred aseptically to a sterile culture medium and incubated to detect any survivors. After an incubation period of two days, the "use dilution" is determined by the greatest dilution of the chemical that kills the organism on 10 carriers in 10 minutes. Testing bacteria from a particular environment by the AOAC use-dilution method can be used to establish effective disinfection procedures. Periodic monitoring of the environment is needed to ensure continued effective sterilization or disinfection procedure.

The Environmental Protection Agency (EPA) regulates use of general purpose disinfectants. Equipment that only comes in contact with a patient's skin or environmental surfaces may be treated with the EPA-regulated general purpose disinfectants. The Federal Drug Administration (FDA) has jurisdiction over chemical sterilants and devices to be introduced into sterile body sites.

Understanding Microbiology

1. Why is asepsis often a goal, rather than an easily accomplished feat?
2. Compare the efficiency of heat and cold as microbicidal and microbiostatic agents.
3. Why is autoclaving a more efficient method of sterilization than boiling or heating in an oven?
4. Name the mode of action of ultraviolet radiation in destroying microorganisms.
5. Why is a "quat" not the most efficient disinfectant to employ for the environment of immunocompromised patients?

Applying Microbiology

6. Obtain a list of three to ten disinfectants and their manufacturers with the help of a local pharmacy. Write to manufacturers and the Environmental Protection Agency for information on their formulations and recommended use in the home or hospital environment. When you have received the information, prepare a report to share with the class on each product.

Chapter 22

Antimicrobial and Chemotherapeutic Agents

Chapter Outline

- **CLASSIFICATION OF ANTIMICROBIAL AGENTS**
  - Antimicrobials Affecting Proteins of Cell Walls and Membranes
  - Antimicrobials Affecting Lipids of Plasma Membranes
  - Antimicrobials Affecting Protein Synthesis
  - Antimicrobials Affecting Synthesis of Nucleic Acids
  - Antimicrobials Affecting Synthesis of Essential Metabolites
  - Antimicrobials Having Lesser Known Mechanisms of Action
- **LABORATORY METHODS**
  - Antimicrobial Susceptibility Tests
- **RESISTANCE TO ANTIMICROBIAL AGENTS**
- **MECHANISMS OF MICROBIAL RESISTANCE**

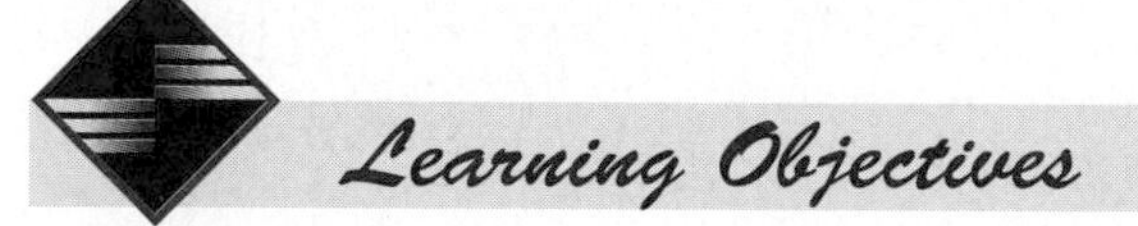

Learning Objectives

After you have read this chapter, you should be able to:

1. Distinguish among natural, semisynthetic, and synthetic antimicrobial agents.
2. List the target sites for the major antimicrobial agents.
3. Explain the significance of beta-lactamases in the choice of treatment for some infectious diseases.
4. Describe three methods of antimicrobial susceptibility testing.
5. Differentiate between the minimum inhibitory concentration (MIC) and the minimum bactericidal concentration (MBC) of an antibiotic.
6. Describe mechanisms in microorganisms that can lead to developing resistance to antimicrobial drugs.

Chemotherapy is the treatment of disease with chemical substances. Paul Erhlich's discovery in 1909 of salvarsan, an arsenic compound that was used to treat syphilis, was the beginning of the modern search for chemicals that would have therapeutic effects on diseases, or **chemotherapeutic** agents. Salvarsan was very toxic for the patient, so the search continued for drugs with a **selective toxicity** for the pathogenic microorganism and not for the human or animal host.

Louis Pasteur had observed that some microorganisms produce substances which inhibit the growth of other microorganisms, a phenomenon called **antibiosis.** Later, Alexander Fleming discovered a *Penicillium* mold producing a substance he called penicillin that killed staphylococci. The large-scale production of penicillin in the 1940s by Howard Florey and Ernst Chain led to widespread use of penicillin and the development of an industry to research and develop other antimicrobial agents. These chemicals derived from microorganisms were called **antibiotics.** Most antibiotics are produced by a few groups of microorganisms from soil: *Streptomyces,* a genus of filamentous bacteria; *Bacillus,* a genus of gram-positive spore-forming rod-shaped bacteria; and the molds of the genera *Penicillium* and *Cephalosporium.*

Most of the antibiotics of medical importance are not essential for the growth of the microorganism producing it. In fact, many antibiotics inhibit the growth of the very organism that produces them. Antibiotics are frequently referred to as **secondary metabolites** because they are usually produced after the organism has already grown and produced a large population of cells.

FOCAL POINT

The Antibiotics in Your Kitchen Cupboard: Allspice

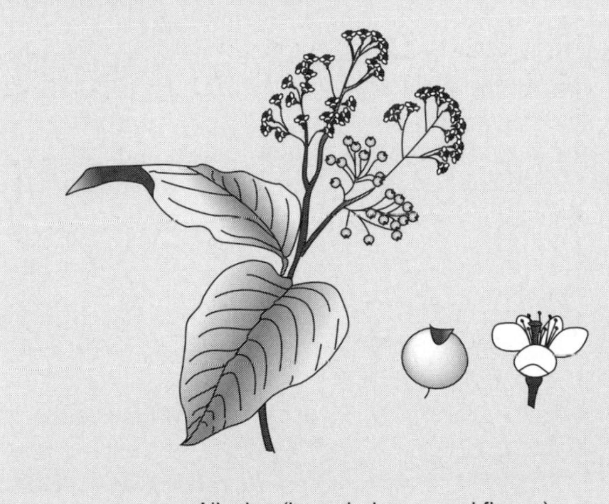

Allspice (branch, berry, and flower)

Despite the technological advances in methods for food preservation, many cultures depend heavily on spices to preserve their food. Paul Sherman and Jennifer Billings of Cornell University in Ithaca, New York, looked at spices used in 31 countries. The most popular spices are allspice, onion, oregano, white pepper, garlic, lemon juice, hot peppers, and ginger. They found that allspice, garlic, onion, and oregano killed all bacteria against which they were tested, including species of *Salmonella* and *Staphylococcus.* Other seasonings destroyed at least 75 percent of the targeted microbes. It appears that the use of spices in cooking not only provides exotic flavors but prevents foodborne illnesses.

Science 277:321, 1997.

Antibiotics derived from microbial sources are **natural** products, while those produced partially or completely by chemical procedures are referred to as **semisynthetic** or **synthetic** antibiotics, respectively. The terms antimicrobics, antimicrobials, antibiotics, antibacterials, and chemotherapeutic agents describe drugs used to treat infectious diseases. The more general term chemotherapeutic agent can describe any chemical substance used to treat disease, but this term frequently refers to drugs for treating a malignant growth, or cancer. The term used to designate all the categories of drugs used to treat infections is **antimicrobial.**

CLASSIFICATION OF ANTIMICROBIAL AGENTS

There are approximately 250 antimicrobial and chemotherapeutic agents in use today. Drug companies assign trade names to their products; thus, a single **generic** drug may have a confusing number of names (Table 22–1). We shall use generic names of drugs to minimize confusion.

Antimicrobial drugs exert either a microbicidal (-cidal, meaning to kill) or a microbiostatic (-static, meaning to inhibit growth) effect on infectious agents. The products with a range of activity limited to one type or group of organisms are called **narrow-spectrum** drugs. **Broad-spectrum** antibiotics are effective against an expanded range of microorganisms. Broad-spectrum drugs are more often prescribed when the exact nature of the infectious agent is unknown.

Despite the advantages of broad-spectrum drugs, one problem connected with their use is the disturbance of normal ecological relationships among microorganisms in the body. If only a few hardy organisms survive, they flourish without competition from their usual neighbor microorganisms and cause **secondary** or **opportunistic infections.** Common **etiologic agents** in such secondary infections are resistant strains of *Proteus, Pseudomonas, Escherichia, Staphylococcus,* and *Candida* species.

Antimicrobial agents may be assigned to one of at least five main groups according to the target site of their interfering activity: action on cell wall and cell membrane proteins, activity on plasma membranes, protein synthesis, nucleic acid synthesis, interference with essential metabolites. The understanding of antimicrobial action on target sites has paralleled the development of molecular biology.

Antimicrobials Affecting Proteins of Cell Walls and Membranes

The cell walls of bacteria contain peptidoglycan, a unique group of molecules not found in eucaryotic cell walls. Peptidoglycan molecules have short chains of amino acids, known as peptides, attached to carbohydrate molecules, or glycan. Antimicrobials affecting the synthesis of these peptides include the natural penicillins and cephalosporins produced by strains of the fungi *Penicillium* and *Cephalosporium,* respectively. The penicillins and cephalosporins work by preventing the action of enzymes, called transpeptidases, which are essential to the formation of peptidoglycan molecules.

Now many of these drugs are produced semisynthetically, but all of them contain a beta-lactam (β-lactam) ring in their chemical structure.

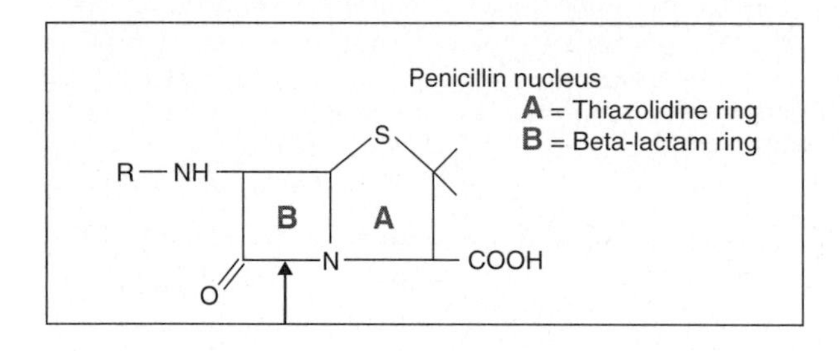

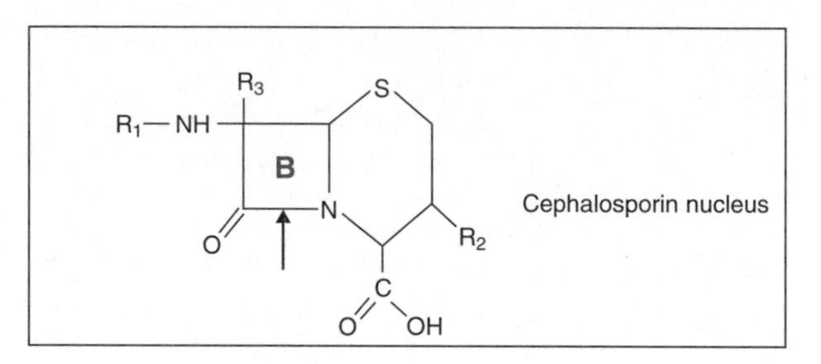

However, the death of cells is explained by multiple actions of the drugs. They also trigger autolytic enzymes that enhance the destruction of the cell.

Table 22–1
GENERIC AND TRADE NAMES OF ANTIMICROBIALS

GENERIC NAME	TRADE NAME
Ampicillin	Omnipen, Polycillin
Penicillin G	Crysticillin
Chlortetracycline	Aureomycin
Oxytetracycline	Terramycin
Tetracycline	Achromycin, Tetracyn
Cephalothin	Keflin
Chloramphenicol	Chloromycetin
Erythromycin	Ilosone
Trimethoprim-sulfamethoxazole	Bactrim, Septra
Chloroquine	Aralen

Cycloserine, another β-lactam drug derived from *Streptomyces orchidaceus,* is more specific in its action; it inhibits the formation of D-alanine from L-alanine, thereby depleting an amino acid component of peptidoglycan.

Because peptidoglycan is a cell wall constituent found only in procaryotic cells, the action of β-lactam drugs have a selective toxicity action on bacteria. The penicillins are extremely valuable to treat infections, but some individuals are allergic to them. The penicillins act as partial antigens and combine with body proteins to produce allergens. Fortunately, most persons who are allergic to the penicillins are not hypersensitive to cephalosporins. The penicillins have a limited spectrum of activity against some strains of staphylococci, *Neisseria gonorrhoeae, Haemophilus influenzae,* and a few other gram-negative bacteria. Ampicillin, a semisynthetic penicillin, is four to eight times more effective against gram-negative bacteria than other penicillins.

Some microorganisms survive the effects of β-

lactam drugs because they produce the enzyme β-lactamase. The natural penicillin molecules are inactivated by β-lactamase as it opens the β-lactam ring. The semisynthetic penicillins, such as methicillin, oxacillin, and nafcillin, usually remain active in the presence of β-lactamase (Fig 22–1). The β-lactam ring of these drugs is protected by specially designed chemical groups chemically added to the penicillin nucleus.

The cephalosporins have a broader spectrum of activity than the penicillins. The synthesis of new cephalosporins has been a rapidly developing field with first-, second-, third-, and fourth-generation drugs. Each generation of drugs increases the spectrum of activity or ability to combat resistance factors of microorganisms. The first-generation drugs, such as cephalothin, are effective against isolates of *Escherichia coli, Klebsiella* species, *Salmonella* species, and streptococci. The second- and third-generation cephalosporins are less active against gram-positive bacteria, but have a broader spectrum of activity against gram-negative bacilli. Unfortunately, some gram-negative bacteria produce β-lactamases by mutation or by an enzyme inducer. Treatment failures may be due to an infection by an organism producing β-lactamases. The fourth generation of drugs show a stability against specific β-lactamases that inactivate penicillins and cephalosporins.

Some bacteria continue to survive in the presence of penicillins or cephalosporins, despite loss of all or part of their cell walls. Cell wall-deficient bacteria have been implicated in the recurrence of an infection (Fig. 22–2). The **protoplast** is the

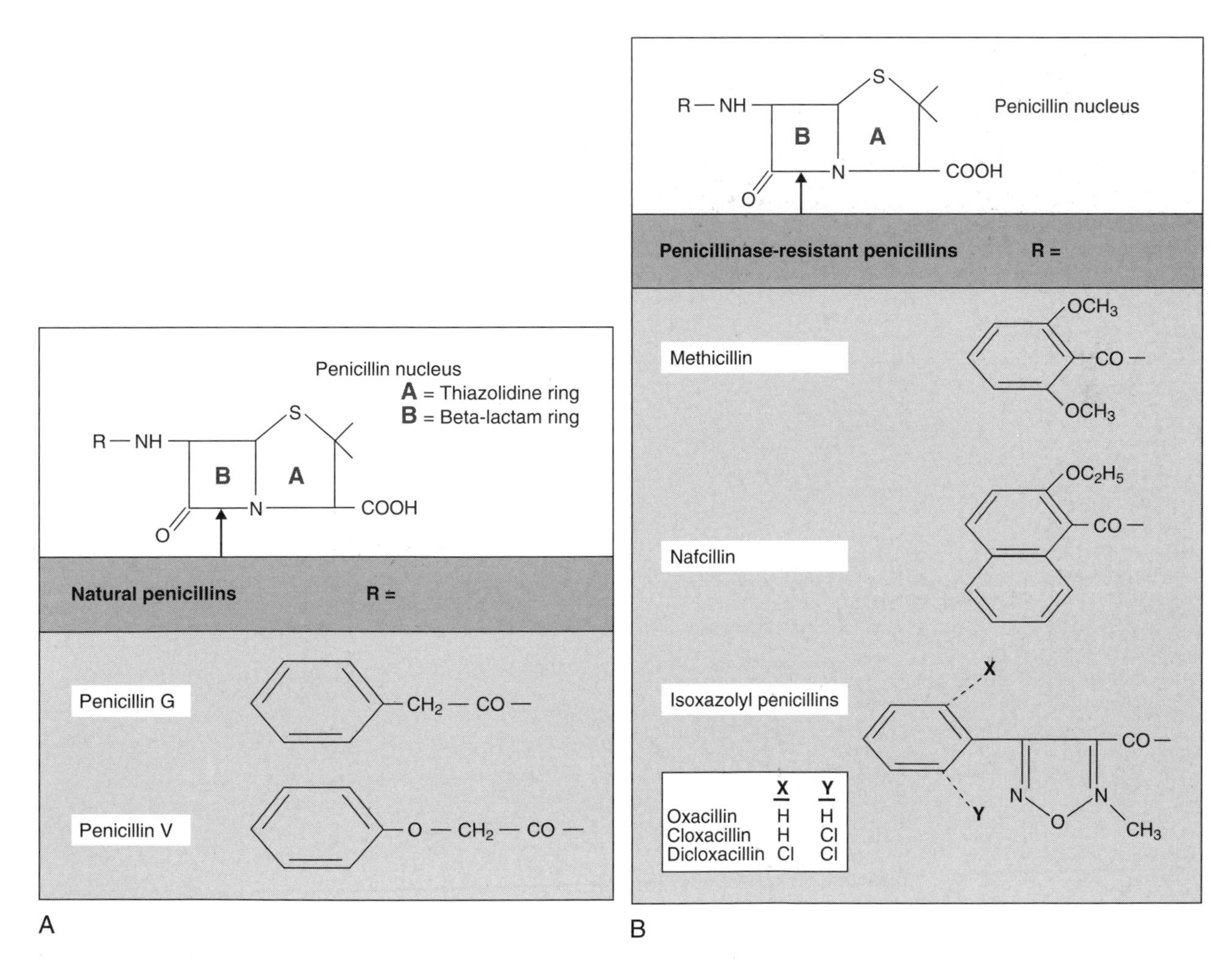

Figure 22–1 ◆ Formulas of some natural (*A*) and semisynthetic (*B*) penicillins. The β-lactam ring is indicated by the arrows. The letter R indicates the location of a chemical group. Penicillin G has an R group that differs from other penicillins.

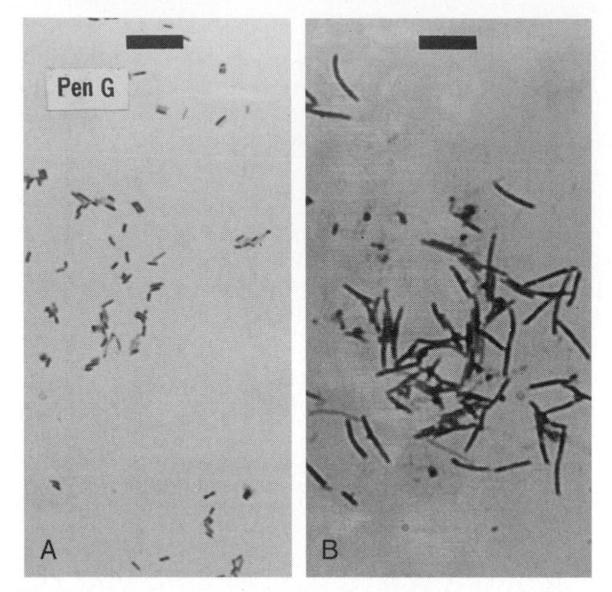

Figure 22–2 ◆ Morphological changes occurring in a bacillus in the presence of penicillin. *A,* Typical rodlike forms. *B,* Conversion to filamentous protoplasts having no cell walls.

cell that has completely lost its cell wall; the **spheroplast** has lost part of the wall.

Micro Check

- Why are most antibiotics called secondary metabolites?
- Why are penicillins and cephalosporins selective for bacteria?
- Explain the advantage of semisynthetic penicillins in therapy?

Antimicrobials Affecting Lipids of Plasma Membranes

Because of the many important functions of the plasma membrane, its destruction is lethal to cells. The membranes of some bacteria and fungi are disrupted by polymyxin and polyene drugs. The subsequent release of cellular fluids causes cell death. The polymyxin and polyene drugs are not as selective in their toxicity for microbial cells. They cause side effects in the human host so that many of them are limited to topical application.

The polymyxins include polymyxin B and colistin or polymyxin E, which are produced by several strains of *Bacillus polymyxa* (Fig. 22–3). These drugs bind to phospholipids of bacterial membranes causing leakage of cell constituents. Polymyxin B and colistin are bactericidal for gram-negative bacteria, but they are primarily used to treat infections caused by multidrug-resistant strains of *Pseudomonas aeruginosa* or superficial infections of the skin or eye caused by gram-negative organisms.

The polyenes, such as amphotericin B, nystatin, and candicidin, are produced by soil bacteria of the *Streptomyces* genus. They bind selectively to the sterol molecules in fungal plasma membranes. The synthetic forms of polyene drugs, such as imidazoles, miconazole, ketoconazole, and clotrimazole, also interact with sterol molecules of membranes. Because sterols are not found in bacterial plasma membranes, with the exception of some mycoplasmas, polyene drugs are not used to treat most bacterial infections.

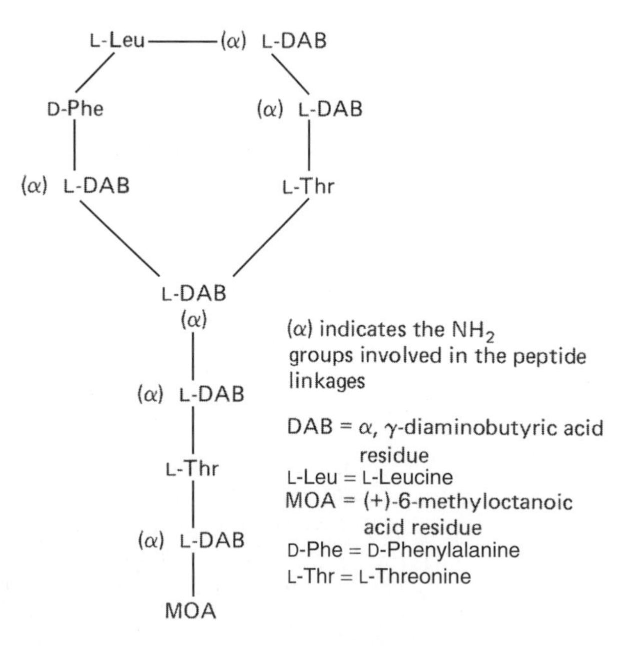

Figure 22–3 ◆ The component molecules of polymyxin B. Polymyxin B binds to phospholipids permitting substances to cross membranes.

Amphotericin B is valuable in the treatment of disseminated coccidioidomycosis or systemic candidiasis. Unfortunately, polyenes bind to sterols of red blood cell membranes. The drug causes hemolytic anemia in patients who require long-term therapy for systemic fungal infections. Nystatin is very effective in controlling intestinal candidiasis. Candicidin is somewhat more effective against *Candida* species than nystatin, but its use has been limited mainly to the treatment of vaginal infections.

The imidazoles are active against superficial *Candida* infections and some systemic mycoses. These drugs are used with some caution because of severe side effects such as gastrointestinal bleeding and renal failure.

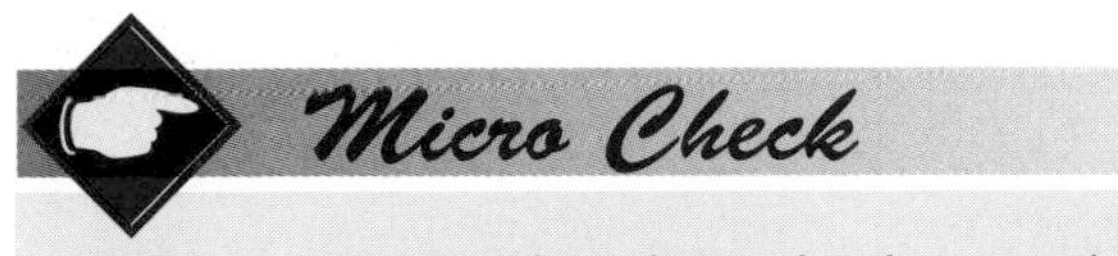

- Why are many polymyxins and polyenes suitable only for topical application?
- Why are polyenes not effective in bacterial infections?
- Why is long-term treatment with polyenes likely to cause hemolytic anemia?

Antimicrobials Affecting Protein Synthesis

Antimicrobial agents may affect one or more of the stages of protein synthesis. The drugs in this category usually have a broad spectrum of activity against a variety of microorganisms; they may also have greater adverse effect on the human host. The drugs include those in the chloramphenicol, tetracycline, and aminoglycoside chemical families.

The soil bacterium, *Streptomyces venezuelae,* was discovered in the 1940s to produce chloramphenicol. This drug is now produced synthetically. Chloramphenicol blocks the attachment of mRNA to the ribosome, stopping protein synthesis. The drug is not recommended for minor infections, but it remains a drug of choice for typhoid fever and other *Salmonella* infections. Adverse side effects include a depressive effect on blood cell production in the bone marrow, and aplastic anemia may occur after prolonged use.

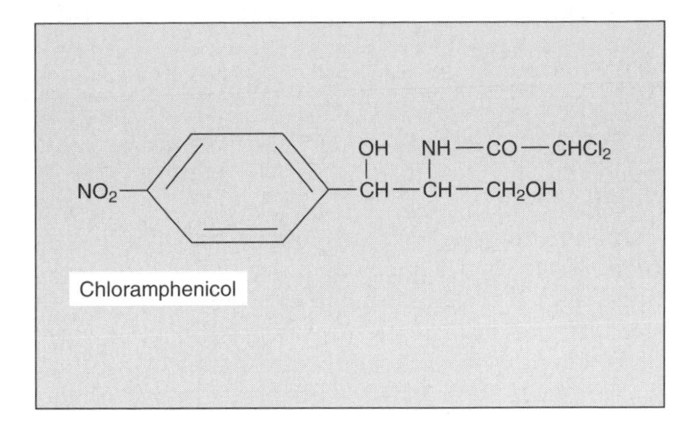

Chloramphenicol

The tetracycline drugs are derived from several *Streptomyces* species. These drugs have four rings attached to different chemical side groups (locations designated by R). They block protein synthesis by preventing the attachment of tRNA molecules carrying amino acids to mRNA on the ribosome. The tetracycline family of drugs have a broad spectrum of activity against bacteria that are gram-positive, gram-negative, and the mycoplasmas, rickettsias, and chlamydias. Although allergic reactions are not common, side effects of prolonged or excessive doses of the tetracyclines include nausea, diarrhea, liver damage, anemia, photosensitivity of skin, and staining of teeth.

Tetracycline nucleus

Natural tetracyclines	R_1 =	R_2 =	R_3 =	R_4 =
Tetracycline	H	OH	CH_3	H
Chlortetracycline	Cl	OH	CH_3	H
Demeclocycline	Cl	OH	H	H
Oxytetracycline	H	OH	CH_3	OH
Semisynthetic tetracyclines	**R_1 =**	**R_2 =**	**R_3 =**	**R_4 =**
Doxycycline	H	H	CH_3	OH
Minocycline	$N(CH_3)_2$	H	H	H

Tetracyline-resistant strains of microorganisms have developed, including some streptococci, *Escherichia, Bacteroides, Shigella,* and *Neisseria* species. The resistance in *Escherichia* and *Shigella* is caused by specific resistance plasmids, called R plasmids, transferred by conjugation.

Other antimicrobials that inhibit the binding of tRNA to the ribosome are erythromycin, azithromycin, and clarithromycin. Erythromycin is effective against many gram-positive and some gram-negative bacteria, mycoplasmas, atypical mycobacteria, and *Legionella pneumophila,* the etiologic agent of Legionnaire's disease. No serious side effects result from the use of the basic form of erythromycin, but alternate forms of erythromycin, such as its esters, can cause liver damage. Some staphylococci are resistant, but the mechanism of the resistance is unclear.

Azithromycin is active against gram-positive and gram-negative bacteria, *Mycoplasma pneumoniae,* and chlamydias. Clarithromycin shows a broad range of activity against some typical and atypical respiratory pathogens, including *M. pneumoniae.*

The aminoglycoside antimicrobials, including streptomycin, kanamycin, neomycin, gentamicin, and tobramycin, are built of two or more sugar residues. The aminoglycosides cause misreading of mRNA, resulting in a defective or missing protein. Many of the aminoglycosides are produced by *Streptomyces* species and usually have the suffix -mycin in their generic names. *Micromonospora* produce some aminoglycosides, which usually carry the suffix -micin in their generic drug name.

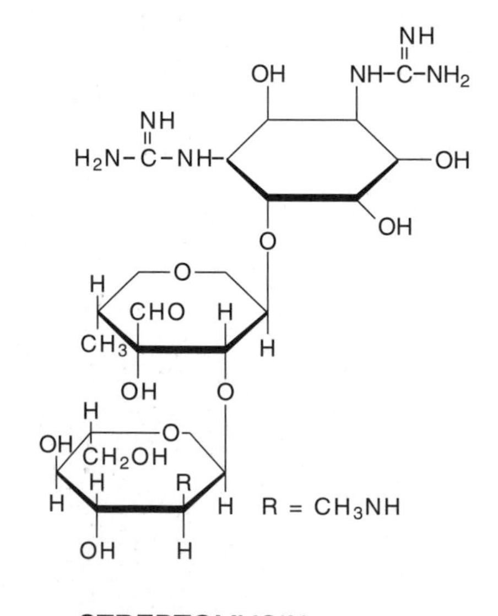

STREPTOMYCIN

Streptomycin, neomycin, and kanamycin are bactericidal for many staphylococci, some gram-negative bacilli, and some mycobacteria. All three drugs are ototoxic. Neomycin and kanamycin may cause deafness, but streptomycin's toxicity is usually limited to vertigo. Streptomycin and penicillin G act together effectively to exert a **synergistic** antibacterial activity against enterococci. In **synergism** the effect of the two drugs used together is greater than the effects expected when their individual actions are totaled. In general, each drug in the combined therapy may be used in a lower dose than would be necessary if used alone. The lower doses may reduce the severity of the side effects on the patient.

Gentamicin and tobramycin are active against many gram-negative bacilli that are often resistant to other antibiotics. In particular, most infections caused by *Proteus, Pseudomonas,* and *Serratia* species respond favorably to these drugs, although a few resistant strains of *Pseudomonas* species have been found. Penicillins and cephalosporins act synergistically with either gentamicin or tobramycin. Like other aminoglycosides, gentamicin and tobramycin can cause vertigo and deafness.

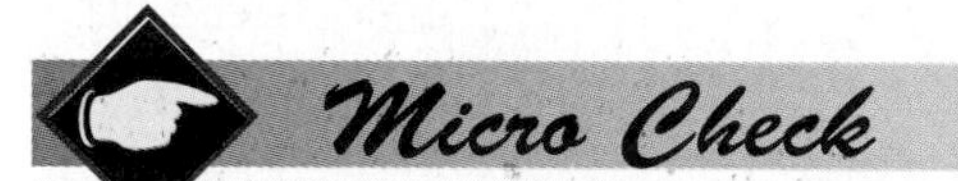

- What are the two ways in which antimicrobial agents can block protein synthesis?
- Why are the tetracyclines so valuable in treatment of infections?
- Why would synergistic action of two or more drugs be useful to treat infections?

Antimicrobials Affecting Synthesis of Nucleic Acids

Many natural products inhibit the synthesis of nucleic acids. Some interfere with the replication of DNA by blocking synthesis of purines and pyrimidines, and others promote fragmentation of DNA. Others limit the transcription of information into mRNA by inhibiting the action of the RNA synthesizing enzyme, RNA polymerase. Several agents useful for treating infections or tumors have a chemical structure similar to the bases in nucleic acids so they are known as base analogs. They act by altering the metabolism of nucleotides such as in nucleic acid synthesis.

Nalidixic acid and the related **quinolone** drugs are potent inhibitors of DNA synthesis. Nalidixic acid is active against most gram-negative bacteria and has been used successfully to treat urinary tract infections. Quinolones, a new group of synthetic drugs containing fluorine, are effective against both gram-positive and gram-negative bacteria. These drugs block DNA gyrase, the enzyme that unwinds DNA before the strands can replicate. Nausea, vomiting, diarrhea, and photosensitization may occur with extended use of either drug. Hypersensitivity and development of resistance do not appear to be significant problems.

Rifampin and rifabutin are examples of drugs that selectively block the action of DNA or RNA polymerase.

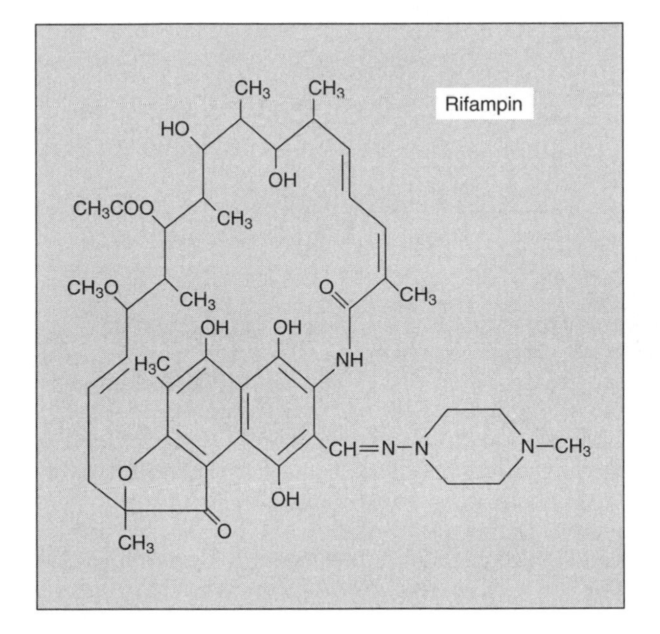

Rifampin inhibits RNA polymerase; it is active against *Mycobacterium tuberculosis* and is tolerated well by most patients. It is most frequently used in combination with other antituberculosis agents, such as isoniazid. Resistance is not usually a problem when the drug combinations are used according to prescribed directions. Rifabutin, an inhibitor of RNA polymerase, is used to prevent dissemination of *Mycobacterium avium* complex (MAC) disease in patients with advanced HIV infection.

The base analog flucytosine was first synthesized for treatment of leukemia where it was not effective; later studies showed it is active against fungal infections. *Cryptococcus neoformans, Candida* species, and a rarer yeast, *Torulopsis glabrata,* are particularly susceptible to flucytosine. Intracellular flucytosine is converted by a fungal enzyme to 5-fluorouracil, a base analog of uracil required for RNA synthesis. The analog is incorporated into RNA in place of uracil resulting in blocked transcription. Flucytosine is less toxic than amphotericin B and is therefore an alternate drug of choice for some fungal infections.

The antiviral drugs, ganciclovir, foscarnet, and ribavirin, interfere with nucleic acid synthesis. Ganciclovir and foscarnet, which inhibit DNA synthesis in cytomegalovirus (CMV), are used to treat CMV retinitis seen in AIDS patients. Ribavirin often affects the synthesis of both DNA and RNA in many viruses. It is only available for aerosol therapy in the United States. Ribavirin is used to treat severe lower respiratory tract infections caused by the respiratory syncytial virus (RSV) in infants and young children.

Idoxuridine (IDU), an analog of thymidine, is active against the herpes simplex virus types 1 and 2 that cause a severe corneal infection. If untreated, the herpes infection can cause ulceration, scarring, and blindness. IDU is applied topically and interferes with viral DNA synthesis. Three other base analogs, acyclovir, cytosine arabinoside (ara-C), and adenine arabinoside (ara-A) as well as IDU, show promise in the treatment of infections caused by herpes simplex and varicella-zoster viruses.

Many of the newly developed drugs interfere with the synthesis of the enzyme reverse transcriptase in the human immunodeficiency virus (HIV). Zidovudine (ZDV), also known as azidothymidine (AZT), is a potent inhibitor of HIV reverse transcriptase, an enzyme important for replicating the virus. A new nucleoside analog, abacavir, which inhibits reverse transcriptase, was approved recently by the FDA for use in AIDS combination therapy. All drugs acting as nucleoside analogs have serious side effects that include bone marrow depression, gastrointestinal disturbances, and peripheral neuropathy (pain in the feet, legs, and hands).

The protease inhibitors saquinavir, indinavir, and ritonavir constitute powerful weapons for inhibiting the replication of HIV. The drugs interfere with the activity of HIV protease, an enzyme required for synthesis of viral proteins. A combined therapy approach using reverse transcriptase and protease inhibitors is dramatically lengthening the lives of AIDS patients. The ingredients of the drug combinations can be altered to make customized "cocktails." A decline in plasma HIV load allows patients to maintain higher counts of their $CD4^+$

lymphocytes. Multiple drug therapy also delays onset of drug resistance in HIV.

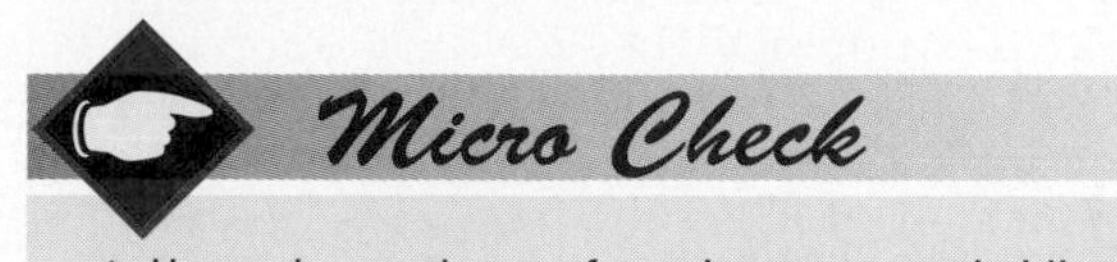

- How do analogs of purines or pyrimidines block synthesis of nucleic acids?
- Why is flucytosine a drug of choice for some fungal infections?
- What benefits do a combined therapy approach have in HIV-infected patients?

Antimicrobials Affecting Synthesis of Essential Metabolites

Microorganisms depend on synthesis of a number of metabolites required for growth. Some antimicrobial drugs inhibit or block the action of enzymes producing essential metabolites. One essential metabolite is folic acid, which is needed by both procaryotic and eucaryotic cells for the synthesis of DNA. Humans and other animals do not synthesize folic acid, but depend on dietary sources. Microorganisms synthesize folic acid by the action of two enzymes on para-aminobenzoic acid (PABA): a synthetase and a reductase.

The sulfonamide drugs competitively inhibit the synthetase because they have chemical structures similar to PABA; they are analogs of PABA and compete with PABA for the active site on the enzyme.

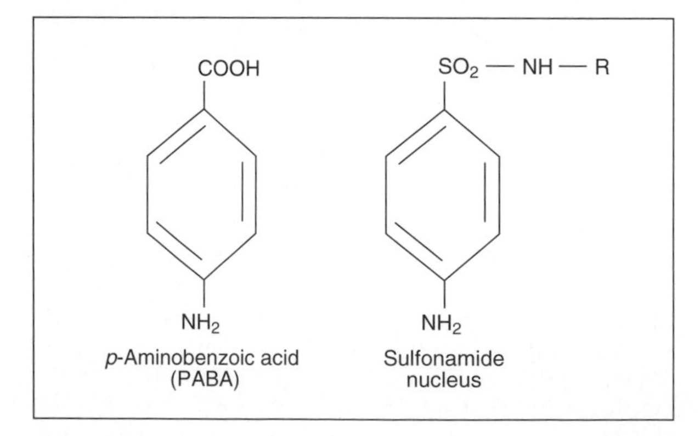

The antimicrobials trimethoprim, chloroguanide, and pyrimethamine limit the action of reductase enzyme. The combination of sulfonamide and trimethoprim is synergistic, producing as much as a tenfold increase in bacteriostatic activity. The protozoan parasites of malaria, *Plasmodium* species, synthesize folic acid; pyrimethamine inhibits its reductase enzyme activity. The drug binds very weakly to the human enzyme.

A combination of trimethoprim and sulfamethoxazole (TMP-SMZ) is especially effective in urinary tract infections caused by gram-negative bacilli and in *Pneumocystis carinii* pneumonia (PCP). All sulfa drugs can produce serious side effects, the most important of which are bone marrow damage and renal failure in the absence of sufficient water. The kidneys and bone marrow may also be impaired as a consequence of an allergic response to the sulfa drugs. Resistance is frequently encountered in long-term sulfa therapy regimens. Trimethoprim is better tolerated than some sulfonamides by adults, but is particularly toxic to fetuses and children and should not be used during pregnancy or for children under 12 years of age.

The antituberculosis drugs isoniazid (INH), ethambutol, and ethionamide inhibit synthesis of essential metabolites, but the details of their action are unclear. Isoniazid, an extremely potent bactericidal agent, is a primary antituberculosis drug generally used in combination with rifampin. INH interferes with the synthesis of mycolic acid, an essential compound in the cell walls of the tuberculosis bacteria. A combination of drugs is usually used to ensure successful treatment since the frequency of drug-resistant mutants is increasing. Isoniazid and ethambutol may be neurotoxic, and ethionamide may be hepatotoxic.

The antituberculosis drug, para-aminosalicylic acid (PAS), has limited bacteriostatic activity against the tubercle bacillus but delays bacterial resistance to streptomycin and isoniazid. Gastrointestinal disturbances and mild-to-severe allergic reactions following PAS administration are not uncommon. Regimens for treating tuberculosis are often complex and are determined both by the severity of disease and the site of the infection.

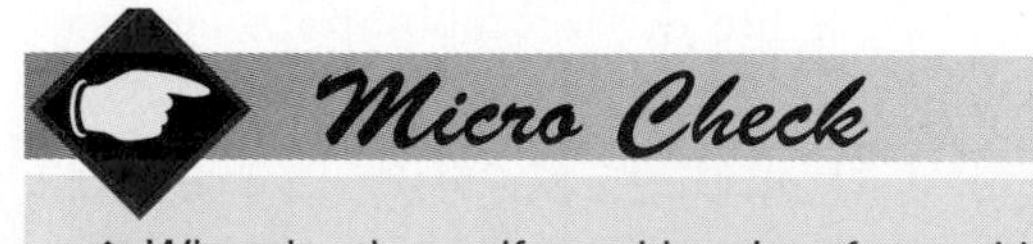

- Why do the sulfonamides interfere with the synthesis of PABA?
- Why is it inadvisable to give children trimethoprim?
- Why is isoniazid often a drug of choice for tuberculosis?

Antimicrobials Having Lesser Known Mechanisms of Action

Quinine, an alkaloid of cinchona bark, has been used for three centuries to treat the protozoan disease malaria; its derivatives chloroquine and primaquine are useful for treatment and prophylaxis of malaria. Although chloroquine inhibits certain enzymes, its activity is directed in part from its interaction with DNA. Primaquine is more effective against the sexual stages and the stages outside the erythrocyte (extra-erythrocytic), but is not indicated in malaria caused by *Plasmodium falciparum*. Although some chloroquine-resistant strains of *Plasmodium falciparum* are sensitive to quinine, other strains encountered along the border between Thailand and Cambodia are resistant to more than one drug.

The parasitic protozoan infections are widely treated by metronidazole, valued for its microbicidal effect on amebas and flagellate protozoans, such as *Entamoeba histolytica* and *Trichomonas vaginalis*. Atovaquone, an analog of ubiquinone, appears to interfere with electron transport in *Plasmodium* species and also inhibits *Pneumocystis carinii* by an unknown mechanism.

Chagas' disease is difficult to treat because the amastigote stage of the protozoan parasite, *Trypanosoma cruzi*, hides in heart muscle cells. Some trypanosomes and plasmodia have developed resistance to antiprotozoal agents, but the mechanisms of drug resistance are unknown.

The most effective antimicrobial against **dermatophytic fungi** is griseofulvin. Produced by fungi of the *Penicillium* genus, it is useful for infections that are not responsive to topical treatment. The drug accumulates in sweat and is deposited onto the epidermis where it acts on the fungal parasite. The drug inhibits cell mitosis and microtubule and cell wall production.

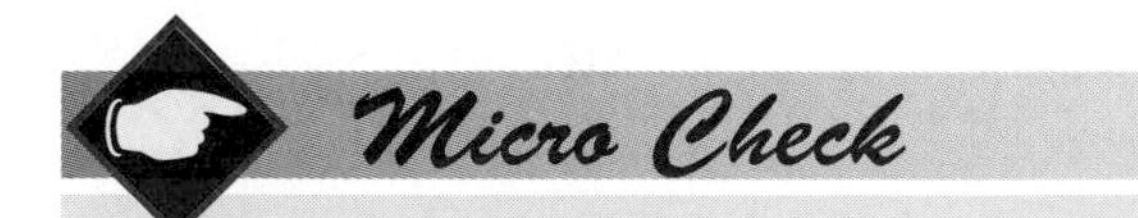

- Name three drugs used to treat protozoan infections.
- Why is Chagas' disease difficult to treat?
- For what type of infections is griseofulvin useful?

LABORATORY METHODS

The goal of drug therapy in infectious disease is to provide the most effective treatment with minimum risk and cost to the patient. This can be accomplished with the aid of the laboratory in identifying the etiologic agent and determining the antimicrobial susceptibilities of the etiologic agent. The patient's clinical symptoms are evaluated, and consideration is given to the pharmacological characteristics of available drugs.

Susceptibility testing to determine which antimicrobial agent will treat an infection is not always required. Some bacteria have a predictable response. For example, group A streptococci and *Neisseria meningitidis* are almost always susceptible to penicillin. The physician may prescribe the drugs without taking a sample for susceptibility testing in the laboratory. Sometimes laboratory tests have not correlated particularly well with actual responses in patients. In one example, *Salmonella typhi* is generally susceptible to cefamandole, a broad-spectrum cephalosporin, in laboratory tests, but it fails to treat the patient's infection.

The laboratory may monitor the effectiveness of antimicrobial therapy by assaying the levels of antibiotics in the patient's serum and by doing culture examinations both during and after drug therapy. The successful treatment of a patient with an antibiotic is the ultimate validity for antimicrobial susceptibility testing.

Antimicrobial Susceptibility Tests

Antimicrobial susceptibility tests are reliable guides for selecting appropriate therapy when the susceptibility of an organism is not predictable. The tests should be performed on pure cultures isolated from the patient. Standardized tests for antibacterial susceptibility are widely used, but current testing for antifungal susceptibility is not yet reliably standardized. If susceptibility tests for particular drugs have not been standardized, it is best not to perform the test because results may be misleading. Each hospital adopts a cost-effective formulary of drugs designed to meet the needs of its patients (Table 22–2).

THE KIRBY-BAUER METHOD

The Kirby-Bauer agar diffusion method is an early method for testing antimicrobial susceptibility of an organism (Fig. 22–4). Mueller-Hinton

Table 22–2
CHOICE OF ANTIMICROBIAL DRUGS FOR SELECTED BACTERIAL, FUNGAL, AND VIRAL PATHOGENS

PATHOGEN	DISEASE	DRUG OF CHOICE
Bacterial pathogens		
Staphylococcus aureus	Staphylococcal infections	
Non-β-lactamase producer		Penicillin
β-lactamase producer		Cefoxitin
Methicillin-resistant		Vancomycin
Streptococcus species	Strep throat, pneumonia, scarlet fever, erysipelas, meningitis	Penicillin
Vibrio cholerae	Cholera	Trimethoprim-sulfamethoxazole or tetracycline
Campylobacter jejuni	Campylobacteriosis	Erythromycin
Neisseria gonorrhoeae	Gonorrhea	Ceftriaxone
Neisseria meningitidis	Meningitis	Penicillin
Escherichia coli	Urinary tract infection	Trimethoprim-sulfamethoxazole
	Bacteremia	Ampicillin/gentamicin
Salmonella species	Typhoid fever, gastroenteritis, septicemia	Ampicillin or chloramphenicol
Shigella species	Shigellosis	Trimethoprim-sulfamethoxazole
Mycobacterium tuberculosis	Tuberculosis	Isoniazid, rifampin, and ethambutol*
Mycobacterium leprae	Leprosy	Dapsone and rifampin*
Mycobacterium avium complex	MAC disease	Rifabutin/ethambutol
Treponema pallidum	Syphilis	Penicillin
Borrelia burgdorferi	Lyme disease	Tetracycline
Rickettsia species	Rocky Mountain spotted fever, typhus fever	Tetracycline
Chlamydia species	Conjunctivitis, urethritis, cervicitis	Tetracycline or erythromycin
Fungal Pathogens		
Coccidioides immitis	Coccidioidomycosis	Amphotericin B
Histoplasma capsulatum	Histoplasmosis	Amphotericin B
Blastomyces dermatiditis	Blastomycosis	Amphotericin B or ketoconazole
Pneumocystis carinii	Pneumonia	Trimethoprim-sulfamethoxazole, pentamidine, or atovaquone
Epidermophyton floccosum	Skin and nail infections	Miconazole
Viruses		
Herpes simplex (Types 1 and 2)	Fever blisters, herpes genitalis	Acyclovir
Epstein-Barr virus	Infectious mononucleosis	Acyclovir
Cytomegalovirus	Encephalitis, systemic disease	Acyclovir
	Retinitis	Foscarnet Ganciclovir
Varicella-zoster virus	Chickenpox, shingles	Acyclovir
Influenza virus A	Influenza	Amantadine
Human immunodeficiency virus	HIV infection, AIDS	Zalcitabine Dideoxyinosine Zidovudine Abacavir
Respiratory syncytial virus	Respiratory tract infections in infants	Ribavirin (aerosol)

* The use of multiple drugs is recommended because of the prevalence of drug-resistant strains.

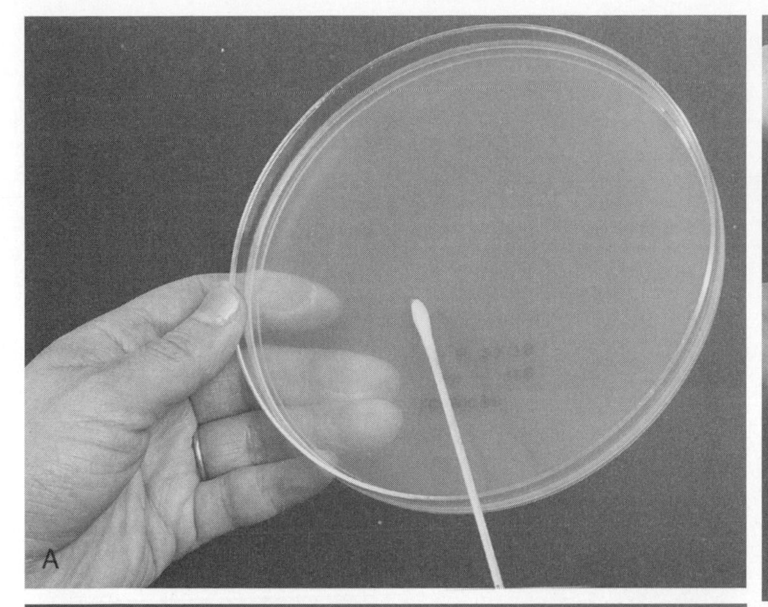

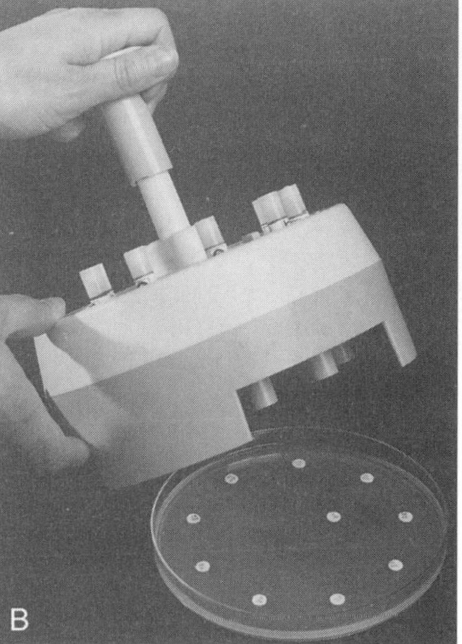

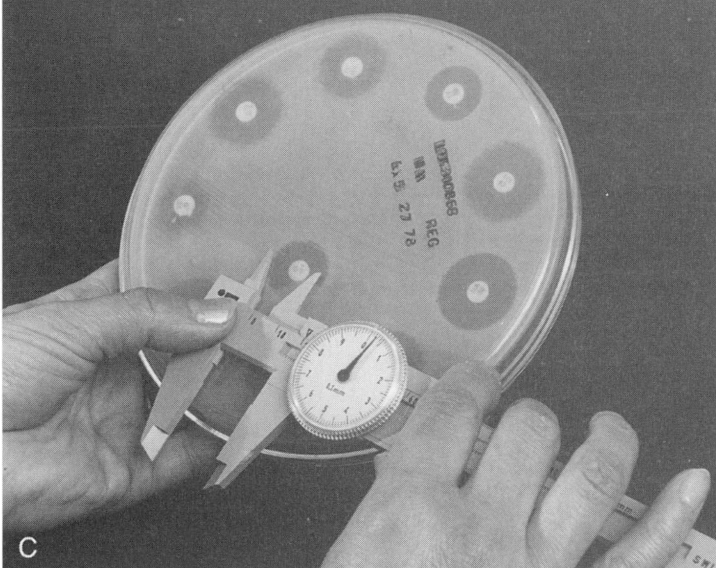

Figure 22–4 ◆ The Kirby-Bauer procedure for antimicrobial susceptibility testing. *A,* The swab is used to inoculate a large plate (150 mm) containing Mueller-Hinton agar. *B,* Antimicrobial disks are dropped onto the plate with a multidisk dispenser. *C,* After incubation the sizes of the zones of inhibition are measured with calipers.

agar, sometimes supplemented with 5 percent sheep red blood cells, is swabbed across its surface with a standardized suspension of a bacterial culture. Antibiotic-containing paper disks are placed on the "lawn" of bacteria using a dispenser or a forceps. After overnight incubation at 35°C, the diameter of each zone of inhibition is measured with calipers; results are recorded in millimeters (see Color Plate 83). A zone-size interpretive chart is consulted to convert the zone diameter into one of three reportable categories: susceptible (S), intermediate (I), or resistant (R) (Table 22–3). The figures on the chart are revised regularly because changes in technology may affect procedures and the standard values.

Susceptibility implies that the organisms should respond favorably to therapeutic doses of the drug. Intermediate zones indicate some susceptibility to therapeutic doses and may be valuable if the patient is allergic to the drugs producing susceptibility. Resistance implies that the usual therapeutic concentrations of antimicrobials would be ineffective. The diameter of the zones of inhibition cannot be directly compared

Table 22–3
ZONE SIZE INTERPRETATIVE CHART FOR THE DISK DIFFUSION SUSCEPTIBILITY TESTING METHOD

ANTIMICROBIAL AGENT	POTENCY OF DISK	INHIBITION ZONE DIAMETER TO NEAREST mm			SELECTED BACTERIAL GROUPS WITH THE SAME ZONE DIAMETER VALUES*
		Resistant	Intermediate	Susceptible	
Amikacin	30 μg	14 or less	15 to 16	17 or more	A, Ent, P, S
Ampicillin					
Enterococci	10 μg	16 or less		17 or more	
Gram-negative rods	10 μg	13 or less	14 to 16	17 or more	Ent, V
Haemophilus	10 μg	18 or less	19 to 21	22 or more	
Staphylococci	10 μg	28 or less		29 or more	
Azithromycin					
Haemophilus	15 μg	10 or less	11 to 12	13 or more	
Staphylococci	15 μg	13 or less	14 to 17	18 or more	Sp
Bacitracin	10 units	8 or less	9 to 12	13 or more	
Cephalothin	30 μg	14 or less	15 to 17	18 or more	Ent, S
Chloramphenicol	30 μg	12 or less	13 to 17	18 or more	A, E, Ent, P, S
Haemophilus	30 μg	25 or less	26 to 28	29 or more	
Clarithromycin					
Haemophilus	15 μg	10 or less	11 to 12	13 or more	
Staphylococci	15 μg	13 or less	14 to 17	18 or more	
Erythromycin	15 μg	13 or less	14 to 22	23 or more	E, S
Gentamicin	10 μg	12 or less	13 to 14	15 or more	A, Ent, P, S
Kanamycin	30 μg	13 or less	14 to 17	18 or more	Ent, S
Methicillin	5 μg	9 or less	10 to 13	14 or more	S
Nafcillin or oxacillin	1 μg	10 or less	11 to 12	13 or more	S
Nalidixic acid	30 μg	13 or less	14 to 18	19 or more	Ent
Neomycin	30 μg	12 or less	13 to 16	17 or more	
Novobiocin	30 μg	17 or less	18 to 21	22 or more	
Penicillin G					
Enterococci	10 units	14 or less		15 or more	
Neisseria gonorrhoeae	10 units	26 or less	27 to 46	47 or more	
Staphylococci	10 units	28 or less		29 or more	
Polymyxin B	300 units	8 or less	9 to 11	12 or more	
Rifampin	5 μg	16 or less	17 to 19	20 or more	E, H, S
Streptomycin	10 μg	11 or less	12 to 14	15 or more	Ent
Sulfonamides	250 or 300 μg	12 or less	13 to 16	17 or more	A, Ent, P, S, V
Tetracycline	30 μg	14 or less	15 to 18	19 or more	A, E, Ent, P, S, V
Haemophilus	30 μg	25 or less	26 to 28	29 or more	
Neisseria gonorrhoeae	30 μg	30 or less	31 to 37	38 or more	
Tobramycin	10 μg	12 or less	13 to 14	15 or more	A, Ent, P, S
Trimethoprim-sulfamethoxazole	1.25/23.75 μg	10 or less	11 to 15	16 or more	A, Ent, H, P, S, V
Vancomycin					
Staphylococci	30 μg			15 or more	
Streptococci, enterococci	30 μg	14 or less	15 to 16	17 or more	

* Symbols: A, *Acinetobacter;* E, enterococci; Ent, enterobacteria; H, *Haemophilus;* P, *Pseudomonas aeruginosa;* S, staphylococci; Sp, *Streptococcus pneumoniae;* V, *Vibrio cholerae.*

Permission to excerpt portions of M100-S9 (Performance Standards for Antimicrobial Susceptibility Testing; Ninth Informational Supplement) has been granted by NCCLS. The interpretive data are valid only if the methodology in NCCLS publication M2-A6 (Performance Standards for Antimicrobial Disk Susceptibility Tests—Sixth Edition; Approved Standard) is followed. NCCLS frequently updates the interpretive tables through new editions of the standard and supplements. Users should refer to the most recent edition. The current standard may be obtained from NCCLS, 940 West Valley Road, Suite 1400, Wayne, PA 19087, U.S.A.

with one another because the rates of diffusion of different drugs and the growth rates of microorganisms vary.

MINIMUM INHIBITORY CONCENTRATION AND MINIMUM BACTERICIDAL CONCENTRATIONS

These tests are valuable for clinical testing of the susceptibility of an organism to antimicrobial drugs. Dilution tests in broth provide a quantitative method for antimicrobial susceptibility testing. Dilution tests require serial twofold dilutions of antibiotics in tubes or wells of plastic plates containing broth and a standardized inoculum (Fig. 22–5). After overnight incubation, tubes or wells are examined for evidence of growth. The lowest concentration of an antimicrobial that inhibits visible growth is reported as the **minimum inhibitory concentration (MIC).**

The **minimum bactericidal concentration (MBC)** is defined as the lowest concentration of an antibiotic that will kill a defined proportion of viable organisms in a bacterial suspension in a specified time period. MBC values are determined by subculturing the clear broths from the MIC test onto an appropriate agar medium. After incubation, the MBC value is the lowest concentration of the antibiotic that fails to produce colonies. The MIC and MBC values may be the same with some bactericidal agents, but in some cases the clear MIC broth will show growth on the agar surface. This quantitative information is important when using particularly toxic antimicrobials and in determining synergism or antagonism between antibiotics. The MIC value is useful for controlling infections in patients with healthy immune systems, but the MBC value is necessary for patients with lowered immune responses, and other serious conditions.

RAPID DETECTION OF BETA-LACTAMASE ACTIVITY

Several methods are available for detecting β-lactamase production directly on colonies of *Staphylococcus aureus, Haemophilus influenzae,* and *Neisseria gonorrhoeae.* In one method, a paper disk

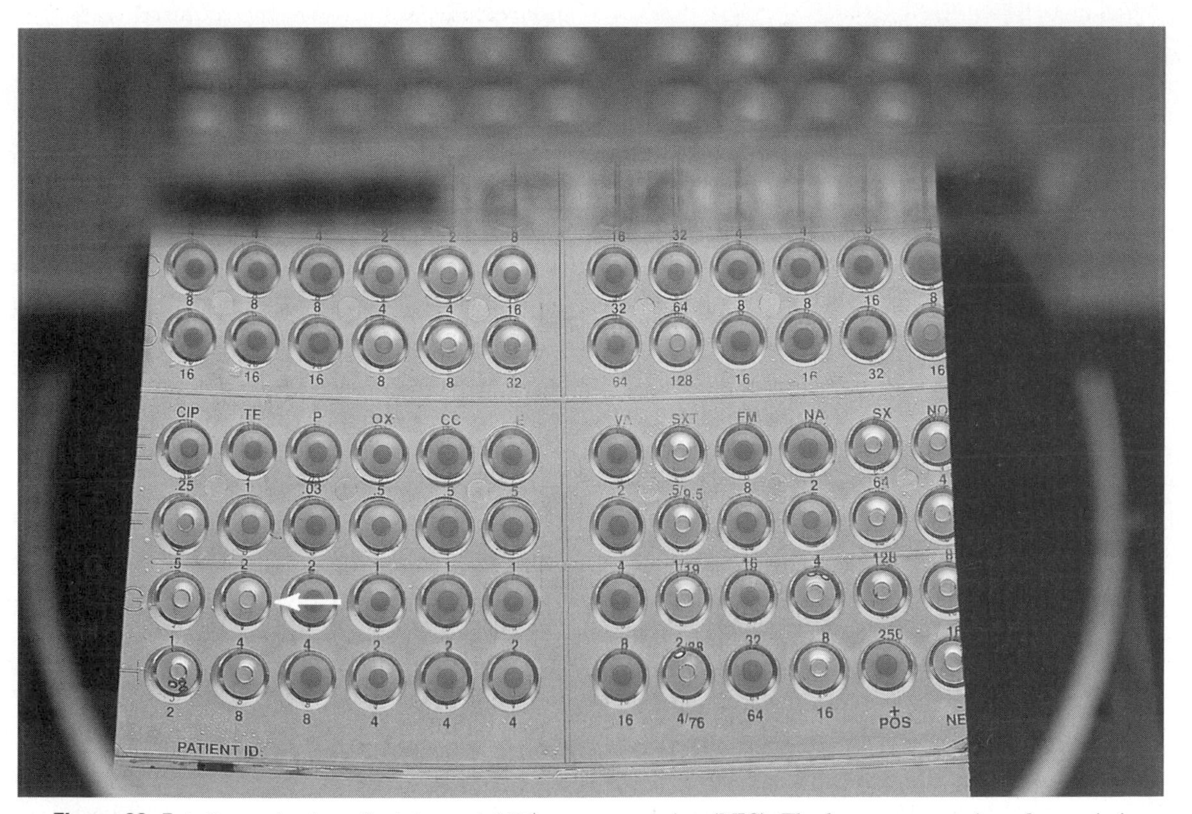

Figure 22–5 ◆ Determination of minimum inhibitory concentration (MIC). The least concentration of an antimicrobial agent inhibiting visible growth is reported in μg/ml as the MIC (*arrow*). The white or cloudy wells show growth of the organism. The dark wells show the concentrations of the antimicrobial agent that inhibit growth.

containing nitrocefin (in the cephalosporin family of antimicrobials) and a dye is moistened (see Color Plate 84). A small amount of a bacterial colony is transferred to the disk. A color change to brownish red indicates a positive result for presence of β-lactamase. The test takes up to 10 minutes for most bacteria or 60 minutes for staphylococci. A positive result confirms the resistance of the microorganism to penicillin, ampicillin, and amoxicillin. Rapid detection of β-lactamase activity assists the physician in prescribing appropriate antimicrobials.

A cefoxitin disk induction test has been designed to detect inducible β-lactamases. Inducible β-lactamase production may be detected in gram-negative bacilli using this disk. The test requires no special equipment and is recommended for certain bacteria that do not ferment sugars, such as *Pseudomonas aeruginosa,* and *Serratia, Morganella, Proteus, Providencia,* and *Enterobacter* species. The information obtained from the cefoxitin-disk method should be included with the results from antimicrobial susceptibility tests.

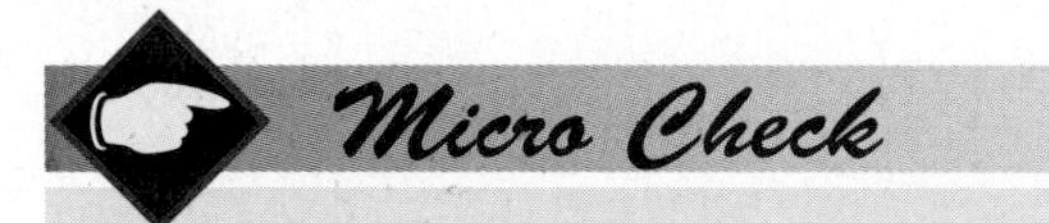

- Define MIC and identify how this value is obtained.
- Define MBC and identify how this value is obtained.
- Why is β-lactamase testing valuable?

RESISTANCE TO ANTIMICROBIAL AGENTS

One of the problems surrounding the widespread use of antimicrobial agents is the development of drug-resistant strains of microorganisms. Resistant strains of some pathogens were isolated in the 1970s, but the problem escalated to frightening dimensions during the 1990s. The occurrence of resistant strains varies globally and even in different regions of the United States. Particularly devastating pathogenic strains of bacteria are resistant to many drugs at once, with the result that the physician has fewer drug choices for treating these diseases.

There is a strong association between the magnitude of the use of antimicrobial agents and the emergence of drug resistance. Both physicians and patients share responsibility for the overuse or abuse of antimicrobial agents. Physicians often prescribe a drug based on their own clinical experience without conducting an antimicrobial susceptibility test. Antimicrobial drugs may be prescribed for a viral infection for which most antimicrobials have no effect.

Multidrug-resistant strains of enterococci present a special challenge to physicians. Enterococci, such as *Enterococcus faecalis* and *E. faecium,* are normal intestinal inhabitants. They sometimes cause urinary tract infections, bacteremias, and surgical wound infections. Vancomycin has been the drug of choice for infections caused by strains of enterococci that are resistant to β-lactam drugs, but many strains are now vancomycin-resistant. The vancomycin-resistant enterococci (VRE) have components in their cell walls which block the action of vancomycin.

The behavior of the patient is very important in reducing the likelihood of survival of drug-resistant strains. Behaviors that may be considered risky in this regard include the decision to stop taking the drug for the prescribed length of time, or by not taking the required daily doses. People sometimes purchase drugs in countries where prescriptions are not required or are not carefully monitored. These people self-medicate and sometimes stockpile antibiotics from previous infections for later use. There is no guarantee that the drug's activity is still high, or that they are using the appropriate drug for their current infection, or that they even need the drug. These practices are not based on an understanding of the antimicrobial susceptibility of the infecting organism. The person faces a risk that an infection is not treated appropriately, that the medication used is unnecessary or dangerous, and that the infection will not clear. In fact, a worse infection by a drug-resistant strain of a microorganism may be selected by these practices.

Animal-rearing practices also contribute to the rise of drug-resistant strains of microorganisms. The addition of antimicrobial agents into livestock feed enhances growth of cattle, pigs, and poultry. However, the feed introduces antimicrobial agents into soil, water, and air. This practice provides opportunities for resistant strains to develop and to spread to human populations.

Indiscriminate use of antibiotics by humans or in animals is a selective pressure that promotes the survival of resistant strains of organisms while killing the antibiotic-sensitive organisms. The range of antimicrobial drugs available and effective to treat disease becomes smaller and smaller.

MECHANISMS OF MICROBIAL RESISTANCE

Microorganisms have acquired several survival strategies over the years. Resistance sometimes occurs when a mutation permits expression of a resistance gene naturally present on a cell's chromosome. Resistance to quinolones, rifampin, and cephalosporin develop as chromosomal changes that are not transferred by gene transfer factors. Other resistance mechanisms develop as a result of gene transfers, such as by conjugation or transformation, from one organism that is resistant to another that is susceptible (Chapter 7). Transferred genes may encode for resistance factors that decrease drug entry into the cell of the microorganism, inactivate drugs, alter antibiotic targets, or produce substitute enzymes which are insensitive to the drug being administered. Penicillin-resistant strains of *Streptococcus pneumoniae* are able to alter penicillin-binding sites after acquiring resistance genes. β-lactamase–producing strains of *Staphylococcus aureus* and *Neisseria gonorrhoeae* inactivate penicillins and cephalosporins.

FOCAL POINT

The Promiscuous Enterococci

Conjugation was once thought to be the most limited process of gene transfer. Recent laboratory studies indicate, however, that some bacteria are quite indiscriminate in their choices for mating. The opportunities for promiscuous gene transfer exist in many natural environments. It is virtually impossible to duplicate complex environments, like soil or the gastrointestinal tract, in the laboratory, so the degree of promiscuity among most bacteria may never be known. What is known is that the conjugative transposons play a major role in antibiotic-resistance gene flux. Enterococcal pathogens, in particular, have been shown to have a large host range. The emergence of vancomycin-resistant enterococci (VRE) has been of major concern in hospitals throughout the United States. The selective pressures from large-scale antibiotic use favors the emergence of resistant strains. Persistent intestinal carriage of vancomycin-resistant *Enterococcus faecium* (VREF) appears to be a significant risk factor for bacteremia, particularly in immunocompromised patients. The survival capacity of enterococci in the hospital environment and poor compliance of hospital personnel in proper handwashing technique are additional factors in VRE nosocomial infections. A minimum of a 30-second handwash with soap is necessary to eliminate the pathogens.

Unfortunately, a single drug resistance may lead to multiple-drug resistance even when only one drug is administered over a period of time. A bacterium may accumulate new genes that code for additional resistance factors or that permit those already present to be expressed.

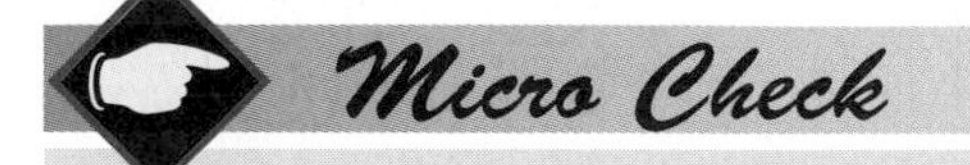

- Name three behaviors of people that may put them at risk of drug-resistant infections.
- Name two practices that a physician could use to avoid drug-resistant infections in patients.
- How might gene transfer processes lead to drug resistance in a bacterium?

Understanding Microbiology

1. Name five natural antimicrobial agents.
2. Name four genera of microorganisms from which major antibiotics are derived.
3. Give two examples of drug combinations that demonstrate synergistic activity.
4. What is the basis of reporting antimicrobial susceptibility tests as susceptible (S), intermediate (I), or resistant (R)?
5. Define minimum inhibitory concentration (MIC) and minimum bactericidal concentration (MBC) and identify their importance in clinical medicine.

Applying Microbiology

6. A prominent toy manufacturer has included a broad-spectrum antimicrobial agent in its plastic toys for infants and toddlers. The drug is embedded in plastic or synthetic fibers during manufacturing. A leading infectious disease specialist has registered his disapproval to using antibiotics in this manner. What objections do you have, if any? Prepare a written explanation of your objections or why you applaud this new material for toys.

Unit 7

Environmental and Food Microbiology

Chapter 23

Microbiology of the Environment

Chapter Outline

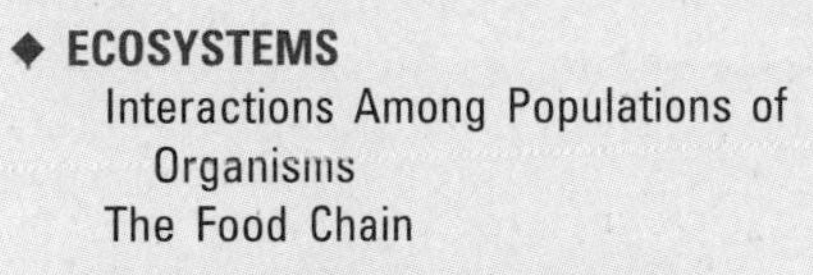

- **ECOSYSTEMS**
  - Interactions Among Populations of Organisms
  - The Food Chain
- **ENERGY FLOW IN ECOSYSTEMS**
- **BIOGEOCHEMICAL CYCLES**
  - The Water Cycle
  - The Oxygen Cycle
  - The Carbon Cycle
  - The Nitrogen Cycle
  - The Sulfur Cycle
  - Cycles of Other Elements
- **TERRESTRIAL ENVIRONMENTS**
  - Microbial Populations of Soil
- **AQUATIC ENVIRONMENTS**
  - Freshwater Environments
  - Marine Environments
- **DRINKING WATER**
  - Methods of Water Purification
  - Microbiological Examination of Water
- **SAFE DISPOSAL OF SEWAGE AND WASTEWATER**
  - Preliminary Treatment
  - Primary Treatment
  - Secondary Treatment
  - Tertiary Treatment
- **HUMAN INTERVENTION IN ECOSYSTEMS**

Learning Objectives

After you have read this chapter, you should be able to:

1. Describe three types of symbiotic relationships involving microorganisms.
2. List specific roles of microorganisms in recycling carbon, nitrogen, and sulfur.
3. Name three major methods used by cities to purify drinking water.
4. Describe methods used in the microbiological examination of water.
5. Describe preliminary, primary, secondary, and tertiary treatments of sewage.
6. Discuss the consequences of human intervention in ecosystems.

The benefits derived from microorganisms on Earth vastly exceed their capacity for causing harm. The role of microorganisms as infectious agents, able to cause massive destruction of humans, animals, or plants, continues to account for much medical research and publicity. Yet, the diverse and abundant population of microorganisms in our environment works quietly as they recycle chemical elements necessary for our very existence. Human activities increasingly are disturbing the balance that permits humans to coexist with plants, animals, and microorganisms. The disappearance or displacement of plants and animals is easily seen, but the assault on microbial populations of the environment is difficult to measure. Some microorganisms, like more resourceful animals and adaptable plants, are surviving in new habitats, but others are probably endangered, because the answers from environmental microbiology are still developing.

ECOSYSTEMS

Ecosystems consist of the **biotic** (living) and **abiotic** (nonliving) components of local environments. The interactions of the biotic and abiotic factors in ecosystems make up the study of **ecology.** Certain plants, animals, and microorganisms are native or indigenous to local environments. Others may be classified as visitors or immigrants to a geographic area.

The physical and chemical properties of terrestrial and aquatic environments determine both the types and numbers of microorganisms present in ecosystems. Species of *Clostridium, Bacillus, Pseudomonas, Nitrobacter, Nitrosomonas,* and many other bacteria and fungi are indigenous to soils. Other microorganisms, including algae, cyanobacteria, protozoa, and bacteria live in moist soils, and fresh water or marine environments.

Some microorganisms are native to exotic environments, such as the hydrothermal vents at the ocean bottom, where temperatures may be as high as 150°C. Thermophilic tubeworms, sea anemones, mussels, clams, and bacteria coexist at these vent regions (Fig. 23–1). All these species probably depend on the chemosynthetic action of the sulfur-metabolizing bacteria to produce food rather than photosynthesis, because sunlight does not reach these depths.

The location of a particular organism and its interactions with other forms of life occupying the same space are called an **ecological niche.** A community consists of the plants, animals, and microorganisms found in that niche. The numbers and types of organisms in a community are affected by changes in the environment. Communities inhabited by more diverse types of life forms tend to be more stable than those containing fewer species.

Interactions Among Populations of Organisms

The organisms in a particular environment are constantly interacting with one another. A close association existing between two organisms within a niche is called **symbiosis.** Symbiotic relationships may be beneficial to one or both organisms or lead to competition for available nutrients. Sometimes one organism does harm to another organism as a result of a close association.

MUTUALISM

Mutualism is a type of symbiosis in which each organism benefits from the relationship. There are many examples of mutualism in nature, but one of the most unique is that which exists between an alga or a cyanobacterium and a fungus.

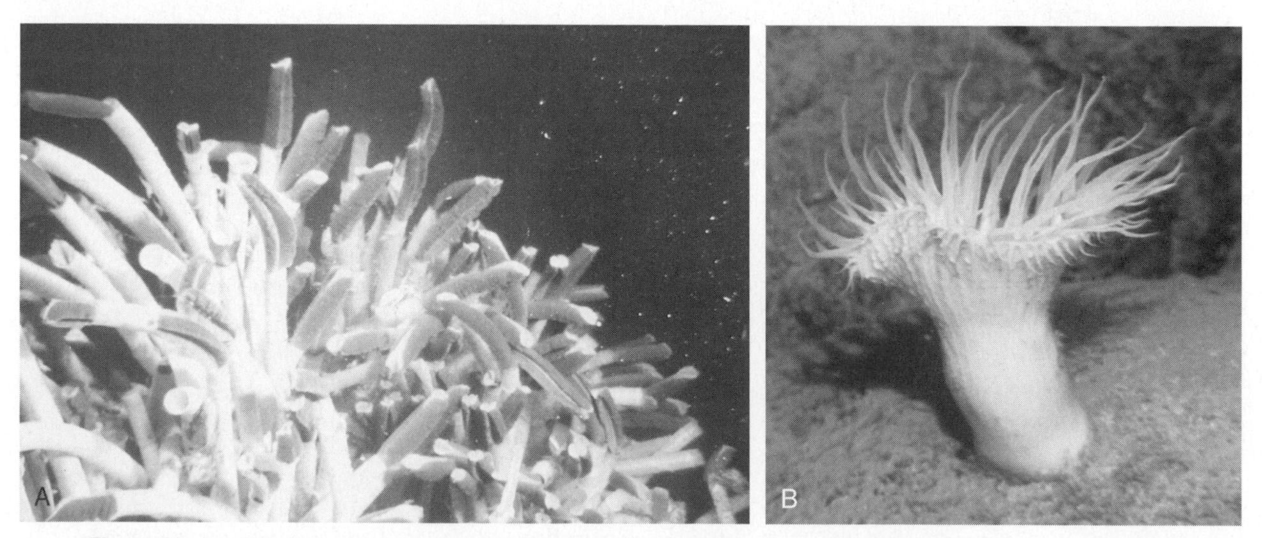

Figure 23–1 ◆ Life forms flourishing near hydrothermal vents on the floor of the ocean more than a mile below the ocean surface are in an ecosystem where the primary producers are bacteria. *A,* Tube worms. *B,* Sea anemones.

The component organisms, known as **lichens,** grow on rocks, on the bark of trees, or in arid soils. Lichens can survive in Arctic regions where they are important food sources for animals.

A typical lichen consists of a layer of fungal mycelia between layers of algal or cyanobacterial cells (Fig. 23–2). The algae or cyanobacteria supply nutrients for the fungi in exchange for the support, moisture, and protection by fungal hyphae. Fungi may absorb inorganic nutrients required by both partners from rocks, bark, or soil (see Color Plates 85 and 86).

The relationships between some plants and nitrogen-fixing bacteria are also examples of mutualism. Species of *Rhizobium* invade root tissue of legumes, such as soy beans, clover, and alfalfa, causing roots to develop **nodules** surrounding and containing the bacteria. Bacteria of the genus *Frankia* induce similar nodules in a variety of nonleguminous plants which grow well on marginal soils. *Rhizobium* and *Frankia* reduce atmospheric nitrogen (N_2) to ammonia (NH_3) by a process known as **nitrogen fixation** (Fig. 23–3). The plants are able to use NH_3 to synthesize essential molecules. The legumes provide nutrients for the bacteria and help to control O_2 levels in nodules.

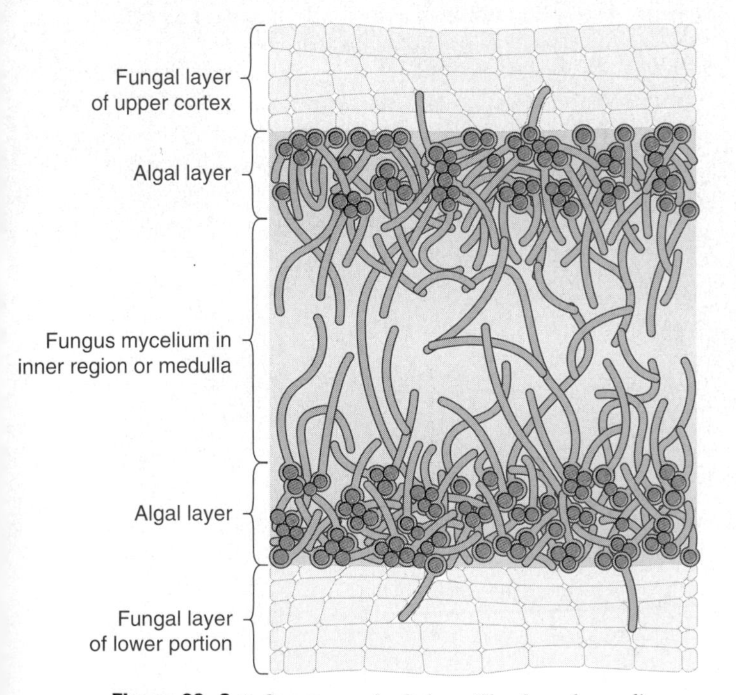

Figure 23–2 ◆ Structure of a lichen. The fungal mycelia provide a support system for the algae. Survival under favorable conditions is possible by a cooperative effort.

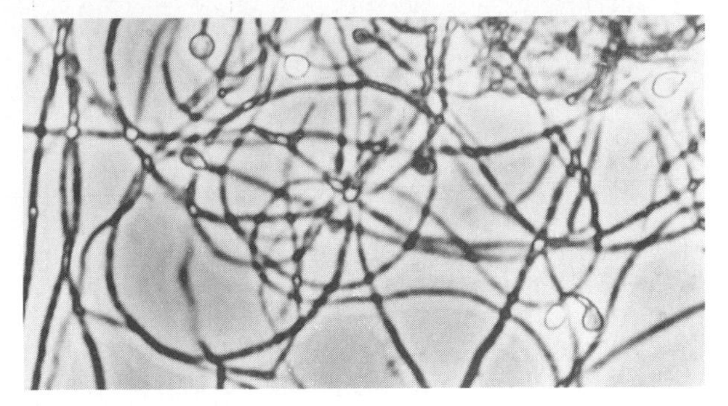

Figure 23–3 ◆ Phase-contrast photomicrograph of *Frankia alni* showing vesicles in which N_2 fixation occurs.

A **mycorrhizal** (fungus-plant root) association of certain fungi with plants is formed when hyphae enter spaces between root cells or penetrate plant cells. Mycorrhizae occur more frequently when roots have large reserves of carbohydrates. Mycorrhizal roots take up nitrogen, phosphorus, and potassium with greater ease than do fungus-free roots, improving the growth of the plant. Some protection may be afforded plants from soil pathogens by this form of mutualism.

Sometimes the partners in a mutualistic association become so dependent on one another that neither can live without the other. The relationship between termites, which cannot digest cellulose in the wood they ingest, and the protozoan flagellates belonging to the genus *Trichonympha,* which have a cellulase enzyme, is one example (Fig. 23–4). The protozoa live in the digestive

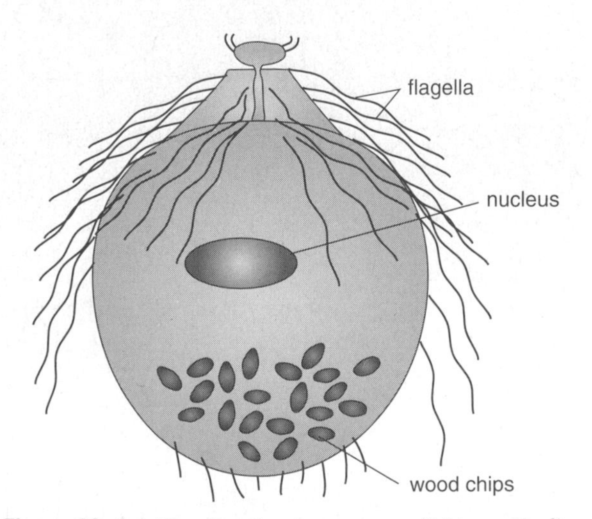

Figure 23–4 ◆ The flagellated protozoan *Trichonympha* lives in the hindgut of a termite.

tract of the termites digesting cellulose, providing the termite host with sugars, while the termite protects *Trichonympha* from predators.

COMMENSALISM

Commensalism is a form of symbiosis in which one partner benefits and the other one appears to be unaffected. Many microorganisms live on the surface of human skin in a commensal relationship. *Staphylococcus epidermidis* and *Propionibacterium acnes* feed on nutrients supplied by the sebaceous glands. In most individuals, the bacteria live in harmony with their hosts. Only in adolescence when hormonal activity causes overproduction of **sebum,** the secretion of sebaceous glands, do the numbers of *P. acnes* become troublesome. The uncontrolled growth of *P. acnes* may be associated with the skin disease acne vulgaris.

PARASITISM

In parasitism, one of the partners in a symbiotic relationship is harmed by the association. The organism responsible for damage is called a **parasite** because it feeds on tissue or products of the host. Plants, animals, and microorganisms may act as hosts to parasites.

The Food Chain

Most species of an ecosystem are not **symbionts** (symbiotic partners), but are nonetheless dependent on activities of other inhabitants. Each member is a part of a **food chain** consisting of different feeding or **trophic** levels. Each organism is in turn both a predator of smaller organisms and a victim of larger predators (Fig. 23–5). Food chains illustrate the relationships and dependence of organisms in ecosystems, but in reality, food chains form **food webs** in which members of more than one food chain interact with one another.

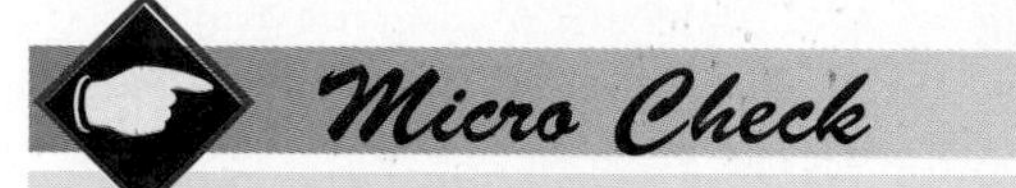

- How are lichens able to survive in nutrient-depleted soils?
- How is the relationship between *Trichonympha* and termites successful?
- What is the definition of commensalism?

ENERGY FLOW IN ECOSYSTEMS

Energy, derived from the sun, is the major source of energy in all ecosystems, with the exception of the hydrothermal vent. The organisms of an ecosystem can be divided into (1) **producers,** (2) **consumers,** and (3) **decomposers.** Producers convert energy from the sun into chemical energy and reducing power by the process of photosynthesis. Producers contain special pigments, such as **chlorophylls,** which absorb light energy to start the process (Chapter 6).

The primary producers of terrestrial ecosystems are the vascular plants. Algae and cyanobacteria make up the producers of aquatic ecosystems. Consumers of both ecosystems require preformed food. **Herbivores** feed on green

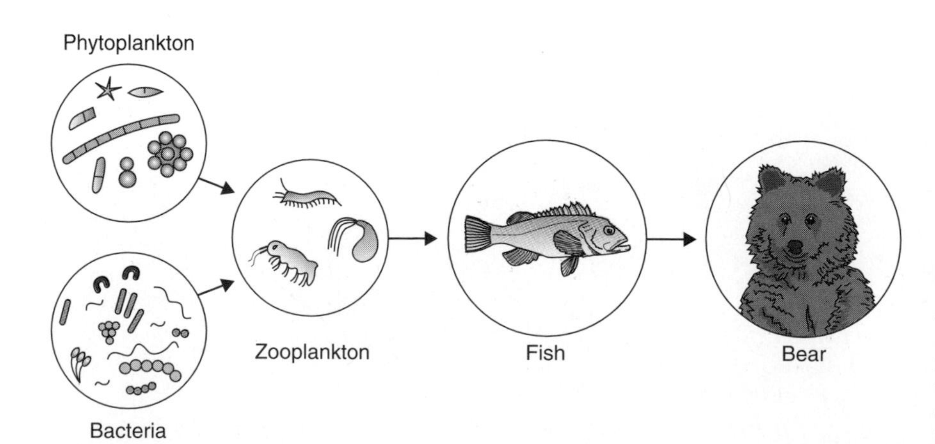

Figure 23–5 ◆ A sample food chain showing primary producers (phytoplankton and some bacteria), primary consumers (zooplankton and other bacteria), a secondary consumer (fish), and a tertiary consumer (bear).

plants; **carnivores** feed on other animals. **Omnivores** eat both plants and animals. **Decomposers** contribute to energy flow by breaking down waste materials of living organisms and the **detritus** (remains) of dead organisms. Fungi, bacteria, some arthropods, and earthworms are the major decomposers.

Energy flows through an ecosystem as consumers feed on producers or other consumers. Some energy is lost as heat during transformations of one form of energy to another. Furthermore, some energy is lost between trophic levels of food chains. Energy from the sun is an essential source for sustaining most life on Earth.

BIOGEOCHEMICAL CYCLES

All forms of life require water and a source of energy. In addition, oxygen (O), carbon (C), nitrogen (N), sulfur (S), phosphorus (P), and iron (Fe) are major nutrients needed to support life. These resources are recycled to maintain life. The biochemical reactions cycling essential elements and the resources contained in the abiotic (nonliving) environment constitute biogeochemical cycles. Microorganisms play major roles in the biogeochemical cycles.

The Water Cycle

Most of us probably consider water a renewable resource because it evaporates and returns as rain or snow (Fig. 23–6). Some water enters the atmosphere as it is lost from leaves and stems of plants by the process of **transpiration.** Most rain or snow falls into the ocean basins. Some water flows from land to the sea as runoff or penetrates soil to establish the ground water. Water vapor is carried by currents from the ocean basins to land where it precipitates as rain, snow, or hail.

Waters of streams, rivers, lakes, and even oceans have become increasingly polluted with organic toxins, raw sewage, industrial wastes, and acid rain. Polluted water causes aquatic organisms to die and interrupts food chains.

The Oxygen Cycle

The cycling of oxygen occurs when gaseous oxygen (O_2) is generated by photosynthetic organisms and consumed by aerobic organisms in the process of respiration. Plants, algae, and cyanobacteria are the primary producers of O_2 on our planet, and animals are the primary consumers of O_2.

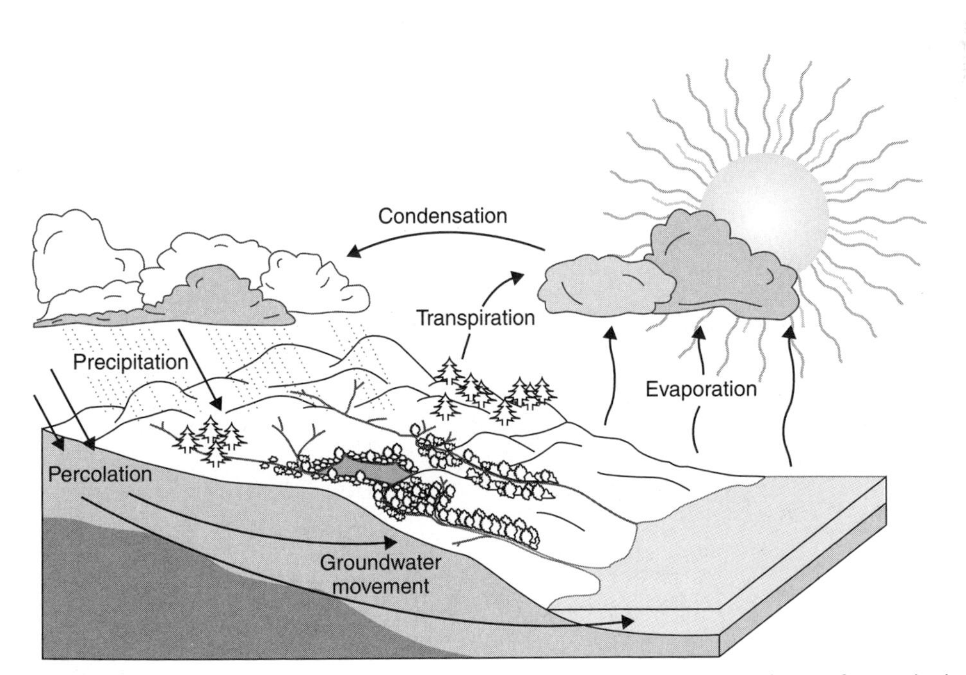

Figure 23–6 ◆ The global water cycle showing directions of precipitation, evaporation, and transpiration.

The Carbon Cycle

Atmospheric and dissolved carbon dioxide (CO_2) are used by primary producers to manufacture nutrients. Vascular plants are the most important producers on land, but **phytoplankton** consisting of free-floating microscopic surface algae are the major producers in aquatic environments. Consumers ingest nutrients and digest them down to raw materials that are converted, in turn, to life-supporting molecules. All aerobic organisms consume O_2 and produce CO_2, returning it to the atmosphere. Smaller amounts of CO_2 are returned to the atmosphere by the weathering of rocks.

The complex carbon-containing molecules synthesized by consumers are broken down by decomposers when the organisms die. It takes many metabolic types and large numbers of microorganisms to completely oxidize the organic compounds. Accumulations of undecomposed organic matter are known as **peat.** Over a period of years, deposits of peat have been transformed into coal. Methane and natural oil are also products of incomplete oxidation of carbon compounds. Interrelationships of the water, oxygen,

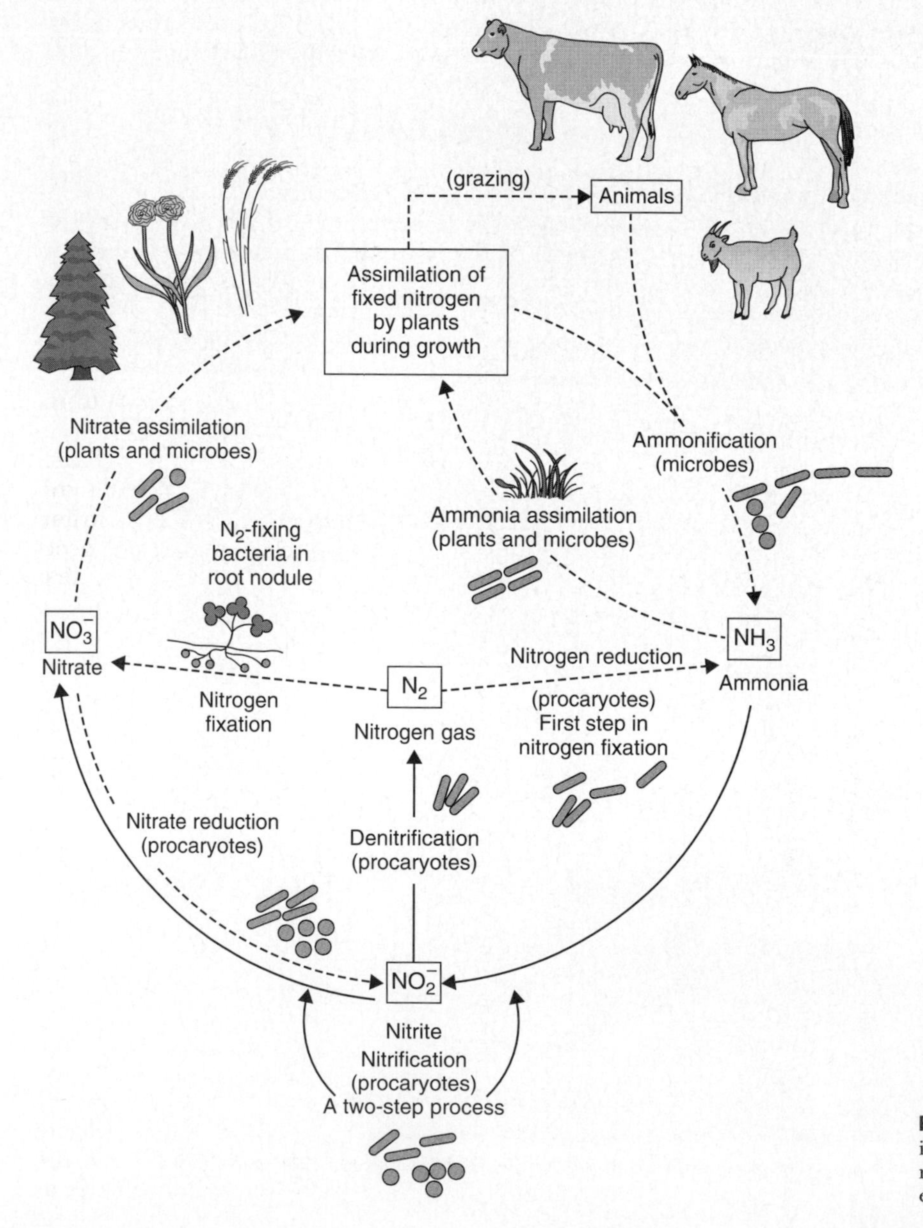

Figure 23–7 ◆ The nitrogen cycle involves animals, plants, and bacteria to keep different nitrogen molecules in continuous circulation.

and carbon cycles are a constant theme in studying life processes, but cycling of other elements is more complex.

The Nitrogen Cycle

Most forms of life cannot use atmospheric nitrogen (N_2) and require N_2 combined with other elements. Approximately 80 percent of the atmosphere is composed of gaseous N_2. Only volcanic disturbances, lightning, and some bacteria can break the triple covalent bonds ($N \equiv N$) of atmospheric N_2 and produce the nitrogenous compounds required by living organisms. About one billion tons of nitrogen gas per year are transformed by the nitrogen cycle. Microorganisms are essential for cycling different forms of nitrogen through four stages: nitrogen fixation, ammonification, nitrification, and denitrification (Fig. 23–7).

NITROGEN FIXATION

Atmospheric nitrogen gas (N_2) is reduced to ammonia (NH_3) or oxidized to nitrate (NO_3^-) by nitrogen fixation processes occurring in bacteria. Some free-living soil bacteria are able to independently fix N_2. Several species of *Clostridium, Azotobacter, Klebsiella, Enterobacter, Citrobacter,* and *Bacillus* are able to produce nitrogenous compounds by a **nonsymbiotic** nitrogen fixation process. Species of *Rhizobium* and *Frankia* fix N_2 only by a symbiotic relationship with roots or stems of certain plants. Nodules develop on the plant roots indicating where N_2-fixing bacteria are located. The bacteria convert N_2 to NO_3^- for improving plant growth (Fig. 23–8). The symbiotic N_2-fixing bacteria are much more efficient in fixing atmospheric N_2 than are the free-living N_2-fixing bacteria.

AMMONIFICATION

Animal wastes and dead animals and plants have organic nitrogen compounds such as proteins and nucleic acids. These organic nitrogen molecules are decomposed to ammonia by soil bacteria and fungi. One of the common waste molecules is urea which is converted by the urease enzyme of microorganisms to ammonia and carbon dioxide gases:

$$\underset{\text{Urea}}{O{=}C(NH_2)_2} + \underset{\text{Water}}{H_2O} \xrightarrow{\text{urease}} \underset{\text{Ammonia}}{2\,NH_3} + \underset{\text{Carbon dioxide}}{CO_2}$$

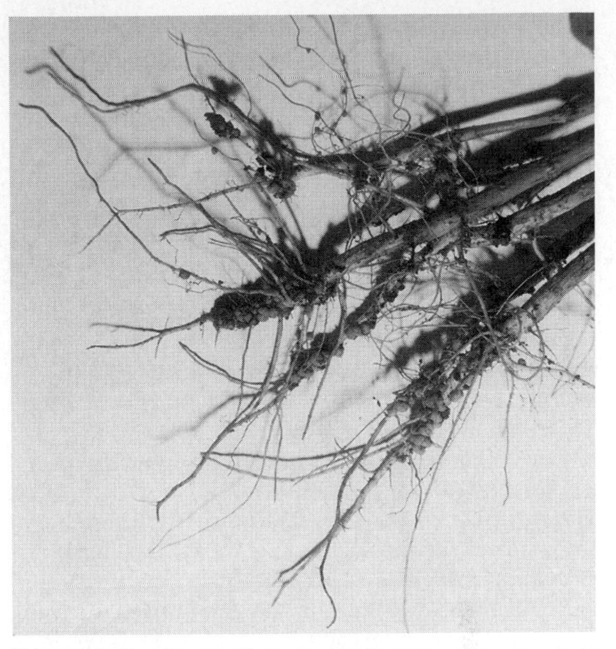

Figure 23–8 ♦ Root nodules on black-eyed pea roots contain abundant N_2-fixing bacteria.

NITRIFICATION

Other bacterial species convert ammonia to nitrite (NO_2^-) and then to nitrate (NO_3^-) in a process called **nitrification.** Gram-negative bacteria belonging to the genera *Nitrosomonas* in soil and *Nitrosococcus* in the ocean are major contributors to the conversion of NH_3 to NO_2^-. The process occurs in the presence of oxygen. The first step produces nitrite or nitrous acid:

$$\underset{\text{Ammonia}}{2NH_3} + \underset{\text{Oxygen}}{3O_2} \longrightarrow \underset{\text{Nitrous acid}}{2HNO_2} + \underset{\text{Water}}{2H_2O}$$

In a second step, nitrites are converted to nitrates (NO_3^-) or nitric acid by gram-negative bacilli belonging to the genus *Nitrobacter* in soil and *Nitrococcus* in marine environments. Nitrates are a major nutrient source of nitrogen for plants.

$$\underset{\text{Nitrous acid}}{2HNO_2} + \underset{\text{Oxygen}}{O_2} \longrightarrow \underset{\text{Nitric acid}}{2HNO_3}$$

DENITRIFICATION

Soil nitrate is converted to nitrogen gas by anaerobic denitrifying bacteria. Many obligate and some facultative anaerobic bacteria use the nitrate ion as a final electron acceptor. Species of

Pseudomonas, Micrococcus, Thiobacillus, Serratia, and *Achromobacter* are able to convert NO_3^- to gaseous N_2. A major cause of nitrogen depletion in soils is a **denitrification** process in which NO_3^- is converted to N_2 through a series of intermediate products:

$$\underset{\text{Nitrate}}{2NO_3^-} \longrightarrow \underset{\text{Nitrite}}{2NO_2^-} \longrightarrow \underset{\text{Nitric oxide}}{2NO} \longrightarrow \underset{\text{Nitrous oxide}}{N_2O} + \underset{\text{Gaseous nitrogen}}{N_2}$$

Denitrification replenishes atmospheric N_2 by removing NO_3^- and NO_2^- from soil and bodies of fresh water.

One increasingly harmful environmental problem results from the pollution of lakes and rivers with fertilizer. The increased use of nitrate and ammonium fertilizers has exceeded the denitrifying capacity of most soils. The subsequent run-off of NH_3 and NO_3^- into streams and lakes fertilizes the water, causing thick mats of algal blooms. When the algae die, the abundance of dead material promotes rapid bacterial growth while consuming most of the dissolved oxygen gas. Fish cannot survive in oxygen-poor aquatic environments, resulting in "fish kills." The oxygen depletion in high nitrogen water with its consequences is called **eutrophication** (see Color Plate 87).

The Sulfur Cycle

A variety of microorganisms are responsible for reduction and oxidation reactions in the cycling of sulfur compounds and elemental sulfur (S). Sulfur is found in the amino acids methionine, cystine, and cysteine and in other molecules. Sulfur that is released from protein breakdown is converted to hydrogen sulfide (H_2S). However, plants require sulfur in the oxidized form of sulfate (SO_4^{2-}).

ANAEROBIC SULFUR REDUCTION AND OXIDATION

Sulfate ions (SO_4^{2-}) may be reduced to hydrogen sulfide (H_2S) by anaerobic soil microorganisms in a process analogous to nonsymbiotic nitrogen fixation. The production of large amounts of hydrogen sulfide (H_2S) often occurs in the blackened bottom sediments of water bodies, where the "rotten egg" odor of H_2S is unmistakable. H_2S can be oxidized to elemental sulfur by the photosynthetic green and purple bacteria belonging to the genera *Chlorobium* and *Chromatium* in anaerobic environments.

$$\underset{\text{Hydrogen sulfide}}{2H_2S} + \underset{\text{Carbon dioxide}}{CO_2} \xrightarrow{\text{light}} \underset{\text{Carbohydrate}}{(CH_2O)} + H_2O + \underset{\text{Elemental sulfur}}{2S}$$

AEROBIC SULFUR OXIDATION

Under aerobic conditions, elemental sulfur is rapidly oxidized to sulfates (SO_4^{2-}) by photosynthetic bacteria and acidophilic bacteria such as *Thiobacillus thiooxidans.*

$$\underset{\text{Sulfur}}{2S} + \underset{\text{Water}}{2H_2O} + \underset{\text{Oxygen gas}}{3O_2} \longrightarrow \underset{\text{Sulfuric acid}}{2H_2SO_4}$$

The sulfuric acid breaks down to sulfates for cellular metabolism or may be excreted into the soil or water as H_2S.

Cycles of Other Elements

Microorganisms are also responsible for cycling of other elements, including phosphorus (P) and iron (Fe), to produce diverse elements used by living organisms. The complete conversions from organic to inorganic molecules represent a cooperative effort of a community of microorganisms.

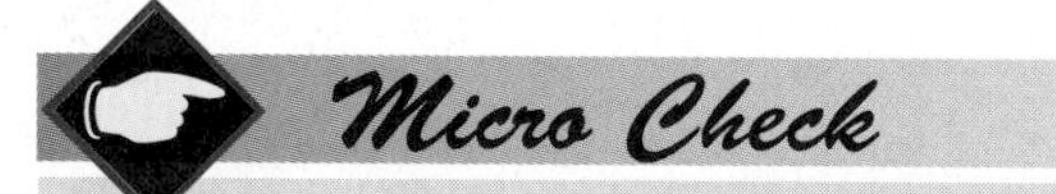

- What organisms are the producers in terrestrial and aquatic environments?
- What is the eutrophication process?
- What forms of nitrogen are used by living organisms?

TERRESTRIAL ENVIRONMENTS

Soil is the product of physical, chemical, and biological processes. Soil scientists divide soil into four layers called **horizons** (Fig. 23–9). The A horizon, or top layer, has an abundance of undecomposed material; it contains a variety of microorganisms. Most minerals and organic matter, known as **humus,** accumulate in the subsoil making up horizon B. The soil base or horizon C originates from underlying bedrock. Horizon D contains unweathered bedrock. There are many variations in soil and the development of a typical profile may take hundreds of years.

Microbial Populations of Soil

The numbers and types of microorganisms present in soil at any one time are dependent on

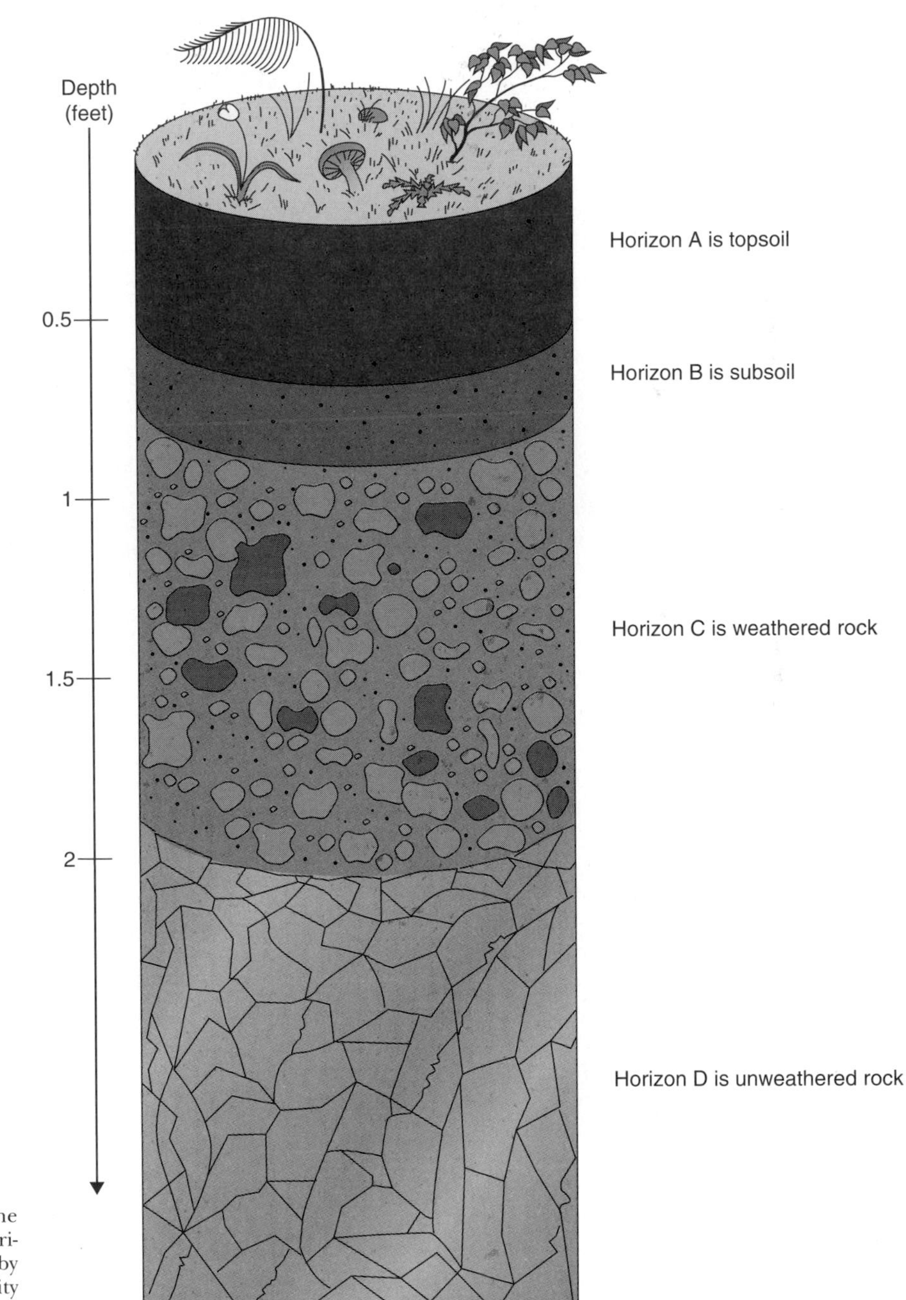

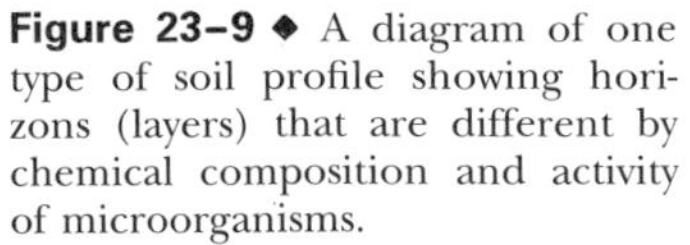
Figure 23–9 ◆ A diagram of one type of soil profile showing horizons (layers) that are different by chemical composition and activity of microorganisms.

Table 23–1
APPROXIMATE NUMBERS OF MICROORGANISMS IN SOIL

TYPE OF ORGANISM	ESTIMATED NUMBERS PER GRAM
Bacteria (other than actinomycetes)	3,000,000–500,000,000
Actinomycetes	1,000,000–20,000,000
Fungi (other than yeasts)	5,000–900,000
Yeasts	1,000–100,000
Algae	1,000–500,000
Protozoa	1,000–500,000

Source: Martin JP, Focht DD: Biological properties of soils. *In* Elliot LF, Stevenson FJ (eds.): Soils for Management of Organic Wastes and Waste Waters. Madison, Wisconsin, American Society of Agronomy, 1977.

factors such as amount of moisture, temperature, pH, availability of nutrients, and degree of aeration. Accurate counts of total microorganisms present in a soil sample are difficult to make, but bacteria are the predominant species (Table 23–1). If soil is examined microscopically, the counts make no distinction between living and dead cells. Standard plate counting methods do not support the growth of all soil species. Bacterial populations, including the mycelial-producing actinomycetes, may be as high as a half billion per gram of soil. Often the actinomycetes are counted separately from the more typical bacteria in soil samples. Several antibiotic-producing species are in the genus *Streptomyces;* typical bacterial genera in soil are: *Clostridium, Bacillus, Pseudomonas, Arthrobacter, Micrococcus, Azotobacter,* and *Rhizobium.*

Fungi counts range from thousands to hundreds of thousands per gram of soil. Molds belonging to the genera *Aspergillus, Penicillium, Mucor, Cladosporium, Rhizopus,* and *Fusarium* are particularly abundant. Yeasts are usually present in smaller numbers, but may be increased in soil of fruit orchards. Mushrooms are a very diverse group that produce the distinctive mushroom cap in warm moist seasons.

The remaining soil microorganisms include algae and protozoa. A variety of arthropods, insects, and nematodes interact with each other and with microbial residents to maintain good soil.

AQUATIC ENVIRONMENTS

Water covers at least 70 percent of the Earth's surface. The oceans contain more than 97 percent of the water on the planet. Only a small fraction of the Earth's total water is contained in lakes, rivers, ponds, and streams, and most of the water on land is unavailable for human use. Freshwater supports the growth of diverse populations on Earth. Marine life is limited by the high salinity, cold temperatures, low nutrient content, and high barometric pressure of the oceans.

Microbial populations are particularly abundant on the surfaces and in bottom sediments of large bodies of water. A collection of microorganisms and small plants or animals on the surface of water is called **plankton.** Water near shore lines receiving treated sewage and industrial wastes have particularly high microbial counts. Some bacteria colonize solid surfaces in **biofilms.** A few microorganisms find refuge in the viscera of fish. One newly discovered "giant" bacterium inhabits the intestinal tract of an Australian fish. The bacterium, which is about a million times bigger than *Escherichia coli,* is one example of a macroscopic bacterium.

A marine alga belonging to the genus *Gonyaulax* may be found in the viscera of mussels and clams. When eutrophication of the marine environment occurs, *Gonyaulax* bloom. These pigmented organisms color the ocean as a red tide when their population is large (see Color Plates 18 and 88). They produce neurotoxins, substances toxic to the human nervous system. If these are present in the shellfish ingested by humans they cause **paralytic shellfish poisoning.**

Freshwater Environments

In freshwater environments, differences in temperature, pH, nutrients, minerals, dissolved oxygen, and depth of light penetration influence the water environment and the types of organisms. Temperatures can vary from 0°C to 80°C, and the pH value ranges from 2 to 9 in particular bodies of water. Nutrients are usually abundant, but O_2 levels are low in stagnant water. The requirement for light by the producers limits their growth to surface waters.

The waters of lakes and ponds are divided into distinct zones that differ in nutrient content, light penetration, and oxygen availability (Fig. 23–10). The **littoral** zone is located along the

FOCAL POINT

Biofilms: A Microbial Survival Strategy

Microorganisms do not exist independently of other microrganisms in nature. Bacteria frequently aggregate in large groups held together by slime in structures called biofilms. Biofilms took on a new notoriety in 1993 and 1994 when hundreds of asthmatic patients developed a mysterious bacterial infection. These asthmatic patients had used the same generic drug albuterol. The bacterium causing serious illness of hundreds of people and killing at least 100 individuals was identified as *Pseudomonas aeruginosa.* Growing in a biofilm in the albuterol processing tank of the manufacturer, the organism had been able to escape chemical disinfection.

Biofilms have been found everywhere from corroding water pipes to computer chips. Dental plaque represents one of the most common biofilms. Biofilms, likewise, have prominent roles in colonization on surfaces of a variety of medical devices. To reduce the amount of colonization, catheters are now treated with antibiotics. It has been estimated that most microbial activities in open ecosystems in nature can be attributed to biofilms colonizing surfaces.

Science, 273:*1795, 1996.*

shores where water is shallow and light penetrates to the bottom. It contains the larger rooted types of vegetation. The **limnetic** zone is the surface layer in open waters beyond the shores. Light penetration is sufficient to promote growth of algae, cyanobacteria, and a variety of aerobic bacteria. The **profundal** zone is located below the area of light penetration. The **benthic** zone is composed of sediment at the bottom of lakes or ponds. The oxygen-deficient benthic environ-

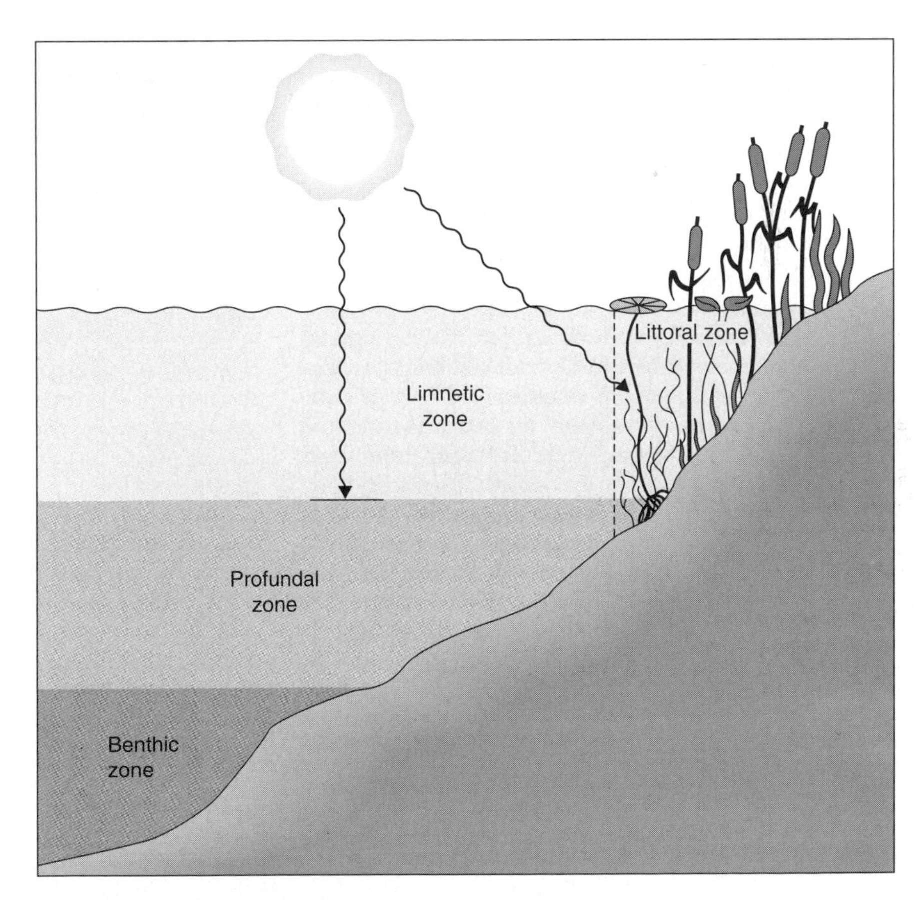

Figure 23–10 ◆ The zones of lakes and ponds.

ment supports the growth of many obligate anaerobes, including some bacteria that produce hydrogen sulfide (H_2S). The unpleasant odor of such sediments can be attributed to high quantities of H_2S.

Microbial populations of rivers and streams are not stable. They reflect the soil populations of the surrounding land. Differences in land usage contribute to the ever-changing indigenous microorganisms of the terrestrial environment and nearby streams. Industrial and agricultural wastes are common pollutants influencing the survival of some species and the probable extinction of others.

Marine Environments

Oceans are the largest habitats on Earth, and the most complex. The geographic boundaries are poorly defined, and waters intermix with one another. Circulation of ocean waters influences the types of organisms found in the marine environment.

Ocean temperatures vary with the location, season, currents, and depths. Temperatures are progressively lower with depth except in the unique hydrothermal vents on the sea floor where the water temperature may be as high as 150°C.

The dissolved salt concentrations of ocean water vary from 3.3 to 3.7 percent. The pH ranges from 6.5 to 8.3. The great depth of the oceans causes hydrostatic pressure to be a limiting factor for some forms of life. Hydrostatic pressure increases at a rate of about 1 atmosphere for every 10 meters of depth.

The discovery of deep-sea hot springs or **hydrothermal vents** on the ocean floor in 1977 introduced biologists to new aquatic ecosystems. Two types of vents, identified as **warm vents** and **hot vents** (black smokers) have been identified. Warm vents release hydrothermal fluid at temperatures of 6 to 23°C; hot vents release hydrothermal fluid of 270° to 380°C. Warm or hot hydrothermal fluid is mixed with the much colder ocean water. Final temperatures after mixing vary, but at least 300 species of life have been discovered capable of living in areas surrounding the vents.

The thermal vents support some diverse invertebrate communities which include large tubeworms, sea anemones, clams, and mussels (see Fig. 23–1). The invertebrates are dependent on chemoautotrophic bacteria, which are able to oxidize inorganic compounds such as H_2S, NH_4^+, and H_2 coming from the vents. In the absence of the primary producers (algae and cyanobacteria), the chemosynthetic bacteria are the primary producers for the animals. The bacteria use the chemical elements to grow and increase their own population. The invertebrate populations of the vents may not feed directly on the living bacteria, but they live on carbon products made by the bacterial cells.

Where the oceans meet the land and mix with fresh water, estuaries are formed. The water of estuaries fluctuates in composition; it reflects the quality of the waters they receive and the land use of surrounding areas. Many marine animals spend the early part of their lives in the protected environment of estuaries. If organic nutrients and wastes are high, enteric bacteria and fungi thrive. In nutrient-poor estuaries, different microorganisms are found, especially the budding or appendaged bacteria.

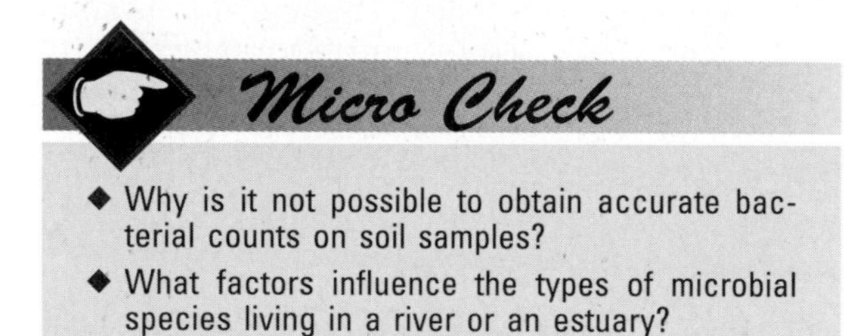

- Why is it not possible to obtain accurate bacterial counts on soil samples?
- What factors influence the types of microbial species living in a river or an estuary?
- What group of organisms are the sole producers in hydrothermal vents?

DRINKING WATER

Most drinking water in urban areas is obtained from rivers, streams, and lakes. Rural areas depend on water from springs or wells for individual residences. Water that meets public health standards for the level of microorganisms and chemicals is fit for human consumption and it is called **potable** water. Municipal water suppliers are responsible for providing safe drinking water. Spring or well water usually must be tested periodically by the user for proof of potability. Many of the world's peoples still do not have potable water, and they suffer gastrointestinal illnesses such as cholera from contaminated water. Cholera, caused by the bacterium *Vibrio cholerae,* is endemic in many parts of the world. In 1992, the epidemic form of cholera devastated Peru and Chile; it was carried to the United States by tourists.

Giardiasis is a form of gastroenteritis that is caused by the protozoan *Giardia lamblia* (see Color Plates 58 and 59). Hikers and campers who drink raw water from rivers or streams are vulnerable to this severe infection. Although surface water may look absolutely clear, it may contain the infective cysts of the protozoan.

The city of Milwaukee experienced a waterborne outbreak of cryptosporidiosis in 1993. The disease was transmitted by oocysts, a dormant stage in the life cycle of the protozoan, *Cryptosporidium* (see Color Plate 62). The presence of the parasite was attributed to runoff from melting snow and the use of an alternative coagulant in the water treatment system. Only boiling, in such instances, can render water safe for drinking.

Methods of Water Purification

The three processes used by cities to purify raw water to a potable level that ensures the delivery of microbiologically acceptable water to consumers are sedimentation, filtration, and chlorination. Sedimentation tanks hold water long enough to allow settling of particulate matter to the bottom. Small quantities of aluminum sulfate (alum) are sometimes added to the reservoir tanks to improve settling of solids. Filtration through sand is another means to remove additional particulate material. Up to 99.5 percent of microorganisms and fine particles can be removed by sedimentation followed by filtration.

Chlorination is the most common method for purifying water. The average amount of chlorine added is about 10 pounds for each million gallons of water. Most microorganisms die within 30 minutes of exposure to chlorine in that dilution. Chlorine also removes foul odors or tastes. A final chlorine level of 0.2 to 0.6 parts per million (ppm) is deemed suitable for consumption. The goal is to reduce survival of pathogenic organisms in water (Table 23–2).

Microbiological Examination of Water

Microbiological examination of water for potability is based on finding evidence of pollution with human or animal feces. It is not practical to attempt to isolate and identify specific pathogens because their numbers are small compared to the indigenous organisms of the intestinal tracts of humans or warm-blooded animals. Furthermore, pathogens do not usually survive for long periods of time outside their hosts.

Table 23–2
EXAMPLES OF WATERBORNE DISEASES

AGENT	DISEASE
Bacteria	
Campylobacter jejuni	Campylobacteriosis
Escherichia coli	Travelers' diarrhea
Salmonella typhi	Typhoid fever
Shigella species	Shigellosis
Vibrio cholerae	Cholera
Protozoa	
Balantidium coli	Balantidiasis
Cryptosporidium parvum	Cryptosporidiosis
Entamoeba histolytica	Amoebic dysentery
Giardia lamblia	Giardiasis
Viruses	
Hepatitis virus, type A	Epidemic hepatitis
Norwalk virus	Gastroenteritis
Rotavirus	Gastroenteritis
Fungi	
Epidermophyton floccosum	Tinea
Microsporum species	Tinea
Trichophyton species	Tinea

The presence of certain **indicator organisms** provides the evidence of fecal contamination in water quality tests approved by the U.S. Public Health Service. One group of indicator organisms are the **coliform** bacteria, which include *Escherichia coli.* Coliforms are gram-negative nonspore-forming, facultatively anaerobic bacilli that ferment lactose with the production of acid and gas within 48 hours at 35°C. Other suitable indicator organisms are *Enterococcus faecalis* and *Clostridium perfringens.*

QUANTITATIVE WATER ANALYSIS

Procedures for the bacteriological analysis of water are published in *Standard Methods for the Examination of Water and Wastewater* developed by the American Public Health Association (APHA), the American Water Works Association (AWWA), and the Water Pollution Control Federation (WPCF). Examination of water samples for numbers of bacteria present per milliliter are useful to indicate general levels of cleanliness. The standard plate count method determines the efficiency of sedimentation, filtration, or chlorination processes for drinking water quality. Potable water should have no more than 100 colony-forming units (CFU) per milliliter of water sample.

QUALITATIVE WATER ANALYSIS

Qualitative tests for water analysis are designed to detect the presence of coliforms. *Escherichia coli* is found in the intestinal tracts of humans and warm-blooded animals. Other coliforms, widely distributed in nature, include *Enterobacter aerogenes* and *Klebsiella* species. Two methods commonly used to detect the presence of coliforms are the (1) membrane filter (MF) method and (2) multiple tube fermentation technique.

Membrane Filter Method. The use of a membrane filter is especially suitable in the field for sampling water from reservoirs, aqueducts, springs, and wells. Samples must be relatively clear because large quantities of suspended material will clog the pores or tear the delicate filter. A water sample is passed through a membrane filter with pores measuring 0.45 μm in diameter to retain bacteria (Fig. 23–11*A*). The filter is transferred aseptically to a plate of eosin, methylene blue (EMB), or Endo agar media selective for gram-negative bacteria. After incubation for 24 hours at 35°C, purple or metallic green colonies on the filter are counted (Fig. 23–11*B*). The presence of more than one coliform colony per 100 ml of water constitutes a positive presumptive test for coliforms and indicates that the water may be unsafe for drinking.

Multiple Tube Fermentation Technique. The multiple tube fermentation technique is a three-part test: presumptive, confirmed, and completed tests. The presumptive test employs between five and 15 tubes of lauryl tryptose or lactose broth in

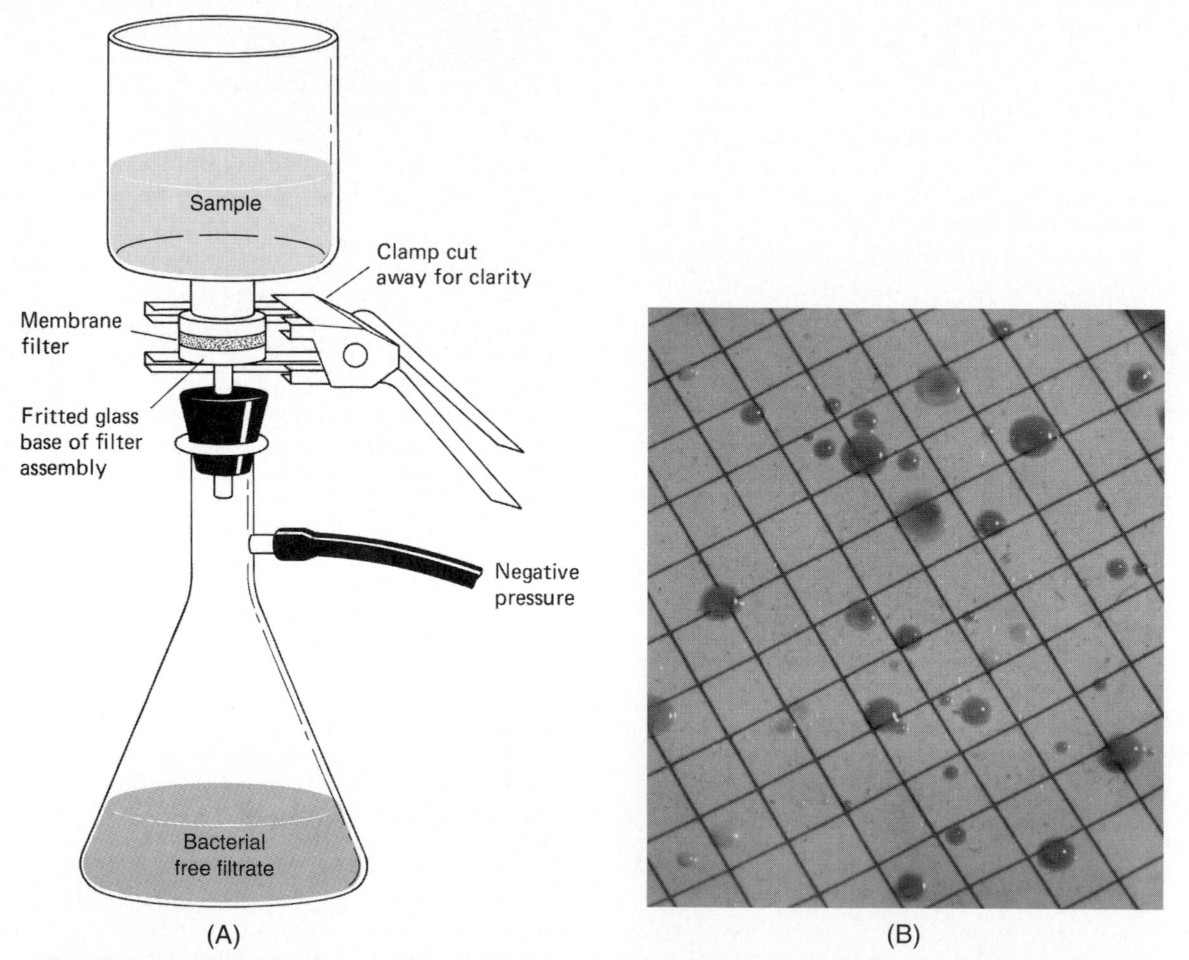

Figure 23–11 ◆ Membrane filter method for detection of coliforms. *A*, A 100-ml sample of water is poured into the sterile membrane filter unit. The filter is removed and placed on an agar medium selective for coliforms, and then incubated. *B*, Any colonies of coliforms are counted.

fermentation tubes (Fig. 23–12). In the 15-tube test, a 100-ml water sample is dispensed into three sets of five tubes. Five of the tubes contain 10 ml of double-strength broth and each tube receives 10 ml of the water sample. Ten tubes contain 10 ml of single-strength broth; five of these tubes receive 1 ml each of the water sample and the final five tubes receive 0.1 ml each of the water sample. The total volume removed from the water sample is 55.5 ml for the 15-tube test.

The tubes are incubated and examined for evidence of gas after incubation at 35°C for 24 and 48 hours. The number of tubes showing gas from lactose fermentation is counted in each set of five tubes as a positive result in the presumptive water test. The count of gas positive tubes is converted to a statistically probable number of bacteria in the water sample by consulting a statistical chart (Table 23–3). The most probable number (MPN) of coliforms per 100 ml of water is determined statistically from the number of tubes showing gas in each set of five tubes.

Table 23–3
MOST PROBABLE NUMBERS (MPN) OF COLIFORMS PER 100 mL OF WATER

POSITIVES WITH			PROBABLE NO. PER	POSITIVES WITH			PROBABLE NO. PER	POSITIVES WITH			PROBABLE NO. PER	POSITIVES WITH			PROBABLE NO. PER
10 mL	1 mL	0.1 mL	100 mL	10 mL	1 mL	0.1 mL	100 mL	10 mL	1 mL	0.1 mL	100 mL	10 mL	1 mL	0.1 mL	100 mL
2	0	0	4.5	3	0	0	7.8	4	0	0	13.0	5	0	0	23.0
2	0	1	6.8	3	0	1	11.0	4	0	1	17.0	5	0	1	31.0
2	0	2	9.1	3	0	2	13.0	4	0	2	21.0	5	0	2	43.0
2	0	3	12.0	3	0	3	16.0	4	0	3	25.0	5	0	3	58.0
2	0	4	14.0	3	0	4	20.0	4	0	4	30.0	5	0	4	76.0
2	0	5	16.0	3	0	5	23.0	4	0	5	36.0	5	0	5	95.0
2	1	0	6.8	3	1	0	11.0	4	1	0	17.0	5	1	0	33.0
2	1	1	9.2	3	1	1	14.0	4	1	1	21.0	5	1	1	46.0
2	1	2	12.0	3	1	2	17.0	4	1	2	26.0	5	1	2	64.0
2	1	3	14.0	3	1	3	20.0	4	1	3	31.0	5	1	3	84.0
2	1	4	17.0	3	1	4	23.0	4	1	4	36.0	5	1	4	110.0
2	1	5	19.0	3	1	5	27.0	4	1	5	42.0	5	1	5	130.0
2	2	0	9.3	3	2	0	14.0	4	2	0	22.0	5	2	0	49.0
2	2	1	12.0	3	2	1	17.0	4	2	1	26.0	5	2	1	70.0
2	2	2	14.0	3	2	2	20.0	4	2	2	32.0	5	2	2	95.0
2	2	3	17.0	3	2	3	24.0	4	2	3	38.0	5	2	3	120.0
2	2	4	19.0	3	2	4	27.0	4	2	4	44.0	5	2	4	150.0
2	2	5	22.0	3	2	5	31.0	4	2	5	50.0	5	2	5	180.0
2	3	0	12.0	3	3	0	17.0	4	3	0	27.0	5	3	0	79.0
2	3	1	14.0	3	3	1	21.0	4	3	1	33.0	5	3	1	110.0
2	3	2	17.0	3	3	2	24.0	4	3	2	39.0	5	3	2	140.0
2	3	3	20.0	3	3	3	28.0	4	3	3	45.0	5	3	3	180.0
2	3	4	22.0	3	3	4	31.0	4	3	4	52.0	5	3	4	210.0
2	3	5	25.0	3	3	5	35.0	4	3	5	59.0	5	3	5	250.0
2	4	0	15.0	3	4	0	21.0	4	4	0	34.0	5	4	0	130.0
2	4	1	17.0	3	4	1	24.0	4	4	1	40.0	5	4	1	170.0
2	4	2	20.0	3	4	2	28.0	4	4	2	47.0	5	4	2	220.0
2	4	3	23.0	3	4	3	32.0	4	4	3	54.0	5	4	3	280.0
2	4	4	25.0	3	4	4	36.0	4	4	4	62.0	5	4	4	350.0
2	4	5	28.0	3	4	5	40.0	4	4	5	69.0	5	4	5	430.0
2	5	0	17.0	3	5	0	25.0	4	5	0	41.0	5	5	0	240.0
2	5	1	20.0	3	5	1	29.0	4	5	1	48.0	5	5	1	350.0
2	5	2	23.0	3	5	2	32.0	4	5	2	56.0	5	5	2	540.0
2	5	3	26.0	3	5	3	37.0	4	5	3	64.0	5	5	3	920.0
2	5	4	29.0	3	5	4	41.0	4	5	4	72.0	5	5	4	1600.0
2	5	5	32.0	3	5	5	45.0	4	5	5	81.0	5	5	5	1800.0

Source: Standard Methods for the Examination of Dairy Products, 16th ed. New York, American Public Health Association, 1992.

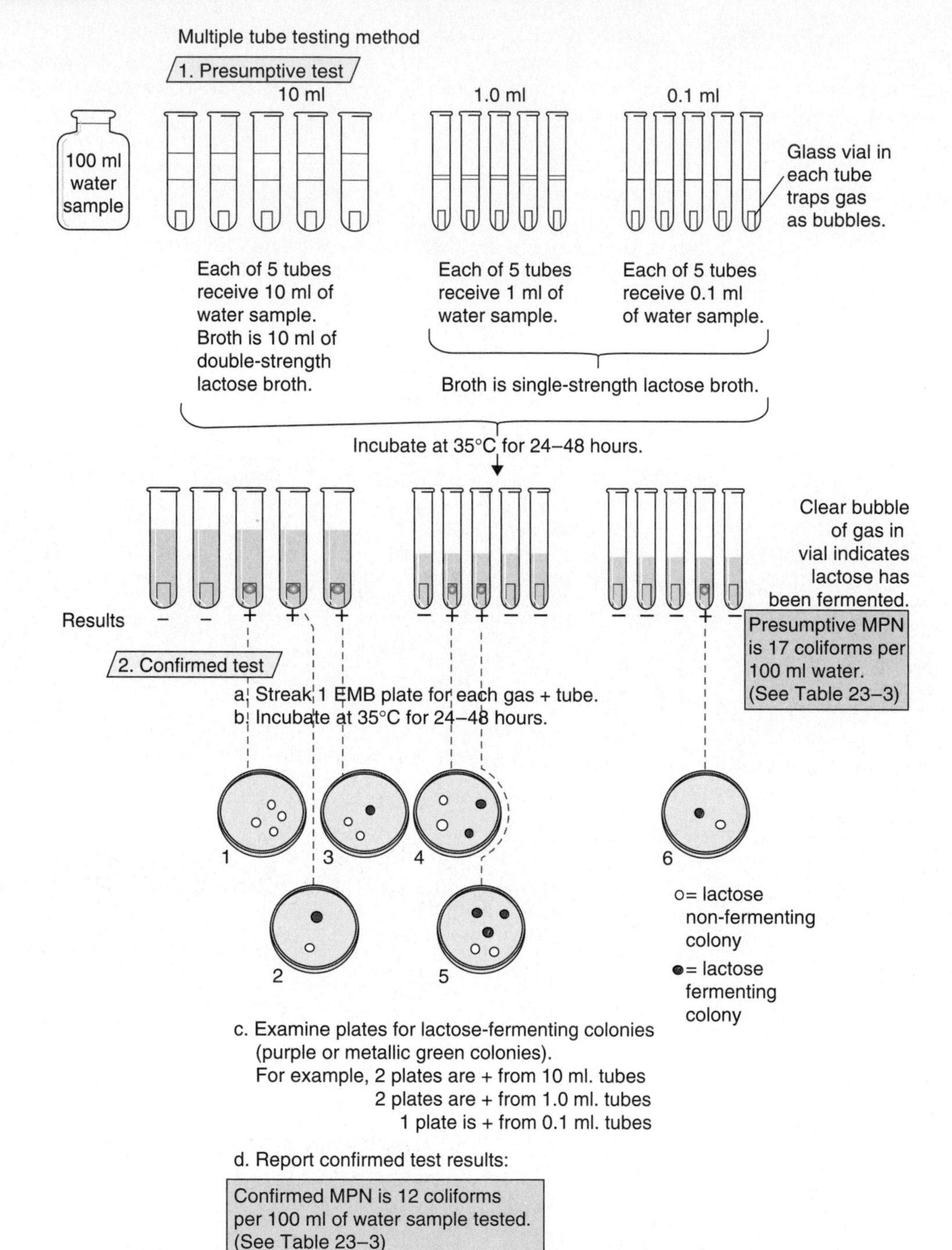

Figure 23–12 ◆ The most probable number (MPN) procedure for determining coliform count in a water sample. The test procedure consists of a presumptive test (1), a confirmed test (2), and a completed test (3).

3. Completed test

a. Inoculate one lactose broth tube and one nutrient agar slant for each plate with one lactose-fermenting colony.
b. Incubate at 35°C for 24–48 hours.

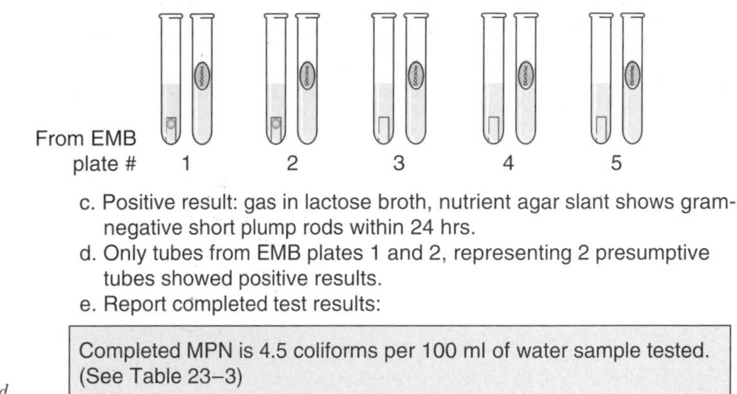

Figure 23–12 ◆ *Continued*

Positive presumptive tubes must be confirmed to be coliform organisms by subculturing each gas positive tube onto plates of EMB agar. Plates are examined after 24 to 48 hours of incubation at 35°C. Positive confirmation of coliforms in the tube is based on the presence of colonies with either a dark metallic green sheen or a pink color with dark centers. The number of plates showing these colonies is tallied. A confirmed MPN value is assigned by using the MPN statistical chart (Table 23–3.)

The third stage of testing is the completed test. A typical coliform colony is transferred from each EMB plate to a tube of lactose broth and a nutrient agar slant. After 24 to 48 hours of incubation at 35°C, gas formation in the lactose broth, accompanied by a Gram stain showing gram-negative, non-spore-forming bacilli from the 24-hour nutrient agar culture constitute a positive result. A completed MPN value is reported based on the number of tubes that tested positive through all three tests.

The presumptive and confirmed tests are more frequently used to determine water potability. The confirmed test is used for water samples that must be verified for legal or other purposes. Since 1991, the Environmental Protection Agency (EPA) has not required enumeration of coliform bacteria in water samples. The present regulations allow reporting of coliforms as present or absent only. The presence/absence (PA) test uses selective media to detect the presence of β-galactosidase and β-glucuronidase and can be completed in 24 hours. Regional standards may be more rigid than those imposed by the EPA. Water quality standards based on coliform content do not preclude the presence of enteropathogenic viruses in a water supply, but viruses may not be present in overwhelming numbers if coliforms are absent.

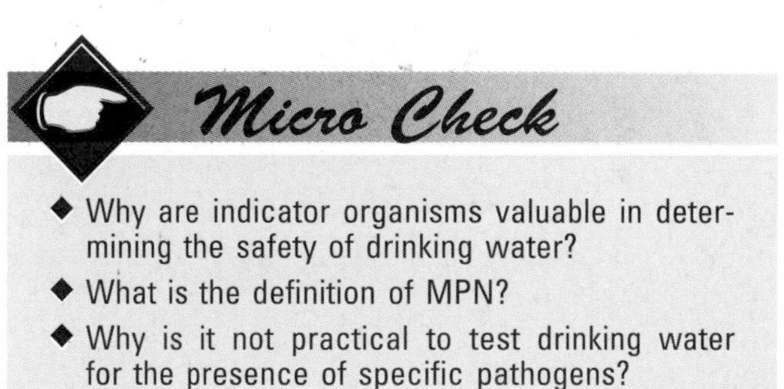

SAFE DISPOSAL OF SEWAGE AND WASTEWATER

Sewage and wastewater includes household, industrial, and agricultural wastewater; it is approximately 99.9 percent water. Most cities in the United States have plants designed to treat sewage before disposing of it in order to reduce its organic matter as **total suspended solids** (**TSS**) and its **biochemical oxygen demand** (**BOD**). BOD is a measure of the oxygen (in milligrams) used by microorganisms to remove the organic matter in 1 liter of polluted water. BOD may also be viewed as a measure of the organic content or the strength of the organics in the wastewater.

Raw **influent** is the wastewater entering a sewage treatment plant with a high BOD value. After treatment, the BOD value of the treated wastewater exiting a process, or **effluent,** must be low to meet public health standards before disposal. Coliform testing of the treated effluent indirectly measures the effectiveness of the treatment processes in removing pathogenic bacteria which may have entered in the raw influent.

Sewage treatment processes include **preliminary, primary, secondary,** and **tertiary** treatments. Many sewage treatment districts use preliminary, primary, and secondary processes only.

Preliminary Treatment

Preliminary treatment of sewage involves a variety of methods to remove solid wastes from the influent. The influent volume is measured and its chemical nature is determined. Rags, plastics, papers, and other large solid debris are trapped by bar screens made of closely spaced metal bars. Mechanical rakes remove the debris from the bars. Chemical processes are used to effect odor control. The water is pumped into a grit chamber so small suspended solids, such as seeds, sand, gravel, and other materials, are settled out. Other processes may include chemical systems such as coagulation and flocculation to clear finely suspended solids.

Primary Treatment

The influent is pumped from the grit chamber to **primary clarifier tanks,** which are often covered for odor control (Fig. 23–13). In the tanks, solid material is removed as it settles to the bottom. Greases and oils are skimmed off the water surface by long arms rotating over the water. Sometimes chemical agents are added in an **advanced primary treatment** process to increase the efficiency of the settling process. Advanced pri-

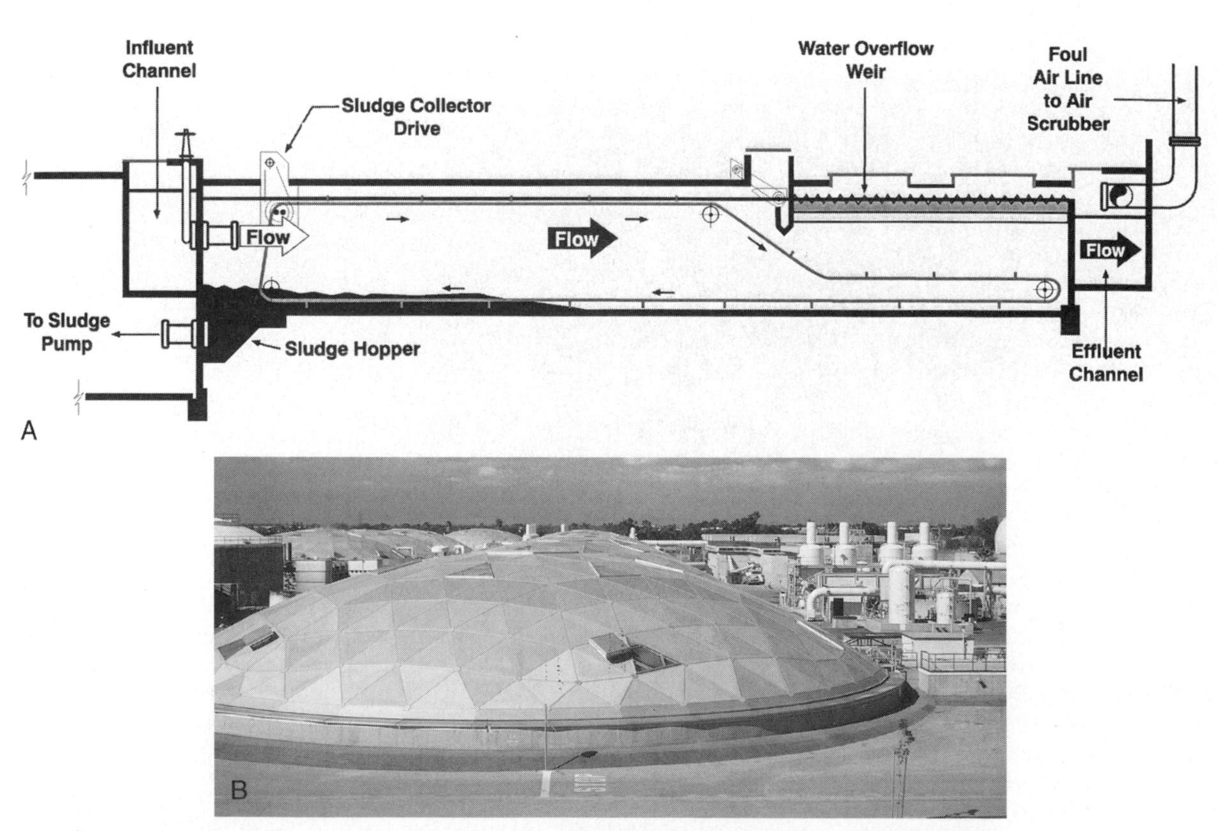

Figure 23–13 ◆ *A,* Cross section of one type of sedimentation basin or primary clarifier. *B,* Basin is covered for odor control.

mary treatment can remove 50 to 75 percent of suspended solids. The residual solids are known as **sludge.** Sludge is removed from primary clarifier tanks and pumped to **anaerobic digester tanks** described below (Fig. 23–14).

Secondary Treatment

The primary effluent enters a secondary treatment, which is an accelerated biological process helping microorganisms to consume organic wastes and to reduce the BOD value by 90 to 98 percent. Secondary treatment processes may involve using combinations of **ponds, lagoons, trickling filter tanks, activated sludge tanks,** and **anaerobic digester tanks.** Aerobic microorganisms are important in the open-air processes, such as trickling filters and activated sludge systems. Acid- and methane-forming anaerobic microorganisms are important to consume organic wastes in the anaerobic digester tanks.

Trickling filter tanks are large tanks filled with river rocks as the media, or in some cases, plastic media (Fig. 23–15). The primary treated water flows up the center column to be sprayed by large rotating sprinkler arms across the surface of the media. Decomposition of organic matter in the water depends on the action of aerobic microorganisms, especially bacteria, attached to the media surfaces. The BOD value of the treated water is reduced by a substantial 85 percent of its original value.

In the activated sludge tanks, a continuous supply of oxygen is provided by bubbling air through diffusers or pure oxygen can be added and dissolved by mixers (Fig. 23–16). The microorganisms, called **activated sludge,** are removed in settling tanks following aeration. Activated sludge and primary effluent are mixed together as a mixed liquor at the head of the tank. The microorganisms include filamentous bacteria and flocculent bacteria, which form **floc particles.** The oxygen pumped into the tank helps the bacteria consume the organic matter rapidly. The temperature and the type of organic matter (nutrients) also influence the rate of consumption by floc bacteria.

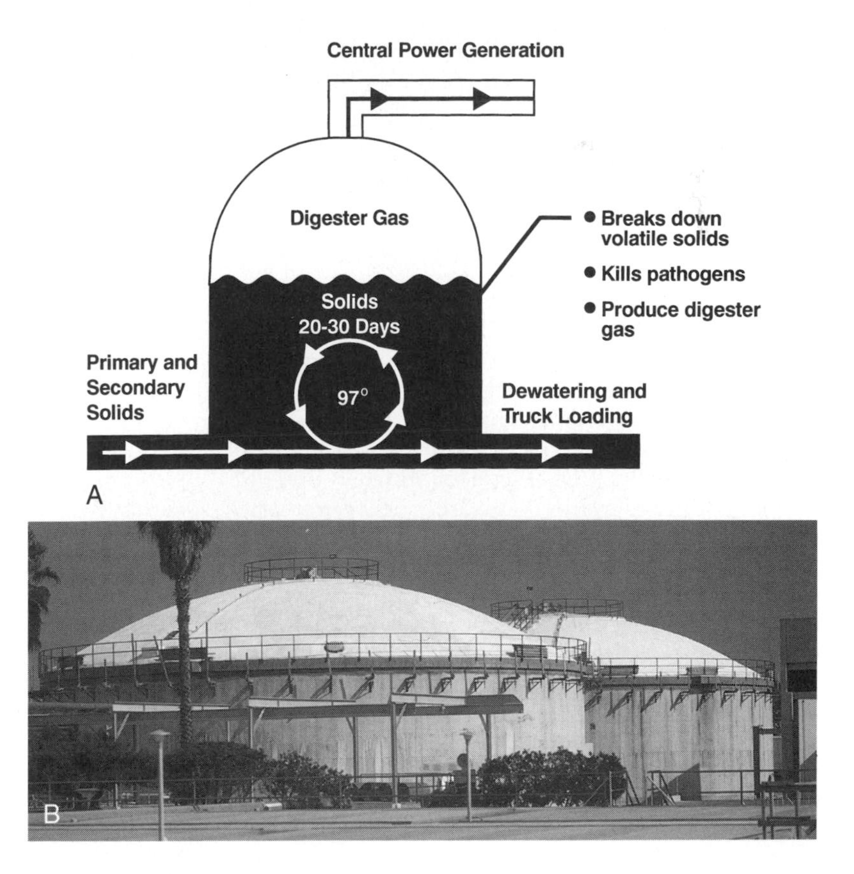

Figure 23–14 ◆ *A,* Cross section of an anaerobic sludge digester tank. Methane (CH_4) gas, a component of the digester gas, is produced by anaerobic bacteria consuming organic wastes. Methane is often used as an energy source to power engines. *B,* Exterior photograph of a digester tank.

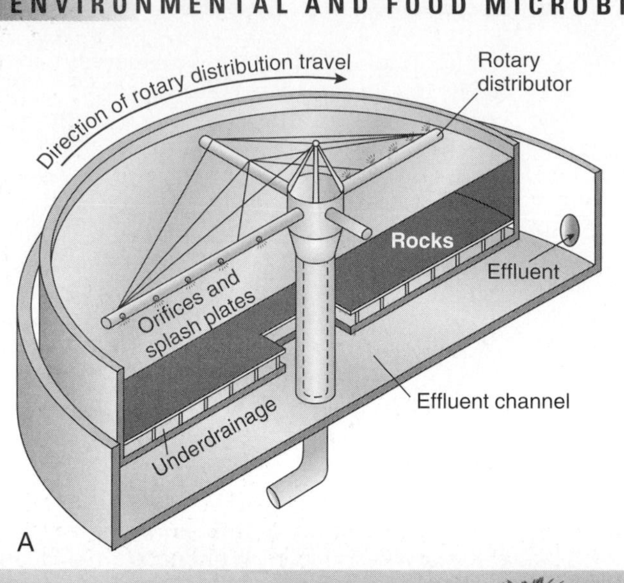

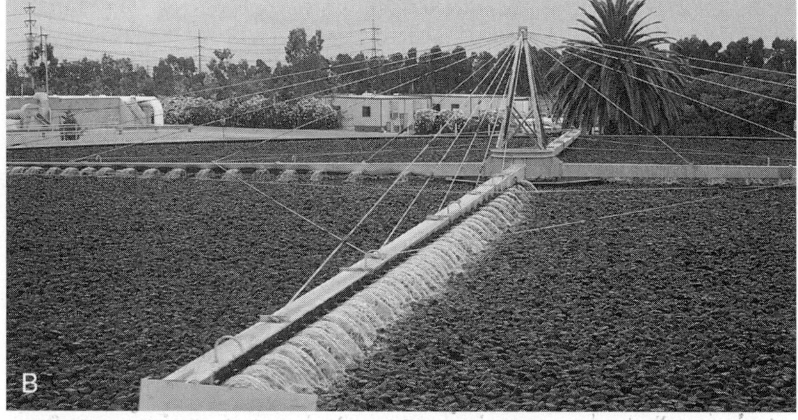

Figure 23–15 ◆ *A,* Cutaway diagram showing spraying arms and rock bed of a trickling filter tank. *B,* Partially treated sewage is sprayed over rocks covered by microorganisms.

The aerobic bacteria increase in numbers as they consume the organic matter and oxygen to form more pinhead-sized visible masses or floc particles. The wastewater travels from one end of the aeration basin to the opposite end while the bacteria lower the BOD value to 90 to 98 percent of the original value. The secondary effluent from these tanks may be released to a receiving body of water, such as a lake, river, or ocean, without causing eutrophication.

The anaerobic digester tanks contain anaerobic microorganisms, which consume the organic contents of sludge and release simple organic compounds, carbon dioxide (CO_2) and methane (CH_4) gases. The mesophilic anaerobic bacteria grow best at 95° to 100°F. The thermophilic organisms grow at 140°F. To meet the temperature requirements of the microorganisms, sludge is subjected to heat produced as steam or hot water passes through heat exchange equipment. Sufficient methane gas may be produced in digester tanks to meet part of the energy needs of the treatment plant. The digested sludge, called biosolids, is dewatered. The dry biosolids may be composted and used to fertilize food crops or applied to nonfood crop farmland as a valuable fertilizer.

Tertiary Treatment

Tertiary treatment processes may produce water for potable or nonpotable use, depending on the processes used to treat secondary effluent. A combination of physical and chemical methods are used to remove residual organic and inor-

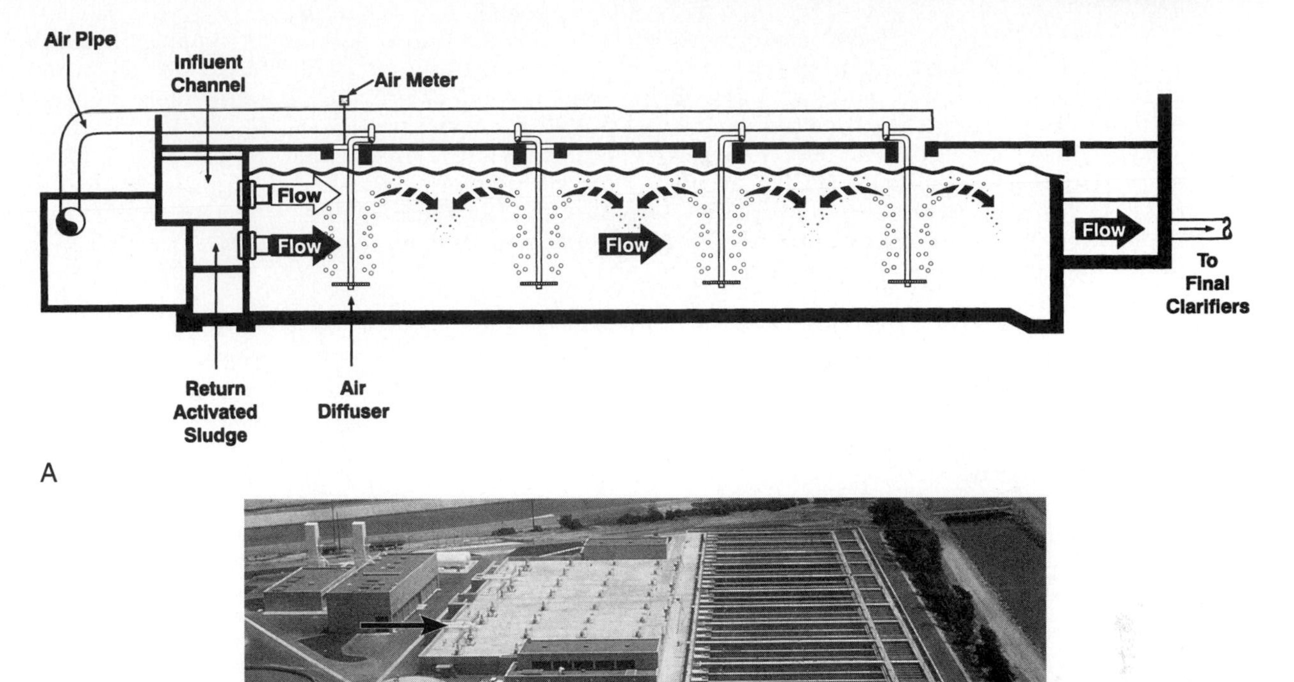

Figure 23–16 ◆ *A,* Interior diagram of an activated sludge tank. Oxygen is bubbled through activated sludge and primary treated sewage to reduce the BOD of the wastewater. *B,* Top view of covered activated sludge tank (arrow) adjacent to clarifier tanks where floc bacteria settle out of the treated water.

ganic components of secondary effluents. Treatment processes may involve additional sedimentation, sand filtration, microfiltration, adsorption by activated carbon, in combination with chlorination, or exposure to heat or ultraviolet light for disinfection. These treatments reduce the odors, colors, and inorganic chemicals that remain after secondary treatment. Effluents from tertiary treatment systems can be used for landscape irrigation and industrial use where human contact is avoided.

If tertiary treatment includes the use of **reverse osmosis** (**RO**) procedures, most minerals are removed including nitrates and phosphates. This RO water is less likely to cause eutrophication if it is released into a body of water. The water quality after tertiary treatment with reverse osmosis generally exceeds potability standards and can be blended with suitable well water for injection into a groundwater basin to restore underground freshwater levels.

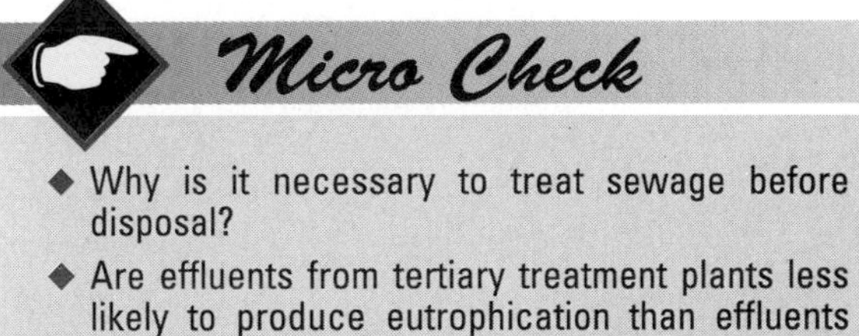

- Why is it necessary to treat sewage before disposal?
- Are effluents from tertiary treatment plants less likely to produce eutrophication than effluents from secondary treatment plants?
- What is the relationship between biochemical oxygen demand (BOD) and organic wastes?

HUMAN INTERVENTION IN ECOSYSTEMS

It is impossible to study any ecosystem without seeing the direct influence of human behaviors. Attempts to prevent blights of crops by harmful microorganisms and transmission of human diseases by vectors have polluted our environment with toxic chemicals. Such synthetic chemicals are not completely selective and, in most instances, harm done to beneficial microorganisms has not been assessed. Most of the chemicals, such as polychlorinated biphenyl (PCB), trichloroethylene (TCE), and dichlorodiphenyltrichloroethane (DDT), have not been around long enough for microorganisms to evolve strategies for degrading them.

A phenomenon, known as **biomagnification,** occurs with PCB and DDT. Once these chemicals enter a food chain, they become more concentrated at each trophic level in aquatic food chains. Such concentrated levels of chemicals may kill fish or be ingested by humans when they eat fish. For these reasons, the use of DDT has been banned in the United States since 1972.

FOCAL POINT

Cellulase 103: An Extraordinary Source for a Million Dollar Product

The secret formulas for hundreds of potentially valuable products lie hidden in the DNA of microbes thriving in extreme environments unsuited for humankind. One such formula is contained in a product that made its debut in May 1997. The detergent additive is an enzyme known as cellulase 103 that promises to make cotton clothes look like new despite hundreds of washings. The enzyme additive was isolated from a *Bacillus* species found in an extreme environment, an alkaline lake. The bacterium is one of more than 100 alkalophiles being discovered annually. Genencor International of Rochester, New York, inserted the cellulase gene into another strain of *Bacillus.* The enzyme, one of many known as extremozymes, is active in hot or cold soapy water; it can remove dirt from cotton textiles with little or no harm to the fabric. The potential market for detergent additives is estimated to be at least 600 billion dollars. Hundreds of other extremophiles have been isolated from high-salt, deep-mud, and hot-temperature environments. It is anticipated that many of their genes can direct enzyme factories of host cells to make products that will revolutionize industrial technology. Kits containing menus of 175 newly discovered extremozyme activities are already as close as your nearest biological supply house.

Science 276:*705, 1997.*

Human behaviors interfere with recycling of elements so essential to life as we know it on Earth. An increasing dependence on nonbiodegradable or slowly biodegradable materials such as plastic and plastic foam boxes used for fast food and convenience items has created challenging problems for society. These materials exceed the decomposing and recycling capabilities of microorganisms.

Deforestation and excessive logging activities in a river basin can cause flood hazards. The rain flows easily off the cut forest causing excessive runoff and soil erosion. Loss of forests often promotes migrations of animals including insect vectors forcing the insects to adapt to new hosts. Excessive deforestation and home building in former forests of the northeastern United States were factors involved in increasing exposure of humans to the deer tick, *Ixodes.* The tick transmits the spirochete of Lyme disease, *Borrelia burgdorferi,* in its bite to humans as well as deer.

On the positive side for human health, purification of water has caused highly virulent strains of enteric pathogens to be replaced by less virulent strains. As water purification measures have been instituted in Third World countries, the incidence of diseases, such as cholera, dysentery, and typhoid fever, have been markedly reduced. An understanding of ecosystems including human behaviors that support the spread of pathogens is necessary to control disease transmission.

Another benefit for our Earth environment is derived from a better understanding of how the metabolism of microorganisms can be directed toward improving environmental pollution. The process of using biological agents to eliminate toxic wastes from the environment is called **bioremediation.** Microorganisms capable of degrading **xenobiotic** (foreign) materials have been isolated from soil or constructed by genetic engineering techniques. Spillage of tons of oil from supertankers into the world's oceans has been cleaned up by a variety of methods including the introduction of oil-degrading bacteria applied to the oil spill surface.

The ability of any one bacterial strain to use complex organic substrates is usually limited. Toxic wastes often contain mixtures of chemicals. It is desirable, therefore, to construct bacterial strains with expanded degradative abilities. Among the promising candidates for such expansion are species of *Pseudomonas* and *Bacillus.* One genetically engineered strain of *Pseudomonas putida,* with the ability to degrade four hydrocarbons present in crude petroleum, was the first organism to be patented in the United States.

Long-term benefits as well as risks involved in managing our resources and preventing infectious diseases need to be evaluated carefully. We all have a responsibility to preserve the environment. There are many steps that individuals can take, but they all begin with an understanding of ecosystems and the role of our microbial allies in sustaining life on Earth.

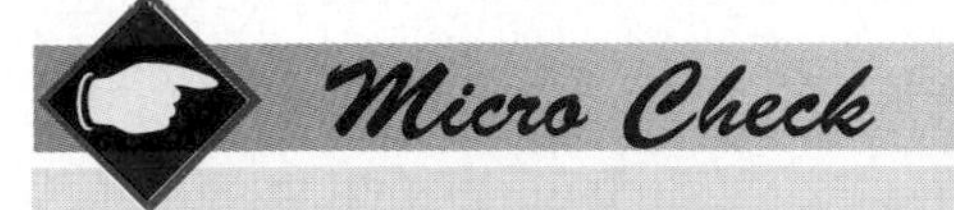

Micro Check

- Name at least three human activities or behaviors that affect the environment.
- What is biomagnification?
- Why must care be taken to preserve beneficial microorganisms on Earth?

Understanding Microbiology

1. Explain human dependence on plants, animals, and microorganisms of the planet Earth.
2. Why are some microorganisms transient residents of ecosystems?
3. How do decomposers contribute to energy flow in ecosystems?
4. Name three main methods used by cities to purify drinking water.
5. Why is drinking water containing coliforms considered unsafe?

Applying Microbiology

6. Devise a four-point program for using television or magazine advertisements to make the public more aware of our growing global ecological problems. Which television stations and magazines would you choose to advertise in? Why?

Chapter 24

Microbiology of Food and Beverages

Chapter Outline

- **METHODS OF FOOD PRESERVATION**
  - Heat
  - Cold
  - Radiatior
  - Chemical Agents
- **MICROORGANISMS IN FOOD PRODUCTION**
  - Vinegar
  - Sauerkraut
  - Cucumber Pickles
  - Milk Products
  - Bread
- **MICROORGANISMS IN THE PRODUCTION OF ALCOHOLIC BEVERAGES**
  - Wine
  - Beer
- **MICROORGANISMS AS A FOOD SOURCE**
- **TRANSGENIC PLANTS AND ANIMALS**
- **FOODBORNE ILLNESSES**
- **MICROBIOLOGICAL EXAMINATION OF FOODS AND DAIRY PRODUCTS**
  - Quantitative Methods
  - Qualitative Methods
  - Dye Reduction Tests
  - Enzyme Assay

Learning Objectives

After you have read this chapter, you should be able to:

1. Describe five methods of food preservation.
2. Differentiate between the high-temperature short time (HTST) and the low-temperature long time (LTLT) methods of pasteurization.
3. Explain why heat is more efficient as a food preservative than cold.
4. Describe the two microbiological stages for making vinegar.
5. Name the type of starter cultures and the type of change they produce when used in the production of butter, yogurt, cottage cheese, wine, beer, and bread.
6. Identify microorganisms commonly involved in foodborne illnesses and the types of food generally implicated.

The accessibility of a safe and flavorful food source for most of us is only as far away as the neighborhood supermarket. The majority of food and dairy products are made safe for human consumption by some form of heat treatment, refrigeration, freezing, radiation, or by the addition of certain chemical agents.

The flavor of many foods is enhanced by microorganisms present in particular foods or those added as **starter cultures** to ferment the natural sugars contained in food. These fermented foods are often preserved by the acids produced in the microbial fermentation process.

Careful surveillance of all processing procedures and of food handlers ensures safe foods of high quality. Microbial or chemical contamination of food and beverages can be the source of pathogens or microbial toxins. In 1997 virus-contaminated frozen strawberries, originally imported from Mexico and processed in California, caused 175 cases of hepatitis A among schoolchildren and teachers from Michigan. The berries were served in school lunch programs in Arizona, California, Georgia, Iowa, and Tennessee. More than 2200 children in Michigan, at least 9000 students in Los Angeles schools, and another 2000 children in Georgia were immunized with immune globulin against hepatitis.

METHODS OF FOOD PRESERVATION

Food preservation methods have developed over thousands of years. The need for fresh food kept early human civilizations on the move as they hunted, fished, and picked wild nuts and berries. With the discovery that drying, smoking, and salting could preserve foods, there was less need to roam. Ultimately, their ability to cultivate grains and to maintain herds of animals provided more stable food sources, allowing them to settle lands. In modern times, a knowledge of the types of microorganisms and naturally occurring enzymes in food and dairy products is essential to select a method of preservation. Some changes occur in food when preservation techniques are used in the manufacturing processes. The magnitude of those changes depends on the method of preservation and times of exposure.

Heat

Originally, the sun was used to dry meats, fruits, and vegetables. Today, foods are dried artificially in hot-air ovens with carefully controlled temperature, humidity, and air flow. As early as 1809, the Frenchman Nicolas Appert devised a method of heating moist foods in sealed containers to prevent spoilage. Appert used cork-stoppered, wide-mouthed glass jars, although most cans today are made of tin-coated steel plate. The first "tin can" was patented by Peter Durand, an Englishman, in 1810. Heat is used to sterilize the canned product or to reduce the total number of microorganisms present.

DRY HEAT

Because moisture is a requirement for microbial growth, any reduction in the moisture content of food delays food spoilage. Yet, complete removal of water would cause foods to be unpalatable and difficult to chew or digest. Dried foods are evaluated by their water content to determine if they are safely preserved. A useful measure to determine dryness is called the water activity, or A_w, of a food (Table 24–1). The A_w indicates the water vapor pressure in a food compared to pure water.

Dehydrated or desiccated food has been used during wartime to feed troops in various parts of the world. Dried foods are also used by hikers, backpackers, and others who want to save weight in carrying supplies into the country. Saving space and reducing weight in shipment of large quantities of food are desirable, but the alterations in flavor are not always popular. The term **evaporated** is applied to a liquid food from which some moisture has been removed. The term **condensed** is usually reserved for a sweetened form of evaporated milk.

Table 24–1
MINIMUM WATER ACTIVITY (a_w) OF FOODS TO PREVENT FOOD SPOILAGE BY MICROORGANISMS

TYPE OF MICROORGANISM	a_w
Most bacteria	0.9
Most yeasts	0.88
Most molds	0.80
Halophilic bacteria*	0.75
Xerophilic molds†	0.61
Osmophilic yeasts‡	0.61

* Halophilic means "salt-loving"; these microorganisms grow when the environment contains at least 15 percent NaCl.

† Xerophilic means "dry-loving"; these microorganisms grow in environments that are extremely low in water.

‡ Osmophilic means "solute-loving"; these microorganisms grow in high concentrations of sugar.

MOIST HEAT

Moist heat methods are more efficient for food preservation because they require lower temperatures and shorter times than dry heat methods. Although the process of boiling requires no special equipment, it is not reliable to sterilize foods that contain bacterial spores. Also, altitude affects the temperature of boiling, and the size and texture of the food mass influence the amount of heat penetration.

Pasteur was the first to use a modified heating process to destroy spoilage microorganisms in wine. The greatest application of the heat treatment, now known as **pasteurization,** is used in the dairy industry. Two common methods of pasteurization reduce the total number of bacteria and destroy pathogens in milk. In the high-temperature short time (HTST) method, the milk is heated to 71.7°C (160°F) for 15 seconds in thin coiled tubes before being cooled. In the low-temperature long time (LTLT) method, the milk is heated to 62.8°C (145°F) for 30 minutes in large vats and then cooled. An ultrahigh temperature process (UHT) is available for heating milk between 140° and 150°C (284°F to 302°F) for a few seconds. The finished milk achieves commercial sterility and may be stored without refrigeration for as long as eight weeks without flavor change. The thermal resistance of pathogens transmitted by contaminated milk, like *Coxiella burnetii* and *Mycobacterium bovis,* serves as the basis for selecting the particular temperatures and times for pasteurization of milk.

Another moist heating method for food preservation is food canning that involves heating food in the sealed can. In industry, this process is known as **commercial sterilization.** A commercially sterile can of food is treated in a manner that will destroy the heat-resistant spores of *Clostridium botulinum* without severe alteration in the consistency of the food. Although not completely sterile, other pathogens and most food-spoilage microorganisms are killed in the process. The temperature used for commercial sterilization varies, depending on the acid content of foods. Although 100°C (212°F) for 2.52 minutes may be sufficient to inactivate botulinal toxins in high-acid foods, temperatures of 121°C (250°F) for the same time is often required for low-acid foods. The time required to destroy 90 percent of the microorganisms or spores is called the D value. The D value is dependent on the type of food and the pH (Table 24–2). Only endospores of obligate thermophilic bacteria can survive, but those endospores will not germinate if canned food is held below 43.3°C (110°F) or at a pH value below 4.5.

Preparation of fresh raw vegetables or fruits for canning involves thorough washing, then **blanching,** a brief scalding process in hot water or steam, and then placing in containers. The containers are evacuated before sealing and heating. The heating is done with or without steam in vessels called retorts.

Most home canning is done in pressure cookers in which a maximum temperature of 121°C at 15 psi (250°F) can be reached and maintained for 15 minutes or more, depending on the quantity (mass) of food. Lower temperatures increase the risk for survival of food-spoilage microorganisms and endospores of *Clostridium botulinum* in low-acid foods. Improperly home-canned foods have frequently caused outbreaks of botulism in the United States.

Cold

Low temperatures inhibit the activity of naturally occurring enzymes and microorganisms in food. Although microbial growth may be slowed by refrigeration temperatures (0° to 7°C) or prevented by freezing temperatures (−18°C or lower), the action of enzymes continues at a low rate. Enzymes and some microorganisms may be inactivated in food by blanching before freezing or by a quick freezing process, but food is not

Table 24–2
EFFECT OF pH ON D VALUES FOR SPORES OF *C. botulinum* SUSPENDED IN SPANISH RICE

pH VALUE	D VALUE (MINUTES)
4.0	0.117
4.2	0.124
4.4	0.149
4.6	0.210
4.8	0.256
5.0	0.266
6.0	0.469
7.0	0.550

Source: Institute of Food Technologists, Chicago, IL.

rendered sterile. Food never should be kept for too long a period of time even at refrigerator temperatures.

Psychrotrophic yeasts, molds, and bacteria grow between 0° and 7°C, so the keeping quality of refrigerated food is limited. Members of the genera *Penicillium, Saccharomyces, Cladosporium, Sporotrichum, Flavobacterium, Pseudomonas, Escherichia, Micrococcus,* and *Achromobacter* exhibit varying degrees of cold tolerance. Unfortunately, *Clostridium botulinum* type E does grow and produce toxin at temperatures as low as 3.3°C. Botulism from type E toxin has most often been associated with fish or fish products. Food containing the botulinum toxin or other toxins is usually tasteless and odorless.

In frozen foods, gram-positive food-poisoning bacteria such as *Staphylococcus aureus* and the clostridia survive better than gram-negative bacteria such as *Salmonella* species.

Radiation

Ultraviolet light, ionizing radiation, and microwave energy are useful in controlling microorganisms in foods and beverages. These electromagnetic waves are tested for their ability to eliminate microbial pathogens and their effects on the nutritional value of foods. Spoilage in some foods is not slowed by irradiation. For example, pears, apples, and citrus fruits spoil rapidly after irradiation. Foods approved for irradiation in the United States appear in Table 24–3.

Table 24–3
FOODS APPROVED FOR IRRADIATION IN THE UNITED STATES

FOOD	PURPOSE
Wheat, wheat flour	To kill insects
White potatoes	To inhibit sprout development
Pork, fresh	To control *Trichinella* worms
Some fruits and vegetables	To delay ripening, spoilage
Poultry	To kill *Salmonella* bacteria
Beef, fresh and frozen	To control enteropathogenic *Escherichia coli*
Dry and dehydrated vegetables, herbs, seeds, spices	To kill insects, to disinfect

Irradiation is considered to be a safe and effective complement to pasteurization, chlorination and immunization as methods for protecting people from foodborne illnesses.

Germany has a total ban and Japan a partial ban on irradiated foods. The issue of irradiation of foods is controversial because the long-term effects of irradiated foods on people are unknown. Currently irradiated food must carry the following symbol.

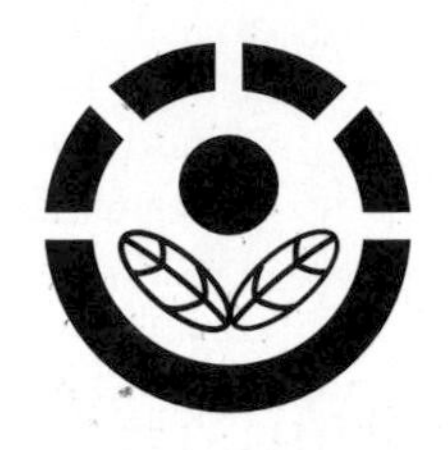

Ultraviolet light (UV) at wavelengths of 260 to 280 nm is powerfully microbicidal when used on the surfaces of some foods. UV light has a limited ability to penetrate the interior of foods. A commercial use of UV light is for the destruction of microorganisms on countertops and utensils used during food preparation.

Ionizing radiation such as x-rays and gamma rays have limited application in food preservation, although low doses can improve the keeping quality of some foods. The dosage required for sterilization often produces undesirable changes in texture, odor, or taste of foods and a substantial reduction in the levels of thiamine, pyridoxine, vitamins B_{12}, C, D, E, and K. Most food spoilage organisms and some pathogens are destroyed by relatively low doses of irradiation, but some spores of *Clostridium botulinum* survive the process.

Irradiation is sometimes combined with modified atmosphere packaging to control microbial growth. Removing the air within a package or substituting a gas, such as nitrogen, can extend the shelf life of a food by limiting the growth of microbial contaminants.

Microwaves have wavelengths between the infrared and radio frequency of the electromagnetic spectrum (see Fig. 21–5). Microwave radiation causes molecules in the food to vibrate extremely rapidly. Vibration of molecules produces friction resulting in heat energy within the food. Microwaves are useful in the food industry not only to cook foods, but to destroy molds in bread, pasteurize beer, and sterilize wine. A successful commercial application of microwaves is in the preparation of potato chips.

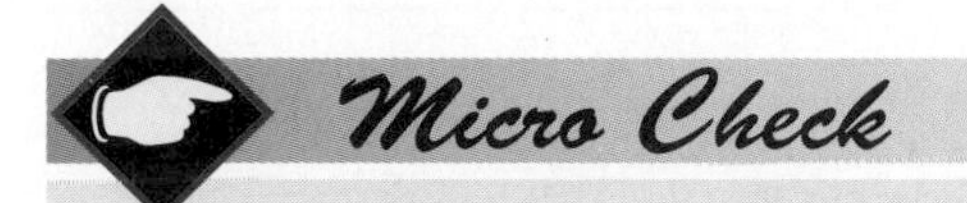

- How does pasteurization improve the keeping quality of milk?
- Why is it undesirable to subject canned food to a process of complete sterilization?
- How do microwaves cause food to become hot?

Chemical Agents

The Food and Drug Administration (FDA) regulations allow the addition of approximately 100 chemicals generally regarded as safe (GRAS) to inhibit growth of some microorganisms. None of these chemicals are antimicrobial agents used to treat infections because they would persist in the cans and they might cause allergic reactions in sensitive individuals. In addition, microorganisms resistant to the antimicrobial agent may survive in the gastrointestinal tract.

Among the most prominent chemical preservatives added to food are sodium propionate, potassium sorbate or sorbic acid, sodium benzoate, sodium nitrate or nitrite, and sulfur dioxide or sulfites. Sodium propionate and potassium sorbate are added to baked goods, beverages, and cheeses to inhibit molds. Both additives are metabolized by humans to produce carbon dioxide and water. Sodium benzoate or benzoic acid prevents spoilage by bacteria in jellies, jams, and margarines. Benzoic acid is metabolized and excreted in the urine.

Sodium nitrate and nitrite are often added to meat particularly to stabilize red meat color, contribute to flavor development, and inhibit food-spoilage organisms and food poisoning organisms, primarily *Clostridium botulinum.* The high levels of these salts cause concern because nitrites can react with amines in the digestive tract, producing highly carcinogenic nitrosamines. Despite the objection to these salts in cured meats, it is unlikely that a suitable substitute for sodium nitrate or nitrite will be found in the near future.

Sulfur dioxide or sodium sulfite has been widely used as a bacterial inhibitor in the processing of dried fruits, fruit juices, and wines. Recently, sulfites have been implicated in some severe allergic reactions, so their status as a safe additive may be reassessed.

Micro Check

- Why are antibiotics not used to a larger extent in the food industry?
- For what purposes are the propionates, sorbates and the benzoates added to foods?
- What is objectionable about using sodium nitrates or nitrites?

MICROORGANISMS IN FOOD PRODUCTION

Many microorganisms found naturally in food are beneficial. Conditions that favor their growth result in such products as vinegar, sauerkraut pickles, fermented milks, cheese, and bread. So called starter cultures of particular bacteria or yeasts are added intentionally to milk to produce desired flavors or textures of fermented dairy products. Naturally occurring microorganisms, or starter cultures, or combinations of them ferment food sugars, creating an acid environment that inhibits growth of spoilage microorganisms.

Vinegar

Vinegar is a condiment made from foods containing starch or sugar. Vinegar was used by Orientals and the Babylonians as early as 1000 B.C. Production of vinegar involves a two-step fermentation process (Fig. 24–1). In the first step, glucose is converted to alcohol and carbon dioxide by yeasts.

$$C_6H_{12}O_6 \longrightarrow 2CO_2 + 2C_2H_5OH$$

The yeast, *Saccharomyces cerevisiae,* is added to apple juice or other raw materials to hasten the anaerobic fermentation process. In the second step, the overall reaction involves the oxidation of alcohol by acetic acid bacteria to form vinegar.

$$C_2H_5OH + O_2 \longrightarrow CH_3COOH + H_2O$$

Mixed cultures of acetic acid bacteria, such as *Acetobacter aceti* and others, are added to the alcohol-containing liquid. The oxidation stage proceeds in generators that are upright wooden

FOCAL POINT

Vinegar—The People's Choice

Although vinegar or vinaigre (vin meaning wine and aigre meaning sour) was used as a food preservative in early history, Hippocrates used the fermented product to treat patients in 400 B.C. The Romans used wine vinegar to purify drinking water. During the First World War, vinegar was used to disinfect wounds. Today, the use of vinegar is largely limited to the preparation of dishes with special culinary appeal and for home pickling of vegetables and fruits. White vinegar is also the people's choice for an all-purpose cleaner. It is nontoxic, inexpensive, and readily available to most consumers. Here are some other uses for vinegar:

Washing baby clothes: Vinegar breaks down uric acid and soapy residue in diapers, leaving them soft and fresh.

Removing smoke odors: A glass of vinegar removes the odor of smoke in a room.

Caring for nylon stockings: Rinsing nylon hose in two quarts of water containing one teaspoon of vinegar will make them last longer.

Cleaning the kitchen: Use vinegar to clean the microwave, cutting board, and kitchen counters.

tanks filled with wood chips. The vinegar bacteria attach to the chips and convert alcohol to acetic acid. Commercial vinegar usually contains a minimum of 4 percent acetic acid or 40 grains. The strength is often expressed in terms of grains which is determined by multiplying the percentage of acetic acid by 10.

In France, vinegar is most often made from

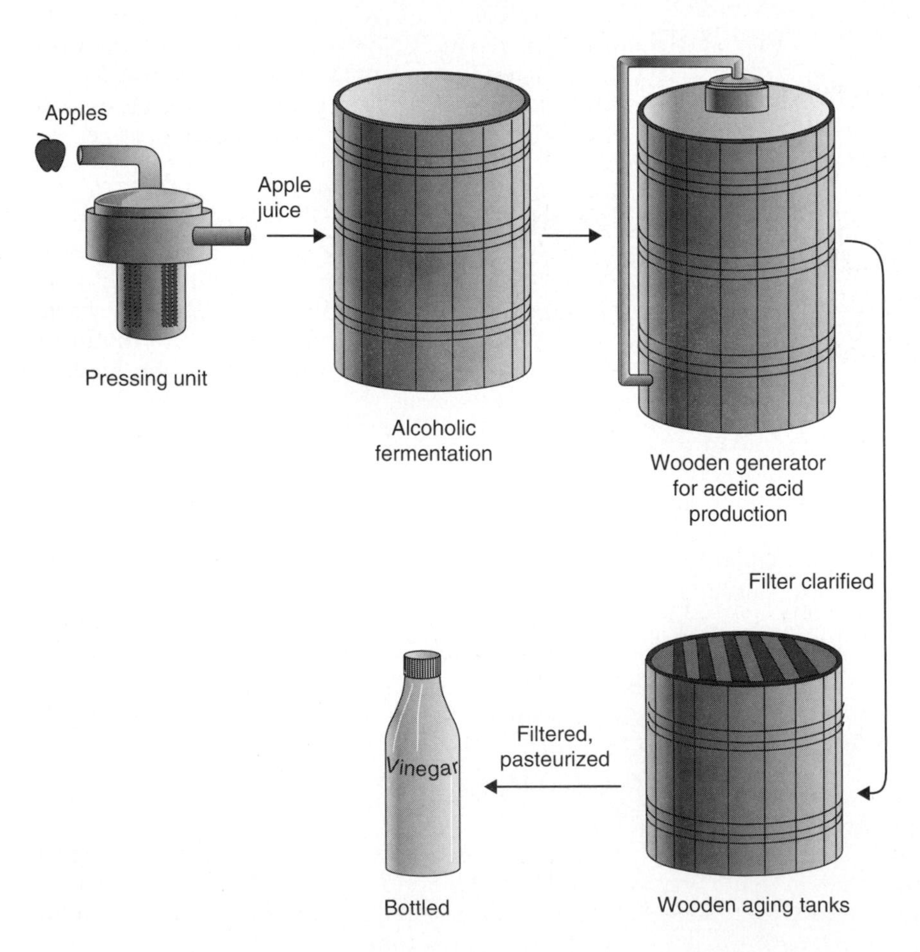

Figure 24–1 ◆ Major steps in the production of apple cider vinegar. Vinegar is also made from grapes and corn.

grapes, and in Great Britain, malted liquors are usually the starter material. Most vinegar is made from apples in the United States and is, therefore, called apple cider vinegar. Although complete fermentation should produce a stable product, vinegar is pasteurized after a filtering process for clarification.

Sauerkraut

Sauerkraut is made from the fermentation of shredded cabbage in the presence of 2.25 to 2.5 percent salt. Packing shredded cabbage tightly in covered vats creates anaerobic conditions. Added salt dehydrates the cabbage and the resulting brine permits the growth of lactic acid bacteria at 15.8°C (70°F) to 23.9°C (75°F). The major bacteria contributing to the fermentation of sugars are species of the gram-positive bacteria *Leuconostoc* and *Lactobacillus*. Most other bacteria cannot tolerate the salty conditions in the fermentation vats. Cabbage is usually colonized with bacteria that act as starter cultures. A tasty final product has a pH value between 3.4 and 4.5, a lactic acid content of approximately 1.25 percent, carbon dioxide, and trace amounts of acetic acid and ethyl alcohol. Sauerkraut is usually canned before it is marketed.

Cucumber Pickles

Cucumber pickles may be products of limited or complete fermentation or may not have undergone fermentation. Most commercially prepared cucumber pickles are subjected to fermentation in the presence of varying concentrations of salt. The desired lactic acid level is reached within six to nine weeks, but depends on the temperature and salting method used. *Lactobacillus plantarum* is the major organism contributing to acidity in both low- and high-salt brines. The final product has a concentration of lactic acid of 0.6 to 0.8 percent.

Milk Products

It has been estimated that about 11 million cows annually produce at least 140 billion pounds of milk in the United States alone. There are several thousand factories employing approximately 150,000 individuals involved in converting milk into a variety of fermented milk products.

Raw milk contains both the fermentable sugar lactose and a variety of acid-producing microorganisms. These microorganisms ferment the lactose to lactic acid, causing the milk to become acidic. The lactic acid causes milk proteins to curdle. However, high quality and safe products are best produced by using starter cultures of lactic acid–producing bacteria. First, the naturally occurring bacteria and any pathogens are destroyed by pasteurization followed by the addition of the desirable starter cultures.

BUTTER, BUTTERMILK, AND SOUR CREAM

Butter is made by adding starter cultures of lactic acid and diacetyl-producing bacteria to pasteurized cream and incubating until the desired acid level is reached. Pasteurization inactivates the enzymes that might interfere with the keeping quality of the final product. The acidified cream is churned to produce solid butter. The remaining fluid is buttermilk and is sold commercially as cultured buttermilk. After removal of excess fluid and salting, butter is packaged. The unique flavor of butter is largely due to diacetyl, a product of butylene glycol fermentation by *Streptococcus diacetylactis* or *Leuconostoc citrovorum*.

Light pasteurized cream and lactic acid bacteria are used to make sour cream. The mixture is incubated until the desired acidity is obtained.

YOGURT

Yogurt is one of the oldest known foods produced by the bacterial fermentation of milk. The lactic acid bacteria ferment lactose, causing milk protein, casein, to curdle resulting in the thick custard-like consistency of yogurt. In traditional cultures, yogurt is made in ordinary households or by nomadic people of the Middle East, Mediterranean countries, and Europe. A small amount of yogurt from a previous batch is added to heated and cooled milk. The yogurt acts as a starter because it contains the necessary lactic acid bacteria.

In the commercial preparation of yogurt, whole or skim milk is usually concentrated to reduce water content. Additional milk proteins

FOCAL POINT

Sour Milk as Fountain of Youth

Elie Metchnikoff (1845–1916), the Russian Nobel Prize winner, was among the first to propose drinking large quantities of "sour" milk to prevent senility and premature death in his book, *The Prolongation of Life.* The longevity of people in the Balkan countries, as well as their passion for fermented milks, were well known at Metchnikoff's time. Metchnikoff's ideas were controversial, but they spurred research on the possible benefits of cultured and culture-containing dairy foods.

Consumption of yogurt and sweet acidophilus milk in the United States has significantly increased in recent times. Cultured dairy foods are good sources of protein, calcium, phosphorus, magnesium, riboflavin, vitamin B_{12}, and niacin. Absorption of nutrients is more rapid because the bacteria have partially digested the milk. Among the other health benefits claimed for fermented milk products are lowering blood cholesterol, preventing colon cancer, and restoring intestinal flora after antimicrobial therapy. The nutritive value of fermented milk products is unquestionable, but there is conflicting data on the other health benefits.

Metchnikoff died at the age of 71 from a cardiac condition, but historical records do not record the amount of sour milk and *friendly* lactic acid bacteria he had consumed. Although the average life span has been lengthened since the time of Metchnikoff, it seems unlikely that it can be directly attributed to consumption of fermented milk products.

Dairy Council Digest, 55:*15, 1984.*

are added to produce a firmer product. The concentrated milk is heated to 82° to 93°C for 30 to 60 minutes to reduce the number of microorganisms. The milk is then cooled to about 45°C before adding the desired starter cultures of *Streptococcus thermophilus* and *Lactobacillus bulgaricus.* During incubation at 45°C for three to five hours the microorganisms rapidly produce lactic acid, which promotes curd formation. The yogurt has a consistency similar to that of a light custard. Fruits or fruit syrups are often added to yogurt to enhance the flavor appeal. The finished yogurt remains fresh for at least one to two weeks when stored at 5°C.

The *S. thermophilus* cells grow first by actively fermenting lactose to produce the majority of the acid. Acid environments encourage the rapid growth of *L. bulgaricus,* which produces the characteristic flavor of yogurt. All fermented milk products are excellent sources of protein, minerals, and some B-complex vitamins.

SWEET ACIDOPHILUS MILK

Lactobacillus acidophilus can be added to low-fat milk to produce sweet acidophilus milk. The milk retains the flavor of sweet pasteurized milk because the lactobacilli are added to cold milk and stored at refrigerator temperatures. Yogurt and sweet acidophilus milk, containing living lactobacilli, are beneficial additions to a diet for many reasons. The lactobacilli have antimicrobial and antitumor activity. Consumption of both products is sometimes recommended for replacement of lactobacilli in the gastrointestinal tract after long-term antibiotic usage.

CHEESES

Cottage cheese is a fresh, unripened cheese; it is made by inoculating whole or skim milk with *Lactococcus lactis* (formerly known as *Streptococcus lactis*) and *Leuconostoc citrovorum* (see Color Plate 89). Rennin, casein coagulase, or chymosin are enzymes that are added to hasten curdling. The liquid portion called **whey** is removed after heating to 37.8°C (100°F) for 30 minutes. The curd is washed, salted, and mixed with cream before the product is marketed.

The manufacture of ripened cheese requires a longer processing time. Additional bacteria or fungi are used as ripening agents to impart characteristic flavors. Ripened cheeses are classified as soft, semisoft, or hard cheeses depending on the water content of the final product (Table 24–4). Ripening of the various cheeses may require six to 16 months or longer. The process requires three steps: curdling, salting, and ripening (see Color Plates 90 to 93).

Curdling is done by lactic acid bacteria and the enzymes rennin, casein coagulase, or chymosin. If whole milk is used, the curd contains fats,

Table 24–4
RIPENING AGENTS OF SELECTED CHEESES

TYPE OF CHEESE	PRIMARY RIPENING AGENT
Soft (50–80 percent water)	
Brie and Camembert	*Penicillium camembertii*
	Penicillium candidum
Limburger	*Brevibacterium linens*
Mozzarella	*Lactobacillus bulgaricus*
	Streptococcus thermophilus
Semisoft (45 percent water)	
Blue	*Penicillium roqueforti*
	Penicillium glaucum
Monterey and Muenster	*Brevibacterium linens*
Roquefort	*Penicillium roqueforti*
	Penicillium glaucum
Hard (20–40 percent water)	
Cheddar	*Lactobacillus casei*
Parmesan	*Lactobacillus bulgaricus*
	Streptococcus thermophilus
Swiss	*Propionibacterium shermanii*
	Propionibacterium freudenreichii

proteins, lactic acid, and some vitamins and minerals. Cheese made from skim or nonfat milk is very low in fat. Curd may be separated from the whey by one or more techniques. The method used depends on the amount of water to be left in the final product. For soft cheeses, the curd may be merely removed and drained on a cheesecloth. For other cheeses, heat and pressure are used to reduce moisture content.

Salt is added to the drained curd for flavor and to prevent the development of spoilage microorganisms. The growth of organisms other than lactic acid bacteria may cause alterations in texture, general appearance, or flavor. Hard cheeses are usually less subject to spoilage than the soft, moister cheeses. The curd is then compressed and molded into particular forms.

Certain cheeses are ripened by adding specific microorganisms to the surface of the curd or by inoculating the interior of the curd. Cheeses requiring long-term processing are often covered with paraffin to prevent contamination during ripening. The fermentative and proteolytic activities of the microorganisms are responsible for the sometimes subtle taste differences in cheeses.

Bread

The so-called baker's yeast sold in yeast cakes or as the lyophilized product, known as active dry yeast, consists of dried cells of *Saccharomyces cerevisiae* strains. Yeast is used in bread making to produce a leavened product that is light in texture. Sometimes the enzyme amylase is also added to convert starch in flour to sugars. The yeast cells rapidly convert the sugar to ethyl alcohol and carbon dioxide by fermentation.

$$C_6H_{12}O_6 \longrightarrow 2C_2H_5OH + 2CO_2$$

The carbon dioxide causes the dough to rise and soften prior to baking while the ethyl alcohol evaporates during baking. If lactic acid starter cultures are inoculated into dough and incubated before baking, a sourdough bread can be obtained.

Micro Check

- What is the purpose of using starter cultures?
- How do soft cheeses differ in content from hard cheeses?
- What is responsible for the taste of sourdough bread?

MICROORGANISMS IN THE PRODUCTION OF ALCOHOLIC BEVERAGES

Alcoholic beverages have been made and consumed by humans for thousands of years. The history of beer making dates back to at least 2000 B.C. The Babylonians brewed some 18 kinds of beer and assigned two goddesses, Ninkasi and Siris, to watch over it. Beer was made at one time by women who fermented flour to produce fresh beer. Many monasteries of the sixteenth and seventeenth centuries also made beer as a source of revenue. The production of wine and beer is often referred to as an art, but the large-scale production of alcoholic beverages is very much an applied science.

Wine

Wine is one of the most popular of the beverages produced by yeast fermentation of freshly harvested grape juice. Fruits or other parts of plants, such as peaches, berries, pears, or dandelions, may be used to make wine, but the name of the plant must appear in the title, such as peach wine. Grapes contain glucose, varying amounts of fructose, water, pigments, proteins, amino acids, organic acids, and minerals. At harvest time in the fall, the sugar content is expected to be at least 24 percent so the final yield of alcohol can reach as much as 12 percent, a stable alcohol content for table wine. The final **aroma** (fragrance), or bouquet, of a wine is related to the contents of particular grapes and the biochemical changes occurring during fermentation and aging.

Wine production begins with the mechanical crushing of the grapes (Fig. 24–2). The grape juice is pumped to a press that separates the juice from skins, stems, and seeds. The pressed grape juice, or **must,** is pumped to vats for fermentation. Undesirable microorganisms are eliminated by the addition of sulfites.

The fermentation vats were made of oak originally, but commercial vats may be made of glass, concrete, or stainless steel. The must is then inoculated with pure cultures of particular yeast strains of *Saccharomyces ellipsoideus*. The mixtures are aerated to allow the initial growth of yeast cells, and then the must becomes anaerobic. For red wines, fermentation proceeds for three to five days at 23.9° to 26.7°C (75° to 80°F) in primary fermentation tanks. Slightly lower temperatures and longer times are used in the production of white wines.

The fermented juice is separated from the residue or **pomace** and pumped to secondary fermentation tanks. Fermentation continues for seven to 11 days at temperatures of 21.1° to 29.4°C (70° to 85°F) and the solid material settles to the bottom of the tanks. Sometimes a series of tanks and fining agents, compounds that attract small suspended solids, causing them to settle, are used to improve the separation of wine from solids. The liquid may be pasteurized or filtered to remove any remaining yeast cells. The clarified wine is pumped into wooden casks or barrels for aging. Aging processes allow time for more complex biochemical changes to develop for enhanced flavor. Red wines may be allowed to age for as long as two to 10 years before bottling.

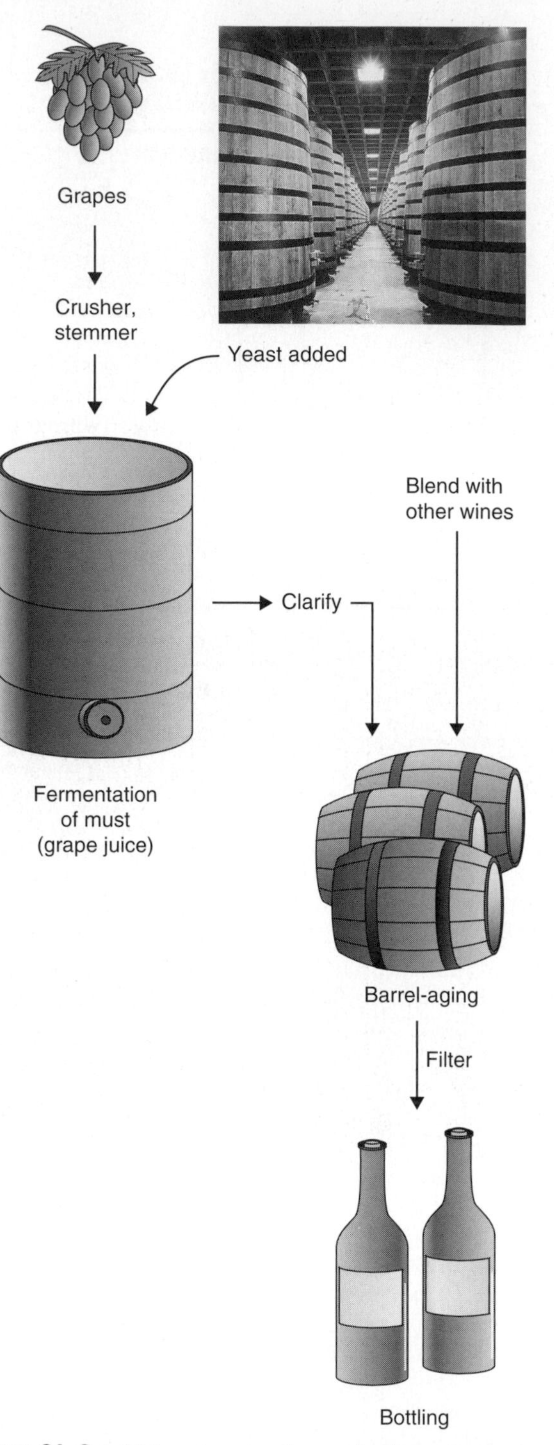

Figure 24–2 ◆ Major steps in the production of red wine. Skins are removed in the making of white wine. *Inset* shows wooden barrels in which wine is aging.

White wines are often aged for up to two years. After cask aging, the wine is bottled and aging may continue before release to consumers. Certain cabernet sauvignon wines are stored for up to 20 years before they are considered ready to drink. **Sparkling wines,** like champagne, are allowed to undergo secondary fermentation in large pressurized vats or in bottles after the addition of sugar or brandy. The additional fermentation creates the high carbon dioxide content. **Dry wines** contain little or no sugar. **Sweet wines** have a residual sugar content because fermentation has been stopped early or because more sugar has been added. Most table wines have about 12 to 15 percent alcohol.

Beer

Barley or another grain is used as the source of fermentable carbohydrate in beer making. A preliminary step, known as **malting,** is required to convert barley starch into sugar (Fig. 24–3). During malting the grain is soaked in water at 10° to 20°C (50° to 68°F) to initiate germination of the grain and for the production of the enzymes amylase and proteinase. Moisture promotes the breakdown of the starch in the presence of amylase.

The grain, called green malt at this state, is dried in a process called kilning and may be stored for future use. Malt is added to corn, rice, or wheat and cooked together in a process known as **mashing.** The mash is filtered to remove solids, and the clear amber liquid is now called **wort.** The wort is boiled for 1.5 to 2.5 hours to kill undesirable microorganisms. **Hops,** the dried flowers of the vine, *Humulus lupulus,* are added to provide color and bitter flavor (see Color Plate 94). The hops also discourage growth of microorganisms, which could interfere with the quality of the final product. They also contribute to forming the foam in beer.

The mixture of wort and hops is cooled and pumped to large fermentation vessels. The addition of the yeast is called **pitching.** Strains of *Saccharomyces cerevisiae* (top yeasts) or *S. carlsber-*

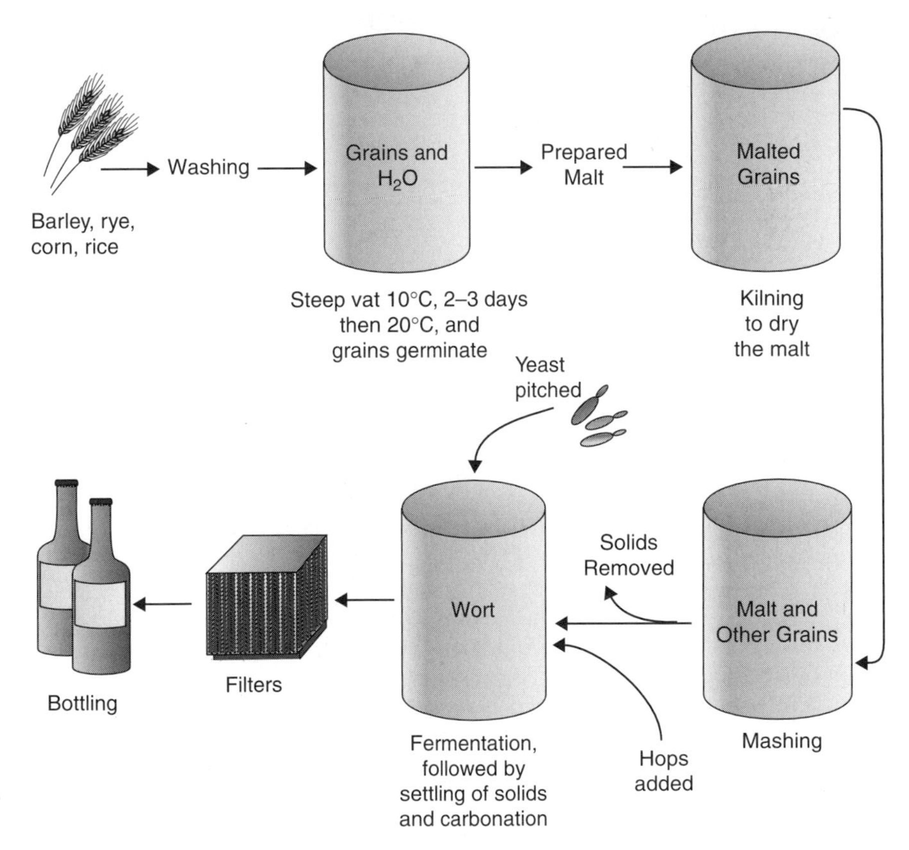

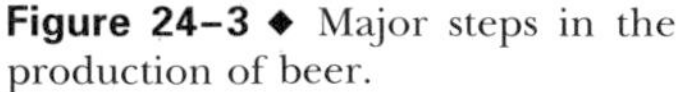
Figure 24–3 ◆ Major steps in the production of beer.

gensis (bottom yeasts) are pitched to the cooled mixture. Top yeasts remain near the surface of the mixture. Bottom yeasts settle out and collect in the bottoms of vessels. The inoculum consists of about 1 pound of yeast per barrel of liquid.

Fermentation is allowed to proceed for eight to 10 days at temperatures ranging from 3.3° to 14°C (38° to 57°F). A large quantity of foam accumulates at the surface of the fermentation vessel. The alcoholic product at this point is known as green beer. Green beer is aged at about 0°C for several weeks or months. Beer is then carbonated so that the final product is about 0.45 to 0.52 percent carbon dioxide. The alcoholic content of commercial beer is approximately 3.8 percent. Beer is pasteurized for 20 minutes at 60° to 61°C (140° to 141.8°F) and filtered before bottling. Light or low-calorie beers have become increasingly popular with consumers. Beer with less calories can be produced by pretreating wort with certain fungal enzymes. The pretreatment converts more carbohydrates to fermentable sugars so that less carbohydrates remain in the final product.

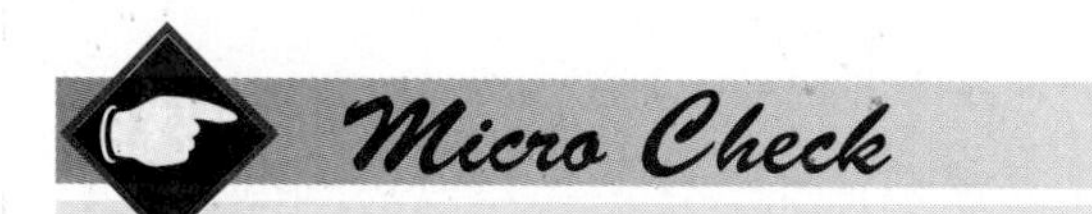

- Why are hops added to wort?
- Describe the fermentation processes for production of wine and beer.
- How are light beers made?

MICROORGANISMS AS A FOOD SOURCE

In 1984, devastating numbers of people died in Africa because of an extended drought. This left the world with a heightened awareness of the havoc caused by climate changes on food production and disease. Attention of world leaders and food scientists was directed toward solutions for food shortages. The high protein content of certain edible microorganisms is considered one potential solution to the protein shortage for an expanding world population. Any high-protein product derived from bacteria, fungi, or algae is called **single-cell protein (SCP),** even though some of these organisms are not unicellular. The photosynthetic algae *Scenedesmus* and *Spirulina* are cost-effective potential sources of SPC. *Spirulina* is commercially available in health food stores as a dietary supplement.

For complete nutrition of humans, all eight of the essential amino acids for human nutrition should be found in SCP. Lysine and methionine are essential amino acids that may be deficient in some SCP. Supplementation with these amino acids would be necessary. One drawback to SCP is its high nucleic acid content which may lead to kidney stone formation or gout in people; animals do not develop these conditions from SCP. Feeding SCP to livestock, therefore, would conserve plant materials for human needs.

TRANSGENIC PLANTS AND ANIMALS

The biotechnology used to create microorganisms for the production of drugs and agricultural products has also been applied to alter the genetic make-up of plants and animals. The modified organisms are called **transgenic** plants and animals meaning genes of another species have been introduced. A novel particle gun is used to insert DNA into plant cells (Fig. 24–4). Genes such as those conferring resistance to insect or viral attack have been transferred to plants. This technology may be another solution in the conserving of plant crops against attack by insects and microbial diseases.

The first transgenic fruit approved by the FDA was a tomato plant in which the ripening enzyme was blocked. Transgenic tomatoes with delayed ripening and improved flavor have been available in many parts of the United States since 1994. The genetic make-up of corn has been engineered to retain sweetness by interfering with the synthesis of starch from glucose. Soybean plants have been altered to produce proteins containing amino acids not naturally found in the native plants. The more complete proteins of modified soybeans are good substitutes in the human diet, for expensive animal proteins.

Transgenic animals are under investigation as potential sources of biological products. Insulin, growth hormone, and plasminogen activator are medical products that may be obtained from the milk of genetically modified cows, goats, and sheep. Although several federal regulatory agencies and state governments do regulate testing and release of genetically engineered foods, the FDA does not require labeling.

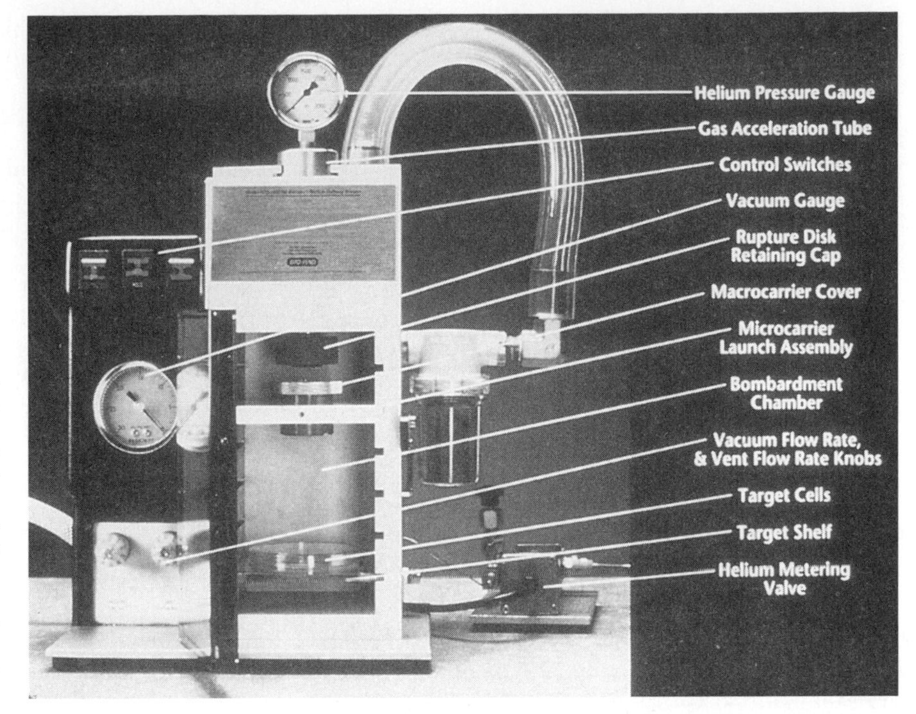

Figure 24–4 ◆ A particle gun used to inject DNA into plant cells. Gold or tungsten spheres measuring 1 to 4 mm are coated with the DNA of interest. Compressed air or helium in the particle gun powerfully launches the DNA-coated spheres into the target cells inside the bombardment chamber. The propulsive force pushes the particles through the plant cell walls and membranes without significant cell damage. The injected DNA integrates into the plant DNA.

Micro Check

- Do you know if you have eaten a transgenic food?
- Do you think genetically altered produce or products should be labeled?
- Why are soybeans with enhanced amino acid composition considered useful for human food?

FOODBORNE ILLNESSES

Many pathogenic organisms may cause serious gastrointestinal disturbances. Foodborne illnesses usually include symptoms such as vomiting, nausea, diarrhea, abdominal cramps, dizziness and others. Diagnosis is made easier by observing the patient's symptoms, taking a food history, and noting the period of time elapsed since eating a suspected food. Foodborne diseases are considered to be either **food infections, food poisonings,** or a combination of both.

Food infections usually involve a food with an excessively large number of microorganisms present. The chemical changes in food brought about by the growth of microorganisms, their enzymes, and other chemicals may be responsible for disease. For example, the bacterium, *Bacillus cereus* grows in starchy foods such as gravies that are kept warm for hours; if eaten, it may produce a food infection. Food poisoning usually involves the growth of an organism that produces one or more toxic compounds in the food. One of the most common bacterial foodborne illnesses is caused by *Staphylococcus aureus* enterotoxin, a heat-stable toxin that causes explosive diarrhea and vomiting. An example of food poisonings caused by a fungus occurs when peanut meal or other grains are stored in a moist environment in which toxin-producing molds, such as *Aspergillus flavus,* may increase rapidly producing **aflatoxin,** a highly carcinogenic toxin (see Color Plate 95).

Organisms may be introduced into food by unsanitary food preparation or by improper handling of food. Some organisms are found normally on the animals, grains, or vegetables. Practices such as not washing fruits and vegetables before cooking or eating them, or using the same knife to cut vegetables to be eaten raw after cutting raw meat, poultry, or fish will expose the consumer to food infections. Food handlers must be careful to wash their hands thoroughly with warm water and soap after using toilet facilities and before handling food. Delicate cream pies must be kept cold. If several hours elapse before leftover food is refrigerated, unwanted microorganisms can grow. If these bacteria produce one or more toxins or destructive enzymes, those who eat the food may develop food poisoning. The most common organisms involved in foodborne illnesses are discussed in Chapter 17 and listed in Table 24–5.

MICROBIOLOGICAL EXAMINATION OF FOODS AND DAIRY PRODUCTS

For the public health, it is important that the food industry make products that are consistently safe and flavorful with a maximal shelf life. Individual food manufacturers monitor food processing from the time of receipt of the raw ingredients to the time the finished product is released for human consumption. To assure high-quality products, acceptable limits of numbers or types of microorganisms called **specifications** are established by a number of regulatory agencies representing the food industry. The responsibility for testing for the microbiological quality of foods and dairy products may be that of a food plant, a dairy, a public health regulatory agency or all of them.

The American Public Health Association publishes standardized methods for the examination of both food and dairy products. The U.S. Department of Agriculture (USDA) and the Food and Drug Administration (FDA) set acceptable

Table 24–5
FOODBORNE ILLNESSES

TYPE OF ORGANISM	COMMON FOODS	COMMENT
Bacteria		
Staphylococcus aureus and other staphylococci	Almost any foods that have been improperly handled since the bacteria are transferred from human and animal skin	Enterotoxin causes GI symptoms; toxin is heat-stable
Clostridium botulinum	Usually improperly canned foods	Neurotoxin is highly toxic, heat-labile
Clostridium perfringens	Improperly handled meats, unsanitary conditions transfer cells and spores from soil, dust to meat	Enterotoxin damages intestinal epithelial cells
Bacillus cereus	Cereals, potatoes, gravy, milk, meat loaf, cooked meat, rice, puddings	Toxins, enzymes, and other chemicals cause diarrhea, vomiting
Listeria monocytogenes	Raw milk, raw meat, poultry, pork, ground beef, some vegetables	Invades tissues, grows from 1°–45°C
Salmonella, Shigella, and *Escherichia*	Poultry, eggs, milk, cake mix, cookie dough, meat, many other foods	Enterotoxins, other chemicals and toxins cause symptoms
Vibrio cholerae	Water, well water, raw oysters, salads	Travelers' diarrhea, epidemic cholera
Molds		
Aspergillus flavus and other species	Peanut meal, fresh beef, ham, bacon, breads, and other foods	Aflatoxin shown to be carcinogenic in animals, mutagenic, damages liver
Marine Dinoflagellates		
Gonyaulax catenella	Mussels, clams, oysters, scallops, other shellfish, raw or cooked	Paralytic shellfish poisoning by saxitoxin, heat-stable, causes cardiovascular collapse, respiratory failure
Viruses		
Polioviruses, enteroviruses, rotaviruses, Norwalk virus, hepatitis A, and others	Water, shellfish, pork, fruits, milk, or foods contaminated by unsanitary methods or food handlers who are infected or are carriers	More documented cases caused by hepatitis A than by any other virus

limits on numbers and types of microorganisms on a raw ingredient or finished product. Those limits are called **standards** and are enforceable under the law. Microbiological testing may include at least quantitative analyses, qualitative analyses, dye-reduction tests, or enzyme assays.

Quantitative Methods

Numbers of microorganisms in food or dairy products are determined by direct microscopic examination or by standard plate count (SPC) techniques. The direct microscopic examination is often used for determining the bacterial quality of raw milk or cream, but the test result is a relative rather than a precise estimation.

For direct examination, 0.01 ml of a milk or cream sample is placed on a glass slide in a 1 cm^2 area and allowed to dry. The smears are stained with a certified solution of methylene blue chloride and xylene or tetrachlorethane for two minutes. Finished smears are examined under oil immersion to obtain estimates of bacteria or body cells from an inflamed udder. The individual cells or small clumps of microbial cells are counted as individual units. The average number of cells or clumps per field is multiplied by a microscopic calibration factor (MCF) to obtain the number of organisms or clumps per ml.

$$MCF = \frac{\text{area of the smear}}{\text{area of the microscopic field}} \times 100$$

Direct microscopic counts of cells or clumps of cells can be made rapidly counting both viable and dead cells. They are most valuable to test milk or cream, in which a relatively high count of cells of certain morphology can be significant.

The standard plate count estimates the total numbers of viable organisms present when standardized test conditions are maintained (see Chapter 5). The SPC is used for grading milk (Table 24–6). In order to comply with established standards, pasteurized or certified raw milk must not contain more than 10 coliforms per ml.

Qualitative Methods

The type of microorganisms in food or dairy products may be of greater significance than the total number of organisms. Certain bacteria, like coliforms, are used as an indicator of possible contamination of a product with human or animal waste materials. Coliforms account for about 10 percent of the intestinal bacteria of humans and other animals. The presumptive, confirmed, and completed tests for coliforms described in Chapter 23 can be modified for food and dairy products.

A test for enterococci, gram-positive cocci that inhabit the intestine, is more reliable in testing the sanitary quality of churned butter, since enterococci have a high salt tolerance. Food quality is evaluated by specific test procedures to detect the number and types of microorganisms frequently found as contaminants. Tests for specific pathogens are less often employed except in the event of outbreaks of foodborne disease.

Dye-Reduction Tests

The number of bacteria in milk can be indirectly estimated by dye-reduction tests. The principle of these tests is based on the ability of microorganisms to transfer electrons to redox dyes, such as methylene blue or resazurin. The dye changes from its colored state to a different color or a colorless state as electrons are accepted. The time of color change is measured. A rapid change of color indicates a high bacterial count.

Table 24–6
STANDARDS FOR DAIRY PRODUCTS

PRODUCT	MAXIMAL SPC	MAXIMAL COLIFORMS
Grade A raw milk (for pasteurization)	100,000/ml	—
Grade A milk (pasteurized)	20,000/ml	10/ml
Certified raw milk	10,000/ml	10/ml
Certified milk (pasteurized)	10,000/ml*	10/ml*

*Before pasteurization

In the testing procedure, a dye is mixed with a milk sample. Methylene blue milk mixtures are blue initially, but they turn colorless quickly in the presence of high numbers of bacteria. Resazurin-milk mixtures are blue initially, but become violet and finally pink or white as resazurin is reduced completely by a high count of bacteria. Poor quality milk produced under unsanitary conditions reduces dye rapidly. Such milk may be unsuitable for pasteurization and may contain potential pathogens.

Enzyme Assay

Alkaline phosphatase is an enzyme that occurs naturally in raw milk, but is inactivated by pasteurization. Measuring phosphatase activity determines if pasteurization was done properly. If raw milk is added to pasteurized milk during manufacturing, phosphatase will be present. Disodium phenylphosphate, the test substrate, is added to a sample of milk. The test measures the amount of phenol released from the substrate; the amount is proportional to the action of the enzyme. The released phenol becomes a blue color when it reacts with an indicator solution of 2,6-dibromoquinone that is added after a 15-minute incubation at 40°C ± 1°C. A positive test is a reliable indicator of phosphatase activity, but a negative test is not an absolute guarantee of adequate pasteurization.

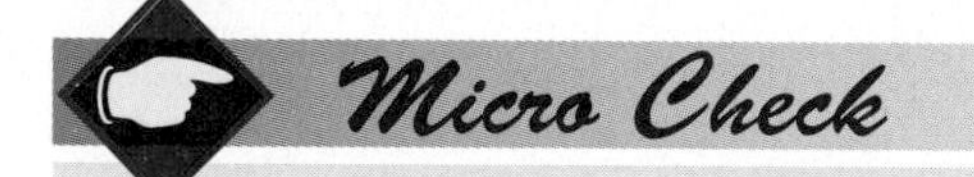

- How does a qualitative microbiological analysis differ from a quantitative microbiological analysis?
- What would be the probable sources for coliforms in a milk sample?
- Why is it more practical to test for coliforms instead of specific intestinal pathogens in food samples?

Understanding Microbiology

1. List five methods of food preservation and explain how each method works.
2. Why is the complete removal of water from food usually undesirable?
3. Why is it important to limit the use of antimicrobial agents as preservatives in foods?
4. Describe the two-stage fermentation process used in the production of vinegar.
5. Identify the times and temperatures for pasteurization of milk and dairy products.

Applying Microbiology

6. Assume you wish to determine the number of viable bacteria per gram of a food sample. What equipment or supplies would you need? What food would you like to test? Why? Do you expect to find microorganisms in the food? Explain why or why not.

Appendixes

Appendix A

Examples of Prefixes, Roots, and Suffixes Used in Microbiology

A prefix is a combining form placed before a word or root to modify its meaning. A root is the main part of the word. A suffix is a combining form placed after a word or root to modify its meaning. Some combining forms can be used as a prefix, root word, or suffix.

PREFIX	MEANING	EXAMPLE
a-, an-	absence of, without	abiotic, anaerobic
amphi-	both	amphibolic
ana-	up	anabolism
anti-	against	antibiotic
archae-	ancient	archaea
arthro-	jointed, segmented	arthroconidium
asco-	sac	ascospore
auto-	self	autotroph
basidio-	base	basidiospore
blasto-	bud	blastoconidium
campylo-	curved	campylobacteriosis
cata-	down	catabolism
caulo-	stalk	caulobacters
chlamydo-	hidden	chlamydoconidium
chromo-	colored	chromosome
co-, con-	with, together	coenzyme, conjugation
coeno-	shared in common	coenocytic
conidio-	dust	conidiophore
cyano-	blue	cyanobacteria
cyst-, cysto-	bladder	cystitis
de-	lack or removal of	dehydration
di-	two	dimorphic
diplo-	double	diplococcus
dys-	bad, painful	dyspnea
ec-, ecto-, exo-	outside, outer	eclipse, ecotoplasm, exoenzyme
em-, en-, endo-	inside, inner	embedded, encephalitis, endospore
epi-	atop, over	epidermis
eu-	true	eucaryote
hetero-	different	heterofermentative
homo-	same	homofermentative
hyper-	above, more than	hyperthyroidism, hypersensitivity
hypo	below, less than	hypogammaglobulinemia, hypotonic

PREFIX	MEANING	EXAMPLE
iso-	same, equal	isograph, isotonic
lopho-	tufted	lophotrichous
macro-	large	macronucleus
micro-	small	microaerophilic
mito-	thread	mitochondria
pan-	all, universal	pandemic, pancytopenia
para-	beside, near	parasite, paratyphoid
peri-	around	peritrichous
photo-	light	photosynthesis
poly-	many	polyarteritis
post-	after, behind	poststreptococcal, posterior
pre-, pro-	before, primary	prenatal, protist
proto-	first	prototroph
pseudo-	false	pseudopodia

ROOT OR COMBINING FORM	MEANING	EXAMPLE
agglutin-	clumping	agglutination
amyl-	starch	amylose
arthr-	joint	arthritis
bacteri-	bacteria	bacteriostatic
bio-	living	microbiology
blephar-	eyelid	blepharitis
carcino-	cancer	carcinogen
ceph-, cephalo-	head or brain	encephalitis
chloro-	green	chlorophyll
crypt-	hidden	cryptococcus
derm-	skin	dermatophyte
electro-	electricity	electrolyte
enter-	intestine	enterococcus
eosino-	rose-colored	eosinophil
eryth-	red	erythrocyte
etio-	cause	etiology
hem-	blood	hemaglobin
hepat-	liver	hepatitis
kerat-	cornea	keratosis
leuk-	white	leukocyte
meningo-	membrane	meningococcus
meso-	middle	mesophil
morph-	shape	morphology
nema-	thread	treponemal
neo-	new	neonatal
nephro-	kidney	nephron
phago-	to eat, engulf	phagocytosis
psychro-	cold	psychrophile
retin-	retina	retinopathy
rhin-	nose	rhinologist
saccharo-	sugar	polysaccharide
sym-	together	symbiosis
taxon-	arrangement	taxonomic

thermo-	heat	thermophile
troph-	feeding, nutrition	auxotroph
undul-	wavelike	undulate

SUFFIX	**MEANING**	**EXAMPLE**
-al	pertaining to	fungal
-algia	pain	myalgia
-ology	study of	protozoology
-ase	enzyme	collagenase
-cyte	cell	monocyte
-ectomy	excision	appendectomy
-emia	blood condition	septicemia
-fy	to become	classify
-genesis	formation	morphogenesis
-gnosis	knowledge	prognosis
-ic	pertaining to	periodic
-ion	process	lesion
-ism	condition of	polymorphism
-itis	inflammation of	pharyngitis
-ity	condition	immunity
-lysis	destruction	hemolysis
-nema	thread	chromonema
-oid	resembling	mucoid
-oma	tumor	myeloma
-osis	condition of	diverticulosis
-otomy	incision	tracheotomy
-pathy	disease	neuropathy
-penia	lack of	leukopenia
-phil	attraction	basophil
-phyte	plant	saprophyte
-scope	instrument	microscope
-scopy	to view, examine	colonoscopy
-some	body	chromosome

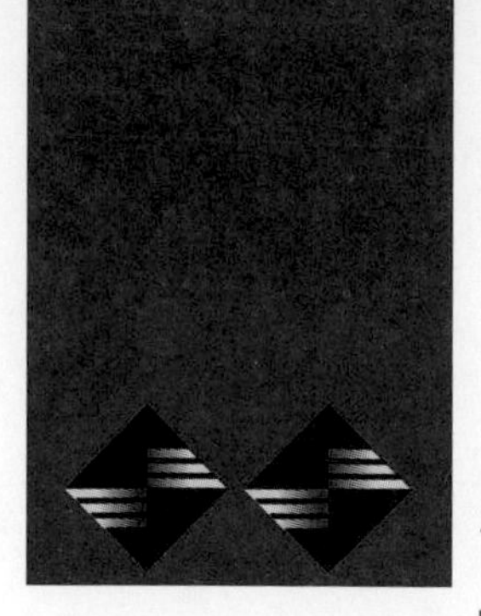

Appendix B

Temperature and Metric System Measurements

TEMPERATURE

degrees Fahrenheit (°F) = 9/5(°C) + 32
degrees Celsius (°C) = 5/9(°F − 32)

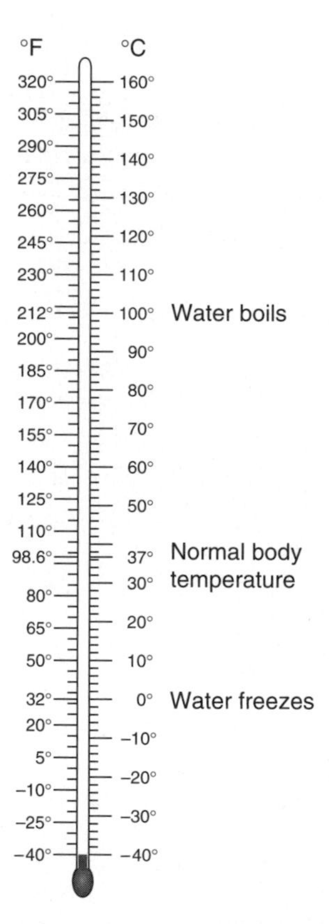

0°C = 32°F (freezing point of water)
100°C = 212°F (boiling point of water)
37°C = 98.6°F (normal body temperature)

METRIC SYSTEM PREFIXES

pico (p) = 10^{-12}
nano (n) = 10^{-9}
micro (μ) = 10^{-6}
milli (m) = 10^{-3}
centi (c) = 10^{-2}
deci (d) = 10^{-1}
kilo (k) = 10^{3}

LENGTH

1 kilometer (km) = 0.62 mile
1 meter = 39.3700 inches = 3.2808 feet
1 meter (m) = 100 centimeters (cm) = 1,000 millimeters (mm)
1 centimeter = 10 millimeters (mm) = 0.394 inch (in.)
1 millimeter = 0.0394 in.
1 micrometer (μm) = 10^{-6} meter
1 nanometer (nm) = 10^{-9} meter
1 angstrom (Å) = 10^{-10} meter

VOLUME

1 liter = 1.0567 quarts
1 liter = 1,000 milliliters (ml)
1 milliliter = 1 cm^3 = 0.061 cubic in.
1 mm^3 = 10^{-3} cm^3 = 10^{-6} liter

MASS

1 kilogram (kg) = 1,000 grams = 2.205 pounds
1 pound = 453.60 g
1 gram (g) = 1,000 milligrams = 0.0353 ounce
1 ounce = 28.35 g
1 milligram (mg) = 10^{-3} g
1 microgram (μg) = 10^{-6} g

Appendix C

Pronunciation Guide

This appendix contains the phonetic pronunciations for selected microorganisms in the text. Names of genera and species often appear intimidating to the novice. A few simple guidelines and examples will allow you to learn to pronounce the scientific names of microorganisms.

1. Thc accent usually falls on the next to the last syllables of short words. Example: *Bacillus* (bah-SIL-us).
2. One or two accents may appear in compound names. Example: *Lactobacillus* (lack-toe-bah-SIL-us) or (LACK-toe-bah-SIL-us).
3. A double i (ii) is pronounced ee-eye. Example *carinii* (kar-IN-ee-eye).
4. An ending of eus is pronounced ee-us. Example: *Proteus* (PRO-tee-us).
5. An ending of ia is pronounced ee-ah. Example: *Escherichia* (esh-er-IK-ee-ah).
6. Correct pronunciation comes with practice.

Acetobacter aceti	a-see-toh-BACT-ter a-SEE-tie
Bacillus stearothermophilus	bah-SIL-lus ste-row-ther-MAH-fil-lus
B. subtilis	B. SAH-til-us
B. thermoacidurans	B. ther-mow-ay-sih-DUR-ans
Bordetella pertussis	bor-de-TEL-lah per-TUSS-sis
Clostridium botulilnum	klos-TREH-dee-um bo-tyoo-LIE-num
C. thermosaccharolyticum	C. ther-mow-sak-ah-row-LIT-ee-kum
Coccidioides immitis	kock-SID-ee-OYE-dees IM-meh-tis
Cryptococcus neoformans	krip-toe-KOCK-kus nee-oh-FOR-mans
Desulfotomaculum nigrificans	dee-sul-foh-toe-MAC-yu-lum NYE-gri-fee-kans
Entamoeba histolytica	en-tah-ME-bah his-toe-LI-tee-kah
Enterococcus faecalis	en-te-roh-KOK-kuss fee-CA-lis
Escherichia coli	esh-er-IK-ee-ah KOH-lee
Giardia lamblia	gee-AR-dee-ah lam-BLEE-ah
Haemophilus influenzae	he-MOF-il-us in-floo-ENZ-eye
Lactobacillus acidophilus	lack-toe-bah-SIL-us ay-seh-DAH-fil-us
L. bulgaricus	L. bul-GAH-reh-kuss
L. plantarum	L. plan-TA-rum
Leuconostoc citrovorum	loo-ko-NOS-tok sit-row-VOR-um
Micrococcus radiodurans	my-krow-KOK-kuss ray-dee-oh-DUR-anz
Morganella morganii	mor-gan-EL-lah mor-GAN-ee-ee
Mycobacterium tuberculosis	my-koh-back-TIR-ee-um too-ber-koo-LOW-sis
Neisseria gonorrhoeae	nye-SEH-ree-ah go-nor-REE-eye
N. meningitidis	N. meh-nin-jit-EE-tid-dis
Pseudomonas aeruginosa	soo-doh-MOH-nass a-ruh-jin-OH-sah
Saccharomyces carlsbergenesis	sak-a-row-MY-sees karlz-ber-JEN-esiss
S. cerevisiae	S. se-ri-VISS-ee-eye
S. ellipsoideus	S. eeh-lip-SOY-dee-us
Salmonella choleraesuis	sal-mon-EL-lah kol-er-ah-SOO-iss
S. typhi	S. TIE-fee
S. typhimurium	S. tie-fee-MUIR-ee-um
Serratia marcescens	ser-RAY-sha mar-SES-sens

Sporothrix schenckii	spo-RO-thriks-SHEN-key-ee
Staphylococcus aureus	staff-il-oh-KOK-kuss ORE-ee-us
Streptococcus diacetylactis	strep-toe-KOK-kuss die-ay-sih-TEEL-lack-tiss
S. mutans	S. MYOO-tans
S. pneumoniae	S. new-MOH-nee-eye
S. thermophilus	S. ther-MAH-fil-us
Toxoplasma gondii	TOK-so-PLAZ-mah GON-dee-ee
Treponema pallidum	tre-poh-NEE-mah PAL-li-dum

Appendix D

Internet Web Sites Useful in Microbiology

One of the most popular, useful, and increasingly accessible tools for searching for information is the Internet. Almost any subject can be accessed by typing keywords into the "Search" line of a directory or search engine service. The computer does not know how to correct an error in typing, so if you mistype keywords or web addresses, the message will be returned with an "error" or sent to the wrong web address.

Sometimes the search engine returns a list containing hundreds of web sites with some relation to your keywords. Finding the most useful sites can be a very daunting task. However, with patience, the search yields web sites that are most useful to you. If you "bookmark" these sites, you can return to them in the future without having to type in a web address. Occasionally, web addresses are changed or dropped. At the time of writing this list, these web addresses were current.

SOME DIRECTORIES AND SEARCH ENGINES WITH GOOD DATABASES FOR MEDICINE AND LIFE SCIENCE

SITE: AltaVista
http://www.altavista.com

SITE: Yahoo
http://www.yahoo.com

SITE: Lycos
http://www.lycos.com

SITE: Internet Sleuth
http://isleuth.com/medi.html

SITE: CliniWeb
http://www.ohsu.edu/cliniweb/search.html

SITE: Matrix
http://www.medmatrix.org

SITE: MedWeb
http://www.medweb.emory.edu

Frequently, when web sites are listed, the address begins with the www. portion assuming that you know http:// precedes www.

SOME WEB SITES SUITABLE FOR BIOLOGY AND MICROBIOLOGY TOPICS

WEB ADDRESS	SITE INFORMATION
www.asmusa.org	***American Society for Microbiology (ASM),*** Washington, D.C. A professional society for life scientists interested in microorganisms, disease, viruses, molecular biology, and immunology. Student membership is offered at a lower membership rate. Multiple professional journals are listed.
www.cdc.gov	***Centers for Disease Control and Prevention (CDC),*** Atlanta, GA The laboratory branch for the U.S. Public Health Service. The site contains guidelines for infection control, immunizations, and hazardous substances. Journals: Morbidity and Mortality Weekly Report (MMWR) and Emerging Infectious Diseases.

FOR SEXUALLY TRANSMITTED DISEASES, AIDS, AND CANCER

SELECT: STDs; recent year's Guidelines for the Treatment of STDs; recent year's STD Surveillance Report
SELECT: HIV/AIDS
SELECT: Chronic Diseases/Cancer Prevention Programs or Environment and Breast Cancer

www.cdc.gov/ncidod/ncid.htm — ***Infectious Diseases***

www.cdc.gov/ncidod/EID/eid.htm — ***Emerging Infectious Diseases***

www.nlm.nih.gov — ***National Library of Medicine, National Institutes of Health (NIH)***

www.nci.nih.gov — ***National Cancer Institute, NIH***

www.biostr.washington.edu/DigitalAnatomist.html — ***Digital Anatomist***
An interactive atlas, with two- and three-dimensional pictures of various regions of the body. Links to text information are included.

www.nasa.gov — ***National Aeronautics and Space Administration***

www.fda.gov — ***Food and Drug Administration***

www.epa.gov — ***Environmental Protection Agency***

www.pasteur.fr — ***Pasteur Institute, Paris, France***
The site is in French, but if you read this language, it contains a wealth of information about the activities of a prestigious medical research organization.

Glossary

Abiotic: nonliving

Abscess: localized collection of pus in any part of the body

Acetyl-CoA: product formed when an acetyl group bonds with coenzyme A

Acid: compound releasing hydrogen ions (H^+) on dissociation

Acid-fast stain: differential staining procedure based on the ability of certain microorganisms to retain carbolfuchsin despite treatment with acid-alcohol

Acidic dye: compound used as a stain in which the negative ion supplies the color

Acidosis: excessive loss of bicarbonate or accumulation of acids

Acquired immunity: see specific immune response

Acquired immunodeficiency syndrome (AIDS): immune dysfunction accompanied by opportunistic diseases

Activated sludge: inoculum of solid waste containing large numbers of sewage-metabolizing microorganisms

Activated sludge tank: a tank with jets to supply oxygen for aerobic decomposition of waste matter by microorganisms

Activation: initiation of cell division of B and T cells

Active: in immunity, the individual produces specific immunoglobulins

Active immunity: resistance obtained from one's own response to a nonself substance

Active site: location on an enzyme molecule that binds substrate

Active transport: movement of molecules or ions from lesser to greater concentrations requiring cellular energy

Actin: flexible protein of microfilaments

Acute glomerulonephritis: inflammatory process affecting glomeruli of the kidney

Adenine: cyclic nitrogen base

Adenosine diphosphate (ADP): product formed by removing a phosphate group from ATP

Adenosine triphosphate (ATP): major molecule for energy transfers in metabolism

Adherence factor: specific receptor site on host tissue that allows the attachment of a particular microorganism

Adhesin: substance enabling microorganisms to adhere to solid surfaces

Adjuvant: chemical substance that enhances antibody production when it is injected with antigen

Advanced primary treatment: addition of chemicals to increase the settling efficiency of solid matter in primary wastewater treatment

Aerobe: organism that grows in the presence of oxygen

Aerobic respiration: series of redox reactions that release energy to generate ATP and use oxygen as a final electron acceptor

Aerosol: droplet containing a fine suspension of particles or a liquid in the air

Affinity: strength of binding between an antigenic determinant and an antibody-combining site

Aflatoxin: chemical produced by *Aspergillus* that is toxic to animals and humans

Agammaglobulinemia: lack of gamma globulin

Agar: solidifying agent used in culturing microorganisms

Agglutination: clumping reaction caused by antibody molecules complexing with the antigens

Agranulocyte: white blood cell having no granules in its cytoplasm

Algae: macroscopic and microscopic photosynthetic organisms belonging to the kingdom Plantae or Protista

Alkylating agent: chemical that adds a methyl or ethyl group to cellular proteins and DNA causing mutations or death of the cell

Allergen: antigen that stimulates an allergic response

Allergy: altered state of immune response; hypersensitivity
Allograft: transplant from a genetically dissimilar donor of the same species as the recipient
Allosteric enzyme: enzyme subject to noncompetitive inhibition
Allosteric modulation: inhibition of an enzyme by the binding of a noncompetitive inhibitor
Allosteric site: site on an enzyme to which a noncompetitive inhibitor binds
Alpha hemolysis: partial destruction of red blood cells surrounding colonies on blood agar
Ames test: procedure for detecting chemical mutagens
Amino acid binding site: position on a tRNA molecule that binds a specific amino acid
Ammonification: biochemical process used by soil bacteria and fungi to convert organic nitrogen molecules to ammonia
Amphibolic pathways: biochemical pathways that participate in catabolic and anabolic reactions
Amphitrichous: type of flagellation with a flagellum at each end of a cell
Amylopectin: major component of starch
Amylose: component of starch that makes up 20 to 25 percent of starch
Anabolism: energy-requiring synthesis of larger molecules from monomers
Anaerobe: organism that grows in the absence of oxygen
Anaerobic digester tank: tank used in wastewater treatment where anaerobic microorganisms decompose organic matter
Anaerobic respiration: series of biochemical reactions that use an inorganic molecule, other than oxygen, as a final electron acceptor
Anal triangle: lower triangular area of perineum
Analgesic: pain-relieving drug
Anamnestic response: rapid and accentuated response after an initial contact with an antigen
Anaphylaxis: immediate hypersensitive response involving IgE, mast cells, and basophils
Anergy: state of nonresponsiveness to nonself antigens
Anion: negatively charged ion
Anionic detergent: molecule that carries a negative charge when dissolved in water
Annealing: recombining nucleic acid strands at low temperatures after separating by heat
Anorexia: loss of appetite
Anoxygenic photosynthesis: photosynthesis occurring under anaerobic conditions
Antibiosis: process of killing or inhibiting the growth of a microorganism by chemicals produced by another microorganism
Antibiotic: chemical substance produced by a microorganism that inhibits or kills other microorganisms; useful in treating infections
Antibody: immunoglobulin produced in response to the presence of an antigen
Antibody-dependent cell-mediated cytotoxicity (ADCC): phenomenon in which target cells coated with antibody are destroyed
Antibody-mediated immunity (AMI): immune defense provided by immunoglobulins
Anticodon: group of three bases on tRNA that binds to a complementary codon on mRNA at the ribosome
Anticodon site: position on a tRNA molecule that contains the anticodon
Antigen: nonself substance that elicits an immune response
Antigen-binding fragment (Fab): the portion of the immunoglobulin molecule that binds to an antigenic epitope
Antigen presentation: introduction of an antigen on the surface of an APC
Antigen-presenting cell (APC): cell that displays antigens on its surface in association with MHC class II molecules
Antigen processing: ingestion, digestion, and return of peptide antigen fragments to the surface of an APC for presentation to T cells
Antigenic drift: a major alteration in viral DNA as a consequence of mutation
Antigenic shift: minor alteration in viral DNA as a consequence of recombinant variance
Antimetabolite: chemical that interferes with the function of an enzyme
Antimicrobial: term for all categories of drugs used to treat infections
Antiseptic: chemical agent that inhibits growth or activity of microorganisms on living tissue
Apocrine: cell that releases part of the cell contents with its secretory products
Apoenzyme: protein portion of an enzyme
Apoptosis: cell death programmed by the dying cell itself
Arachnoid: middle membrane of brain and spinal cord
Archaea: domain of procaryotes lacking peptidoglycan in their cell walls
Aroma: fragrance of volatile chemicals detected by the sense of smell
Arthroconidium: cylindrical or cask-shaped asexual reproductive structure of some fungi

Arthus reaction: local reaction after repeated intradermal injections of antigen

Artificially acquired active immunity: immune defense developed by an individual who receives microbial antigens

Artificially acquired passive immunity: immune defense in an individual receiving antibodies

Ascospore: sexual spore of some fungi

Ascus: spore-bearing sac of ascospores

Asepsis: absence of any form of life

Aspiration: withdrawal of fluid from a cavity

Asthma: localized anaphylactic response to an inhaled allergen characterized by difficulty in breathing

Astrocyte: type of neuron

Ataxia: irregularity in muscle coordination

Atom: smallest particle of an element that can exist

Atomic number: number equal to the number of protons in an atom

Atopic allergies: allergies with a genetic basis

ATP-driven transport: movement of molecules or ions from an area of lesser to greater concentration by expenditure of cellular energy

Attenuated: less virulent form of an infectious agent

Attenuation: process exerting fine control of gene expression; method of decreasing virulence of a pathogen

Attenuator: genetic code stopping transcription of operon

Autoantibody: antibody produced by a person that reacts with self antigens

Autoantigen: a self antigen that stimulates an immune response

Autoclave: instrument using moist heat under pressure to destroy microorganisms

Autograft: skin graft from one site to another site on the same individual

Autoimmune disease: tissue or organ damage caused by the immune response directed against self antigens

Autotroph: organism that obtains carbon from atmospheric CO_2

Auxotroph: nutritional mutant requiring one or more growth factors

A_w: water activity of a food expressing the water vapor pressure of a food compared with water vapor pressure of pure water

Axon: projection of the cell body of the neuron

B cell: a class of lymphocytes

B-cell receptor: surface protein on B cells that binds to antigen

β-galactosidase: enzyme that hydrolyzes lactose to galactose and glucose

β-lactam ring: part of the structure of the penicillin molecule

β-lactamase: microbial enzyme that breaks the β-lactam ring of penicillins and cephalosporins

Bacille Calmette-Guérin (BCG) vaccine: live attenuated strain of *Mycobacterium bovis* used as an immunizing agent for tuberculosis

Bacilli: rod-shaped bacteria

Back mutation: mutation reversing an earlier mutation

Bacteremia: presence of viable bacteria in blood

Bacteria: domain of procaryotes containing peptidoglycan in their cell walls

Bacteriophage: virus that infects bacteria

Barophile: organism that grows in the presence of high hydrostatic pressure

Barotolerant: organism that can withstand high hydrostatic pressure

Base: compound releasing hydroxyl ions (OH^-) on dissociation

Base analog: nitrogen-containing compound similar in structure to one of the nitrogen bases of nucleic acid

Base-pair: two complementary nitrogen bases that form hydrogen bonds between them

Base-substitution: mutation resulting by replacing one base with another

Basic dye: ionic compound used as a stain in which the positive ion supplies the color

Basidiocarp: fruiting body of some fungi

Basidiospore: sexual reproductive structure of some fungi

Basidium: spore-bearing clublike structure of some fungi

Basophil: polymorphonuclear white blood cell that releases mediators of immediate hypersensitivity

Benthic: sediment and rocky formations on bottom of a body of water

Beta hemolysis: complete destruction of red blood cells surrounding colonies on blood agar

Binomial system of nomenclature: a system by which two names are assigned to every organism

Biochemical Oxygen Demand (BOD): amount of oxygen required for biological processes in an aquatic environment

Biocide: chemical agents with antiseptic, disinfectant, or preservative activities

Biofilm: layers of living metabolizing bacteria and other microrganisms attached to a solid surface

Bioluminescence: emission of light by living organisms

Biomagnification: increasing concentrations of a chemical in successively higher members of a food chain

Bioremediation: use of microorganisms, enzymes, or other living organisms to reduce or remove hazardous materials from an environment

Biotechnology: manipulation of genes to produce commercially valuable products

Biotic: living

Blackwater fever: acute hemolytic form of malaria

Blanching: process of scalding fresh raw food in hot water or steam for a brief period

Blastoconidium: asexual reproductive structure of some fungi

Blooms: abundance of phytoplankton on the surface of a body of water

Boiling: using heat to cause a liquid to bubble vigorously

Broad spectrum: refers to the activity range of drugs against a variety of gram-positive and gram-negative bacteria and some fungi

Brownian movement: random movement of molecules

Bubo: inflamed, swollen, or enlarged lymph node

Buffer: mixture of a weak acid or a weak base and its salt that resists changes in pH in a solution

Bullae: blisters of congenital syphilis

Caliper: instrument used to measure diameter of zones of inhibition

Calorie: amount of energy needed to raise the temperature of one gram of water by 1° C

Calvin-Benson cycle: series of light-independent reactions of photosynthesis

cAMP: form of adenosine monophosphate containing a circular ring formed by the phosphate group binding to both the 3′ and 5′ carbons of ribose

Cancerous cell: cell demonstrating abnormalities associated with malignant cells

Candling: process used to detect defects in shelled eggs

Cannibalism: custom in which human flesh is eaten by other humans

Capsid: protein coat of a virus

Capsomere: subunits of the protein coat of a virus

Capsule: layer of lipopolysaccharides surrounding a bacterial cell

Carboxylation: reaction transferring a carboxyl (—COOH) group of atoms to a molecule

Carbuncle: cutaneous pus-producing lesion of multicentric origin

Carcinogenic: tumor-producing

Cariogenic: caries-producing

Carnivore: meat-eater

Carrier: individual harboring an infectious agent but showing no evidence of disease

Catabolism: energy-releasing breakdown of complex molecules into smaller molecules

Catabolite activator protein (CAP): allosteric protein that turns on operons when bound to cAMP in presence of substrate

Catabolite repression: inhibition of inducible enzymes in the presence of glucose

Catalyst: chemical or physical agent that increases the rate of a chemical reaction without being changed itself

Catalytic site: see active site

Catalyze: to speed up the rate of a chemical reaction without changing the catalyst

Catarrhal phase: initial phase of pertussis characterized by a nonproductive cough and a watery discharge from the nose

Catecholamines: adrenal hormones inhibiting an anaphylactic response

Cation: positively charged ion

Cationic detergents: chemicals that carry a positive charge when dissolved in water

CD4+ cell: cell containing the CD4+ surface marker (helper T cells)

CD8+ cell: cell containing the CD8+ surface marker (suppressor or cytolytic T cells)

Cellular immunity: immune response requiring action of T cells

Cellulitis: inflammation of dermal cells

Cementum: thin layer of bone below the gumline

Cerebrospinal fluid (CSF): protective layer of fluid surrounding brain and spinal cord

Certified raw milk: nonpasteurized milk produced by cows that are certified to be in good health by federal or state veterinarians

Chancre: lesion of primary syphilis

Chancroid: rare sexually transmitted bacterial disease

Chemical bond: attraction between electrons of atoms

Chemiluminescence: property of generating light in a chemical reaction

Chemiosmosis: process by which energy from respiration generates and pumps hydrogen ions across a membrane producing a potential difference that fuels formation of ATP

Chemoautotroph: autotroph that obtains energy from inorganic substances

Chemoheterotroph: heterotroph that obtains energy from organic substances
Chemostat: growth apparatus used for keeping cells in a continuous logarithmic phase
Chemotaxis: movement toward or away from a chemical
Chemotaxonomy: method of classification based on chemical composition
Chemotherapeutic: descriptive for any chemical used to treat disease
Chemotroph: organism that obtains energy from chemical sources
Chitin: chemical present in cell walls of most fungi
Chlamydoconidium: asexual reproductive structure of some fungi
Chlorophyll: green pigment found in some cells that converts light energy to chemical energy in photosynthesis
Chloroplast: membranous organelle where photosynthesis occurs in eucaryotic cells
Chromatid: one of a connected chromosome pair
Chromosome: units of DNA responsible for inherited characteristics of cells
Chronic carrier: long-term carrier of an infectious agent
Chronic disease: disease that persists for months or years
Chronic granulomatous disease (CGD): primary deficiency in oxidase production by phagocytes
Cilia: short, hairlike appendages responsible for motility in some protozoa
Cisternae: membranes of the Golgi complex
Citric acid cycle: cyclic series of redox reactions releasing carbon dioxide and producing reduced coenzymes
Classes: taxonomic groups of related orders
Clonal selection theory: proposal suggesting how a specific B cell line is activated by an antigen
Clone: population of genetically identical cells
Clue cells: vaginal epithelial cells stippled with *Gardnerella vaginalis*
Cluster of differentiation (CD): surface proteins that serve as identifying markers on lymphocytes
Coagulase: microbial enzyme that promotes clotting of plasma
Cocci: spherical-shaped bacteria
Coccidia: members of the protozoan order Coccidiorida
Coccobacilli: small, oval-shaped bacilli
Codon: three-base sequence on mRNA molecules that designates a specific amino acid
Coenocytic: having aseptate hyphae with multiple nuclei
Coenzyme: nonprotein carrier that transports atoms or functional groups
Coenzyme Q (CoQ): nonprotein carrier that transports electrons in the electron transport chain
Cohorts: control group matched with a study group except for the factor being studied
Cold sore: fever blister caused by herpesvirus
Coliform: facultatively anaerobic, gram-negative bacillus that ferments lactose with the production of gas
Colitis: inflammation of the colon
Collagenase: microbial enzyme that dissolves collagen, a substance found in skin, bone, and cartilage
Colonization: ability of an organism to adhere, grow, and multiply on a surface
Colony-forming unit (CFU): quantitative unit expressing the number of colonies growing on a particular medium under standard conditions
Commensalism: close relationship between two organisms in which one organism benefits and the other one is unaffected
Commercial sterilization: application of heat to destroy or reduce numbers of microorganisms in canned foods
Communicable disease: disease capable of being transmitted from one individual to another
Community-acquired disease: disease originating outside a hospital
Competitive inhibition: interference with the rate of an enzyme reaction by a chemical structurally similar to the substrate
Complement: 30 or more proteins that are active in the immune response (also called complement system)
Complement cascade: orderly activation of complement components
Complementary base: base that always pairs with the same base on double-stranded DNA or RNA
Complementarity: pairing of bases on double-stranded DNA or RNA
Complementary DNA (cDNA): DNA synthesized from an RNA template
Complex media: media containing ill-defined mixtures of ingredients
Compound: two or more elements chemically combined in definite proportions
Compound microscope: instrument with more than one lens used for viewing small objects

Concentration gradient: differences in concentrations of molecules on either side of a plasma membrane

Condensed milk: sweetened form of evaporated milk

Congenital rubella syndrome: birth defects caused by rubella virus crossing the placenta

Conidium: asexual reproductive structure of some fungi

Conjugated protein: protein combined with a nonprotein

Conjugation: transfer of genes from one bacterium to another by a mating process involving cell-to-cell contact

Conjunctivitis: inflammation of the mucous membrane lining an eyelid

Constant: unchanged order of amino acid sequences on immunoglobulin molecules

Constitutive enzyme: enzyme produced in the absence or presence of a substrate

Consumer: an organism that obtains energy and nutrients from another organism

Contact dermatitis: allergic condition caused by touching irritating chemicals resulting in a mild rash, erythema of the skin, or weeping lesions

Contiguous: touching

Continuous cell line: cell line capable of an unlimited number of transfers

Continuous culture: open system for growing cells with conditions designed to support the logarithmic growth phase

Contractile vacuole: specialized vacuole able to expel water

Convalescent phase: terminal phase of pertussis characterized by gradual disappearance of the cough

Convulsions: involuntary contractions and relaxations of muscles

Cortex: protective layer surrounding an endospore

Corticosteroid: steroid hormone released by adrenal glands

Cosmid: phage-hybrid plasmid

Counterstain: stain of a contrasting color applied in a differential staining technique

Coupled reactions: two reactions occurring simultaneously

Covalent bond: chemical attraction formed by sharing of electrons by atoms

Covalent modification: alteration of eucaryotic enzymes by addition of modifying chemical groups

Cranium: bones enclosing the brain

Creutzfeld-Jakob disease (CJD): rare neuromuscular degenerative disease

Cribriform plate: part of the ethmoid bone forming the anterior floor of the cranium and the roof of the nasal cavity

Cristae: inner membranes of mitochondria

Crithidial form (epimastigote): extracellular, motile form of a *Leishmania* parasite that develops in sandflies

Crossing over: process in which one portion of a chromatid is exchanged with a portion of another chromatid

Crypt: small sac or cavity extending into an epithelial surface

Cyclic AMP (cAMP): molecule important in inducing the synthesis of regulated enzymes

Cyst: resistant stage of some protozoa and bacteria

Cystitis: inflammation of the urinary bladder

Cytochrome: a protein that acts as an electron donor and recipient in the electron transport chain

Cytokine: protein secreted by cells that regulates the immune response

Cytolytic T cell: lymphocyte that lyses virus-infected cells and tumor cells and activates macrophages

Cytopathic effect: morphological change in virus-infected cells

Cytoplasmic streaming: flowing movement of cytoplasm observable in eucaryotic cells

Cytosine: cyclic nitrogen base

Cytoskeleton: network of microtubules and microfilaments in eucaryotes

D value: time in minutes required to kill 90 percent of microorganisms or spores by heat vapor pressure

Dark reaction of photosynthesis: fixation (reduction) of CO_2 by light-independent reactions of photosynthesis

Dark repair: action of enzymes that replace thymine dimers in DNA with normal basepairs

Data: information including facts and figures from which conclusions can be drawn

Deamination: removal of an amino ($—NH_2$) group from a molecule

Death phase: last phase of a bacterial growth curve in which cells are dying at an exponential rate

Decarboxylation: removal of a carboxyl (—COOH) group from a molecule

Decolorizer: chemical applied to remove stain from microorganisms

Decomposer: microorganism that breaks down complex dead organic matter into simpler compounds

Decubitus: cutaneous ulcer caused by pressure obstructing capillary blood flow

Deep mycoses: fungal infections of deep tissues or internal organs

Defined media: media in which all components are known

Degeneracy: specification of the same amino acid by two or more codons

Dehydrogenase: enzyme that removes hydrogen atoms from a molecule

Delayed hypersensitivity: cell-mediated response to antigen occurring hours to days after release of cytokines

Deletion: loss of a base in the DNA sequence causing a frame shift mutation

Delta agent: defective virus sometimes found in hepatitis B infections

Denaturation: loss of structural integrity of a molecule by heat or chemical action

Denatured: altered conformation of a molecule

Dendritic cell: one type of antigen-presenting cell

Dendrogram: treelike diagram based on phenotypes

Denitrification: chemical process used by microorganisms to reduce nitrate (NO_3^-) to nitrogen gas

Dental caries: decay of the teeth

Dental plaque: accumulation of dissolved food, saliva, and bacteria on the exposed enamel surfaces of teeth

Dentin: main tissue of a tooth

Dentition: number and kind of teeth

Deoxyribonucleotide: building block of DNA composed of a phosphate group, deoxyribose sugar, and one of four nitrogen bases

Deoxyribose: five-carbon sugar found in nucleotides of DNA

Dermatitis: inflammatory response of the skin

Dermatophytic fungi: fungi that infect the skin, hair, or nails

Desiccation: process of removing moisture

Desquamation: shedding of the surface epithelium

Detritus: remains of dead organisms

DiGeorge syndrome: error in embryonic development of thymus and parathyroid

Diaminopimelic acid (DAP): amino acid found in cell walls of bacteria

Diatomaceous earth: remnants of silica from diatoms on the ocean floor

Diauxic: having two phases of growth

Differential medium: medium containing ingredients that distinguish between groups of bacteria

Differential stain: staining techniques using two or more dyes that distinguish between groups of bacteria or cell structures

Diffusion: movement of molecules from an area of greater concentration to an area of lesser concentration

Diglyceride: lipid containing two ester bonds

Dimorphism: two forms of growth, shapes, or size

Diphtheroid: non–toxin-producing pleomorphic bacillus resembling etiologic agent of diphtheria

Diplococci: pairs of cocci

Diploid: cell or organism with two of each type of chromosome

Direct contact: transmission of an infectious agent from contact with an infected person or carrier

Direct immunofluorescence: fluorescence obtained with an antigen and a fluorescent-labeled antibody

Disease: any departure from normal body function

Disinfectant: chemical agent that destroys infectious agents

Disinfection: process that destroys infectious agents exclusive of endospores and viruses

Disseminated disease: disease that has spread to many parts of the body

Disulfide bond: bond occurring between two sulfur atoms of cysteine side chains

Diverticulum: pouch in the walls of a canal or organ

DNA ligase: enzyme that forms a covalent bond to link one nucleotide with the phosphate of another nucleotide

DNA polymerase: enzyme catalyzing the synthesis of DNA

DNA-RNA hybrid: molecule containing one strand each of DNA and RNA

Döderlein's bacilli: vaginal lactobacilli

Donor: cell that contributes genes to another cell

Double bond: sharing of two pairs of electrons by two atoms

Droplet nuclei: dried remnants of aerosols

Dry wine: wine with a low content of sugar

Dura mater: outer membrane of brain and spinal cord

Dysentery: acute gastrointestinal disease characterized by diarrhea accompanied by mucus and blood in stool

Dysuria: painful or difficult urination

Eclipse period: period in which viruses infecting a cell cannot be detected

Ecological niche: see Niche

Ecology: study of the relationships between living organisms and nonliving components of an environment

Ecosystem: living and nonliving components of a local environment

Edema: swelling

Effector: end phase of an immune response

Efficiency of plating (EOP): A numerical expression of the ID_{50} compared with an electron microscope count of viral suspensions

Effluent: water leaving a treatment plant

Elastase: microbial enzyme that degrades elastin in tissues

Electron: negatively charged subatomic particle that orbits the nucleus of an atom

Electron micrograph: photograph of an image taken through an electron microscope

Electron microscope: microscope using a beam of electrons as an energy source and magnetic fields to produce an image

Electron transport chain: series of energy-liberating reactions in which electrons are transferred to coenzymes and cytochromes to a final electron acceptor

Element: substance that cannot be broken down into simpler components

Elongation: process in which a group of atoms or molecules is added to a sequence of chemical compounds

Embden-Meyerhof-Parnas (EMP) pathway: glycolytic pathway for the breakdown of glucose to pyruvic acid producing ATP and reducing NAD

Encephalitis: inflammation of the brain

End product repression: inhibition of a metabolic pathway by accumulation of an end product

Endemic: presence of a limited number of cases of a disease at all times within a geographic area

Endergonic: chemical reaction that requires energy

Endocytosis: process whereby materials move into a eucaryotic cell

Endoenzyme: enzyme that catalyzes reactions within cells

Endogenous: originating from inside

Endoplasmic reticulum: system of membrane-enclosed channels in a eucaryotic cell

Endospore: dormant form of bacteria with enhanced resistance to heat, staining, and disinfection

Endosymbiont: organism that sets up a mutually beneficial association within another organism

Endosymbiosis: mutually beneficial relationship between two organisms living together

Endotoxin: lipopolysaccharide (LPS) portion on the surface of gram-negative bacteria released on cell death

Energy-liberating: chemical reaction yielding energy

Energy of activation: amount of energy required to trigger the reaction between an enzyme and its substrate

Energy-requiring: chemical reaction needing energy

Enriched media: media containing specific growth factors or ingredients

Enteric: relating to the intestinal tract

Enterotoxin: an exotoxin secreted by microorganisms that produces gastrointestinal disease

Enzyme: protein catalyst specific in its action on a substrate

Enzyme-linked immunosorbent assay (ELISA): method for quantifying antigen or antibody in a specimen using an antibody labeled with an enzyme

Eosinophil: white blood cell containing granules whose numbers are increased in allergies

Eosinophil chemotactic factor: substance attracting eosinophils to site of an immediate-type hypersensitivity

Epidemic: unusually large number of cases of a disease occurring in a community within a short time

Epidemiology: study of the nature and circumstances (the how, when, and where) of diseases

Epimerase: enzyme that converts D- to L- isomers

Epitope: specific portion of an antigen stimulating an immune response (antigenic determinant)

Equation: shorthand expression for a chemical reaction

Erysipelas: streptococcal skin infection of young children

Erythema: diffused redness of the skin

Erythroblast: immature nucleated red blood cells

Erythrocyte: red blood cell

Erythrocytic: pertaining to stages of parasitemia in which parasites are inside red blood cells

Erythrogenic: redness-producing

Eschar: skin lesion of miteborne typhus fever

Espundia: form of leishmaniasis characterized by ulcerative metastases

Essential ions: inorganic ions necessary for enzyme activity

Ester bond: bond that links an alcohol and a fatty acid when a molecule of water is lost
Ethanolamine: major constituent of many bacterial phospholipids derived from activated glycerol
Etiologic agent: organism that causes an infection
Eucarya: domain of eucaryotes whose cells contain membrane-bound nuclei and divide by mitosis
Eucaryotes: cells with membrane-bound nuclei
Eutrophication: growth of algae and bacteria caused by an oversupply of nutrients in freshwater resulting in oxygen depletion
Evaporated milk: milk from which some moisture has been removed
Exergonic: chemical reaction that releases energy
Exocytosis: process whereby materials move out of a eucaryotic cell
Exoenzyme: enzyme that catalyzes reactions outside cells
Exofolin: virulence factor produced by microorganisms that promotes shedding of epidermal cells
Exogenous: originating from outside
Exon: DNA segment in eucaryotes that codes for mRNA
Exonuclease: dark repair enzyme that removes the thymine dimers formed in DNA after exposure to ultraviolet radiation
Exosporium: outermost protective layer of an endospore
Exotoxin: microbial poison secreted by living microorganisms
Extraerythrocytic: pertaining to stages of parasites outside red blood cells
Exudate: pus-containing fluid at a site of inflammation
F factor: extrachromosomal or chromosomal fertility factor responsible for mating in some bacteria
Facilitated diffusion: movement of molecules or ions from greater to lesser concentrations by carrier molecules
Facultative: having ability to tolerate the presence or absence of a growth condition
Families: taxonomic groups of related genera
Farmer's lung disease: Type III hypersensitivity response in persons sensitive to fungi or bacteria in the air
Febrile: pertaining to a fever
Feedback inhibition: metabolic control mechanism in which the first enzyme of a metabolic pathway is blocked by the end product
Fermentation: energy-liberating process in which an organic molecule is both an electron donor and an electron acceptor
Fever blister: cold sore caused by a herpesvirus
Filamentous bacilli: threadlike bacilli
Fingerprinting: method of DNA typing based on detecting unique short repetitive sequences in DNA
First Law of Thermodynamics: principle stating that energy is neither created nor destroyed by conversions from one form to another
Fistula: a channel to the skin or between two hollow organs
Fix: process of fastening a specimen to a glass slide
Flagella: filamentous appendages of some microorganisms responsible for movement
Flagellin: protein of a flagellum
Flaming: heating process to sterilize metal wires or loops by placing them in a burner flame
Flatulence: presence of gas in the stomach or intestines
Flavoproteins: coenzymes containing a derivative of riboflavin
Floc particle: small, finely suspended solid material containing live bacteria used as activated sludge
Flowing steam: sterilizing method that requires three or more intermittent periods of steaming
Fluid mosaic model: structure of plasma membrane having an inner bilayer of phospholipids and embedded proteins surrounded by peripheral proteins
Fluorescence: emission of a brilliant color in the presence of ultraviolet radiation
Fluorescence-activated cell sorter (FACS): method of separating classes of lymphocytes using fluorescent-labeled antibodies
Focal length: working distance between an objective lens and a specimen needed to bring an object into focus
Foci: small, localized areas of infection
Fomite: inanimate object responsible for transmission of an infectious agent
Food chain: sequence of who eats whom in an ecosystem
Food infection: disease produced by consuming food with a large number of microorganisms and/or their products
Food poisoning: disease produced by consuming food with toxic chemicals produced by microorganisms

Food web: complex interaction of many food chains within an ecosystem

Foramen magnum: opening in the skull through which the spinal cord passes

Forespore: initial structure of an endospore

Fragment crystallizable (Fc): constant portion of the immunoglobulin molecule that forms crystals when released by papain digestion

Frameshift mutation: insertion or deletion of one or more nitrogen bases of DNA causing misreading of an entire sequence of DNA

Friedlander's bacillus: another name for *Klebsiella pneumoniae*

Frustule: two-part cell wall of a diatom

Fucoxanthin: brown accessory pigment of some algae

Functional group: combination of atoms differing in behavior from that of atoms of which it is composed

Fungi: unicellular or multicellular nonphotosynthetic organisms belonging to the kingdom Fungi

Furuncle: pus-producing lesion of a hair follicle

Fusiform bacilli: bacilli with tapered ends

Gamma globulin: type of blood plasma proteins that include the immunoglobulin molecules

Gamete: sex cell

Gene: segment of a DNA molecule constituting a unit of heredity

Gene cloning: cultivating recombinant cells to increase the number of cells with copies of a particular gene

Generalized transduction: form of gene transfer in which a virus carries any combination of genes from one bacterium to another

Generation time: time required for a population of organisms to double in number

Generic: common chemical name for a drug

Genetic code: three-base sequence that is translated into a specific amino acid

Genetic engineering: process of combining genetic material from different sources

Genital warts: lesions of the genital organs caused by papilloma viruses

Genome: full complement of genes of an organism

Genotype: sum total of genetic material of an organism

Genus: latinized first name of an organism

Germ tubes: short, lateral hyphal filaments

Germicide: see biocide

Gingivitis: inflammation of the gums

Global repressor: chemical that blocks the synthesis of several enzymes

Glucose effect: form of energy conservation in which a bacterium does not synthesize enzymes until glucose is depleted

Glycocalyx: extracellular layer of polysaccharides surrounding procaryotic cells

Glycolipid: compound lipid containing a carbohydrate derivative

Glycolysis: series of oxidation reactions that convert glucose to pyruvic acid

Glycosidic bond: bond that links two monosaccharides when a molecule of water is lost

Golgi complex: membranous organelle that modifies and packages chemical compounds and produces lysosomes

Gonorrhea: sexually transmitted infection of genital mucous membranes

Graft-versus-host (GVH) reaction: the destructive assault of a host by the immunocompetent cells of a graft

Gram molecular weight: sum of the atomic masses of atoms of a molecule expressed in grams

Gram-negative bacteria: bacteria with thin cell walls and an outer membrane that stain red in the Gram stain procedure

Gram-positive bacteria: bacteria with thick cell walls that retain the purple color in the Gram stain procedure

Gram stain: differential staining procedure that divides bacteria into two major groups

Granule: inclusion in cytoplasm containing reserve materials

Granulocyte: white blood cell that has granules in its cytoplasm

Granulocyte-macrophage colony-stimulating factor (GM-CSF): spleen product that stimulates bone marrow to produce more white blood cells

Granulocytic: having cytoplasmic granules

Granuloma inguinale: ulcerative genital infection

Granulomatous: type of granular tissue or tumors formed in some infectious diseases

Granulomatous hypersensitivity: clustering of large macrophages around antigens promoting an inflammatory response

Graves' hyperthyroidism: autoimmune disease characterized by presence of antibodies to thyroid cells

Group translocation: movement of nutrients into cells after chemical modification of molecules

Guanine: cyclic nitrogen base

Guillain-Barré syndrome: inflammation of nerves and mild paralysis following a viral infection

Gumma: lesion of tertiary syphilis
Halophile: salt-loving organism
Haploid: eucaryotic cell with one of each type of chromosome
Hapten: incomplete antigen
Hay fever: localized anaphylactic response to an inhaled allergen characterized by irritation of mucous membranes
Head: anterior end of a bacteriophage
Heavy-chain disease: B-cell malignancy characterized by excess production of heavy chains of IgG, IgA, or IgM
Hematuria: blood in the urine
Hemolysin: microbial enzyme that destroys red blood cells
Hemolysis: destruction of red blood cells
Hemolytic disease of the newborn: disease of the newborn caused by incompatibility of an Rh^+ fetus and an Rh^- mother
Hemolytic uremic syndrome: life-threatening kidney disease occurring as a complication of an *E. coli* 0157:H7 infection
Hemorrhagic: associated with bleeding
Hepatosplenomegaly: enlargement of the liver and spleen
Herbivore: animal that eats plant material
Herd immunity: immunity of most individuals in a particular population
Heterofermentative: ability to produce a variety of end products from fermentation of a sugar
Heterotroph: organism that obtains carbon from organic compounds
High frequency of recombination (Hfr): strain of donor cells of *Escherichia coli* in which the F plasmid is a part of the bacterial chromosome
Histamine: primary mediator of anaphylactic hypersensitivity
Histone: protein associated with DNA of eucaryotic cells
Holdfast: structure that anchors some macroscopic algae
Homofermentative: ability to produce a single end product from fermentation of a sugar
Hops: female flower of *Humulus* species used in brewing beer
Hospital-acquired disease: disease originating from a hospital stay
Host cell: cell that harbors infectious agents
Hot vent: hydrothermal vent on the deep ocean floor that releases hot water with temperatures of 270° to 380° C
Human leukocyte antigens: group of chemical substances on cell surface that make up the major histocompatibility complex
Humoral: referring to immunoglobulins in body fluids
Humus: accumulated minerals and organic matter in the subsoil region
Hyaluronidase: microbial enzyme that dissolves hyaluronic acid in human connective tissue
Hybridoma: product resulting from fusion of an antibody-producing cell and a myeloma cell
Hydrogen bond: weak chemical attraction formed by sharing of hydrogen atoms between two molecules or parts of the same molecule
Hydrolase: enzyme catalyzing hydrolytic reactions
Hydrolysis: enzyme reaction in which a complex substance is broken down to simpler ones in the presence of water
Hydrophilic: water-loving
Hydrophobic: water-hating
Hydrostatic pressure: pressure exerted by water
Hydrothermal vent: any type of hot spring found on the deep ocean floor
Hyperbaric oxygen therapy: treatment in an atmosphere of high oxygen tension
Hypersensitive pneumonitis: inflammation of lungs caused by inhaled allergens
Hypersensitivity: altered or exaggerated immune response on repeated exposure to an allergen
Hypertension: high blood pressure
Hypertonic: solution with a higher osmotic pressure than that of the cell
Hypha: tubular filament of a mold
Hypogammaglobulinemia: deficiency of IgG
Hypotension: low blood pressure
Hypothalamus: region in diencephalon of brain below the thalamus with regulatory functions
Hypotonic: solution with an osmotic pressure less than that of the cell
Icosahedron: geometric figure with multiple plane surfaces
ID_{50}: reciprocal of the highest dilution of a viral suspension causing an infection in 50 percent of test animals
Immediate hypersensitivity: allergic response occurring within minutes after exposure to an allergen
Immune adherence: process in which microorganisms are coated with antibodies (opsonization)
Immune complex: a combination of antigen and antibody
Immune modulators: chemicals that influence the activity of immune cells
Immune response: activities of cells and their

products for defense against pathogenic organisms and foreign molecules
Immunity: resistance to an infectious disease
Immunofluorescence (IF): technique used in fluorescence microscopy to detect presence of specific antigens or antibodies
Immunogen: substance that stimulates an immune response
Immunoglobulin: protein having antibody activity
Immunological memory: ability of the immune system to recall previous exposure to an antigen
Impedance: opposition of an electric current to the flow of an alternating current of a single frequency
Impetigo: highly contagious staphylococcal disease of the skin
In utero: within the uterus
In vitro: outside a living organism
In vivo: inside a living organism
Incidence: numbers of cases of a disease in a total population within a given period of time
Incineration: process of burning an object until it is reduced to ashes
Incubation time: time period between exposure and first symptoms of disease
Indicator organism: organism detected in test procedures that indicates fecal pollution
Indigenous: occurring naturally in a particular environment
Indirect immunofluorescence: fluorescence obtained with an antibody and a fluorescent-labeled anti-immunoglobulin
Induced mutation: use of chemicals or radiation to cause change in DNA
Inducible enzyme: enzyme synthesized only in the presence of a particular substrate
Induction: activation of a gene in the presence of a particular substrate
Induration: hardening of a tissue
Infection: invasion of the body by a pathogenic microorganism
Infectious: capable of producing an infection
Inflammation: nonspecific response to injury or infection characterized by heat, redness, pain, and swelling
Influent: raw sewage entering a treatment plant
Initiation: chemical processes that occur at the beginning of a synthetic pathway
Innate: immunity present from birth (nonspecific immunity)
Insertion sequence element: segment of DNA that can move from plasmid to plasmid or become inserted in the chromosome (transposon)
Insulin-dependent diabetes mellitus (IDDM): disease characterized by deficiency of insulin
Interferons: proteins produced by cells in response to viral agents, their products, or synthetic polymers
Interleukin-1: cytokine produced by phagocytes that promotes an inflammatory response and T-cell proliferation
Interleukins: cytokines produced by antigenically stimulated immune cells that activate and regulate activities of other immune cells
Intron: noncoding segment of DNA that intervenes within an exon
Invasiveness: ability of a microorganism to gain entry and spread in a host
Inversion: reversal of positions of adjacent bases on DNA
Iodophor: disinfectant with iodine in its structure
Ion: atom or group of atoms with an electric charge
Ionic bond: chemical bond formed when atoms gain or lose electrons
Iron-sulfur enzyme: enzyme containing iron and sulfur found in the electron transport chain
Irradiation: exposure to a radiant form of electromagnetic energy
Isograft: tissue transplant from a donor that is genetically identical to the recipient
Isomer: chemical compound containing the same types and numbers of atoms as another chemical compound in different positions
Isomerase: enzyme that rearranges atoms in a molecule
Isomerization: rearrangement of atoms within a molecule
Isotonic: solution having an osmotic pressure the same as that of the cell
Isotope: variant form of an element having a different number of neutrons in the nucleus
Isotype switching: process in which the receptor of an IgM-bearing B cell changes to IgG, IgE, or IgA
Kala azar: visceral form of leishmaniasis
Karyosome: spherical mass of chromatin within the nucleus of a cell
Keratin: protein made by epidermal cells of the skin
Kilocalorie: 1000 calories
Kilorad: 1000 rads
Kinase: microbial enzyme that dissolves fibrin in a blood clot
Kinetoplast: point of origin of flagella in protozoa

Krebs cycle: biochemical pathway in which organic acids are decarboxylated and NAD and FAD are reduced

Kuru: degenerative disease of the cerebellum

Labeled antibodies: antibodies bound to indicator molecules, making them sensitive to detection at low concentrations

Lactose operon: sequence of regulatory and structural genes that control degradation of lactose

Lag phase: initial phase of a bacterial growth curve in which bacteria grow in size but not in number

Lagoon: large body of wastewater open to the air where microorganisms decompose organic matter

Latency: ability of a virus to remain dormant within a host cell

Latent disease: inactive state of a disease

Latent syphilis: stage of syphilis having no apparent signs of infection

LD_{50}: lethal dose of microorganisms or toxins for 50 percent of test animals or tissue cultures

Lecithinase: microbial enzyme that dissolves tissue lecithin

Legume: plant associated with symbiotic nitrogen-fixing bacteria

Leguminous: belonging to a plant group participating in symbiotic nitrogen fixation

Leishman-Donovan (LD) bodies: intracellular oval forms of leishmanial parasites

Leishmanial form (amastigote): intracellular, nonmotile form of a *Leishmania* species that lives in macrophages of a vertebrate host

Leproma: cutaneous mass of granulomatous tissue in leprosy

Lepromatous: pertaining to the cutaneous form of leprosy

Lepromin: product of *Mycobacterium leprae* used in skin testing

Leptomonas form (promastigote): extracellular, motile form of a *Leishmania* species that lives in the intestinal tract of sandflies and spleen or liver of vertebrate hosts

Leptospirosis: multisystem disease caused by a spirochete that frequently localizes in the kidney

Lethal mutation: alteration in DNA resulting in the death of an organism

Leukocidin: microbial enzyme that destroys certain white blood cells

Leukocyte: white blood cell

Leukopenia: lack of white blood cells

Leukotriene: slow-reacting substance of anaphylactic hypersensitivity

Lichen: organism that results from a symbiotic association of a fungus with an algal partner

Ligase: enzyme that bonds two molecules

Light-independent reaction: dark reaction of photosynthesis

Limnetic: open water beyond the shore

Linkage map: representation of gene sequence on the DNA molecule of cells

Liquid media: nutrient-containing broths

Littoral: water along a shore

Local disease: disease confined to one area of the body

Localized anaphylaxis: respiratory, conjunctival, or intestinal mucosal allergic reaction involving IgE

Locus: place

Logarithmic phase: second phase of a bacterial growth curve in which cells are increasing at an exponential rate

Lophotrichous: type of flagellation with a tuft of flagella at one or both ends of a cell

Lyase: enzyme that removes or adds a functional group to a molecule

Lymphocyte: mononuclear white blood cell that responds to the presence of an antigen

Lymphogranuloma inguinale: ulcerative genital infection caused by a bacterium

Lymphogranuloma venereum (LGV): tropical, sexually transmitted chlamydial disease

Lyophilization: process of rapidly freezing a substance while removing water by using a vacuum pump

Lysis: dissolution of cells

Lysogenic conversion: conversion of a non–toxin-producing bacterium into a toxin-producing bacterium by integration of viral DNA into the DNA of a bacterial host

Lysogeny: state exhibited by a phage-infected bacterium in which the phage coexists with the bacterial genome

Lysosome: membrane-bound organelle containing digestive enzymes of eucaryotes

Lysozyme: enzyme of biological fluids with antimicrobial activity

M protein: surface protein that contributes to the virulence of *Streptococcus pyogenes*

Macroconidium: multicellular asexual spore of some fungi

Macrogametocyte: sexually differentiated cell of a malarial parasite capable of producing a female sex cell

Macroglobulinemia: B-cell malignancy characterized by large amounts of IgM

Macrolesion: mutational event that involves several base-pairs

Macromolecule: molecule containing large numbers of monomers
Macrophage: phagocytic mononuclear cell that processes antigens
Macropinocytosis: indiscriminate uptake of extracellular fluid by dendritic cells
Magnification: enlarging power of a lens or a lens system
Major histocompatibility complex (MHC): set of linked genes coding for cell surface markers making each individual unique
Major histocompatibility complex class I (MHC-I): cell surface proteins expressed by nearly all nucleated cells
Major histocompatibility complex class II (MHC-II): cell surface proteins expressed mainly on dendritic cells, B cells, and macrophages
Malting: preliminary step in brewing that is required to convert starch of barley into sugars
Mantoux test: skin test based on delayed hypersensitivity to tuberculin
Marker: genetically determined chemical unique to the surface of a cell
Mashing: process of cooking grains and malt in preparation for fermentation to beer
Mast cell: noncirculating mononuclear granulocyte found in connective tissue
Matter: anything that occupies space and has mass
Maximal growth temperature: highest temperature at which an organism will grow
Mediator: biologically active chemical
Medium: combination of nutrients that support microbial growth
Medulla oblongata: inferior portion of brain stem
Megakaryocyte: giant cell in bone marrow from which platelets are derived
Meiosis: process of cell division in which the number of chromosomes is reduced by one half
Membrane attack complex (MAC): association of several complement components that act together to create a channel through the membrane of a cell
Membrane-filter count: method for determining numbers of coliform bacteria in water samples using a membrane filter and a selective medium
Memory cell: partially activated B or T cell generated during an immune response
Meningitis: inflammation of the meninges
Merozoite: stage of a malarial parasite produced by fragmentation within a red blood cell
Mesophile: organism that grows best between 20° and 45° C
Messenger RNA (mRNA): type of RNA that codes for particular amino acids
Metabolism: sum total of the biochemical reactions occurring in a cell
Metachromatic granules: cytoplasmic inclusions that appear to change color when stained with basic dyes
Methanogen: archaea generating methane from metabolic activities
Microaerophilic: requiring less oxygen than that found in the atmosphere
Microbicidal: having the ability to kill a microorganism
Microbiostatic: having the ability to inhibit the growth of a microorganism
Microbiota: microscopic forms of life
Microconidium: single-celled asexual reproductive structure of some fungi
Microgametocyte: sexually differentiated cell of a malarial parasite capable of producing a male sex cell
Microlesion: damage to a single pair of nitrogen bases caused by mutation
Microscope: instrument used to magnify and resolve objects too small to be seen with the naked eye
Microscopic calibration factor (MCF): a factor used to measure microorganisms per milliliter of milk or cream
Microtubule: flexible protein cylinder of eucaryotic cells
Minimal broth: nutritional medium that supplies only the essential ingredients to cultivate a species
Minimal growth temperature: lowest temperature at which an organism will grow
Minimum bactericidal concentration (MBC): lowest concentration of an antimicrobial that kills a defined proportion of bacteria in a specific time period
Minimum inhibitory concentration (MIC): lowest concentration of an antimicrobial that inhibits growth of a microorganism
Mitochondria: membranous organelles where respiration and fatty acid synthesis occurs in eucaryotic cells
Moist heat: term that includes boiling, pasteurizing, and autoclaving methods for controlling the growth of microorganisms
Mold: multicellular fungus

Molecular mimicry: similarity of microbial and host surface

Molecule: smallest part of a compound that can exist

Monoclonal antibodies: homogeneous population of antibodies derived from a hybrid of a plasma cell and a myeloma cell

Monocyte: mononuclear phagocytic white blood cell

Monoglyceride: lipid containing a single ester bond

Monolayer: single layer of eucaryotic cells used in culturing viruses, rickettsias, or chlamydias

Monomer: basic unit of which larger molecules are composed

Monotrichous: type of flagellation with a single flagellum at one end of a cell

Morbidity: illnesses occurring in a geographic area or population

Mordant: chemical used to promote or fix a staining reaction

Mortality: deaths occurring in a geographic area or population

Most probable number: statistical measure of the most probable number of coliform bacteria in a 100-ml sample of water

Multiple tube fermentation technique: water quality testing procedure using a standard number of broth tubes inoculated with specific volumes of a water sample

Multiple sclerosis (MS): degenerative neurological disease affecting myelin sheaths

Must: juice from pressed grapes used in making wine

Mutagen: chemical or physical agent that causes a mutation

Mutant: organism differing from the parent cell by at least one inheritable characteristic

Mutant frequency: number of a particular mutational type within a population of cells

Mutation: sudden inheritable change in the DNA molecule of an organism

Mutation rate: probability that a certain average number of mutations will occur per cell per generation

Mutualism: close relationship between two organisms in which each organism benefits

Myasthenia gravis: autoimmune disease characterized by antibodies to acetylcholine receptors

Mycelium: filamentous vegetative structure of a mold

Mycorrhiza: mutually beneficial associations of fungi and roots of plants

Mycoses: infections caused by fungi

Mycotoxin: toxic product of fungi

Narrow spectrum: activity range of drugs against a small group of microorganisms

Natural: in antimicrobials, the molecule produced by a living microorganism

Natural killer (NK) cell: large granular lymphocyte that destroys virus-infected cells, tumor cells, and cells of transplants

Naturally acquired active immunity: protection against reinfection provided by antibodies made by an individual

Naturally acquired passive immunity: protection against infection provided to a fetus by placental transfer and breast milk

Necrosis: death of tissue

Negative control: metabolic control mechanism that operates in the absence of a substrate by a repressor molecule binding to the operator gene blocking the function of the operon

Negative sense RNA: strand of RNA that is transcribed to form a complementary strand of DNA

Neutral fat: triglyceride containing mixed fatty acids

Neutron: subatomic particle with no charge found in the nucleus of an atom

Neutrophil: phagocytic polymorphonuclear white blood cell

Niche: location and interactions of a particular organism with others in the same space

Nitrification: chemical process used by some bacteria to convert nitrites (NO_2^-) to nitrates (NO_3^-) or nitric acid

Nitrogen-fixation: process of converting gaseous nitrogen into nitrogenous compounds

Nodule: enlargement on the roots of a legume containing bacteria that fix nitrogen

Noncompetitive inhibition: interference with the rate of a reaction by a chemical that binds to a site other than an active site on an enzyme

Nongonococcal urethritis: nongonococcal infection of the urethra

Nonionic detergent: chemical that carries no net electrical charge when dissolved in water

Nonpolar: equal distribution of charges on shared electrons

Nonpolar covalent bond: bond in which atoms exert a pull of the same magnitude on shared electrons

Nonself antigen: antigen that does not occur on host cells

Nonspecific vaginitis (NSV): infection of the

vagina often caused by organisms normally present in the vagina

Normal flora: those species of microorganisms that dwell on or in the human host without causing infection

Nosocomial disease: hospital-acquired disease

Nucleic acid hybridization: technique for identifying single strands of DNA or RNA by mixing them with known DNA or RNA fragments

Nucleocapsid: nucleic acid and protein coat of a virus

Nucleoid: DNA-containing region of procaryotic cells

Nucleoli: RNA-containing portions of nuclei

Nucleoside: a two-part unit of a nucleic acid containing a nitrogen base linked to ribose or deoxyribose

Nucleosome: spherical subunit of DNA and histones

Nucleotide: three-part unit of a nucleic acid containing a sugar, a phosphate group, and a nitrogen base

Numerical aperture: mathematical expression of the light-gathering ability of a lens

Numerical taxonomy: computer-based method for classifying organisms

Objective lens: lens of a microscope closer to the object being viewed

Obligate: requiring an environmental condition

Octet principle: tendency of atoms of elements in a compound to lose, gain, or share electrons to produce an arrangement of eight electrons in the outer shell

Ocular lens: lens of a microscope closer to the viewer

Omnivore: organism that eats plants and animals

Oncogene: gene associated with cancer

Oocyst: encysted form of a malarial parasite

Ookinete: elongated, motile stage of a malarial parasite

Operational taxonomic unit (OTU): unit (usually a strain) expressing phenotypic relatedness

Operator gene: gene that acts as the "on-off" switch of an operon

Operon: set of genes that control one function

Ophthalmia neonatorum: conjunctivitis of the newborn

Opportunistic infection: infection caused by a microorganism in an immunosuppressed host

Opportunistic pathogen: microorganism causing disease in an immunosuppressed host

Opsonin: antibody or complement protein that coats microorganisms and enhances phagocytosis

Opsonization: process by which a microorganism is coated, enhancing its susceptibility to phagocytosis

Optimal growth temperature: temperature at which an organism grows best

Oral groove: food-gathering structure of some protozoa

Orchitis: inflammation of a testicle

Order: taxonomic group of related families

Organelle: subcellular structure with a specialized function

Organic compound: compound containing carbon atoms linked covalently to hydrogen atoms

Organism: a living plant, animal, or microorganism

Oriental sore: form of cutaneous leishmaniasis

Osmophile: organism that requires high solute concentrations

Osmosis: movement of water molecules from an area of greater concentration to an area of lesser concentration across a selectively permeable membrane

Osmotic pressure: force exerted by water on a plasma membrane

Osmotolerant: organisms that survive or grow in environments with high solute concentrations

Otitis media: inflammation of the middle ear

Ototoxicity: detrimental effect on hearing

Outer membrane: portion of plasma membrane occurring outside the cell wall in gram-negative bacteria

Outgrowth: early vegetative stage occurring after breakage of spore coat

Ovum: egg

Oxidation: loss of electrons and hydrogen from a molecule

Oxidative phosphorylation: process that occurs in the electron transport chain to form ATP during oxidation reactions

Oxidoreductase: enzyme that catalyzes an oxidation-reduction reaction

Oxygenic photosynthesis: photosynthetic process that produces oxygen as a final product

Palisade: steplike arrangement of bacilli

Pandemic: a worldwide epidemic

Papillary hyperplasia: an elevation produced by a larger than usual number of cells on conjunctiva

Paralytic shellfish poisoning: food-borne disease in humans caused by eating shellfish contaminated with dinoflagellates that produce neurotoxins

Parasite: organism that benefits from an association with a host organism while causing harm to it

Parasitemia: presence of viable parasites in the blood

Parasitism: symbiotic relationship in which one organism benefits and one organism is harmed

Parenteral: pertaining to transmission by injection

Parfocal: ability of a microscope to remain in approximate focus with different lenses

Paroxysmal phase: secondary phase of pertussis characterized by periodic, severe, productive coughing spells

Passive immunity: type of immunity an individual receives from antibodies from another person

Passive transport: movement of molecules or ions from an area of greater concentration to an area of lesser concentration with no cellular expenditure of energy

Pasteurization: heat process employed to reduce total numbers of bacteria and destroy pathogens

Pasteurized milk: milk that has been heat treated to reduce the numbers of microorganisms and to destroy pathogens

Pathogen: a disease-producing microorganism

Pathogenicity: ability of a microorganism to cause disease

Pathogenicity island: large DNA segments that encode for virulence properties of a pathogen

Peat: undecomposed organic matter

Pellicle: flexible outer layer of some unicellular microorganisms

Pelvic inflammatory disease (PID): infection of the pelvic cavity usually occurring in women of childbearing age

Peptide bond: bond that links amino acids when a molecule of water is lost

Peptidoglycan: chemical component of bacterial cell walls

Peptococci: anaerobic cocci occurring singly or in pairs, tetrads, or clusters

Perforin: protein that produces holes in target cells

Periodicity: recurrence at regular intervals

Periodontal: surrounding a tooth

Periodontal disease: disease of the supportive tissue of teeth

Perineum: region comprising the skin, muscles, and fascia between the vulva or scrotum and the anus

Periplasm: space between the plasma membrane and the outer membrane of gram-negative bacteria

Peritrichous: type of flagellation with flagella surrounding an entire cell

Petechiae: tiny hemorrhages into the skin appearing as small purple spots

Petroff-Hauser chamber: calibrated glass slide used for counting bacteria

Peyer's patches: lymphatic nodules distributed in the lining of the small intestine

pH: measurement of hydrogen ions (H^+) in a solution

Phage: shortened version of bacteriophage

Phagocyte: immune cell having the ability to engulf solid particles

Phagocytosis: the process of engulfing nonself solid particles

Pharyngitis: inflammation of the pharynx

Phenol coefficient: testing procedure to evaluate the ability of various chemicals to kill microorganisms compared with the ability of phenol

Phenotype: sum total of expressed characteristics of an organism

Phosphatase: enzyme found in raw milk used by the dairy industry to monitor efficiency of pasteurization

Phospholipid: lipid linked to a phosphate group

Photoautotroph: autotroph that obtains energy from light

Photoheterotroph: phototroph that obtains energy from light

Photooxidation: chemical changes induced by visible light in the presence of oxygen

Photophosphorylation: chemical reaction that forms ATP from light energy

Photoreactivation: process for repairing ultraviolet damage to DNA by enzymes that are activated by visible light

Photosynthesis: conversion of light energy to chemical energy in the presence of a reducing agent, CO_2, and chlorophyll

Phototaxis: movement toward or away from a light source

Phototroph: organism that obtains energy from the sun

Phycobilins: accessory pigments of algae

Phycoerythrin: red accessory pigment of some algae

Phycomycoses: fungal diseases caused by rapidly growing fungi

Phyla: taxonomic groups of related classes

Phylogenetic: referring to a natural classification based on evolutionary relationships

Phytoplankton: microscopic plant life that lives on aquatic surfaces

Pia mater: inner membrane covering the brain and spinal cord

Pili: filamentous appendages of some bacteria responsible for adherence to solid surfaces or that take part in conjugation

Pimple: superficial lesion caused by infection of a hair follicle

Pitching: addition of yeast to fermentation vessels in the making of beer

Plankton: community of microscopic protozoa and algae in water

Plaque: slime layer consisting of bacteria and organic matter on teeth

Plaque-forming unit (PFU): quantitative expression of the number of bacteriophages on a lawn of bacteria

Plasma: liquid component of whole blood

Plasma cell: mature B cell that produces antibodies

Plasma membrane: lipoprotein bilayer that surrounds the cytoplasm of a cell

Plasmid: small extrachromosomal circular molecule of DNA

Plasmodium: streaming mass of cytoplasm of acellular slime molds

Platelet: cell fragment that promotes blood clotting

Pleomorphism: variation in size and shape

Pneumonic plague: infection of the lungs caused by the plague bacillus

Pneumonitis: inflammation of the lungs

Point mutation: change in a single nitrogen base-pair

Polar: unequal distribution of charges on shared electrons

Polar covalent bond: bond in which atoms exert a pull of unequal magnitude on shared atoms

Polyarteritis nodosa: arterial disease caused by deposits of immune complexes

Poly-β-hydroxybutyric acid: major energy reserve molecule for bacteria

Polyhedral: having more than six plane surfaces

Polymer: molecule made of many chemical units

Polymerase chain reaction (PCR): process of rapid synthesis of copies of DNA using repeated cycles of heating and cooling

Polymorphism: presence of a larger than expected number of variants at a particular chromosomal locus

Polymorphonuclear granulocyte: alternate term for neutrophil

Polyploidy: increase in normal numbers of chromosomes within a cell

Pomace: solid pulp of fruit pressed for juice

Pond: small open-air wastewater treatment system for decomposition of organic matter by microorganisms

Positive control mechanism: process regulating action of an operon in which a represser protein is bound to the substrate

Positive sense RNA: strand of RNA that acts as messenger RNA

Potable: suitable for drinking

Pour plate: method for obtaining isolated colonies using serial dilutions of a test sample

Precipitation: formation of complexes by soluble antigens and specific antibodies

Preliminary treatment: procedure to remove solid wastes and aromatic compounds in wastewater treatment

Prevalence: numbers of cases of a disease in a population at a specific time

Primary cell line: cell line capable of a limited number of transfers

Primary clarifier tank: large tank used in wastewater treatment to settle solid sludge and remove fats and greases

Primary disease: initial disease in a previously healthy person

Primary immune response: the rise in antibody levels that occurs on the first exposure to an antigen

Primary lymphoid organs: bone marrow and thymus

Primary metabolite: chemical required by an organism

Primary stain: initial stain applied in a differential staining procedure

Primary syphilis: first stage of syphilis characterized by a chancre

Primary treatment: physical removal from wastewater of settled solids, fats, and greases in a clarifying tank

Primer RNA: segment of RNA formed initially during replication of DNA

Prion: infectious protein particle associated with chronic diseases of the central nervous system

Privileged site: site, isolated from B- or T-cell activity, that does not generate an immune response to a transplant

Probe: radioactively labeled single strand sequence of DNA

Procaryote: cell without membrane-bound nuclear material

Prodigiosin: red pigment produced by *Serratia marcescens*

Producer: organism in an ecological niche that uses photosynthesis or chemosynthesis to provide its own food

Product: substance resulting from a chemical reaction

Profundal: water not penetrated by light

Progeny: offspring or replicated forms of a nucleic acid

Progressive multifocal leukoencephalopathy (PMC): rare complication of polyoma virus infection

Proinflammatory cytokine: chemical released by macrophages to attract other immune cells to a site of microbial invasion

Proliferation: process of rapid reproduction

Promoter site: location of the gene in an operon where RNA polymerase binds before transcribing the structural genes

Prontosil: dye from which sulfa drugs were derived

Properdin: major mediator of alternative pathway of complement activation

Prophage: nucleic acid of a temperate phage integrated into host-cell DNA

Prospective study: study based on data to be collected

Prostaglandin: biologically active chemical produced by many cells of the body

Proton: positively charged subatomic particle that is found in the nucleus of an atom

Proton gradient: electrical and concentration differences that develop across a membrane as protons are pumped out

Protoplast: cell without a cell wall

Protoplast fusion: method of producing hybrid plant cells after removal of cell walls and introduction of donor DNA

Prototroph: organism that can synthesize growth factors; wild type

Prototype: reference strain of a genus and species

Protozoa: single-celled nonphotosynthetic organisms belonging to the kingdom Protista

Provirus: viral DNA integrated into host-cell chromosome

Provocative dose: second or subsequent encounter with an allergen

Pseudocyst: cyst-like structure containing microorganisms

Pseudoplasmodium: aggregate of ameboid cellular slime molds

Pseudopodia: temporary extensions of cytoplasm responsible for motility in some protozoa

Psychrophile: organism that grows best at 20° C or below

Psychrotroph: food-spoilage organism that grows at 0° C but has an optimal temperature range between 25° and 30° C

Ptomaine: nitrogenous product derived from putrefactive action of bacteria

Puerperium: period during or after delivery

Purified protein derivative (PPD): proteins extracted from *Mycobacterium tuberculosis* used in tuberculin skin testing

Purine: six-sided cyclic nitrogen base fused to an imidazole ring

Purulent exudate: thick fluid containing white blood cells, bacteria, and serum produced in infections; also known as pus

Putrefaction: partial decomposition of proteins by microorganisms producing disagreeable odors

Pyelonephritis: inflammation of the kidney

Pyrimidine: cyclic six-sided nitrogen base

Pyrogenic: fever-producing

Quaternary ammonium compound (quat): cationic detergent composed of four organic groups attached to a nitrogen atom

Quaternary structure: fourth level of organization of a protein

Racemase: enzyme that alters the light rotation properties of a molecule

Rad: unit equivalent to the absorption of 100 ergs of radiation energy per gram of matter

Radiation: propagation of energy through space as electromagnetic waves

Radioimmunoassay (RIA): quantitative diagnostic method using an antibody labeled with a radioactive isotope

Radiolytic: chemical changes caused by radiation

Raw milk: standard term for milk obtained directly from the animal before pasteurization

Receptor site: attachment site on the surface of a host cell

Recipient: cell that receives the transferred DNA in genetic transfer processes

Recombinant cell: cell that has incorporated genes from another strain or species

Recombinant DNA: product of joining two segments of DNA to form a new DNA molecule

Recombinant DNA technology: manipulation of genes to produce commercially valuable products

Recombination: process of joining DNA segments from two sources

Redox reaction: chemical reaction involving the coupled reaction of oxidation and reduction

Reduction: gain of electrons by a molecule
Reflux: return or backward flow
Regimen: regulated form of treatment
Replica plating: technique for separating nutritionally deficient mutants from mixed populations
Replication: process by which a particle or molecule duplicates itself
Replication fork: initial Y-shaped opening occurring during initiation of DNA replication
Replicative intermediate: intervening compound necessary for duplication of a nucleic acid
Repression: inhibition of gene activity in the absence of a particular substrate
Repressor protein: product of regulator gene of an operon
Reservoir: environment or host that supports growth and multiplication of an infectious agent
Resistance: lack of microbial susceptibility to an antimicrobial agent
Resolving power: ability of a microscope to distinguish between two points that are closely spaced
Respiration: sum total of energy-liberating reactions within cells in which inorganic molecules act as the final electron acceptors
Restriction enzyme: enzyme that produces "nicks" or cuts in both strands of DNA at specific sites
Retrograde axonal transport: reverse movement along axons
Reverse osmosis: filtration procedure that removes chemicals dissolved in water
Reverse transcriptase: enzyme of retroviruses that catalyzes the replication of DNA from RNA
Reversion: mutation that restores a mutant's original genotype; a back-mutation
Rheumatic fever: inflammatory process affecting connective tissue of many organs
Rheumatoid arthritis: chronic inflammatory condition of joints
Rhinorrhea: thin, watery discharge from the nose
Ribonucleotide: building block of RNA containing a phosphate group, ribose sugar, and one of four nitrogen bases
Ribosomal RNA (rRNA): type of RNA associated with ribosomes
Ribosome: site of protein synthesis in cells
Ropy: viscous, thickened milk formed usually as a result of microbial growth producing slimy compounds
Runt disease: disease of small size; in transplantation, occurs when allogenic spleen cells are injected into newborn animals
Saccharophilic: sugar-loving
Salt: compound dissociating in water that produces cations other than H^+ and anions other than OH^-
Salvarsan: arsenic-containing drug first used to treat syphilis
Sanitizer: chemical agent that reduces the number of microorganisms present
Saprophyte: organism that grows on decaying organic matter
Sarcinae: cocci occurring in packets
Saturated fatty acid: fatty acid having no double bonds
Scalded skin syndrome: staphylococcal infection of the skin occurring in young infants
Schizogony: asexual cycle of malarial parasites
Sebum: secretion from sebaceous glands
Second Law of Thermodynamics: principle that states that the amount of energy released as heat energy during chemical conversions is less than 100 percent efficient
Secondary disease: disease occurring in a person with a primary disease
Secondary immune organs: spleen, lymph nodes, mucosal sites such as Peyer's patches
Secondary immune response: rise in antibody level that occurs on second exposure to an antigen
Secondary metabolite: compound that is nonessential for the growth of an organism
Secondary syphilis: second stage of syphilis characterized by a rash
Secondary treatment: use of microorganisms in wastewater treatment to reduce organic matter
Selective medium: medium that permits one type of microorganism to grow and inhibits the growth of other microorganisms
Selective permeability: characteristic of plasma membranes that allows only certain molecules or ions to enter or leave cells
Selective toxicity: property of a chemical to be toxic to a pathogen without harming the human or animal host
Self: referring to antigens of one's own tissues
Self-tolerance: lacking the ability to mount an immune response against one's own antigens
Semiconservative replication: method for copying DNA so that the two new DNA molecules contain one strand of the original DNA and one newly synthesized strand

Semisolid medium: medium containing 0.4 percent of a solidifying agent
Semisynthetic: refers to an antimicrobial agent that has a portion of its structure chemically modified
Sense strand: DNA strand containing a gene to be transcribed
Sensitizing dose: initial encounter with an allergen
Septate: having cross walls
Septicemia: infection of the blood
Septum: cell wall
Sequela: consequence of a disease
Serous exudate: thin watery fluid discharged usually during inflammation
Serum: liquid portion of clotted blood
Serum sickness: inflammatory process caused by circulating immune responses
Severe combined immunodeficiency disease (SCID): inability to mount B-cell and T-cell defenses against infectious diseases
Sex pilus: appendage connecting two cells during conjugation
Shell: orbit containing electrons surrounding the nucleus of an atom
Siderophore: substance that complexes with iron and makes ferric ions available to bacteria
Sign: objective finding in illness
Signal transduction: process by which a signal is transmitted from the outside of the cell to the inside resulting in alterations of cell behavior
Silent mutation: change or substitution of one base for another producing a new codon for the same amino acid
Simple microscope: single-lens instrument used for viewing small objects
Simple stain: use of a single dye to stain a smear or tissue
Single cell protein (SCP): protein food supplement extracted from microorganisms
Sinusitis: inflammation of a paranasal sinus
Slime layer: layer of glycoproteins surrounding a bacterial cell
Slow-reacting substances of anaphylaxis (SRS-A): chemicals released by mast cells and basophils in anaphylaxis
Sludge: sedimented solid wastes of sewage
Slug: association of slime mold cells
Smear: thin layer of a liquid specimen spread on a glass slide
Snapping division: type of binary fission leaving cells partially attached
Soil horizon: layers of different types of materials in soil
Solid medium: medium containing 1.5 percent of a solidifying agent
Solute: substance dissolved in a solvent to make a solution
Solvent: chemical having the ability to dissolve solutes
Sparkling wine: type of wine that contains tiny carbon dioxide bubbles creating a "sparkle"
Specialized transduction: process in which a virus transfers a specific gene from one bacterium to another
Species: latinized second name of an organism
Specific immunity: immunity derived from particular antibodies (acquired immunity)
Specifications: acceptable limits of numbers and types of microorganisms in food
Specificity: ability to react with particular chemicals
Sperm: male sex cell
Spheroplast: cell with some parts of its cell wall removed
Spike: surface projection on an envelope of a virus
Spirilla: spiral-shaped bacteria
Spirochete: tightly coiled spiral bacterium
Spontaneous generation: origin of life from nonliving sources
Spontaneous mutation: change in the base sequence of DNA occurring with no known cause
Sporadic: occurrence of a disease without regularity in a community
Sporangioconidium: asexual spore of some fungi
Sporangium: enlarged cell containing sporangioconidia
Spore: sexual reproductive structure of fungi
Spore coat: protective layer between the cortex and spore coat
Spore germination: return to the vegetative stage of a spore-forming bacterium
Sporogony: sexual cycle of malarial parasites
Sporozoite: infective stage of malarial parasite
Spread plate: method for obtaining isolated colonies using a bent glass rod
Standard: legal limit set by government regulatory agencies on acceptable numbers or types of microorganisms on raw ingredients and finished food products
Standard plate count (SPC): method for determining numbers of bacteria present in milk, water, and foods
Staphylococci: clusters of cocci
Starter culture: desirable microorganisms added to a food to initiate a fermentation

Stationary phase: third phase of a bacterial growth curve in which the rate of cell death equals the rate of cell division

Steady-state growth: growth sustained in the logarithmic growth phase

Steam under pressure: technique of heating water higher than its boiling point by increasing pressure

Stem cell: primitive multipotential cell in the bone marrow that can give rise to all of the cellular elements of the immune system and blood

Sterilization: process of destroying all microorganisms

Steroid: structurally complex lipid containing an alcohol group

Sterol: organic molecules having four interlocking rings of carbon and one or more —OH groups

Stigma: red eyespot of some algae

Strain: members of the same genus and species differing in one or more characteristics from the reference strain

Streak plate: method for obtaining isolated colonies using a bacteriological loop

Streptococci: chains of cocci

Structural gene: a gene containing a sequence of bases coding for the amino acid sequence of a protein

Subacute sclerosing panencephalitis (SSPE): rare complication after measles

Substrate: substance acted on by an enzyme

Substrate phosphorylation: process of forming ATP during a reaction between a substrate and enzyme

Sulfa drug: compound derived from the dye prontosil

Superantigen: peptides of certain bacterial toxins and viruses that elicit an excessive, often harmful, T-cell response

Suppressor T cell: lymphocyte carrying $CD8^+$ marker

Suppuration: process of pus formation

Sweet wine: wine that contains between 0.5 and 32% residual sugar

Symbiosis: mutually beneficial relationship between two organisms

Symbiotic nitrogen fixation: mutually beneficial association of certain bacteria living in nodules on plant roots

Symmetry: similarity of form or arrangement on both sides of a dividing line

Symptom: complaint in illness described by a person

Synchronized culture: growth system designed to sustain cells in the same stage of cell cycles

Syndrome: collection of signs and symptoms characteristic of a disease

Synergism: effect of two drugs used together is greater than the total effects of each drug when used alone

Synthetic: pertaining to an antimicrobial agent that has been completely compounded artificially

Systemic anaphylaxis: sudden, sometimes fatal, vasomotor collapse induced by a second or subsequent exposure to an antigen

Systemic lupus erythematosus: immune-complex disease caused by antinuclear antibodies

T cell: lymphocyte that functions in cell-mediated immunity

T-cell receptor (TCR): molecule on T cell that binds to an antigen-MHC complex on an antigen-presenting cell

T helper cell (TH): T lymphocyte having a $CD4^+$ marker on cell surface

T helper cell type 1 (TH1): T helper cell participating in cell-mediated immunity

T helper cell type 2 (TH2): T helper cell participating in antibody-mediated immunity

Table wine: wine that has an average alcoholic content of 12 to 12 1/2 percent

Tachycardia: rapid heart beat

Tail: appendage of a bacteriophage

Taxon: unit used in classifying organisms

Taxonomy: study of classification

Teichoic acid: polysaccharide found in walls of some gram-positive bacteria

Temperate phage: bacteriophage that can be integrated into the genome of a bacterium

Termination: action of the stop codon on mRNA to end protein synthesis and release the protein from the ribosome

Tertiary syphilis: third stage of syphilis characterized by gummas

Tertiary treatment: combination of physical and chemical methods to remove chemicals from wastewater after secondary treatment

Thermal death point: temperature required to kill a particular microorganism within 10 minutes

Thermal death time: time required to kill a particular microorganism at a specific temperature

Thermal denaturation: change in molecular structure caused by heat

Thermoacidophile: organism that grows best at 45° C or above under acid conditions

Thermophile: organism that grows best at 45° C or above

Thrombocyte: alternate term for platelet

Thrombocytopenia: abnormally low platelet count in blood

Thrush: oral infection caused by a yeast

Thylakoid: inner pigment-containing membrane of chloroplasts

Thymine: cyclic nitrogen base

Thymus: lymphoid organ located behind the sternum responsible for maturation of T lymphocytes

Tinea: superficial fungal infection of the skin

Titer: quantitative expression of antibodies present in serum

Tolerance: lacking the ability to mount an immune response

Tonsillitis: inflammation of a tonsil

Total suspended solids (TSS): total organic matter contained in wastewater

Toxic-shock syndrome: multisystemic infection caused by toxin-producing staphylococci

Toxigenicity: capacity to produce a toxin

Toxins: poisons produced by some infectious agents

Toxoid: inactivated toxin

Tracheotomy: incision and insertion of tube into the trachea to overcome obstruction

Transcription: process for synthesizing RNA from a DNA template

Transduction: transfer of genes from one bacterium to another by a virus

Transducing particles: viruses that transfer bacterial genes to other bacteria

Transduction: process by which a virus carries bacterial genes from one bacterium to another

Transfer RNA (tRNA): type of RNA that transports amino acids to ribosomes

Transferase: enzyme that moves one group of atoms from one molecule to another

Transformation: transfer of genes as soluble DNA from one bacterium to another

Transgenic: genetically engineered organisms containing genes from another species

Transient carrier: a short-term carrier of an infectious agent

Transition: mutation in which a purine replaces another purine or a pyrimidine replaces another pyrimidine on a DNA molecule

Translation: process for synthesis of a protein from an mRNA molecule

Transpiration: evaporative water loss from leaves and stems of plants

Transplant rejection: the destruction of a transplanted tissue or graft by the immune system

Transposon: gene or cluster of genes having the ability to move to another segment on a chromosome, plasmid, or viral nucleic acid

Transudate: noncellular fluids of blood or lymph leaking into surrounding tissue

Transversion: process of mutation involving the substitution of a purine for a pyrimidine or a pyrimidine for a purine in DNA

Tricarboxylic acid cycle: alternate name for Krebs cycle

Trichomoniasis: inflammation of the vagina caused by a protozoan

Trickling filter tank: large rock or plastic media-filled tank onto which primary treated wastewater is sprinkled to allow the decomposition of organic matter by aerobic microorganisms

Triglyceride: a lipid containing three ester bonds

Trophic level: feeding level within a food chain or web

Trophozoite: vegetative feeding stage of some protozoa

Trypanosomal form (trypomastigote): extracellular, motile form of a *Leishmania* parasite that develops in sandflies

Tubercle: calcified lesion of the lung containing viable cells of *Mycobacterium tuberculosis*

Tuberculoid: resembling tuberculosis or a tubercle

Tubulin: protein making up microtubules that alternates between assembled and disassembled states

Tumor necrosis factor (TNF): cytokine that induces local inflammation

Twiddles: tumbling movements made by bacteria

Tympanocentesis: puncture of the eardrum

Tyndallization: process of killing endospore-forming bacteria by intermittent exposure to flowing steam

Universal precautions: recommendations of the Centers for Disease Control and Prevention for preventing transmission of pathogens in body fluids

Unsaturated fatty acid: fatty acid having one to four double bonds

Uracil: cyclic nitrogen base

Urea breath test (UBT): noninvasive diagnostic test for *Helicobacter* infection

Urogenital triangle: upper triangular area of the perineum

Urticaria: localized type response to an inhaled, ingested, or contact allergen characterized by the appearance of red, raised skin lesions

Use-dilution method: method for evaluating a

chemical for its effectiveness in killing microorganisms

Vaccination: inoculation of microbial antigens

Vaccine: antigenic preparation used to stimulate an immune response

Vacuole: membrane-bound inclusion in cytoplasm containing liquid or gas

Variable: differing order of amino acid sequences of an immunoglobulin

Variable number of tandem repeats (VNTR): unique number of short repetitive sequences in a DNA molecule

Vector: plasmid, phage, or a cosmid that acts as a carrier of foreign DNA into a cell

Vegetative: growing, reproducing stage of a microorganism

Vertebrae: bones enclosing the spinal cord

Vertigo: dizziness

Vesicle: transitory infoldings of plasma membrane containing liquid or gas; open blister containing fluid

Viable: capable of reproducing

Vibrios: short, slightly curved rods

Viral load: quantitative expression of circulating human immunodeficiency virus

Virion: extracellular phase of a virus

Viroid: subcellular RNA particle that infects plant cells

Viropexis: process by which a virus enters a cell

Virulence: degree of pathogenicity

Virulent phage: bacteriophage causing a lytic cycle in a host bacterium

Viruses: submicroscopic acellular particles containing DNA or RNA surrounded by protein

Vulvovaginal candidiasis: inflammation of the vulva and vagina caused by a yeast

Warm vent: hydrothermal crack or opening on the deep ocean floor that releases water with a temperature of 6 to 23° C

Weil-Felix reaction: agglutination of certain strains of *Proteus* by rickettsial antibodies

Western blot assay: method for identifying proteins in a mixture using gel separation, membrane transfer, and labeled antibodies to identify proteins

Wiscott-Aldrich syndrome: deficiency of B cells, T cells, and platelets

Wort: the liquid resulting from cooking grains, malt, and hops in preparation for beer fermentation

Xenobiotic: foreign chemical or poison

Xenograft: transplant from a donor of a different species from the recipient

Xerophilic: having the capacity to grow in environments that are extremely low in water

Yeast: unicellular fungus

Zoonosis: disease of animals that can be transmitted to humans

Zygospore: sexual reproductive structure of some fungi

Zygote: cell formed by union of male and female sex cells

Zygotic induction: process by which a prophage becomes virulent

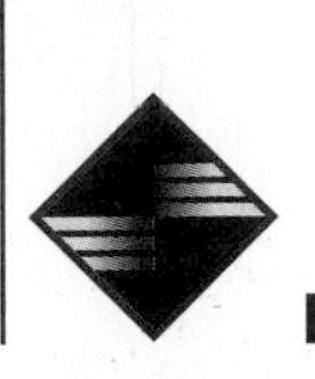

ILLUSTRATION CREDITS

Chapter 1

Figure 1–2. *A*, Parke-Davis, a division of Warner-Lambert, Morris Plains, NJ. ©1959.

Figure 1–4. Parke-Davis, a division of Warner-Lambert, Morris Plains, NJ. ©1962.

Figure 1–6. Parke-Davis, a division of Warner-Lambert, Morris Plains, NJ. ©1959.

Figure 1–7. Becton Dickinson Microbiological Systems, Sparks, MD.

Figure 1–8. National Library of Medicine, Bethesda, MD.

Figure 1–9. Photo 16583, World Health Organization, Geneva, Switzerland.

Figure 1–11. National Library of Medicine, Bethesda, MD.

Figure 1–12. National Library of Medicine, Bethesda, MD.

Figure 1–14. Evans EH, Foulds I, Carr NG: J Gen Microbiol *92:*149, 1976.

Figure 1–15. U.S. Department of Agriculture.

Figure 1–16. Horne RW: Virus Structure. San Diego, Academic Press, 1974.

Chapter 3

Figure 3–1. Leica, Inc., Deerfield, IL.

Figure 3–4. Leica, Inc., Deerfield, IL.

Figure 3–6. Beckman Diagnostics, Fullerton, CA.

Figure 3–7. GD Roberts, Rochester, MN.

Figure 3–8. CK Stumm, University of Nijmegen, The Netherlands.

Figure 3–9. Philips Electronic Instruments, Inc., Mahwah, NJ.

Figure 3–11. Horne RW, Waterson AP, Farnham A, Wildy P: Virology *11:*79, 1960.

Figure 3–12. Bayer ME, Leive L: Effect of ethylenediaminetetraacetate upon the surface of *Escherichia coli.* J Bacteriol *130:*1367, 1977.

Figure 3–13. *A* and *B*, K Amako, Fukuoka, Japan; *C*, WP Reed, Albuquerque, NM.

Figure 3–17. CK Kwan, White Memorial Medical Center, Los Angeles, CA.

Chapter 4

Figure 4–2. *A*, Providence Saint Joseph Medical Center, Burbank, CA. *B* and *C*, Carolina Biological Supply Company, Burlington, NC.

Figure 4–15. DiPersio JR: J Gen Microbiol 83:355, 1974, Cambridge University Press.

Figure 4–16. Reprinted with permission, Kingsbury EW, Voelz H: Science 166:768, 1969. Copyright © 1969 by the American Association for the Advancement of Science.

Figure 4–17. L Archer and GB Chapman, Washington, DC.

Figure 4–18. S Decker, Cincinnati, OH.

Figure 4–19. Amako F, Umeda A: J Electron Microscopy *26*(2):155, 1977.

Figure 4–20. PE Hargroves, Kingston, RI.

Figure 4–23. GH Rose, Houston, TX.

Figure 4–24. Pappas GD, Brandt J: Biophys Biochem Cytol 6:85, 1959.

Figure 4–25. Wergin WP: Sci Am *223*(24):24, 1970.

Figure 4–26. RT Moore, The New University of Ulster, Coleraine, Northern Ireland.

Figure 4–27. H Beaudry, Brussels, Belgium.

Figure 4–28. Sugihara R, et al.: Electron Microscopy, Vol 2. Tokyo, Maruzen, 1966.

Chapter 5

Figure 5–5. Becton Coulter Inc., Fullerton, CA.

Figure 5–6. Toucan Technologies Inc., Cincinnati, OH.

Figure 5–10. C Luckenbach, Valley Glen, CA.

Figure 5–16. New Brunswick Scientific Co., Edison, NJ.

Figure 5–17. Reprinted with permission of Millipore Corporation, Bedford, MA.

Chapter 7

Figure 7–2. Elmer W. Koneman, Instructional Design Consultants, Denver, CO.

Figure 7–3. Belas MR: The swarming phenomenon of *Proteus mirabilis*. ASM News *58*:19, 1992.

Figure 7–10. Adapted from Sokatch JR, Ferretti JJ: Basic Bacteriology and Genetics. Wilmette, IL, Mosby–Year Book, 1976.

Figure 7–15. Reprinted from Mutation Research, *31*, Ames BN, McCann J, Yamasaki E: Methods for detecting carcinogens and mutagens with the *Salmonella*/mammalian-microsome mutagenicity test. 347, 1975, with permission of Elsevier Science.

Figure 7–19. Adapted from Boyd RF: Basic Medical Microbiology, 5th ed. Boston, Little, Brown & Co, 1995, Fig. 5–8a.

Figure 7–20. Adapted from Boyd RF: Basic Medical Microbiology, 5th ed. Boston, Little, Brown & Co, 1995, Fig. 5–8b.

Chapter 8

Figure 8–1. Kline MW, Mason EO Jr, Kaplan SL: J Clin Microbiol *27*:1793, 1989.

Figure 8–5. Krieg NR, Holt JG, eds: Bergey's Manual of Systematic Bacteriology, Vol. 1, Baltimore, Williams & Wilkins, 1975.

Figure 8–6. M Shilo, Jerusalem, Israel.

Figure 8–7. L Nesbitt, National Research Council of Canada, Saskatoon, Saskatchewan, Canada.

Figure 8–8. Berg HC: Sci Am *233*(2):36, 1975.

Figure 8–9. Rocky Mountain Laboratory, U.S. Public Health Service, Hamilton, MT.

Figure 8–10. ES Boatman, University of Washington, Seattle, WA.

Figure 8–11. Davis BD, et al.: Microbiology, 2nd ed. New York, Harper & Row, 1973.

Figure 8–12. Centers for Disease Control and Prevention, Atlanta, GA.

Figure 8–13. PD Mitchell, Marshfield, WI.

Figure 8–14. Zeikus JG, Ward JC: Science *184*:1181, 1974.

Figure 8–15. Carolina Biological Supply Co., Burlington, NC.

Chapter 9

Figure 9–1. Bold HC, Wynne MJ: Introduction to the Algae—Structure and Reproduction, 2nd ed. Upper Saddle River, NJ, Prentice-Hall, 1985.

Figure 9–2. Redrawn from Palmer CW: Algae in Water Supplies. Washington, DC, US Department of Health, Education, and Welfare, 1962.

Figure 9–4. Fisher Scientific Co., Chicago, IL.

Figure 9–5. © R Calentine/Visuals Unlimited.

Figure 9–6. Carolina Biological Supply Co., Burlington, NC.

Figure 9–7. © Veronica Burmeister/Visuals Unlimited.

Figure 9–8. Redrawn from Standard Methods for the Examination of Water and Wastewater, 13th ed. New York, American Public Health Association, 1971.

Figure 9–13. G Svihla, Portage, IN.

Figure 9–18. USDA Photo No. BN 9384.

Chapter 10

Figure 10–1. Knight CA: Chemistry of Viruses, 2nd ed. New York, Springer Verlag, 1975.

Figure 10–3. Horne RW: Virus Structure. New York, Academic Press, 1974.

Figure 10–5. Horne RW: Virus Structure. New York, Academic Press, 1974.

Figure 10–7. Chardonnet Y, Dales S: Virology *40*:462, 1970.

Figure 10–8. GB Chapman and J Pisani, Washington, DC.

Figure 10–10. Maruyama K, Oboshi S: Electron Microscopy, Vol 2. Tokyo, Maruzen, 1966.

Figure 10–13. Armed Forces Institute of Pathology, No. 58-13966-4.

Figure 10–14. Volkman LE, Summers MD: J Virol *16*:1632, 1975.

Figure 10–15. Frankel JW, West MK: Proc Soc Exp Biol Med *97*:741, 1958.

Figure 10–16. PI Marcus, Storrs, CT.

Figure 10–17. Yamada M, Commoner B, Symington J: Proc Natl Acad Sci *48*:1675, 1962.

Figure 10–18. Biolabs, Inc., Northbrook, IL.

Figure 10–19. Acton JD, et al.: Fundamentals of Medical Virology. Philadelphia, Lea & Febiger, 1974.

Figure 10–20. Acton JD, et al.: Fundamentals of Medical Virology. Philadelphia, Lea & Febiger, 1974.

Figure 10–21. RW Horne, P Wildy, John Innes Institute, Norwich, England.

Figure 10–22. Acton D, et al.: Fundamentals of Medical Virology. Philadelphia, Lea & Febiger, 1974.

Figure 10–23. Acton D, et al.: Fundamentals of Medical Virology. Philadelphia, Lea & Febiger, 1974.

Figure 10–24. Acton D, et al.: Fundamentals of Medical Virology. Philadelphia, Lea & Febiger, 1974.

Figure 10–26. Acton D, et al.: Fundamentals of Medical Virology. Philadelphia, Lea & Febiger, 1974.

Chapter 11

Figure 11–3. MMWR *46*(21):473, 1997.

Figure 11–7. Centers for Disease Control and Prevention, Atlanta, GA.

Chapter 12

Figure 12–1. P Patrick Cleary, Minneapolis, MN.

Figure 12–2. JWF Costerton, Bozeman, MT.

Figure 12–4. Walker TS: Microbiology. Philadelphia, WB Saunders, 1998.

Figure 12–5. Aly R: Infect Immun *17*:547, 1977.

Figure 12–6. Applegate EJ: The Anatomy and Physiology Learning System. Philadelphia, WB Saunders, 1995.

Chapter 13

Figure 13–1. Applegate EJ: The Anatomy and Physiology Learning System. Philadelphia, WB Saunders, 1995, Figure 14–5, page 292.

Figure 13–3. Applegate EJ: The Anatomy and Physiology Learning System. Philadelphia, WB Saunders, 1995, Figure 14–8, page 296.

Figure 13–4. Applegate EJ: The Anatomy and Physiology Learning System. Philadelphia, WB Saunders, 1995, Figure 11–2, page 231.

Figure 13–5. Applegate EJ: The Anatomy and Physiology Learning System. Philadelphia, WB Saunders, 1995, Figure 14–7, page 295.

Figure 13–7. MR Talluto.

Figure 13–8. Applegate EJ: The Anatomy and Physiology Learning System. Philadelphia, WB Saunders, 1995, Figure 14–6, page 294.

Figure 13–12. Applegate EJ: The Anatomy and Physiology Learning System. Philadelphia, WB Saunders, 1995, Figure 14–10, page 298.

Figure 13–17. Applegate EJ: The Anatomy and Physiology Learning System. Philadelphia, WB Saunders, 1995, Figure 14–9, page 297.

Figure 13–19. Damjanov I: Pathology for the Health-Related Professions. Philadelphia, WB Saunders, 1996, Figure 3–8, page 52.

Figure 13–20. Applegate EJ: The Anatomy and Physiology Learning System. Philadelphia, WB Saunders, 1995, Figure 14–12, page 300.

Chapter 14

Figure 14–1. Baylor College of Medicine, Houston, TX.

Figure 14–2. Damjanov I: Pathology for the Health Related Professions. Philadelphia, WB Saunders, 1996, Figure 3–11, page 55.

Figure 14–3. Damjanov I: Pathology for the Health Related Professions. Philadelphia, WB Saunders, 1996, Figure 3–12, page 56.

Figure 14–4. Damjanov I: Pathology for the Health Related Professions. Philadelphia, WB Saunders, 1996, Figure 3–20, page 63.

Figure 14–5. Damjanov I: Pathology for the Health Related Professions. Philadelphia, WB Saunders, 1996, Figure 3–21, page 64.

Figure 14–6. Damjanov I: Pathology for the Health Related Professions. Philadelphia, WB Saunders, 1996, Figure 3–14, page 57.

Figure 14–7. Damjanov I: Pathology for the Health Related Professions. Philadelphia, WB Saunders, 1996, Figure 3–15, page 58.

Figure 14–8. Frazier MS, Drzymkowski JA, Doty JS: Essentials of Human Diseases and Conditions. Philadelphia, WB Saunders, 1996, Figure 3–5, page 62.

Figure 14–9. Kahana and A/V Services, McMaster University, Hamilton, Ontario, Canada.

Figure 14–10. Damjanov I: Pathology for the Health Related Professions. Philadelphia, WB Saunders, 1996, Figure 3–18, page 60.

Figure 14–13. Male D: Immunology—An Illustrated Outline, 3rd ed. St. Louis, CV Mosby, 1998, Figure 5–12.

Figure 14–14. Barrett JT: Textbook of Immunology, 2nd ed. St. Louis, CV Mosby, 1974.

Figure 14–16. de la Maza LM, Pezzlo MT, Baron EJ: Color Atlas of Diagnostic Microbiology. St. Louis, CV Mosby, 1997, Figure 17–5.

Figure 14–17. de la Maza LM, Pezzlo MT, Baron EJ: Color Atlas of Diagnostic Microbiology. St. Louis, CV Mosby, 1997, Figure 17–6, page 196.

Figure 14–18. de la Maza LM. Pezzlo MT, Baron EJ: Color Atlas of Diagnostic Microbiology. St. Louis, CV Mosby, 1997, Figure 17–7, page 196.

Figure 14–19. de la Maza LM, Pezzlo MT, Baron EJ: Color Atlas of Diagnostic Microbiology. St. Louis, CV Mosby, 1997, Figure 17–3, page 195.

Figure 14–20. de la Maza LM, Pezzlo MT, Baron EJ: Color Atlas of Diagostic Microbiology. St. Louis, CV Mosby, 1997, Figure 17–4, page 195.

Figure 14–21. Roitt I, Brostoff J, Male D: Immunology, 3rd ed. London, Mosby–Year Book International, 1993, page 25.5.

Figure 14–22. RL Hodinka, Philadelphia, PA.

Chapter 15

Figure 15–2. Armed Forces Institute of Pathology, Neg. No. DET B-525-B.

Figure 15–3. Armed Forces Institute of Pathology, Neg. No. 68-13506.

Figure 15–4. Thomas SW, Baird IM, Frazier RD: Toxic shock syndrome following submucous resection and rhinoplasty. JAMA *247*:2402, 1982, copyright ©1982, American Medical Association.

Figure 15–5. Courtesy of Mrs. Eloise Nelson, Burbank, CA.

Figure 15–6. Armed Forces Institute of Pathology, Neg. No. 58-6180.

Figure 15–7. Low DE, Toronto, Ontario, Canada.

Figure 15–8. Laboratory Identification of Pyogenic Cocci, Part I. Baltimore, University Park Press, 1975.

Figure 15–9. Armed Forces Institute of Pathology, Neg. No. 75-4203-9.

Figure 15–10. Groman N, Chambers V: Basic Laboratory Techniques for Microbiology. New York, Harper & Row, 1972.

Figure 15–11. World Health Organization, Geneva, Switzerland.

Figure 15–12. Armed Forces Institute of Pathology, Neg. No. 55-12646.

Figure 15–13. Conant NF, Smith DT, Baker RD, Callaway JL: Manual of Clinical Mycology, 3rd ed. Philadelphia, WB Saunders, 1971.

Figure 15–14. EW Koneman, Denver, CO.

Figure 15–15. EW Koneman, Denver, CO.

Figure 15–16. EW Koneman, Denver, CO.

Figure 15–17. Conant NF, Smith DT, Baker RD, Callaway JL: Manual of Clinical Mycology, 3rd ed. Philadelphia, WB Saunders, 1971.

Figure 15–18. Bowman PI, Ahearn DG: J Clin Microbiol *2*:356, 1975.

Figure 15–19. Conant NF, Smith DT, Baker RD, Callaway JL: Manual of Clinical Mycology, 3rd ed. Philadelphia, WB Saunders, 1971.

Figure 15–20. Emmons CW, Binford CH, Utz JP: Medical Mycology, 2nd ed. Philadelphia, Lea & Febiger, 1970.

Figure 15–21. DH Koobs, Department of Pediatrics, Loma Linda School of Medicine, Loma Linda, CA.

Figure 15–22. White DO, Fenner F: Medical Virology, 3rd ed. Orlando, Academic Press, 1986.

Figure 15–23. Armed Forces Institute of Pathology, Neg. No. 55-11961.

Figure 15–24. Armed Forces Institute of Pathology, Neg. No. ACC 219482-16013.

Figure 15–25. GW Korting, Mainz, Germany.

Chapter 16

Figure 16–2. Armed Forces Institute of Pathology, Neg. No. 55-6150.

Figure 16–3. C Luckenbach, Valley Glen, CA.

Figure 16–4. JJ Le Beau, University of Illinois Medical Center, Chicago, IL.

Figure 16–5. Providence Saint Joseph Medical Center, Burbank, CA.

Figure 16–6. Abbott Laboratories, Atlas of Diagnostic Microbiology, July 1974.

Figure 16–7. FLA Buckmere, Department of Microbiology, The Medical College of Wisconsin, Madison, WI.

Figure 16–8. Abbott Laboratories, Atlas of Diagnostic Microbiology, July 1974.

Figure 16–9. SM Gibson, General Bacteriology Laboratory, Texas Department of Health Resources, Austin, TX.

Figure 16–10. Centers for Disease Control and Prevention, Atlanta, GA. Summary of Notifiable Diseases in the United States, 1996.

Figure 16–11. Harris HW, McClement JH: *In* Hoeprich PD: Infectious Diseases, 2nd ed. New York, Harper & Row, 1977.

Figure 16–12. GD Roberts, Rochester, MN.

Figure 16–13. Liu C: *In* Hoeprich PD: Infectious Diseases, 2nd ed. New York, Harper & Row, 1977.

Figure 16–14. Centers for Disease Control and Prevention, Atlanta, GA.

Figure 16–15. Lattimer GL, Ormsbee RA: Legionnaires' Disease. New York, Marcel Dekker, 1981.

Figure 16–16. Nikon Instrument Division, Garden City, NY. Photomicrograph by JP Vetter, Western Pennsylvania Hospital, Pittsburgh, PA.

Figure 16–17. NL Goodman, University of Kentucky Medical College, Lexington, KY.

Figure 16–18. Larsh HW, Goodman NL: *In* Lennette EH, et al.: Manual of Clinical Microbiology, 4th ed. Washington, DC, American Society for Microbiology, 1985.

Figure 16–19. Larsh HW, Goodman NL: *In* Lennette EH, et al.: Manual of Clinical Microbiology, 4th ed. Washington, DC, American Society for Microbiology, 1985.

Figure 16–20. Larsh HW, Goodman NL: *In* Lennette EH, et al.: Manual of Clinical Microbiology, 4th ed. Washington, DC, American Society for Microbiology, 1985.

Figure 16–21. Larsh HW, Goodman NL: *In* Lennette EH, et al.: Manual of Clinical Microbiology, 4th ed. Washington, DC, American Society for Microbiology, 1985.

Figure 16–22. Hazen EL, Gordon MA, Reed FC: Laboratory Identification of Pathogenic Fungi Simplified, 3rd ed. Springfield, IL, Charles C Thomas, 1970.

Figure 16–23. H Sepp, Toronto, Ontario, Canada.

Figure 16–24. Norrby E, Marusyk H, Örvell C: J Virol *6:*240, 1970.

Chapter 17

Figure 17–2. PD Mitchell, Marshfield, WI.

Figure 17–3. Gottlieb DS, Miller LH: J Periodontol *42:* 412, 1971.

Figure 17–4. Hoeprich PD (ed.): Infectious Diseases, 2nd ed. New York, Harper & Row, 1977.

Figure 17–5. Listgarten MA: J Periodontol *47:*1, 1976.

Figure 17–6. Bergquist LM: Changing Patterns of Infectious Disease. Philadelphia, Lea & Febiger, 1984. Photograph by RL Guerrant, Charlottesville, VA.

Figure 17–7. Groman N, Chambers V: Basic Laboratory Techniques for Microbiology. New York, Harper & Row, 1972.

Figure 17–8. Kaplan RL: *In* Lennette EH (ed.): Manual of Clinical Microbiology, 3rd ed. Washington, DC, American Society for Microbiology, 1981.

Figure 17–9. Marcy SM, Kibrick S: Mumps. *In* Hoeprich PD (ed.): Infectious Diseases, 2nd ed. New York, Harper & Row, 1977.

Figure 17–10. JS Nelson, St. Louis, MO.

Figure 17–12. Brandt H: *In* Marcial-Rojas RA (ed.): Pathology of Protozoal and Helminthic Diseases with Clinical Correlation. Baltimore, Williams & Wilkins, 1971.

Figure 17–13. Reese NC, Current WL, Ernst JV, Bailey WS: Cryptosporidiosis of man and calf: A case report and results of experimental infections in mice and rats. Am J Trop Hyg *31:*226, 1982.

Figure 17–14. DGW Berlin, University of California, Los Angeles, CA.

Figure 17–19. IG Kagan, Centers for Disease Control and Prevention, Atlanta, GA.

Figure 17–20. IG Kagan, Centers for Disease Control and Prevention, Atlanta, GA.

Chapter 18

Figure 18–6. MC Shepard, Camp Lejeune, NC.

Figure 18–7. DA Kuhn, Northridge, CA.

Figure 18–8. Morbidity and Mortality Weekly Report Supplement 45(53). Centers for Disease Control and Prevention, Atlanta, GA, 1997.

Figure 18–9. Morbidity and Mortality Weekly Report Supplement 45(53). Centers for Disease Control and Prevention, Atlanta, GA, 1997.

Figure 18–10. Abbott Laboratories, Atlas of Diagnostic Microbiology, July 1974.

Figure 18–11. Morbidity and Mortality Weekly Report Supplement 45(53). Centers for Disease Control and Prevention, Atlanta, GA, 1997.

Figure 18–12. Armed Forces Institute of Pathology, Neg. No. 78-1413.

Figure 18–13. Armed Forces Institute of Pathology, Neg. No. 53-19638.

Figure 18–14. Armed Forces Institute of Pathology, Neg. No. 78-1412.

Figure 18–16. Nahmias AJ, Starr SE: *In* Hoeprich PD (ed.): Infectious Diseases, 3rd ed. New York, Harper & Row, 1977.

Chapter 19

Figure 19–5. Centers for Disease Control and Prevention, Atlanta, GA.

Figure 19–6. Armed Forces Institute of Pathology, Neg. No. N-33470.

Figure 19–7. Davis BD, et al.: Microbiology, 2nd ed. New York, Harper & Row, 1973.

Figure 19–8. World Health Organization, Geneva, Switzerland.

Figure 19–9. L Ajello, Centers for Disease Control and Prevention, Atlanta, GA.

Figure 19–10. Prier JE, Friedman H (eds.): Opportunistic Pathogens. Baltimore, University Park Press, 1974.

Figure 19–11. Frenkel JK: *In* Hammond DM, Long PL (eds.): The Coccidia. Baltimore, University Park Press, 1973.

Figure 19–12. Estelle Doheny Eye Foundation, Los Angeles, CA.

Figure 19–16. Hess AD, Holden P: Ann NY Acad Sci *70:*294, 1958.

Figure 19–17. P Atansiu and J Sisman, Pasteur Institute, Paris, France.

Figure 19–18. DC Gajdusek, Bethesda, MD.

Chapter 20

Figure 20–1. R Steinman, The Rockefeller University, New York, NY.

Figure 20–5. Centers for Disease Control and Prevention, Atlanta, GA.

Figure 20–6. Bibel DJ, Chen TH: Bacteriol Rev *40*:633–651, 1976.

Figure 20–7. CT Taylor, Rocky Mountain Laboratory, Hamilton, MT.

Figure 20–8. CT Taylor, Rocky Mountain Laboratory, Hamilton, MT.

Figure 20–9. Steere AC, et al.: Ann Intern Med *86*:685, 1977.

Figure 20–10. Centers for Disease Control and Prevention, Atlanta, GA.

Figure 20–11. HG Cramblett, Ohio State University Medical Illustrations, Columbus, OH.

Figure 20–12. Radetsky MA: Pediatr Infect Dis *1*:425, 1982.

Figure 20–16. Brown HW: Basic Clinical Parasitology, 4th ed. Englewood Cliffs, NJ, Prentice Hall, 1975.

Figure 20–17. Carolina Biological Supply Company, Burlington, NC.

Figure 20–19. Zaiman H: A Pictorial Presentation of Parasites, Valley City, ND.

Figure 20–20. Centers for Disease Control and Prevention, Atlanta, GA.

Figure 20–21. RC Rau, Columbus, OH.

Figure 20–22. R Yaeger, New Orleans, LA.

Chapter 21

Figure 21–1. Chick H: Process of disinfection by chemical agents and hot water. J Hyg *10*:237, 1910.

Figure 21–3. *A*, Block SS: Disinfection, Sterilization, and Preservation, 2nd ed. Philadelphia, Lippincott Williams & Wilkins, 1977.

Figure 21–4. American Type Culture Collection, Manassas, VA.

Figure 21–5. Joklik WK, Willett HP, Amos DB (eds.): Zinsser Microbiology, 18th ed. Norwalk, CT, Appleton Century Crofts, 1984.

Figure 21–7. Block SS: Disinfection, Sterilization, and Preservation, 4th ed. Philadelphia, Lippincott Williams & Wilkins, 1991.

Figure 21–8. Steris Corporation, Mentor, OH.

Chapter 22

Figure 22–1. Walker TS: Microbiology. Philadelphia, WB Saunders, 1998.

Figure 22–2. Onishi HR, Zimmerman SB, Stapley EO: Observations on mode of action of cefoxitin. Ann NY Acad Sci *235*:406, 1974.

Figure 22–4. Providence Saint Joseph Medical Center, Burbank, CA.

Figure 22–5. Forbes BA, et al.: Bailey & Scott's Diagnostic Microbiology, 10th ed. St. Louis, Mosby–Year Book, 1998, page 256.

The molecular structures on page 154 for the penicillin nucleus and the cephalosporin nucleus, the molecular structures on page 157 for chloramphenicol and the tetracyclines, the molecular structure on page 159 for rifampin, and the molecular structures on page 160 for *p*-aminobenzoic acid and sulfonamide are redrawn from Walker TS: Microbiology. Philadelphia, WB Saunders, 1998.

Chapter 23

Figure 23–1. H Jannasch, Woods Hole Oceanographic Institute.

Figure 23–3. DR Benson, Storrs, CT.

Figure 23–8. SCS USDA. Photo by Morrison W. Liston.

Figure 23–11. Millipore Corp., Bedford, MA.

Figures 23–13 to 23–16. Orange County Sanitation District, Fountain Valley, CA.

Chapter 24

Figure 24–2. Ernest and Julio Gallo Winery, California.

Figure 24–4. Monsanto Company, St. Louis, MO.

Color Plates

Color Plate 1. © T. E. Adams/Visuals Unlimited.

Color Plate 2. © Cabisco/Visuals Unlimited.

Color Plate 3. © Tom Adams/Visuals Unlimited.

Color Plate 4. © A. M. Siegelman/Visuals Unlimited.

Color Plate 5. C Luckenbach, Valley Glen, CA.

Color Plate 6. C Luckenbach, Valley Glen, CA.

Color Plate 7. Chan FTH, MacKenzie MR: Enrichment medium and control system for isolation of *Campylobacter fetus* subsp. *jejuni* from stools. J Clin Microbiol *15*:12, 1982.

Color Plate 8. C Luckenbach, Valley Glen, CA.

Color Plate 9. Forbes BA, Sahm DF, Weissfeld AS: Bailey & Scott's Diagnostic Microbiology, 10th ed. St. Louis, CV Mosby, 1998, Figure 12–1A, page 151.

Color Plate 10. Biomerieux, Inc., Hazelwood, MO.

Color Plate 11. Forbes BA, Sahm DF, Weissfeld AS: Bailey & Scott's Diagnostic Microbiology, 10th ed. St. Louis, CV Mosby, 1998, Figure 66–6, page 981.

Color Plate 12. Forbes BA, Sahm DF, Weissfeld AS: Bailey & Scott's Diagnostic Microbiology, 10th ed. St. Louis, CV Mosby, 1998, Figure 37–3, page 516.

Color Plate 13. © Cabisco/Visuals Unlimited.

Color Plate 14. © Philip Sze/Visuals Unlimited.

Color Plate 15. © A. M. Siegelman/Visuals Unlimited.

Color Plate 16. © T. E. Adams/Visuals Unlimited.

Color Plate 17. © Philip Sze/Visuals Unlimited.

Color Plate 18. © David M. Phillips/Visuals Unlimited.

Color Plate 19. © M. Abbey/Visuals Unlimited.

Color Plate 20. © Cabisco/Visuals Unlimited.

Color Plate 21. © M. Eichelberger/Visuals Unlimited.

Color Plate 22. © George Loun/Visuals Unlimited.

Color Plate 23. Forbes BA, Sahm DF, Weissfeld AS: Bailey & Scott's Diagnostic Microbiology, 10th ed. St. Louis, CV Mosby, 1998, Figure 66–7, page 981.

Color Plate 24. Courtesy of Centers for Disease Control and Prevention, slide 21.

Color Plate 25. Lehman CA (ed): Saunders Manual of Clinical Laboratory Science. Philadelphia, WB Saunders, 1998, page 854.

Color Plate 26. Lehman CA (ed): Saunders Manual of Clinical Laboratory Science. Philadelphia, WB Saunders, 1998, page 859.

Color Plate 27. Stevens ML: Fundamentals of Clinical Hematology. Philadelphia, WB Saunders, 1997, Figure 10–2, page 207.

Color Plate 28. Margulies DH: The major histocompatibility complex. In Paul WE (ed): Fundamental Immunology, 4th ed. Philadelphia, Lippincott–Raven, 1999, Chapter 8, Colorplate 4.

Color Plate 29. Reprinted by permission from *Nature,* Stern LJ, Brown JH, Jardetzky TS, et al: Crystal structure of the human class II MHC protein HLA-DR1 complexed with an influenza virus peptide. Nature *368:*215–221, 1994, Macmillan Magazines, Limited.

Color Plate 30. Reprinted by permission from *Nature,* Fields BA, Malchiodi EL, Li H, et al.: Crystal structure of a T-cell receptor beta-chain complexed with a superantigen. Nature *384:*188–192, 1996, Macmillan Magazines, Limited.

Color Plate 31. Armed Forces Institute of Pathology, Negative No. 55-18251.

Color Plate 32. Forbes BA, Sahm DF, Weissfeld AS: Bailey & Scott's Diagnostic Microbiology, 10th ed. St. Louis, CV Mosby, 1998, Figure 28–7, page 408.

Color Plate 33. Mahon CR, Manuselis G: Textbook of Diagnostic Microbiology. Philadelphia, WB Saunders, 1995, Figure 11–3, page 342.

Color Plate 34. Armed Forces Institute of Pathology, negative No. 68-13583-2.

Color Plate 35. Armed Forces Institute of Pathology, negative No. 75-4203-7.

Color Plate 36. Armed Forces Institute of Pathology, negative No. 76-19180.

Color Plate 37. Forbes BA, Sahm DF, Weissfeld AS: Bailey & Scott's Diagnostic Microbiology, 10th ed. St. Louis, CV Mosby, 1998, Figure 31–1, page 455.

Color Plate 38. Forbes BA, Sahm DF, Weissfeld AS: Bailey & Scott's Diagnostic Microbiology, 10th ed. St. Louis, CV Mosby, 1998, Figure 1–3B, page 17.

Color Plate 39. Elmer W. Koneman, MD, Industrial Design Consultants, Denver, CO.

Color Plate 40. Elmer W. Koneman, MD, Industrial Design Consultants, Denver, CO.

Color Plate 41. Mahon CR, Manuselis G: Textbook of Diagnostic Microbiology. Philadelphia, WB Saunders, 1995, Figure 11–19, page 359.

Color Plate 42. Mahon CR, Manuselis G: Textbook of Diagnostic Microbiology. Philadelphia, WB Saunders, 1995, Figure 16–3, page 457.

Color Plate 43. Mahon CR, Manuselis G: Textbook of Diagnostic Microbiology. Philadelphia, WB Saunders, 1995, Figure 15–8, page 425.

Color Plate 44. Forbes BA, Sahm DF, Weissfeld AS: Bailey & Scott's Diagnostic Microbiology, 10th ed. St. Louis, CV Mosby, 1998, Figure 43–1, page 559.

Color Plate 45. Forbes BA, Sahm DF, Weissfeld AS: Bailey & Scott's Diagnostic Microbiology, 10th ed. St. Louis, CV Mosby, 1998, Figure 48–1, page 588.

Color Plate 46. Forbes BA, Sahm DF, Weissfeld AS: Bailey & Scott's Diagnostic Microbiology, 10th ed. St. Louis, CV Mosby, 1998, Figure 11–15B, page 147.

Color Plate 47. Susan Gibson, Austin, TX.

Color Plate 48. Forbes BA, Sahm DF, Weissfeld AS: Bailey & Scott's Diagnostic Microbiology, 10th ed. St. Louis, CV Mosby, 1998, Figure 60–3A, page 732.

Color Plate 49. Forbes BA, Sahm DF, Weissfeld AS: Bailey & Scott's Diagnostic Microbiology, 10th ed. St. Louis, CV Mosby, 1998, Figure 11–15A, page 147.

Color Plate 50. Forbes BA, Sahm DF, Weissfeld AS: Bailey & Scott's Diagnostic Microbiology, 10th ed. St. Louis, CV Mosby, 1998, Figure 57–3A, page 680.

Color Plate 51. Elmer W. Koneman, MD, Industrial Design Consultants, Denver, CO.

Color Plate 52. Elmer W. Koneman, MD, Industrial Design Consultants, Denver, CO.

Color Plate 53. Elmer W. Koneman, MD, Industrial Design Consultants, Denver, CO.

Color Plate 54. Elmer W. Koneman, MD, Industrial Design Consultants, Denver, CO.

Color Plate 55. Forbes BA, Sahm DF, Weissfeld AS: Bailey & Scott's Diagnostic Microbiology, 10th ed. St. Louis, CV Mosby, 1998, Figure 1–3A, page 17.

Color Plate 56. Bostick Maurer C: Laboratory detection of CMV. Microbiology Tech Sample No. MB-3. American Society of Clinical Pathologists, 1995, page 5.

Color Plate 57. Linda A. Smith, San Antonio, TX.

Color Plate 58. Forbes BA, Sahm DF, Weissfeld AS: Bailey & Scott's Diagnostic Microbiology, 10th ed. St. Louis, CV Mosby, 1998, Figure 64–33 left, page 830.

Color Plate 59. Forbes BA, Sahm DF, Weissfeld AS: Bailey & Scott's Diagnostic Microbiology, 10th ed. St. Louis, CV Mosby, 1998, Figure 64–33 right, page 830.

Color Plate 60. Meridian Diagnostics, Cincinnati, OH.

Color Plate 61. Lynne S. Garcia, Santa Monica, CA.

Color Plate 62. Pearl Ma, PhD.

Color Plate 63. OGW Berlin, Los Angeles, CA.

Color Plate 64. Mahon CR, Manuselis G: Textbook of Diagnostic Microbiology. Philadelphia, WB Saunders, 1995, Figure 11–8, page 348.

Color Plate 65. Reproduction of photograph from Schneierson SS (ed.): Schneierson's Atlas of Diagnostic Microbiology, 9th ed., Abbott Park, IL, Abbott Laboratories, Inc., has been granted with approval of Abbott Laboratories, Inc., all rights reserved by Abbott Laboratories, Inc.

Color Plate 66. Mahon CR, Manuselis G: Textbook of Diagnostic Microbiology. Philadelphia, WB Saunders, 1995, Figure 14–9, page 403.

Color Plate 67. Lois M. Bergquist.

Color Plate 68. Elmer W. Koneman, MD, Industrial Design Consultants, Denver, CO.

Color Plate 69. Forbes BA, Sahm DF, Weissfeld AS: Bailey & Scott's Diagnostic Microbiology, 10th ed. St. Louis, CV Mosby, 1998, Figure 66–9H, page 990.

Color Plate 70. Forbes BA, Sahm DF, Weissfeld AS: Bailey & Scott's Diagnostic Microbiology, 10th ed. St. Louis, CV Mosby, 1998, Figure 28–5, page 407.

Color Plate 71. Friedman-Kien AE: Color Atlas of AIDS. Philadelphia, WB Saunders, 1989, Figure 2–19, page 18.

Color Plate 72. Linda A. Smith, San Antonio, TX.

Color Plate 73. Lynne S. Garcia, Santa Monica, CA.

Color Plate 74. Armed Forces Institute of Pathology, negative No. 72-2312-6.

Color Plate 75. Armed Forces Institute of Pathology, negative No. 58-2952-3.

Color Plate 76. Armed Forces Institute of Pathology, negative No. 58-2952-1.

Color Plate 77. Armed Forces Institute of Pathology, negative No. 54-26364 (A).

Color Plate 78. Laurel Woodley, Rancho Palos Verdes, CA.

Color Plate 79. Zaiman H: A Pictorial Presentation of Parasites, Valley City, ND.

Color Plate 80. Zaiman H: A Pictorial Presentation of Parasites, Valley City, ND.

Color Plate 81. Armed Forces Institute of Pathology, negative No. 54-26364(B).

Color Plate 82. Molecular Probes, Inc., Eugene, OR.

Color Plate 83. Forbes BA, Sahm DF, Weissfeld AS: Bailey & Scott's Diagnostic Microbiology, 10th ed. St. Louis, CV Mosby, 1998, Figure 18–5A,B, page 259.

Color Plate 84. Forbes BA, Sahm DF, Weissfeld AS: Bailey & Scott's Diagnostic Microbiology, 10th ed. St. Louis, CV Mosby, 1998, Figure 18–15, page 268.

Color Plate 85. © Doug Sokell/Visuals Unlimited.

Color Plate 86. © John D. Cunningham/Visuals Unlimited.

Color Plate 87. © Doug Sokell/Visuals Unlimited.

Color Plate 88. © Sanford Berry/Visuals Unlimited.

Color Plate 89. Lois M. Bergquist.

Color Plate 90. Tillamook County Creamery Association.

Color Plate 91. Tillamook County Creamery Association.

Color Plate 92. Tillamook County Creamery Association.

Color Plate 93. Tillamook County Creamery Association.

Color Plate 94. © Gerald and Buff Corsi/Visuals Unlimited.

Color Plate 95. © Science VU/Visuals Unlimited.

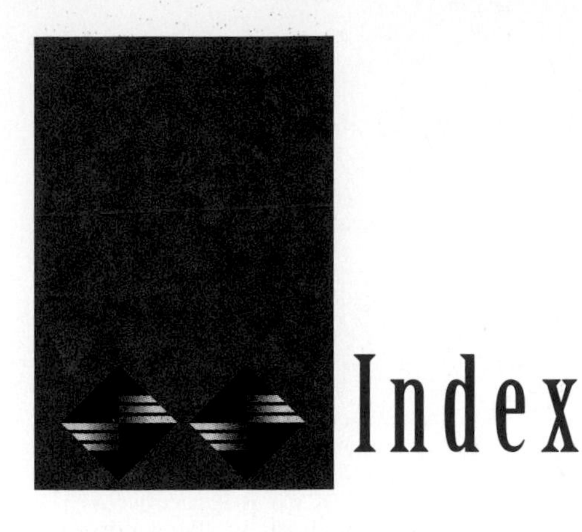

Index

Note: Page numbers in *italics* refer to illustrations; page numbers followed by (t) refer to tables; and page numbers followed by (d) refer to definitions.